Clinical Practice
of
Blood Transfusion

CLINICAL PRACTICE
OF
BLOOD TRANSFUSION

Edited by

Lawrence D. Petz, M.D.
Chairman, Division of Medicine
City of Hope National Medical Center
Duarte, California

and

Scott N. Swisher, M.D.
Professor of Medicine
Associate Dean for Research
Michigan State University
College of Human Medicine
East Lansing, Michigan

Churchill Livingstone
New York, Edinburgh, London, and Melbourne 1981

Distributed in the United Kingdom by Churchill Livingstone, Robert Stevenson House, 1–3 Baxter's Place, Leith Walk, Edinburgh EH1 3AF and by associated companies, branches and representatives throughout the world.

First published in 1981

Printed in USA

ISBN 0 443 08067 4

7   6   5   4   3   2   1

Library of Congress Cataloging in Publication Data
Main entry under title:
Clinical practice of blood transfusion.
    Bibliography: p.
    Includes index.
    1. Blood—Transfusion.   I. Petz,
Lawrence D.   II. Swisher, Scott N.
[DNLM: 1. Blood transfusion.   WB 356 P513c]
RM171.C5   615'.65   81-6158
ISBN 0-443-08067-4   AACR2

Contributors

Joseph Aisner, M.D., F.A.C.P.
Chief
Section of Medical Oncology
Baltimore Cancer Research Program
Division of Cancer Treatment
National Cancer Institute
Associate Professor of Medicine
University of Maryland
School of Medicine
Baltimore, Maryland

Lewellys F. Barker, M.D.
Vice President
Blood Services
American Red Cross
Washington, D.C.

**G.W.G. Bird, D.Sc., Ph.D.,
M.M.B.S., F.R.C. Path.**
Director
Regional Blood Transfusion Centre
Birmingham
England

Donald Branch, MT (ASCP) SBB
Research Associate
Division of Medicine
City of Hope Medical Center
Duarte, California

Hugh Chaplin, Jr., M.D.
Professor of Medicine & Preventive
  Medicine
Department of Preventive Medicine
  and Public Health
Washington University School of
  Medicine
St. Louis, Missouri

John A. Collins, M.D.
Professor and Chairman
Department of Surgery
Stanford University
Stanford, California

Dennis M. Donohue, M.D.
Director
Division of Blood Products
Food and Drug Administration
Bethesda, Maryland

Harold L. Engel, M.D., J.D.
Associate Clinical Professor of
  Anesthesiology
School of Medicine
University of Southern California
Member of Law Firm
Bonne, Jones, Bridges, Mueller and
  O'Keefe
Los Angeles, California

Patricia Giardina, M.D.
Assistant Clinical Professor of
  Pediatrics
Cornell University Medical College
Assistant Attending Pediatrician
The New York Hospital
Cornell Medical Center
New York, New York

Paul V. Holland, M.D.
Chief
Blood Bank Department
Clinical Center
National Institutes of Health
Bethesda, Maryland

William S. Howland, M.D.
Chairman
Department of Critical Care
Vice President for Clinical Affairs
Memorial Hospital
New York, New York

Ernst R. Jaffé, M.D.
Professor of Medicine
Head
Division of Hematology
Senior Associate Dean
Associate Dean for Faculty
Albert Einstein College of Medicine
Yeshiva University
Bronx, New York

Donald B. Kaufman, M.D.
Associate Professor
Department of Pediatrics and Human
  Development
Director of Clinical Immunology
College of Human Medicine
Michigan State University
East Lansing, Michigan

Aaron Kellner, M.D.
President
New York Blood Center
New York, New York

Martin R. Klemperer, M.D.
Professor and Chairman
Department of Pediatrics
Marshall University
School of Medicine
Huntington, West Virginia

**W. Laurence Marsh, F.I.M.L.S.,
  M.I. Biol., M.R.C. Path.**
Immunohematologist
The New York Blood Center
New York, New York

Harold T. Meryman, M.D.
Assistant Medical Director
Blood Services
Head
Cryobiology Laboratory
American Red Cross
Bethesda, Maryland

Denis R. Miller, M.D.
Chairman, Department of Pediatrics
Memorial Sloan-Kettering Cancer
  Center
Enid A. Haupt Professor of Pediatrics
Cornell University Medical College
New York, New York

William V. Miller, M.D.
Executive Vice President
Director of Blood Services
Missouri/Illinois Regional Red Cross
  Blood Services
St. Louis, Missouri

Cynthia Murray, MT (ASCP) SBB
Director
Technical Services
American Red Cross Blood Service
Great Lakes Region
Lansing, Michigan

Jacob Nusbacher, M.D.
Director
American Red Cross Blood Services
Rochester Region
Associate Professor
Departments of Medicine and
  Pathology
University of Rochester School of
  Medicine
Rochester, New York

Harold A. Oberman, M.D.
Professor
Department of Pathology
Head
Section of Clinical Pathology
University of Michigan Medical
  School
Director
Clinical Laboratories and Blood Bank
University Hospital
Ann Arbor, Michigan

John Penner, M.D.
Professor of Medicine
Head, Hematology Oncology Unit
College of Human Medicine
Michigan State University
East Lansing, Michigan

Herbert A. Perkins, M.D.
Scientific Director
Irwin Memorial Blood Bank
Clinical Professor of Medicine
University of California
San Francisco, California

Lawrence D. Petz, M.D.
Chairman, Division of Medicine
City of Hope National Medical
    Center
Duarte, California

Johanna Pindyck, M.D.
Vice President and Director
Greater New York Blood Program
New York Blood Center
New York, New York

Charles A. Schiffer, M.D.
Head
Cell Component Therapy Section
Baltimore Cancer Research Program
Associate Professor of Medicine
University of Maryland
School of Medicine
Baltimore, Maryland

William C. Sherwood, M.D.
Director
Penn-Jersey Regional Red Cross
    Blood Service
Associate Professor of Medicine
Jefferson Medical College
Philadelphia, Pennsylvania

Rainer Storb, M.D.
Professor of Medicine
Department of Medicine
Division of Oncology
University of Washington
The Fred Hutchinson Cancer
    Research Center
Seattle, Washington

Scott N. Swisher, M. D.
Professor
Department of Medicine
Associate Dean for Research
College of Human Medicine
Michigan State University
East Lansing, Michigan

Garson H. Tishkoff, M.D., Ph.D.
Professor
Department of Medicine
College of Human Medicine
Michigan State University
East Lansing, Michigan

Peter A. Tomasulo, M.D.
Medical Director
John Elliott Community Blood Center
Associate Professor
Clinical Pathology
Associate Professor of Medicine
University of Miami School of
    Medicine
Miami, Florida

Paul Weiden, M.D.
Physician
Department of Hematology/Oncology
Mason Clinic
Virginia Mason Hospital
Seattle, Washington

Carl F.W. Wolf, M.D.
Director
Blood Bank and Transfusion Service
Associate Attending Pathologist
The New York Hospital
Associate Clinical Professor of
    Pathology
Department of Pathology
Cornell University Medical College
New York, New York

Preface

This book is directed primarily toward an audience of clinicians involved in the everyday care of patients who require transfusion. It is also directed toward those students and residents who are in training for careers that will involve the management of transfusion problems in their patients. The book attempts insofar as possible to present blood transfusion as part of an overall integrated therapeutic plan for the individual patient. Blood transfusion is widely employed in medicine, pediatrics, surgery, and obstetrics and gynecology, as well as in other clinical disciplines. It is impossible to present in the available pages comprehensive clinical discussions of all the disorders treated with transfusion, as well as their management with drugs, surgical procedures, and other therapies. The reader must integrate the information presented here with other significant knowledge related to the treatment of the patient—knowledge derived from many sources. The book does, however, attempt to relate those areas in which there are major issues of transfusion therapy with other approaches to treatment that are of signal importance.

This book is not intended to be primarily a technically oriented book for the use of the blood banker. However, blood bank directors are increasingly involved with decision making in clinical medicine. Indeed, physician directors should not serve merely as administrators of blood banks. More importantly, they should function as directors of blood transfusion services; as such, they should frequently serve as clinical consultants on a wide variety of transfusion problems. The book is directed to blood bank directors and blood bank personnel in this sense. There are a number of excellent sources of the information of a primarily technical nature which is necessary to operate a blood bank or transfusion service. There is no need to restate much of this information in the present book.

The authors also hope that this volume will be of use to personnel of transfusion services and transfusion committee members of hospitals. Many hospitals have only pro forma transfusion committees which function intermittently and have little impact on transfusion practices of the institution. Formally organized transfusion services are infrequently found today in American medical institutions, even in the large centers. It is our hope that this volume will not only indicate the usefulness of a transfusion service and an active transfusion committee of the hospital staff, but also provide a resource for those carrying out these activities by providing clinical guidance to the best of practice in connection with blood transfusion.

The work of Patrick L. Mollison, *Blood Transfusion in Clinical Medicine* (Blackwell Scientific Publications, Oxford, Sixth Ed, 1979), has been and continues to be an excellent reference source for information about the laboratory investigations that form the scientific basis of the field of blood transfusion today. The present volume makes no effort to deal with the field of blood transfusion in the same way as does Mollison. Rather, we have set as our purpose to speak to the student and clinician primarily in their own largely clinical terms in the context of both common and uncommon transfusion problems. There are, of course, many other excellent reference sources and a large and diverse medical literature devoted to this topic. Each chapter lists many additional references pertinent to the subject material discussed, and the interested reader will find these sources useful for further study.

The present volume is, with one exception, contributed by authors from the United States. They were selected from a list of well-qualified clinicians and researchers in this field, many from other countries; our choice of contributors was based largely upon our feeling that close contact with contributors would ensure a more cohesive work. We had the opportunity to meet with the contributors to discuss the contents of their chapters at a number of meetings during the past several years. The long-distance telephone was employed liberally in developing these contributions. All of the contributors are relatively close acquaintances, present or former colleagues, or clinicians and researchers whose work is well-known to the editors of this volume. We feel that the book reflects the current state-of-the-art and that it will be of value not only in the United States but in the international clinical community as well.

This book is divided into three major sections. The first section is an introduction. The second section deals with those scientific and technological matters which provide the basic science and resources of clinical blood transfusion. The third section is devoted to clinical uses of blood transfusion in the context of modern clinical medicine. In some instances, a disciplinary viewpoint is presented—as, for example, transfusion in relation to anesthesiology. In other instances, specific problems such as massive acute blood loss and the management of the patient with thrombocytopenia are considered.

The bibliography is designed to direct the reader to the current major references related to each chapter. It is not designed to provide an exhaustive list of every reference in the field. The reader who wishes to delve further into a topic will find additional references in the bibliographies of further readings.

A number of contributions overlap in their scope of coverage to a significant degree. This has been done deliberately for two reasons. We wished to provide the reader with a relatively comprehensive review of the topic in one place in the book. This was felt to be preferable to constantly referring the reader throughout the book to various aspects of the topic being discussed. Even more importantly, we found that in some areas, differences of opinion about a variety of issues still remain. We wanted to permit the individual contributors to present their formulations of these issues, along with the data which they feel justify the positions they have taken. The reader can then judge the merits of the controversies that still exist in this field. Individual contributions have been read critically by both editors and found to lie well within the range of informed opinion in the field; in most instances they are in accord with our own personal views.

The topic of massive transfusion and its consequences deserves specific comment. This subject is dealt with in a number of chapters, each from a somewhat different perspective. Chapters 22, 23, and 24 deal with the problems of massive transfusion as seen by a surgeon (Chapter 22), an anesthesiologist (Chapter 23), and an internist-hematologist blood bank director (Chapter 24). The same problems are considered, again from somewhat different viewpoints, in Chapter 12 (Characteristics of Red Cell Products for Transfusion) and in Chapter 25 (Transfusion Therapy in Patients with Coagulation Disorders).

Massive transfusion remains a central problem in clinical medicine—a problem which has been difficult to study in man, where it is virtually always encountered in a setting of trauma, major surgery, or complicating medical illness. Animal models have been found frequently to be misleading. Although ultimately these somewhat different perspectives and interpretations of available data must converge upon a common set of facts, that time has not yet arrived. It is not surprising that differences of opinion and practice persist. Practice may reasonably be based upon experience as well as investigation in such situations. The opinions presented here on this important topic reflect both disciplinary views of the best management of the problem based upon experience as well as somewhat variable interpretations of the currently available data.

The authors feel that the opinions presented in this book are authoritative but not authoritarian. Be prepared for recommendations and opinions which vary from your own and which may not even be in complete accord with others in the book. The reader will realize more than ever that the clinical practice of blood transfusion is not an exact science; it is the informed and intelligent reader who must in final analysis apply the available information to the solution of patient care problems.

Lawrence D. Petz, M.D.
Scott N. Swisher, M.D.

Contents

I. Introduction

1

An Overview of Blood Transfusion

Scott N. Swisher, M.D., and Lawrence D. Petz, M.D.

AN OVERVIEW OF THE PRACTICE OF TRANSFUSION IN CLINICAL MEDICINE TODAY

In the United States alone, it has been estimated that about 10 million units of blood are collected annually in addition to some 5 million liters of plasma for the production of plasma protein derivatives by fractionation. Exact figures on the level of activity in the field of blood transfusion are difficult to obtain in the U.S. because there is as yet no centralized data-gathering system to collect this information. This may well change in the near future with the establishment of a national blood service data center under the auspices of the American Blood Commission. It is essential to know the levels of blood transfusion-related activities for appropriate management of this important human resource as well as for health care planning, which has become increasingly important in this country and throughout the world.

Component Therapy

The introduction during the 1960s of component therapy—in which the donated unit of whole blood is broken down into sedimented red cells, platelets, cryoprecipitated antihemophilic factor, or fresh frozen plasma—has had a major impact upon the practice of blood transfusion in the last 15 years. A much larger number of useful therapeutic units are now derived from a single donation. There is little comprehensive information about the impact of component therapy on transfusion practice throughout the entire country, because of a similar lack of appropriate data. It is known that the effective practice of component therapy varies widely throughout the country, seemingly depending upon the level of organization, sophistication, and effectiveness of the available transfusion services in a region. Although transfusion of components has been highly developed in many areas, a great deal of additional educational effort will be required before the benefits of these techniques are universally available.

Component therapy has been of major significance in two ways. It has provided more specific replacement of the blood component(s) that the patient needs. As a corollary, it has also made unnecessary the administration of components of whole blood which the patient does not require. This has improved both the safety and the efficacy of blood transfusion. Of almost equal importance has been the impact of component therapy on the national blood supply. It has permitted much more efficient utilization of available donor resources to meet an ever-expanding need for transfusion.

The National Blood Supply

It has been suggested that, if component therapy were employed in a maximally useful way in the United States and if overuses of blood transfusions not well justified by clinical or scientific data were greatly reduced, the blood supply of the United States currently available would be in very close balance with the real needs of the American population. Further growth in the need for blood would, in effect, then depend largely upon the introduction of new therapeutic procedures that require blood or one or more of its components. A relatively modest rate of future growth can be predicted on the basis of increasing population and increasing participation of those segments of the American population that are currently underserved in the health care service system. Other changes in medical practice might reduce the need for blood.

Impact of New Medical Technology

The introduction of major new medical and surgical techniques may increase the requirement for blood transfusions on a major scale. However, plans to develop an increased blood supply are rarely undertaken prior to the appearance of the increased need in a relatively acute form. In this respect, it is of interest to examine the impact of the introduction of cardiac surgery—and of coronary artery bypass surgery in particular—on the national blood supply. These procedures depended very directly upon the availability of blood transfusions for their development. This has been true of many surgical developments in this century, as well as a number of medical procedures such as renal dialysis.

Taken together with advances in anesthesiology and a better physiological understanding of the surgical patient, enormous advances in surgery in all areas have occurred since 1945. Up until the introduction of cardiac surgery, with its requirement for cardiac bypass pump priming and substantial intraoperative and postoperative blood replacement during the developmental phase, the growth of the base of blood donors in the United States was able to keep reasonably well apace with needs for blood.

The sudden, almost explosive rise in cardiac surgical procedures that occurred in the early 1970s seriously depleted the blood supply of the country. For example, in Milwaukee at that time it was found that well over one-third of the blood supply of that area was directed to cardiac surgical patients, and it was difficult for a well-organized blood bank to keep pace with the demand. Their carefully constructed volunteer donor base was again threatened by calls from hospitals and surgeons for recruitment of professional donors. It was probably only the threat of hepatitis associated with professional blood donation that prevented reemergence of substantial commercial blood banking activity in this country at that time.

As new medical technologies that depend upon blood transfusion are introduced in the future, it would be wise to examine first their impact upon the blood supply. Plans could then be made for further development of the donor base, if this is necessary, or for more efficient utilization of blood resources already available. Newer medical approaches to remaining serious health problems in some instances might have quite the opposite effect upon the national blood supply. At the present time, for example, large numbers of blood platelets are being administered to patients undergoing chemotherapy for malignant diseases, particularly acute leukemia. If a more effective treatment of these disorders were to be discovered, it would have an immediate effect upon the demand for platelets, an effect which would have major economic effects upon the national blood supply and cause a readjustment of pricing policies for other blood components in order to meet the costs of operating the system as a whole. At present, there is controversy about the use of platelet transfusions given prophylactically to prevent bleeding in severely thrombocytopenic patients undergoing intensive chemotherapy; the alternative approach is administration of platelets at the onset of clinically significant bleeding. When this question can be resolved on the basis of adequate data, it may have a major effect upon the blood supply and upon the economics of blood services. Even without new technology, changes in established practice based upon better information will affect blood services in ways that are not easy to predict.

It is possible that a number of additional components of plasma—specifically alpha-1 antitrypsin, antithrombin-III and alpha-2 macroglobulin enzyme inhibitor—may be isolated and found to be clinically useful. If this were to occur, additional products with economic value and unknown demand and need would then be available from plasma and again result in a restructuring of the needs, demands, and economics of plasma derivative production. At present, there is increasing evidence that serum albumin is overutilized in the United States, as well as in many countries of Western Europe. If this results in a declining market for serum albumin and albumin products, it will presumably have an effect upon the price and availability of antihemophilic factor—the other component of plasma which currently is of major economic importance, and in which there is a relatively narrower balance between need and supply at the present time. The uses for plasma immunoglobulins might change suddenly and dramatically, although this seems somewhat unlikely at the present time, with similar effects upon the operation of the total blood services system of the country and the Western world.

For these and other reasons, there would appear to be a need for a more integrated management of the national blood resource than the present system, or nonsystem, permits. There is widespread opinion that this management should be exerted outside of the complete control of government, but the specific agency which might carry out such a program effectively is uncertain at present and unlikely to appear in the present climate. There are those who would argue for a return to a more or less completely free market situation as the most effective and efficient way of achieving the best relationship between costs and availability of blood and blood products. This is equally unlikely to happen in view of the past experiences in the United States and the Western world. The free market approach is incompatible with the increasingly widely accepted concept that the blood service complex is, in fact, a human service, and not primarily a commercial enterprise. How these matters ultimately will be resolved in the United States and other countries will be of great interest during the next 20 years.

PROBLEMS OF MEDICAL EDUCATION AND PUBLIC EDUCATION

By any assessment, the systematic exposure of medical students and residents to even fundamental information about blood transfusion at the clinical level is totally inadequate. Transfusion practice and related research has not had widespread acceptance in academic circles until very recently. As a result, many medical students and residents learn what they do know about blood transfusion by the process of "chaining." The chief resident passes along what he has learned, gathered in an entirely unsystematic way, to the assistant residents, who then in turn teach the interns and medical students as they rotate through the various clinical services. The teaching is usually unsystematic, and entirely in the context of the transfusion management of individual patients. It is little wonder that physicians emerge into their definitive careers with little understanding in either depth or breadth about the appropriate management of one of their most important therapeutic tools. This is partly a reflection of the fact that, in most medical institutions, the blood transfusion service is regarded as primarily a laboratory service. The laboratory aspects of blood transfusion service are, of course, of great importance. Without them in their highly developed present state, little of modern transfusion practice could be done. Unfortunately, clinical pathologists and laboratory directors have not been particularly well informed about the clinical management of blood transfusion. Many of the standard textbooks in medicine, surgery, pediatrics, obstetrics and gynecology have in the past had little to say about blood transfusion at the clinical level, although this is slowly improving.

One of the major tasks for the future should be to improve the education of medical students, medical residents, and the senior staffs of all medical institutions in the proper management of blood transfusion in clinical practice. To accomplish this, this audience would have to be convinced of the importance of such knowledge for the patient's welfare. Their performance in this area will have to be subjected to the same scrutiny by peers as are their performances of surgical procedures themselves or the management of complex medical therapies. A number of the now outmoded concepts and indeed some of the myths about blood transfusion therapy will have to be abandoned and replaced by what we now know on a reasonably firm scientific basis. This will result not only in better patient care, but in a more intelligent, rational, and cost-effective use of this precious human resource. This is the arena in which we should look for improvements in blood services in this country in the near future, rather than to startling new scientific "breakthroughs."

THE FUTURE

Blood transfusion now enjoys a relatively well-developed and mature technology capable of meeting most of the major demands placed upon the system at the present time. At least these needs can be met within the current biologically imposed limitations on the effectiveness of transfusion of red cells, platelets, leukocytes, and the currently available plasma derivatives.

REQUIREMENTS FOR COST EFFECTIVENESS

This is not to say that present technologies cannot still be substantially improved. But one must now examine the marginal value of these improvements. For example, improvement of the period of in vitro storage of red cells from the present 35-day limit to 40 or 45 days would have relatively little value, if we are to judge by the impact that the change from a 21-day limit to a 35-day limit has had in recent years. On the other hand, improvement of in vitro storage to beyond 60 days, particularly if this could be accomplished with a higher level of viability of the transfused cells beyond the current limit of 70 percent, might have a substantial value. The value would have to be judged also in terms of the cost of the new system before it might be expected to replace the present technology. Almost any improvement in the in vitro storage life of blood platelets will be of value at the present time. Other improvements in the technology of production, storage, and distribution of blood components will have to be subjected to the same comparisons with the current methods and the marginal value of the improvements estimated. With increasingly tight controls on all health care-related costs, relatively higher cost-benefit ratios will probably be required in the future than have been in the past, when the tendency has been to introduce any innovation carrying even a very small improvement in efficacy without regard to cost.

TECHNOLOGICAL IMPROVEMENTS

Of all the new technologies in prospect for blood services, widespread introduction of automation holds the most promise. It should soon be possible to employ automated data processing for control of every step in the transfusion sequence from donor to recipient; this should improve safety by marked reduction of clinical errors, a continuing hazard. Improvements will have to be demonstrated by initial analysis of field experience, first on a pilot trial basis and later in more general application. What work has already been accomplished in this area is promising. Automated testing is already an established and proven procedure, but it requires a large base of activity in order to be economically feasible. This may result in consolidation of laboratory procedures over large areas, by employing rapid transportation and electronic communication techniques. Not only does this type of automation improve control of data, but it also provides the information necessary for a sophisticated program of blood inventory management. Improved utilization, better product quality, and decreased losses by outdating are already proven benefits of the best of these systems. Although they require substantial capital costs and some operating expenses as well, it seems probable that these systems, when they are of adequate size, will prove to be cost-effective. Indeed, there may be no other feasible way to manage large-scale blood service programs in the absence of automation.

The impact of recently developed oxygen-carrying artificial compounds in the circulation has been the subject of wide speculation. These may well find their way into clinical use for a number of specific purposes where they may be of great value; however, the most informed opinion in the field—that of the researchers working on these substances—tends to be very conservative in predicting a significant impact upon blood services as we now know them. There is relatively little interest at present in artificial substitutes for plasma proteins, based upon a better understanding of the effect of adequate crystalloid therapy and the small margin of additional benefit to be obtained in many clinical circumstances even from the use of albumin, the physiological intravascular oncotic protein.

Further development of blood transfusion equipment—both the disposable materials and the machinery—can be expected. This will probably be based upon refinements of most of the current concepts behind these systems as they are presently employed. There is certainly room for major innovations in the field of blood transfusion equipment. Vigorous participation of industry, slowly broadening now to include some of the United States' most technologically sophisticated industries, will probably lead to improved biocompatible materials, equipment, and technology. Again, the marginal value of these improved items will have to be evaluated in terms of their cost. Costs always seem to rise; an approach that would significantly lower costs, even at the present level of capability of our equipment systems, would be equally attractive for the future.

Autologous transfusion in which a patient predeposits blood in anticipation of a need—for example, scheduled surgery—is now a well-developed technology. Its use has not as yet grown to the point where it has had a significant impact upon the blood supply of the country. This may occur, depending upon a number of economic, social, and professional factors which are impossible to evaluate. On the other hand, use of intraoperative and perioperative blood salvage does appear to be expanding and will probably continue to do so, given continuing improvements of the needed technology. It is difficult to decide whether the use of these procedures should be promoted in the absence of adequate information on which to evaluate their cost effectiveness. Current opinion and experience seem to favor further development of blood salvage procedures and their use.

The blood transfusion complex of the United States—including the industrial sector, which has been so important—can take real satisfaction from the fact that it has met quite well the challenges presented to it in the past. One can confidently expect the same kind of performance in the future.

ORGANIZATIONAL IMPROVEMENTS

Improved organization of blood services, with better coordination between its various elements and improved professional utilization of the products of the blood transfusion services of the country, presents major opportunities for improvements in overall patient care at the present time. Improved approaches to donor recruitment, particularly those which tend to level the blood supply around the year, can be expected at some point to contribute to resolution of nagging problems of blood availability. Resource sharing by which supply and demand are adjusted over wide areas and nationally will contribute to the security of the blood supply for individual institutions and the patients they serve. There is need for a clear, coherent, and unified message to blood donors of the country. These changes are possible without additional costs in most instances, and they have the possibility of reducing costs by improving efficiency.

2

The History of Blood Transfusion

Harold A. Oberman, M.D.

The therapeutic benefits of blood have been recognized for centuries; however, blood transfusion as we know it today is of comparatively recent vintage. Not until the present century was there full appreciation of the scientific rationale for blood transfusion, nor was there complete realization of its consequences.

The evolution of blood transfusion is a fascinating story, ranging from mysticism and pseudoscience to present-day rational therapy. It also reflects the parallel expansion of knowledge in bioengineering, physiology, immunology, mechanical engineering, biochemistry, and genetics. The history is enhanced by the role of a variety of personages who became famous in other areas, both medical and nonmedical, yet all of whom played a role in the dramatic story of transfusion.

EARLY BEGINNINGS

One of the first references to blood transfusion is contained in the seventh book of the *Metamorphoses* by Ovid.[1] Jason pleaded that Medea restore the youth of his father, King Aeson. She complied as follows:

Medea took her unsheathed knife and cut the old man's throat, letting all of his old blood out of him. She filled his ancient veins with a rich elixir. Received it through his lips and wound, his beard and hair no longer white with age, turned quickly to their natural vigor, dark and lustrous; and his wasted form renewed, appeared in all the vigor of bright youth.

Medea's remarkable success was achieved with an elixir, brewed in a bronze cauldron, containing:

root herbs, seeds and flowers, strong juices, and pebbles from the farthest shores of oceans east and west, hoar-frost taken at the full of the moon, a hoot owl's wings and flesh, a werewolf's entrails, the fillet of a snake, the liver of a stag, and the eggs and head of a crow which had been alive for nine centuries.

Medea's practice as a transfusionist was not confined to this single event. Later, when she wished to kill Pelias, she pretended to perform a similar miracle on him. Before killing Pelias, Medea gained his confidence by changing an aged sheep into a lamb.

There are several citations in the *Old Testament* indirectly bearing on blood transfusion which have had a social impact to the present day. Denial of blood transfusion on religious grounds has its foundation in passages such as the following:

For the life of the flesh is in the blood; and I have given it to you upon the altar to make atonement for your souls; for it is the blood that maketh atonement by reason of the life. Therefore, I said unto the children of Israel: No soul of you shall eat blood, neither shall any stranger that sojourneth among you eat blood.[2]

Only flesh with the life thereof, which is the blood thereof, shall ye not eat.[3]

Be steadfast in not eating the blood; for the blood is the life; and thou shalt not eat the life with the flesh. Thou shalt not eat it; thou shalt pour it out upon the earth as water.[4]

There are many ancient references to the use of blood. For example, Pliny described the drinking of the blood of dying gladiators "as if out of loving cups" as a cure of epilepsy, and also noted the practice of Egyptian kings bathing in blood as a cure for elephantiasis. Galen advised the drinking of the blood of a weasel, or of a dog, for the cure of rabies. Similarly, ancient Norwegians drank the blood of seals and whales as a remedy for epilepsy and scurvy.[5] Whereas these references refer to the drinking of blood, or the application of blood to the skin, an ancient reference to the possible transfusion of blood is contained in an ancient Hebrew manuscript:

Naam, leader of the armies of Ben-Adad, King of Syria, afflicted with leprosy, consulted physicians, who, in order to kill him, drew out the blood from his veins and put in that of another.[6]

In the thirteenth century, Petro de Abano described the management of an adverse reaction occasioned by ingestion of blood:

He who drinks of menstrual blood or that of a leper will be seen to be distracted and lunatic, evil-minded and forgetful, and his cure is to drink of daisies powdered and mixed with water of honey, and to bathe in tepid water and to copulate with girls according the law natural, and to play with pretty girls and young boys; and the anti-dote is to eat serpents whose heads and tails have been cut off with the edge of a palm frond.[5]

Aside from other significant events of 1492, did the first transfusion also occur in that year? In 1492, Pope Innocent VIII was terminally ill with chronic renal disease. A mystic arrived in Rome and promised to cure the Pope by exchanging his blood with that of three young boys.

Three ten-year-old boys were selected, paid one ducat apiece, and the procedure was instituted. Villary states that the blood of the dying Pope was cast into the veins of the boys, who gave him their own in exchange.[7] Each boy died shortly after the procedure, and there was no modification of the Pope's illness.

It seems probable that this presumed transfusion stems from an incorrect translation of an earlier account of the Pope's illness. What most likely happened is that the blood of the three young boys was intended for use in preparation of a potion for the Pope. However, when the Pope heard of this he condemned the practice, refused the potion, and ordered the mystic punished.[8]

TRANSFUSION IN THE SEVENTEENTH CENTURY

The event which first kindled interest in blood transfusion was the description of the circulation of blood by William Harvey, in 1613, and subsequently published in his *De Motu Cordis* in 1628. This occasioned considerable speculation regarding the possibility of blood transfusion and also pertaining to the infusion of other medications. For example, in 1628 Giovanni Colle suggested transfusion as a means of prolonging life,[9] and a decade earlier, in 1615, Andreas Libavius, the renowned chemist, postulated the following in a satirical sense while defending his theories against his critics:

Let there be a young man, robust, full of spirituous blood, and also an old man, thin, emaciated, his strength exhausted, hardly able to retain his own soul. Let the performer of the operation have two silver tubes fitting into each other. Let him open the artery of the young man and put into it one of the tubes, fastening it in. Let him immediately after open the artery of the old man, and put the female tube into it, and then the two tubes be joined together, the hot and spirituous blood of the young man will pour into the old one as if it were from a fountain of life, and all of his weaknesses will be dispelled. Now, in order that the young man may not suffer from weakness, to him is to be given good care and food, but to the doctor, hellebore.[5]

In the middle of the seventeenth century, several claimants presented themselves for the honor of being the first to transfuse blood. Based upon his reading of Ovid's story of Medea, Frances Potter may have been the first to conceive of transfusion on a practical basis. Potter was a recluse whose efforts were documented in the writings of his contemporary, John Aubrey. Apparently, Potter originated the idea of transfusion as early as 1639, and devised quills and tubes for the purpose. In 1649 he reportedly attempted the procedure of transfusion on a pullet; however, likely because of the size of the bird, it proved unsuccessful.[10]

Sir Christopher Wren, who achieved lasting fame as an astronomer and architect, in 1656 first proposed the intravenous administration of medications into the veins of dogs.[11] For this purpose he devised an animal bladder attached to quills. Wren was assisted in this endeavor by his contemporary, Robert Boyle. Four years later Johannes Elsholz, a physician in Brandenburg, began his experiments on the intravenous injection of wine and emetics into the veins of dogs. These were summarized in his book, *Chlysmatica Nova,* published in 1667.[12] Other seventeenth century experiments in intravenous medication

administration were performed using nitric acid, sulfuric acid, beer, or water.

In a book published in 1660, Francesco Folli of Florence described techniques for transfusion using silver tubes inserted into the vein of the recipient, connected with the artery of an animal. He also stated that he demonstrated this procedure in 1654, although there was never a public presentation.[5]

At a meeting of a learned society held in Paris in July, 1658, Robert des Gabets, a Benedictine monk, enunciated the concept of transfusion, and noted that seven years earlier a friar, Pichot, had prepared an instrument consisting of two small silver cannulae connected by a small leather bag, which could be used for this purpose.[13]

It seems most likely that the first public demonstration of transfusion was presented by the English physician, Richard Lower, who began his experiments at Oxford in late February, 1665 (Fig. 2-1). Lower initially attempted to join the jugular veins of two dogs, but the blood promptly clotted in the tubing. He thereupon cannulated a cervical artery in one dog, and attached it to the jugular vein of the recipient, thereupon exsanguinating the donor animal. Boyle invited Lower to demonstrate this before the Royal Society, and it was subsequently documented in its *Philosophical Transactions* in December, 1666.[14]

It seems clear that Lower was the first to define the appropriateness of transfusional replacement of blood in severe hemorrhage, since he was able to demonstrate that a dog could be exsanguinated to the point of death and then be completely restored by transfusion. It is interesting to note that a contemporary record of this experiment is contained in the diary of Samuel Pepys. His entry of November 14, 1666 notes:

> Dr. Croone told me that, at the meeting at Gresham College tonight there was a pretty experiment of the blood of one dog let out till he died, into the body of another on one side, while all his own run out on the other

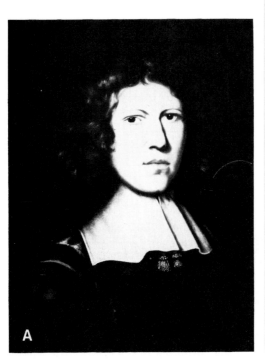

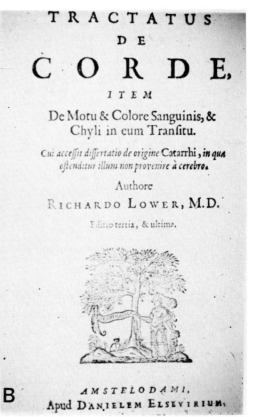

Fig. 2-1. (*A*) Portrait of Richard Lower. (Courtesy of Wellcome Museum of History of Medicine, London). (*B*) Title page of Lower's book, *Tractatus de Corde* (1669), in which transfusion of blood is described in detail.

side. The first died upon the place, and the other very well and likely to do well. This did give occasion to many pretty wishes, as of the blood of a Quaker to be let into an Archbishop, and such like; but, as Dr. Croone says, may if it takes, be of mighty use to man's health, for the amendment of bad blood by borrowing from a better body.[15]

Lower's efforts were the stimulus for a series of experiments upon animals by a multitude of workers throughout Europe, and eventually led to the transfusion of blood from animal into man. The priority for the latter procedure occasioned a rancorous debate across the English Channel.

On November 23, 1667, Lower, assisted by Dr. Edmund King, transfused a man named Author Coga, described by Pepys as "a man that is a little frantic, that hath been a kind of minister, that the College hath hired for twenty shillings" (Fig. 2-2*A*). Pepys observed that the members of the Royal College "differ in the opinion they have of the effects (of the transfusion); some think it may have a good effect upon the man as a frantic man by cooling his blood, others that it will not have any effect at all." The experiment, using blood of a lamb, apparently proceeded without mishap, and afterwards, Coga allowed that he felt better, although Pepys observed that "he is cracked a little in the head."[16]

A second, and uneventful, transfusion of Coga took place the following month; however, it was never recorded in the Transac-

(489) *Numb.* 27.

A LETTER

Concerning a new way of curing sundry diseases by Transfusion of Blood, Written to Monsieur de MONTMOR, *Counsellor to the* French King, *and Master of Requests.*

By J: DENIS *Professor of* Philosophy, *and the* Mathematicks.

Munday July 22. 1667.

SIR,

 HE project of causing the Blood of a healthy animal to passe into the veins of one diseased, having been conceived about ten years agoe, in the illustrious Society of *Virtuosi* which assembles at your house, and your goodness having received M. *Emmerez* & my self, very favorably at such times as we have presum'd to entertain you either with discourse concerning it, or the sight of some not inconsiderable effects of it : You will not think it strange that I now take the liberty of troubling you with this Letter, and design to inform you fully of what pursuances and successes we have made in this Operation; wherein you are justly intitled to a greater share than any other, considering that it was first spoken of in your *Academy,* & that the Publick

A

An Account
Of the Experiment of *Transfusion,* practised upon a
Man in *London.*

This was perform'd, Novemb. 23. 1667. *upon one Mr.* Arthur Coga, *at* Arundel-House, *in the presence of many considerable and intelligent persons, by the management of those two Learned Physitians and dextrous Anatomists Dr.* Richard Lower, *and Dr.* Edmund King, *the latter of whom communicated the Relation of it, as followeth.*

THe Experiment of Transfusion of Blood into an *humane* Veine was made by Us in this manner. Having prepared
M m m   the

B

Fig. 2-2. (*A*) Account of Denis and Emmerez's first human transfusion in the *Philosophical Transactions.* (*B*) Lower's report of human transfusion in the *Philosophical Transactions* four months later.

---

tions because of events which expired almost simultaneously in France.

Jean Denis, a young physician on the large staff attached to King Louis XIV, read of Lower's experiments in the *Journal des Savants* of January 31, 1667. In association with a surgeon, Paul Emmerez, Denis initiated his own trials approximately a month later, performing numerous dog-to-dog transfusions. Eventually, on June 15, 1667, Denis transfused a 15-year-old boy who had a febrile illness of unknown nature with associated extreme weakness, likely related to multiple bloodlettings. The youngster was relieved following the transfusion (Fig. 2-2*B*). Denis' second human transfusion was performed on a 45-year-old man, apparently with little clinical indication. Denis reported that this individual felt stronger than before the transfusion. Shortly thereafter, the son of the

Minister of State to the King of Sweden became seriously ill while traveling in Paris and was transfused twice by Denis. Denis subsequently transfused a hemiplegic woman during the autumn of 1667.[17, 18]

Denis submitted the report of his transfusion of the teenage boy to Henry Oldenburg, editor of the *Philosophical Transactions,* in July, 1667, and the letter was published in the July 22, 1667 issue. However, because of Oldenburg's confinement in the Tower of London at that time, he did not formally recognize it until the issue of September 23, 1667.[19] Nevertheless, considering that Lower did not perform his first human transfusion until November of that year, there seems little question that Denis was the first to perform transfusion of a human being.

Denis favored use of animal blood for his transfusion experiments because he believed it less likely "to be rendered impure by passion or vice." In contrast to Lower, he favored use of a femoral artery in the donor animal, rather than the cervical vessels used by Lower.[17]

Following transfusion of the four individuals described above, Denis and his associate performed a fifth transfusion later in 1667 which was to have far-reaching repercussions. A 34-year-old man, Antoine Mauroy, had had a severe "phrensy" for seven or eight years, ostensibly occasioned by an unfortunate love affair. His madness was manifest by his running through the streets of Paris naked. Denis's patron, Monsieur de Montmor, proposed transfusion, believing it would allay the "heat of his blood." Following removal of 10 ounces of blood from a vein in the man's right arm, 5 or 6 ounces of blood from a calf were administered without event.[20]

Two days later a second transfusion of Mauroy took place, more plentiful than the first. This resulted in what we would now recognize as a hemolytic transfusion reaction. Denis' description can be considered a medical classic:

> As soon as the blood began to enter into his veins, he felt the heat along his arm and under his armpits. His pulse rose and soon after we observed a plentiful sweat over all his face. His pulse varied extremely at this instant and he complained of great pains in his kidneys, and that he was not well in his stomach, and that he was ready to choke unless given his liberty. He was made to lie down and fell asleep, and slept all night without awakening until morning. When he awakened he made a great glass full of urine, of a color as black as if it had been mixed with the soot of chimneys.[21]

Denis recounted that the following morning the subject also manifested hemoglobinuria and had epistaxis. However, by the third day his urine cleared, and he improved his mental status and returned to his wife. Denis attributed the color of the urine to a "black choler" which had been retained in the body and had sent vapors to the brain, causing the subject's mental disturbance.[21] Several months later Mauroy again became violent and irrational, and his wife persuaded Denis and Emmerez to repeat the transfusion. Transfusion was attempted; however, mechanical difficulties precluded its performance. Mauroy died the following night.

Through their experiments of the previous year, Denis and Emmerez had acquired many enemies among the physicians of Paris. Three of these persuaded Mauroy's widow to accuse Denis and Emmerez of contributing to the death of her husband by the transfusion. Moreover, other physicians published pamphlets condemning the work of Denis and Emmerez. At one time the widow offered to withdraw the law suit provided she would receive payment from Denis; however, he responded, "that those physicians, and herself, stood more in need of the transfusion than ever her husband had done.[20] Denis lodged a counter-complaint against the widow. At the subsequent trial he was exonerated, and the widow was subsequently shown to have poisoned her husband with arsenic.

Most important, the Faculty of Medicine of Paris issued a decree based on the results of the trial, stating that the procedure of transfusion was a criminal act unless given sanction by the Faculty of Medicine.[5] It must be recalled that the Faculty was an extremely conservative body, which had refused for many years to recognize Harvey's theory of circulation.

By 1678 an edict of the French parliament specifically forbade transfusion in France, and the procedure also was outlawed by the Royal Society in London. In 1679, the Pope joined the outcry and banned the procedure. Therefore, interest in transfusion quickly waned.[22]

It is of interest that, aside from Lower's comments associated with his initial dog experiments, in the seventeenth century little consideration was given to the use of transfusion for replacement of blood loss. Most popular was the possibility of altering mental aberration through transfusion. Considerable importance was attached in contemporary writings to the possibility of restoring youth to the aged, and even suggesting that marital discord might be settled by reciprocal transfusions of the blood of husband and wife. In line with the mysticism associated with transfusion, it was speculated that a dog transfused with sheep blood might grow wool, cloven hooves, and horns. There was even an account of a young girl who received blood from a cat and was quickly endowed with feline characteristics.[5]

Only sporadic efforts at transfusion were undertaken during the remainder of the seventeenth and throughout the eighteenth century, all representing instances of transfusion of animal blood to humans. Not until 1749 did a member of the Faculty of Medicine of Paris, Cantwell, state that transfusion was valuable and advocate its use as a procedure in extreme emergencies.[6]

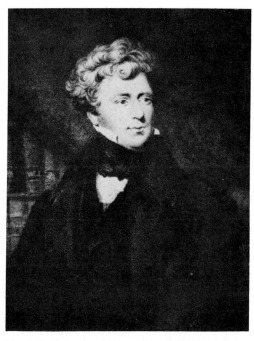

Fig. 2-3. Portrait of James Blundell (1790-1877). (Jones, W.H. and Mackmull, G.: The influence of James Blundell on the development of blood transfusion. Ann. Med. Hist. 10:242, 1928.)

TRANSFUSION IN THE NINETEENTH CENTURY

James Blundell and the Rebirth of Transfusion

Blood transfusion lay dormant for a century and a half. The credit for rekindling interest in the procedure and providing it with a semblance of a rational approach must be given to James Blundell. Blundell, born in 1790, was a physician with far-reaching interests (Fig. 2-3). He was one of the outstanding obstetricians of his day, and between 1816 and 1834 he delivered the lectures on midwifery at Guy's Hospital in London. These were printed in *Lancet* and subsequently were published in book form both in England and in the United States. Among the new operations which Blundell proposed were: operative reduction of intussusception; sterilization by bilateral partial salpingectomy; bilateral oophorectomy for severe dysmen-

orrhea; a method for removal of the cancerous uterus either through the abdominal wall or per vagina; and Cesarean hysterectomy.[23] It should be noted that, although he suggested these procedures, he did not actually perform all of them.

Blundell's interest in blood transfusion stemmed from his perception that this would be an appropriate treatment for postpartum hemorrhage. He initially experimented on dogs, exsanguinating them and subsequently reviving them by transfusion of arterial blood obtained from other dogs.[24] From his experiments he concluded that the blood of one animal could not be substituted for that of another with impunity, and he thereupon turned to use of human blood for human transfusion.

It should be appreciated that Blundell received his medical degree from the University of Edinburgh and undoubtedly was influenced in his early experiments by the experiments of John Leacock.[25] Although Leacock's manuscript on the subject was written while he was in Barbados, his experiments were performed during his tenure in Edinburgh, where one of his contemporaries was Blundell. Utilizing a 6-inch length of ox ureter with crow-quills attached to each end, Leacock operated on dogs, resuscitating exsanguinated animals by transfusion. Although Leacock did not perform human transfusion, he argued against mixing blood of different species, and his experiments quite clearly pointed to the efficacy of such treatment.

Blundell initially advocated direct transfusions; however, he showed that blood was still satisfactory if allowed to remain in a container for only a few seconds and then injected by syringe. Blundell described transfusion by syringe in several papers, noting the necessity of removing air from the instrument before the transfusion.

Following his experiments with animals, Blundell turned to transfusing humans with human blood. On December 22, 1818, Blundell transfused a 35-year-old man with gastric carcinoma (Fig. 2-4). When first seen by Blundell, the patient was severely wasted and near death. Approximately 14 ounces of blood were administered by syringe in small amounts at intervals of 5 to 6 minutes; however, despite temporary improvement, the patient died 56 hours later.[26]

This transfusion is generally accepted as the first transfusion of a human with human blood. However, a footnote in an American journal, coupled with a report of a transfusion in England, notes that Dr. Philip Syng Physick performed the procedure "under precisely the same circumstances" in 1795.[27] It is impossible to verify this citation, for, in contrast to Blundell's numerous publications, Physick never recorded this event. His biographer notes that Physick "maintained a most invincible repugnance to appear before the public in the shape of an author; and this feeling induced him to exact the promise that

SOME ACCOUNT OF A CASE

OF

OBSTINATE VOMITING,

IN WHICH

AN ATTEMPT WAS MADE

TO PROLONG LIFE,

BY THE

INJECTION OF BLOOD INTO THE VEINS.

By JAMES BLUNDELL, M.D.

LECTURER, IN CONJUNCTION WITH DR. HAIGHTON, ON PHYSIOLOGY AND MIDWIFERY, AT GUY'S HOSPITAL.

Read Dec. 22, 1818.

Fig. 2-4. Report of Blundell's first transfusion. (Blundell, J.: Some account of a case of obstinate vomiting in which an attempt was made to prolong life by the injection of blood into the veins. Med. Chir. Trans. 10:296, 1819.)

none of his manuscripts, lectures or letters should be published."[28]

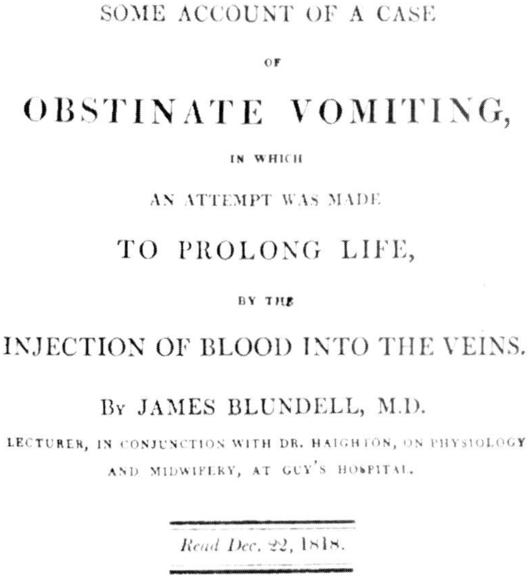

Blundell subsequently transfused several women with postpartum hemorrhage, and consulted in numerous other transfusions at that time. In 1828, defending the use of human, rather than animal blood for transfusion, he noted the impracticality of animal blood because of the difficulty of finding the appropriate animal in an emergency:

> "What is to be done in an emergency? A dog might come when you whistled, but the animal is small; a calf might have appeared fitter for the purpose, but then it had not been taught to walk properly up the stairs."[29]

Blundell was also aware that the operation might be performed needlessly, and emphasized that it should be reserved for desperately ill patients.

Blundell stimulated his contemporaries to practice transfusion. For the most part, these were obstetricians who utilized the procedure

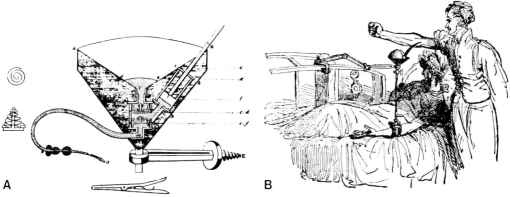

Fig. 2-5. (*A*) Blundell's "impellor." Blood is indicated by dots, surrounded by warm water indicated by horizontal lines. (Jones, H.W. and Mackmull, G.: The influence of James Blundell on the development of blood transfusion. Ann. Med. Hist. 10:242, 1928.) (*B*) Sketch of Blundell's gravitator. (Blundell, J.: Observations on transfusion of blood. Lancet 2:321, 1828-1829.)

in cases of postpartum hemorrhage. Two of the most active transfusionists were Doubleday and Waller.[30] The medical writing of the time is remarkably descriptive, as exemplified by Doubleday's description of his transfusion of a woman with postpartum hemorrhage with her husband's blood. After 6 ounces had been administered, the woman, previously semicomatose, suddenly exclaimed, "by Jesus, I feel strong as a bull."[31]

Similarly, Blundell, in 1829, describing a transfusion for postpartum hemorrhage, claimed that "the patient expresses herself very strongly on the benefits resulting from the injection of the blood; her observations are equivalent to this—that she felt as if life were infused into her body."[32] It is of interest that this report, in *Lancet*, is in apposition to the thorough documentation of the murder trial of the notorious resurrectionists, Burke and Hare.

Blundell developed several different methods of transfusion. Following his demonstration of the effectiveness of a syringe, he devised an "impellor," an instrument in which the blood was collected in a metal cup surrounded by warm water, and then injected into the vein of the recipient with the aid of an attached syringe (Fig. 2-5*A*). He also fabricated a piston-syringe-cup device, a tube for direct transfusion, and a gravitator (Fig. 2-5*B*). In the gravitator technique, blood from the donor dripped into a cup several feet above the arm of the recipient and flowed through tubing into the recipient vein.[33]

Apparently Blundell performed transfusion on ten different occasions, five being successful. In three of the unsuccessful cases, the patient was moribund when transfused. Blundell also served as a consultant in many other cases. One of these, in 1840, was most significant, for it was the first demonstration that a freshly drawn blood product could correct the bleeding tendency in Hemophilia A.[34] In this situation, the patient was an 11-year-old boy who had persistent hemorrhage after operative correction of strabismus (Fig. 2-6).

Although Blundell was remarkably progressive in developing his techniques of transfusion, it should be noted that he commonly applied leeches to the skin of the donor and recipient in an effort to prevent inflammation of the veins.[35] After 1830, his interest in transfusion waned. He retired from medical practice in 1847, undoubtedly facilitated by a fortune of a half million pounds sterling he had accumulated in practice and in bequests. Blundell lived in comparative obscurity until his death in 1878. He was a contro-

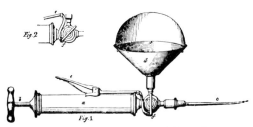

Fig. 2-6. Syringe used by Samuel Lane for transfusion in 1840. (Lane, S.: Hemorrhagic diathesis. Successful transfusion of blood. Lancet 1:185, 1840.)

versial figure, frequently at odds with the Medical Society of London and with the Directors of Guy's Hospital. His retirement from Guy's, in 1838, was occasioned by the appointment of a successor as chairman of obstetrics during Blundell's temporary absence. A heated dispute ensued, leading to his severance of all relations with the hospital.[36]

Considerable debate occupied London during the mid-nineteenth century regarding the use of transfusion, as evidenced by the minutes of the Medical Society. Many felt that the procedure was dangerous and that it may have hastened the death of some of the patients in whom it was used. Furthermore, it was claimed that most of the patients who benefited from the procedure would have recovered without its use. Conversely, Blundell argued strenuously on its behalf, noting that the danger of hemorrhage in these patients far outweighed the possible danger resulting from transfusion.[29]

This debate was still raging in 1849 when Routh reviewed all of the transfusions published to that date.[37] He was only able to find 48 recorded cases, of which 18 had a fatal outcome. This gave a mortality "rather less than that of hernia, or about the same as the average amputation." Furthermore, he noted that the mortality rate was unjustly high, for in many of these patients death was due to causes other than the transfusion. Routh concluded that the greatest danger was transmission of air, and he suggested that the

quantity of blood transfused should not be less than 6 ounces nor more than 16 ounces.

Among the indications for transfusion cited by Routh were severe hemorrhage, extreme exhaustion from dyspepsia, stricture of the esophagus, collapse following fever, and severe diarrhea or dysentery.

Early Transfusion in the United States

Aside from the unproven transfusion by Physick, it is doubtful that transfusion was practiced in the United States before 1830. The citations of transfusions in the early American literature most likely were culled from foreign journals, often without appropriate credit. As late as 1853, Benedict, in a review of the subject, stated that he had no knowledge of the procedure being performed in the United States.[38] The following year, an anonymous report of a transfusion in New Orleans was published.[39] The recipient was a patient with cholera who received 10 ounces of human blood by syringe but died a few minutes later. Four years later, Benedict transfused a young woman with yellow fever.[40] Austin Flint reviewed the subject in 1874 and noted that his son had performed the procedure in New Orleans during the winter of 1860-1861.[41] However, during the entire Civil War, only four transfusions are recorded.[42] It is of interest that two of these took place within a ten-day interval in 1864, one in Louisville, Kentucky, and the other in Alexandria, Virginia.[43]

Although never published, George McClellan was said to have transfused a patient with cholera in 1832, and William Hammond, an army surgeon, transfused soldiers with cholera in New Mexico in 1849.[42] Hammond subsequently became Surgeon General of the Union Army during the Civil War. There is no record of the use of transfusion by the Confederate forces during the Civil War.

Anticoagulation—Early Efforts

It is obvious that one of the problems that had to be solved before blood transfusion could be placed on a practical basis was the prevention of coagulation. Attempts to achieve this took several forms in the nineteenth century. Blundell observed in his writings the need for rapid performance of transfusion to avoid coagulation, and initiated the use of a syringe to overcome this problem. He also noted the impracticality of vein-to-vein direct transfusion, and encouraged the use of direct transfusion using the artery of the donor attached to the vein of the recipient.

In 1835 Bischoff proposed the use of defibrinated blood.[44] A variety of techniques were used for this purpose, the majority incorporating some form of a stirring proccess. One of the first to use an anticoagulant additive was Neudorfer, who, in 1860, recommended the addition of sodium bicarbonate as an anticoagulant.[45] Two physicians who were to achieve fame in other areas actively sought an answer to the problem of blood coagulation. Braxton Hicks utilized a solution of sodium phosphate as an anticoagulant in six unsuccessful transfusions,[46] while Brown-Sequard used defibrinated blood for his experiments performed in the early 1850s.[47] Nevertheless, half a century was to elapse before a practical means of anticoagulation was derived.

Late Nineteenth Century Transfusion

During the remainder of the nineteenth century, efforts were directed toward improvement of devices for indirect transfusion or refinement of surgical techniques to facilitate direct transfusion (Figs. 2.7-2.9). Nevertheless, indiscriminate use of transfusion resulted in increasing numbers of untoward reactions in recipients, so that the procedure fell into disfavor. Once again, transfusion of animal blood to humans was attempted; however, the experiments of Ponfick and Landois, in effect, put an end to heterologous blood transfusion.[9] Ponfick also was the first to note that the dark urine following an incompatible blood transfusion was hemoglobinuria, not hematuria, and resulted from destruction of the donor red cells and not those of the recipient.

During the final quarter of the nineteenth century, frustration and discouragement with blood as a transfusion product resulted in a brief wave of enthusiasm for transfusion of milk as a blood substitute.[48] This form of treatment achieved its greatest popularity in the United States between 1873 and 1880, with milk from cows, goats, and humans being used. The most outspoken advocate of milk transfusion was Thomas, who discouraged use of blood transfusion because of "the inherent difficulties and dangers of the operation, almost all of which arise from the tendency to coagulation."[49] Prout supported

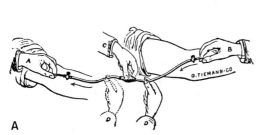
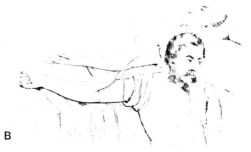

A

B

Fig. 2-7. (*A*) Direct transfusion as practiced by Aveling in 1872. (*B*) The donor artery was connected to the recipient vein, and pumping action was provided by a rubber bulb. (Aveling, J.H.: Immediate transfusion in England. Obst. J. Gt. Britain and Ireland 5:289, 1873.)

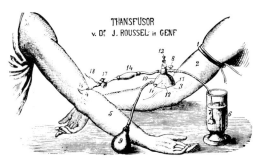

Fig. 2-8. Roussel's method of direct transfusion. In this technique, a lancet was inserted into the donor's vein and a suction cup, as well as an in-line rubber bulb, were used to maintain adequate flow. (Roussel, J.: Leçons sur la transfusion directe du sang. Asselin et Houzeau. Paris, 1885.)

Thomas, and even postulated a medical-legal use for milk transfusion in that it might prolong life for a sufficient time to permit "the victim of an assault to identify his assailant."[50]

By 1878 Brinton predicted that transfusion of milk would entirely supersede transfusion of blood.[51] However, by 1880 increasing numbers of adverse reactions associated with its administration led to its abandonment. This was hastened by the advent of saline infusion as a "blood substitute" in 1884.[52]

THE ADVENT OF MODERN BLOOD TRANSFUSION

At the end of the nineteenth century, blood transfusion was only slightly less primitive than at its inception two and a half centuries earlier. The principal accomplishment during this interval was the recognition of the inappropriateness of animal blood for human transfusion. Beyond that, solutions to such problems as anticoagulation, immune destruction of transfused red cells, long-term preservation of blood for transfusion, recognition of the serologic heterogeneity of red cells, and component preparation awaited developments of the twentieth century.

The Discovery of Blood Groups

The modern era of blood transfusion was initiated with the epochal work of Landsteiner, who demonstrated the presence of A, B, and O isoagglutinins in serum in 1900, and in the following year divided human blood into three groups on the basis of the serologic reactions of red cells with these agglutinins. Landsteiner's initial publication was in the form of a footnote to an article on bacterial fermentation.[53] In his 1901 article, Landsteiner indicated the importance of taking into account these blood differences for the successful outcome of transfusion.[54] Unfortunately, several years were to pass until such a practice was introduced. In 1902 the fourth blood group, AB, was described by Sturli and De Castello. Following these initial studies, Landsteiner abandoned his work on blood groups for over 20 years to pursue other interests.

In 1907 Richard Weil, a pathologist at German Hospital in New York, alerted his intern, Reuben Ottenberg, to the importance of Landsteiner's discovery.[55] Ottenberg was the first to perform ABO typing of patient and donor before blood transfusion, and also was the first to use compatibility testing before transfusion. Furthermore, he first suggested inheritance of the ABO types, and noted the relatively minor role of donor antibodies in transfusion therapy.

While the ABO blood types were defined in the first years of this century, considerable debate ensued relative to their appropriate terminology. In his original paper, Landsteiner identified the three groups as A, B, and C. Working independently, Jansky, of Czechoslovakia, in 1907, and Moss, of the United States, in 1910, described four blood groups, using Roman numeral designations. Unfortunately, Moss was unaware of Jansky's work and, in classifying the groups, transposed the order of the Roman numeral designations. In 1927 the American Association of Immunologists, in an effort to resolve

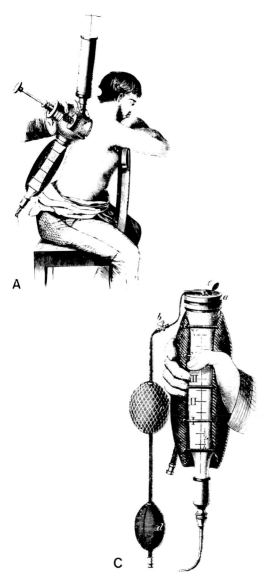

A

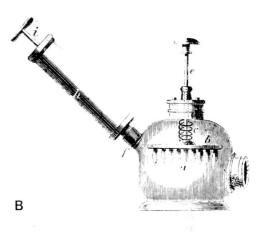

B

C

Fig. 2-9. (*A*) Collection and transfusion of capillary blood by the method of Gesellius. (*B*) An evacuated suction cup was placed over the back of donor, and multiple lancets were plunged into skin. (*C*) A graduated cylinder surrounded by warm water was disconnected from donor apparatus and used for the transfusion. (Gesellius, F.: Die Transfusion des Blutes. E. Hoppe. St. Petersburg and Leipzig, 1873.)

the resultant terminologic confusion, sponsored a new classification, suggested by Landsteiner, which is the present one used for the ABO system.

Although Moss is remembered for his efforts in classifying the ABO group, his most important contribution may have been his demonstration that isohemolysis was parallel to isoagglutination. This permitted determination of blood groups by agglutination reactions rather than by the more laborious hemolysis tests.[56]

Blood Preservation and the Advent of the Blood Bank

The second major problem to be solved in the twentieth century was that of anticoagulation and preservation of blood for transfu-

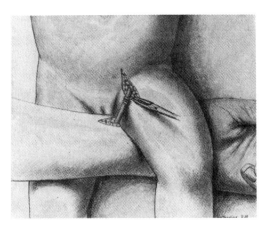

Fig. 2-10. Direct transfusion using artery-vein anastomosis by Crile's technique for hemorrhagic disease of newborn. (Lespinasse, V.D.: The Treatment of hemorrhagic disease of the newborn by direct transfusion of blood. J.A.M.A. 62:1868, 1914. Copyright, 1914, American Medical Association.)

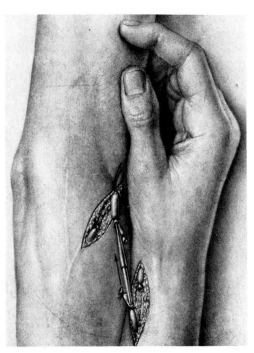

Fig. 2-11. Artery-vein anastomosis using paired tubes, as devised by Bernheim. (Bernheim, B.M.: Blood transfusion, hemorrhage and the anemias. J.B. Lippincott, Philadelphia, 1917.)

sion. In the early years of the century, coagulation was prevented by improved methods of direct transfusion. Anastomosis of blood vessels for direct transfusion, first performed by Alexis Carrel, was refined and popularized in 1907 by George Crile, who utilized a cannula through which the vein of the recipient and the artery of the donor were drawn (Fig. 2-10). Although other methods for direct transfusion were devised (Fig. 2-11), such procedures necessitated sacrifice of the two vessels; therefore, these operations did not have long-lasting popularity.

Various paraffin-coated tubes were employed for direct transfusion in an effort to forestall coagulation; however, of greater significance was the comparatively simple multiple syringe method, proposed in 1913 by Edward Lindeman, representing a rediscovery of a method which had been described in 1892 by von Zeimssen.[57] The syringe procedures effectively put an end to direct vessel anastomosis transfusion.

The principal advantage of the Lindeman technique was the elimination of the need for dissection of blood vessels in either the donor or the recipient.[58] The direct anastomosis procedure often proved more difficult than the operation it was intended to support. Furthermore, with use of syringes the exact quantity of blood transfused was known; however, repeated filling and washing of syringes required several operators, because rapid injection of the blood was essential to avoid coagulation. Two years later Unger devised a simple syringe method using a four-way stopcock which overcame many of the difficulties of the Lindeman procedure.[59] Dozens of variations of Unger's syringe technique appeared during the following two decades, as did mechanical devices for direct transfusion (Fig. 2-12).

In 1914 and 1915, use of sodium citrate as an anticoagulant was proposed independently from four different sources. In March of 1914, Albert Hustin, a Belgian, apparently was the first to use citrate, in a solution containing salt and glucose.[55] His solution ren-

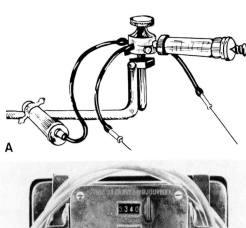

A

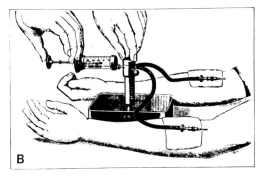

B

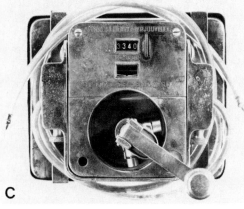

C

Fig. 2-12. (*A*) Unger's device for transfusion by syringe, using four-way stopcock. (Killduffe, R.A.: and DeBakey, M.: The blood bank and the technique and therapeutics of transfusion. The C. V. Mosby Company, St. Louis, 1942.) (*B*) Tzanck's modification of the Unger technique. (Tzanck, A.: Techniques de transfusion sanguine. Paris Med. 59:301, 1925. As drawn in: Jeanneney, G. and Ringenbach, G.: Traite de la transfusion sanguine. Masson et cie. Paris, 1940.) (*C*) Device of Henry and Jouvelet (1934) for direct transfusion using manual roller pump. (From author's collection)

dered the red cells so dilute as to be impractical. In November of the same year, Luis Agote, of Buenos Aires, performed a transfusion in which citrate alone was used. Rather than publishing his report in a medical journal, Agote gave the story to *La Prensa,* the leading newspaper of Buenos Aires, and it was also published in detail in the *New York Herald.*[60] Two months later, two New York physicians independently provided the most significant impetus for the use of citrate as an anticoagulant.

Richard Lewisohn, a surgeon at Mount Sinai Hospital, used citrate for human blood transfusion only after performing multiple studies of citrate toxicity in dogs (Fig. 2-13). He carefully demonstrated the optimal citrate dose for anticoagulation. Simultaneously, Richard Weil, the pathologist who had served as a stimulus for Ottenberg, noted that citrated blood could be stored in a refrigerator for several days before use.[61]

Based upon Weil's and Lewisohn's work, Rous and Turner prepared a solution of salt, isocitrate, and glucose to accomplish both anticoagulation and preservation of blood.[62] This was a most cumbersome method, in that there was a tremendous excess of anticoagulant solution to blood volume, requiring removal of the anticoagulant before transfusion. However, it was the only such solution available for almost 25 years.

The availability of the Rous-Turner solution permitted an American physician attached to the British Army to perform the first transfusions with preserved blood during World War I. Oswald Robertson transfused 20 casualties on 22 occasions during the Battle of Cambrai in November, 1917. The blood units had been preserved for 10 to 26 days before transfusion. Robertson used only group O blood.[63]

By March, 1918, citrated blood had become the official method for combating shock in both the British and American armies.[64] Prior to that time, the majority of transfusions in the War were by syringe or by related techniques such as the Kimpton-Brown tube (Fig. 2-14). The Kimpton-Brown tube, which was devised in 1913, was a paraffin-coated grad-

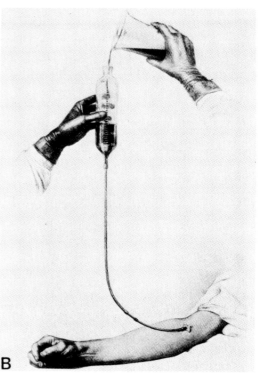

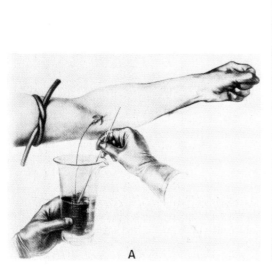

Fig. 2-13. Lewisohn's method of transfusion of citrated blood. (*A*) Blood is collected in graduated flask containing citrate and (*B*) is promptly transfused to patient. (Lewisohn R.: The citrate method of blood transfusion after ten years. Boston Med. and Surg. J. [N. Engl. J. Med.] 190:733, 1924. Reprinted by permission from the New England Journal of Medicine.)

uated glass cylinder with a horizontal side tube for suction. The bottom of the cylinder was drawn into an S-shaped cannula for use both in the donor and recipient veins.[65] A combination of the paraffin-coated cylinder with a syringe technique is shown in Fig. 2-15.

Blood preservation in the United States

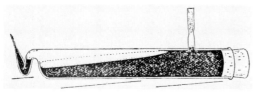

Fig. 2-14. Kimpton-Brown tube. Blood has been drawn from the donor and the tube has been kept horizontal until transfusion. (Kimpton A.R. and Brown J.H.: A new and simple method of transfusion. J.A.M.A. 61:117, 1913. Copyright 1913, American Medical Association.)

following World War I largely was through use of the Rous-Turner solution or subsequent minor modifications introduced in the early 1940s by DeGowin, Alsever, and their colleagues.[66-67] All of these solutions had the disadvantage of having a large volume of preservative solution in relation to the amount of blood. Blood preserved in this manner was used during most of World War II.

In December, 1943, Loutit and Mollison introduced ACD as a preservative having the advantage of a reduced volume of solution.[68] Whereas the blood-preservative ratio of Alsever solution was 1:1, that of ACD as initially formulated was 4:1, and it was later reduced to 6:1. Moreover, ACD was simpler to prepare and to autoclave than the Alsever solution. However, because of the need for testing the new preservative, as well as ob-

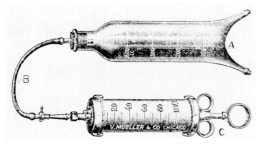

Fig. 2-15. Combination of syringe and paraffin-lined cylinder for transfusion, as devised by Davis and Curtis. The cannula tips at *A* are attached to the recipient and donor veins. (Davis, V.C. and Curtis, A.H.: Recent experiences with blood transfusion. J.A.M.A. 62:775, 1914. Copyright 1914, American Medical Association.)

taining new bottles and transporting materials, ACD solution was not adopted by the United States Army until April, 1945.[64]

Preserved blood originally was collected in glass bottles with rubber seals and tubing, and steel needles. All these products were reused after sterilization. Lack of removal of all of the blood or proteins from the apparatus, as well as contamination by rinsing solutions, often resulted in pyrogenic reactions in the recipients of subsequent units. Not until 1933 was the incidence of such reactions reduced through greater attention to bottle cleaning.[69] Moreover, evacuated blood-collection bottles resulted in foaming of the collected blood with the attendant possibility of coagulation. Also, gravity-draw bottles carried the risk of air embolism for the donor, while a similar risk existed for the recipient transfused with blood in glass bottles when air was pumped into the bottle to hasten transfusion.

A most significant expansion of the horizons of blood banking was the advent of plastic transfusion equipment. By 1949 trials of such equipment were conducted by the American National Red Cross and a few hospital blood banks; however, more than ten years were to elapse before such equipment was incorporated into transfusion programs.[70] The use of plastic transfusion equipment facilitated the advent of blood component therapy, primarily a development of the 1950s and 1960s.

A major impetus for further development of blood component therapy was the revival of interest in the technique of plasmapheresis in the sixth and seventh decades of this century. This had been initially described in 1914 at Johns Hopkins Hospital by Abel, Rowntree, and Turner, who proposed the technique as a method of increasing the yield of antitoxic sera from hyperimmune animals.[71]

The availability of preservative solutions, coupled with the development of electrical refrigeration equipment, permitted the development of organized programs for blood preservation. While the first blood bank likely was formulated in Leningrad in 1932, the first functional blood bank was instituted in Barcelona in 1936, in association with the need for blood in the Spanish Civil War.[72] Fantus organized the first blood bank in the United States, at Cook County Hospital in Chicago, in 1937. However, even in the early 1940s, direct or indirect transfusion of unmodified blood was favored in many hospitals.

Other Developments of the Twentieth Century

During the early years of the twentieth century, the difficulty of direct transfusion and the relative impracticality of transfusion with citrated blood, led to attempts to identify alternate sources of blood for transfusion. For example, in Moscow, Yudin initiated the use of cadaver blood for transfusion.[73] By 1938 he had accomplished 2500 such transfusions. However, cadaver blood transfusion, even in Russia, never achieved significant popularity. Another alternate source of blood was placental blood, although there is no record that it ever achieved significant use in the United States.[74]

The development of blood banking in the third quarter of the twentieth century has been phenomenal. Whereas only a handful of blood group systems had been identified by 1950, over 200 are now recognized. This expansion of knowledge of blood group serology has been reflected in enhancement of the safety of blood transfusion through pretransfusion testing.

One of the primary factors facilitating such testing was the advent of the antiglobulin reaction. Although originally described by Moreschi in 1908, current use of this test stems from the 1945 work of Coombs, Mourant, and Race.[75] Not only has pretransfusion testing mitigated the risk of immune hemolysis of the transfused red cells, it also has optimized the survival of such cells through recognition of antibodies which occasion more protracted removal of the transfused erythrocytes.

The expansion of knowledge of blood group antigens is indicated by the fact that only the ABO system, the MN, and P antigens were recognized by 1935. Landsteiner and Wiener described Rh polymorphism in 1940,[76] and in 1941 Levine and associates demonstrated that isoimmunization to the Rh antigen was the principal cause of hemolytic disease of the newborn.[77] Prior to that time, the latter disease often had been attributed to seronegative syphilis. The profusion of newly identified blood group systems was intimately related to the development of new methods of detection of IgG antibody. This included not only the antiglobulin test, but also the use of high protein medium and of enzyme techniques for serologic testing.[78]

Developments during the last decade have further enhanced the safe and effective utilization of blood as a therapeutic resource. For example, storage of blood has been prolonged by the development of newer blood preservative solutions. Moreover, through use of automated and semiautomated equipment, the procurement of platelets and granulocytes for transfusion has been facilitated. Improvement of methods for enhancement of agglutination in serologic testing has expedited provision of blood for transfusion. The safety of transfusion has been greatly enhanced through the advent of serologic testing for hepatitis B antigen, the recognition of the danger of blood obtained from commercial donors, the advent of quality control programs, and the promulgation of minimum performance standards with associated inspection programs. Automation also has greatly expanded the efficiency and accuracy of serologic testing in blood donor centers.

It is obvious that clinical acceptance of blood transfusion has been achieved only over the past several decades. The scope of blood banking has now broadened to include diagnostic and therapeutic implications which could not have been envisioned when the term was first used. One can only wonder what the future holds in store for this rapidly changing field.

REFERENCES

1. Ovid's Metamorphoses. Vol. 2. Cornhill Publishing Co., Boston, 1941.
2. Leviticus. 17:11-12.
3. Genesis. 9:4.
4. Deuteronomy. 12:23-4.
5. Brown, H.M.: The beginnings of intravenous medication. Ann. Med. Hist. 1:177, 1917.
6. Dutton, W.F.: Intravenous Therapy: Its Application in the Modern Practice of Medicine. F. A. Davis Co., Philadelphia, 1925.
7. Villari, P.: The Life and Times of Giralamo Savonarola. T. Fisher Unwin Ltd., London, 1888.
8. Lindeboom, G.A.: The story of a blood transfusion to a pope. J. Hist. Med. 9:455, 1954.
9. Maluf, M.F.R.: History of blood transfusion. J. Hist. Med. 9:59, 1954.
10. Webster, C.: The origins of blood transfusion. Med. Hist. 15:387, 1971.
11. Wren, C.: Philos. Trans. R. Soc. Lond. 1:128, 1665.
12. Gladstone, E.: Johann Sigmund Elsholtz. Calif. and West. Med. 38:432; 39:45, 1933.
13. Jennings, C.E.: Transfusion. Leonard and Co., New York, 1883.
14. Lower, R.: Philos. Trans. R. Soc. Lond. 1:353, 1666.

15. Pepys, S.: The Diary of Samuel Pepys. Henry Wheatley, ed. G. Bell and Sons, Ltd., London, 6:64, 1896.
16. Ibid. 7:208.
17. Brown, H.: Jean Denis and transfusion of blood, Paris, 1667-1668. Isis. 39:15, 1948.
18. Keynes, G.: Tercentenary of blood transfusion. Br. Med. J. 4:410, 1967.
19. Denis, J.: Philos. Trans. R. Soc. Lond. 3:489, 1667.
20. Denis, J.: Philos. Trans. R. Soc. Lond. 4:710, 1668.
21. Denis, J.: Philos. Trans. R. Soc. Lond. 4:617, 1668.
22. Hoff, H.E. and Guillemin, R.: The tercentenary of transfusion in man. Cardiovasc. Res. Center Bull. 6:47, 1967.
23. Young, J.H.: James Blundell (1790-1878): Experimental physiologist and obstetrician. Med. Hist. 8:159, 1964.
24. Blundell, J.: Experiments on the transfusion of blood by the syringe. Med. Chir. Trans. 9:56, 1818.
25. Leacock, J.H.: On the transfusion of blood in extreme cases of hemorrhage. Med. Chir. J. & Rev. 3:276, 1816.
26. Blundell, J.: Some account of a case of obstinate vomiting in which an attempt was made to prolong life by the injection of blood into the veins. Med. Chir. Trans. 10:296, 1819.
27. Editorial: Transfusion of blood. Phila. J. M. Phys. Sci. 9:205, 1825.
28. Randolph, J.: Memoir of Dr. P. S. Physick. Am. J. Med. Sci. 24:93, 1839.
29. Blundell, J.: The after-management of floodings, and on transfusion. Lancet 13:673, 1828.
30. Waller, C.: Successful transfusion. Lancet 11:457, 1827.
31. Doubleday, E.: Another successful case of transfusion. Lancet 1:111, 1825.
32. Blundell, J.: Successful case of transfusion. Lancet 1:431, 1829.
33. Ibid.: Observations on transfusion of blood. Lancet 2:321, 1828-1829.
34. Lane, S.: Hemorrhagic diathesis. Successful transfusion of blood. Lancet 1:185, 1840.
35. Blundell, J.: Lectures on the theory and practice of midwifery. Lancet 2:513, 1827-1828.
36. Jones, H.W. and Mackmull, G.: The influence of James Blundell on the development of blood transfusion. Ann. Med. Hist. 10:242, 1928.
37. Routh, C.: Remarks statistical and general on transfusion of blood. Med. Times 20:114, 1849.
38. Benedict, N.B.: On the operation of transfusion, being the report of a committee. New Orleans M. and S. J., 10:191, 1853.
39. Charity Hospital Reports. New Orleans Med. News and Hosp. Gaz. 1:216, 1854.
40. Benedict, N.B.: Transfusion in yellow fever—successful case. New Orleans Med. News and Hosp. Gaz. 5:721, 1859.
41. Flint, A.: Transfusion. Med. Record. 1:187, 1874.
42. Schmidt, P.J.: Transfusion in America in the eighteenth and nineteenth centuries. N. Engl. J. Med. 279:1319, 1968.
43. Kuhns, W.J.: Blood transfusion in the Civil War. Transfusion 5:92, 1965.
44. Bischoff, T.L.W.: Beitrage zur Lehre von dem Blute und der Transfusion desselben. Arch. f. Anat. Physiol. p. 347, 1835.
45. Neudorfer: Uber Transfusionen bei Anaemischen. Oesterr. Ztschr. f. prakt. Heild. 6:124, 1860.
46. Braxton-Hicks, J.: On transfusion and new mode of management. Br. Med. J. 3:151, 1868.
47. Brown-Sequard, E.: Experimental researches on the faculty possessed by certain elements of the blood of regenerating the vital properties. Med. Times and Gaz. 11:492, 1855.
48. Oberman, H.A.: Early history of blood substitutes. Transfusion of milk. Transfusion 9:74, 1969.
49. Thomas, T.G.: The intravenous injection of milk as a substitute for the transfusion of blood. Illustrated by seven operations. New York Med. J. 27:449, 1878.
50. Prout, J.S.: Intravenous injection of milk. Med. Rec. 13:378, 1878.
51. Brinton, J.H.: The transfusion of blood and the intravenous injection of milk. Med. Rec. 14:344, 1878.
52. Bull, W.T.: On the intravenous injection of saline solutions as a substitute for blood. Med. Rec. 25:6, 1884.
53. Landsteiner, K.: Zur kenntnis der antifermentativen, lytischen und agglutinierenden wirkungen des blutserums und der lymphe. Zbl. Bakt. 27:361, 1900.
54. Landsteiner, K.: Uber agglutinationserscheinungen normalen meuschlichen blutes. Wein. Klin. Wochenschr. 14:1132, 1901.

55. Rosenfield, R.: Early twentieth century origins of modern blood transfusion therapy. Mt. Sinai J. Med. 41:626, 1974.

56. Moss, W.L.: Studies on isoagglutinins and isohemolysins. Bull. J. Hopk. Hosp. 21:63, 1910.

57. von Ziemssen, H.: Uber die subcutane Blutinjection und uber eine neue einfache Methode der Intravenoson Transfusion. Munch. Med. Wschr. 39:1, 1892.

58. Lindeman, E.: Simple syringe transfusion with special cannulas. Am. J. Dis. Child. 6:28, 1913.

59. Unger, L.J.: A new method of syringe transfusion. J.A.M.A. 64:582, 1915.

60. Kyle, R.A. and Shampo, M.A.: Louis Agote. J.A.M.A. 228:860, 1974.

61. Weil, R.: Sodium citrate in the transfusion of blood. J.A.M.A. 64:425, 1915.

62. Rous, P. and Turner, P.: The preservation of living red blood cells in vitro. II. The transfusion of kept cells. J. Exper. Med. 23:239, 1916.

63. Robertson, O.: Transfusion with preserved red blood cells. Br. Med. J. 1:691, 1918.

64. Kendrick, D.B., Ed.: Blood programs in World War II. Dept. of the Army. Wash., D.C., 1964.

65. Kimpton, A.R. and Brown, J.H.: A new and simple method of transfusion. J.A.M.A. 61:117, 1913.

66. De Gowin, E.L., Harris, J.E. and Plass, E.D.: Studies on preserved human blood. I. Various factors inducing haemolysis. J.A.M.A. 114:850, 1940.

67. Alsever, J.B. and Ainslee, R.B.: A new method for the preparation of dilute plasma and the operation of a complete transfusion service. N.Y. State Med. J. 41:126, 1941.

68. Loutit, J.F. and Mollison, P.L.: Advantages of a disodium-citrate-glucose mixture as a blood preservative. Br. Med. J. 2:744, 1943.

69. Lewisohn, R. and Rosenthal, N.: Prevention of chills following the transfusion of citrated blood. J.A.M.A. 100:467, 1933.

70. Diamond, L.K.: History of blood banking in the United States. J.A.M.A. 193:140, 1965.

71. Abel, J.J., Rowntree, L.G. and Turner, B.B.: Plasma removal with return of corpuscles. J. Pharmacol. Exp. Ther. 5:625, 1914.

72. Jorda, J.D.: The Barcelona blood transfusion service. Lancet 1:773, 1939.

73. Swan, H. and Schechter, D.C.: The transfusion of blood from cadavers: a historical review. Surgery 52:545, 1962.

74. Hawkins, J. and Brewer, H.: Placental blood for transfusion. Lancet 1:132, 1939.

75. Coombs, R.R.A., Mourant, A.E. and Race, R.R.: A new test for the detection of weak and "incomplete" Rh agglutinins. Br. J. Exp. Pathol. 26:225, 1945.

76. Landsteiner, K. and Wiener, A.S.: An agglutinable factor in human blood recognized by immune serum for Rhesus blood. Proc. Soc. Exp. Biol. 43:223, 1940.

77. Levine, P., Burnham, L., Katzin, E.M. and Vogel, P.: The role of isoimmunization in the pathogenesis of erythroblastosis fetasis. Am. J. Obstet. Gynecol. 42:925, 1941.

78. Rosenfield, R.E.: The past and future of immunohematology. Am. J. Clin. Pathol. 64:569, 1975.

II. Biology, Technology, and Organization of Blood Transfusion

3

Immunology and Its Relation to Blood Transfusion

Lawrence D. Petz, M.D., and Scott N. Swisher, M.D.

INTRODUCTION

The purpose of this chapter is to provide a brief review of selected aspects of immunology that have relevance to the practice of blood transfusion. A number of clinical applications of these immunological principles are pointed out throughout the chapter. Although some of the basic immunology discussed does not yet have direct application to the practice of transfusion, the information will nevertheless allow the interested reader to develop greater depth of knowledge in these selected areas; it will provide a basis for understanding some of the phenomenology of blood transfusion, enable the reader to cope with much of the modern medical literature, and point toward future developments in transfusion and transplantation biology.

THE IMMUNE SYSTEM

THE CELLULAR SYSTEM OF THE IMMUNE RESPONSE

The immune system has two major components: humoral immunity and cellular immunity. These components, or "limbs" as they are frequently called, develop along separate but related pathways of differentiation involving several types of cells and tissues. The cells of the immune system include T and B lymphocytes, and macrophages (Fig. 3-1). Initiation of either type of immune response requires the direct interaction of an antigen with a lymphocyte. In some responses, the macrophage plays a role in processing the antigen before contact with the lymphocyte.

Immunocompetent cells are lymphocytes that can be functionally divided into two components: those involved in humoral immunity and those involved in cellular immunity. Although early work indicated that the lymphocyte was involved in antibody production[1-6] and in cellular immune reactions,[7-9] the division of lymphocytes into these functional compartments received an enormous impetus from the work of Glick et al.[10] which was reported in 1956 in the journal *Poultry Science*. They reported that removal of the bursa of Fabricius from neonatal chicks resulted in loss of their ability to produce antibody when challenged with various bacterial antigens. Subsequent work by Cooper et al.[11,12] indicated a definite separa-

31

CELLS INVOLVED IN IMMUNE RESPONSES

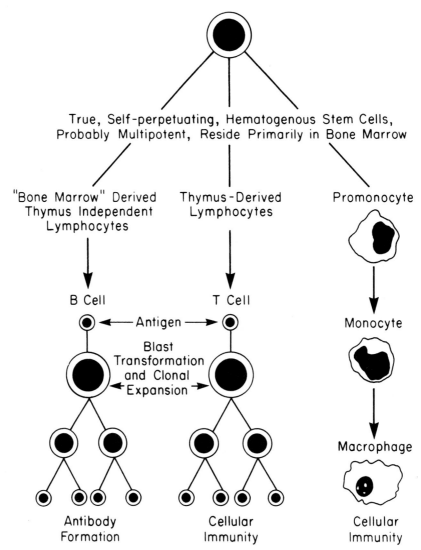

True, Self-perpetuating, Hematogenous Stem Cells,
Probably Multipotent, Reside Primarily in Bone Marrow

"Bone Marrow" Derived
Thymus Independent
Lymphocytes

Thymus-Derived
Lymphocytes

Promonocyte

B Cell

T Cell

←—— Antigen ——→

Monocyte

Blast
Transformation
and Clonal
←Expansion→

Antibody
Formation

Cellular
Immunity

Macrophage

Cellular
Immunity

Fig. 3-1. Cells involved in immune responses.

tion of lymphocyte immunological functions; it established that lymphocytes depending on the thymus for maturation mediate cellular immunity while lymphocytes dependent on the bursa mediate humoral immunity.

In man, there are congenital immunodeficiency states comparable to the experimental immunodeficient states in animal models. Bruton's agammaglobulinemia, in which there is normal thymic development and intact cellular immunity, is characterized by absence of plasma cells and circulating antibody. This disease is strikingly similar to the model of bursectomized chicks. The DiGeorge syndrome is a deficiency of thymic development and lack of cellular immunity; however, plasma cells and circulating antibody are present. This disease is the clinical counterpart of thymectomized experimental animals.

T LYMPHOCYTES AND B LYMPHOCYTES

It has been possible to define characteristic cell surface markers for the detection of B and T lymphocytes, using immunofluorescence microscopy, radioautography, or rosette formation with erythrocytes coated with immunoproteins. Certain generalizations can be made from these studies. It should be pointed out, however, that: (1) overlapping cell populations exist; (2) the specificity of these markers requires further investigation; and (3) the identification of subpopulations of B and T cells is still more complex, although monoclonal antibodies for this purpose are now being developed for T cell subpopulations of man and animals.

The B lymphocyte in humans and most mammalian species is characterized by the presence of readily detectable surface immunoglobulin. Surface immunoglobulin can be demonstrated using fluoresceinated polyvalent or monovalent antisera directed against various immunoglobulin classes. The major immunoglobulin class present on circulating B lymphocytes is IgM, present in monomeric form. IgD, IgG, and IgA may also be present on B lymphocyte membranes. Under some circumstances, IgM and IgD have both been detected on the same lymphocyte.

In addition, most of the B lymphocytes have a membrane receptor for antigen-antibody complexes, or aggregated immunoglobulin. This receptor appears to be specific for a site on the Fc portion of the immunoglobulin molecule (see Structure of Immunoglobulins) and is known as the Fc receptor. It has been possible to demonstrate a receptor for the third component of complement (C3) on some B cells, using erythrocytes coated with antibody and complement. Lymphocytes bearing this receptor have been called complement receptor lymphocytes. The complement receptor is not a single molecular species; there are distinct membrane-binding sites for C3b, C3d, and C4. The complement receptors have been shown to be distinct from the Fc receptor.

In mice, several characteristic antigens have been demonstrated on T lymphocytes. These include: the theta (θ) antigen; antigens known as thymus-leukemia (TL) antigens which appear on normal thymocytes in some strains and on leukemic cells of all strains; and antigens known as Ly antigens (lymphocyte alloantigens). The Ly antigen system has made it possible to define T cells subsets in the mouse which are related to helper, suppressor, and killer functions.

In humans, T lymphocytes have the property of forming rosettes with sheep erythrocytes, and this property is used to identify human T cells. Many human peripheral T lymphocytes have membrane receptors for the Fc portion of IgG and of monomeric IgM. These markers may identify functionally distinct T cell subsets in humans. In addition, antisera prepared against brain tissue react with T cells, as do antisera prepared in rabbits injected with thymocytes. Various markers have been used to determine the distribution of B and T lymphocytes in various tissues.

T lymphocytes are essential for the full expression of immunity and, as such, are involved in many functions for which they have received special names:

1. T cells function as regulatory cells modulating the activities of B cells (or other T cells). The regulatory function of T cells can be expressed in two ways: positively (helper) or negatively (suppressor). Helper T cells are those that need to interact with antigen in order for other lymphocytes to fully respond. Suppressor T cells, as their name indicates, are capable of suppressing a given immune function.

2. T cells are involved in cellular immune reactions, which include reactions of delayed sensitivity, contact sensitivity, and resistance to infection with certain bacteria, such as the

facultative intracellular bacteria, and viruses. T cells perform part of these functions by elaborating a number of molecules that can affect the inflammatory response or the behavior of other inflammatory cells—principally, macrophages. Such molecules are termed lymphocyte mediators or lymphokines.

3. T cells are the major cells involved in transplantation immunity and as such are involved in allograft rejection and graft-versus-host reactions which consist of the reaction of a set of immunocompetent T cells against cells or tissues bearing different histocompatibility antigens.

4. T cells can act as cytotoxic T cells; that is to say, they have the capacity to kill other cells. This phenomenon is best seen as part of the immune response against tumors. The name, cytotoxic T cells, is synonymous with cytolytic or killer T cells.

A subpopulation of peripheral lymphocytes in humans has been described which lacks typical B and T cell markers. These cells are called "null cells." Some of these null cells bear Fc receptors and function as killer cells (K cells) in antibody-dependent, cell-mediated cytotoxicity.

Several reagents known as mitogens stimulate lymphocytes in vitro, including plant lectins, bacterial products, polymeric substances, and enzymes. Morphologic transformation occurs following stimulation, with the formation of blast cells or in some instances plasma cells. Lymphocyte transformation may also be assessed biochemically by the measurement of RNA, DNA, or protein synthesis. Some characteristics of B and T cells are summarized in Table 3-1.

MONONUCLEAR PHAGOCYTES (MONOCYTE-MACROPHAGES)

The mononuclear phagocytes include the circulating peripheral blood monocytes, promonocytes, precursor cells in the bone marrow, and tissue macrophages. The tissue macrophages are present in several tissues, organs, and serous cavities. The organization of the mononuclear phagocyte system is shown in Table 3-2. Mononuclear phagocytes

Table 3-1. Characteristics of B and T Subclasses of Lymphocytes

Properties	B-cells	T-Cells
Cell surface receptors and antigens		
Ig	+	−
C3	+	−
Fc	+	−
Thy 1 (θ) (mouse)	−	+
Immune function		
Humoral	Antibody-forming cell	−
Cell-mediated	−	"Helper" cells "Suppressor" cells Regulatory cells Cytotoxic cells Lymphokines
Derivation	Avian bursa Bone marrow Fetal liver Spleen	Thymus
Responsiveness to mitogens in soluble form		
Concanavalin A	−	+
Phytohemagglutinin	−	+
Pokeweed mitogen	+	+
Lipopolysaccharide	+	−

Table 3-2. The Mononuclear Phagocyte System

Development of Macrophages	Location of Cells
PRECURSOR CELLS ↓	bone marrow
PROMONOCYTES ↓	bone marrow
MONOCYTES ↓	bone marrow, blood
MACROPHAGES	connective tissue (histiocytes) liver (Kupffer cells) lung (alveolar macrophages) spleen (free and fixed macrophages) lymph node (free and fixed macrophages) bone marrow (macrophages) serous cavity (pleural and peritoneal macrophages) bone tissue (osteoclasts?) nervous system (microglial cells?)

(Van Furth, R., Cohn, Z. A. Hirsch, J. G. Humphrey, J. H. Spector, W. G., and Langevoort, H. L.: The mononuclear phagocyte system: A new classification of macrophages, monocytes, and their precursor cells. Bull. Wld. Hlth. Org. *46*:845, 1972.)

originate from precursor cells in the bone marrow. They circulate in the peripheral blood as monocytes. The tissue macrophages are derived from both blood monocytes and local proliferation of macrophages.

The monocyte-macrophage is capable of both nonimmunologic and immunologic phagocytosis. Monocyte-macrophages have a plasma membrane receptor which recognizes two of the four subclasses of human IgG (IgG1 and IgG3); this binding site on the IgG molecule has been localized to the C_H3 domain of the immunoglobulin molecule. The monocyte-macrophage also has an independent receptor system which recognizes the activated third component of complement (C3). Cells of the monocyte-macrophage series are active in killing bacteria, fungi, and tumor cells.

Mononuclear phagocytes have the capacity to bind antigen and antigen-antibody complexes. The monocyte-macrophage frequently degrades antigen which binds to its surface. There is evidence that small amounts of antigen bound to macrophage surfaces are important in the induction phase of the immune response.

Most experimental investigations of macrophage function have employed macrophages of bone marrow monocyte origin. It should be recalled, however, that macrophages of reticuloendothelial origin exist as both fixed and free forms throughout the lymphoreticular organs. These macrophages are much more difficult to obtain and isolate for studies in vitro. Thus, less is known of their surface sites and physiological function; these are important fields for further investigation.

OTHER CELLS INVOLVED IN IMMUNOLOGIC PHENOMENA

Other cell types participate in a very important way in immunity—(1) by carrying out crucial effector functions such as phagocytosis; (2) by increasing vascular permeability; and/or (3) by processing antigen during immune induction (i.e., during the time the antigen is introduced and T and B lymphocytes are being stimulated). Thus, polymorphonuclear neutrophils, eosinophils, basophils, and mast cells participate in the inflammatory response mediated by antibodies. The mononuclear phagocytes participate both as effector cells in cellular immunity reactions and as auxiliary cells during immune induction.

IMMUNOGLOBULINS

The immunoglobulins are protein molecules that carry antibody activity; that is, the property of specific combination with the substance that elicited their formation (antigen). Immunoglobulins, or antibodies, carry out the functions of humoral immunity and are produced by B cells and their progeny, plasma cells.

STRUCTURE OF IMMUNOGLOBULINS

The core or monomeric unit structure of immunoglobulin (Ig) molecules consists of four polypeptide chains—two identical heavy (H) chains and two identical light (L) chains (Fig. 3-2). In each molecule, the H and L chains are held together by disulfide bonds and by noncovalent hydrophobic interactions. Superimposed upon this basic prototype four-chain structure are differences in chain length, carbohydrate content, biologic activity, and antigenicity (Table 3-3). These differences, found primarily on the heavy chains, can be used to identify five major classes of immunoglobulins—IgG, IgA, IgM,

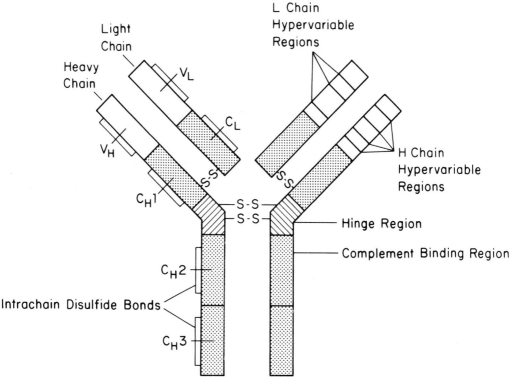

Fig. 3-2. A simplified diagram of an IgG immunoglobulin molecule showing the four chain basic structure and domains. V_H and V_L are the variable domains of the heavy and light chains, respectively. C_H1, C_H2, and C_H3 are the domains in the constant region of the heavy chains. The interchain disulfide bonds are indicated by the symbol -S-S-. The molecule may be cleaved in the hinge region by certain enzymes into Fab and Fc fragments (see text).

Table 3-3. Characteristics of Human Immunoglobulins

Characteristics	IgG	IgA	IgM	IgD	IgE
			Class		
Molecular formula	$(\kappa_2\gamma_2)$	$(\kappa_2\alpha_2)_n$**	$(\kappa_2\mu_2)_5$	$(\kappa_2\delta_2)$	$(\kappa_2\epsilon_2)$
	or	or	or	or	or
	$(\lambda_2\gamma_2)$	$(\lambda_2\alpha_2)_n$**	$(\lambda_2\mu_2)_5$	$(\lambda_2\delta_2)$	$(\lambda_2\epsilon_2)$
Molecular weight	150,000	$(160,000)_n$**	900,000	180,000	200,000
Heavy Chains					
Class	γ	α	μ	δ	ϵ
Subclasses	γ1, 2, 3, 4	α1, 2	μ1, 2	—	—
Molecular weight	53,000	58,000	70,000	65,000	72,000
Allotypes	Gm	Am	—	—	—
Light Chains					
Type	κ, λ	κ,λ	κ,λ	κ,λ	κ,λ
Molecular weight	22,500	22,500	22,500	22,500	22,500
Allotypes	Inv	Inv	Inv	Inv	Inv
J Chain	—	+	+	—	—
Secretory piece	—	+*	+*	—	—
Placental passage	yes	no	no	no	no
Blood Group Antibody Activity Described	yes	yes	yes	no	no
Serum level (mg/dl)	600 to 1800	200 to 500	60 to 200	0.1 to 4.0	0.01 to 0.9

* Found on secretory IgM or IgA
** $_n$ usually = 1–3

IgD, and IgE. The heavy chains of the immunoglobulin molecules are referred to by Greek letters, as follows: IgG by γ, IgM by μ, IgA by α, IgD by δ, and IgE by ϵ. The class of immunoglobulins is determined by the nature of the heavy chain, the light chains being common to all classes of immunoglobulin. Light chains occur as two immunologically distinct types designated kappa (κ) or lambda (λ). A given immunoglobulin molecule always contains identical κ or λ chains, never a mixture of the two.

Figure 3-2 depicts the basic structural unit of all antibody molecules. Some antibody molecules exist as monomers, whereas other antibody molecules are composed of more than one of these basic structural units. IgA may occur in a variety of polymeric forms including dimers, trimers, or even higher multimers.IgM most often exists in the pentameric form. Polymeric antibody molecules contain an extra component, the J, or joining chain.

Each polypeptide chain contains an amino terminal portion (the variable or V region) and a carboxyl terminal portion (the constant or C region). These terms denote the considerable heterogeneity or variability in the amino acid residues in the V region compared to the C region. The polypeptide chains do not exist as linear sequences of amino acids; instead, they are folded by disulfide bonds into globular regions called domains. The domains in H chains are designated V_H and C_H1, C_H2, C_H3, and C_H4; those in L chains are designated V_L and C_L. The part of the antibody molecule which binds antigen is formed by only small numbers of amino acids in the V regions of H and L chains. Variability of the V_L or V_H segments is constrained: certain residues do not change from one protein species to another; only a limited number of different amino acids occur at certain other positions; but some positions of the variable region show great variability in sequence composition (hypervariable regions).

The area of the H chains between the first and second C region domains is the "hinge" region. It is more flexible than the other segments and is more exposed to enzymes and chemicals. Papain and trypsin attack the heavy chain at the N or amino terminal side of the interheavy chain disulfide bonds, liberating the Fc fragment and two Fab fragments. The Fc fragment is a dimer of the C- or carboxy-terminal portion of the heavy chain, whereas the two Fab fragments consist of an intact light chain and an amino-terminal half or Fd fragment of the heavy chain linked together by a single interchain disulfide bond. It is the Fab fragments that contain the antigen-combining sites of the antibody molecules; hence, the IgG immunoglobulin molecule is divalent. The Fc fragment, containing most of the carbohydrate of the IgG molecule, has a tendency to crystallize but does not have the capacity to combine with antigen. Pepsin, unlike papain or trypsin, hydrolyzes the immunoglobulin molecule on the C-terminal side of the inter-heavy chain disulfide bonds, liberating a single bivalent antibody fragment called $F(ab')_2$. The fragment has a molecular weight of 110,000 daltons.

Studies of the biologic properties of Fab and Fc fragments have shown that the immunoglobulin molecule can be divided into two distinct functional regions. The region of the molecule encompassing the Fab fragment is responsible for specific antigen binding while the Fc portion of the heavy chain determines the effector functions of antibody molecules such as complement-fixation, transplacental passage, and binding to mast cells.

According to current concepts, the V_H and V_L regions contribute to the formation of the antigen-binding pocket or cleft in the Fab portion of the antibody molecule. Extensive folding of the V_H and V_L segments serves to bring the hypervariable regions into close spatial proximity so as to form a structure complementary to that of a given antigenic determinant. The remaining amino acid sequences of the V_H and V_L domains are now viewed as maintaining the hypervariable re-gions in appropriate alignment in the antigen-binding site. Hence, these residues constitute the framework of the combining site. Amino acid substitutions, and additions or deletions in the hypervariable regions, make it possible to generate the large number of unique antigen-binding sites required to interact with the vast diversity of potential antigens.

SUBCLASSES OF IMMUNOGLOBULINS

Distinct antigenic differences can be detected within classes of immunoglobulins by using antisera prepared in heterologous species, and after suitable cross-absorption. Thus, the heavy chains of individual immunoglobulin molecules can be grouped into subclasses based primarily on structural and antigenic differences within their heavy chain Fc fragments. A number of biologic properties of immunoglobulins are associated with specific molecular subclasses.

The most extensively studied subclasses are those found in the IgG class immunoglobulins (Table 3-4). Four such subclasses called IgG1, IgG2, IgG3, and IgG4 have been identified, and their distinctive heavy chains have been classified γ1, γ2, γ3 and γ4. IgG1 molecules represent about 70 percent of all immunoglobulin molecules. Proteins within each IgG subclass possess a distinctive set of genetically inherited antigens of the type referred to as Gm. Only the IgG1 and IgG3 molecules readily fix complement.

Two distinct subclasses of IgA molecules—IgA1 and IgA2—have been defined. In the circulation, 90 percent of the molecules belong to the IgA1 class while in exocrine secretions the majority appear to be IgA2 molecules. Two subclasses of IgM have been identified on the basis of antigenic or immunochemical differences, and by differences in tryptic peptide maps. Unique effector functions for those subclasses have yet to be established. No subclasses have been defined for either IgD or IgE molecules.

Table 3-4. Biologic Properties of Subclasses of Human IgG

	IgG1	IgG2	IgG3	IgG4
Complement fixation (at Cl step)	+	+	+	−
Passive cutaneous anaphylaxis*	+	0	+	+
Binding to Fc receptors on neutrophils	+	+	+	+
Binding to Fc receptors on monocytes	+	−	+	−
Placental transfer	+	+	+	+
Antigen for Rheumatoid Factor	+	+	−	+
Rheumatoid Factor Antibody	+	+	+	+
serum concentration (mg/ml)	5 to 12	2 to 6	0.5 to 1	0.2 to 1

* In guinea pigs

ANTIGENIC MARKERS ON IMMUNOGLOBULINS

Several different types of antigenic determinants may be recognized on immunoglobulin molecules. First, there are antigenic determinants which characterize all γ, μ, α, δ, or ϵ heavy chains and all κ or λ light chains. These antigenic determinants are termed *isotypic determinants*. A rabbit antiserum directed against the isotypic determinants on the γ heavy chain, for example, will "recognize" the IgG molecules present in all normal human sera.

Second, there are antigenic determinants which are present on the γ heavy chains and κ light chains of some but not all normal people. For example, a substitution of a single amino acid, either leucine or valine, at position 191 in the C segment of κ light chains produces a change in the protein sufficient to result in a unique antigenic determinant recognizable by appropriate antisera. These antigenic determinants are called *allotypic determinants*. Kappa chains with leucine at position 191 bear the InV (1, 2) allotypic determinants; those with valine in this position bear the InV (3) allotype. Approximately 20 allotypic determinants have been recognized on γ heavy chains; these are termed Gm markers and are found chiefly on the Fc segment of the γ chains. Each subclass of IgG has its own allotypic markers which are under genetic control by codominant alleles.

A third type of marker is the *idiotypic antigenic determinant*. The term idiotype denotes the unique V region sequences produced by each clone of antibody-forming cells. Idiotypic antigenic determinants of immunoglobulin molecules were first identified by immunizing animals with specific antibodies raised against a particular antigen in genetically similar animals. The only antigenic differences between the immunoglobulins of the donor and recipient were the unique V region sequences related to the specificity of the antibody. Thus, responses were restricted to such determinants. It is also possible to immunize across species lines to obtain anti-idiotype antisera, but in this case the antisera must be carefully absorbed with immunoglobulins from the donor species to render them specific for idiotypic markers.

KINETICS OF ANTIBODY FORMATION

Following antigenic challenge, after a latent period of 4 to 24 hours, antibody-forming cells appear, proliferate, and begin to produce antibody. The level of serum antibody over the next few days rises exponentially in direct proportion to the number of antibody-forming cells. However, as the immune response continues, the recruitment of new cells declines, possibly due to regulation by T cells and macrophages, or to an inhibitory effect of circulating antibodies. The existence of this latter form of feedback inhibition is based on the observation that small amounts of IgG antibody tend to depress the immune response to the corresponding antigen. This is probably the mechanism whereby Rh alloimmunization is suppressed by the administration of small quantities of anti-Rh_o(D) antibody (see Ch. 39). Thus, as a result of depletion of antigen and failure to recruit new antibody-forming cells, antibody synthesis gradually declines and antibody titers fall.

The first molecular species of antibody to appear in the circulation in response to primary antigenic stimulation belongs mainly to the IgM class of immunoglobulins. After continued antigenic exposure or reexposure to the same antigen, the IgM antibodies are usually replaced by IgG in much larger amounts. Thus, the primary antibody response is characterized by a relatively low titer of antibodies which are primarily IgM, whereas the secondary response is characterized by a much higher titer of antibodies which are primarily IgG. An exception to this pattern is the case of thymus-independent antigens; the IgA class of antibody then appears after the IgG response. The kinetics of antibody production may be explained by an antigen-driven switch of B lymphocytes from IgM-producing to IgG-producing cells followed by a second switch from IgG-producing to IgA-producing cells. The second, or late, Ig response is also characterized by antibodies (especially of the IgG class) that are of higher affinity than those in the primary response, with greater cross reactivity with related antigenic determinants. In addition, the secondary response is more rapid in appearance, a phenomenon related to immunologic memory.

develops a much higher antibody titer than a nonresponder strain. Genetic control of the immune response may be observed in either primary or secondary antibody responses, or in the production of a certain antibody class. In a few cases, the specificity of the antibody may be genetically affected.

There are other types of immune responses in which genetic control may be manifested: the rejection of skin allografts, resistance to virus infections or autoimmune disease. Also under genetic control are the proliferation (doubling time) and differentiation of precursor B cells to antibody-forming cells. Some, but not all, Ir genes are linked to the major histocompatibility (H) locus that codes for the strongest H antigens expressed on the surface of cells. In the inbred mouse, the I region which contains Ir genes is located within the H-2 complex.

Using alloantisera prepared in congeneic strains of mice that have only I region differences, a complex system of antigens termed Ia (I region-associated) has recently been defined serologically. These gene products are expressed on almost all B lymphocytes, on some T lymphocytes, and on certain other cells including macrophages and epidermal cells. Genes coding for Ia antigens are distributed throughout the I region. The relationship between the functionally defined Ir genes and the serologically defined Ia antigens has not yet been established.

GENETIC CONTROL OF IMMUNE RESPONSES

In recent years, it has become apparent that the ability to respond specifically to a wide variety of antigens is under genetic control. Genes that specifically control immune responses are termed immune response (Ir) genes. Most of the Ir genes studied to date appear to control the amount of antibody formed against a specific antigen. For example, in inbred mice immunized with a synthetic polypeptide, a responder strain of mice

IMMUNE RESPONSES TO RED CELL ANTIGENS

CLASSES OF IMMUNOGLOBULIN PRODUCED

Although the primary immune response characteristically results initially in development of IgM antibodies, with a later switch to synthesis of IgG antibodies, it has been difficult to prove that this generalization applies to the production of red cell alloantibodies in man.[13] It is not known with certainty whether IgM antibody is the first to be made in human subjects responding to the Rh antigen, but it is quite clear that, in the majority of people, IgG anti-Rh_o(D) antibody soon predominates and is often the only type which can be identified at any time. In a minority of challenged subjects, IgM anti-Rh_o(D) is also produced in substantial amounts. In hyperimmunized donors with anti-Rh in their serum, "boosting" with small amounts of Rh-positive red cells is often followed by the production of IgM as well as IgG anti-Rh. In these hyperimmunized antibody donors, anti-Rh is also quite often partly IgA.[13] Responses to several other red cell antigens— e.g., K, Fy^a and Jk^a—appear to be similar to responses to Rh; that is to say, most antibodies are predominantly IgG, although in some subjects alloimmunized to these antigens a mixture of IgM and IgG antibodies is found.[14]

Within the ABO system, perhaps all humans should be regarded as immunized. Moreover, ABO-incompatible pregnancies and injections of various animal products cause both quantitative and qualitative changes in anti-A and anti-B. Perhaps the most interesting fact about antibody production in the ABO system is that immune anti-A and anti-B are predominantly IgM in A or B subjects but may be largely IgG (and partly IgA) in group O subjects.

RELATIVE POTENCY OF DIFFERENT RED CELL ALLOANTIGENS

An estimate of the relative potency of different red cell alloantigens can be obtained by comparing the actual frequency with which particular alloantibodies are encountered with the calculated frequency of the opportunity for immunization.[15] The relative opportunities for immunization to K and Fy^a can be estimated by simply comparing the frequency of the combination K-positive donor/K-negative recipient; i.e., $0.09 \times 0.91 = 0.08$, with the frequency of the combination Fy^a-positive donor/Fy^a-negative recipient; i.e., $0.66 \times 0.34 = 0.22$. Thus, the opportunity for immunization to Fy^a is about 3.5 times greater than that for K (0.22 vs. 0.08). Although opportunities for immunization to Fy^a are 3.5 times more frequent than those to K, anti-K is in fact found 2.5 times more commonly than anti-Fy^a; overall, K can be said to be 9 times more potent than Fy^a. If a single transfusion of K-positive blood to a K-negative subject induces the formation of serologically detectable anti-K in 10 percent of cases, it can be predicted that the transfusion of a single unit of Fy(a+) blood to a Fy^a-negative subject would induce the formation of serologically detectable anti-Fy^a in about 1 percent of cases. Giblett[15] calculated that c and E of the Rh system were about one third as potent as K; Fy^a was calculated to be about one twenty-fifth as potent, and Jk^a one fiftieth to one one-hundredth as potent as K.

THE EFFECT OF Rh_o(D) ALLOIMMUNIZATION ON THE FORMATION OF OTHER RED CELL ALLOANTIBODIES

Among Rh-negative volunteers deliberately injected with Rh-positive red cells, those who form anti-D also tend to form alloantibodies outside the Rh system, whereas those who do not form anti-D seldom form any red cell alloantibodies. In one series, of 73 subjects who formed anti-D, 6 formed anti-Fy^a, 4 formed anti-Jk^a, and 4 formed other alloantibodies; by contrast, among 48 subjects who failed to form anti-D, not one made any detectable alloantibodies.[16]

Several studies in which Rh-negative subjects have been deliberately immunized with Rh-positive red cells are available for analysis. The data indicate a tremendously increased response to antigens outside the Rh system in subjects responding to the D antigen. In subjects who formed anti-D and were also exposed to other potentially immunogenic antigens, 50 percent formed anti-K. The incidence of anti-Fy[a], anti-Jk[a], and anti-s in those who were challenged was about 20 percent in each instance.

RESPONDERS AND NONRESPONDERS

It has long been apparent that it is very difficult to elicit the formation of anti-D in some D-negative subjects; despite repeated injections of Rh-positive red cells, about one-third of Rh-negative subjects fail to form anti-Rh.[13]

Krevans et al.[17] and Woodrow et al.[18] made an observation of great interest when they found that, within 6 weeks (sometimes longer) after a first injection of Rh-positive red cells, Rh-negative subjects could be divided into two classes: (1) those in whom the second and subsequent injections of ^{51}Cr-labeled Rh-positive red cells were rapidly eliminated and who formed anti-Rh after a few more injections, and (2) those in whom the second and subsequent injections of Rh-positive red cells survived normally and who did not subsequently form anti-Rh. Although most Rh-negative responders produce serologically detectable anti-Rh after two injections of Rh-positive red cells given at an interval of 3 to 6 months, a few do not; such subjects can be classified as nonresponders only if the survival of Rh-positive red cells is measured or if several further injections of Rh-positive cells are given.

A few subjects produce trace amounts of anti-Rh after a few injections of Rh-positive cells, but increased antibody levels do not occur after further injections. The antibody may even become undetectable. Subjects who take a long time to produce anti-Rh tend to produce low-titer antibody: of 116 subjects who produced anti-Rh within 9 months of the first immunization, the agglutination titer (in albumin) eventually reached 512 or more in all cases. In those in whom anti-Rh was first detected 12 months or more after the first injection, the titer reached a maximum of 128 or less in 8 out of 18 cases.[13]

The genetic differences between individuals who are responders or nonresponders are not well understood. No consistent differences in HLA antigens have been identified. In a study of the relation between responsiveness to Rh antigen and to certain bacterial and other antigens, no relationship could be found.[19]

SUPPRESSION OF ANTIBODY RESPONSE BY PASSIVELY ADMINISTERED ANTIBODY

Practical aspects of suppression of Rh immunization by passively administered antibody are discussed in Chapter 39. Some theoretical aspects of the subject will be briefly considered here.

The immune response to soluble antigens can be suppressed by giving "excess" antibody.[13] "Excess" in this context is usually thought of as literally an outnumbering of antigenic determinant groups by antibody molecules. The response to antigens carried on red cells can be suppressed by very much smaller amounts of antibody. For example, 25 μg anti-D is generally effective in suppressing immunization when 1 ml of D-positive red cells is injected into an Rh-negative recipient. Assuming that the antibody is distributed within a space about twice as great as the plasma volume, it can be calculated that, at equilibrium, only 5 percent of antigen and about 1 percent of antibody will be in the bound state. Similarly, the amount of passively administered antibody required to suppress the immune response of mice to sheep red cells was calculated to be one one-hundredth the amount required to saturate the antigen sites.[13]

A further apparent difference between the suppressive effect of passively acquired antibody against soluble antigens and cell-bound antigens lies in the specificity of the phenomenon. For example, in an experiment with soluble antigen, it was shown that with a molecule carrying two antigenic determinants the response to one could be suppressed without affecting the response to the other.[20] On the other hand, in the only parallel experiment so far reported with human red cells, when cells carrying both D and K were injected together with anti-K, the response both to K and D was suppressed.[21] Volunteers, all of whom were D-negative and K-negative, were given an injection of 1 ml of D-positive, K-positive red cells. In addition, half the subjects were given an injection of 14 μg of IgG anti-K, which was sufficient to clear the K-positive, D-positive red cells from the circulation into the spleen within 24 h. At 6 months, 7 of 31 control subjects but only one of 31 antibody treated subjects had formed anti-D. After a further antigenic stimulus, four more control subjects but no more treated subjects developed anti-D.

The fact that ABO-incompatible Rh-positive red cells induce Rh immunization far less frequently than ABO-compatible Rh-positive cells is consistent with these obervations. Immunization to Rh during pregnancy is less common when the father is "ABO-incompatible" with the mother, as first noted by Levine.[22] In a series of matings between Rh-positive fathers and Rh-negative mothers who had given birth to infants affected with hemolytic disease of the newborn, 24.7 percent were ABO-incompatible (father's red cells versus mother's serum) compared with 35 percent of ABO-incompatible matings expected in the general population.

Race and Sanger[23] suggested that this phenomenon might be explained by the ABO-incompatible Rh-positive red cells being rapidly destroyed in the mother's circulation and accordingly incapable of inducing Rh immunization. The essential correctness of this interpretation was later demonstrated experimentally, and these observations ultimately led to the use of anti-D for suppression of Rh-immunization of the mother which may occur as a result of Rh-incompatible pregnancies (see Ch. 39).

AUTOIMMUNITY

The mechanisms of immunologic unresponsiveness afford the body tissues a large measure of protection against potential destruction by an immune system developed for the elimination of antigenically foreign substances. Nevertheless, a number of well-established clinical syndromes exist in which the self-recognition process apparently fails and the immune response is directed against autologous antigens. The autoantibodies which appear in these disease states demonstrate different degrees of specificity with respect to the target tissue and the range of species with which the autoantibody will react.

Four general mechanisms have been hypothesized in the pathogenesis of autoantibody production. They are: (1) release of sequestered antigens; (2) abnormalities of the lymphoid system; (3) alterations in the structure of autoantigens; and (4) cross-reactive antigens.

SEQUESTERED ANTIGENS

Since continued exposure of the immune system to antigen is necessary for the maintenance of immunologic unresponsiveness, tolerance may be lost to sequestered antigens, such as those of the lens of the eye, spermatozoa, and brain tissue, that are not accessible to the blood and lymphatic circulation. Tissue damage leading to exposure to the sequestered components, with or without molecular modification, might then be associated with autoantibody production, since these products would no longer be looked upon as "self." Moreover, a vicious cycle might develop in which autoantibody production leading to tissue destruction might further augment the autoantibody response by release of more antigen.

ABNORMALITIES OF THE LYMPHOID SYSTEM

Multiple autoantibodies are detected in certain disease states. Unless a general mechanism that could alter numerous tissue constituents simultaneously is postulated, the events leading to autoantibody production might be more easily explained on the basis of an alteration of the immune apparatus. Loss of suppressor T cell immunoregulatory function could constitute such a mechanism and be responsible for the development of multiple autoimmune disorders. Evidence for this theory is found in certain mouse strains which undergo early thymic atrophy; they show demonstrable loss of suppressor T cell activity with increasing age, accompanied by concomitant development of autoimmune disease. Enhanced T cell inducer/helper function might have the same effect.

A number of other suggestions have been made based on the original "forbidden clone" theory of autoimmunity which postulated the emergence of clones of self-reactive lymphocytes which should normally be eliminated early in their development. A breakdown of this hypothetical elimination mechanism or development of mutant lymphocytes resistant to this process might lead to autoantibody formation. Present interest is focused largely on abnormalities of T cell immunoregulation as the basis for autoimmunity.

ALTERATIONS IN THE STRUCTURE OF AUTOANTIGENS

The interaction of normal body constituents with a variety of exogenous agents may lead to modifications in their antigenic structure. Possible inciting agents include microorganisms, radiation, thermal changes, and chemicals or drugs. In general, any form of tissue destruction may be associated with antigenic alteration. A drastic change in antigen structure is unlikely to result in the formation of autoantibodies which will cross react with normal body constituents. More subtle nongenetic molecular modifications, such as those induced on cell surfaces by certain viral infections or by drugs, are more likely to evoke an immune response in which the autoantibodies will cross-react with native tissue constituents and may result in tissue damage. The autoantibody production may be a temporary phenomenon, extending only for that period of time during which the agent is present. It is possible, however, that exposure to the modified material may result in a permanent loss of tolerance to the native component.

Chronic autoantibody production might also be elicited by a permanent change in the structure of native components. Some viral infections, irradiation, and mutagenic drugs are capable of altering the genetic information of cells which, in turn, may result in the synthesis of abnormal macromolecules. In addition, some drugs may alter cellular metabolism, leading to abnormal cell surface structures.

CROSS-REACTIVE ANTIGENS

The fortuitous antigenic similarity between constituents of infecting microorganisms and components of the body might, during chronic infection, lead to a persistent state of autoantibody production. The idea that cross-reactive or altered autoantigens can be instrumental in the development of autoimmune disease is made more credible by findings regarding the kinetics of T and B cell tolerance. Tolerance to autoantigens that are present in low concentration in body fluids may only extend to the T cell population. Therefore, potentially self-reactive B lymphocytes might exist that could be stimulated fairly early to produce autoantibodies if the T cell requirement were to be circumvented in some manner. For instance, an altered autoantigen might activate a different set of T lymphocytes able to cooperate with preexisting B cells. There is considerable circumstantial evidence in support of this theory. Neonatal tolerance to bovine serum albumin (BSA) in rabbits can be broken by administering a cross-reacting albumin such as human serum albumin (HSA), but the antibodies obtained against BSA are only those directed against determinants shared by both antigens. Thus, nontolerant B lymphocytes appear to be activated by T cells reactive with carrier determinants of HSA to make antibodies against shared determinants of BSA and HSA.

COMPLEMENT

Complement (C) is a multimolecular biological system which constitutes the primary humoral mediator of antigen-antibody reactions.[24] It consists of at least 17 serum proteins including inhibitor and inactivator components. Most familiar among the biologic activities of the complement system is its ability to effect lysis of a spectrum of different kinds of cells, including erythrocytes, lymphocytes, platelets, tumor cells, bacteria, viruses, and artificial phospholipid membranes.[25] In addition to such direct cytopathic effects, reaction products of complement components have the potential of modifying and triggering specialized cellular functions. Thus, activation may result in: membrane damage (e.g., lysis); the production of biologically active fragments of complement molecules (e.g., C3a and C5a anaphylatoxins); and formation of membrane-bound complement components that will then interact with specific receptors on cells (e.g., red cell-bound C3b will interact with the specific C3b receptor on macrophages). The biomedical significance of complement includes its role in the induction of inflammation, in the contribution of its components to various aspects of host defense, and in the pathogenesis of various im-

munologically mediated diseases.[26] Complement reactions also are of particular significance in blood transfusion laboratories, since these reactions are important in the detection and differential diagnosis of immune hemolytic anemias and are of significance in the detection of some red cell alloantibodies.

Two pathways of complement protein activation have been identified, each comprising several functional units. The classical pathway proceeds through the sequential activation of C1, C4, and C2 to the activation of C3 and the later components of the complement sequence. Its eleven proteins have been grouped into three functional units: the recognition unit—C1q, C1r, and C1s; the activation unit—C2, C3 and C4; and the membrane attack system—C5, C6, C7, C8, and C9.[24] The alternative or properdin pathway[27] bypasses C1, C4, and C2 and proceeds directly to the activation of C3. Although the pathways differ in their mechanism of activation, they both lead to the generation of biologically active complement fragments.

NOMENCLATURE

The components of the classical system are designated numerically, C1 to C9; the three subcomponents of C1 are referred to as C1q, C1r, and C1s.[24,28,29] Individual polypeptide chains of proteins with quaternary structure are denoted with Greek letters—e.g., $C3\alpha$ and $C3\beta$. Fragments of components are produced by enzymatic cleavage during complement activation and are denoted by small Arabic letters. For example, the fragments of C4 are C4a, C4b, C4c, and C4d. A transiently activated binding site of a nascent fragment is indicated by an asterisk (e.g., C3b*), its inactivated state is indicated by a subscript i (e.g., $C3b_i$). Enzyme activity is indicated by placing a bar above the designation of the component in which the activity resides. For example, the symbol for enzymatically active C1 is $\overline{C1}$. In composite reaction products, fragments are indicated—e.g., $\overline{C4b, 2a}$.

Terminology of the alternative pathway currently includes both trivial names and symbols—e.g., properdin(P), proactivator (B), and proactivator convertase (D). The respective activated forms are indicated by a bar, e.g., $\bar{B}$.

THE MOLECULAR DYNAMICS OF COMPLEMENT ACTIVATION

The Classical Pathway

The proteins of the complement system circulate throughout the extracellular compartment as inactive precursors until they are activated. Some of the physicochemical characteristics of the proteins participating in the classical pathway of activation are listed in Table 3-5.

Activation is the term applied to the process which enables the inactive circulating forms of the complement components to participate in the complement reaction; it is a prerequisite for the manifestation of cytolytic activity and for the other biological activities of the complement system. The activation of the classical pathway can be initiated by a number of substances, including: immunoglobulins; enzymes such as trypsin, plasmin, and lysosomal enzymes; endotoxins; lymphocyte membranes; enveloped viruses; and artificial low-ionic-strength media. Only one

molecule of IgM on a cell membrane is necessary to activate the complement system;[30,31] it is thought that two of the IgM subunits have to attach to the membrane before activation occurs. In contrast, it is thought that IgG needs to form a "doublet"—that is to say, two IgG molecules have to combine with antigens on the cell membrane as close together as 250-400Å before they are able to activate C1.[31] Only IgG1, IgG2, and IgG3 subclasses can activate complement. Their activity is in the order of IgG3 > IgG1 > IgG2.[32]

The interaction of antibody with antigen—as, for example, on an erythrocyte (the abbreviation EA is commonly used for the erythrocyte-antibody complex)—leads to the activation of the complement system, often ending in cytolysis. This process involves a series of protein-protein interactions resulting in the generation of a series of cellular intermediates bearing bound complement components designated by numbers (e.g., EAC1, EAC1, 4). The activation process is usually achieved by the cleavage of the next complement molecule into fragments. The activated products usually have enzymatic properties; thus, the pathway is an enzymatic cascade similar to the coagulation cascade. The system is held in check by the instability of the complexes formed and the naturally occurring inhibitors and inactivators present in normal plasma.

Table 3-5. Proteins Participating in the Classical Pathway of Complement Activation

Protein	Molecular Weight	Number of Chains	Electrophoretic Mobility	Serum Concentration μg/ml)
C1q	400,000	18	$\gamma2$	180
C1r	190,000	2	$\beta1$	100
C1s	85,000	1	α	80
C2	115,000	1	$\beta1$	25
C3	180,000	2	$\beta2$	1500
C4	206,000	3	$\beta1$	450
C5	180,000	2	$\beta1$	75
C6	128,000	1	$\beta2$	60
C7	121,000	1	$\beta2$	60
C8	154,000	3	γ	80
C9	80,000	1	α	150

* Not including activated forms and reaction products.
(Petz, L.D. and Garratty, G.: Acquired Immune Hemolytic Anemias. Churchill Livingstone, New York, 1980.)

The Recognition Unit. C1q is a collagen-like protein with binding sites for IgG and IgM. When C1 collides with an antigen-antibody complex (e.g., EA) it is bound to the C_H2 domain of the Fc fragment of the immunoglobulin molecule through the C1q subunit. This process activates C1r ($C\overline{1r}$) and C1s ($C\overline{1s}$) sequentially, each by the cleavage of a single polypeptide chain (Fig. 3-3). Two regulatory proteins are involved in this stage of the reaction. C1q inhibitor (C1q INH) prevents the attachment of complement to the immunoglobulin molecule. C1 inhibitor (C1 INH) abrogates the enzymatic activity of activated C1r and C1s.

The Activation Unit. This unit is assembled in two steps: activated C1 ($C\overline{1s}$) acts on native C4 by cleaving the molecule into C4a

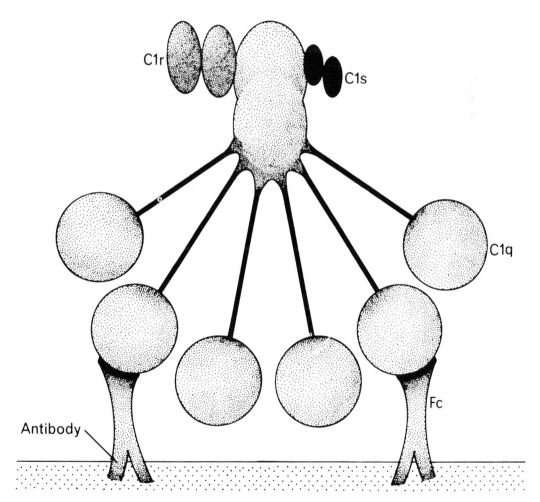

Fig. 3-3. C1q can interact with the Fc portion of immunoglobulin molecules (an IgG doublet is illustrated). Once a suitable interaction occurs, C1r is activated and finally C1s, which possesses esterase activity; its natural substrates are C4 and C2. (Petz, L.D. and Garratty, G.: Acquired Immune Hemolytic Anemias. Churchill Livingstone, New York, 1980.)

and C4b. The major fragment C4b binds to the cell membrane. A shower of C4 fragments is produced by a single C$\overline{1s}$ enzyme, so that many C4b molecules may cluster around the EAC1 site on the cell. The binding site on C4b is short-lived and rapidly decays; if the C4b molecule does not attach to the membrane quickly, it loses its ability to do so.

C$\overline{1s}$ also cleaves native C2 into two fragments. The major C2 fragment, C2a, combines with C4b on the cell membrane to form an active complex C$\overline{4b2a}$ (C3 convertase) that has enzymatic activity directed against C3. Magnesium ions are necessary for the formation of the C$\overline{4b2a}$ complex (Fig. 3-4).

C3 is cleaved by the C$\overline{4b2a}$ complex into two molecules, C3a, and C3b. The smaller C3a molecule (MW 10,000) does not bind to the cell membrane but is released into the fluid phase as a mediator of inflammation (anaphylatoxin I).

The C3b molecule (MW 171,000) binds to the cell membrane and can also bind to its own activation enzyme, C$\overline{4b2a}$ (Fig. 3-5). Because the C$\overline{4b2a}$ complex is an enzyme, it can react with its substrate repeatedly and produce a shower of C3b fragments. However, only the C3b fragments that become

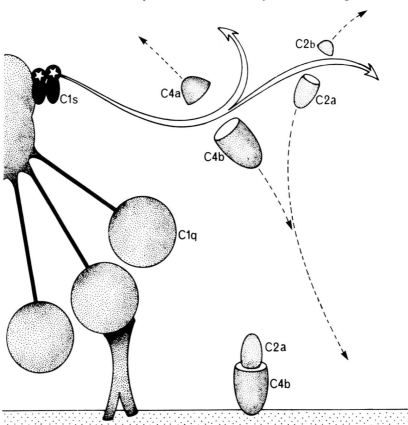

Fig. 3-4. If inhibition is overcome, then activated C1 (C$\overline{1}$) is capable of cleaving the C4 molecule into two fragments; C4a, which does not attach to cells and C4b, which can attach to cell membranes. C1 also cleaves C2 molecules into C2b, which does not combine with membranes and C2a, which may combine with cell bound C4b to form a complex C$\overline{4b2a}$. This complex (C3 convertase) is enzymatic, having C3 as its natural substrate. (Petz, L.D. and Garratty, G.: Acquired Immune Hemolytic Anemias. Churchill Livingstone, New York, 1980.)

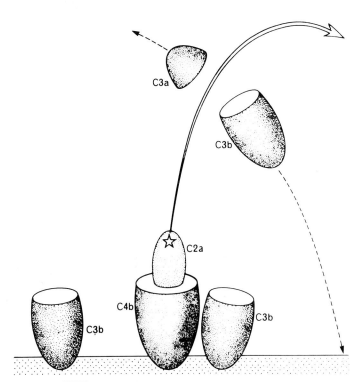

Fig. 3-5. C3 convertase (C$\overline{\text{4b2a}}$) cleaves C3 into fragments, C3a anaphylatoxin, which circulates in the plasma and C3b, which can attach to cell membranes. Some C3b molecules will fall close to C$\overline{\text{4b2a}}$ complexes and will form a new enzyme, C$\overline{\text{4b2a3b}}$ or C5 convertase. (Petz, L.D. and Garratty, G.: Acquired Immune Hemolytic Anemias. Churchill Livingstone, New York, 1980.)

bound adjacent to the C$\overline{\text{4b2a}}$ enzyme are believed to participate in the next reaction, in which C5 is cleaved. Some of the C3b molecules combine with C4b2a to form C$\overline{\text{4b,2a,3b}}$ (C5 convertase), which will cleave to C5 molecule into C5a (anaphylatoxin II), and C5b (Fig. 3-6). This is the last enzymatic reaction in the pathway. During the enzymatic cascade, only about 5 to 20 percent of molecules activated by C2, C3, C4, and C5 become bound to the cell membrane.

When C3b and/or C4b-sensitized red cells are allowed to incubate in normal plasma or serum, they are acted upon by a naturally occurring enzyme, C3b inactivator (C3bINA). This occurs in vivo or after prolonged incubation in vitro. The C3b and C4b molecules are cleaved, releasing C3c and/or C4c into the plasma and leaving C3d and/or C4d on the red cell membrane. β1H is necessary for the efficient activity of C3b INA (Fig. 3-7).

Membrane Attack Complex. C5b appears to bind C6 and C7 by absorption (Fig. 3-6). The resulting trimolecular complex attaches to the cell membrane and binds C8 and C9 (Fig. 3-8). Fully assembled, the membrane attack complex (MAC) consists of a dimer of C5b-9.[33,34] The end result of the pathway is lysis of the cell.

The ring-shaped ultrastructural membrane lesions induced by complement[35] have been identified as membrane-bound MAC.[33,36] Tranum-Jensen et al.[36] as well as Dourmashkin[37] have described the MAC as a hollow cylinder projecting from the cell membrane

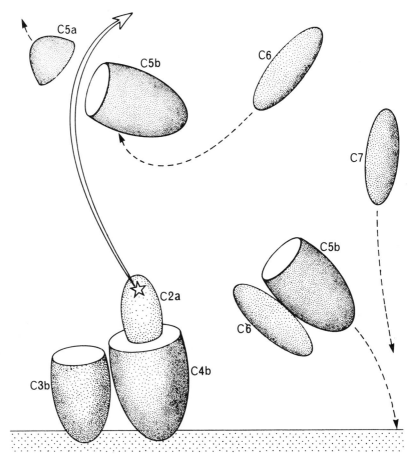

Fig. 3-6. C5 convertase (C4b2a3b) cleaves C5 into two fragments, C5a anaphylatoxin which circulates in the plasma and C5b that is capable of adsorbing C6 and C7. The trimolecular complex can attach to cell membranes, initiating the formation of the membrane attack complex (MAC). (Petz, L.D. and Garratty, G.: Acquired Immune Hemolytic Anemias. Churchill Livingstone, New York, 1980.)

and partly penetrating it. The hollow cylinder model has been linked to Mayer's[38] "doughnut" hypothesis of complement-dependent cell lysis, according to which C5b-9 produces a hydrophilic transmembrane protein channel. The cytolytic activity of the MAC appears to be due to its ability to bind phospholipids and to form mixed protein-phospholipid micelles and thus hydrophilic lipid channels in its immediate vicinity.[39] This causes a disruption of the normal permeability barrier of cell membranes with resultant lysis.[34]

The Alternative Pathway

In 1954, Pillemer published the results of a series of experiments that led him to believe there was a mechanism capable of mediating the bactericidal and opsonic effects of complement which did not require specific antibody.[40] He believed that this mechanism might be important in providing protection for the unimmunized host. Pillemer's concept of host defense grew out of a series of experiments in which zymosan, the insoluble residue remaining after the proteolytic digestion

REACTION PRODUCTS OF C3

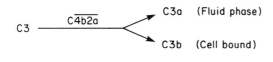

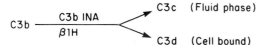

Fig. 3-7. The reaction products of C3. Cell-bound C3b is cleaved by C3b inactivator (C3bINA). This occurs in vivo or after prolonged incubation in vitro and is facilitated by β1H. After fragmentation, only C3d remains on the cell surface. Similar fragmentation of the C4 molecule occurs resulting in sensitization of cells with C4d.

of yeast, was reacted with serum. The interaction of zymosan with serum led to the depletion of the late components of the complement cascade. This depletion was not mediated by the classical complement pathway but required the presence of another serum protein which he termed "properdin." However, the then relatively primitive technology of protein chemistry frustrated efforts by other investigators to reproduce Pillemer's work, and it became quite modish to discount it. After a while, properdin was all but abandoned by investigators, and the field lay largely dormant. Later work by several investigators gradually led to the recognition that an alternative pathway of activation did, indeed, exist.[41-48] It has been renamed the alternative pathway because properdin is no longer felt to play a central role in its function.

The proteins that participate in the alternative pathway are listed in Table 3-6. The pathway may be activated by antibody under certain circumstances,[49,50] but it is also acti-

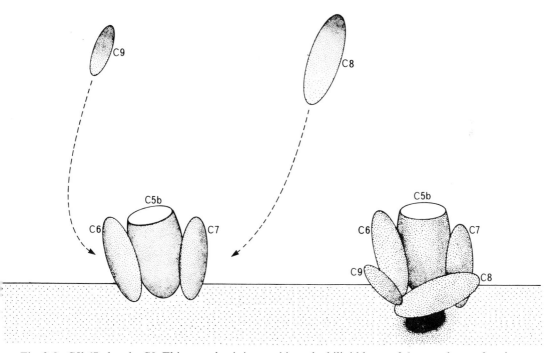

Fig. 3-8. C5b67 absorbs C8. This complex is inserted into the bilipid layer of the membrane, forming a channel through the membrane. Finally C9 is absorbed, forming the final membrane attack complex (MAC), leading to lysis of the cell. (Petz, L.D. and Garratty, G.: Acquired Immune Hemolytic Anemias. Churchill Livingstone, New York, 1980.)

Table 3-6. Proteins Participating in the Alternative Pathway

Component	Symbol	Molecular Weight	Electrophoretic Mobility	Synonyms
Properdin	P	184,000	γ	—
Activated P	$\bar{\text{P}}$	184,000	γ	—
Proactivator	B	93,000	β	PA,GBG
Activated B Proactivator	$\bar{\text{B}}$	63,000	γ	C3A,GGG,2ll,Bb
Convertase	D	24,000	α	PAse, GBGase
C3	C3	180,000	β	Factor A, HSF
C3b	C3b	171,000	$\alpha 2$	HSFa
C3b Inactivator	C3b INA	88,000	β	—
β1H	β1H	180,000	β	—

(Petz, L.D. and Garratty, G.: Acquired Immune Hemolytic Anemias. Churchill Livingstone, New York, 1980.)

vated by bacterial cells, complex polysaccharides, or lipopolysaccharides in the absence of detectable antibody.[50]

This pathway has now been clearly shown to bypass C1, C4, and C2 of the classical system and to proceed to the activation of C3 by the interaction of alternative pathway proteins. Present concepts[27,51] indicate that six proteins are responsible for alternative pathway activity of serum. Only five of these proteins are essential for initiation and amplification, because these events can occur in the absence of one of them, properdin. Of the five essential proteins, three (C3, Factor B, and Factor D) are required for the generation of the initial enzyme and the amplifying enzyme of the pathway. The other two proteins (β1H and C3bINA) are regulators of the C3 convertase; they suppress C3 convertase formation in the fluid phase and confine enzyme formation to the surface of activators.

Initiation of the alternative pathway appears to be a two-step process involving, first, random binding of C3b through its labile binding site to an activator and, second, discriminatory interaction of the bound C3b with surrounding surface structures. The random event is the result of the action of the initial C3 convertase, which is a fluid-phase enzyme. It is envisaged that native C3 and Factor B form a reversible complex which, if activated by Factor D, becomes the initial C3 cleaving enzyme $\overline{\text{C3,Bb}}$. This complex constitutes a transient C3 convertase, splitting

serum C3 into C3a and C3b; the latter can then attach to the cell surface. Once on the surface, C3b can combine with more Factor B and D, forming another C3 convertase (Fig. 3-9). The magnitude of the resultant C3b deposition is low, due to the small amount of enzyme produced at any given time and to the low efficiency of binding that is characteristic of C3b surface deposition from the fluid phase.

The discriminatory interaction occurs after binding of C3b. When bound to a nonactivator, C3b is able to bind β1H and becomes inactivated through the combined effects of C3bINA and β1H. When bound to an activator, control is restricted because β1H binding to C3b is decreased. As a consequence of the discriminatory phase of initiation, C3 convertase formation on the activator occurs, and amplification through the solid-phase C3 convertase commences (Fig. 3-10). Through the additional enzymatic cleavage of C3, more C3b attaches to the membrane; receptor function is thought to reside in at least two critically oriented and closely spaced C3b molecules. Binding of activated Factor B to the receptor results in the generation of the labile C5 convertase, $\overline{\text{C3b,B}}$, which also acts on C3. Upon the collision of native properdin (P) with the complex, P undergoes a transition to its bound form, $\bar{\text{P}}$. $\bar{\text{P}}$ confers an increased degree of stability on $\overline{\text{C3b,B}}$, converting it to the $\overline{\text{C3b,B,P}}$ enzyme. The $\bar{\text{P}}$-enzyme effects activation of C5 and self-

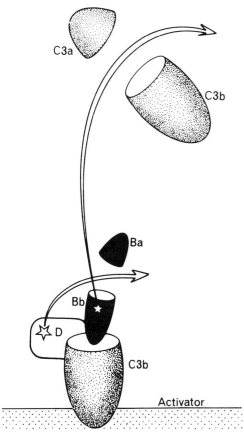

Fig. 3-9. C3b is formed through initial fluid phase cleavage of C3 (possibly by a C3, Factor B complex, which when activated by Factor D, becomes the initial fluid phase C3 convertase $\overline{C3bBb}$). If C3b attaches to a surface containing structures capable of activating the alternative pathway then the C3b will combine with Factor B. Factor D will cleave Factor B, releasing a fragment Ba into the plasma. The resulting complex $\overline{C3bBb}$ will cleave more C3, resulting in the formation of additional C3b. (Petz, L.D. and Garratty, G.: Acquired Immune Hemolytic Anemias. Churchill Livingstone, New York, 1980.)

assembly of the membrane attack complex C5b-9.

Once C3 is activated in the alternative pathway, the molecular consequences seem to be identical to those of the classical pathway. The alternative pathway has not yet been incriminated in many immunohemato-logic problems; this may be due to the fact that it is very inefficient in the lysis of human red cells when compared with the classical pathway.[52] It is of interest to note that the red cells of patients suffering with paroxysmal nocturnal hemoglobinuria (PNH) can be shown to hemolyse through the alternative pathway as well as by the classical pathway.[53] Also, activation of the alternative pathway by autologous red cell stroma has been described.[54]

BIOLOGICAL ACTIVITIES OF COMPLEMENT

Apart from the end result of cytolysis, the complement cascade is associated with other important biological activities. Most of these other activities, unlike cytolysis, do not need all the complement components to participate (see Tables 3-7 & 3-8).

As a result of these biologic activities, complement plays a role in the body's defense mechanism against infectious agents; it is also a mediator of inflammation and of tissue damage in immunopathologic processes. Complement abnormalities are of importance in a wide range of human disorders, some of which are listed in Tables 3-9 and 3-10. However, a detailed discussion of complement in these disorders is beyond the scope of this chapter.

COMPLEMENT RECEPTORS

Receptors for activated complement components are widely distributed on tissue cells of most mammalian species. In addition, the genetic control of certain complement components appears to be linked to the genes that code for the major histocompatibility complex (MHC). Many of these components are also present on cell surfaces. In fact, it has been suggested that the functions of the complement system and the major histocompatibility complex may be related.[55]

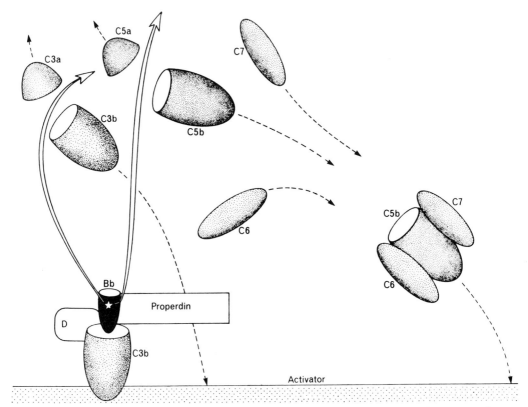

Fig. 3-10. The C3b,Bb complex (C3 convertase), by cleaving C3, will allow more C3b to accumulate on the surface. Properdin binds to the C3b,Bb complex, stabilizing the enzyme. The enzyme is also capable of cleaving C5 into C5a anaphylatoxin and C5b, which can combine with C6, C7, and attach to the membrane. Finally, C8 and C9 are adsorbed, causing lysis of the cell. (Petz, L.D. and Garratty, G.: Acquired Immune Hemolytic Anemias. Churchill Livingstone, New York, 1980.)

C1q

Receptors for C1q have been reported on both T and B lymphocytes as well as on certain lymphoblastoid cells.[56,57] Platelets have also been reported to have C1q receptors.[58]

C3b

Receptors for C3b (immune adherence receptor) have been detected on the membrane of human and subhuman primate red cells, granulocytes, monocytes, macrophages, a subpopulation of lymphocytes, epithelial cells of normal renal glomeruli, and nonprimate platelets.[59] The C3b receptors have also

been shown to also react with C4b, perhaps due to their structural similarity.[60]

C3d

Receptors to C3d are found on a small population of normal B lymphocytes and certain lymphoblastoid cells, but there are differences of opinion as to their presence on monocytes and macrophages. Certainly, if they are present they appear to have very little, if any, biological activity in the process of immune red cell destruction by macrophages.

It has been suggested that the complement receptors may be involved in three functions; control of the traffic of immune complexes

Table 3-7. Biologic Activities of Complement Components

C1	Increases association of Ag-Ab complexes
C4b	Virus neutralization
	Adherence via receptor on lymphocytes and phagocytic cells. ?Physiologic significance
C2 fragment	?C2 kinin
C3b	Adherence via receptor on lymphocytes and phagocytic cells—opsonin
	Activation of alternative pathway
	Triggers B lymphocytes to make mediators
	Triggers bone marrow leukocyte release
	Triggers release of Ag-Ab complexes from leukocyte surfaces
	Triggers more rapid division of tumor cells
C3d	Adherence via receptor on lymphocytes and macrophages opsonically active in association with IgG
C3a	Chemotactic factor, anaphylatoxin I
C5a	Chemotactic factor, anaphylatoxin II
C5b67	Chemotactic factor, may attack unsensitized cells
C8	Slow membrane damage
C9	Rapid membrane damage

(Petz, L. D. and Garratty, G.: Acquired Immune Hemolytic Anemias. Churchill Livingstone, New York, 1980.)

and cells, control of the fate of immune complexes, and the triggering of cellular functions (e.g., the immune response).[61]

CELL-ASSOCIATED COMPLEMENT COMPONENTS

The genes controlling the serum expression of certain complement components, notably C2, C4, C8, and Factor B, are now known to be linked to the genes coding for the major histocompatibility complex.[55] Some of these components are also present on cell membranes (e.g., C4, C8, and Factor B are present

Table 3-8. Biologic Functions That Can Result from Alternative-Pathway Activation

Cobra-venom-mediated lysis of unsensitized erthrocytes
Erythrocyte lysis in paroxysmal nocturnal hemoglobinuria
Bactericidal activity
Phagocytosis
Anaphylatoxin production
Platelet histamine release, lysis, and promotion of blood clotting in animals
Leukotaxis
Mediation of Arthus vasculitis
Proteinuria of experimentally induced glomerulonephritis
Participation in renal damage of hypocomplementemic glomerulonephritis

(Petz, L.D. and Garratty, G.: Acquired Immune Hemolytic Anemias. Churchill Livingstone, New York, 1980.)

on lymphocytes). By contrast, genes controlling C1, C4, C6, and C7 are not linked to the major histocompatibility complex, and none of these components are present on cells.

A recent finding has been that Chido and Rodgers blood group antigens appear to be immunologically identical to antigenic determinants on the C4 complement component.[62] Chido (Ch^a) and Rodgers (Rg^a) were described as new blood group antigens in 1967[63] and 1976,[64] respectively. The antibodies to these antigens often caused weak and unreliable reactions with red cells. Both Ch^a and Rg^a were found to be present in plasma; in fact, the typing of patients was more accurately determined by using plasma in inhibition procedures than by using the red cells. Approximately 98 percent of random white donors were found to be Ch(a+) and Rg(a+). Neither of the antibodies appeared to be capable of destroying red cells in vivo. The Chido and Rodgers loci were shown to be very close to HLA on chromosome 6.[65,66] In 1978, O'Neill and his coworkers showed that Chido and Rodgers are distinct components of human C4.[62] Further studies have shown that both Ch and Rg antigens reside on the C4d fragment of C4.[66]

Other workers have also detected complement components on normal red cells. Graham et al.[67] showed that a high proportion of normal red cells have small amounts of C3d

Table 3-9. Genetically Determined Complement Deficiencies in Humans

Deficient Component	Associated Clinical Findings
C1q (?)	SCID,* hypogammaglobulinemia
C1r	CGN,† SLE syndrome, frequent infections
C1s	SLE syndrome
C4	SLE syndrome, SLE‡
C2	No disease, SLE syndrome, MPGN, § H-S purpura.‖ dermatomyositis, discoid lupus, infections, chronic vasculitis, Hodgkin's disease
C3	Pyogenic infections, absence of expected neutrophilia
C5	Pyogenic infections, SLE
C5 dysfunction?	Infections, Leiner's disease
C6	No disease, meningococcal infections
C7	No disease. Raynaud's phenomenon, sclerodactyly, gonococcal infections
C8	No disease, gonococcal infections, SLE
C1-INH	Hereditary angioedema, SLE
C3b-INA	Pyogenic infections

* Severe combined immunodeficiency disease
† Chronic glomerulonephritis
‡ Systemic lupus erythematosus
§ Membranoproliterative glomerulonephritis
‖ Henoch-Schönlein purpura
(Petz, L.D. and Garratty, G.: Acquired Immune Hemolytic Anemias. Churchill Livingstone, New York, 1980.)

on their surface. Using a PVP-Augmented AutoAnalyzer System, Rosenfield and Jagathambal[68] showed that C3 and C4 (possibly in the form of C3d and C4d) are present on normal red cells; they suggested that this varied from <5 to 40 molecules per red cell, which would be below the threshold of the usual laboratory antiglobulin test.

Table 3-10. Some Diseases Associated with Acquired Abnormalities of Complement

1. Connective tissue disease
   A. Systemic lupus erythematosus
   B. Rheumatoid arthritis
2. Immune hemolytic anemias
3. Renal disease
   A. Post-streptococcal glomerulonephritis
   B. Membranoproliferative glomerulonephritis
   C. Lupus nephritis
   D. Goodpasture's syndrome
   E. Bacterial endocarditis, malaria, etc.
4. Infectious hepatitis with arthritis
5. Malaria
6. Cryoglobulinemia
7. Dermatologic disorders
   A. Systemic lupus erythematosus
   B. Bullous pemphigoid
   C. Discoid lupus
   D. Pemphigus vulgaris
   E. Herpes gestationis
8. Septic shock
9. Severe liver disease
10. Serum sickness

SENSITIZATION OF RED CELLS WITH COMPLEMENT COMPONENTS

Complement Activation by Red Cell Antibodies

Complement may be activated by autoantibodies or alloantibodies of the IgM class, or by IgG antibodies of IgG3, IgG1, or IgG2 subclasses. Some blood group alloantibodies commonly cause complement-dependent lysis of normal red cells in vitro—e.g., anti-A, -B, -Vel, $-PP_1P^k(Tj^a)$; others may sensitize the red cells with complement components, often not causing lysis unless they have been enzyme-treated—e.g., some anti-Lewis and anti-Kidd. Still other examples of anti-Lewis, -Kidd, -Kell, -Duffy, -S, -s, -I, -i, -H, -P, $-Gy^a$, and -Jr may sensitize red cells with complement components without causing lysis of untreated or enzyme-treated cells. It is not understood why some antibodies sensitize red cells with enough C3 to give strongly positive antiglobulin tests yet do not proceed to lysis. Red cells that become sensitized with complement components without proceeding to lysis may have C3 (C3d), C4 (C4d), C5, C6 and C8 bound to their membrane, as demonstrated by specific complement component antiglobulin tests.[69-71]

It is not understood why some alloantibodies, such as anti-Rh, which may be IgG1, IgG3, or IgM, do not activate complement. It has been suggested that the ability to fix complement might relate to the number of antigenic sites present on the red cell.[13] It has been calculated that 1000 IgG molecules would be necessary to form one IgG doublet on a red cell with 800,000 antigenic sites (e.g., A or B). There are only about 10,000 to 30,000 Rh sites per red cell; thus, the chance of two IgG molecules falling close enough together to form a doublet is remote. However, some other antibodies (e.g., anti-K[72]) can activate complement, yet there are only about 3,000 to 6,000 K antigenic sites per red cell. Further, a few anti-Rh antibodies have been described that do sensitize red cells with complement.[73,74]

Although antigen site number per red cell has been investigated in some detail, notably by Masouredis et al., little is known about antigen site distribution.[75] This may be of importance in connection with the probability that a "doublet" of two antigen sites in close proximity will be occupied by either IgG antibody molecules or two subunits of an IgM molecule; in turn, this may determine the ability of a given antigen and its antibody to fix complement. Antigen site distribution may also be important in a variety of cell-cell interactions of red cells with lymphoreticular cells and their derivatives.

Antigen sites might be uniformly or randomly distributed; in either case, site density would be a function of total site number. If sites are grouped relatively tightly, closely spaced doublets could occur even in the face of a low total number of sites. It is also possible that antigen sites are not fixed in location but are mobile in the relatively fluid red cell membrane. This problem has been difficult to investigate with ferritin-labeled alloantibodies. The possibility that artifacts may be introduced in processing either intact labeled red cells or red cell membranes for electron microscopic examination has made the interpretation of many studies equivocal or unreliable.[76]

Knowledge of the possible biochemical and physiological functions of antigen sites might also lead to better understanding of red cell destruction initiated by antibodies. A number of alterations in red cell membrane function might occur as a result of interaction with antibodies, which could then lead indirectly to loss of viability.

Complement Activation by Immune Complexes

Red cells can become sensitized with complement from the activation of the complement cascade by immune complexes in plasma. A good example of this is the formation of immune complexes by certain drugs, e.g., phenacetin or quinidine.[77] The drug-antidrug complex can attach temporarily and nonspecifically to the red cells and cause activation of complement, with subsequent attachment of complement components to the red cell membrane. It is possible that other immune complexes such as DNA-anti-DNA, bacteria-anti-bacteria, and virus-anti-virus may also result in red cells becoming sensitized with complement.

Nonimmune Sensitization of Red Cells with Complement

Attachment of complement to red cell membranes by nonimmunologic mechanisms occurs as a result of the action of cephalosporin antibiotics which modify the red cell membrane and result in nonspecific adsorption of many proteins.[77,78]

THE SIGNIFICANCE OF COMPLEMENT SENSITIZATION OF RED CELLS IN THE DIAGNOSIS OF IMMUNE HEMOLYTIC ANEMIAS AND IN ALLOANTIBODY DETECTION

Evaluating the red cells of patients with acquired hemolytic anemias for the presence or absence of complement components by the direct antiglobulin test is of distinct value in developing a precise diagnosis.[71] In patients with the warm antibody type of autoimmune hemolytic anemia, the direct antiglobulin test will reveal IgG and C3d in about 62 percent of patients, IgG only in 20 percent, and C3d only in 13 percent. The red cells of patients with cold agglutinin syndrome are sensitized with C3d but not with IgG. Patients with drug-induced immune hemolytic anemia caused by penicillin and methyldopa typically have red cells strongly sensitized by IgG but without fixation of complement. Other drug-induced immune hemolytic anemias are usually characterized by weak-to-moderate sensitization of red cells by complement components without detectable immune globulins. However, some such patients do have IgG on their red cells, more often in association with complement. Table 3-11 summarizes the characteristic antiglobulin test results in various hemolytic anemias (see also Tables 31-3 and 31-14).

A point that must be emphasized is that about 26 percent of patients with immune hemolytic anemias will appear to have a negative direct antiglobulin test unless the antiglobulin serum used contains antibodies against complement components[71] (Table 3-12).

Although the results of the direct antiglobulin test provide valuable information if performed as described above, they must be in-

Table 3-11. Direct Antiglobulin Test Results in Immune Hemolytic Anemias Using Anti-IgG and Anti-C3 Antisera

	IgG	C3*
Warm antibody AIHA		
(67%)	+	+
(20%)	+	0
(13%)	0	+
Cold agglutinin syndrome	0	+
Paroxysmal cold hemoglobinuria	0	+
Penicillin or methyldopa-induced†	+	0
Other drug-induced immune hemolytic anemias‡	0	+
Warm antibody AIHA associated with systemic lupus erythematosus	+	+

* Such cells are primarily sensitized with the C3d component of C3 (see text).

† Weakly positive reactions with anti-C3 may occur; invariably, reactions are strongly positive with anti-IgG.

‡ The most common pattern of red cell sensitization is indicated, but occasionally IgG may be detected with or without C3

(Petz, L.D. and Garratty, G.: Acquired Immune Hemolytic Anemias. Churchill Livingstone, New York, 1980.)

terpreted in conjunction with clinical and other laboratory data to avoid erroneous conclusions. A positive direct antiglobulin test occurs in situations other than immune hemolytic anemias. A positive direct antiglobulin test does not necessarily indicate the presence of autoantibody; furthermore, even if autoantibody is present, the patient may or may not have a hemolytic anemia. Thus, an independent clinical assessment must be made to determine the presence or absence of hemolytic anemia; the role of the direct anti-

Table 3-12. Results of direct Anti-Globulin Test with Anti-IgG and Anti-C3 in 347 Patients with AIHA and Drug-Induced Immune Hemolytic Anemias

	Percent*	
IgG (no C3)	23	73% have IgG on RBC
IgG + C3	50	76.4% have C3 on RBC
C3 (no IgG)	26.4	

* Two patients (0.6%) had only IgA present on their red blood cells.

(Petz, L.D. and Garratty, G.: Acquired Immune Hemolytic Anemias. Churchill Livingstone, New York, 1980.)

globulin test is to aid in the evaluation of the etiology of hemolysis when present.[71] (The significance of complement fixation by alloantibodies in reference to compatibility testing is discussed in Chapter 7.)

THE PATHOPHYSIOLOGY OF IMMUNE HEMOLYSIS

Lysis in vivo of red cells injured by immune mechanisms can result directly from the effects of complement on the red cell membrane or from the interaction of cells of the reticuloendothelial system with red cells sensitized with antibody and/or complement.[79] The former is often referred to as "intravascular" hemolysis and the latter as "extravascular" hemolysis. Clinical indications of intravascular hemolysis include increased plasma hemoglobin, methemalbuminemia, hemoglobinuria, and hemosiderinuria; even with only minimal intravascular hemolysis, the serum haptoglobin will be low or absent.[71, 80, 81] Prototype disorders that are primarily associated with intravascular hemolysis are ABO hemolytic transfusion reactions, mechanical hemolytic anemia, paroxysmal nocturnal hemoglobinuria, and paroxysmal cold hemoglobinuria. Extravascular hemolysis results in an increase in serum bilirubin and in bilirubin degradation products in the urine and stool without causing evidence of release of free hemoglobin into the blood. Hemolysis in hereditary spherocytosis, or that induced by Rh antibodies or warm autoantibodies, is characteristically extravascular in nature.

It is useful to discuss intravascular and extravascular hemolysis separately, even though a sharp distinction between the two is not always justified either on clinical grounds or in regard to the pathophysiology involved.[82] Indeed, with brisk hemolysis of any etiology, some manifestations of intravascular hemolysis may be present, especially low-serum haptoglobin. Also, complement may participate in red cell lysis by both mechanisms. Finally, it should be pointed out that in many instances of immune hemolysis the process of red cell destruction is multimodal, and it is currently impossible to separate and quantitate the several processes going on simultaneously.[79]

INTRAVASCULAR IMMUNE RED CELL DESTRUCTION

This type of immune red cell destruction is complement-mediated. Not many alloantibodies are able to destroy red cells intravascularly; among the alloantibodies that do destroy red cells through this mechanism, anti-A and anti-B are the best examples; anti-Kidd, -Vel, -Tj^a and -Le^a sometimes can also activate the complement cascade. Thus, on rare occasions, they are capable of causing the intravascular lysis of donor red cells. Intravascular hemolysis is also uncommon in autoimmune hemolytic anemia. When it occurs it is usually associated with paroxysmal cold hemoglobinuria, and less commonly with cold agglutinin syndrome and with cases of drug-induced hemolytic anemia due to immune-complex formation. Intravascular hemolysis is less common in warm antibody autoimmune hemolytic anemia, but does occur particularly in the hyperacute form of the disease.

Complement-mediated immune hemolysis occurs by way of the classical pathway of complement activation, which has been described in the preceding section. Theoretically, any of the many substances that can activate the alternative pathway could cause intravascular hemolysis, but there is at present no evidence to suggest that antibody-mediated red cell lysis occurs as a result of this pathway of complement activation. Indeed, studies by May et al.[52] on antibody-mediated cytolysis of erythrocytes and nucleated cells have indicated that the alternative pathway mediates cell lysis inefficiently or not at all.

EXTRAVASCULAR IMMUNE RED CELL DESTRUCTION

The second major mode of in vivo erythrocyte destruction is mediated by a mechanism of temporary or permanent sequestration of erythrocytes within portions of the reticuloendothelial system, primarily in the liver and spleen. If red cells become sensitized with IgG, or if cells are sensitized with complement but do not proceed through the entire cascade to lysis, they may then be destroyed or damaged within the reticuloendothelial system. This system is capable of removing up to about 400 ml of red cells per day.[13]

It is believed that red cells sensitized with antibody and/or complement are destroyed within the reticuloendothelial system by interaction with mononuclear phagocytes. The most important phagocyte participating in immune red cell destruction is the macrophage. Macrophages arise primarily from bone marrow precursors, probably the promonocyte. After a short period of maturation in the bone marrow, monocytes are released into the blood. After spending a few days in the peripheral circulation, they migrate to the tissues, and there they mature functionally and morphologically to become typical histiocytic or exudative macrophages.[84] They are particularly prominent in the liver (Kupffer cells), lung (alveolar macrophages), spleen, and bone marrow (Table 3-2). The survival time of mature tissue macrophages is thought to be several weeks, or even months.[85]

Macrophage Receptors

Macrophages have receptors on their membranes that specifically recognize certain classes of immunoglobulins (either free or as part of an immune complex) and certain complement components.[86] One type of receptor is capable of interaction with the Fc portion of the IgG molecule, specifically with a portion of the molecule in the domain nearest the carboxyl terminus of the heavy chain.[87] This site appears to be found on human IgG molecules of only the IgG1 and IgG3 subgroups.[88] It is not present on the IgM molecule.[89] Such receptor sites on the macrophages are relatively insensitive to digestion by proteolytic enzymes[90] and appear to be present on granulocytes as well as monocytes. Qualitatively similar sites are demonstrable on certain lymphocytes as well.[91] Quantitative studies have indicated that there are approximately 1×10^6 IgG receptors on the membrane of each macrophage.[92] The number of receptor sites seems to increase during macrophage activation,[93] a finding that may have important clinical implications.

In addition, there appear to be receptors for a biologically active fragment of C3, C3b.[90,94] When C3b is enzymatically degraded by C3b inactivator, interaction with this receptor no longer occurs.[95] Other investigators have described receptors for C3c,[96] C4,[97,98] and C3d.[99,100]

Mechanisms of Extravascular Immune Hemolysis and Red Cell Fragmentation

Red cells sensitized by antibody and/or complement may fragment in vivo in several ways.[101] If two red cells approach each other closely enough to result in contact of their membranes, a small area of membrane fusion may result. When mechanical forces such as those found in the circulation force the cells apart, a long membrane thread may be drawn out and break off to form a small membrane fragment. This fragment was termed a "myelin form" by Ponder, who first observed the phenomenon.[102,103] The process is enhanced by antibody and probably by complement components bound to the red cell membrane; it is easily observed in patients with autoimmune acquired hemolytic disease who are actively hemolyzing and who have spherocytes in their peripheral blood. Microspherocyte formation results from this loss of membrane material without loss of cell contents, thereby leading to a decrease in the ratio of surface area to volume. This causes the membrane of the spherocytic cell to be rigid and results in its being unable to change its shape readily to traverse the fine channels of the spleen; the membrane is thus susceptible to early destruction by trapping.[104-106]

A second type of red cell fragmentation which may be induced by sensitization with antibody has been termed phagocytic frag-

mentation.[107] The attachment of appropriately sensitized red cells to macrophages can be visualized in vitro by so-called rosette formation; the macrophage becomes ringed by sensitized red cells, like petals on a flower (Fig. 3-11). On attachment to the macrophage, the red cells usually undergo considerable distortion and deformity in the region of attachments.[108] Sensitized red cells may become completely engulfed by the macrophage and destroyed internally (Fig. 3-12). However, in some instances a red cell is only partially engulfed by a phagocytic cell (Figs. 3-13 & 3-14); it is then fragmented into two relatively large pieces, with the unengulfed

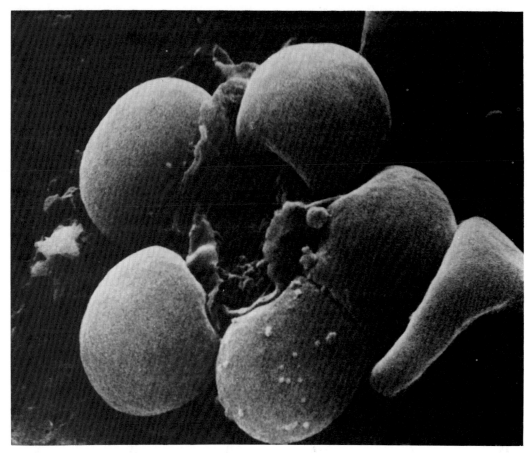

Fig. 3-11. Scanning electron micrograph illustrating the interaction of antibody coated red cells and a phagocytic white cell. The white cell is surrounded by sensitized red cells forming a rosette. (Courtesy of Dr. W. Rosse. Petz, L.D. and Garratty, G.: Acquired Immune Hemolytic Anemias. Churchill Livingstone, New York. 1980.)

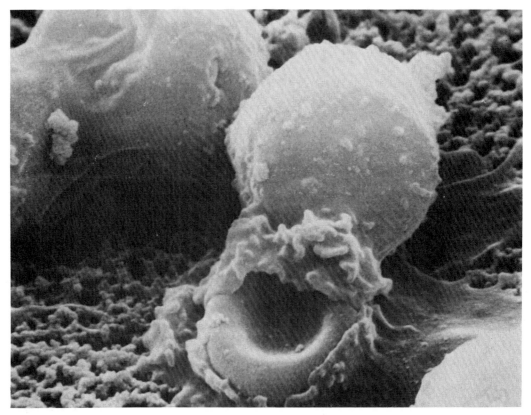

Fig. 3-12. Scanning electron micrograph illustrating the reaction of a phagocytic white cell with an antibody coated red cell. Only a small exposed area remains of a nearly ingested red cell. (Rosse, W.F. and de Boisfleury, A.: The interaction of phagocytic cells and red cells following alteration of their form or deformability. Blood Cells, 1:359, 1975.)

fragment escaping into the circulation possibly as a result of simple mechanical forces. This process results in small, variably shaped poikilocytic and spherocytic red cell fragments[109] (Fig. 3-15) which are presumably rapidly removed by subsequent phagocytosis or filtration in the spleen. Red cell-phagocyte interaction may also result in loss of small membrane fragments if the red cells are swept away by circulatory forces after they are attached but before phagocytic engulfment.

Although extravascular red cell destruction typically leads to the appearance in the plasma and urine of breakdown products of hemoglobin, such as bilirubin and urobilinogen, laboratory tests may show some results that are associated with intravascular lysis.

For instance, hemoglobinemia and hemoglobinuria may occur following Rh-incompatible tranfusions.[13] The Rh antibodies in these cases have not been shown to fix complement, and it therefore seems likely that hemoglobin may be released into the blood following fragmentation of the red cells during macrophage-mediated cell damage, particularly when large amounts of blood are rapidly destroyed (e.g., several units). Recent evidence has suggested that macrophages (and possibly lymphocytes) may destroy sensitized red cells by extracellular cytotoxicity[110] in addition to phagocytosis; this phenomenon may be an alternative explanation for hemoglobinemia and hemoglobinuria associated with extravascular lysis.

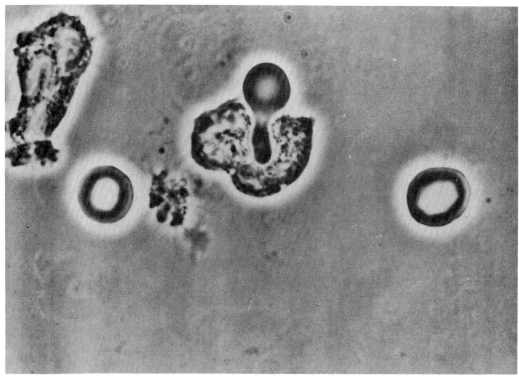

Fig. 3-13. Phase-contrast photomicrograph illustrating the interaction of an antibody coated red cell and a phagocytic white cell. The red cell, having been taken by the metapod, is deformed as the metapod flows along its sides. (Rosse, W.F., de Boisfleury, A., and Bessis, M.: The interaction of phagocytic cells and red cells modified by immune reactions. Comparison of antibody and complement coated red cells. Blood Cells, 1:345, 1975.)

Factors Affecting Extravascular Immune Hemolysis

Quantitative Factors. Most studies have indicated that there is a correlation between the amount of IgG on the red cells and the rate of red cell destruction. Mollison et al.[111] performed red cell survival studies using erythrocytes sensitized with 12 different concentrations of a single anti-D antibody over the range of 1.6 to 47 μg antibody per ml of red cells. The rate of clearance of red cells increased with the amount of antibody on the cells. When there was less than approximately 20 μg of antibody per ml, destruction took place predominantly in the spleen; above this value there was also appreciable destruction in the liver. Rosse[112] studied the concentration of cell-bound antibody in a series of patients with warm antibody autoimmune hemolytic anemia. The rate of hemolysis was, in general, proportional to the concentration of cell-bound antibody.

However, exceptions to this correlation are rather frequent, and the reasons for such exceptions are not well understood. For example, most patients who have a positive direct antiglobulin test caused by methyldopa administration have normal red cell survival, although these cells can be extremely strongly sensitized with IgG.[71,77] Similarly, a small porportion of normal persons have a strongly positive direct antiglobulin test but have normal red cell survival.[113] At the other end of the spectrum are patients with acquired immune hemolytic anemias who have

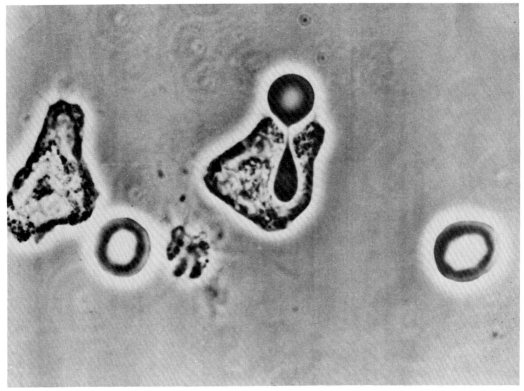

Fig. 3-14. Further interaction between the phagocytic white cell and the antibody coated red cell results in internalization of a portion of red cell. (Rosse, W.F., de Boisfleury, A., and Bessis, M.: The interaction of phagocytic cells and red cells modified by immune reactions. Comparison of antibody and complement coated red cells. Blood Cells, 1:345, 1975.)

marked hemolysis but very weakly positive or negative direct antiglobulin tests[71,114] (see Ch. 7). Studies of the IgG subclasses of antibodies [115-118] or the ability of macrophages to interact with red cells coated with various antibodies have not offered an explanation for the wide discrepancy in their ability to cause red cell destruction in vivo.[71]

Antibody Class. *IgG.* Erythrocytes sensitized with IgG antibodies that do not fix complement (e.g., Rh antibodies) appear to be destroyed as a result of the interaction of the IgG on the red cell and the Fc receptor on macrophages. However, this interaction is markedly inhibited in vitro by physiologic concentrations of normal human IgG.[94,108] It has been suggested that a unique splenic microenvironment is present which allows

erythrocyte-bound IgG to mediate this effect, and there is evidence that the inhibition of interaction by normal serum globulin is minimal in the presence of hemoconcentration as found in the red pulp of the spleen.[108,119]

A second factor that has a strong influence on the inhibitory effect of IgG is the number of sensitized red cells per monocyte.[119] When the number of sensitized red cells per monocyte in in vitro tests is increased from 1 to 32, the percentage of inhibition by a fixed amount of IgG (50 μg/ml) decreases significantly. Since considerable hemoconcentration occurs in the spleen, it is conceivable that a highly sensitized red cell-to-macrophage ratio is accomplished. A high ratio may allow interaction between weakly sensitized red cells and splenic macrophages, despite the

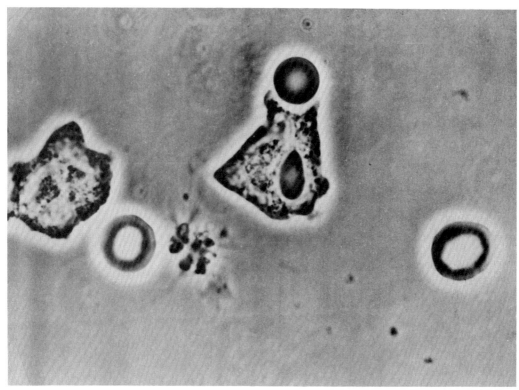

Fig. 3-15. The separation of the internal and external portions of the red cell is complete; the portion of the red cell outside the macrophage may escape and circulate as a spherocyto. (Rosse, W.F., de Bois-fleury, A., and Bessis, M.: The interaction of phagocytic cells and red cells modified by immune reactions. Comparison of antibody and complement coated red cells. Blood Cells, 1:345, 1975.)

presence in vivo of a high concentration of IgG.

Not all workers accept this explanation. Scornik et al.[120] showed that IgG-sensitized red cells are rapidly cleared from the circulation of patiens with myelomas in spite of serum IgG concentrations several times higher than normal. They concluded that the current explanations derived from in vitro experiments are insufficient to explain the IgG-dependent clearance of red cells in the presence of free IgG.

Another explanation has been offered to explain destruction of red cells by IgG antibodies.[100] Anti-Rh-sensitized ^{51}Cr-labeled red cells were infused into normal volunteers or into patients with low serum C4 (<0.1 percent of normal). Each of six patients with

low complement levels had a marked reduction in red cell clearance rates, even though they had normal reticuloendothelial clearance of ^{125}I-aggregated human albumin. On the basis of these and other data, the authors suggest that complement may participate in Rh-antibody-mediated clearance in vivo in spite of the fact that the antibodies could not be shown to fix complement by in vitro techniques.

IgM. IgM red cell antibodies usually activate complement; the erythrocytes are then hemolyzed intravascularly or removed extravascularly through C3b/macrophage interaction. Schreiber and Frank demonstrated that red cells sensitized with IgM antibody survived normally when given to guinea pigs genetically deficient in the fourth component of complement[121] and to humans with complement deficiencies.[122] In contrast, Cutbush and Mollison[123] and Burton and Mollison[124] have described examples of noncomplement-binding IgM alloantibodies that led to a shortened red cell survival. Mollison[13] has suggested that this observation might be explained by red cell agglutinates being trapped in small blood vessels and eventually suffering metabolic damage. It should be noted that Schreiber and Frank[121,122] used relatively weakly sensitized red cells in their experiments.

IgA. Receptors for IgA have not been demonstrated on macrophages or monocytes. There are few experimental data on the survival of IgA sensitized red cells. Indeed, IgA serum alloantibodies and autoantibodies are uncommon, and it is rare for them to be found as the only immunoglobulin class present in an alloantibody. Nevertheless, a number of examples of autoimmune hemolytic anemia have been described in which the direct antiglobulin test was positive only with anti-IgA antiglobulin serum.[71,125] It is possible that a small number of IgG molecules were also present on the patient's red cells in these cases; indeed, this has been demonstrated in one instance.[71]

Complement. Huber et al.[94] were the first to show that human monocytes have a receptor for C3 and that it may function independently of IgG, or cooperatively in the induction of phagocytosis. They showed that, if red cells were sensitized with complement in addition to IgG, the previously described inhibitory effect of free IgG was diminished considerably. In fact, in experiments in vitro in which red cells sensitized with IgG only or IgG + C3 were added to monocytes in the presence of IgG in the fluid phase, only 100 molecules of bound C3 per red cell were sufficient to overcome the inhibitory effect of IgG on the monocyte-sensitized red cell reaction. In addition, C3 sensitization of the red cells alone was not sufficient to induce the ingestion of red cells by monocytes; when IgG antibodies were present, C3 appeared to initiate

ingestion, suggesting a cooperative function in phagocytosis. Other workers have confirmed and extended these observations.[126-128]

Complement sensitized red cells are destroyed mainly in the liver.[13,129] In contrast to sensitization with IgG, the complement receptor/complement-sensitized red cell interaction is not inhibited by plasma or serum. This phenomenon can be explained by the fact that the receptor is specific for C3b, and normal plasma or serum does not contain C3b, which is an activation product of C3. As the liver is a much larger organ with a larger blood flow, proportionally more macrophage interactions will occur in the liver than in the spleen.

In some patients, red cells that are coated with complement may have no detectable immunoglobulins on their surface. There are several possible explanations for apparent red cell sensitization only by complement components. The antibody may be present in concentrations too low to be detected by serologic techniques, or complement may be fixed by a transient interaction with a cold-reactive antibody which subsequently elutes when the cells are warmed. Also, complement may be activated by immune complexes in the serum, with subsequent adherence of activated components to the red cell membrane. Finally, complement may be fixed by immune complexes loosely adsorbed on the surface of red cells or by allo- or autoantibodies of very low avidity which subsequently elute from the cell.

The fate of complement-sensitized red cells in vivo is variable.[130] If sufficient complement is attached to the red cell membrane, intravascular lysis will occur. More often the complement activation leads to extravascular sequestration of the sensitized erythrocytes by hepatic macrophages.

Lewis et al.[131] and Mollison[132] demonstrated that red cells coated with complement components may be temporarily sequestered in the liver but then reenter the circulation and survive normally. Brown et al.[129] elaborated on these experiments and demonstrated that

that red cells sensitized with IgM antibody and complement attach to hepatic macrophages (Kupffer cells), presumably through the specific C3b macrophage receptor, where some are immediately ingested. To activate the hepatic clearance mechanism, approximately 550 to 800 C3b molecules per red cell are required.[133,134] With time, unphagocytized red cells returned to the circulation at a slow exponential rate (half time 25 to 100 min). It was suggested that the return of the EC43 cells to the circulation from sites of attachment on fixed macrophages resulted from the progressive in vivo inactivation of fixed C3. The cell-bound C3b is acted on by the C3 inactivator in plasma; the molecule is cleaved into C3c and C3d, the latter remaining attached to the red cell. The macrophage

does not seem to interact efficiently, if at all, with C3d in vivo. Thus, the red cell may now survive relatively normally, although giving a strongly positive direct antiglobulin test due to a bound-complement degradation product (C3d).

Schreiber and Frank[121,122] confirmed these data by using C4-deficient guinea pigs and complement-deficient humans (Fig. 3-16). These authors further demonstrated that, although IgG is less efficient in initiating complement fixation, it appears to cause relatively more red cell damage than IgM. In their studies in guinea pigs, at least 60 molecules of IgM per red cell (60 complement-fixing sites) were required to initiate immune clearance; although several thousand IgG molecules per red cell were needed to form one C1-fixing

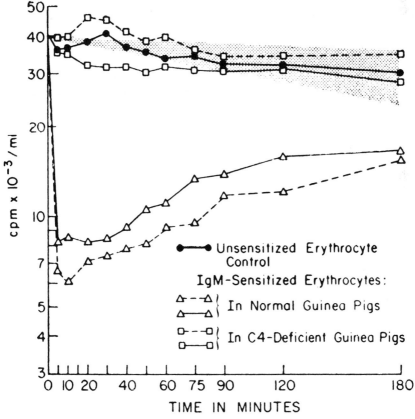

Fig. 3-16. Survival of ^{51}Cr-labeled erythrocytes with 234 IgM C1-fixing sites/erythrocyte in two normal and two C4-deficient guinea pigs. (Schreiber, Alan D. and Frank, Michael M.: Role of antibody and complement in the immune clearance and destruction of erythrocytes. J. Clin. Invest. 51:575, 1972.)

site, as few as 1.4 IgG complement-fixing sites per cell would effectively mediate in vivo clearance. Also, red cells sensitized by complement-fixing IgG antibodies are progressively removed from the circulation, and there is no evidence of immediate sequestration of sensitized cells with subsequent release (Fig. 3-17).

Thus, complement sensitization of red cells may result in: (1) intravascular lysis; (2) sequestration of red cells in the reticuloendothelial system with ingestion by phago-cytes; (3) sequestration with later return to the circulation, where the red cells may have normal survival or perhaps become damaged poikilocytic or spherocytic cells with somewhat shortened survival; or (4) essentially normal red cell survival. Critical determinants of red cell survival are: (1) the rate of complement sensitization; (2) the extent of complement sensitization; (3) the nature of the antibody causing complement sensitization, including its immunoglobulin class; (4) the number of antigen sites on the red cell

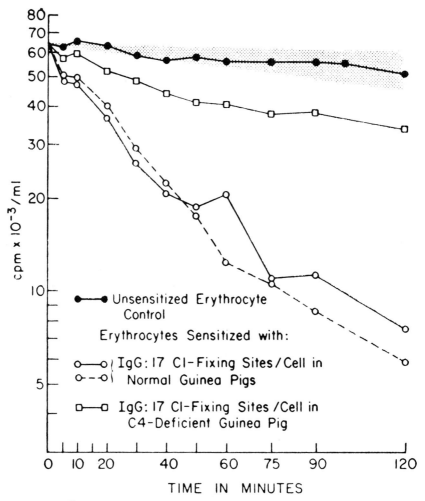

Fig. 3-17. Survival of ^{51}Cr-labeled erythrocytes with 17 IgG C1-fixing sites/erythrocyte in two normal and one C4-deficient guinea pigs. (Schreiber, Alan D. and Frank, Michael M.: Role of antibody and complement in the immune clearance and destruction of erythrocytes. J. Clin. Invest. 51:575, 1972.)

membrane; and (5) the biologic activity of the complement components.

Variation in Macrophage Activity. There are few data available correlating variations in macrophage activity with red cell destruction. However, this would seem to be an important area to study, as variation in macrophage activity may well explain some of the discrepancies between strength of red cell sensitization and red cell survival.

MacKenzie[135] found that monocytes from patients with autoimmune hemolytic anemia showed 40 to 80 percent ingestion of IgG-sensitized red cells, compared with 10 to 15 percent when normal donors were used. Patients with nonhemolytic anemias and microangiopathic hemolytic anemia did not show such differences.

Kay and Douglas[136] studied 21 patients with immune hemolytic anemia; four were studied sequentially. Fifteen of 17 patients showed enhanced monocyte activity (i.e., rosetting and phagocytosis) with autologous sensitized red cells, as compared with normal monocytes exposed to the same sensitized red cells. The most consistently elevated monocyte activity was found in patients with both IgG and complement-sensitized red cells.

Similarly, Atkinson and Frank[137] showed increased clearance of IgG-sensitized red cells in BCG-infected animals; they hypothesized that increased macrophage activation in such animals is responsible for the shortened in vivo red cell survival. Arend and Mannik[138] demonstrated an approximate doubling of IgG receptors and an increase in IgG association constants for rabbit alveolar macrophages following maximal stimulation of the animal with complete Freud's adjuvant. Thus, the relative activity of the macrophage system may play a significant role in controlling the rate of immune red cell destruction.

In contrast, macrophages may be decreased in activity by a number of physiological and pharmacological effects.[139-141] For example, phagocytic monocytes and granulocytes have been shown to be inhibitable by corticosteroids in an antibody dependent erythrophagocytic test system in vitro.[142] These same agents are also inhibitory when administered to the donor of leukocytes for the tests.[143] Their value in controlling the rate of hemolysis in autoimmune hemolytic anemia may be related to this activity. Corticosteroid drugs are apparently not of value in preventing hemolytic transfusion reactions where donor erythrocytes are rapidly destroyed. Other drugs which have cytostatic properties and which are employed as so-called immunosuppressive agents may also exert suppressive effects directly upon macrophage activity.

Possible Role of Lymphocytes. The role, if any, of lymphocytes in immune red cell destruction is controversial. Lymphocytes are known to have receptors for IgG (Fc) and complement (C3b, C3d, and C4). They have been found to be capable of destroying sensitized nucleated cells (e.g., other lymphocytes, tumor cells, and chicken red cells).[144] The mechanism of cell destruction involved is cell-mediated cytotoxicity. Before the cell is damaged, contact between the lymphocyte and target cell has to occur; complement may or may not be involved. In vitro cell-mediated lysis requires several hours to occur, even under optimal conditions. The exact mechanism is unclear but could be an enzymatic process.

Cell-mediated cytotoxicity can be independent of antibody. In this case, direct cell-mediated cytolysis by presensitized lymphocytes occurs. The effector cells are thought to be cytotoxic T-lymphocytes which do not require IgG antibodies as specific recognition factors for target cell antigens. Cell-mediated cytotoxicity can also be antibody-dependent, where the target cells have to be sensitized with antibody for identification. The effector cells for this reaction have been described as possibly "null" lymphocytes (i.e., those lacking sheep red cell receptors and surface Ig, but with IgG and complement receptors),[145] or "killer" lymphocytes (K cells), which are nonphagocytic and nonadherent lymphocytic cells.[144] Hinz and Chickosky,[146] using lymphocyte preparations containing less than 1 percent neutrophils and virtually no monocytes, were able to demonstrate cytotoxic reactions between lymphocytes and A- and Rh-positive red cells in the presence of anti-A and anti-Rh, respectively. In the experiments with Rh antibodies, only lymphocytes from an Rh-hyperimmune donor would cause lysis of the red cells. Normal lymphocytes from both Rh-positive and Rh-negative donors were completely without effect, even in the presence of a powerful anti-Rh. In contrast, Urbaniak[147] was able to show that normal or autologous lymphoid cells would lyse Rh-sensitized red cells, and that killing occurred at a very low antibody concentration. Recently, other workers have also reported antibody-dependent, cell-mediated cytotoxicity against human red cells, mediated by anti-A[148] and anti-Rh.[149-151]

The lymphocyte-induced, antibody-dependent, cell-mediated cytotoxicity demonstrated with human blood group alloantibodies was almost as efficient as that obtained with monocytes. In addition, antibody-dependent, cell-mediated cytotoxicity involving lymphocytes is not inhibited by free IgG (e.g., normal plasma), although it can be inhibited by aggregated IgG. Thus, it is possible that antibody-dependent, cell-mediated cytotoxicity by lymphocytes may play an important role in immune hemolysis.

Macrophage/Monocyte Cytotoxicity. Since the incrimination of macrophages as the major effector cell in immune red cell destruction, the emphasis has been on the phagocytic properties of the cell. Recent studies have suggested that an extracellular mechanism is operative, and perhaps the cytotoxic properties of the macrophage may be more important than first thought.

Holm and Hammarstrom[152] showed that purified human monocytes were able to lyse red cells treated with hyperimmune anti-A. In fact, one monocyte was able to lyse 2 or 3 red cells within an 18-hour incubation period.

Complement was not necessary for this reaction.

Actual lysis of the cell may result from a heat-labile cytotoxin designated by McIvor et al.[153] as specific macrophage cytotoxin. Most of the interactions are similar to those described previously for antibody-dependent, cell-mediated cytotoxicity by lymphocytes.

Kurlander et al.[149] demonstrated monocyte-mediated lysis in vitro of human red cells sensitized with IgG anti-Rh(D) and anti-A or -B. Cells sensitized only with human complement components (even up to 80,000 molecules per red cell) were not lysed, but C3b or C3d sensitization augmented IgG-mediated lysis and reduced the amount of IgG necessary to produce lysis.

Fleer et al.[154-156] have suggested that cytotoxicity may play a more important role than phagocytosis in immune red cell destruction. Using ^{51}Cr-labeled human red cells sensitized with anti-D, they were able to demonstrate cytotoxicity by monocytes, independent of phagocytosis.

Unlike other workers,[157-160] Fleer et al.[154-156] were not able to demonstrate lysis of Rh-sensitized cells by lymphocytes. Another important effect noted by Fleer et al.[161] was the development of an increased osmotic fragility of a considerable part of the non-lysed Rh-sensitized red cells. In fact, they found that the osmotically more fragile cells considerably outnumbered lysed and ingested red cells. A correlation with increased osmotic fragility and severity of autoimmune hemolytic anemia has been described previously.[162] The presence of spherocytes has, for years, been said to be a hallmark of autoimmune hemolytic anemia; the spherocytes are now thought to be formed through fragmentation of the sensitized red cells by macrophages. It has also been assumed that the increased osmotic fragility is due to the presence of spherocytes, but it may well be that the damage to the red cell membrane caused by cytotoxicity without fragmentation may also contribute to the increased fragility.

REFERENCES

1. McMaster, P.D. and Hudack, S.S.: The formation of agglutinins within the lymph node. J. Exp. Med. 61:783, 1935.
2. Fagraeus, A.: Antibody production in relation to the development of plasma cells. Acta. Med. Scand. 132:3, 1948.
3. Coons, A.L., Deduc, E.H., and Connoly, J.M.: Studies on antibody production. I. A method of histochemical demonstration of specific antibody and its application to the study of hyperimmune rabbits. J. Exp. Med. 102:49, 1955.
4. Attardi, G., Cohn, M., and Horibata, K., et al.: Antibody formation in the rabbit lymph node cell. J. Immunol. 92:346, 1964.
5. Hullinger, L. and Sorkin, E.: Synthesis of antibodies by blood leukocytes of the rabbit. Nature 198:229, 1963.
6. Landy, M., Sanderson, R.R., and Berstein, M.T., et al.: Antibody production in leukocytes in peripheral blood. Nature 204:1320, 1964.
7. Landsteiner, K. and Chase, M.: Experiments on transfer of cutaneous sensitivity to simple compounds. Proc. Soc. Exp. Biol. Med. 49:688, 1942.
8. Mitchison, N.A.: Passive transfer of transplantation immunity. Proc. Roy. Soc. Exp. Biol. Med. 142:7, 1954.
9. Algire, G.H., Weaver, J.M., and Prehn, R.T.: Studies on tissue homotransplantation in mice, using diffusion chamber methods. Ann. N.Y. Acad. Sci. 64:1009, 1957.
10. Glick, B., Chang, T.S., and Jaap, R.G.: The bursa of Fabricius and antibody production. Poultry Sci. 35:224, 1956.
11. Cooper, M.D., Peterson, R.D.A., and Good, R.A.: Delineation of the thymic and bursal lymphoid systems in the chicken. Nature 205:143, 1965.
12. Cooper, M.D., Peterson, R.D.A., and South, M.A., et al.: The function of the thymus system and the bursa system in the chicken. J. Exp. Med. 123:75, 1966.
13. Mollison, P.L.: Blood Transfusion in Clinical Medicine, 6th Edition. Blackwell Scientific Publications, Oxford, 1979.
14. Polley, M.J., Mollison, P.L., and Soothill, J.F.: The role of 19s gamma globulin blood group antibodies in the antiglobulin reaction. Br. J. Haematol. 8:149, 1962.
15. Giblett, E.R.: A critique of the theoretical hazard of inter- vs. intra-racial transfusion. Transfusion (Philad.) 1:233, 1961.
16. Archer, G.T., Cooke, B.R., Mitchell, K., and Parry, P.: Hyperimmunisation des donneurs de sang pour la production des gamma-globulines anti-Rh(D). Rev. Frac. Transfus. 12:341, 1969.
17. Krevans, J.R., Woodrow, J.C., Nosenzo, C., and Finn, R.: Patterns of Rh-immunization. Commun. 10th Congr. Int. Soc. Haematol. Stockholm, 1964.
18. Woodrow, J.C., Finn, R., and Krevans, J.R.: Rapid clearance of Rh positive blood during experimental Rh immunization. Vox Sang. 17:349, 1969.
19. de Wit, C.D. and Borst-Eilers, E.: Lack of relationship between the response to the D-antigen and to some other antigens. Vox Sang. 16:222, 1969.
20. Brody, N.I., Walker, J.G., and Siskind, G.W.: Studies on the control of antibody synthesis: interaction of antigenic competition and suppression of antibody formation by passive antibody on the immune response. J. Exp. Med. 126:81, 1967.
21. Woodruff, J.C., Clarke, C.A., Donohof, W.T.A., Finn, R., McConnel, R.B., Sheppard, P.M., Lehane, D., Roberts, Freda M., and Gimlette, T.M.D.: Mechanism of Rh prophylaxis: an experimental study on specificity of immunosuppression. Br. Med. J. 2:57, 1975.
22. Levine, P.: Serological factors as possible causes in spontaneous abortions. J. Hered. 34:71, 1943.
23. Race, R.R. and Sanger, Ruth: Blood Groups in Man. Blackwell Scientific Publications, Oxford, 1950.
24. Müller-Eberhard, H.J.: Complement, Annu. Rev. Biochem. 44:697, 1975.
25. Cooper, N.R.: Complement in cell survival and destruction. In: Progress in Transfusion and Transplantation. Schmidt, P.J., ed., American Association of Blood Banks, 1972, p. 191.
26. Frank, M.M. and Atkinson, J.P.: Complement in clinical medicine. Disease-a-Month, Year Book Medical Publishers, Chicago, January, 1975.

27. Fearon, D.T. and Austen, K.F.: Current concepts in immunology: The alternative pathway of complement—A system for host resistance to microbial infection. N. Engl. J. Med. 303:259, 1980.

28. Austen, K.F., Becker, E.L., Borsos, T., Lachmann, P.J., Lepow, I.H., Mayer, M.M., Müller-Eberhard, H.J., Nelson, R.A., Rapp, H.J., Rosen, F.S., and Trnka, Z.: Nomenclature of complement. Immunochemistry 7:137, 1970.

29. Ruddy, S., Gigli, I., and Austen, K.F.: The complement system of man (four parts). N. Engl. J. Med. 287, 489, 545, 592, 642, 1972.

30. Borsos, T. and Rapp, H.R.: Hemolysin titration based on fixation of the activated first component of complement: Evidence that one molecule of hemolysin suffices to sensitize an erythrocyte. J. Immunol. 95:559, 1965.

31. Humphrey, J.H. and Dourmashkin, R.R.: Electron microscope studies of immune cell lysis, in CIBA Foundation Symposium. Complement. J. & A. Churchill, London, 1965.

32. Augener, W., Grey, H.M., Cooper, N.R., and Müller-Eberhard, H.J.: The reaction of monomeric and aggregated immunoglobulins with C1. Immunochem. 8:1011, 1971.

33. Bieseker, G., Podack, E.R., Halverson, C.A., and Müller-Eberhard, H.J.: C5b-9 dimer: isolation from complement lysed cells and ultrastructural identification with complement-dependent membrane lesions. J. Exp. Med. 149:448, 1979.

34. Podack, E.R., Esser, A.F., Biesecker, G., and Müller-Eberhard, H.J.: Membrane attack complex of complement: A structural analysis of its assembly. J. Exp. Med. 151:301, 1980.

35. Borsos, T., Dourmashkin, R.R., and Humphrey, J.H.: Lesions in erythrocyte membranes caused by immune hemolysis. Nature (Lond.) 202:251, 1964.

36. Tranum-Jensen, J., Bhakdi, S., Bhakdi-Lehnen, B., Bjerrum, O.J., and Speth, V.: Complement lysis: the ultrastructure and orientation of the C5b-9 complex on target sheep erythrocyte membranes. Scand. J. Immunol. 7:45, 1978.

37. Dourmashkin, R.R.: The structural events associated with the attachment of complement components in reactive lysis. Immunology 35:205, 1978.

38. Mayer, M.M.: Mechanism of cytolysis by complement. Proc. Natl. Acad. Sci. U.S.A. 69:2954, 1972.

39. Podack, E.R., Biesecker, G., and Müller-Eberhard, H.J.: Membrane attack complex of complement: Generation of high affinity phospholipid binding sites by fusion of five hydrophilic plasma proteins. Proc. Natl. Acad. Sci. U.S.A., 76:897, 1979.

40. Pillemer, L., Blum, L., and Lepow, I.H.: The properdin system and immunity. I. Demonstration and isolation of a new serum protein, properdin, and its role in immune phenomena. Science 120:279, 1954.

41. Schur, P.H. and Becker, E.L.: Pepsin digestion of rabbit and sheep antibodies. The effect on complement fixation. J. Exp. Med. 118:891, 1963.

42. Gerwurz, H., Shin, H.S., and Mergenhagen, S.E.: Interactions of the complement system with endotoxin lipopolysaccharides: Consumption of each of the six terminal complement components. J. Exp. Med. 128:1049, 1968.

43. Sandberg, A.L., Oliveira, B., and Osler, A.G.: Two complement interaction sites in guinea pig immunoglobulins. J. Immunol. 106:282, 1971.

44. Frank, M.M., May, J.E., Gaither, T., and Ellman, L.: In vitro studies of complement function in sera of C4 deficient guinea pigs. J. Exp. Med. 134:176, 1971.

45. Götze, O. and Müller-Eberhard, H.J.: The C3-activator system: An alternate pathway of complement activation. J. Exp. Med. 134:Suppl. 90, 1971.

46. Götze, O. and Müller-Eberhard, H.J.: The alternative pathway of complement activation. Adv. Immunol. 24:1, 1976.

47. Schreiber, R.D. and Müller-Eberhard, H.J.: Assembly of the cytolytic alternative pathway of complement form 11 isolated plasma proteins. J. Exp. Med. 148:1722, 1978.

48. Brade, V.: The properdin system: Composition and function. Vox Sang. 35:1, 1978.

49. Perrin, L.H., Joseph, B.S., Cooper, N.R., and Oldstone, M.B.A.: Mechanism of injury of virus infected cells by antiviral antibody and complement: participation of IgG, F(ab')$_2$ and the alternative complement pathway. J. Exp. Med. 143:1027, 1976.

50. Lawley, T.J. and Frank, M.M.: The comple-

ment system in clinical diagnosis. Internat. J. Dermatol. 18:673, 1979.

51. Schreiber, R.D., Pangburn, M.K., Lesavre, P.H., and Müller-Eberhard, H.J.: Initiation of the alternative pathway of complement: Recognition of activators by bound C3b and assembly of the entire pathway from six isolated proteins. Proc. Nat. Acad. Sci. U.S.A. 75:3948, 1978.

52. May, J.E., Green, I., and Frank, M.M.: The alternate complement pathway in cell damage: Antibody-mediated cytolysis of erythrocytes and nucleated cells. J. Immunol. 109:595, 1972.

53. Götze, O. and Müller-Eberhard, H.J.: Paroxysmal nocturnal hemoglobinuria: Hemolysis initiated by the C3 activator system. N. Engl. J. Med. 286:180, 1972.

54. Poskitt, T.R., Fortwengler, H.P., and Lunskis, B.J.: Activation of the alternative complement pathway by autologous red cell stroma. J. Exp. Med. 138:715, 1973.

55. Hobart, M.J. and Lachman, P.J.: Allotypes of complement components in man. Transpl. Rev. 32:26, 1976.

56. Dickler, H.B. and Kunkel, H.G.: Interaction of aggregated γ-globulin with B lymphocytes. J. Exp. Med. 136:191, 1972.

57. Sobel, A.T. and Bokisch, V.A.: Receptor for C1q on peripheral human lymphocytes and human lymphoblastoid cells. Fed. Proc. 34:965, 1975.

58. Suba, E.A. and Csako, G.: C1q(C1) receptor on human platelets: Inhibition of collagen-induced platelet aggregation by C1q(C1) molecules. J. Immunol. 117:304, 1976.

59. Nelson, D.S.: Immune adherence. Adv. Immunol. 3:131, 1963.

60. Nussenzweig, V.: Receptors for immune complexes on lymphocyte. Adv. Immunol. 19:217, 1974.

61. Bianco, C.: Plasma membrane receptors for complement. In: Comprehensive Immunology. Good, R. and Day, S.B., eds. Plenum Press, New York, 1975.

62. O'Neill, G.J., Yang, S.Y., Tegoli, J., Berger, R., and Dupont, B.: Chido and Rodgers blood groups are distinct antigenic components of human complement C4. Nature 273:668, 1978.

63. Harris, J.P., Tegoli, J., Swanson, J., Fischer, N., Gavin, J., and Noades, J.: A nebulous an-

tibody responsible for cross-matching difficulties (Chido). Vox Sang. 12:140, 1967.

64. Longster, G. and Giles, C.M.: A new antibody specificity, anti-Rg[a], reacting with a red cell and serum antigen. Vox Sang. 30:175, 1976.

65. Middleton, J., Crookston, M.C., Falk, J.A., Robson, E.B., Cook, P.J.L., Batchelor, J.R., Bodmer, J., Ferrara, G.B., Festenstein, H., Harris, R., Kissmeyer-Nielson, F., Lawler, S.D., Sachs, J.A., and Wolf, E.: Linkage of Chido and HL-A. Tissue Antigens 4:366, 1974.

66. Tilley, C.A., Romans, D.G., and Crookston, M.C.: Localization of Chido and Rodgers determinants to a tryptic C4d fragment of human C4. Transfusion 18:622, 1978.

67. Graham, H.A., Davies, D.M., Jr., and Brower, C.E.: Detection of C3b and C3d on red cell membranes. Proceedings of an International Symposium on "The Nature and Significance of Complement Activation." Pollack, W., Mollison, P.L., and Reiss, A.M., eds. Ortho Research Institute of Medical Sciences, Raritan, New Jersey, 1977.

68. Rosenfield, R.E. and Jagathambal: Antigenic determinants of C3 and C4 complement components on washed erythrocytes from normal persons. Transfusion 18:517, 1978.

69. Kerr, R.O., Dalmasso, A.P., and Kaplan, M.E.: Erythrocyte-bound C5 and C6 in autoimmune hemolytic anemia. J. Immunol. 107:1209, 1971.

70. Pondman, K.W., Rosenfield, R.E., Tallal, L., and Wasserman, L.R.: The specificity of the complement antiglobulin test. Vox Sang. 5:297, 1960.

71. Petz, L.D. and Garratty, G.: Acquired Immune Hemolytic Anemias, Churchill Livingstone, New York, 1980.

72. Petz, L.D.: Complement in immunohematology and in neurologic disorders. In: International Symposium on The Nature and Significance of Complement Activation. Pollack, W., Mollison, P. L., and Reiss, A.M., Eds. Raritan, New Jersey. Ortho Research Institute of Medical Sciences, 1977, p. 87.

73. Ayland, J., Horton, M.A., Tippett, P., and Waters, A.H.: Complement binding anti-D made in a D[u] variant woman. Vox Sang. 34:40, 1978.

74. Waller, M. and Lawler, S.D.: A study of the properties of the rhesus antibody (Ri) diagnostic for rheumatoid factor and its application to Gm grouping. Vox Sang. 7:591, 1962.

75. Masouredis, S.: Quantitative and Ultrastructural Aspects of Red Cell Membrane Rh Antigens. In: A Seminar on Recent Advances in Immunohematology. American Association of Blood Banks, Washington, D.C., 1973, pp. 41-62.

76. Masouredis, S.: Personal Communications, 1980.

77. Petz, L.D.: Drug-Induced Immune Haemolytic Anaemia. Clinics in Haematology, 9:455, 1980.

78. Spath, P., Garratty, G., and Petz, L.: Studies on the immune response to penicillin and cephalothin in humans. I. Optimal conditions for titration of hemagglutinating penicillin and cephalothin antibodies. II. Immunohematologic reactions to cephalothin administration. J. Immunol. 107:854, 1971.

79. Swisher, S.N.: Cell Survival in the Presence of Antibody. N.Y. Acad. Sci. 127:901, 1965.

80. Andersen, M.N., Gabrieli, E., and Zizzi, J.A.: Chronic hemolysis in patients with ball-valve prostheses. J. Thorac. Cardiovasc. Surg. 50:501, 1965.

81. Brus, I. and Lewis, S.M.: The haptoglobin content of serum in haemolytic anaemia. Br. J. Haematol. 5:348, 1959.

82. Petz, L.D.: The Diagnosis of Hemolytic Anemia. In: A Seminar on Laboratory Management of Hemolysis. American Association of Blood Banks, Washington D.C., 1979, pp. 1–27.

83. Petz, L.D., and Garratty, G.: Complement in immunohematology. Prog. Clin. Immunol. 2:175, 1974.

84. Van Furth, R., Cohn, Z.A., Hirsch, J.G., Humphrey, J.H., Spector, W.G., and Langevoort, H.L.: The mononuclear phagocyte system: A new classification of macrophages, monocytes, and their precursor cells. Bull. Wld. Hlth. Org. 46:845, 1972.

85. Van Furth, R.: Origin and kinetics of monocytes and macrophages. Seminars Hematol. 7:125, 1970.

86. Huber, H. and Fudenberg, H.H.: Receptor sites of human monocytes for IgG. Int. Arch. Allergy. 34:18, 1968.

87. Yasmeen, E., Ellerson, J.R., Dorrington, K.J., and Painter, R.H.: Location of the site of cytophilic activity toward guinea pig macrophages in the CH3 homology region of human immunoglobulin. G.J. Immunol. 110:1706, 1973.

88. Huber, H., Douglas, S.D., Nusbacher, J., Kochwa, S., and Rosenfield, R.F.: IgG subclass specificity of human monocyte receptor sites. Nature (Lond.) 229:419, 1970.

89. Rosse, W.F., de Boisfleury, A., and Bessis, M.: The interaction of phagocytic cells and red cells modified by immune reactions. Comparison of antibody and complement coated red cells. Blood Cells 1:345, 1975.

90. Lay, W.H. and Nussenzweig, V.: Receptors for complement on leukocytes. J. Exp. Med. 128:991, 1968.

91. Dickler, H.B.: Studies of the human lymphocyte receptor for heat-aggregated or antigen-complexed immunoglobulin. J. Exp. Med. 140:508, 1974.

92. Arend, W.P. and Mannik, M.: Quantitative studies on IgG receptors on monocytes. In: Mononuclear Phagocytes in Immunity, Infection, and Pathology. Van Furth, R., ed., Blackwell Scientific Publications, Oxford, 1975.

93. Arend, W.P. and Mannik, M.: The macrophage receptor for IgG: Number and affinity of binding sites. J. Immunol. 110:1455, 1973.

94. Huber, H., Polley, M., Linscott, W., Fudenberg, H.H., and Müller-Eberhard, H.: Human monocytes: Distinct receptor sites for the third component of complement and for immunoglobulin. G. Science 162:1281, 1968.

95. Logue, G.L., Rosse, W.F., and Adams, J.P.: Complement-dependent immune adherence measured with human granulocytes: Changes in the antigenic nature of red cell-bound C3 produced by incubation in human serum. Clin. Immunol. Immunopath. 1:398, 1973.

96. Polley, M.J. and Ross, Gordon D.: Macrophage and Lymphocyte Receptor Sites for Complement (C3) and for Immunoglobulin (IgG). Proceedings of an International Symposium on "The Nature and Significances of Complement Activation." Ortho Diagnostics, Raritan, New Jersey, 1976.

97. Cooper, R.A.: Loss of membrane components in the pathogenesis of antibody-induced spherocytosis. J. Clin. Invest. 51:16, 1972.

98. Ross, G.D. and Polley, M.J.: Specificity of human lymphocyte complement receptors. J. Exp. Med. 141:1163, 1975.

99. Munn, I.R. and Chaplin, H., Jr.: Rosette formation by sensitized human red cells— Effects of source of peripheral leukocyte monolayers. Vox Sang. 33:129, 1977.

100. Atkinson, J.P. and Frank, M.M.: Role of complement in the pathophysiology of hemotologic diseases. Progr. Hematol. 10:211, 1977.

101. Weed, R.I. and Reed, C.F.: Membrane Alterations Leading to Red Cell Destruction. Am. J. Med. 41:681, 1966.

102. Ponder, E.: Hemolysis and Related Phenomena. Grune & Stratton, New York, 1948, p. 132.

103. Bessis, M.: Living Blood Cells and Their Ultrastructure. Springer Verlag, New York, Heidelberg, Berlin, 1973, pp. 165–169.

104. Cooper, R.A.: Loss of membrane components in the pathogenesis of antibody-induced spherocytosis. J. Clin. Invest. 51:16, 1972.

105. Mohandas, N. and de Boisfleury, A.: Antibody-induced spherocytic anemia. I. Changes in red cell deformity. Blood Cells 3:187, 1977.

106. Weed, R.I.: The importance of erythrocyte deformability. Am. J. Med. 49:147, 1970.

107. Bessis, M.: Living Blood Cells and Their Ultrastructure. Springer Verlag, New York, Heidelberg, Berlin, 1973, p. 104.

108. Lo Buglio, A.F., Cotran, R., and Jandl, J.H.: Red cells coated with immunoglobulin G: Binding and sphering by mononuclear cells in man. Science 158:1582, 1967.

109. Brown, D.L. and Nelson, D.A.: Surface microfragmentation of red cells as a mechanism for complement-mediated immune spherocytosis. Br. J. Haematol. 24:301, 1973.

110. Fleer, A., Van Schaik, M.L.J., Borne, A.E.G.Kr. von dem, and Engelfriet, C.P.: Destruction of sensitized erythrocytes by human monocytes in vitro. Effects of cytochalasin B. Hydrocortisone and Colchicine. Scand. J. Immunol. 8:515, 1978.

111. Mollison, P.L., Crome, P., Hughes-Jones, N.C., and Rochna, E.: Rate of removal from the circulation of red cells sensitized with different amounts of antibody. Br. J. Haematol. 11:461, 1965.

112. Rosse, W.F.: Quantitative Immunology of Immune Hemolytic Anemia. II. The relationship of cell-bound antibody to hemolysis and the effect of treatment. J. Clin. Invest. 50:734, 1971.

113. Weiner, W.: "Coombs-positive" "normal" people. Proceedings of the 10th International Society of Blood Transfusion, Stockholm, 1964, p. 35.

114. Gilliland, B.C.: Coombs-negative immune hemolytic anemia. Semin. in Hematol. 13:267, 1976.

115. Natvig, J.B. and Kunkel, H.G.: Detection of genetic antigens utilizing gamma globulin coupled to red blood cells. Nature 215:68, 1967.

116. Abramson, N. and Schur, P.: The IgG subclasses of red cell antibodies and relationship to monocyte binding. Blood 40:500, 1972.

117. Frame, M., Mollison, P.L., and Terry, W.D.: Anti-Rh activity of human γG4 proteins. Nature 225:641, 1970.

118. Engelfriet, C.P., Borne, A.E.G. Kr von dem, Beckers, D., and Van Loghem, J.J.: Autoimmune haemolytic anaemia: Serological and immunochemical characteristics of the autoantibodies: Mechanisms of cell destruction. Series Hematologica. VII:328, 1974.

119. Fleer, A., Van Der Meulen, F.W., Linthout, E., and Borne, A.E.G.Kr.von dem.: Destruction of IgG-sensitized erythrocytes by human blood monocytes: Modulation of inhibition by IgG. Br. J. Haematol. 39:425, 1978.

120. Scornik, J.C., Salinas, M.C., and Drewinko, B.: IgG-dependent clearance of red blood cells in IgG myeloma patients. J. Immunol. 115:901, 1975.

121. Schreiber, A.D. and Frank, M.M.: Role of antibody and complement in the immune clearance and destruction of erythrocytes. 1. In vivo effects of IgG and IgM complement fixing sites. J. Clin. Invest. 51:575, 1972.

122. Schreiber, A.D. and Frank, M.M.: Role of antibody and complement in the immune clearance and destruction of erythrocytes. II. Molecular nature of IgG and IgM complement-fixing sites and effects of their interaction with serum. J. Clin. Invest. 51:583, 1972.

123. Cutbush, M. and Mollison, P.L.: Relation between characteristics of blood-group antibodies in vitro and associated patterns of red

cell destruction *in vivo*. Br. J. Haematol. 4:115, 1958.

124. Burton, M.S. and Mollison, P.L.: Effect of IgM and IgG iso-antibody on red cell clearance. Immunol. 14:861, 1968.

125. Worlledge, S.M. and Blajchman, M.A.: The autoimmune haemolytic anaemias. Br. J. Haematol. 23:(Suppl.)61 1972.

126. Bianco, C., Griffin, F.M., Jr., and Silverstein, S.C.: Studies of the macrophage complement receptor. J. Exp. Med. 141:1278, 1975.

127. Ehlenberger, A.G. and Nussenzweig, V.: Immunologically-mediated phagocytosis: Role of C3 and Fc receptors. In: Clinical Evaluation of Immune Function in Man. Litwin, S.D., Christian, C.L., and Siskind, G.W., eds. Grune & Stratton, New York, 1976.

128. Mantovani, B., Rabinovitch, M., and Nussenzweig, V.: Phagocytosis of immune complexes by macrophages. Different roles of the macrophage receptor sites for complement (C3) and for immunoglobulin (IgG). J. Exp. Med. 135:780, 1972.

129. Brown, D.L., Lachmann, P.J., and Dacie, J.V.: The *in vivo* behavior of complement-coated red cells: Studies in C6-depleted and normal rabbits. Clin. Exp. Immunol. 7:401, 1970.

130. Petz, L.D. and Garratty, G.: Complement in Immunohematology. Prog. Clin. Immunol. 2:175, 1974.

131. Lewis, S.M., Dacie, J.V., and Szur, L.: Mechanisms of haemolysis in the cold-haemagglutinin syndrome. Br. J. Hematol. 6:154, 1960.

132. Mollison, P.L.: The role of complement in haemolytic processes *in vivo*. In: Complement. Wolstenholme, G.E.W. and Knight, J., eds. J. & A. Churchill, London, 1965, p. 323.

133. Atkinson, J.P. and Frank, M.M.: Studies on the *in vivo* effects of antibody interaction of IgM antibody and complement in the immune clearance and destruction of erythrocytes in man. J. Clin. Invest. 54:339, 1974.

134. Jaffe, C.H., Atkinson, J.P., and Frank, M.M.: The role of complement in the clearance of cold agglutinin-sensitized erythrocytes in man. J. Clin. Invest. 58:942, 1976.

135. MacKenzie, M.R.: Monocytic sensitization in autoimmune hemolytic anemia. Clin. Res. 23:132A, 1975 (Abstr.).

136. Kay, N.E. and Douglas, S.D.: Monocyte-erythrocyte interaction in vitro in immune hemolytic anemias. Blood 50:889, 1977.

137. Atkinson, J.P. and Frank, M.M.: The effect of Bacillus Calmette-Guerin-induced macrophage activation on the in vivo clearance of sensitized erythrocytes. J. Clin. Invest. 53:1742, 1974.

138. Arend, W.P. and Mannik, M.: The macrophage receptor for IgG: Number and affinity of binding sites. J. Immunol. 110:1455, 1973.

139. Greendyke, R., Swisher, S.N., and Trabold, N.: Studies of the mechanism of erythrophagocytosis. Proc. 9th Congress of the Internat. Soc. of Hematology 1:293, 1963.

140. Greendyke, R., Brierty, R., and Swisher, S.N.: In vitro studies on erythrophagocytosis. Blood 22:295, 1963.

141. Greendyke, R.M., Brierty, R.E., and Swisher, S.N.: In vitro studies on erythrophagocytosis. II. Effects of incubating leukocytes with selected cell metabolites. J. Lab. Clin. Med. 63:1016, 1964.

142. Packer, J.T., Greendyke, R.M., and Swisher, S.N.: The inhibition of erythrophagocytosis in vitro by corticosteroids. Trans. Assoc. Am. Phys. 73:93, 1960.

143. Greendyke, R.M., Bradley, E.M., and Swisher, S.N.: Studies of the effects of administration of ACTH and adrenal corticosteroids on erythrophagocytosis. JCI 44:746, 1965.

144. Perlmann, P. and Holm, G.: Cytotoxic effects of lymphoid cells in vitro. Adv. Immunol. 11:117, 1969.

145. Brier, A.M., Chess, L., and Schlossman, S.F.: Human antibody-dependent cellular cytotoxicity. Isolation and identification of subpopulation of peripheral blood lymphocytes which kill antibody-coated autologous target cells. J. Clin. Invest. 56:1580, 1975.

146. Hinz, C.F., Jr. and Chickosky, J.F.: Lymphocyte Cytotoxicity for Human Erythrocytes. Schwarz, M.R., ed. Leukocyte Culture Conference, University of Washington, 1972.

147. Urbaniak, S.J.: Lymphoid cell dependent (K-cell) lysis of human erythrocytes sensitized with rhesus alloantibodies. Br. J. Haematol. 33:409, 1976.

148. Northoff, H., Kluge, A., and Resch, K.: Antibody dependent cellular cytotoxicity (ADCC) against human erythrocytes, mediated by blood group alloantibodies: A

model for the role of antigen density in target cell lysis. Z. Immun. Forsch. 154:15, 1978.

149. Kurlander, R.J., Rosse, W.F., and Logue, W.L.: Quantitative influence of antibody and complement coating of red cells on monocyte-mediated cell lysis. J. Clin. Invest. 61:1309, 1978.

150. Milgrom, H. and Shore, S.L.: Lysis of antibody-coated human red cells by peripheral blood mononuclear cells. Altered effector cell profile after treatment of target cells with enzymes. Cellular Immunol. 39:178, 1978.

151. Handwerger, B.S., Kay, N.W., and Douglas, S.D.: Lymphocyte-mediated antibody-dependent cytolysis: Role in immune hemolysis. Vox Sang. 34:276, 1978.

152. Holm, G. and Hammarstrom, S.: Haemolytic activity of human blood monocytes: Lysis of human erythrocytes treated with anti-A serum. Clin. Exp. Immunol. 13:29, 1973.

153. McIvor, K.L., Piper, C.E., and Bell, R.B.: Mechanisms of target cell destruction by alloimmune peritoneal macrophages. In: The Macrophage in Neoplasia. Fink, M.A., ed. Academic Press, Inc., New York, 1976, p. 135.

154. Fleer, A., van der Hart, M., Borne, A.E.G. Kr. von dem, and Engelfriet, C.P.: (Abstract) Mechanism of antibody-dependent cytotoxicity by human blood monocytes towards IgG-sensitized erythrocytes. Europ. J. Clin. Invest. 6:333, 1976.

155. Fleer, A., van der Hart, M., Borne, A.E.G. Kr. von dem, and Engelfriet, C.P.: Monocyte-mediated lysis of human eryghrocytes. In: Leucocyte Membrane Determinants Regulating Immune Reactivity. Eijsvoogal, V.P., Roos, D., and Zeijlemaker,W. P., eds. New York, Academic Press, 1976, p. 673.

156. Fleer, A., Van Schaik, M.L.J., Borne, A.E.G.Kr. von dem, and Engelfriet, C.P.: Destruction of sensitized erythrocytes by human monocytes *in vitro*. Effects of Cytochalasin B. Hydrocortisone and Colchicine. Scand. J. Immunol. 8:515, 1978.

157. Handwerger, B.S., Kay, N.W., and Douglas, S.D.: Lymphocyte-mediated antibody-dependent cytolysis: Role in immune hemolysis. Vox Sang. 34:276, 1978.

158. Hinz, C.F., Jr. and Chickosky, J.F.: Lymphocyte Cytotoxicity for Human Erythrocytes. Schwarz, M.R., ed. Leukocyte Culture Conference, University of Washington, Seattle, 1972.

159. Northoff, H., Kluge, A., and Resch, K.: Antibody dependent cellular cytotoxicity (ACDD) against human erythrocytes, mediated by blood group alloantibodies: A model for the role of antigen density in target cell lysis. Z. Immun. Forsch. 154:15, 1978.

160. Urbaniak, S.J.: Lymphoid cell dependent (K-cell) lysis of human erythrocytes sensitized with rhesus alloantibodies. Br. J. Haematol. 33:409, 1976.

161. Fleer, A., Koopman, M.G., Borne, A.E.G.Kr. von dem, and Engelfriet, C.P.: Monocyte-induced increase in osmotic fragility of human red cells sensitized with anti-D alloantibodies. Br. J. Haematol. 40:439, 1978.

162. Borne, A.E.G.Kr. von dem, Engelfriet, C.P., Beckers, D., and Van Loghem, J.J.: Autoimmune haemolytic anemias. Biochemical studies of red cells from patients with autoimmune haemolytic anemia with incomplete warm autoantibodies. Clin. Exp. Immunol. 8:377, 1971.

4

Blood Groups of Human Red Cells

W. Laurence Marsh, F.I.M.L.S., M.I. Biol., M.R.C. Path.

Discovery of the human ABO blood group was an essential step in the development of safe blood transfusion techniques.[1] Rapid expansion in the use of blood transfusion, and the development of sensitive serological methods, led to the recognition of more antibodies and further blood group systems. At present, nearly 400 antigenic markers on human red cells are known,[2] and the number continues to grow. Blood group studies contribute to ethnology, anthropology, forensic science, and genetics, but it is in clinical blood transfusion and the recognition and treatment of hemolytic disease of the newborn that knowledge of the blood groups has made the greatest impact.

DISCOVERY OF BLOOD GROUP ANTIGENS AND ANTIBODIES

Recognition of a blood group begins with discovery of an antibody. Such an antibody may be stimulated by a blood transfusion, may arise through fetal-maternal blood group incompatibility, or may appear spontaneously, presumably by exposure to some environmental immunogenic agent. Antibodies react in a recognizable manner with red cells carrying the appropriate antigen. Depending upon the nature of the antibody, and to some extent also upon the number and to-

pography of antigen receptors on the cell membrane, the reaction may be agglutination, sensitization without agglutination, complement-mediated hemolysis; or, the antibody may activate the first stages of the complement cascade and attach complement components to the cell membrane without leading to hemolysis. If the antigen is in a soluble form, the result of the interaction may be precipitation of insoluble antibody-antigen complexes. In blood group serology, most procedures utilize agglutination techniques.

Alloantibodies of the human blood groups are produced by people who lack the corresponding antigen. They are active against antigens on red cells from different members of the same species. In some blood-group systems spontaneous or "naturally occurring" antibodies occur commonly. In the ABO system, for example, anti-A or anti-B are found in the serum of all normal adult individuals who lack the antigens. A-like and B-like antigens are widely distributed in nature and are present on many bacterial cells.[3, 4] It is probable that immunization to microbial A-like or B-like antigen is responsible for anti-A and anti-B in human serum.[5] Because of the regular occurrence of ABO antibodies in the serum of people who lack the antigens, accidental transfusion of blood that is incompatible in its ABO type is a matter for grave concern. Most fatal hemolytic transfusion reactions are caused by ABO incompatibility between the recipient and donor.

Anti-P_1 may be found as a naturally occurring antibody in the serum of people who lack the P_1 antigen, although only a minority of these individuals have detectable antibody. P_2 people with hydatid disease may produce potent anti-P_1. The fluid from hydatid cysts contains P_1 substance,[6] and extracts of certain worms also have P_1 activity.[7] It seems possible that immunization to P_1-like antigens of parasitic origin may be an explanation for some examples of naturally occurring anti-P_1.

On occasion, other blood group antibodies may be found having apparent natural occurrence in individuals who have not knowingly been exposed to antigen, but the origin of these antibodies is uncertain. However, demonstration that an example of naturally occurring anti-Kell (anti-K) in an infant was caused by infection with a coliform organism having a Kell-like antigen[8] suggests that immunization by bacterial antigens may be the explanation for some other blood group antibodies.

Naturally occurring antibodies are frequently IgM saline-reactive agglutinins, but they may also occur as IgG proteins. Thus, natural anti-A or anti-B often has both IgM and IgG components, and some examples of natural anti-K may be exclusively IgG. Anti-Wr^a, found in some normal sera, may be either IgM or IgG. Some natural antibodies, such as anti-M^g or anti-To^a, may be fairly common, while individuals whose red cells carry the reactive antigen are rare. Antibodies against low-incidence red cell antigens are found frequently in people who have warm-antibody autoimmune hemolytic anemia,[9] and also in people who have been hyperimmunized against Rh antigens.[10] It has been suggested (although there is no proof) that subdetectable levels of these antibodies may be very common, but a nonspecific immunological boost in hyperimmune states increases their activity to a level that allows their detection. Red cell typing sera are often obtained from hyperimmunized donors. The presence of antibodies against low-incidence antigens in some of these sera is a cause of occasional false positive results.[11] Certain blood group antibodies are found only after immunization by blood transfusion or pregnancy. These include antibodies in the Duffy or Kidd systems and the great majority of those in the Rhesus or Kell systems.

BLOOD GROUP GENETICS

Almost all red-cell antigens are inherited characteristics. The only exceptions are the acquired A and acquired B antigens, and possibly certain types of cryptantigen involved in polyagglutination. Even cryptantigens must be under genetic control, however, for they are concealed below the surface of all red cells; in most cases it is their uncovering by microbial enzymes that converts a latent antigen into an active receptor.

Genetic Terms

Genes that are on the same chromosome and within recognizable distance of each other are said to be linked. Linked genes will be transmitted together through different generations of a family, but will be separated occasionally by the phenomenon of crossing over. This occurs at the meiosis phase of spermatogenesis or oogenesis when homologous portions of a pair of chromosomes are exchanged. For linked genes to be separated by crossing over, the break point in the chromosome must be between them; the closer they are the less likely it is that this will happen. The frequency of crossing over, in studies of informative families, can be used, therefore, as a measure of the distance between the genes.

Genes that are on the same chromosome but so widely separated that linkage cannot be recognized by family studies are said to be syntenic. Alternative forms of a gene that can occupy the same position (or locus) on a chromosome are called alleles. Genes that are on different chromosomes, or are widely separated on the same chromosome, segregate independently; their simultaneous inheritance will be a matter of chance.

Sex-linked genes are those carried on the X or Y chromosomes. Many X-borne genes are known, including those of the Xg and Xk (Kell-related) blood groups. Little is known concerning genes on the Y chromosome—apart from those determining testicular differentiation, the H-Y cell surface antigen,[12] and probably a gene for the hairy ear phenomenon in which harmless, but exuberant, hair growth takes place from the ear rims of affected males.[13]

Blood Group Genes

Most blood group genes are clearly expressed and seem to obey simple laws of Mendelian inheritance. They thus provide excellent markers for use in genetic studies. If different populations are tested for many genetic markers, an almost infinite variety of permutations is seen. But a population could be identified as African, Asian, or Caucasian, and even neighboring tribes within a population would differ, although less strikingly. These differences are of great anthropological interest. The similarity between different people, however, is even more striking than the differences. For example, almost everyone has the antigens Rh29, Lu^b, Kp^b, Co^a, and Di^b. No population has been found that lacks any of the blood group systems, a finding that must surely reflect the unity of the human species.

Although much progress has been made in understanding genetic phenomena in *E. coli,* relatively little is known of the exact genetic mechanisms that operate in mammalian cells. However, the conclusions of Jacob and Monod[14] on the mode of gene activation and regulation in *E. coli* seem to be tailor-made for the complex human blood groups. A genetic model for Rh based on conjugated operons has been described,[15] and the concept of regulators, operators, and structural genes can be invoked to explain observed phenomena in other groups.

In the broad field of blood group antigens, it has slowly become clear that some antigens are present on several kinds of cells. Thus, A and B, and certain HLA antigens are present on both red cells and leukocytes. All nucleated somatic cells of the body carry the complete genetic blueprint of the individual, although in differentiated cells the great majority of structural genes are inactive. Therefore, it should not come as a surprise to find that red cells have genes for "leukocyte" antigens.

Genes can only be recognized by observing their phenotypic effects, and there is no way of identifying the gene itself. A blood group in which antigenicity is determined by the nature of a protein on the cell membrane is a direct product of the particular gene, which must code for amino acid sequences of the peptide. If antigenicity is determined by the nature of an immunodominant sugar, the antigen cannot be a direct product of the gene. In this circumstance, the protein specified by the gene must be a transferase enzyme that attaches the group-specific sugar to a component of the cell membrane. Blood group genes are usually codominant characters and produce their phenotypic effect in both homozygous and heterozygous individuals. In some systems, quantitative differences in cell antigenicity can be recognized that reflect a double or single dose of the particular gene.

A blood group system comprises a group of related antigens that are determined by a single gene. A gene, in this context, is defined as a DNA sequence short enough that linkage disequilibrium (i.e., divergence from random frequency) is apparent on analysis of populations in Hardy-Weinberg equilibrium. Chromosomal crossovers that separate components of this DNA sequence are so uncommon that some combinations of antigens are more frequent than would otherwise be expected. Linkage disequilibrium is illustrated in the Rh blood group by the finding that most D+ people are also C+, while most D− people are C−.

Many of the antigens on red cells belong to one of about 20 systems. There is at present no means of establishing the number of blood group systems, and it has yet to be shown that some of the named systems are independent of one another. For example, no one has yet been found who is both a Diego (Di^a) and Wright (Wr^a) positive. The children of such a person would demonstrate whether *Di^a* and *Wr^a* segregate independently and are thus markers of independent systems. These two antigens do not appear to be related, for it is known that people of the rare En(a−) type are unable to express their Wright genes; they are Wr(a−b−).[16] But such cells react strongly with anti-Di^b.[17] Despite this evidence that the antigens are not associated, it is still necessary to have pedigree data showing genetic independence.

Maximum information during genetic studies would be provided by an antiserum having a reaction frequency of 50 percent. Anti-A in the ABO system is close to this, with 45 percent positive. Many blood group antigens have frequencies greater than 99 percent or less than 1 percent. These provide little help in recognizing genetic relationships in population studies.

Gene Interaction

In most blood groups, there appears to be a one-to-one relationship between gene and antigen, and synthesis of each antigen is ordered by one structural gene. However, a few antigens are known that arise by interaction between the products of more than one independent gene. For example, Le^b in the Lewis system requires interaction between the *Le, Secretor,* and *H* genes to produce the Le^b configuration. Development of IA, IB, or IH antigens requires contributions by the *I* and *ABO* genes, while IP$_1$ appears to reflect interaction between the *I* and *P$_1$* genes. The antigen Fy5 is only present on red cells that have functional *Rh* and *Duffy* genes and thus appears to be an interaction product of the two

systems. These interactions possibly occur on the red cell membrane when two or more antigen structures, under separate genetic control, have a steric relationship that creates a unique determinant.

Modifying Genes

Independent modifying genes may affect the expression of blood group genes (Fig. 4-1). Modifiers may have either dominant or recessive inheritance. At one time it was believed that genes like *h,* the rare allele at the H locus, exerted a positive inhibitory effect when in the homozygous state. But it now seems more likely that such a genotype represents absence of a normal allele (in this case *H*), the presence of which is needed for continuation of a biosynthetic sequence. On rare occasions, proper expression of a blood group gene is prevented by absence of an essential precursor structure that is involved in the biosynthetic pathway. In these cases, production of the precursor is determined by other independent genes. In a broad sense, genes controlling production of precursors can be regarded as inherited modifiers of the blood group gene.

In some Melanesian populations, up to 15 percent of individuals have hereditary erythrocyte ovalocytosis. Recent studies[18] show that red cells from these people have depressed activity for a wide range of antigens including D, S, s, U, Jk^a, Xg^a, and En^a. These changes cannot result from direct interference at the gene level but are, presumably, a reflection of a membrane anomaly. There is no evidence, thus far, that this kind of ovalocytosis is accompanied by hemolytic anemia.

Independence of Blood Group Systems

When a new blood group antigen is discovered, it has to be determined whether it is an

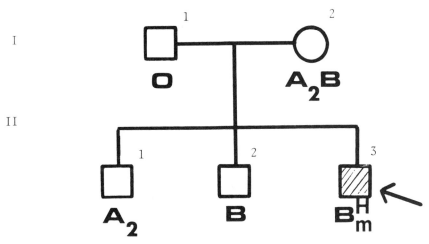

Fig. 4-1. A pedigree showing inheritance of an independent modifier preventing proper expressing of B. I-2 and II-2 are normal B. II-3 must have received the same *B* gene but an independent modifier is preventing its proper expression. (Marsh, W.L., Ferrari, M., Nichols, M.E., Fernandez, G., and Cooper, K.: B_m^H: a weak B variant. Vox Sang. 25:341, 1973).

extension of a known system or whether it is independent. Genetic independence of blood groups is most easily shown, once data are available, by 2 × 2 contingency tables. Independence of the ABO and Duffy systems is shown by the observed phenotype frequencies shown in Table 4-1. The frequencies are so close to randomness that there can be little doubt. However, demonstration that the ABO gene is on the long arm of chromosome 9 [19, 20] while the Duffy gene is near the centromere of chromosome 1 [21, 22] has now added cytogenetic authority to the independence of the two loci. Observations such as these do not mean that there can be no relationship between the products of the two genes but only that the loci themselves are independent.

Sometimes a 2 × 2 contingency table reveals an association between a new antigen and an existing blood group system. For example, when anti-S was found, it was first thought to recognize an antigen independent of other groups.[23] However, a 2 × 2 table established that the frequency of positive reactions among M and N bloods was not random; too many M bloods were reactive.[23, 24] The new antibody was not anti-M but recognized an antigen that was associated with the

MN system. Family studies subsequently established that the *S* gene segregated with the *MN* genes.

CHARACTERISTICS OF BLOOD ANTIGENS

Antigenicity may be a characteristic of a membrane protein, a sugar that is attached to a protein, or a complex formed between a protein and a lipid. Biochemical studies on antigens of the ABO, Lewis, and I groups have shown that in these systems specificity is dependent upon immunodominant sugars.[25, 26] Rh labels a membrane protein, although lipid is required for the antigenicity to become manifest.[27] Red cell membranes so-

Table 4-1. Independence of the ABO and Duffy Systems

	A	Non-A	Total
Fy(a+)	277	381	685
Fy(a−)	142	200	342
Total	419	581	1000

The frequencies of A and Fy^a in 1000 individuals are shown in this 2 × 2 contingency table. The frequency of Fy^a is almost identical in both the A's and the non-A's.

lubilized with detergent lose Rh activity but it is restored by addition of Ca^+ or Mg^+. Electron microscopy of such reactivated preparations show the formation of numerous vesicles or tubules about 50 to 100 nm in diameter.[28] It appears that Rh is a protein but that it must be in an organized structure with a proper protein:lipid relationship for Rh antigenicity to be detectable. A new light on Rh may be shed by recent biochemical studies on solubilized and separated cell membrane components. In these investigations, comparable amounts of Rh(D) antigen were demonstrated in solubilized preparations from Rh-positive and Rh-negative cells.[29] The implication from this is that the structural gene, and the Rh antigenic protein, are present in both types of cell, but in Rh-negative cells the protein is not exposed on the outer surface where it would be accessible to antibody. The presence of D antigen on both Rh-positive and Rh-negative cells would provide an explanation for the failure to find anti-d.

MN and Kell antigens are glycoproteins. Early studies on MN suggested that specificity was determined by the sugar-like substance sialic acid, but recent work indicates that M and N reflect different aminoacid sequences of the peptide component of the glycoprotein. P antigens are glycosphingolipids; their biochemistry is considered later in this chapter. Little is known concerning the nature of other blood group antigens.

Estimates of the number of antigen receptors on red cells can be obtained by immunoelectronmicroscopy using antibody molecules coupled covalently with an electron-dense marker (usually ferritin), or by measuring the uptake of antibody labeled with radioactive iodine (^{125}I). Studies using either, or both, of these techniques indicate that a group A_1 cell has between 810,000 and 1,170,000 A antigen sites and a B cell 610,000 to 850,000 B sites.[30] An Rh-positive red cell of ordinary phenotype has from 10,000 to 36,-700 D sites,[31] a heterozygous K-positive cell has 2,750 to 3,900 K antigen sites,[32] and a Duffy positive cell between 10,000 and 14,500

Fy^a sites.[33] The membrane of a human red cell has at least nine major polypeptides and an indeterminate number of minor components. The wide variation in number of receptors for the different blood groups may be evidence that the antigens mark different membrane components.

MATURATION OF BLOOD GROUP ANTIGENS AND ANTIBODIES

Red cells from newborn infants are deficient in some blood group antigens. This deficiency may have a protective effect, for immature antigens are not usually involved in hemolytic disease of the newborn. A and B antigens are usually somewhat deficient at birth, but it is noticeable that newborn infants affected by ABO hemolytic disease always have exceptionally well-developed A or B antigens. There appears to be a general correlation between the nature of antigens and their presence on fetal red cells. Antigens that are proteins are well-developed at birth, while antigens that are sugars and, therefore, require transferase enzymes for their appearance, may not be fully active.

Newborn infants are grossly deficient in I antigen but have greatly increased activity of the antithetical i antigen. The cells lack Lewis antigens, all newborns being Le(a−b−), and they are deficient in P_1, Lutheran, Sd^a, Sd^x, and Bg. All antigens of the Rh complex and antigens of the MN, Kell, Kidd, and Duffy systems are comparable to those found on red cells from adults.

Newborn infants seldom have anti-A or anti-B of their own manufacture; they usually develop them, according to their ABO type, within 6 months of birth. Somewhat surprisingly, the serum of newborns usually contains cold-reacting auto anti-I.[34] The antibody is an IgM protein and appears to be synthesized by the fetus in utero. Serum from cord blood samples usually lacks anti-T and other polyagglutinins.

SHARED ANTIGENS OF RED CELLS, LEUKOCYTES, AND TISSUES

A and B antigens are present on red cells, leukocytes, platelets, certain tissue cells, in plasma, and in gastric and salivary mucoids.[35-38] A or B antigens on red cells are mainly synthesized by the cells themselves, although small amounts of antigen are acquired by absorption from the plasma. Group O donor red cells that have been in the circulation of an A or B recipient for several days absorb some A or B antigen from the plasma of the host. The separated cells may be weakly agglutinated by potent ABO antisera,[39] and will give a positive absorption/elution test with the same antibodies. In contrast to the situation in red cells, it has been shown that group A lymphocytes acquire their antigen by absorption of A substance from the plasma.[40]

Not all individuals have the ability to secrete A, B, or H antigens in a water-soluble form in their saliva. The characteristic is under control of an autosomal dominant gene called *Se*, which seems to act as a regulator of the *H* gene in secretions. *Se* segregates independently of the *H* and *AB* genes.[37] About 77 percent of North American Caucasians and about 70 percent of North American Negroes are ABH secretors. The *Se* gene also seems to play a role in the synthesis of ABH by red cells, for in secretors both glycoproteins and glycolipids carry the determinants, while in nonsecretors they are present only as glycolipids.[41]

Some other blood group antigens are not exclusive properties of the red cells. Thus, I substance is present in saliva,[42] human milk,[43] and some other body fluids, and i antigen occurs as a soluble glycoprotein in plasma[44] and is also present on lymphocytes.[45] Le^a, Le^b,[46] and Sd^a [47] antigens are also present in plasma, and Le^a is taken up by lymphocytes.[48] In some blood group systems, a single, high-incidence antigen has been demonstrated on phagocytic leukocytes,

using an antibody absorption technique. Thus, anti-U,[49] anti-Jk3,[50] anti-Sc1, anti-Di^b,[51] and anti-Gerbich[52] are absorbed by both red cells and leukocytes. Kx antigen, which is related to the Kell blood group system, has been demonstrated on normal neutrophil leukocytes and monocytes. Absence of leukocyte Kx is a rare event, but the deficiency is of more than genetic interest because such leukocytes have a defect in bactericidal function and owners of the cells have chronic granulomatous disease.[53]

Certain HLA antigens are now known to be present on red cells, but red-cell workers call them by different names. Bg^a, Bg^b, and Bg^c on red cells are the same as HLA-B7, −B17, and −A28,[54, 55] respectively, on leukocytes. Thus, the same antibody would be reported by a leukocyte laboratory as anti-HLA-B7 and by a red cell laboratory as anti-Bg^a. Shared antigenicity is not restricted to these, for further studies have shown that other antileukocyte antibodies may react to cause hemagglutination.[56]

Chido, Rodgers, and Complement

An exciting area of commonality has been opened by recent studies on the Chido (Ch^a)[57] and Rodgers (Rg^a)[58] antigens. Both are high-incidence characters present on red cells, lymphocytes,[59] and in plasma.[58, 60] Different studies have established that the Ch^a and Rg^a loci are closely linked to the HLA locus on chromosome 6,[61, 62] and that the locus for the C4 component of complement is also linked to HLA.[63] Correlation of these findings has been a collaborative triumph, for it now appears that Ch^a and Rg^a are markers on the fourth component of complement.[64, 65] Ch(a−) red cells become Ch(a+) if they are allowed to bind C4 from serum of a Ch(a+) person, and the same happens with Rg^a.[66] Rare individuals who have a congenital lack of C4 are both Ch(a−) and Rg(a−).[66] Thus, Ch^a and Rg^a are polymorphisms of C4, viewed from the perspective of a red-cell grouper. These findings provide convincing evidence that normal red cells have complement components on their surface.

ACQUIRED CHANGES IN RED CELL ANTIGENS

Blood group antigens are generally constant characteristics of the individual that are unaffected by disease or environment. On rare occasions, however, changes in a red cell blood group do occur, either through acquisition or loss of an antigen.

Polyagglutination

All sera from normal adults contain antibodies with specificity for cryptantigens that are usually hidden below the red cell surface. The uncovering of such an antigen leaves the cell susceptible to agglutination by the appropriate polyagglutinin. The most well characterized of these mechanisms is the Hubener-Thomsen-Freidenriech, or T-active, type of polyagglutination.[67] In this condition, neuraminidase, of microbial origin, removes sialic acid from the red cell surface to expose an underlying β-galactose residue that has T specificity.[68] The changed cells are agglutinated by anti-T present in all adult serum samples. T-activation of red cells may occur as an in vitro phenomenon through infection of a blood sample, or as an in vivo phenomenon in a patient with an infection.

Anti-T is present in most red cell typing sera of human origin and may cause false positive results when they are used to test polyagglutinable cells. Sera from some other species of animal also contain polyagglutinins. Rabbit serum, for example, contains anti-T. The antibody may be present as a contaminant in rabbit anti-human globulin reagents and give rise to false positive results against T-active red cells. Some commercial reagents are processed to remove polyagglutinins.

Other forms of polyagglutination are called Tn, Tk, and Va.[69, 70] Each type represents a distinct specificity and has its own serological characteristics. Tn polyagglutinable red cells, for instance, usually show mixed agglutination in tests with sera containing anti-Tn.[71, 72] Certain lectins have specificity for these polyagglutinogens and can be used to classify polyagglutinable red cells. The most useful is anti-T extracted from peanuts (*Arachis hypogeae*).[73, 73a] Other lectins with polyagglutinin activity are obtained from different varieties of *Salvia*.[74]

Although in most patients with polyagglutination it is an acquired phenomenon, on rare occasions the condition may be inherited. The susceptibility of red cells from HEMPAS patients to lysis by acidified normal serum may be regarded as a kind of inherited polyagglutination.[75, 76] Cad, at first believed to be an inherited type of polyagglutination,[77] is now considered to be an exceptionally strong Sd^a antigen that reacts with anti-Sd^a present in most normal sera.[78]

Tn polyagglutinability[70] does not seem to arise by enzymatic degradation of the red cell membrane. Instead it appears that somatic mutation changes activity of a gene involved in formation of the membrane glycoprotein that carries the Tn structure.[75] The mutation prevents completion of a carbohydrate chain, a block that leaves N-acetyl-D-galactosamine α-linked to serine or threonine as the terminal (Tn-active) sugar.[73a, 79] Exposure of this A-like sugar explains why Tn blood samples are sometimes called acquired A.[73a, 80] Both T and Tn activity may appear on leukocytes and platelets as well as on red cells. Individuals who manifest Tn polyagglutination sometimes have hemolytic anemia, leukopenia, and thrombocytopenia.[70, 75]

The Acquired B Antigen

An interesting change of cellular antigenicity is that found in the acquired B phenomenon. On rare occasions, group A people acquire a weak B antigen on their red cells as a temporary characteristic.[81] For a variable period of time they become AB. A few examples have been seen in healthy people, but the acquired B antigen is usually found in people with infections or lesions (particularly cancer) of the intestinal tract. The acquired antigen arises through action of a microbial enzyme,[82] an intestinal lesion possibly facilitating its absorption. The mechanism is believed to be one in which bacterial deacetylase converts *N*-acetyl galactosamine, the A-specific sugar on the red cell membrane, to galactosamine.[83] This is sufficiently close to D-galactose, the B-specific sugar, that anti-B serum gives a positive reaction. Red cells with acquired B antigens are frequently also polyagglutinable, usually with the Tk variety.[84]

Chromosomal Changes Affecting Blood Groups

Loss of a specific antigen from red cells could occur through somatic mutation affecting the controlling gene, although no convincing example has been documented. However, cytogenetic changes with deletion, translocation, or inversion of a portion of chromosome carrying a blood group gene may result in a change of phenotype. Correlation of such findings may provide important information. Thus, loss of the end of the short arm of a number 1 chromosome in one patient was accompanied by loss of an Rh gene;[85] in another, loss of the end of the long arm of a number 9 chromosome was associated with loss of an ABO gene.[19] In each case, the chromosome carrying the gene was already known, but the deletion studies allowed each locus to be assigned to a specific position. This technique of genetic assignment is called deletion mapping. The procedure may also provide information from the other direction. Thus, in an individual who has a chromosomal deletion, it can be concluded that none of the genes for which he, or she, is recognizably heterozygous can be on the deleted portion.

BLOOD GROUPS AND DISEASE

Apart from their role in hemolytic disease of the newborn, blood groups have other involvements with disease. In some cases antigens appear to label functional structures on the cell membrane. It is unlikely that complex genes such as those of the blood groups would persist during evolution if their products did not play some advantageous functional role on the cell. But only recently has it been demonstrated that there are associations between certain antigens and cell function.

Anthropologists have speculated for many years over reasons for the marked variation in frequency that occurs with some blood groups in different populations. Are they the result of natural selection, in which possession of a certain phenotype confers an advantage on the individual, or are they the result of random processes operating during prehistoric tribal migrations? If possession of a certain blood group phenotype confers an advantage in a particular environment, then the antigenic structures, or the antibodies that an individual can produce, must have some functional importance. Many organisms possess A–, B–, or H–like antigens, and it is possible that common antigens may adversely affect an individual's ability to produce antibody against the organism. Because of this, it has been suggested that individuals of certain ABH types may have been better able to survive during past great epidemics.[86]

Malaria and the Duffy Blood Group

The only instance recognized thus far where natural selection appears to favor a particular blood type is in the association between the Duffy blood group and susceptibility to benign tertian (BT) malaria. Almost all

Caucasians have Fy^a or Fy^b, or both, antigens of the Duffy system, but the great majority of African Negroes lack both antigens and have the phenotype Fy(a−b−).[87] The highest frequency has been found in Pygmies, all of whom appear to be Fy(a−b−).[88] It has been known for over 20 years that the great majority of Negroes are resistant to infection by the parasite of benign tertian malaria (*Plasmodium vivax*).[89] Development of an effective technique for the in vitro culture of *Pl. knowlesi* (a simian parasite that can infect man) allowed correlation of these two frequency observations. Repeated in vitro experiments showed that the malaria parasite invaded Fy(a+) or Fy(b+) red cells without difficulty, but did not invade Fy(a−b−) cells.[90] Furthermore, coating Fy(a+) red cells with anti-Fy^a largely protected them from invasion by the parasite.[91] Retrospective study of volunteers used in previous infectivity experiments showed that six Negroes who were Fy(a+) or Fy(b+) were all infected after exposure to mosquitoes carrying *Pl. vivax* while five volunteers who were Fy(a−b−) showed no evidence of infection.[92] Very rare Fy(a−b−) Caucasians are known. Red cells from these people are also resistant to invasion by the BT malaria parasite.[93] This suggests that the resistance factor is associated with Duffy and is not an effect on an independent gene closely linked to the Duffy locus in Negroes. A good deal of additional evidence has confirmed that possession of the Fy(a−b−) phenotype protects against benign tertian malaria, and the Duffy antigen, or a membrane structure related to it, must be a receptor utilized by the parasite during its invasion of red cells.[93] The relationship between malaria and the Duffy blood group is summarized in Table 4-2. It is likely that a number of genetic phenomena are involved in population differences in blood group frequencies, but the association between Duffy and malaria indicates that natural selection is one of them.

The parasite of malignant tertian malaria (*Pl. falciparum*) infects Fy(a−b−) and Fy(a+b+) red cells with equal facility and does not seem to utilize the Duffy antigen for its invasion. It is assumed that some other cell receptor is involved, although its nature is at present unknown.

Rh_{null} Syndrome

In 1961, an Australian aboriginal woman was found during an anthropological survey, whose red cells lacked detectable antigens of the Rh complex.[94] Other examples of this rare phenotype, which was subsequently named Rh_{null}, have been discovered,[95] together with another rare Rh variant, called Rh_{mod}, in which mere traces of Rh antigens can be detected.[96] Subsequent studies have established that gross deficiency of Rh antigens in these individuals is associated with changes in red cell morphology, in which stomatocytosis is a prominent feature, and reduced in vivo cell survival.[97-99] These serological and hematological changes are usually accompanied by the biochemical changes expected in a modest hemolytic condition.

Table 4-2. The Duffy Blood Group in Benign Tertian Malaria

Duffy Phenotype	Frequency In: Europe and N. America	Africa	Susceptibility to B.T. Malaria
Fy(a+b−)	common	rare	Yes
Fy(a+b+)	common	uncommon	Yes
Fy(a−b+)	common	infrequent	Yes
Fy(a−b−)	very rare	common	No*

* In vitro tests show that the parasite does not invade Fy(a−b−) red cells.

Although phenotypic characteristics of unrelated Rh_{null} individuals may be the same, there is considerable variation in the extent to which the red cells are compromised. In some people, the hematological defect is so mild that it is recognized only through a slight reduction of in vivo red cell survival.

Rh antigens label a protein component of the red cell membrane. However, while antigenicity is determined by a protein structure, phospholipid is required for the antigenicity to be detectable.[27] Rh_{null} red cells lack the Rh protein, and the cells have altered permeability in which passive and active K^+ and Na^+ transport are increased.[100, 101] However, it does not appear that Rh antigen and the Na^+K^+ pump share common structural components;[100] despite extensive biochemical studies, the exact nature of the membrane defect in Rh_{null} red cells is unknown.

Chronic Granulomatous Disease and the McLeod Syndrome

The Kell blood group has expanded in the last few years until its complexity now approaches that of Rh. Two rare phenotypes of particular interest in the system are K_o[102], in which all antigens produced by the Kell autosomal gene are missing, and McLeod, in which very weak forms of Kell antigens are present.[103] Blood transfusions of common Kell type given to patients of McLeod phenotype may stimulate antibody that was first called anti-KL,[104] but which is now known to contain two separable components called anti-Kx (anti-K15)[53] and anti-Km (anti-K20).[105] Normal red cells of common Kell type have both Kx and Km antigens.

Some boys with X-linked chronic granulomatous disease (CGD)[106] have red cells of the McLeod type.[107, 108] These two conditions are so rare that their association cannot be coincidental. Chronic granulomatous disease is caused by a defect in the bactericidal activity of phagocytic leukocytes of the blood.[109]

As a consequence, the individual has a long history of repeated, and sometimes overwhelming, infections by organisms of low-grade pathogenicity.

Both CGD and the McLeod phenotype have an X-linked mode of inheritance.[110, 111] More than 20 examples of the McLeod type are known, and all are males. The conditions are transmitted by a carrier mother to those sons who receive her X-chromosome carrying the responsible gene.

The link that associated phagocytic leukocytes and the Kell blood group of red cells proved to be Kx.[110] Normal leukocytes do not have antigens of the Kell system but do have Kx. However, leukocytes from boys with X-linked CGD are Kx negative.[108] The exact nature of the complex biochemical lesion present in CGD leukocytes is unknown, although it seems to center on a defect in activation of NADH-oxidase in the plasma membrane.[112] It seems possible that Kx labels a leukocyte membrane structure that is involved in activation of oxidative enzymes.

In normal red cells, Kx is believed to mark a precursor necessary for proper expression of Kell. McLeod red cells lack Kx antigen, a deficiency that is probably responsible for the weakened Kell antigens. McLeod red cells have marked acanthocytic morphological changes which are accompanied by reticulocytosis, reduced haptoglobins, and clinical evidence of a hemolytic state.[113] These related blood group and hematological changes are called the McLeod syndrome.[110] Severity of the clinical effect in unrelated McLeod individuals ranges from a mild well-compensated hemolytic process to a severe condition, with possible bone marrow exhaustion, that may be fatal.[114] McLeod red cells have a slight defect in osmotic water permeability and normal electrolyte transport.[115] Biochemical studies have not yet revealed the nature of the membrane abnormality.

Recent studies have shown that individuals who have McLeod syndrome without CGD have a high level of serum creatine phosphokinase and a muscle cell anomaly.[115a] Patients are usually, but not always, asymptomatic. The serum enzyme is the MM isoenzyme variant derived from skeletal muscle or cardiac muscle, and muscle biopsy shows evidence of structural changes. It seems probable that the gene producing Kx antigen is also involved in normal muscle cell function, and, as in red cells, inheritance of a variant allele compromises that function.

The conclusion from these data is that synthesis of Kx is controlled by an X-linked gene and that the antigen labels a membrane structure of considerable biological importance.

Genetics of Kx

The X-borne locus that directs production of Kx is called Xk.[53] In healthy people of normal Kell antigenicity, a common allele called X^1k orders synthesis of Kx by leukocyte and red cells. Three rare variants at the same locus, called X^2k, X^3k, and X^4k, are each responsible for a different permutation of Kx antigenicity between the two cell types.[108] Lack of leukocyte Kx is associated with chronic granulomatous disease, while lack of Kx on red cells is associated with

McLeod syndrome. The X^2k variant produces no Kx in either cell type; these unfortunate boys have both CGD and McLeod syndrome. Table 4-3 summarizes these antigenic patterns and their associated clinical effects.

Phenotypic Changes in Leukemia

On rare occasions, red cells from patients with leukemia or an allied condition show reduction in A, B, H, or I agglutinability,[116,117] although the cells usually retain a good capacity to absorb appropriate antibodies. The magnitude of the antigenic change may fluctuate in parallel with the clinical course of the disease, and the antigens sometimes reappear during remission.[118] The cause of the change is unknown. It appears to reflect defective synthesis by the cells themselves and not degradation by some agent in the plasma, for A_1 red cells injected into leukemia-weakened group A patients retain their strong A antigenicity.[119] For various reasons, somatic mutation of the blood group gene is unlikely to be the cause of the change, but there does seem to be interference at the genetic level, for activity of appropriate serum transferases is markedly reduced.[120]

Table 4-3. Phenotypic Effects That Result from Inheritance of Variant Xk Alleles

Xk Allele	Kx Antigenicity		Clinical Features
	Leukocytes	Red Cells	
X^1k	Strong	Weak	Normal people of common Kell type.*
X^2k	None	None	Type II CGD and McLeod syndrome.
X^3k	None	Weak	Type I CGD. Normal red cells of common Kell type.
X^4k	Strong	None	Normal leukocytes and McLeod syndrome.

* K_o individuals have normal leukocyte Kx and an excess of red cell Kx.

Associations Between Blood Group Frequency and Disease

Although many associations between blood group frequency and disease have been reported, most of the early studies can be criticized on technical and statistical grounds,[121] and few have been confirmed.

Some imaginative, but unlikely, associations involving blood groups include the suggestions that group A people have more severe hangovers[122] and group O people have better teeth.[123] The claim that group O people have a higher IQ[124] is obviously true. Some confirmed positive associations exist, although the way in which they operate is unknown. Numerous studies have confirmed that group A people have about a 20 percent greater chance of developing cancer of the stomach than group O people,[125] while group O people have a 20 percent greater chance of developing duodenal ulcer than people of other ABO types.[126, 127] In addition, there is good evidence that duodenal ulceration is about 50 percent more frequent in people who are ABH nonsecretors than in those who are secretors.[128] It may be significant that these correlations all involve lesions of the intestinal tract, where large quantities of secreted ABH substances may be present. Simple postulates that soluble blood-group-active substances have a direct protective effect are unlikely to be true, however, for ABH secretors and nonsecretors have about the same amount of secreted mucopolysaccharides, the specificity difference reflecting variations only in a few terminal sugars.

THE BLOOD GROUPS

Each year, more antigens are recognized on human red cells. Many represent subspecificities within known blood group systems. Blood groups such as Rh, MN, Lutheran, and Kell are now seen to be highly complex, but others, such as Kidd, appear to be relatively simple. The appearance of simplicity may, however, only reflect our present inability to recognize complexity. Blood group antigens are recognized by discovery of an antibody, and complexities in which the resulting membrane structure had low immunogenicity would pass unrecognized. Complex genes, such as those of some of the blood groups, are believed to arise during evolution through uneven crossing-over between pairs of chromosomes. As a result, the same gene is present on both portions of a chromosome that subsequently recombines. Mutation of one of the duplicated genes leads to recognizable complexity; over a long period of time, further duplication and mutation continue the process. It has been suggested that crossing-over is not a random process and that it may occur more frequently in specific chromosome regions.[129] It is possible, therefore, that development of complexity in a blood group gene may be influenced by its position on the chromosome.

Close study of a rare variant blood group often provides information that illuminates the whole system. For example, discovery and investigation of the O_h (Bombay) phenotype[130, 131] in the ABO system was a vital stage is understanding the biosynthetic sequence that produces normal A and B antigens.

Blood group notation has evolved during the past 70 years and, not surprisingly, its evolution has produced some oddities. In the MN system, for example, M and N are regarded as alleles, but so also are S and s in the same system. Despite these inconsistencies in terminology, there is general agreement on the order of presentation. Phenotypes, either in a pedigree or in a text, are written in the sequence that the groups were discovered.

THE ABO SYSTEM

Although 80 years have passed since discovery of the ABO groups,[1] knowledge of the system is still incomplete. Three independent loci, ABO, H, and Se, and possibly a fourth called Y, are involved in expression of ABO. The *O* allele at the ABO locus is believed to be an amorph having no recognizable product, and the rare *h* allele at the H locus also appears to be silent. The ABO gene is located near the end of the long arm of chromosome 9, where it provides a useful cytogenetic marker.[19, 20] ABO is one of a linked group of genes that includes *Np*, a dominant gene that determines nail-patella syndrome,[132] and the gene for the enzyme adenylate kinase (*AK₁*). *H* and *Se* are both autosomal genes, but neither has been mapped, although the Se locus is closely linked to the locus for the Lutheran blood group.[133] The *Y* gene segregates independently of other ABO associated genes, and appears to be necessary for full expression of A. Homozygosity for recessive *y* genes results in marked depression of A antigen of the red cells, although the saliva, if the subject is a secretor, contains A substance.[134]

The Nature of ABH Antigens

A, B, and H specificities are determined by specific immunodominant sugars attached to a precursor structure.[25, 26] Two kinds of precursor chains, called type 1 and type 2, have slight structural differences, but both have acceptors for ABH sugars. The antigens cannot be direct gene products but must reflect activity of products that are transferase enzymes, responsible for attachment of the sugars. The genes must function in the correct sequence for synthesis of normal ABH antigens. The *H* gene acts first and produces an α-2-fucosyltransferase that adds L-fucose to the precursor, while the *A* and *B* genes order transferases that then add *N*-acetylgalactosamine and D-galactose, respectively, to the same structure. These transferases are present in various body fluids and can be demonstrated in plasma from persons of appropriate blood type. The origin of plasma transferases is unknown; they are not responsible for the ABH antigens of red cells. Group O red cells do not have a specific O antigen, but the absence of

A or B sugars leaves exposed a considerable amount of H-specific sugar.

On rare occasions, individuals are found who are homozygous for a silent *h* allele at the H locus. The first example was found in India, which explains why the variant is called the Bombay (or O_h) phenotype.[130] The H antigen structure is necessary for attachment of A or B sugars; because of this, red cells of Bombay type are not agglutinated by anti-H, anti-A, or anti-B. These rare individuals always have anti-A, anti-B, and anti-H in their serum and can only be transfused with red cells of Bombay type.[135] Although Bombay cells are not agglutinated by anti-H, absorption and elution studies show that they will take up the agglutinin from selected anti-H reagents.[136] Antibody absorption and elution tests can also be used to demonstrate traces of A or B antigens on some Bombay red cell samples.[137] Bombay cells treated with neuraminidase become strongly H active,[138] and studies on solubilized components of Bombay red cell membranes show considerable amounts of H activity. These observations emphasize that blood group antibodies only recognize surface-active structures on red cells. The precise nature of the biochemical change that occurs in the Bombay phenotype remains to be established. The sugars that determine ABH specificities do not seem to be vital for membrane integrity or function, and Bombay red cells have normal morphology and normal in vivo survival.

Inheritance of ABO Groups

Inheritance of the ABO groups was first demonstrated in 1910,[139] but another 14 years elapsed before the three-allele *A*, *B*, and *O* hypothesis was shown to be the most likely genetic explanation.[140] As *O* is considered to be an amorph, both *A* and *B* are fully expressed in people of the *AO* and *BO* genotypes. The presence of *O* in these individuals can only be demonstrated by tests on informative members of their family. A mating between an O and AB person produces only A or B children. An AB individual does not, under normal circumstances, have an O parent or an O child. Patterns of inheritance in families in which some members are of Bombay type are more complicated. As the ABO and H loci are independent, a Bombay (*hh*) person will have normal, but unexpressed, genes at the ABO locus.[131] His, or her, children will usually inherit an *H* gene from the other parent and as a result an A or B gene inherited from the Bombay parent will be expressed normally. This will sometimes be mistaken for evidence of nonparentage, particularly if the Bombay individual is mistyped as group O.

Many phenotypes characterized by weak A or B antigens have been described. The first hint that a weakly reacting A or B antigen is present in a blood sample is often the finding that an expected ABO antibody is missing. Thus, a "group O" sample that has anti-B but no anti-A may well prove to be a weak A variant. Most of these phenotypes arise by inheritance of variant alleles at the ABO locus, but some are caused by inheritance of independently segregating modifying genes that interfere with expression of a normal *A* or *B* gene. Both recessive[134, 141] and dominant[142] modifiers have been reported. Figure 4-1 shows the ABO phenotypes in a pedigree that includes an independently segregating modifier of a *B* gene.[143]

Investigation of variant phenotypes will include tests on the red cells with a range of potent A-, B-, and H-specific antisera, studies by absorption and elution technique to determine whether the cells have the capacity to bind antibodies, tests for A, B, and H substances in saliva, and studies on members of the family.

ABO on Tissue Cells

ABO antigens have been demonstrated in many tissues, and they are important from the transplantation viewpoint. In malignancy, tissues lose their ABH antigens,[144] a change that is believed to reflect dedifferentiation in malignant cells. Tests for tissue ABO antigens in histological preparations have been claimed to be of help in the early diagnosis of certain cancers.[144] Leukemic leukocytes have been reported to lose their A and H antigens[145]. Loss of red cell antigens in leukemia is discussed under *Phenotypic Changes in Leukemia.*

Cis-AB

The recognition that some AB people are able to transmit both *A* and *B* genes to a single child was a discovery of considerable theoretical importance.[146, 147] In these cases, an AB person married to an O partner may produce either AB or O children. The A and B antigens in these people are usually, but not always, weaker than normal, and some examples have weak anti-B in the serum. Red cells from cis-AB people have enhanced H, reacting more strongly with anti-H than do cells from A_2B individuals.[148] The phenomenon is very rare in Caucasians but more common in Japan and other countries of the East, where it has been estimated that 1 in 5,000 group AB people is of this type.[149] The explanation for cis-AB may be mutation at the ABO locus to give a gene producing a transferase able to add both *N*-acetylgalactosamine and D-galactose to the ABO precursor substance. It is also possible that uneven crossing-over at the ABO locus has duplicated an ABO gene. Cytogenetic studies of chromosome 9 (which carries the ABO locus) from cis-AB people have not shown any recognizable change,[150] but current cytogenetic techniques are not sufficiently sensitive to reveal small duplications. The importance of the phenotype lies in the belief that complex blood group genes have arisen during evolution by gene duplication through uneven crossing over. Cis-AB, with the possibility that *A* and *B* genes are together on one chromosome, may be an example of this evolutionary phenomenon in progress.

THE MN SYSTEM

Blood group antibodies may be of natural occurrence in human sera or may appear as an immune response to blood transfusion or pregnancy. Some animals may make antibodies of new specificity if they are injected with human red cells. Serum of rabbits, immunized in this way, will contain strong species antibodies that react with all human red cells. But after absorption with selected human red cell samples, specific antibodies may remain. Such a procedure resulted in discovery of the MN blood groups.[151] Two antibodies, called anti-M and anti-N, were made by rabbits injected with red cells from different people. Three cell phenotypes, M+N−, M+N+, and M−N+, were defined. Tests of families indicated that M and N were inherited as codominant characters.

M and N are good immunogens in rabbits, but they have very little immunogenicity in man. Although many human anti-M antibodies have been found, most of them appear to be of natural occurrence. However, examples of immune anti-M have been reported, and on rare occasions the antibody has been responsible for hemolytic disease in a newborn child. Anti-M is usually a saline-reactive agglutinin. Somewhat surprisingly, studies of its immunoglobulin nature have shown that most anti-M antibodies are IgG rather than IgM proteins.[152]

Anti-N is much rarer than anti-M. Most examples of anti-N appear to be naturally occurring, but some have a demonstrably immune origin. About 20 percent of hemodialysis patients who use a formaldehyde-sterilized dialyzer develop an anti-N-like antibody.[153] The antibody is not related to blood transfusion but appears to be a response to a change in the patient's MN antigens induced by formaldehyde.[154,155] The patients may be M, MN, or N. Laboratory tests show that the antibody, which is a saline-reactive cold agglutinin, reacts most strongly against N red cells that have been exposed to formaldehyde.[155]

Complications in the MN system began with the discovery of anti-S[23,24] and anti-s,[156] which define a second pair of alleles. S is more often associated with M than with N, while s occurs most frequently in company with N. This linkage disequilibrium is evidence that the *MN* and *Ss* genes are related, and family studies show that the *Ss* genes segregate with *MN*. Figure 4-2 is a pedigree that illustrates inheritance in the MN system. Very rare examples of recombination between *MN* and *Ss* have been reported, and it is a matter of semantics whether they should be considered as separate loci and different systems or whether both should be placed in one operon. From the practical viewpoint, the loci are certainly very close together. There is evidence that the *MNSs* genes are carried on chromosome 4.[157]

No blood sample that is undoubtedly M-negative and N-negative has been found, but about 1 percent of American Negro bloods are S−s−. Some of these individuals, if immunized, make an antibody called anti-U,[158] which is compatible only with other examples of the Negro S−s−U− phenotype. Despite numerous extensive testing programs, no example of the S−s−U− phenotype has been found in a Caucasian. Anti-U was originally viewed as inseparable anti-S plus anti-s. However, about 16 percent of S−s− Negro blood samples are U+, and U must represent a distinct specificity.[159] Support for this conclusion is provided by the observation that leukocytes from U+ people have U antigen but lack S and s.[49] The frequency of U− people varies widely in different parts of Africa; Congo Pygmies hold the present record, with a frequency of about 35 percent.[160]

Many additional antigens related to the MN blood group have been described. Most of these are of low frequency and are sometimes called satellite antigens of the MN system. Five of these uncommon antigens are

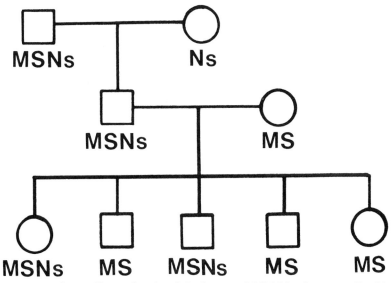

Fig. 4-2. A representative pedigree showing inheritance of MN blood groups. In this family S is segregating with M and s with N.

related to one another in the Miltenberger subsystem (Mi Class I-V).[159] Antibodies directed against low-incidence MN antigens are not uncommon in human sera, but the source of their stimulation is unknown.

The MN antigens are not of great clinical importance because of their low immunogenicity. Anti-S and, less commonly, anti-s, have been responsible for a few transfusion reactions. Although anti-U is rare, it is usually a powerful IgG immune antibody and has been a cause of hemolytic transfusion reactions and hemolytic disease of the newborn. The main interest in the MN system is because of its contribution to genetics. If the four antisera are used in family studies, the system is the most discriminating of all of the red cell blood group systems. Table 4-4 shows frequencies of some antigens in the MN system.

Biochemistry of MN

MN antigens are carried on the major sialoglycoprotein (also called Glycophorin A) of the red cell membrane. Early studies suggested that specificity was dependent upon

Table 4-4. Some Antigens of the MN System

Antigen	Date of Discovery	Percent Frequency N. American Negroes	Caucasians
M	1927	74	72
N	1927	75	72
Hu	1934	7	0.1
Vw(Gr)	1946	1	0.1
S	1947	30	55
s	1951	92	89
He	1951	3	0.1
Mi[a]	1951	1	0.1
U	1953	98.5	>99

N-acetylneuraminic acid (sialic acid) linked to β-D galactosyl residues.[160a] The primary M gene product was believed to be a sialyl transferase that attached sialic acid to a preformed N-specific precursor structure. Apparent support for this was provided by the observation that red cells lose MN activity when treated with certain proteases or with neuraminidase, which remove sialic acid. However, it is now clear that some examples of anti-M do not require intact sialic acid residues on red cells for activity of the specific receptor.[161,162] Biochemical views on the structure of MN have moved toward the concept that the MN genes place the stamp of specificity upon the protein moiety of the glycoprotein,[163, 164] and there is good evidence that the genes code for amino-acid sequences. The oligosaccharides represent important, but nonspecific, components of the immunodeterminants. They are possibly present in different steric configurations on M and N glycoproteins due to the differences in amino-acid sequence.

THE P SYSTEM

The first antibodies in the P system were produced by injecting rabbits with human red cells. Absorption of other antibodies from the immune rabbit sera left a new antibody that agglutinated about 78 percent of human red cell samples.[165] The reactive antigen was named P. Subsequent studies have shown that the same antibody, now called anti-P_1, is present in many animal bloods and is not uncommon in human sera. Human anti-P_1 is nearly always a naturally occurring cold agglutinin with very little clinical significance.[166] Transfusion of P_1 blood to a person whose serum contains anti-P_1 demonstrable only below body temperature does not cause any recognizable clinical complications, or any change in the serological characteristics of the antibody. On very rare occasions, anti-P_1 has been a cause of a hemolytic reaction to a blood transfusion, but these antibod-

ies are usually IgG proteins active at $37\,^\circ$C, and usually with the capability of causing in vitro hemolysis of P_1 red cells. The distinct serological characteristics of the rare anti-P_1 antibodies that are clinically important allows their differentiation from the many innocuous antibodies of the same specificity. The P_1 antigen is not well developed on fetal red cells, and anti-P_1 does not cause hemolytic disease of the newborn.

Anti-TJ^a, discovered in 1951,[167] reacts with an almost universal antigen that was later seen to be part of the P system.[168] One rare and two common phenotypes have to be included on a basic level of understanding. The first, called p, or Tj(a−), is rare. In Northern Sweden, the p phenotype occurs once in about every 7,000 people,[169] but in other parts of the world it is very much rarer. Serum from p people always contains antibody against other P system antigens (anti-P + P_1 + P^k), and it is usually because of the serological problems caused by the antibody that p people are recognized. The second basic phenotype, called P_2 (previously P-negative), occurs in about 22 percent of random people. Red cells of these individuals have basic P antigen, and their serum may contain anti-P_1. The third and most common phenotype, P_1, has a frequency of about 78 percent in Caucasians; serum of these people contains no P-related antibodies. The frequency of P_1 varies in different parts of the world. It is lowest in the East, where about 88 percent of Chinese are P_2.

The reaction strength of red cells from different P_1 people varies widely. Some weak P_1 cell samples are only agglutinated by strong anti-P_1 sera. This variation in P_1 antigenicity is due in part to inheritance of a weak P_1 gene, and partly to zygosity (heterozygous red cells in many blood group systems are known to be less reactive than homozygous cells). The dominant inhibitor gene, called *In(Lu)*, which does not allow expression of the Lutheran genes, also prevents proper expression of P_1. In this circumstance, cells of P_1 genotype type as P_2.[170]

A further complication of the P system was revealed in 1959 by the discovery of P^k.[171] The antigen is unusual in that it appears to have recessive inheritance, since P^k-negative parents may have P^k-positive children. Although P^k red cells lack P antigen, the majority have P_1 (the P_1^k phenotype). The P^k antigen is very rare. About 30 P^k propositi have been found, half of them in Finland. The serum from P^k people contains anti-P that reacts with all bloods except those of P^k or p types.

Biochemistry of the P System

Biochemical studies on red cells have now provided an explanation for P system interrelationships, and for the curious pattern of P^k inheritance. Antigens of the P system are glycosphingolipids.[172] In the biosynthetic pathway, lactosyl ceramide is converted to trihexosyl ceramide, to give a structure with P^k specificity[82,173] in which α-galactose is the immunodominant sugar.[174] This in turn is converted to globoside by addition of a nonreducing β-galactosaminyl residue. Globoside, the most abundant glycosphingolipid of common erythrocytes,[175] has P specificity. P^k red cells have a genetically determined deficiency in the transferase that adds the P-specific galactosaminyl residue; as a result, trihexosyl ceramide with P^k specificity accumulates in the cells. In an alternative pathway, lactosyl ceramide is converted to paragloboside and then, by addition of α-linked galactose, to P_1 substance. In people of p type, a primary transferase deficiency blocks synthesis of trihexosyl ceramide (preventing development of P^k and P antigens), and the cells also have a block in the second pathway that produces the P_1 active structure.[173] As might be expected, the membrane of p and P^k red cells contains only trace amounts of globoside.[173a] These biochemical studies change the thinking of the P system because, with two separate branches in the biosynthetic pathway, producing P and P_1,

respectively, the concept that P_1 and P (P_2) are allelic genes is no longer tenable.

Very rare antibodies have been found that react most strongly with p red cells. However, it seems probable that these antibodies react with sialosylparagloboside. This is not part of the P system biosynthetic pathway, but is related to it. The inability of p cells to synthesize trihexosyl ceramide results in accumulation of sialosylparagloboside, which accounts for the serological reactions given by "anti-p."[176]

P antigens are not restricted to red cells but have been demonstrated on fibroblasts, where it has been found that all cells are P^k irrespective of the red cell type of the donor.[177] The Donath-Landsteiner cold-reactive hemolysin that causes cold hemoglobinuria usually has P specificity.[178]

THE RH SYSTEM

The Rhesus blood group system[179,180] is next to ABO in terms of its clinical importance for, even with the advent of Rh immune globulin prophylaxis, it is still the most commonly involved blood group in pregnancy-associated immunization. Rh incompatibility can cause severe hemolytic disease of the newborn or fetal death in utero.[181] About a third of severely affected infants have an associated hemorrhagic disorder with defibrination and deficiency of multiple coagulation factors.[182] One of the most important contributions of immunohematology to medicine is the demonstration that active blood group incompatibility between a mother and child is the cause of hemolytic disease, and that the Rh antigen is usually involved. The Rh system is named after the monkey whose red cells stimulated the first antibodies when they were injected into rabbits and guinea pigs. Subsequent investigations have indicated that, although the Rhesus monkey antigen is similar to the Rh(D) antigen of human red cells, it is not identical. Most human red cells have both the monkey antigen and a separate, but related, Rh antigen.[159] The name LW, to honor Landsteiner and Weiner, has been given to the antigen shared by monkeys and humans. Studies on informative families have established that the *Rh* and *LW* genes segregate independently. LW is now known to include a number of subtle complexities. Clinical transfusion problems associated with Rh nearly always involve variants within the human Rh system, and only rarely is LW implicated.

In clinical practice, the terms Rh-positive and Rh-negative refer to the presence or absence of detectable D antigen on the red cell membrane. About 85 percent of Caucasians are Rh positive. From the practical viewpoint, D is a strong immunogen and will provoke anti-D in about 50 percent of D negative people given one unit of D positive blood.[183] Almost all specificities in the Rh system have been responsible for hemolytic disease of the newborn, and for hemolytic transfusion reactions. However, while many Rh-related transfusion reactions have occurred, fatal reactions are almost unknown.

Although rare examples of naturally occurring Rh antibodies are known, the great majority of these antibodies follow immunization by transfusion or pregnancy. Immune Rh antibodies are usually IgG proteins of the IgG1 or IgG3 subclasses and, with very rare exceptions, do not bind complement. All Rh antibodies react well by the indirect antiglobulin technique and even more effectively by proteolytic enzyme methods.

D Fractions

During the past four decades Rh has grown into a system of great complexity. More than 30 antibody specificities are now known. While the most important of these is still D, it is now clear that D itself consists of a cluster of antigenically separate components.[184,185] Six D fraction categories have been described, but subtle variations shown by bloods within different categories indicate

that in reality the situation is more complex. Red cells lacking different components of the D mosaic have been recognized. In some cases, blood lacking such a component may have in its place an alternative antigen. Anti-Go[a] and anti-D[w], for example, react with uncommon antigens that are substitutions for missing D components in category IV and category V, respectively.[159] These D-fraction problem bloods are usually revealed by finding people who appear to be D positive but who have an immune anti-D antibody in their serum that does not react with their own red cells.

Rh Genetics

Early studies on Rh suggested that three closely linked genes are responsible for production of three antigens called C, D, and E.[186] Evidence from several directions indicates that the linear sequence of the genes is probably *D*, *C*, and *E*. Numerous alternatives have been identified at the C and E loci, but nothing corresponding to d has been found; most workers consider d to represent an absence of D. Recent work on solubilized red cell membranes indicates that Rh-negative cells have D antigen but that it is not exposed on the surface of the cell.[29] If further work confirms this finding it would seem that the difference between Rh-positive and Rh-negative red cells lies in a changed membrane configuration of a common Rh-labeled protein.

Much controversy has existed over the exact genetic mechanism that governs Rh. But whether one super gene that produces an agglutinogen comprised of multiple blood factors,[187,188] or three separate, but closely linked, genes[186] are involved, is of no importance from the practical viewpoint. On the conversational level, the C, D, E nomenclature has certain advantages, and the complexities in Rh that have become apparent may be viewed simplistically as variations on the basic three-gene theme. However, the CDE model cannot accommodate some of

Table 4-5. Equivalent Notations for Some Rh Antigens

Fisher-Race	Wiener	Numerical	Percent Frequency in Caucasians
D	Rh_o	Rh1	84
C	rh′	Rh2	70
E	rh″	Rh3	30
c	hr′	Rh4	80
e	hr″	Rh5	98
f	hr	Rh6	64
C^W	$rh^{W'}$	Rh8	1
G	rh^G	Rh12	85
Total Rh	—	Rh29	>99

the subtle findings, and the concept of a single supergene is more likely to be correct. Certainly it is true that an individual always contributes an intact Rh gene complex to his or her offspring. A genetic model for the Rh system has been proposed, which consists of a conjugated operon with four operators, each with a structural gene.[15] In an attempt to circumvent these ideological problems, a numerical system of Rh notation that corresponds only with phenotypic characteristics has been devised.[189] Table 4-5 shows equivalent notation for some Rh antigens.

The Rh gene is located near the end of the short arm of chromosome 1.[85,190] It is one of a linked group of genes that includes El_1, which determines a type of erythrocyte elliptocytosis, and genes for the enzymes phosphoglucomutase (PGM_1), 6-phosphogluconate dehydrogenase (6-PGD), and peptidase C (PepC).[159]

The D^u Antigen

In addition to D fraction bloods, a weak form of D, called D^u, also exists.[191] D^u antigens exist in different grades. High-grade D^u red cells are agglutinated quite readily by most anti-D testing sera, while low-grade D^u cells only react weakly with selected potent anti-D typing reagents using a sensitive technique such as the indirect antiglobulin test. Some automated methods that combine the

use of enzymes with a high molecular weight additive are sufficiently sensitive that the antiglobulin test is not necessary. High-grade D^u donor blood can stimulate anti-D if given to an Rh-negative recipient, but there is good evidence that low-grade D^u blood has little immunogenicity.[192]

The D^u phenotype may arise by inheritance of a weak D gene.[191] Alternatively, it may arise by inheritance of a modifying r′(Cde) gene complex that, for an unknown reason, prevents full expression of a normal D gene received from the other parent.[193] The depressed D gene is expressed normally again in the next generation when it segregates from the r′ modifier.

C, E, and G

Either of two common alleles called C and c are present in most Rh gene complexes. However, other rare variants at the C locus are also known. Similarly, each Rh gene complex will have a representative at the E locus, usually E or e, and again rare Ee variants have been described. There is evidence that Ee variants are highly complex, in a way that seems to be analogous to the more well-defined D fractions.[194] Complex Rh problems in Negroes often involve Ee variants.

Some Rh-negative people immunized with cDE red cells make antibody that reacts as anti-C plus anti-D. However, the description of G antigen provided an explanation for this puzzling finding.[195] Most Rh gene complexes that produce C or D also make an antigen called G. The phenotype of the immunizing red cells in the above case is cDEG, and the antibody is in reality anti-D plus anti-G. Like most aspects of Rh, G is now known to include subtle complexities.

Rh Deletion Phenotypes

One of the most interesting and informative aspects of Rh has been the discovery of partially deleted and fully deleted phenotypes. Rare red cell samples may lack all antigens of the C or E variety, a phenotype called −D−/−D−.[196] The −D− samples have greatly increased amounts of D antigen, and the owners of such cells are prone to make antibody (called anti-Rh17) that is compatible only with homozygous −D− or Rh_{null} red cells. Other partially deleted phenotypes include cD− and $C^wD−$. A deletion phenotype called ·D· resembles −D−[197] but possesses a rare antigen called Evans.[198] The immune antibody made by immunized ·D·/·D· people may be indistinguishable from anti-Rh17. A number of other phenotypes with markedly depressed, but not quite aberrant, expression of parts of the Rh complex are also known.

Rh_{null} cells lack all antigens produced by the Rh gene.[94] The phenotype may arise by homozygous inheritance of independently segregating modifying genes (called $X°r$) that prevent expression of the Rh gene,[95] or by inheritance of silent alleles at the Rh locus itself.[199] Rh_{null} people may make an antibody (called anti-Rh29) that is compatible only with other Rh_{null} blood samples, if they are immunized by red cells of ordinary Rh type. An important contribution to knowledge made through studies on Rh_{null} blood is that Rh antigen is necessary for maintenance of red cell membrane integrity. Rh_{null} red cells are stomatocytes and have reduced in vivo survival.[97,99] For details, see *Blood Groups and Disease.*

Rh and Autoimmune Hemolytic Anemia

IgG autoantibodies responsible for warm antibody autoimmune hemolytic anemia (AIHA) may have recognizable specificity. When this occurs, Rh is the blood group most commonly involved. Mechanisms that regulate autoantibody and alloantibody responses are different and antigens involved in autoimmunity do not have to be highly immunogenic in alloimmune situations. Thus, Rh e antigen has low immunogenicity in e-negative people, yet anti-e is the most frequent specific autoantibody seen in patients with AIHA.[200] Other autoantibody specificities that may be found include c, f, E, rh_i, and G.[194] In many cases, the specific antibody has an associated "nonspecific" component that reacts with all other blood samples. Some autoantibodies react strongly only with Rh-positive red cells, but critical studies show that in most cases the specificity is anti-LW and not anti-D.[201] Use of Rh-deleted, or partially deleted, test cells allows demonstration of Rh-related specificity in some other cases.[202] About 34 percent of IgG autoantibodies fail to react with Rh_{null} red cells, an observation that is of academic interest only, for Rh_{null} blood is too rare to be used in transfusing patients with AIHA.

THE LUTHERAN SYSTEM

For 15 years after its recognition, the Lutheran system comprised the antigens Lu^a, with a frequency of about 8 percent in Caucasians,[203] and Lu^b, which is present in more than 99 percent of random bloods.[204] In many of the blood groups, discovery of a null phenotype has allowed advances in knowledge; perhaps nowhere has this been more striking than in Lutheran. The key discovery of the Lu(a−b−) phenotype was made by the proposita herself when testing her own red cells; they were not agglutinated by either anti-Lu^a or anti-Lu^b.[205] Family studies were surprising, for they showed that the phenotype had a dominant mode of inheritance. A child of the dominant Lu(a−b−) type always has an Lu(a−b−) parent. Many such families are now known. Inheritance of an independently segregating dominant inhibitor gene, called *In(Lu)*, prevents expression of the Lutheran gene.[206] The inhibitor is not aimed exclusively at Lutheran, for it also prevents proper expression of Auberger (Au^a), P$_1$, and i.[170]

More recently, families have been found in which the Lu(a−b−) phenotype is inherited as a recessive characteristic, through a silent (*Lu*) allele at the Lutheran locus.[207,208] Thus, two genetic mechanisms can give rise to the Lu(a−b−) phenotype. However, critical studies show that the phenotypes are subtly different. Traces of Lutheran antigens on dominant Lu(a−b−) cells can be demonstrated by antibody absorption-elution technique, but cells of recessive type are devoid of Lutheran antigens. This slight difference seems to have some practical importance, for individuals of dominant Lu(a−b−) type are not prone to make Lutheran antibodies, but recessives may make an antibody called anti-Lu3 (anti-Lu^{a}Lu^b) if they are transfused with blood of common Lutheran type.[208]

Lutheran-Related Antigens

Discovery of anti-Lu4 in 1971 began a considerable expansion of the Lutheran system.[209] Anti-Lu4 reacts with nearly all Lu(a−b+), Lu(a+b+), and Lu(a+b−) cell samples but does not agglutinate any that are Lu(a−b−). Further investigations have established that Lu4 is a high-incidence antigen absent from cells of dominant or recessive Lu(a−b−) type. A number of similar antibodies are known that identify different high-incidence antigens related to the Lutheran system. These have been named anti-Lu5, anti-Lu6, anti-Lu7, anti-Lu8, anti-Lu11, anti-Lu12 (Much) and anti-Lu13.[210-212] In addition, two antibodies recognizing low-incidence Lutheran antigens have been reported. Anti-Lu9 (Mull) recognizes an uncommon antigen (frequency 2 percent) that has an allelic relationship to Lu6,[213] while anti-Lu14 defines an antigen (frequency 2.5 percent) that is produced by an allele of *Lu8*.[214] These antigenic pairs have a relationship in the Lutheran blood group that is analogous to Kp^a-Kp^b and Js^a-Js^b in the Kell blood group. At the present time, therefore, the Lutheran system comprises three pairs of antigens, a number of related high-incidence antigens about which little genetic information is available, and an independent locus involved in expression of the Lutheran gene. One of the high-incidence antigens, Lu12 (Much), appears not to be a product of the Lutheran gene.[212] These relationships are summarized in Table 4-6.

Lutheran is inherited as an autosomal dominant characteristic. The Lutheran locus and the ABH secretor locus are closely linked,[133] but there are no data to show which autosome is the carrier. The expansion of Lutheran is of considerable genetic interest, but antibodies in the system are usually weak, and only on very rare occasions have they caused transfusion reactions or hemolytic disease in newborn infants.

THE KELL SYSTEM

Discovery of the Kell blood group was an early bonus that followed development and utilization of the antiglobulin test in 1946.[215] Since that time, Kell has expanded into a system that bids to rival MN and Rh in its

Table 4-6. Antigens Associated with the Lutheran Blood Group

Uncommon antigens	Lu^a	Lu9	Lu14							
Common antigens	Lu^b	Lu6	Lu8	Lu3	Lu4	Lu5	Lu7	Lu11	Lu12*	Lu13

* Lu12 is probably not produced by the Lutheran gene.

complexity. Twenty-one related antigens have been recognized thus far.

The Kell gene is an autosomal character that segregates independently of other blood group systems. An interesting close linkage between the Kell locus and the locus for *PTC*, a gene determining the ability to taste dilute solutions of phenylthiocarbamide, may prove to be informative.[216] Studies on Kell-variant families should always include tests to determine their "taster" status, for segregation with *PTC* would suggest that the variant reflects an allele at the Kell locus.

Anti-k (anti-Cellano) defines a high-incidence antigen that has an allelic relationship to K.[217] Further expansion of the Kell system began with the discovery of anti-Kp^a and anti-Kp^b,[218, 219] which define a second pair of alleles at the Kell locus. The discovery that a third Kp allele, called *Kp^c* (K21), exists came as a recent surprise.[220] Rare Japanese have been found who are Kp(a−b−c+) but otherwise of common Kell type. Just as interesting was the finding that Levay, the first "private" antigen known, is the same as Kp^c.[221] So, more than 30 years after its discovery, Levay can now be fitted into the Kell system. No Kp^c-positive was found in testing more than 1,000 Caucasians, but it seems likely that the antigen is more common in Japanese.

Two more pairs of alleles at the Kell locus have also been recognized. Js^a is essentially a Negroid characteristic with a frequency of about 14 percent;[222] its partner, Js^b, is of high incidence.[223] K17 (Wk^a) is a rare antigen (frequency 0.3 percent) in Caucasians and is partnered by the very common antigen K11.[224] A rare antigen called Ul^a, found almost exclusively in Finnish people (frequency about 2.5 percent), is also part of the Kell system,[225] but no antibody with anti-Ul^b specificity has been found.

Numerical notation is now used quite commonly for blood groups. Most of the Kell-related antigens found in the last few years have been numbered.[226] In numerical notation, a positive phenotype would be written K:1, a negative phenotype as K:−1, the antibody as anti-K1, and the gene as *K^1*.

The K$_o$ Phenotype

The null phenotype of the Kell system is called K$_o$ and lacks all antigens that are known to be products of the Kell gene.[102] The phenotype arises by inheritance from both parents of a silent *K^o* gene. In the Kell system, and indeed in other blood group systems, it is useful to borrow the Jacob-Monod[14] concept of gene regulation and imagine that the silent allele represents mutation at the operator region of the gene while the many associated antigens of the blood group system itself reflect different mutational sites in the structural gene. K$_o$ cells have normal morphology and normal in vivo survival, and Kell antigens do not seem to be essential for membrane integrity. K$_o$ individuals pose difficulties if they are recipients of blood transfusions, for the antibody that they may make, anti-Ku,[227] is compatible only with other examples of the K$_o$ type.

A number of other antibodies have been found that react with "public" (very common) antigens but do not react with K$_o$ cells. Anti-K12, anti-K13, anti-K14, anti-K18, and anti-K19 detect five different antigens of this kind.[110] The serological reactions given by these antibodies are characteristic of the Kell system, but there is, as yet, no direct proof from family studies that the antigens are produced by the Kell gene. Table 4-7 shows antigens that are related to the Kell blood group.

Biosynthesis of Kell Antigens

Kell antigens are glycoproteins, but it is not known whether the protein or the carbohydrate moiety of the glycoprotein determines specificity. Recent investigations have suggested that synthesis of Kell antigens takes

Table 4-7. Antigens Associated with the Kell Blood Group

Uncommon antigens	K	Kp^a	Kp^c	Js^a	K17	Ul^a		
Common Antigens	k		Kp^b	Js^b	K11			
High-incidence related antigens	K12	K13	K14	K18	K19	Ku	Km	Kx*

* Kx is a related antigen but is not produced by the Kell gene.

place in two stages.[108] The first involves production of an essential precursor substance which carries an antigenic marker called Kx(K15). The gene producing Kx is X-linked and is called X^1k[53]. In the second stage, the Kell autosomal gene puts the stamp of Kell specificity upon the precursor. Kell phenotypes thus reflect the result of interaction between the products of two independently segregating genes. Variations in either gene affect Kell antigens. This sequential process is shown in Figure 4-3.

The McLeod Phenotype

One of the rarest and most interesting Kell phenotypes is called McLeod, after the donor in whom it was first found.[103] The red cells have antigens produced by common Kell genes, but all of them in a markedly depressed form. The phenotype is an X-linked characteristic and arises through inheritance of a variant allele at the Xk locus.[108] All known examples of the McLeod phenotype have occurred in males. It seems probable that lack of Kx precursor substance prevents proper expression of a normal Kell gene, thus producing the effect seen as the McLeod phenotype. If transfused with blood of common Kell type, some CGD males of McLeod type make antibody that was originally called anti-KL,[104] but which is now known to comprise two separable specificities called anti-Kx (anti K15)[53] and anti-Km (anti-K20).[105] Kx seems to label an essential membrane structure, for McLeod red cells have acanthocytic morphology and reduced in vivo survival,[113] a condition called McLeod syndrome. Kx is also present on normal phagocytic leukocytes of the blood, but it is absent from leukocytes of boys with X-linked chronic granulomatous disease. Further details of these clinical associations will be found under *Blood Groups and Disease*.

Km antigen appears to be a product of all fully functional Kell genes. It is not present on McLeod cells, in which expression of the Kell gene is modified, or on K_o cells. Non-

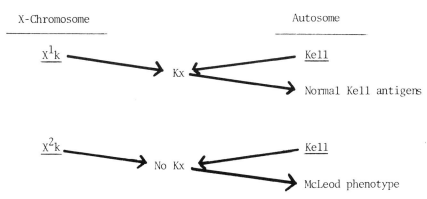

Fig. 4-3. Possible biosynthetic events in the Kell blood groups.

CGD McLeod subjects may make monospecific anti-Km if they are transfused with blood of common Kell type.[228]

The Xk locus is inactivated by the Lyon phenomenon of X-chromosome inactivation; because of this, female carriers of certain Xk variant genes are mosaics with a mixed red-cell population of McLeod acanthocytes and normal red cells of common Kell type.[113,114]

Alloantibodies in the Kell System

The first reported example of anti-K caused hemolytic disease in a newborn infant.[215] Other examples of the antibody have caused hemolytic transfusion reactions. The K antigen has strong immunogenicity and about 1 in 20 K-negative people make anti-K if they are given one unit of K-positive blood.[229] Other Kell specificities may be stimulated by transfusion or by pregnancy, and most have the capability of causing in vivo red cell destruction. Kell system antibodies are usually IgG proteins reactive by the antiglobulin test. Some examples of anti-K or anti-Kp^a are naturally occurring. The pathogenic coliform *E. coli* O_{125} has a K-like antigen; coliform enterocolitis involving this organism has been responsible for production of apparently naturally occurring anti-K.[8]

AUTOIMMUNE HEMOLYTIC ANEMIA AND THE KELL SYSTEM

The Kell blood groups are involved in rare cases of IgG warm antibody autoimmune hemolytic anemia. In about 1 in every 250 patients, the causative autoantibody has clearly defined specificity for a high-incidence Kell antigen.[230] Auto-anti-Kp^b, auto-anti-K13, and auto-anti-K12 have been recognized thus far.[230-232] Red cells of these patients have acquired temporary depression of their Kell antigens, and the patient's serum frequently contains allo anti-K. Although

there is no proof, it has been suggested that in these cases the acquired loss of Kell antigens reflects enzymatic degradation, possibly of bacterial origin, and that the change in cell membrane configuration precipitates the Kell-specific autoimmune response.[230]

THE LEWIS SYSTEM

Lewis is usually considered to be an independent system,[233] but two other loci, H and Secretor, play an important part in production of Lewis antigens. In addition, the immunodominant sugars that determine Le^a and Le^b specificities are attached to the same precursor as that utilized for ABH antigenicity. Antigens of the I system also have a biochemical relationship to ABO and Lewis, and it may be easier from the conceptual viewpoint to consider AB, H, Lewis, and I as parts of one highly complex multigenic system. An important difference between Lewis and most other blood groups is that Lewis is not primarily a red cell antigen. Lewis substances are found in abundance in the plasma of persons of appropriate genotype and are passively absorbed from the plasma by any red cells that are present.[234] As a result, red cells from an Le(a−) person transfused to an Le(a+) recipient become Le(a+) within about 72 hours. The first experiment of this kind was made by nature in a pair of chimeric twins.[235] Each twin had a double population of red cells that differed in several blood group systems, and they were of different genetic Lewis types. But all red cells in each twin were of the Lewis type of the host. Thus, inheritance must determine the type of plasma Lewis substance produced by an individual, but passive absorption is responsible for its appearance on red cells. Lewis substances in plasma are glycoproteins and glycosphingolipids.[236] They are not produced by red cell precursors, and the site of production is unknown. Soluble Lewis substances are also present in saliva, urine, milk, amniotic fluid, seminal fluid, and gastric juice. Absorption of plasma antigen to give a positive red cell phenotype is not peculiar to man. Similar systems are known in sheep (R system),[237] cattle (J system),[238] and pigs (O and A system).[239]

The Genetics of Lewis

Three independently segregating genes are involved in the synthesis of Lewis antigens. The Lewis (*Le*) gene codes for an α-4-fucosyl-transferase that attaches L-fucose to the ABO precursor structure, but in a different position from the fucose added by the *H* gene enzyme. The Lewis-specified transferase gives Le^a specificity to the molecule. The silent allele of *Le* is called *le*. The Secretor gene allows expression of *H* in secretory tissues, and the Lewis- and H-specified fucoses together give a structural configuration that has Le^b specificity.

Le^a and Le^b are not present on red cells of infants at birth, as all newborns type as Le(a−b−). Within 10 days of birth, the Le^a antigen appears; by 8 weeks after birth, most infants are Le(a+).[240] At about two years of age, the red cell and plasma antigens have settled into the pattern that will be maintained for life.[46] About 22 percent of adult group O or A_2 people are Le(a+b−), and 72 percent are Le(a−b+). In Caucasians, only about 6 percent of random people are Le(a−b−) but the incidence may be up to 40 percent in some Negro populations.

Because Lewis phenotypes reflect interaction between the products of several independent genes, inheritance is somewhat complicated. Children who will be Le(a+) at maturity can be born to Le(a−) parents, and Le(b+) children can have Le(b−) parents. In plasma, Le^a will be present if *Le* is inherited, while *Le, Se,* and *H* must be inherited for Le^b to appear.

Le^a substance can be demonstrated on lymphocytes by means of selected cytotoxic anti-Le^a sera.[48] As with red cells, the lympho-

cyte antigen is acquired by passive absorption of Lewis substance from plasma.

Lewis Antibodies

Lewis antibodies are nearly always of natural occurrence. Apart from anti-A, anti-B, and anti-I, they probably represent the most common specificity seen in blood group serology. In laboratory tests, they may show activity over a thermal range from 0°C to 37°C, and some sera have complement-binding properties. Many examples of anti-Le^b react well only with group O or A_2 red cells. Because newborn infants are Le(a−b−), Lewis antibodies do not cause hemolytic disease of the newborn. On rare occasions, strong hemolytic anti-Le^a has been responsible for a transfusion reaction, but clinical hemolytic reactions due to anti-Le^b are unknown, although large numbers of Le(b+) bloods have been transfused to recipients with anti-Le^b. Transfusion of plasma containing Le^b substance to such a recipient neutralizes the Lewis antibody, and Le(b+) red cells can subsequently be transfused without complications.[241] The fact that Lewis antigens are only passengers on red cells probably accounts, in part at least, for the effectiveness of this procedure. Transfused Le(b+) red cells soon lose their Le^b antigen and become Le(b−) like the cells of the recipient.[242]

Three additional antibodies in the Lewis system have been described. Anti-Le^x gives the reactions expected of anti-Le^a plus anti-Le^b, except that anti-Le^x reacts strongly against red cells from most newborn infants.[243] Anti-Le^c is a rare antibody that reacts with red cells from Le(a−b−), H nonsecretor people.[244] Anti-Le^d was produced by injecting a goat with saliva from a group O, Le(a−b+) person. After the immune serum was absorbed with Le(a+b−) red cells, the antibodies that remained were anti-Le^b and the new anti-Le^d, which reacted only with red cells from Le(a−b−) secretors.[245] The reactions of anti-Le^d are also consistent with the reactive antigen being an H determinant on Type 1 ABO precursor that is taken up by red cells from the plasma.[246]

THE DUFFY SYSTEM

The first example of anti-Fy^a was found in the serum of a much-tranfused patient named Mr. Duffy.[247] The notation Fy was chosen to avoid confusion with D of the Rh system. The antibody reacts with about 66 percent of Caucasian blood samples, and is not uncommon in patients who have received multiple blood transfusions. Anti-Fy^b, which recognizes the product of an allele of *Fy^a*, is a much rarer antibody.[248]

Duffy group frequencies vary greatly in different populations of the world. In Japanese, Chinese, and Koreans, Fy^a is by far the more common antigen, while in Europeans Fy^b has the higher frequency. A weak form of Fy^b, called Fy^x, is present in a small number of Caucasians.[249] About 80 percent of Negroes have the phenotype Fy(a−b−).[87] This seems to be the result of natural selection, for recent studies have shown that Duffy antigens are associated with the receptor utilized by the parasite of benign tertian malaria during its invasion of red cells.[91] Fy(a−b−) cells are not invaded by this parasite, and the owners of such cells are resistant to this kind of malaria. (See *Blood Groups and Disease*). The Fy(a−b−) phenotype occurs as a great rarity in Caucasians, and a silent *Fy* gene has to be invoked to explain apparent anomalies of Duffy inheritance in a few Caucasian families.

Duffy antibodies are almost always IgG proteins reactive only by the antiglobulin test. They may cause a hemolytic reaction to an incompatible blood transfusion, and on rare occasions anti-Fy^a has been responsible for hemolytic disease in a newborn infant. Fy^a and Fy^b antigens are denatured if red cells are treated with the enzymes papain, bromelin, or ficin. The antigens are not affected by

neuraminidase, however, and the denaturing effect of the plant latex enzymes must be a result of their protease activity.

Fy3, Fy4, and Fy5

Three other Duffy-related antibodies are known. Anti-Fy3 is found on rare occasions in the serum of Fy(a−b) people.[250] Fy3 antigen has, so far, always accompanied Fy^a or Fy^b. However, Fy3 appears to be a distinct entity, and anti-Fy3 is not simply anti-Fy^a plus anti-Fy^b. Fy4 is present on all Fy(a−b−) red cells and on some that are Fy(a+b−) or Fy(a−b+).[251] The genetic background has yet to be established and it is not known whether *Fy^4* is an allele of *Fy^3*, or whether it is a third allele at the *Fy^{a}Fy^b* locus.

The Fy5 antigen appears to be related to both the Duffy and Rh groups, for both systems have an influence on its production.[252] Fy5 is present on Fy(a+) and Fy(b+) red cells and is absent from Fy(a−b−) cells. Thus, Fy5 resembles Fy3. However, Rh$_{null}$ red cells of common Duffy type lack Fy5, and −D− cells have a reduced amount of the antigen. It appears that contributions by the products of both the Duffy and Rh genes are necessary for formation of the structure that has Fy5 antigenicity.

The Fy3, Fy4, and Fy5 antigens are not denatured by papain, bromelin, or ficin, a finding which supports the conclusion that, although they are related to Fy^a and Fy^b, they are distinct specificities.

Duffy and Gene Mapping

Duffy has the distinction of being the first human gene to be assigned to a specific autosome. In 1968, an inherited structural variation of chromosome 1, called Uncoiler-1 (Un-1), was described.[22] It was also shown that the Un-1 cytogenetic marker was linked to the Duffy blood group, thus placing the Duffy locus on chromosome 1. Chromosome

1 is the largest and most extensively mapped of the human autosomes. In addition to Duffy and Rh, it also carries the genes for the Scianna and probably the Dombrock blood groups. The fact that Duffy and Rh are syntenic is unlikely to be a factor in the production of Fy5 antigen, for genes do not have to be on the same chromosome for their products to interact.

No other blood group makes such distinctions betwen different populations of the world as the Duffy group. Although not a major cause of clinical transfusion problems, its role in benign tertian malaria infection makes it a system of considerable importance.

THE KIDD SYSTEM

The Kidd system takes its name from the maker of the "first" antibody, which caused hemolytic disease in her newborn infant.[253] Many examples of anti-Jk^a have been found, and it has been incriminated in numerous hemolytic transfusion reactions. Anti-Jk^b,[254] which defines an antigen that is antithetical to Jk^a, has also been a cause of severe hemolytic reactions to blood transfusions.

Antibodies in the Kidd system are often difficult to work with for, although they are IgG proteins, they may not react well in the antiglobulin test. With both antibodies, a feature sometimes encountered is a dramatic clinical effect from an antibody of apparent low potency as judged by in vitro tests.

The Kidd gene is inherited as an autosomal dominant characteristic. There is evidence that the locus is on chromosome 7 and that it may be linked to Colton, which is believed to be on the same chromosome.[255] About 76 percent of Caucasians are Jk(a+), and about 74 percent are Jk(b+).

Rare individuals have red cells that are Jk(a−b−),[256] a null phenotype found mainly in Chinese, Polynesians, and South American Indians. It is assumed to arise by homozygous inheritance of a silent *Jk* allele at the Kidd locus, although there is, as yet, no proof of this. A silent *Jk* gene also seems to occur as a rarity in Caucasian populations, for its presence has to be invoked to explain anomalies of Kidd inheritance in some families. Blood transfusions of common Kidd type given to Jk(a−b−) recipients may provoke an antibody called anti-Jk3 (anti-Jk^{a}Jk^b), which is compatible only with other Jk(a−b−) bloods.[256] The Jk3 antigen has always accompanied Jk^a or Jk^b on red cells, but it appears to be a distinct specificity.[257] Support for this is provided by the finding that phagocytic leukocytes have Jk3 but lack Jk^a and Jk^b.[50]

THE I SYSTEM

Most human sera from birth onwards contain a weak antibody that agglutinates the individual's own and most random red cell samples, at low temperature. These normal "nonspecific cold agglutinins" are not active at 37° C, but they have been a nuisance to blood group serologists for many years. It was assumed by early workers that some kind of universal receptor on red cells was involved. In 1956 it was shown that powerful examples of these cold agglutinins may cause hemolytic anemia, and the reactive antigen was named I.[258]

Progress in understanding the nature of I antigen came with the discovery that soluble forms of I substance are present in saliva,[42] milk,[43] and some other body fluids. Biochemical studies on these substances have shown that I is heterogeneous and that antigenicity is determined by immunodominant sugars attached to the same precursor structure as that involved in the development of ABH and Lewis antigens.[259]

It is not known whether the temperature requirement of anti-I is imposed by some thermally-dependent aspect of the antibody molecule, or by a change in configuration, orientation, or mobility of the cell membrane receptor. If low temperature unfolds a surface structure on the red cell to expose a receptor that is masked at 37° C, it might be more appropriate to view I as a system of cold-active receptors.

Anti-i, a cold autoagglutinin defining an antigen that is reciprocally related to I, is a much rarer antibody.[260] Red cells that are rich in I have very little i, and vice versa, but the exact nature of the relationship between the two antigens is unknown. The rare adults who are almost lacking in I have a large amount of i on their red cells, and are called i adults. Very rare people are known whose cells are weak in both I and i.

Red cells from newborn infants are markedly deficient in I antigen and have an excess of i. Cells taken from umbilical cord blood are a useful aid in identifying Ii system antibodies. About 18 months is needed for infants to acquire their normal adult quota of red cell I antigen.[260]

The Genetics of I

The genetics of I are different to other blood groups, for some I and i antigen are present on all human red cells. The different phenotypes represent genetically determined quantitative variations. All fetal bloods have strong i, and conventional genetic explanations in which *I* and *i* are allelic genes cannot be applied. The i adult phenotype is inherited, but it seems to arise by failure to inherit a common gene, *Z*, that superimposes I specificity onto fetal i.[261] Without this gene (i.e., the genotype *zz*) the fetal relationship of Ii antigens persists for life.

Clinical Aspects of the I System

In adults, maturation of I antigen takes place during normal erythropoeisis. In hemorrhagic or hemolytic conditions where there is erythropoietic hyperplasia, transit time of maturing red cell precursors in the bone marrow is reduced, and red cells from these people often have increased i antigen.[262,263]

Cold antibody hemolytic anemia caused by

anti-I may be a transient or a chronic condition. In both instances, the antibody has demonstrable activity at 31°C and binds complement. The antibody usually, but not always, has a high titer in tests at low temperature. The most important feature from the clinical viewpoint, however, is not the serological characteristics at low temperature, but whether the antibody is active at physiological temperature.

Strong anti-i may be found in patients with reticuloendothelial neoplasias and some other pathological conditions.[260] Weaker forms of the antibody are found commonly in patients with infectious mononucleosis.[264] In any of these conditions, anti-i may be of sufficient potency to cause hemolytic anemia. Anti-i has not been found as a naturally occurring antibody in a healthy person.

Other Sources of I Antigens and Antibodies

Cellular I antigen is not restricted to red cells but has been identified on epithelial cells and on T and B lymphocytes.[45]

Antigens of the I system are widely distributed in nature. They are present in many animal species[265] and in certain bacteria. Rabbits appear to have the strongest I antigen of any species. Some primates, rhesus monkeys in particular, have very strong i antigens, and their red cells are useful in identifying weak examples of anti-i. I antibodies are also widely distributed and are responsible for most instances of cold autoagglutination encountered in other species.

Other Cold Autoantibody Systems

Three other cold-reactive autoantibody specificities, which are not related to I, have been recognized.

Anti-Sp₁. Anti-Sp_1 defines a universal antigen on human red cells.[266] Despite extensive testing programs, no cell sample lacking the antigen has been found. Fetal red cells and i adult cells have strong Sp_1 antigen. Red cells treated with proteases or with neuraminidase lose their Sp_1 antigen; sialic acid is an essential component of the membrane receptor. This provides a useful means of distinguishing between cold antibodies of the I and Sp_1 systems, for I system antibodies give enhanced reactions against protease-treated red cells. Anti-Sp_1 has also been called anti-Pr, and under this terminology a number of subspecificities have been described.[267] Anti-Sp_1 may show enhanced reactions in laboratory tests in a low pH medium, and the antibody may cause cold antibody hemolytic anemia.

Anti-Gd. Two examples of cold agglutinin disease caused by a cold-reactive autoagglutinin called anti-Gd have been described.[268] The Gd antigen is a membrane glycolipid and is well developed on fetal red cells and on i adult cells. The antigen is denatured by neuraminidase but is not by proteases. Thus, the Gd receptor requires sialic acid for its activity, but it is not carried on a protease-sensitive component of the membrane.

Anti-Sd^x. Anti-Sd^x is a cold-reactive autoagglutinin that appears to be related to the Sd^a blood group.[269] Two examples have been reported, and both were responsible for in vivo hemolysis. In laboratory tests, the antibodies hemolyse enzyme-treated red cells, give optimum reactions at room temperature, and are most active in a medium at pH 6.5. Red cells from i adults have strong Sd^x, but fetal cells have slightly reduced amounts of the antigen. Like other cold autoagglutinins, anti-Sd^x defines a public antigen. Red cells that are Sd(a−), Sd(a+), or Sd(a++) are equally reactive, and the relationship to Sd^a is shown by inhibition studies, for urine from Sd(a+) people inhibits anti-Sd^x but Sd(a−) urine does not. Guinea pig urine, which is a potent source of Sd^a substance, has strong inhibitory activity against anti-Sd^x. The antibody is not the same as anti-Sd^a, but it appears to recognize a related antigenic determinant.

THE Xg^a BLOOD GROUP

One of the most interesting and informative blood groups is the X-linked Xg^a.[270] Only one specificity, anti-Xg^a, has been found, but numerous examples of the antibody are known. Rare examples of auto anti-Xg^a in Xg(a+) people have also been reported. Frequency of the Xg(a+) phenotype is higher in females (89 percent) than in males (67 percent) because females, having two X chromosomes, have twice the chance of inheriting an X chromosome carrying the *Xg^a* gene. No antibody that recognizes an antithetical antigen has been found; the Xg(a−) phenotype is recognized only by the absence of Xg^a. The currently silent allele is called *Xg*. If an antibody is found that recognizes a product of this gene, it will be promoted to Xg^b.

In family studies, Xg^a obeys the fairly complicated rules of inheritance for dominant X-borne characters. The best proof of X-linkage comes from a family in which the father is positive, the mother is negative, and all of the sons are negative while all of the daughters are positive. This is illustrated in Figure 4-4.

The Xg^a antigen is present on the red cells of newborn infants, although it seems to be a little weaker than in adults, and it has been identified in cultured fibroblasts.[271] The antigen, or at least one closely similar to it, is present on red cells from some gibbons, where again it appears to be an X-linked character.[272]

Discovery of Xg^a, with its useful frequency, stimulated early hopes that linkages with other X-linked characters would follow quickly. However, the harvest of information has been slower to accumulate than was anticipated. A number of prominent loci on the X-chromosome, including G6PD, hemophilia, Christmas disease, deuton and proton

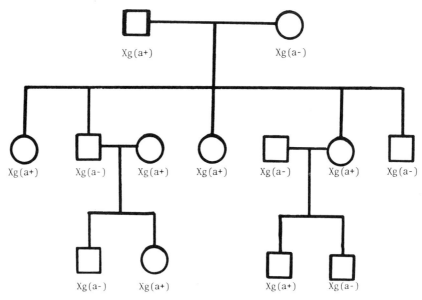

Fig. 4-4. A pedigree illustrating inheritance of the X-borne Xg^a blood group.

color blindness, and Duchenne's muscular dystrophy are not linked to Xg, but the loci for ichthyosis, occular albinism, and retinoschisis are.[159] Recent studies indicate, with good probability, that the Xk locus, which is responsible for chronic granulomatosis disease and the McLeod syndrome, is linked to Xg.[273]

One of the most useful applications of Xg^a has been to sex chromosome aneuploidy, in which there is an abnormal number of X chromosomes. The results in XO patients with Turner's syndrome, for example, show a male distribution of Xg^a, providing confirmation, if it were needed, that Xg^a is indeed X-borne. In individuals with an excess of X chromosomes, Xg^a typing may show whether the nondisjunction took place during spermatogenesis or oogenesis.

Lyon Effect and the Xg Locus

In females one of the two X chromosomes of somatic cells is inactivated, at an early stage of cell differentiation and maturation,[274] a phenomenon called Lyon effect.

Lyonization may produce mosaicism in mature cells if the woman is heterozygous for certain X-borne genes. However, not all genes on the inactivated X chromosome are silent.

Xg^a antigen has been detected using a radioimmunoassay technique; extension of the method to include autoradiography has allowed demonstration of Xg^a on individual red cells.[275] Data from these studies have confirmed earlier conclusions that the Xg locus escapes inactivation during lyonization.[276] All red cells from heterozygous Xg(a+) females have Xg^a antigen. It is of interest that Xk (which produces Kx antigen) is probably linked to Xg and is inactivated by Lyon effect. Female carriers of certain Xk variant genes have a double population of Kx-positive and Kx-negative red cells (see the Kell blood groups).

THE En^a BLOOD GROUP

The antibody called anti-En^a reacts with nearly all red cell samples. En(a−) red cells have remarkable properties, for they behave in many ways as though they have been treated with proteolytic enzymes.[277] The cells have less than half of the normal sialic acid content, show changes in their electrophoretic mobility (which is a charge-dependent phenomenon), and can be agglutinated while resuspended in saline by certain IgG blood group antibodies.[278] En(a−) cells have markedly depressed M and N antigens and lack the major sialoglycoprotein (Glycophorin A) of the red cell membrane.[279] The notation, En, in fact stands for envelope,[277] signifying the involvement of En with membrane structure. Somewhat surprisingly, En(a−) red cells have normal morphology and appear to have normal in vivo survival.

The En(a−) phenotype is inherited as an autosomal recessive characteristic, although *En* heterozygotes can be recognized by modest changes in the sialic acid level and electrophoretic mobility of their red cells.[278] Details of En[a] genetics have been elusive. The *En[a]* gene segregates independently of most known blood group systems but there are data which suggest that *En[a]* is a gene at the MN locus.[280] En(a−) red cells are also Wr(a−b−),[16] which establishes a phenotypic association with the Wright system.

The few examples of anti-En[a] have been immune IgG antibodies which were stimulated by transfusion and possibly by pregnancy. Untransfused En(a−) people do not have naturally occurring anti-En[a].

THE SID BLOOD GROUP

Anti-Sd[a], which defines the only antigen known in this system, is often difficult to work with, for the reaction strength of cell samples from different positive individuals varies greatly.[281,282] However, Sd[a] substance is present in various body fluids, particularly urine, and it is sometimes easier to categorize apparent weak Sd(a+) people by tests on their urine. Using this technique, about 4 percent of random people are Sd(a−). Rare blood samples having an enhanced red cell antigen, called Sd(a++) or "Super Sid," are known, and an even more exalted form of Sd[a] antigen,[78] named Cad, was originally thought to be a form of inherited polyagglutinability.[77] Encounters with weak examples of anti-Sd[a] are not uncommon in blood bank laboratories. Such antibodies do not cause hemolytic transfusion reactions if incompatible blood is transfused, and they can be ignored from the practical transfusion viewpoint. Strong examples of anti-Sd[a] may, however, cause a reaction if blood of a "Super Sid" donor is inadvertently transfused, but the coincidence of such rare events is highly unlikely. The main structural determinant of Sd[a] is *N*-acetyl-D-galactosamine; and because of this, Sd(a++) and Cad red cells are agglutinated by *Dolichos bifloris* lectin, which has specificity for this sugar.

Body fluids from some other animal species also contain Sd[a] substance; urine from moles, hedgehogs, or guinea pigs is a particularly rich source.[47] The successful pursuit of a guinea pig should yield a prized laboratory reagent.

The Sd[a] antigen is inherited as an autosomal dominant character and appears to be genetically independent of most other blood group systems.

An autoantibody named anti-Sd[x] has been described,[269] which seems to define a red-cell receptor related to Sd[a]. The antibody, which is inhibited by Sd(a+) urine but not by Sd(a−) urine, has been responsible for rare cases of cold antibody autoimmune hemolytic anemia.

OTHER BLOOD GROUP SYSTEMS

A large number of blood group antigens are known that cannot be fitted into any of the established systems. Many of these have a frequency of more than 99 percent, and, with such a high incidence, genetic relationships are difficult to recognize. Very few laboratories have comprehensive collections of bloods of rare types for cross-testing and, despite careful investigation, it is possible that some antigens published under different names are the same. For example, recent studies have shown that the high-incidence antigen Gn[a] is the same as Lan,[283] and that the rare antigen Far is the same as Kam.[284] Use of red cells of different null phenotypes in the investigation of antibodies to high-incidence antigens may be informative. It can be concluded, for example, that an antibody which reacts strongly with Rh_{null} or Jk(a−b−) cells is unlikely to be related to the Rh or Kidd systems.

The Diego, Dombrock, Scianna, and Colton groups are four blood group systems that, although well characterized, are rarely involved in problems of clinical blood transfusion.

Diego

The Di[a] antigen of Diego is mainly a Mongoloid characteristic.[285] Up to 35 percent of American Indians, or a smaller proportion of Orientals, are Di(a+). Only rarely has the antigen been found in a Caucasian blood sample. Anti-Di[b] [286] recognizes an antigen that is produced by an allele of *Di[a]*, and, as would be expected, it is made only by immunized people of Mongoloid origin who are homozygous for *Di[a]*. All Caucasians are Di(b+). The Diego system is of no *clinical* importance in Caucasians; the main interest lies in the field of anthropology. Di[a] has not been found in Eskimos; therefore, it is difficult to explain how the gene can be present in widely separated areas of the Mongoloid world but absent in the region of the Behring Straits, which is believed to be the topographical link between North America and Asia.

Diego has achieved full status as an independent blood group system, for it has been shown recently that it is not part of Lutheran, which was the last hurdle in its claim for independence.[287]

Dombrock

The Dombrock system has two antigens, Do[a] (frequency 66 percent),[288] and Do[b] (frequency 82 percent).[289] Few examples of anti-Do[a] or anti-Do[b] have been found. Most are IgG in nature, and they are usually fastidious in their choice of suitable antiglobulin reagents. Both Do[a] and Do[b] are well developed on fetal red cells. Dombrock is genetically independent of other blood group systems. There is evidence that the Do locus may be on chromosome 1.[290]

Scianna

Scianna is the name given to a system that resulted from a marriage between a very common antigen called Sm (frequency greater than 99.9 percent)[291] and a rare antigen called Bu[a] (frequency about 0.8 percent).[292] The discovery that an Sm negative person was Bu(a+) led to investigations which established that the antigens are, in all probability, controlled by allelic genes.[293] In a new notation, Sm is called Sc1 and Bu[a] is called Sc2. The separate identity of Scianna is almost established. The last obstacle in this claim to independent status will be difficult to clear, for it has yet to be shown that Scianna is not part of Diego. Chromosome 1 has also claimed another blood group, for it is known that it carries the Sc locus.[294] A null phenotype blood sample called Sc:−1,−2 has been found, the serum of which contains an immune antibody that reacts with all other red cell phenotypes.[295]

Colton

The Colton system has similarities to Scianna, for it has two antigens, Co[a] [296] and Co[b] [297] with the former being very common (frequency 99.8 percent) and the latter uncommon (frequency about 9 percent). Its independence from Diego also remains to be

Table 4-8. Characteristics of Some Other Red-Cell Antigens

Antigen	Frequency	Notes
Auberger (Au[a])	82 percent of Europeans are Au (a+)	Two examples of anti-Au[a] are known. The antigen has a relationship to Lutheran for dominant Lu(a−b−) red cells are Au(a−).
Cartwright (Yt[a],Yt[b])	About 0.3 percent of Caucasians are Yt (a−b+), 8 percent are Yt(a+b+), and 91.7 percent are Yt(a+b−).	Immune anti-Yt[a] is often found in the serum of Yt(a−) people.
York (Yk[a])	About 95 percent of random people are Yk(a+).	York is related to the high-incidence antigen Cs[a]. Neither is of significance from the transfusion viewpoint.
Gerbich (Ge)	Less than 0.1 percent of Caucasians are Ge(−). In New Guinea, the incidence is much higher (more than 40 percent in some areas).	Three subspecificities anti-Ge-1,-2,-3 have been described.
Langereis (Lan)	About 1 in 3000 random people is Lan negative.	There are no reported complexities.
Vel	About 1 in 4000 people is Vel negative.	Anti-Vel may be hemolytic. Subdivisions designated Vel:1 and Vel:2 have been described.
Gregory (Gy[a]) Holley (Hy)	These antigens are related. Both are of high incidence (1 in 10,000 bloods is negative).	
Jr[a]	A high-incidence antigen. Negatives were first thought to be more common in Japanese; it is now known that frequencies in Caucasians are about the same.	Anti-Jr[a] may be a strong IgG antibody.

shown. A rare null phenotype in the Colton system, Co(a−b−), was brought to light by discovery of an antibody in the serum of the propositus that reacted with all other blood samples.[298] Colton is inherited as an autosomal dominant characteristic; the locus has been provisionally assigned to chromosome 7. Examples of anti-Co[a] have been identified in many blood group reference laboratories.

A large number of other blood group antigens are known, but space does not permit their consideration. Characteristics of some of them have been summarized in Table 4-8.

BLOOD GROUPS IN CLINICAL MEDICINE

Active blood group incompatibility between the recipient of a blood transfusion and red cells of the donor may be the cause of a hemolytic reaction. Similarly, incompatibility between a mother and red cells of her fetus may be responsible for hemolytic disease in the infant at birth or in utero fetal death. A hemolytic reaction is a largely preventable complication of blood transfusion, and the responsibility for doing so falls mainly on the blood bank laboratory.

The significance of blood group antibodies in relationship to blood transfusion depends upon the conditions under which they are active and, to some extent, their specificity. Almost all antibodies of clinical significance are IgG proteins. hemolytic reactions due to incompatibility involving IgM antibodies are extremely rare. While a great number of blood group antigens are known, it is important for practical blood bankers to realize that many of them have little significance from the blood transfusion viewpoint. Clinical reactions, if incompatible blood is transfused, are almost unknown with some antibody specificities. Many antibodies to high-incidence antigens such as Ch[a], Rg[a], Bg, Yk[a], Kn[a], Cs[a], and JMH come into this category.[299-303] Antibodies of the Rhesus, Kell, Duffy, Kidd, and Ss groups have all been involved in transfusion reactions and must be considered as potentially harmful if they are found in the serum of a recipient. However, it is worth remembering that, even in these cases, if incompatible blood is inadvertently transfused, frank hemolytic reactions with obvious clinical signs are uncommon. A reaction may be shown only by laboratory tests which show premature elimination of the transfused cells. On many occasions, incompatibility that is missed by the blood bank also passes unnoticed by the clinician. These observations are not, of course, a recommendation for the casual use of incompatible blood. They are included to allow those who find themselves involved in these situations to keep a proper perspective.

Immunogenicity of Blood Group Antigens

Most clinical problems of blood transfusion are associated with antigens having high immunogenicity together with a fairly high incidence of negative (i.e., susceptible) individuals in the population. Antigens of high immunogenicity and high positive frequency do not commonly cause problems, for few people have the capability of mounting an immune response to them. Thus, Tj[a] of the P system is a potent immunogen, but only about one person in a million is Tj(a−). Similarly, rare antigens of high immunogenicity present little problem for, if an antibody to such an antigen is encountered, most donors will be compatible.

Blood group antigens vary greatly in their ability to provoke an antibody response. Some have greater immunogenicity in other animal species. For example, M and N are good immunogens in rabbits but only rarely provoke an immune response in man. Apart from A and B, the Rh D antigen has the greatest immunogenicity of the common blood

groups. At least 50 percent of Rh negative people given one unit of Rh positive blood make anti-Rh.[183,304] However, about 30 percent of Rh negative people appear to be nonresponders and do not make Rh antibody, even after repeated transfusions with Rh positive red cells.[183] The Rh C or E antigens have low immunogenicity in D negative recipients,[305] and there is little justification for C or E typing of blood donors who are found to be D negative.

Studies on hospital patients, correlating phenotype frequencies with the incidence of antibodies encountered, have allowed the calculation of the relative potency, or immunization potential, of various other blood group antigens. Anti-K is one of the most common immune antibodies encountered in transfused patients, and about 5 percent of K-negative people given one unit of K-positive blood make antibody.[229] The K antigen has about 2.5 times greater immunogenicity than c of the Rh system, about 3 times greater than E, and at least 20 times greater than any other moderately common blood group antigen.[229] Fortunately, the K antigen has a relatively low frequency (9 percent), and there is no difficulty in locating K negative donors.

Cold Agglutinins

Antibodies that are only active below physiological temperature do not cause reactions if incompatible blood is transfused.[166,306] Normal anti-I and most examples of anti-P_1, anti-A_1, and anti-H come into this category. Inclusion of a saline test at ambient or lower temperature does not contribute information of clinical significance to routine compatibility procedures. Cold agglutinins may require consideration, however, if the patient is to be subjected to hypothemia. In these cases, strong cold agglutinins should be characterized for their specificity, highest reaction temperature, and ability to bind complement. If it is not possible to supply compatible blood, it may be necessary to compromise on the extent to which the patient's temperature is lowered.

It is apparent that it is not sufficient to merely detect antibodies in recipients and to reject donors as incompatible if they possess the reactive antigen. The blood bank policy should be to assess the significance of any antibodies that are found, and then transfuse appropriate blood which may, or may not, be serologically compatible.

Antibodies in Donor Blood

When antibodies are present in the plasma of donor blood, they present little hazard. Even when the recipient's red cells carry the reactive antigen, dilution of the plasma that takes place in the recipient's circulation is sufficient to prevent recognizable complications of an antibody-antigen reaction. Only when the antibody in the donor plasma is an IgG protein of high titer does the possibility of a reaction occur. If an A or B recipient is transfused with group O blood containing potent hemolytic IgG anti-A or anti-B, the transfusion is occasionally followed by biochemical evidence of destruction of some of the recipient's red cells.[242] Severe reactions are extremely rare. It is advisable, and usually possible, to transfuse patients with blood of homologous ABO type. But, with patients having complex blood group antibodies, only group O compatible blood may be available. Use of such blood as packed red cells virtually eliminates all possibility of a reaction caused by donor anti-A or anti-B. Group O red cells that have been preserved frozen, or have been washed, may be safely transfused to recipients of any ABO type, for such cells are free of antibody.

There are no well-substantiated clinical cases in which a donor antibody with specificity outside of the ABO system has caused hemolysis of a recipient's red cells. Experimentally, 800 μg of anti-Rh immunoglobulin given to an Rh positive subject over a period of 8 days produced only a slight transient increase in serum lactate dehydrogenase but no other detectable clinical effects.[307] Transfusion of 250 ml of plasma containing moderately potent anti-Rh or anti-Kell into incompatible volunteers produced no definite evidence of red cell destruction.[308] However, transfusion of plasma containing anti-Rh with an antiglobulin titer of 1000 caused a slow fall in the recipient's packed cell volume and mild hemoglobinemia.[309] On rare occasions, a coincidence of unusual transfusion events may produce hemolysis in a recipient. For example, a K-negative patient given several units of blood—one of which was K-positive and one containing exceptionally potent anti-K (titer 2048)—suffered a transfusion reaction.[310]

It is apparent that only potent IgG antibodies have any potential for harm if they are present in donor plasma. Many blood-processing laboratories engage in the *unnecessary* practice of screening donors for antibodies using multiple procedures, which include saline tests at room or lower temperature, and then not issuing any with positive results. A test for IgG blood group antibodies that are active at 37° C will detect all antibodies of clinical importance.

PATERNITY TESTING

With rare exceptions, blood group antigens are inherited characters. In the great majority of instances an antigen will only appear on the red cells of a child if it is present on the cells of one of the parents. Providing appropriate antisera are available, determination of a blood group phenotype is usually a simple exercise with no problems in interpretation. The discovery of many new genetic markers during the past 20 years has greatly enhanced the ability to identify particular people by testing their blood. The frequency of the most common combination of phenotypes—O,

R$_1$r, MNSs, P$_1$, K−k+, Lu(a−b+) HLA1, 2, 8, 12, etc.—in Caucasians, if the 18 most commonly used red cell, leukocyte, and serum-protein markers are used, is about 1 in 60 million. As more polymorphic markers are recognized and utilized, it will undoubtedly become clear that no two unrelated individuals are alike. By utilizing these 18 markers, nonfathers can be excluded by blood tests in about 98 percent of paternity cases. Because of the large number of haplotypes, HLA typing of leukocytes is the single most useful system.

While in most cases blood group genes obey simple Mendelian laws, the existence of rare variants necessitates caution in the interpretation of family data where there is a question of disputed parentage. Silent genes are known in most of the blood group systems, but they tend to be overlooked when testing families. For example, a situation where putative parents are Lu(a+b+) and Lu(a−b+) and a child is Lu(a+b−) may not be an exclusion of parentage, for the Lu(a−b+) parent may carry a rare silent *Lu* gene. With the great increase in number of genetic markers that can be used, it is unlikely that an exclusion of parentage needs to rest on one marker.

From the opposite viewpoint, with the ability to exonerate falsely accused men has come the capability to establish, with a high degree of confidence, that ostensible parents of a particular child are in fact the biological parents. Depending upon the gene frequencies, the probability that an uninvolved man would contribute the same array of genes to the child is highly unlikely. If, after all of these tests, he is not exonerated, he is highly likely to be the father.

CONCLUSION

The great fascination of the human blood groups stems partly from their applications to anthropology, genetics, membrane structure, and forensic science, and partly from their involvement in clinical medicine. Most of the mechanisms of inheritance have models in the blood groups, for in different systems intricacies of inheritance reflect activity of recessive genes, silent alleles, independent modifiers, or gene interaction.

The mapping of autosomal genes in man began with the assignment of Duffy to chromosome 1. A large number of genes have now found homes. In linkage studies, blood groups have a particularly important place because of their potential value in genetic counseling. The genes of Duffy, Rh, Scianna, Chido, Rodgers, ABO, Xg, Xk, and probably Colton, MN, and Kidd, have been mapped so far. There may be encouragement in the fact that no other blood group genes are linked to them. This may mean that other blood group genes are spread widely over the autosomes to make a net which, in due time, will trap other linkages.

Blood group frequencies may vary greatly in different populations, but reasons for such variation are not now entirely speculative. A plausible explanation can be provided to explain population differences in Duffy blood group frequencies. The Duffy antigen, or a membrane structure related to it, is utilized by the parasite of benign tertian malaria during its invasion of the red cell. The pressure of natural selection has, presumably, caused the near elimination of Fy^a and Fy^b antigens that is seen in most African populations. At first sight it may seem surprising that a mild type of malaria could exert such selective pressure. However, evolution has probably attenuated the virulence of the parasite to give the improved host-parasite relationship that is seen today.

Some other blood group antigens have now been shown to have recognizable functional roles. Certainly the Rh$_{null}$ syndrome and the McLeod syndrome tell us that membrane affairs do not proceed properly without *Rh* or *X'k* (Kx) gene products. These blood group genes cannot be neutral from the evolutionary viewpoint. From the broad view, it seems that lack of an antigen in which specificity is determined by an immunodominant sugar carried above the membrane does not compromise the cell. But absence of an antigen that is an integral part of a membrane protein may alter the cell morphology and prevent proper cell function.[311]

The illumination that may result from collaboration between scientists in different disciplines is exemplified by the triumphant demonstration that Chido and Rodgers are markers on the fourth component of complement. But this is surely only a beginning. As rabbits can be persuaded to make antibodies to a wide range of human proteins, it is possible that the same proteins are also immunogenic in the right man, and that some of these may also masquerade as blood groups.

Although blood group antibodies signpost different components of the red cell membrane, proper understanding follows only when the curiosity of biochemists is aroused. In some systems, biochemical analysis of the antigenic structures has provided explanations for membrane relationships and for the mode of genetic control. Biochemical studies on MN antigen, for example, have led to the view that, while sugar (sialic acid) is involved in the immunodeterminants, the *MN* gene itself codes for amino acid sequences of the protein backbone. Although there are, as yet, no definitive data, it is tempting to speculate that the same model may apply to Kell. Here again it seems that sugars are involved, but it is easier to imagine that the many antigens coded for by the Kell gene reflect differences in amino-acid sequences of the peptide component of a membrane glycoprotein.

There seems to be no limit to the number of blood group specificities. Indeed, if gene duplication followed by mutation is responsible for the bewildering array of antigens that have been recognized, then the process will continue. Most large reference laboratories have collections of antibodies to either high-incidence or low-incidence antigens of unknown specificity. These antibodies may react with all random blood samples, or perhaps with only a single blood. They are, presumably, heralds of further complexities in the human blood groups.

This general overview of the blood groups is, inevitably, far from complete; it is only an appetizer. Authoritative texts, in particular the 6th edition of *Blood Groups in Man* by Race and Sanger,[159] will supply further details.

REFERENCES

1. Landsteiner, K.: Über Agglutinationserscheinungen normalen menschlichen Blutes. Wien. Klin. Wschr. 14:1132, 1901.
2. Issitt, P.D. and Issitt, C.H.: Applied blood group serology, 2nd ed., Spectra Biologicals, Oxnard, Ca 1975.
3. Springer, G.F.: Inhibition of blood-group agglutinins by substances occurring in plants. J. Immunol. 76:399, 1956.
4. Williamson, P. and Springer, G.F.: Blood group B active somatic antigen of *E. coli* O_{86}. Fed. Proc. 18:604, 1959.
5. Springer, G.F., Horton, R.E., and Forbes, M.: Origin of anti-human blood group B agglutinins in white leghorn chicks. J. Exp. Med. 110:221, 1959.
6. Cameron, G.L. and Staveley, J.M.: Blood group P substance in hydatid cyst fluids. Nature (Lond.) 179:147, 1957.
7. Prokop, O. and Schlesinger, D.: Über das vorkommen von P_1,—Blutgruppensubstanz bei einigen Metazoen, insbesondere Ascaris suum und Lumbris terrestris. Z. Immuno-Forsch. 129:344, 1965.
8. Marsh, W.L., Nichols, M.E., Øyen, R., Thayer, R.S., Deere, W.L., Freed, P.J., and Schmelter, S.E.: Naturally occurring anti-Kell stimulated by E. coli enterocolitis in a 20-day-old child. Transfusion 18:149, 1978.
9. Cleghorn, T.E.: The occurrence of certain rare blood group factors in Britain with information on their clinical importance, mode of inheritance, and relation to other established blood group systems. M.D. Thesis, University of Sheffield, 1961.
10. Contreras, M., Barbolla, L., Lubenko, A., and Armitage, S.E.: The incidence of antibodies to low frequency antigens (LFA) in

plasmapheresis donors with hyperimmune Rh antisera. Br. J. Haematol. 41:413, 1979.

11. Pavone, B.G. and Issitt, P.D.: Anti-Bg antibodies in sera used for red cell typing. Br. J. Haematol. 27:607, 1974.

12. Koo, G.C., Wachtel, S.S., Breg, W.R., and Miller, O.J.: Mapping the locus of the H-Y antigen. Cytogenet. Cell. Genet. 16:175, 1975.

13. Fraser-Roberts, J.A.: An introduction to medical genetics. 4th ed., Oxford University Press, London, 1967, p. 104.

14. Jacob, F. and Monod, J.: Genetic regulatory mechanisms in the synthesis of proteins. J. Molec. Biol. 3:318, 1961.

15. Rosenfield, R.E., Allen, F.H., Jr., and Rubinstein, P.: Genetic model for the Rh blood-group system. Proc. Natl. Acad. Sci. USA 70:1303, 1973.

16. Issitt, P.D., Pavone, B.G., Goldfinger, D., and Zwicker, H.: An En (a−) red cell sample that types as Wr (a−b−). Transfusion 15:353, 1975.

17. Pavone, B.G., Issitt, P.D., and Wagstaff, W.: Independence of Wright from many other blood group systems. Transfusion 17:47, 1977.

18. Booth, P.B., Serjeantson, S., Woodfield, D.G., and Amato, D.: Selective depression of blood group antigens associated with hereditary ovalocytosis among Melanesians. Vox Sang. 32:99, 1977.

19. Ferguson-Smith, M.A., Aitken, D.A., Turleau, C., and de Grouchy, J.: Localization of the human ABO: Np-1: AK-1 linkage group by regional assignment of AK-1 to 9q34. Hum. Genet. 34:35, 1976.

20. Westerveld, A., Jongsma, A.P.M., Meera Khan, P., Someren, H. van, and Bootsma, D.: Assignment of the AK_1; Np: ABO linkage group to chromosome 9. Proc. Natl. Acad. Sci. 73:895, 1976.

21. Cook, P.J.L., Page, B.M., Johnson, A.W., Stanford, W.K., and Gavin, J.: Four further families informative for lq and the Duffy blood group. Cytogenet. Cell Genet. 22:378, 1978.

22. Donahue, R.P., Bias, W.B., Renwick, J.H., and McKusick, V.A.: Probable assignment of the Duffy blood group locus to chromosome 1 in man. Proc. Nat. Acad. Sci. 61:949, 1968.

23. Walsh, R.J. and Montgomery, C.: A new human isoagglutinin subdividing the MN blood groups. Nature (Lond.) 160:504, 1947.

24. Sanger, R. and Race, R.R.: Subdivisions of the MN groups in man. Nature (Lond.) 160:505, 1947.

25. Watkins, W.M.: Blood group substances. Science 152:172, 1966.

26. Watkins, W.M. and Morgan, W.T.J.: Possible genetical pathways for the biosynthesis of blood group mucopolysaccharides. Vox Sang. 4:97, 1959.

27. Green, F.A.: Erythrocyte membrane lipids and Rh antigen activity. J. Biol. Chem. 247:871, 1972.

28. Lorusso, D.J., Binette, J.P., and Green, F.A.: Solubilized human erythrocytic membranes and the Rh antigen system. In: Human Blood Groups, 5th Int. Convoc. Immunol., Buffalo, N.Y., Mohn, J.F., Plunkett, R.W., Cunningham, R.K., and Lambert, R.M., eds. Karger, Basel, 1977, pp. 226–235.

29. Plapp, F.V., Kowalski, M.M., Tilzer, L., Brown, P.J., Evans, J., and Chiga, M.: Partial purification of $Rh_o(D)$ antigen from Rh positive and negative erythrocytes. Proc. Natl. Acad. Sci. 76:2964, 1979.

30. Economidou, J., Hughes-Jones, N.C., and Gardner, B.: Quantitative measurements concerning A and B antigen sites. Vox Sang. 12:321, 1967.

31. Hughes-Jones, N.C., Gardner, B., and Lincoln, P.J.: Observations of the number of available c, D, and E antigen sites on red cells. Vox Sang. 21:210, 1971.

32. Hughes-Jones, N.C. and Gardner, B.: The Kell system studied with radioactively labelled anti-K. Vox Sang. 21:154, 1971.

33. Masouredis, S.P.: Red cell membrane blood group antigens. In: Membrane structure and function of human blood cells. Am. Assoc. Blood Banks, Washington, D.C., 1976, p. 43.

34. Adinolfi, M.: Anti-I in normal newborn infants. Immunology 9:43, 1965.

35. Berroche, L., Maupin, B., Hervier, P. and Dausset, J.: Mise en evidence des antigenes A et B dans les leucocytes humains pars les epreuves d'absorption et d'elution. Vox Sang. 5:82, 1955.

36. Gurevitch, J. and Nelken, D.: A B O groups in blood platelets. Nature (Lond.) 173:356, 1954.

37. Schiff, F. and Sasaki, H.: Der Ausschei-

dungstypus, ein auf serologischem Wege nachweisbares mendelndes Merkmal. Klin. Wochenschr. 11:1426, 1932. (Translated in Secretion of Blood Group Substances and Lewis System, Vol. II, Fort Knox, U.S. Army Medical Research Lab, 1970, p. 336.)

38. Thomsen, O.: Untersuchungen über die serologische Gruppen differenzierung des Organismus. Acta Pathol. Microbiol. Scand. 7:250, 1930.

39. Renton, P.H. and Hancock, J.A.: Uptake of A and B antigens by transfused group O erythrocytes. Vox Sang. 7:33, 1962.

40. Rachkewich, R.A., Crookston, M.C., Tilley, C.A., and Wherrett, J.R.: Evidence that the A antigen on lymphocytes is derived from the plasma. Abstracts of Volunteer papers. Am. Assoc. Blood Banks, 30th Ann. Meet., 1977, p. 32.

41. Gardas, A. and Koscielak, J.: A, B, and H blood group specificities in glycoprotein and glycolipid fractions of human erythrocyte membranes. Absence of blood group active glycoproteins in the membranes of non-secretors. Vox Sang. 20:137, 1971.

42. Dzierzkowa-Borodej, W., Seyfried, H., Nichols, M., Reid, M., and Marsh, W.L.: The recognition of water soluble I blood group substance. Vox Sang. 18:222, 1970.

43. Marsh, W.L., Nichols, M.E., and Allen, F.H.: Inhibition of anti-I sera by human milk. Vox Sang. 18:149, 1970.

44. Boissezon, J.F. de, Marty, Y., Ducos, J., and Abbal, M.: Presence constante d'une substance inhibitrice de l'anticorps anti-i dans le serum humain normal. C.R. Acad. Sci. Paris 271:1448, 1970.

45. Shumak, K.H., Rachkewich, R.A., Crookston, M.C., and Crookston, J.H.: Antigens of the Ii system on lymphocytes. Nature New Biol. 231:148, 1971.

46. Grubb, R. and Morgan, W.T.J.: The 'Lewis' blood group characters of erythrocytes and body fluids. Br. J. Exp. Path. 30:198, 1949.

47. Morton, J.A., Pickles, M.M., and Terry, A.M.: The Sd^a blood group antigens in tissues and body fluids. Vox Sang. 19:472, 1970.

48. Dorf, M.E., Eguro, S.Y., Cabrera, G., Yunis, E.J., Swanson, J., and Amos, D.B.: Detection of cytotoxic non-HL-A antisera. I. relationship to anti-Le^a. Vox Sang. 22:447, 1972.

49. Marsh, W.L., Øyen, R., Nichols, M.E., and Charles, H.: Studies of MNSsU antigen activity on leukocytes and platelets. Transfusion 14:462, 1974.

50. Marsh, W.L., Øyen, R., and Nichols, M.E.: Kidd blood-group antigens of leukocytes and platelets. Transfusion 14:378, 1974.

51. Kuriyan, M.A., Øyen, R., and Marsh, W.L. (1978): Demonstration of Diego (Di^b) and Scianna (ScI) antigens on phagocytic leukocytes of the blood. Transfusion 18:361, 1978.

52. Marsh, W.L. and Øyen, R.: Demonstration of the Gerbich antigenic determinant on neutrophil leukocytes. Vox Sang. 29:69, 1975.

53. Marsh, W.L., Øyen, R., Nichols, M.E., and Allen, F.H., Jr.: Chronic granulomatous disease and the Kell blood groups. Br. J. Haematol. 29:247, 1975.

54. Morton, J.A., Pickles, M.M., and Sutton, L.: The correlation of the Bg^a blood group with the HL-A7 leukocyte group: demonstration of antigenic sites on red cells and leukocytes. Vox Sang. 17:536, 1969.

55. Morton, J.A., Pickles, M.M., Sutton, L., and Skov, F.: Identification of further antigens on red cells and lymphocytes. Association of Bg^b with W17 (Te57) and Bg^c with W28 (Da15, Ba*). Vox Sang. 21:141, 1971.

56. Nordhagen, R.: Association between HLA and red cell antigens. IV. Further studies of haemagglutinins in cytotoxic HLA antisera. Vox Sang. 32:82, 1977.

57. Harris, P.J., Tegoli, J., Swanson, J., Fischer, N., Gavin, J., and Noades, J.: A nebulous antibody responsible for cross-matching difficulties (Chido). Vox Sang. 12:140, 1967.

58. Longster, G. and Giles, C.M.: A new antibody specificity, anti-Rg^a, reacting with a red cell and serum antigen. Vox Sang. 30:175, 1976.

59. Swanson, J.: Laboratory problems associated with leukocyte antibodies. In: A seminar on recent advances in immunohematology. Amer. Assoc. Blood Banks, 1973. pp. 121–155.

60. Middleton, J.: Anti-Chido: a crossmatching problem. Canad. J. Med. Tech. 34:41, 1972.

61. Giles, C.M., Gedde-Dahl, T., Jr., Robson, E.B., Thorsby, E., Olaisen, B., Arnason, A., Kissmeyer-Nielsen, F., and Schreuder, I.: Rg^a (Rodgers) and the HLA region. Linkage

and associations. Tissue Antigens 8:143, 1976.

62. Middleton, J., Crookston, M.C., Falk, J.A., Robson, E.B., Cook, P.J.L., Batchelor, J.R., Bodmer, J., Ferrara, G.B., Festenstein, H., Harris, R., Kissmeyer-Nielsen, F., Lawler, S.D., Sachs, J.A., and Wolf, E.: Linkage of Chido and HL-A. Tissue Antigens 4:366, 1974.

63. Ochs, H.D., Rosenfeld, S.I., Thomas, E.D., Giblett, E.R., Alper, C.A., Dupont, B., Schaller, J.G., Gilliland, B.C., Hansen, J.A., and Wedgewood, R.J.: Linkage between the gene (or genes) controlling synthesis of the fourth component of complement and the major histocompatibility complex. N. Engl. J. Med. 296:470, 1977.

64. O'Neill, G.J., Yang, S.F., Berger, R., Tegoli, J., and Dupont, B.: Chido and Rodgers are distinct antigenic components of complement C4. Fed. Proc. 37:1269, 1978.

65. Tilley, C.A., Romans, D.G., and Crookston, M.C.: Localisation of Chido and Rodgers determinants to a trypic C4d fragment of human C4. P. 685 abstracts. Joint Cong. Int. Soc. Haem./Int. Soc. Blood Trans. Paris, 1978.

66. O'Neill, G.J., Yang, S.F., Tegoli, J., Berger, R., and Dupont, B.: Chido and Rodgers blood groups are distinct antigenic components of human complement C4. Nature 273:668, 1978.

67. Friedenreich, V.: The Thomsen Hemagglutination Phenomenon, Levin and Munksgaard, Copenhagen, 1930, p. 128.

68. Uhlenbruck, G., Pardoe, G.I., and Bird, G.W.G.: On the specificity of lectins with a broad agglutination spectrum. II. Studies on the nature of the T antigen and the specific receptors for the lectin of Arachis hypogaea (goundnut). Z. Immun. Forsch. 138:423, 1969.

69. Bird, G.W.G.: Significant advances in lectins and polyagglutinable red cells, p. 87. Plenary session. Joint. Cong. Int. Soc. Haem./Int. Soc. Blood Trans., Paris, 1978.

70. Moreau, R., Dausset, J., Bernard, J., and Moullec, J.: Anémie hémolytique acquise avec polyagglutinabilité des hématies par un nouveau facteur présent dans le sérum humain normal (anti-Tn). Bull. Soc. Med. Hôp. Paris. Séance, May 17th, 1957, p. 569.

71. Haynes, C.R., Dorner I., Leonard, G.L., Arrowsmith, W.R., and Chaplin, H.: Persistent polyagglutinability *in vivo* unrelated to T-antigen activation. Transfusion, 101:43, 1970.

72. Myllylä, G., Furuhjelm, U., Nordling, S., Pirkola, A., Tippett, P., and Gavin, J.: Persistent mixed field polyagglutinability: electrokinetic and serological aspects. Vox Sang. 20:7, 1971.

73. Bird, G.W.G.: Anti-T in peanuts. Vox Sang. 9:748, 1964.

73a. Bird, G.W.G.: Comparative serological studies of the T, Tn, and Cad receptors. Blut. 21:366, 1970.

74. Bird, G.W.G. and Wingham, J.: Haemagglutinins from Salvia Vox Sang. 26:183, 1974.

75. Bird, G.W.G.: Erythrocyte polyagglutination. In: CRC hand book series in clinical laboratory science. Vol. 1, section D, Blood banking, Seligson, D., ed., CRC Press, Cleveland, 1977, p 443.

76. Crookston, J.H., Crookston, M.C., Burnie, K.L., Francombe, W.H., Dacie, J.V., Davis, J.A., and Lewis, S.M.: Hereditary erythrocytic multinuclearity with a positive acid serum test. Br. J. Haematol. 23:83, 1972.

77. Cazal, P., Monis, M., Caubel, J., and Brives, J.: Polyagglutinabilité héréditaire dominante: antigene prive (Cad) correspondent a un anticorps public et à une lectine de *Dolichos biflorus*. Rev. Franc. Transfus. 11:209, 1968.

78. Sanger, R., Gavin, J., Tippett, P., Teesdale, P., and Eldon, K.: Plant agglutinin for another human blood group. Lancet i:1130, 1971.

79. Dahr, W., Uhlenbruck, G., and Bird, G.W.G.: Cryptic A-like receptor sites in human erythrocyte glyoproteins: proposed nature of Tn antigen. Vox Sang. 27:29, 1974.

80. Berman, H.J., Smarto, J., Issitt, C.H., Issitt, P.D., Marsh, W.L., and Jensen, L.: Tn activation with acquired A-like antigen. Tranfusion 12:35, 1972.

81. Cameron, C., Graham, F., Dunsford, I., Sickles, G., MacPherson, C.R., Cahan, A., Sanger, R., and Race, R.: Acquisition of a B-like antigen by red blood cells. Br. Med. J. ii:29, 1959.

82. Marsh, W.L., Jenkins, W.J., and Walther, W.W.: Pseudo B: an acquired group antigen. Br. Med. J. ii:63, 1959.

83. Gerbal, A., Maslet, C., and Salmon, C.: Immunological aspects of the acquired B antigen. Vox Sang. 28:398, 1975.

84. Judd, W.J., Beck, M.L., Hicklin, B.L., Shankar Iyer, P.N., and Goldstein, I.J.: B S II lectin: a second hemagglutinin isolated from *Bandeiraea simplicifolia* seeds with affinity for type III polyagglutinable red cells. Vox Sang. 33:246, 1977.

85. Marsh, W.L., Chaganti, R.S.K., Gardner, F.H., Mayer, K., Nowell, P.C., and German, J.: Mapping human autosomes: evidence supporting assignment of Rhesus to the short arm of chromosome 1. Science 183:966, 1974.

86. Mourant, A.E., Kopec, A., and Domaniewska-Sobczak, K.: The distribution of the human blood groups, 2nd ed. Oxford University Press, London, 1976.

87. Sanger, R., Race, R.R., and Jack, J.: The Duffy blood groups of New York Negroes: the phenotype Fy(a−b−). Br. J. Haematol. 1:370, 1955.

88. Cavalli-Sforza, L.L., Zonta, L.A., Nuzzo, F., Bernini, L., Jong, W.W.W.de, Kahn, P.M., Ray, A.K., Went, L.N., Siniscalco, M., Nijenhuis, L.E., Loghem, E. van, and Modiano, G.: Studies on African Pygmies. i. A pilot investigation of Babinga Pygmies in the Central African Republic (with an analysis of genetic diseases), Am. J. Hum. Genet. 21:252, 1969.

89. Young, M.D. and Eyles, D.E.: Experimental testing of the immunity of Negroes to *Plasmodium vivax*. J. Parasitol. 41:315, 1955.

90. Miller, L.H., Mason, S.J., Dvorak, J.A., McGinnis, M.H., and Rothman, I.K.: Erythrocyte receptors for (*Plasmodiuim Knowlesi*) malaria: Duffy blood group determinants. Science 189:561, 1975.

91. Miller, L.H., Mason, S.J., Clyde, D.F., and McGinniss, M.H.: The resistance factor to *Plasmodium vivax* in Blacks. N. Engl. J. Med. 295:302, 1976

92. McGinniss, M.H. and Miller, L.H.: Malaria, erythrocyte receptors and the Duffy blood group system. In: Cellular Antigens and disease. Am. Assoc. Blood Banks, Washington, D.C., 1977, p. 74.

93. Miller, L.H., Mason, S.J., Dvorak, J.A., Shiroishi, T., and McGinnis, M.H.: Erythrocytic receptors for malarial merozoites and the Duffy blood group system. In: Human blood groups. 5th Int. Convoc. Immunol., Buffalo, N.Y., 1976. Karger, Basel, 1977, p. 394.

94. Vos, G.H., Vos, D., Kirk, R.L., and Sanger, R.: A sample of blood with no detectable Rh antigens. Lancet i:14, 1961.

95. Levine, P., Celano, M.J., Falkowski, F., Chambers, J.W., Hunter, O.B., Jr., and English, C.T.: A second example of ---/--- or Rh$_{null}$ blood. Transfusion 5:492, 1965.

96. Chown, B., Lewis, M., Kaita, H., and Lowen, B.: An unlinked modifier of Rh blood groups: Effects when heterozygous and when homozygous. Am. J. Hum. Genet. 24:623, 1972.

97. Schmidt, P.J. and Vos, G.H.: Multiple phenotypic abnormalities, associated with Rh$_{null}$ (---/---). Vox Sang. 13:18, 1967.

98. Schmidt, P.J., Lostumbo, M.M., English, C.T., and Hunter, O.B., Jr.: Aberrant U blood group accompanying Rh$_{null}$. Transfusion 7:33, 1967.

99. Sturgeon, P.: Hematological observations on the anemia associated with blood type Rh$_{null}$. Blood 36:310, 1970.

100. Lauf, P.K.: Blood group antigens and membrane permeability in erythrocytes of man and ruminants. In: Human Blood Groups, 5th Int. Convoc. Immunol., Buffalo, N.Y., Mohn, J.F., Plunkett, R.W., Cunningham, R.K., and Lambert, R.M., eds. Karger, Basel, 1977, pp. 383–393.

101. Lauf, P.K. and Joiner, C.H.: Increased potassium transport and ouabain binding in human Rh$_{null}$ red blood cells. Blood 48:457, 1976.

102. Chown, B., Lewis, M., and Kaita, H.: A 'new' Kell blood-group phenotype. Nature (Lond.) 180:711, 1957.

103. Allen, F.H., Krabbe, S.M.R., and Corcoran, P.A.: A new phenotype (McLeod) in the Kell blood-group system. Vox Sang. 6:555, 1961.

104. van der Hart, M., Szaloky, A., van Loghem, J.J.: A "new" antibody associated with the Kell blood group system. Vox Sang. 15:456, 1968.

105. Marsh, W.L.: Revised notation for "Anti-KL" in the Kell blood group system. Vox Sang. 36:375, 1979.

106. Bridges, R.A., Berendes, H., Good, R.A.: A fatal granulomatous disease of childhood. Am. J. Dis. Child 97:387, 1959.

107. Giblett, E.R., Klebanoff, S.J., Pincus, S.H., Swanson, J., Park, B.H., and McCullough, J.: Kell phenotypes in chronic granulomatous disease: A potential transfusion hazard. Lancet i:1235, 1971.

108. Marsh, W.L., Øyen, R., and Nichols, M.E.: Kx antigen, the McLeod phenotype, and chronic granulomatous disease: further studies. Vox Sang. 31:356, 1976.

109. Quie, P.G., White, J.G., Holmes, B., and Good, R.A.: *In vitro* bactericidal activity of human polymorphonuclear leukocytes: diminished activity in chronic granulomatous disease of childhood. J. Clin. Invest. 46:668, 1967.

110. Marsh, W.L.: The Kell bloods and their relationship to chronic granulomatous disease. In: Cellular antigens and disease. Am. Assoc. Blood Banks, Washington, D.C., 1977, p. 52.

111. Windhorst, D.B., Holmes, B., and Good, R.A.: Newly defined X-linked trait in man with demonstration of the Lyon effect in carrier females. Lancet i:737, 1968.

112. Segal, A.W. and Peters, T.J.: Characterization of the enzyme defect in chronic granulomatous disease. Lancet i:1363, 1976.

113. Wimer, B.M., Marsh, W.L., Taswell, H.F., and Galey, W.R.: Haematological changes associated with the McLeod phenotype of the Kell blood group system. Br. J. Haematol. 36:219, 1977.

114. Symmans, W.A., Shepherd, C.S., Marsh, W.L., Øyen, R., Shohet, S.B., and Linehan, B.J.: Hereditary acanthocytosis associated with the McLeod phenotype of the Kell blood group system. Br. J. Haematol. 42:575, 1979.

115. Galey, W.R., Evan, A.P., Van Nice, P.S., Dail, W.G., Wimer, B.M., and Cooper, R.A.: Morphology and physiology of the McLeod erythrocyte. Vox Sang. 34:152, 1978.

115a. Marsh, W.L., Marsh, N.J., Moore, A., Symmans, W.A., Johnson, C.L., and Redman, C.M.: Evidence for an associated muscular defect in subjects with McLeod Syndrome. Vox Sang. In Press.

116. Stratton, F., Renton, P.H., and Hancock, J.A.: Red cell agglutinability affected by disease. Nature (Lond.) 181:62, 1958.

117. van Loghem, J.J., Dorfmeier, H., and van der Hart, M.: Two A antigens with abnormal serologic properties. Vox Sang. 2:16, 1957.

118. Gold, E.R., Tovey, G.H., Benney, W.E., and Lewis, F.J.W.: Changes in the group A antigen in a case of leukemia. Nature (Lond.) 183:892, 1959.

119. Salmon, C., André, R., and Philippan, J.: Agglutinabilité normale des hématies A_1 transfusées à 3 malades leucémiques de phénotype A modifié. Revue Fr. Etud. Clin. Biol. 8:792, 1961.

120. Ropars, C. and Cartron, J.P. personal communication cited by Salmon, Ch. and Cartron, J.P.: ABH blood group changes. In: Handbook series in clinical laboratory science. Section D. Blood Banking. Vol. 1, Seligson, D., ed., CRC Press, Cleveland 1977 p 201

121. Wiener, A.S.: Blood groups and disease. A critical review. Lancet, 1:813, 1962.

122. Warnowsky, J.: Über beziehung der Blutgruppen zu Krankheiten. Heterohämagglutination. Münch med. Wschr. 1758, 1927.

123. Suk, V.: Faultless teeth and blood groups (with remarks on decay and the care of teeth in whites) in Spisy lék, Fak. masaryck. Univ. Brno (Czech) 125:1, 1930.

124. Gibson, J.B., Harrison, G.A., Clarke, V.A., and Hiorns, R.W.: IQ and the ABO blood groups. Nature (Lond.) 246:498, 1973.

125. Aird, I., Bentall, H.H. and Roberts, J.A.F.: A relationship between cancer of the stomach and the ABO Blood Groups. Br. Med. J. i:799, 1953.

126. Aird, I., Bentall, H.H., Mehigan, J.H., and Roberts, J.A.F.: The blood groups in relation to peptic ulceration and carcinoma of colon, rectum, breast and bronchus: an association between the ABO groups and peptic ulceration. Br. Med. J. ii:315, 1953.

127. Clarke, C.A., Edwards, J.W., Haddock, D.R.W., Howel-Evans, A.W., and McConnell, R.B.: ABO groups and secretor character in duodenal ulcer. Population and sibship studies. Br. Med. J. ii:725, 1956.

128. Wallace, J., Brown, D.A.P., Cook, I.A., and Melrose, A.G.: The secretor status in duodenal ulcer. Scot. Med. J. 3:105, 1958.

129. Hultén, M., Luciani, J.M., Kirtan, V., Devictor-Vuillet, M.: The use and limitations of chiasma scoring with reference to human genetic mapping. Cytogenet. Cell Genet. 22:37, 1978.

130. Bhende, Y.M., Deshpande, C.K., Bhatia, H.M., Sanger, R., Race, R.R., Morgan,

W.T.J., and Watkins, W.: A "new" blood-group character related to the ABO system. Lancet i:903, 1952.

131. Levine, P., Robinson, E., Celano, M., Briggs, O., and Falkinburg, L.: Gene interaction resulting in suppression of blood group substance B. Blood 10:1100, 1955.

132. Renwick, J.H. and Lawler, S.D.: Linkage between the ABO and nail patella loci. Ann. Hum. Genet. 19:312, 1955.

133. Mohr, J.: A search for linkage between the Lutheran blood group and other hereditary characters. Acta Path. Microbiol. Scand. 28:207, 1951.

134. Weiner, W., Lewis, H.B.M., Moores, P., Sanger, R., and Race, R.R.: A gene, y, modifying the blood group antigen A. Vox Sang. 2:25, 1957.

135. Davey, R.J., Tourault, M.A., and Holland, P.V.: The clinical significance of anti-H in an individual with the O_h (Bombay) phenotype. Transfusion 18:738, 1978.

136. Dzierzkowa-Borodej, W., Meinhard, W., Nestorowicz, S., and Pirog, J.: Successful elution of anti-A and certain anti-H reagents from two Bombay (O_h^a) blood samples and investigation of isoagglutinins in their sera. Arch. Immunol. Ther. Exp. 20:841, 1972.

137. Lanset, S., Ropartz, C., Rousseau, P.-Y., Guerbet, Y., and Salmon, C.: Une famille comportante les phénotypes Bombay: O_h^a et O_h^b. Transfusion (Paris) 9:255, 1966.

138. Dodd, B.E. and Lincoln, P.J.: Serological studies of the H activity of O_h red cells with various anti-H reagents. Vox Sang. 35:168, 1978.

139. Von Dungern, E. and Hirszfeld, L.: Über Vererbung gruppenspezifischer Strukturen des Blutes. Strukturen des blutes. Z. Immun. Forsch. 6:284, 1910.

140. Bernstein, F.: Ergebnisse einer biostatischen zusammerfassenden Betrachtung über die erblichen Blutstrukturen des Menschen. Klin. Wschr 3:1495, 1924.

141. Gundolf, F. and Andersen, J.: Variant of B lacking the B antigen on the red cells. Vox Sang. 18:216, 1970.

142. Rubinstein, P., Allen, F.H., Jr., and Rosenfield, R.E.: A dominant suppressor of A and B. Vox Sang. 25:377, 1973.

143. Marsh, W.L., Ferrari, M., Nichols, M.E.,

Fernandez, G., and Cooper, K.: B_m^H: a weak B variant. Vox Sang. 25:341, 1973.

144. Davidsohn, I.: Early immunologic diagnosis and prognosis of carcinoma. Am. J. Clin. Pathol. 57:715, 1972.

145. Kassulke, J.T., Hallgren, H.M., and Yunis, E.J.: Studies of red cell isoantigens on peripheral leukocytes from normal and leukemic individuals. Am. J. Pathol. 56:333, 1969.

146. Hirzfeld, L.: *Translated in* Selected contributions to the literature of blood groups and immunology. Vol. 3, Part I, p. 109. (U.S. Army Medical Research Laboratory), F.R. Camp and F.R. Ellis, editors, 1969.

147. Seyfried, H., Walewska, I., and Weblinska, B.: Unusual inheritance of ABO group in a family with weak B antigens. Vox Sang. 9:268, 1964.

148. Lopez, M.: Le groupe sanguin cis AB. Etude quantitative et qualitative des antigènes ABH. Rev. Fr. Transfus. 19:1, 1976.

149. Yamaguchi, H.: A review of cis-AB blood. Jpn. J. Hum. Genet. 18:1, 1973.

150. Sabo, B.H., Bush, M., German, J., Carne, L.R., Yates, A.D., and Watkins, W.M.: The cis-AB phenotype in three generations of one family: serological, enzymatic, and cytogenetic studies. J. Immunogenet. 5:87, 1978.

151. Landsteiner, K. and Levine, P.: A new agglutinable factor differentiating individual human bloods. Proc. Soc. Exp. Biol. N.Y. 24:600, 1927.

152. Smith, M.L. and Beck, M.L.: The immunoglobulin structure of human anti-M agglutinins. Transfusion 19:472, 1979.

153. Howell, E.D. and Perkins, H.A.: Anti-N-like antibodies in the sera of patients undergoing chronic hemodialysis. Vox Sang. 23:291, 1972.

154. Fassbinder, W., Seidl, S., and Koch, K.M.: The role of formaldehyde in the formation of haemodialysis-associated anti-N-like antibodies. Vox Sang. 35:41, 1978.

155. White, W.L., Miller, G.E., and Kaehny, W.D.: Formaldehyde in the pathogenesis of hemodialysis-related anti-N antibodies. Transfusion 17:443, 1977.

156. Levine, P., Kuhmichel, A.B., Wigod, M., and Koch, E.: A new blood factor, s, allelic to S. Proc. Soc. Exp. Biol. N.Y. 78:218, 1951.

157. German, J., Walker, M.E. Stiefel, F.H., and

Allen, F.H.: MN blood group locus: data concerning the possible chromosomal location. Science 162:1014, 1968.

158. Wiener, A.S., Unger, L.J., and Gordon, E.B.: Fatal hemolytic transfusion reaction caused by sensitization to a new blood factor, U. J.A.M.A. 153:1444, 1953.

159. Race, R.R. and Sanger, R.: Blood groups in man. 6th ed., Blackwell, Oxford, 1975.

160. Fraser, G.R., Giblett, E.R., and Motulsky, A.G.: Population genetic studies in the Congo. III. Blood groups (ABO, MNSs, Rh, Js^a). Am. J. Hum. Genet. 18:546, 1966.

160a. Springer, G.F. and Huprika, S.V.: On the biochemical and genetic basis of the blood-group MN specificities. Haematologica 6:81, 1972.

161. Judd, W.J., Issitt, P.D., Pavone, B.G., Anderson, J., and Aminoff, D.: Antibodies that define NANA-independent MN-system antigens. Transfusion 19:12, 1979.

162. Lisowska, E. and Kordowicz, M.: Specific antibodies for desialized M and N blood group antigens. Vox Sang. 33:164, 1977.

163. Dahr, W., Uhlenbruck, G., and Knott, H.: Immunochemical aspects of the MNSs blood group system. J. Immunogenet. 2:87, 1975.

164. Walker, M.N., Rubinstein, P., and Allen, F.H.: Biochemical genetics of MN. Vox Sang. 32:111, 1977.

165. Landsteiner, K. and Levine, P.: Further observations on individual differences of human blood. Proc. Soc. Exp. Biol. N.Y. 24:941, 1927.

166. Giblett, E.R.: Blood group alloantibodies. An assessment of some laboratory practices. Transfusion 17:299, 1977.

167. Levine, P., Bobbitt, O.B., Waller, R.K., and Kuhmichel, A.: Iso immunization by a new blood factor in tumor cells. Proc. Soc. Exp. Biol. N.Y. 77:403, 1951.

168. Sanger, R.: An association between the P and Jay systems of blood groups. Nature (Lond.) 176:1163, 1955.

169. Cedergren, B.: Population studies in northern Sweden. IV. Frequency of the blood type p. Hereditas. 73:27, 1973.

170. Crawford, M.N., Tippett, P., and Sanger, R.: The antigens Au^a, i, and P$_1$ of cells of the dominant type of (Lu)a−b−). Vox Sang. 26:283, 1974.

171. Matson, G.A., Swanson, J., Noades, J.,

Sanger, R., and Race, R.R.: A "new" antigen and antibody belonging to the P blood group system. Am. J. Hum. Genet. 11:26, 1959.

172. Naiki, M. and Marcus, D.M.: Human erythrocyte P and P^k blood group antigens: identification as glycosphingolipids. Biochim. Biophys. Res. Commun. 60:1105, 1974.

173. Marcus, D.M., Naiki, M., Kundu, S.K., and Schwarting, G.A.: Immunochemical studies of the human blood group P system. In: Human Blood Groups, 5th Int. Convoc. Immunol., Buffalo, N.Y., Mohn, J.F., Plunkett, R.W., Cunningham, R.K., and Lambert, R.M., Eds. Karger, Basel, 1977, pp. 206–215.

173a. Marcus, D.M., Naiki, M., and Kundu, S.K.: Abnormalities in the glycosphingolipid content of human P^k and p erythrocytes. Proc. Natl. Acad. Sci. U.S.A. 73:3263, 1976.

174. Voak, D., Anstee, D., and Pardoe, G.: The α-galactose specificity of anti-P^k. Vox Sang. 25:263, 1973.

175. Vance, D.E. and Smeeley, C.: Quantitative determination of the neutral glycosyl ceramides in human blood. J. Lipid Res. 8:621, 1967.

176. Schwarting, G.A., Marcus, D.M., and Metaxas, M.: Identification of sialosylparagloboside as the erythrocyte receptor for an "anti-p" antibody. Vox Sang. 32:257, 1977.

177. Fellous, M., Gerbal, A., Tessier, C., Frézal, J., Dausset, J., and Salmon, C.: Studies on the biosynthetic pathway of human P erythrocyte antigens using somatic cells in culture. Vox Sang. 26:518, 1974.

178. Levine, P., Celano, M.J., and Falkowski, F.: The specificity of the antibody in paroxysmal cold hemoglobinuria (PCH). Transfusion 3:278, 1963.

179. Landsteiner, K. and Wiener, A.S.: An agglutinable factor in human blood recognized by immune sera for rhesus blood. Proc. Soc. Exp. Biol. N.Y. 43:223, 1940.

180. Levine, P. and Stetson, R.E.: An unusual case of intragroup agglutination. J.A.M.A. 113:126, 1939.

181. Diamond, L.K.: Erythroblastosis foetalis or haemolytic disease of the newborn. Proc. Roy. Soc. Med. 40:546, 1947.

182. Hey, E. and Jones, P.: Coagulation failure in babies with Rhesus immunization. Br. J. Haematol. 42:441, 1979.

183. Archer, G.T., Cooke, R.R., Mitchell, K., and

Parry, P.: Hyperimmunization of blood donors for the production of anti-Rh (D) gammaglobulin. Proc. 12th Cong. Int. Soc. Blood Trans. Moscow, 1971.

184. Tippett, P. and Sanger, R.: Observations on subdivisions of the Rh antigen D. Vox Sang. 7:9, 1962.

185. Wiener, A.S. and Unger, L.J.: Rh factors related to the Rh_0 factor as a source of clinical problems. J.A.M.A. 169:696, 1959.

186. Race, R.R.: The Rh genotypes and Fishers theory. Blood (suppl. 2):27, 1948.

187. Wiener, A.S.: Genetic theory of the Rh blood types. Proc. Soc. Exp. Biol. N.Y. 54:316, 1973.

188. Wiener, A.S.: Blood groups and transfusion. 3rd ed., Thomas, Springfield, 1943.

189. Rosenfield, R.E., Allen, F.H., Jr., Swisher, S.N., and Kochwa, S.: A review of Rh serology and presentation of a new terminology. Transfusion 2:287, 1962.

190. Ruddle, F., Riccuiti, F., McMorris, F.A., Tischfield, J., Creagen, R., Darlington, G., and Chen, T.: Somatic cell genetic assignment of peptidase C and the Rh linkage group to chromosome A-1 in man. Science 176:1429, 1972.

191. Stratton, F.: A new Rh allelomorph. Nature (Lond.) 158:25, 1946.

192. Schmidt, P.J., Morrison, E.G., and Shohl, J.: The antigenicity of the Rho (D^u) blood factor. Blood 20:196, 1962.

193. Ceppellini, R., Dunn, L.C., and Turri, M.: An interaction between alleles at the Rh locus in man which weakens the reactivity of the Rh_0 factor (D^u). Proc. Nat. Acad. Sci. Wash. 41:283, 1955.

194. Issitt, P.D.: Serology and genetics of the Rhesus blood group system. Montgomery Scientific Publications, 1979.

195. Allen, F.H. and Tippett, P.: A new Rh blood type which reveals the Rh antigen G. Vox Sang. 3:321, 1958.

196. Race, R.R., Sanger, R., and Selwyn, J.G.: A probable deletion in a human Rh chromosome. Nature (Lond.) 166:520, 1950.

197. Contreras, M., Armitage, S., Daniels, G.L., and Tippett, P.: Homozygous •D• Vox Sang. 36:81, 1979.

198. Contreras, M., Stebbing, B., Blessing, M., and Gavin, J.: The Rh antigen Evans. Vox Sang. 34:208, 1978.

199. Ishimori, T. and Hasekura, H.: A case of a Japanese blood with no detectable Rh blood group antigen. Proc. Japn. Acad. 42:658, 1966.

200. Weiner, W., Battey, D.A., Cleghorn, T., Marson, F.G.W., and Meynell, M.J.: Serological findings in a case of hemolytic anemia with some general observations on the pathogenesis of this syndrome. Br. Med. J. ii:125, 1953.

201. Celano, M.J. and Levine, P.: Anti-LW specificity in autoimmune acquired hemolytic anemia. Transfusion 7:265, 1967.

202. Weiner, W. and Vos, G.H.: Serology of acquired hemolytic anemias. Blood 22:606, 1963.

203. Callender, S.T. and Race, R.R.: A serological and genetical study of multiple antibodies formed in response to blood transfusion by a patient with lupus erythematosus diffusus. Ann. Eugen. (Lond.) 13:102, 1946.

204. Cutbush, M. and Chanarin, I.: The expected blood-group antibody, anti-Lu^b. Nature (Lond.) 178:855, 1956.

205. Crawford, M.N., Greenwalt, T.J., Sasaki, T., Tippett, P.A., Sanger, R., and Race, R.R.: The phenotype Lu(a−b−) together with unconventional Kidd groups in one family. Transfusion 1:228, 1961.

206. Taliano, V., Guévin, R.M., and Tippett, P.: The genetics of a dominant inhibitor of the Lutheran antigens. Vox Sang. 24:42, 1973.

207. Brown, F., Simpson, S., Cornwall, S., Moore, B.P.L., Øyen, R., and Marsh, W.L.: The recessive Lu(a−b−) phenotype: a family study. Vox Sang. 26:259, 1974.

208. Darnborough, J., Firth, R., Giles, C.M., Goldsmith, K.L.G., and Crawford, M.N.: A "new" antibody, anti-Lu^aLu^b, and two further examples of the genotype Lu(a−b−). Nature (Lond.) 198:796, 1963.

209. Bove, J.R., Allen, F.H., Jr., Chiewsilp, P., Marsh, W.L., and Cleghorn, T.E.: Anti-Lu4, a new antibody related to the Lutheran blood group system. Vox Sang. 21:302, 1971.

210. MacIlroy, M., McCreary, J., and Stroup, M.: Anti-Lu8, an antibody recognizing another Lutheran-related antigen. Vox Sang. 23:455, 1972.

211. Marsh, W.L.: Anti-Lu5, anti-Lu6, and anti-Lu7. Three antibodies defining high frequency antigens related to the Lutheran

blood group system. Transfusion 12:27, 1972.

212. Sinclair, M., Buchanan, D.I., Tippett, P., and Sanger, R.: Another antibody related to the Lutheran blood group system (Much). Vox Sang. 25:156, 1973.

213. Molthan, L., Crawford, M.N., Marsh, W.L., and Allen, F.H.: Lu9, another new antigen of the Lutheran blood-group system. Vox Sang. 24:468, 1973.

214. Judd, W.J., Marsh, W.L., Øyen, R., Nichols, M.E., Allen, F.H., Contreras, M., and Stroup, M.: Anti-Lu14: A Lutheran antibody defining the product of an allele at the Lu8 blood group locus. Vox Sang. 32:214, 1977.

215. Coombs, R.R.A., Mourant, A.E., and Race, R.R.: *In vivo* isosensitization of red cells in babies with hemolytic disease. Lancet i:264, 1946.

216. Conneally, P.M., Dumont-Driscoll, M., Hartzinger, R.S., Nance, W.E., and Jackson, C.E.: Linkage relations of the loci for Kell and Phenylthiocarbamide. Hum. Hered. 26:276, 1976.

217. Levine, P., Backer, M., Wigod, M., and Ponder, R.: A new human hereditary blood property (Cellano) present in 99.8% of all bloods. Science 109:464, 1949.

218. Allen, F.H., and Lewis, S.J.: Kp^a (Penney) a new antigen in the Kell blood group system. Vox Sang. 2:81, 1957.

219. Allen, F.H., Lewis, S.J., and Fudenberg, H.: Studies of anti-Kp^b, a new antibody in the Kell blood group system. Vox Sang. 3:1, 1958.

220. Yamaguchi, H., Okubo, Y., Seno, T., Matsushita, K., and Daniels, G.L.: A "new" allele, Kp^c, at the Kell complex locus. Vox Sang. 36:29, 1979.

221. Gavin, J., Daniels, G.L., Yamaguchi, H., Okubo, Y., and Seno, T.: The red cell antigen once called Levay is the antigen Kp^c of the Kell system. Vox Sang. 36:31, 1979.

222. Giblett, E.R.: Js, A "new" blood antigen found in Negroes. Nature (Lond.) 181:1221, 1958.

223. Walker, R.H., Argall, C.I., Steane, E.A., Sasaki, T.T., and Greenwalt, T.J.: Anti-Js^b, the expected antithetical antibody of the Sutter blood group system. Nature (Lond.) 197:295, 1963.

224. Sabo, B., McCreary, J., Gellerman, M., Stroup, M., Neale, P., and Bell, C.B.: Confirmation of K^{11} and K^{17} as alleles in the Kell blood group system. Vox Sang. 29:450, 1975.

225. Furuhjelm, U., Nevanlinna, H.R., Nurkka, R., Gavin, J., Tippett, P., Gooch, A., and Sanger, R.: The blood group antigen Ul^a (Karhula) Vox Sang. 15:118, 1968.

226. Allen, F.H., and Rosenfield, R.E.: Notation for the Kell blood group system. Transfusion 1:305, 1961.

227. Corcoran, P., Allen, F.H., Lewis, M., and Chown, B.: A new antibody, anti-Ku (anti-Peltz), in the Kell blood group system. Transfusion 1:181, 1961.

228. White, W., Washington, E.D., Sabo, B.H., Stroup, M., McCreary, J., Øyen, R., and Marsh, W.L.: Anti-Km in a transfused man with McLeod Syndrome. Blood Transf. Immunohematol. 23:305, 1980.

229. Giblett, E.R.: A critique of the theoretical hazard of inter *vs* intraracial transfusion. Transfusion 1:233, 1961.

230. Marsh, W.L., Øyen, R., Alicea, E., Linter, M., and Horton, S.: The Kell blood groups and autoimmune hemolytic anemia. Am. J. Hematol. 7:155, 1979.

231. Beck, M.L., Marsh, W.L., Pierce, S.R., DiNapoli, J., Øyen, R., and Nichols. M.E.: Auto anti-Kp^b associated with weakened antigenity in the Kell blood group system: a second example. Transfusion 19:197, 1979.

232. Seyfried, H., Górska, B., Maj, S., Sylwestrowicz, T., Giles, C.M., and Goldsmith, K.L.G.: Apparent depression of antigens of the Kell blood group system associated with auto immune hemolytic anemia. Vox Sang. 23:528, 1972.

233. Mourant, A.E.: A "new" human blood group antigen of frequent occurrence. Nature (Lond.) 158:237, 1946.

234. Sneath, J.S. and Sneath, P.H.A.: Transformation of the Lewis group of human red cells. Nature (Lond.) 176:172, 1955.

235. Nicholas, J.W., Jenkins, W.J., and Marsh, W.L.: Human blood chimeras: a study of surviving twins. Br. Med. J. i:1458, 1957.

236. Crookston, M.C. and Tilley, C.A.: A and B and Lewis antigens in plasma. In: Human Blood Groups. 5th Int. Convoc. Immunol.

Buffalo, N.Y., Mohn, J.F., Plunkett, R.W., Cunningham, R.K., and Lambert, R.M., Eds. Karger, Basel, 1977, pp. 246–256.

237. Rendel, J., Sorensen, A.N., and Irwin, M.R.: Evidence for epistatic action of genes for antigenic substances in sheep. Genetics 39:396, 1954.

238. Stormont, C.: Acquisition of the J-substance by bovine erythrocytes. Proc. Natl. Acad. Sci. 35:232, 1949.

239. Saison, R. and Ingram, D.G.: A report on blood groups in pigs. Ann. N.Y. Acad. Sci. 97:226, 1962.

240. Andresen, P.H.: Blood groups with characteristic phenotypical aspects. Acta. Path. Microbiol. Scand. 24:616, 1948.

241. Mollison, P.L. and Polley, M.J.: Temporary suppression of Lewis blood-group antibodies to permit incompatible transfusion. Lancet i:909, 1963.

242. Mollison, P.L.: Blood transfusion in clinical medicine. 6th ed. Blackwell, Oxford, 1979.

243. Andresen, P.H., and Jordal, K.: An incomplete agglutinin related to the L (Lewis) system. Acta Path. Microbiol. Scand. 26:636, 1949.

244. Gunson, H.H. and Latham, V.: An agglutinin in human serum reacting with cells from Le(a−b−) non-secretor individuals. Vox Sang. 22:344, 1972.

245. Potapov, M.I.: Detection of the antigen of the Lewis system, characteristic of the erythrocytes of the secretory group Le(a−b−). Probl. Haemathol. (Moscow) No. 11, 45, 1970.

246. Graham, H.A., Hirsch, H.F., and Davies, D.M.: Genetic and immunochemical relationships between soluble and cell-bound antigens of the Lewis system. In: Human Blood Groups. 5th Int. Convoc. Immunol. Buffalo, N.Y., Mohn, J.F., Plunkett, R.W., Cunningham, R.K., and Lambert, R.M., Eds. Karger, Basel, 1977, pp. 257–267.

247. Cutbush, M., Mollison, P.L., and Parkin, D.M.: A new human blood group. Nature (Lond.) 165:188, 1950.

248. Ikin, E.W., Mourant, A.E., Pettenkofer, H.J., and Blumenthal, G.: Discovery of the expected haemagglutinin anti-Fy[b]. Nature (Lond.) 168:1077, 1951.

249. Chown, B., Lewis, M., and Kaita, H.: The Duffy blood group in Caucasians: evidence for a new allele. Am. J. Hum. Genet. 17:384, 1965.

250. Albrey, J.A., Vincent, E.E.R., Hutchinson, J., Marsh, W.L., Allen, F.H., Jr., Gavin, J., and Sanger, R.: A new antibody, anti-Fy3, in the Duffy blood-group system. Vox Sang. 20:29, 1971.

251. Behzad, O., Lee, C.L., Gavin, J. and Marsh, W.L.: A new anti-erythrocyte antibody in the Duffy system: anti-Fy4. Vox Sang. 24:337, 1973.

252. Colledge, K.I., Pezzulich, M., and Marsh, W.L.: Anti-Fy5, an antibody disclosing a probable association between the Rhesus and Duffy blood group genes. Vox Sang. 24:193, 1973.

253. Allen, F.H., Diamond, L.K., and Niedziela, B.: A new blood-group antigen. Nature (Lond.) 167:482, 1951.

254. Plaut, G., Ikin, E.W., Mourant, A.E., Sanger, R., and Race, R.R.: A new blood group antibody: anti-Jk[b]. Nature (Lond.) 171:431, 1953.

255. Keats, B.J.B., Morton, N.E., and Rao, D.C.: Possible linkages (lod score over 1.5) and a tentative map of the *JK-Km* linkage group. Cytogenet. Cell Genet. 22:304, 1978.

256. Pinkerton, F.J., Mermod, L.E., Liles, B.A., Jack, J., Jr., and Noades, J.: The phenotype Jk(a−b−) in the Kidd blood group system. Vox Sang. 4:155, 1959.

257. Humphrey, A.J. and Morel, P.A.: Further evidence of heterogeneity within the Kidd blood group system. Transfusion 16:242, 1976.

258. Wiener, A.S., Unger, L.J., Cohen, L., and Feldman, J.: Type-specific cold autoantibodies as a cause of acquired hemolytic anemia and hemolytic transfusion reactions. Biologic test with bovine red cells. Ann. Intern. Med. 44:221, 1956.

259. Feizi, T., Kabat, E.A., Vicari, G., Anderson, B., and Marsh, W.L.: Immunochemical studies on blood groups. XLVII. The I antigen complex-precursors in the A, B, H, Le[a] and Le[b] blood group system—hemagglutination-inhibition studies. J. Exp. Med. 133:39, 1971.

260. Marsh, W.L.: Anti-i: a cold antibody defining the Ii relationship in human red cells. Br. J. Haematol. 7:200, 1961.

261. Jenkins, W.J. and Marsh, W.L.: Unpublished observations cited by Race, R.R. and Sanger,

R. (1975) Blood Groups in man. 6th ed., Blackwell, Oxford, 1961.

262. Giblett, E.R. and Crookston, M.C.: Agglutinability of red cells by anti-i in patients with Thalassaemia major and other haematological disorders. Nature (Lond.) 201:1138, 1964.

263. Hillman, R.S. and Giblett, E.R.: Red cell membrane alteration associated with marrow stress. J. Clin. Invest. 44:1730, 1965.

264. Jenkins, W.J., Koster, H.G., Marsh, W.L., and Carter, R.L.: Infectious mononucleosis: an unsuspected source of anti-i. Br. J. Haematol. ii:480, 1965.

265. Wiener, A.S., Moor-Jankowski, J., Gordon, E.B., Davis, J.: The blood factors I and i in primates including man, and in lower species. Am. J. Phys. Anthrop. 23:389, 1965.

266. Marsh, W.L. and Jenkins, W.J.: Anti-Sp₁: the recognition of a new cold auto-antibody. Vox Sang. 15:177, 1968.

267. Roelcke, D.: A review. Cold agglutination. Antibodies and antigens. Clin. Immunol. Immunopathol. 2:266, 1974.

268. Roelcke, D., Riesen, W., Geisen, H.P., and Ebert, W.: Serological identification of the new cold agglutinin specificity anti-Gd. Vox Sang. 33:304, 1977.

269. Marsh, W.L., Johnson, C.L., Øyen, R., Nichols, M.E., DiNapoli, J., Young, H., Brassel, J., Cusumano, I., Bazaz, G.R., Haber, J., and Wolf, C.F.W.: Anti-Sd^x: a "new" auto agglutinin related to the Sd^a blood group. Transfusion 20:1, 1980.

270. Mann, J.D., Cahan, A., Gelb, A.G., Fisher, N., Hamper, J., Tippett, P., Sanger, R., and Race, R.R.: A sex linked blood group. Lancet i:8, 1962.

271. Fellous, M., Bengtsson, B., Finnegan, D., and Bodmer, W.F.: Expression of the Xg^a antigen on cells in culture and its segregation in somatic cell hybrids. Ann. Hum. Genet. 37:421, 1974.

272. Gavin, J., Noades, J., Tippett, P., Sanger, R., and Race, R.R.: Blood group antigen Xg^a in gibbons. Nature (Lond.) 204:1322, 1964.

273. Marsh, W.L.: Linkage relationship of the Xg and Xk loci. Cytogenet. Cell Genet. 22:531, 1978.

274. Lyon, M.F.: Genetic factors on the X chromosome. Lancet ii:434, 1961.

275. Szabo, P., Campana, T., and Siniscalco, M.:

Radioimmune assay for the Xg(a) surface antigen at the individual red cell level. Biochem. Biophys. Res. Commun. 78:655, 1977.

276. Race, R.R.: Is the Xg blood group locus subject to inactivation? Proc. 4th Int. Cong. Hum. Genet., Excerpta Medica, Amsterdam, 1971, p. 311.

277. Darnborough, J., Dunsford, I., and Wallace, J.A.: The En factor. A genetic modification of human red cells affecting their blood grouping reactions. Program Brit. Soc. Haemat. Meet., 1975, p. 28.

278. Furuhjelm, U., Myllylä, G., Nevanlinna, H.R., Nordling, S., Pirkola, A., Gavin, J., Gooch, A., Sanger, R., and Tippett, P.: The red cell phenotype En(a−) and anti-En^a: serological and physiochemical aspects. Vox Sang. 17:256, 1969.

279. Tanner, M.J.A. and Anstee, D.J.: The membrane change in En(a−) human erythrocytes. Biochem. J. 153:271, 1976.

280. Metaxas, M.N. and Metaxas-Bühler, M.: Rare genes of the MNSs system affecting the red cell membrane. In: Human Blood Groups, 5th Int. Convoc. Immunol., Buffalo, N.Y., Mohn, J.F., Plunkett, R.W., Cunningham, R.K., and Lambert, R.M., eds. Karger, Basel, 1977, pp. 344–352.

281. Macvie, S.I., Morton, J.A., and Pickles, M.M.: The reactions and inheritance of a new blood group antigen, Sd^a. Vox Sang. 13:485, 1967.

282. Renton, P.H., Howell, P., Ikin, E.W., Giles, C.M., and Goldsmith, K.L.G.: Anti-Sd^a a, a new blood group antibody. Vox Sang. 13:493, 1967.

283. Nesbit, R.: The red cell antigen Gn^a. Transfusion, 19:354, 1979.

284. Giles, C.M.: The identity of Kamhuber and Far antigens. Vox Sang. 32:269, 1977.

285. Layrisse, M., Arends, T., and Sisco, R.D.: Nuevo grupo sanguineo encontrado en descendientes de Indios. Acta Med. Venez. 3:132, 1955.

286. Thompson, P.R., Childers, D.M., and Hatcher, D.E.: Anti-Di^b—first and second examples. Vox Sang. 13:314, 1967.

287. Buchanan, D.I., Makelki, D., Marsh, S., and Gangopadhyay, K.C.: Genetic independence of the Lutheran and Diego blood group loci. Transfusion 17:277, 1977.

288. Swanson, J., Polesky, H.F., Tippett, P., and Sanger, R.: A new blood group antigen, Do[a]. Nature 206:313, 1965.

289. Molthan, L., Crawford, M.N., and Tippett, P.: Enlargement of the Dombrock blood group system: the finding of anti-Do[b]. Vox Sang. 24:382, 1973.

290. Lewis, M., Kaita, H., Giblett, E.R., and Anderson, J.E.: Genetic linkage analysis of the Dombrock (Do) blood group locus. Cytogenet. Cell Genet. 22:313, 1978.

291. Schmidt, R.P., Griffitts, J.J., and Northman, F.F.: A new antibody, anti-Sm, reacting with a high incidence antigen. Transfusion 2:338, 1962.

292. Anderson, C., Hunter, J., Zipursky, A., Lewis, M., and Chown, B.: An antibody defining a new blood group antigen, Bu[a]. Transfusion 3:30, 1963.

293. Lewis, M., Kaita, H., and Chown, B.: Scianna blood group system. Vox Sang. 27:261, 1974.

294. Lewis, M., Kaita, H., and Chown, B.: Genetic linkage between the human blood group loci *Rh* and *Sc*. Am. J. Hum. Genet. 28:619, 1976.

295. McCreary, J., Vogler, A.L., Sabo, B., Eckstein, E.G., and Smith, T.R.: Another minus-minus phenotype: Bu(a−) Sm− two examples in one family. Transfusion 13:350, 1973.

296. Heistö, H., van der Hart, M., Madsen, G., Moes, M., Noades, J., Pickles, M.M., Race, R.R., Sanger, R., and Swanson, J.: Three examples of a new red cell antibody, anti-Co[a]. Vox Sang. 12:18, 1967.

297. Giles, C.M., Damborough, J., Aspinall, P., and Fletton, M.W.: Identification of the first example of anti-Co[b]. Br. J. Haematol. 19:267, 1970.

298. Rogers, M.J., Stiles, P.A., and Wright, J.: A new minus-minus phenotype: three Co(a−b−) individuals in one family. Abstracts of Volunteer papers. Am. Assoc. Blood Banks 27th Ann. Meet., 1974, p. 95.

299. Moore, H.C., Issitt, P.D., and Pavone, B.G.: Successful transfusion of Chido opositive blood to two patients with anti-Chido. Transfusion 15:266, 1975.

300. Nordhagen, R. and Aas, M.: Association between HLA and red cell antigens. VII. Survival studies of incompatible red cells in a patient with HLA-associated haemagglutinins. Vox Sang. 35:319, 1978.

301. Sabo, B., Moulds, J., and McCreary, J.: Anti-JMH: another high titer low avidity antibody against a high frequency antigen. Abstracts of Volunteer papers. Am. Assoc. Blood Banks, 30th Ann. Meet., 1977, p. 25.

302. Shore, G.M. and Steane, E.A.: Survival of incompatible cells in a patient with anti-Cs[a] and three other patients with antibodies to high-frequency red cell antigens. Abstracts of volunteer papers. Am. Assoc. Blood Banks. 30th Ann. Meet., 1977, p. 26.

303. Tilley, C.A., Crookston, M.C., Haddad, S.A., and Shumak, K.H.: Red blood cell survival studies in patients with anti-Ch[a], anti-Yk[a], anti-Ge, and anti-Vel. Transfusion 17:169, 1977.

304. Archer, G.T., Cooke, R.R., Mitchell, K. and Parry, P.: Hyper-immunization des donneurs de sang pour la production des gamma-globulines anti-Rh (D). Rev. Franc. Transfus. 12:341, 1969.

305. Schorr, J.B., Schorr, P.T., Francis, R., Spierer, G., and Dugan, E.: The antigenicity of C and E antigens when transfused into Rh-negative and Rh-positive recipients. Prog. 24th Ann. Meet. Am. Assoc. Blood Banks, 1971, p. 100.

306. Mollison, P.L.: Factors determining the relative clinical importance of different blood-group antibodies. Br. Med. Bull. 15:92, 1959.

307. Hoppe, H.: Personal communication cited by Mollison, P.L. Blood transfusion in clinical medicine. 6th ed. Blackwell, Oxford, 1979, p. 556.

308. Mohn, J.F., Bowman, H.S., Lambert, R.M., and Brason, F.W.: Experimental transfusion of donor plasma containing blood-group antibodies into incompatible normal human recipients. I. Absence of destruction of red cell mass with anti-Rh, anti-Kell and anti-M. Br. J. Haematol. 7:112, 1961.

309. Bowman, H.S., Brason, F.W., Mohn, J.F., and Lambert, R.M.: Experimental transfusion of donor plasma containing blood group antibodies into incompatible normal recipients. II. Induction of iso-immune hemolytic anemia by a transfusion of plasma containing exceptional anti-CD antibodies. Br. J. Haematol. 7:130, 1961.

310. Zettner, A. and Bove, J.R.: Hemolytic transfusion reaction due to interdonor incompatibility. Transfusion 3:48, 1963.
311. Levine, P., Tripodi, D., Struck, J., Jr., Zmijewski, C.M., and Pollack, W.: Hemolytic anemia associated Rh_{null} but not with Bombay blood. Vox Sang. 24:417, 1973.

5

Lectins and Polyagglutination

G.W.G. Bird, D.Sc., Ph.D., M.B.B.S., F.R.C. Path.

Lectins are proteins present in plants (usually in their seeds); in the hemolymph, albumin glands, or eggs of some invertebrate animals; and in the plasma of some lower vertebrate animals.[1] Lectins now have a leading place in biological research in a wide variety of scientific applications,[2,3,4] including: blood grouping and blood group research; the elucidation of erythrocyte polyagglutination; studies of cell-membrane structure; research in tumor immunology; and, because of the mitogenic properties of some extracts, routine cytogenetics. Indeed, mitogenic stimulation of lymphocytes by lectins has completely revolutionized cytogenetics and its application to clinical problems.

This chapter is devoted to those lectins—many of which are highly specific for red cell membrane receptors—which have found useful application in blood grouping and blood group research, with particular reference to the identification and characterization of erythrocyte polyagglutination.

BASIS OF LECTIN SPECIFICITY

Lectins combine with sugars, for which they have a strong affinity, and therefore react only with cell membrane receptors or body fluid constituents, which are carbohydrate, glycolipid, or glycoprotein. They combine with single sugars or only parts of single sugars. Many lectins are highly specific; however, their specificity is not entirely dependent on the mere presence of reactive sugar in terminal (or sometimes subterminal) position in the carbohydrate chain, but is also influenced by various other factors such as anomeric conformation; the nature of the carrier sugar, lipid, or protein; the site of attachment of the reactive sugar to the carrier structure; the number and distribution of reactive sites on the red surface; and the amount of steric hindrance from vicinal structures. The most important factor is the outward conformational display of the receptor site, which may depend on its carbohydrate configuration alone, or on the configuration imparted to the carbohydrate chain by the structure of the protein or lipid to which it is attached.

There are only seven sugar constituents of the human red cell membrane: galactose, mannose, fucose, glucose, acetylglucosamine, acetylgalactosamine, and N-acetylneuraminic (sialic) acid. Red cell membrane carbohydrates are therefore combinations of these seven sugars and differ in the serial order of the sugar constituents, in their sites of attachment to each other or to protein or lipid, and in the anomeric nature of the linkage between them. Since there is inevitably some similarity in these various combinations it is not surprising that many lectins cross-react. What is surprising however is the high degree of specificity of some lectins.

Early studies of lectin specificity were conducted with conventional panels of human red blood cells. Recently however several new specificities have been detected by the use of exotic panels of various polyagglutinable erythrocytes.

LECTINS SPECIFIC FOR ERYTHROCYTE ANTIGENS

Many lectins specific for various red cell antigens are now known (Table 5-1). Some of these lectins are established as useful reagents in routine blood grouping and in blood group research. The most useful and widely used is the remarkable lectin from the seeds of *Dolichos biflorus*[5] which reacts much more strongly and quickly on A_1 or A_1B cells than on those of the weaker subgroups of A or AB and therefore provides a reliable and avid specific anti-A_1 reagent. The *Dolichos* lectin and the anti-A lectin from the albumin gland or eggs of *Helix pomatia*[6] or other snails are also reliable when used in automated blood grouping machines.

The *Dolichos biflorus* and other lectins are ideal for separating mixtures of red cells of different blood groups in the investigation of mosaics and chimeras. For example a mixture of A_1 and O red cells can be separated by means of the *Dolichos* lectin which forms dense agglutinates of A_1 cells which fall to the bottom of the tube, either by gravity or after slow centrifugation, leaving O cells in the supernatant. The agglutinated A_1 cells are washed and resuspended in isotonic saline solution. The A_1 cells are then readily disagglutinated by neutralizing the lectin with a one percent aqueous solution of N-acetyl-D-galactosamine or a solution of purified group A-specific substance. The disagglutinated A_1 cells are washed and resuspended, apparently without adverse effect on their A-receptor sites.

The anti-H lectin from *Ulex europaeus* seeds is a good reagent for distinguishing group O secretors from non-secretors, because it is very readily inhibited by H-blood group active substance present in the saliva of secretors. The anti-N lectin from *Vicia graminea* seeds has been useful in research studies of the biosynthesis of the M and N antigens. Many other lectins have proved to be very valuable in the investigation of erythrocyte polyagglutination as described below. This application has helped to increase our

Table 5-1. Specific Lectins for Human Red Blood Cells

Predominant specificity[a]	Selected example of source of lectin
Anti-A	*Helix pomatia*
Anti-A_1, −Tn, −Cad	*Dolichos biflorus*
Anti-B	*Fomes fomentarius*
Anti-H	*Cytisus glabrescens*
Anti-A+B	*Phlomis fruticosa*
Anti-N[b]	*Vicia graminea*
Anti-A+N	*Moluccella laevis*
Anti-T, −Tk, −Th	*Arachis hypogaea*
Anti-Tk	*Bandeiraea simplicifolia II* (BS II)
Anti-Tn	*Salvia sclarea*
Anti-Cad	*Leonurus cardiaca*

[a] Lectin specificity is not exactly the same as the specificity of the corresponding human antibody.
[b] Could be visualized as anti-N+T

knowledge of red cell membrane structure.[7]

Many lectins also act as specific precipitins and form dense precipitates with the corresponding antigens in solution. For example, *Dolichos biflorus* is a powerful precipitin for A-substance in solution, and forms dense precipitates when added to the saliva of a group A_1 secretor.

It is easy to prepare seed extracts and it is easy to do hemagglutination tests. However, the potency of seed lectins may vary with the source of seed and the technique of extraction, so that unreliable information is often published by workers who are not sufficiently experienced in blood group serology.

Crude seed extracts are suitable for most purposes. Purified preparations of some lectins are commercially available, which are clear and stable and are ideal for precipitation studies.

Lectins for red blood cells act best on slides or tiles because the "rocking" movement essential to the tile technique is ideal for lectin agglutination. Avidity studies on tiles give a more rapid and clear indication of lectin selectivity than titration studies in tubes.

ERYTHROCYTE POLYAGGLUTINATION

Erythrocyte polyagglutination is generally defined as the agglutination of red cells, irrespective of blood group, by many sera. The abnormality is a property of the red cells, not the sera. The polyagglutinable cells may be altered, defective or otherwise abnormal.[4,8,9] Interest in the subject has been revived in recent years and several studies have contributed very usefully not only to Clinical Pathology but also to knowledge of red cell membrane structure and of lectin specificity. Indeed a "symbiotic relationship"[4] between lectins and polyagglutination has been formed in recent years because increasing use of lectins has led to the demonstration of new forms of polyagglutination, and the new forms of polyagglutination have led to the discovery of new lectin specificities.[4,10]

Classification of Polyagglutination

There are two broad classes of polyagglutinable red cells; acquired and inherited; the acquired forms are conveniently subdivided into microbial and non-microbial classes (Table 5-2).

Acquired Polyagglutination (Microbial)

There are two ways in which bacteria can produce polyagglutinable red cells: first by the passive coating of red cells with bacteria or their products, and second by the action of bacterial or viral enzymes on the red cell surface. Polyagglutination due to the second mechanism is much more commonly observed.

Table 5-2. Classification of Red Cell Polyagglutination

MICROBIAL	
Acquired	
a. Passive	Adsorption of bacteria or bacterial products by red cells
b. Enzymic	T, Tk, Acquired B
c. Probably enzymic	VA, Th
NONMICROBIAL	
Acquired (by somatic mutation)	Tn
Inherited	Cad, HEMPAS

Passive Microbial Polyagglutination

Bacterial antigens are adsorbed by red cells, which are then agglutinated by sera which contain the specific antibacterial antibody.[11,12] In many examples there is direct agglutination of the red cells; in others the red cells are not agglutinated directly, but give positive antiglobulin tests, which demonstrate that antibacterial antibody has combined with bacteria or bacterial product adherent to the red cell surface.[13]

Enzymic Microbial Polyagglutination

T- and Tk-polyagglutination, and the acquired B state, definitely belong to this category, which probably also includes Th- and VA-polyagglutination.

Acquired Polyagglutination (Nonmicrobial)

The only known form of acquired nonmicrobial polyagglutination is the interesting phenomenon of Tn-polyagglutination.

Inherited Polyagglutination

This category consists of Cad-polyagglutination and the polyagglutination associated with the hematological disorder known as HEMPAS.

T-POLYAGGLUTINATION

T-polyagglutination was observed by Hübener,[14] Schiff and Halberstädter,[15] and Thomsen,[16] and extensively studied by Friedenreich[17] (for a recent review see[18]). The normally latent red cell receptor T is exposed by microbial neuraminidase, an enzyme, correctly a group of enzymes, which specifically split N-acetylneuraminic acid from cell surfaces. Many microbes make neuraminidase: the best known are *Vibrio cholerae*, *Clostridium perfringens*, *Diplococcus pneumoniae*, and the influenza virus. The substrate for neuraminidase in humans is N-acetylneuraminic acid (NANA), also known as sialic acid, which is an important constituent of the red cell membrane. NANA contributes largely to the net negative charge of red cells, and therefore to the maintenance of their separate state.

T-transformed red cells are polyagglutinable because most adult sera contain naturally occurring (IgM) anti-T antibodies which can fix complement.[19] T-transformation is usually observed as an in vitro condition when blood specimens sent for laboratory investigation are contaminated by neuraminidase-producing bacteria. The red cells from such contaminated blood specimens give anomalous blood grouping results because of the presence of anti-T in grouping sera. More interestingly T-transformation may occur as an in vivo state; the earlier literature on in vivo T-polyagglutination has been reviewed by Chorpenning and Hayes.[20] For in vivo T-polyagglutination to occur, neuraminidase, derived from bacteria in the blood or which enter the bloodstream from septic lesions or inflamed organs, must be present in sufficient amounts to first neutralize enzyme-inhibitors normally present in plasma. The same is true for other forms of polyagglutination due to microbial enzymes.

The identification of T-transformed cells is rapidly and reliably made with the peanut (*Arachis hypogaea*)[21] lectin and other lectins as mentioned below.

Clinical Aspects of in vivo T-Polyagglutination

In vivo T-polyagglutination may be associated with hemolytic anemia.[22-26] It may also be associated with hemolytic transfusion reactions, especially in children, due to anti-T in donor plasma.[24,27]

Anti-T may also be responsible for some examples of the hemolytic-uremic syndrome, in which hemolytic anemia, thrombocytopenia and renal impairment are the consequence of exposure of T-receptors of red cells, platelets and renal glomeruli respectively. Klein et al.[28] have described two examples of the hemolytic uremic syndrome in pneumococcal pneumonia in which exposure of the T-antigen was demonstrated by immunofluorescence techniques using fluorescein-labelled peanut lectin.

In vivo T-polyagglutination is particularly prone to occur in children[29] with lung or bowel disease. Rickard et al.[22] reported polyagglutination with acute hemolysis in a 14-month-old child with bilateral bronchopneumonia and Obeid et al.[30] described two children, one with congenital megacolon (Hirschsprungs's Disease) and one with *volvulus neonatorum* in which T-transformation, ordinarily a transient condition, persisted for months. Seger et al.[31] have described erythrocyte T-transformation in a premature baby with fulminant necrotizing enterocolitis with *Clostridium perfringens* bacteremia. Both Obeid et al.[29] and Seger et al.[31] drew attention to the importance of using washed cells for blood transfusions to patients with in vivo T-polyagglutination, and Obeid et al.[29] emphasized that all blood group AB findings in very young babies be carefully checked to exclude polyagglutination as a source of error.

A possible example of prenatal T-transformation has been described by Jørgensen,[32] in which cord blood cells were found to be polyagglutinable. The infant became jaundiced, but this was probably unrelated to polyagglutinability because newborn children lack antibodies, and maternal anti-T, an IgM antibody, could not have been responsible. The serological findings were not compatible with a diagnosis of T-transformation. This example may really have been another form of erythrocyte polyagglutination e.g. Tk or Th, which was unknown at the time. The association of the T-antigen with breast cancer and with the MN biosynthetic pathway is discussed below.

Tk-Polyagglutination

For many years T-transformation was the only known form of erythrocyte polyagglutination which was clearly the result of exposure of a latent red cell membrane receptor through the action of a microbial enzyme.

In 1972 however Bird and Wingham[33] described a new form of polyagglutination, clearly different to T, which they named Tk. Tk cells are agglutinated by the peanut lectin, but have normal levels of sialic acid. Tk cells are agglutinated by sera from which anti-T has been absorbed. Agglutination of Tk cells by the peanut lectin is enhanced after the red cells are treated with papain. An example of co-existent T- and Tk-polyagglutination was investigated by Inglis et al.[34] which suggested that *Bacteroides fragilis* was probably responsible. This possibility was soon confirmed when Bird et al.[35] found that the red cells of a patient with *Bacteroides fragilis* septicemia were strongly Tk-polyagglutinable. In another example of *Bacteroides fragilis* septicemia the red cells were not Tk-polyagglutinable. This was however shown by Inglis to be due to a powerful inhibitor in the patient's serum.[10] Further studies of the effect of *Bacteroides fragilis* on the red cell membrane[36,37] have shown that early recognition of Tk may be an aid to the diagnosis of *Bacteroides fragilis* infection strong enough to neutralize enzyme inhibitor usually present in plasma. Furthermore it was shown that various strains of *Bacteroides fragilis* secrete a number of enzymes including neuraminidase, α-fucosidase and the hitherto unidentified Tk-producing enzyme. Some strains of *Bacteroides fragilis* are capable of exposing the Tk-receptors only, so that, by use of their culture supernatants, Tk-polyagglutinable red cells can readily be produced for laboratory use.

Tk-polyagglutination may be associated with T-polyagglutination, VA-polyagglutination or the acquired B state. Furthermore, it is invariably associated with depressed H-receptors,[37,38,39] and sometimes with depressed A,[37] or depressed I- and i-antigens.[39] The enzyme responsible for Tk may therefore be a glycosidase which acts at a point on the carbohydrate precursor chain common to the ABH and Ii antigens.

Some examples previously reported as T-polyagglutination may have actually been Tk or one of the "newer" forms of polyagglutination described below.

The finding of Tk-polyagglutination led to the discovery of a very useful specific anti-Tk lectin, BSII, isolated from the seeds of *Bandeiraea simplicifolia.*[40] The lectin is specifically inhibited by N-acetyl-D-glucosamine;[40] the precise significance of this observation has not yet been determined.

Acquired B

If polyagglutination is defined as in the beginning of this section, acquired B does not qualify for inclusion under this heading. Nevertheless it is usually classified as a form of polyagglutination, on an "honorary" basis because its mechanisms of production are similar to those of various forms of microbial polyagglutination and because it is often present together with one or more of them.

Passively Acquired B. It is possible in vitro to coat group O or A cells with bacterial lipopolysaccharides, e.g. from *E. coli* O_{86} and *Proteus vulgaris* OX19[41,42] structurally similar to the human blood group antigen B, so that they appear to have acquired a B antigen. *E. coli* O_{86} and *Proteus vulgaris* OX19 have some A-activity as well[42,43] which may be too weak to be noticed on O cells and would not be noticed at all on A_1 cells. An *in vivo* example of acquired B in a *Proteus vulgaris* infection has been described;[44] it is not clear however whether it was passively acquired or of enzymic origin.

Enzymic Acquired B. This type of acquired B is the one usually found as an in vivo condition and occurs only in group A persons. It was first described by Cameron et al. in 1959.[45] The condition usually occurs in cancer of the colon and sometimes in other cancers, chiefly those of the alimentary tract, and in various infections.[46] However it is also found in perfectly healthy persons.[46]

Studies by Gerbal et al.[47,48] have shown that the in vivo acquired B state is probably due to the action of a microbial deacetylase which converts N-acetyl-D-galactosamine, the immunodominant sugar of A-specificity to D-galactosamine, which crossreacts with D-galactose, the immunodominant sugar of B-specificity. Acquired B activity increases as A-reactivity declines. This process is reversed during recovery.

Acquired B red cells react with an anti-B antibody in human sera which is not identical with that which agglutinates normal B cells. Acquired B is best detected by the use of anti-B serum from an A_2 person.[47]

The acquired B state may be associated with a form of polyagglutination peculiar to itself or with other forms of polyagglutination e.g. T, Tk. the polyagglutination peculiar to acquired B is enhanced after the red cells are treated with papain.

Theoretically acquired B should be commoner than it is. Its incidence however is low because the sera of 95 percent of group A_1 and of all group A_2 persons destroys acquired B cells. Furthermore most strains of *E. coli* lack deacetylase, and the action of enzyme inhibitors would still further reduce the incidence.[10]

VA-Polyagglutination

VA-polyagglutination, so named because the first example was found in Vienna[50,51] in a patient with hemolytic anemia, is characterized by a significant depression of erythrocyte H-receptors, probably due to the action of microbial α-fucosidase. VA-cells also show a characteristic stippled appearance in immunofluorescence tests using the lectin from *Helix pomatia*;[51] this appearance was also demonstrated with the red cells of a patient who had a hemolytic anemia associated with infection with influenza A_2 virus,[51] VA has also been found in combination with Tk.[37,38] Tk-polyagglutination is itself associated with depressed H- and other receptors (see above). VA is however clearly different to Tk because the original VA patient had a normal amount of anti-Tk in his serum.

Th-Polyagglutination

A new form of polyagglutination named Th was described by Bird et al. in 1978[52] in a patient who developed peritonitis after perforation of a Meckel's diverticulum. Tests with a battery of lectins showed that whereas the red cells were agglutinated by the peanut lectin they were neither T- nor Tk-transformed because they were agglutinated neither by the *Glycine soja* (Soya Bean) lectin, which strongly agglutinates T-transformed cells, nor by BSII, which is Tk-specific (see also Table 5-6) and the patient's serum contained both anti-T and anti-Tk. Red cell sialic levels were normal. Treatment of the red cells with papain greatly reduced Th-polyagglutinability.

Several further examples have already been found. Veneziano et al.[53] described Th-polyagglutination in a three-year-old girl with a yolk sac tumor, and also in her mother. Bird and Wingham have detected this form of polyagglutination in blood samples from six more cases referred to them. In one blood specimen referred by Professor F. Stratton of Manchester, the Th-polyagglutination was weak; nevertheless, the patient was anemic, and her red cells were shown to have fixed complement.[54] However, other stronger Th-polyagglutinable erythrocytes apparently did not fix complement. The cause of Th-polyagglutination, which is probably due to a microbial enzyme, has not yet been established.

Some examples of polyagglutination, previously reported as T- or Tk-transformation, may have really been Th.

Simultaneous Occurrence of More Than One Form of Polyagglutination

More than one form of erythrocyte polyagglutination may occur simultaneously and cause problems in elucidation.[3] This situation is usually associated with microbial polyagglutination of the enzymic type. A single bacterial species often produces more than one enzyme, capable of modifying the surface of the red cell membrane, or more than one bacterial species may be responsible for the infection with which the polyagglutination is associated.

These factors are no doubt responsible for the various combinations reported—e.g., T and Tk, T and acquired B, Tk and acquired B, Tk and VA etc.[3]

Microbial polyagglutination can of course occur in persons with other forms of poly agglutinable red cells. For example, T-polyagglutination has occurred in an individual whose red cells were known to be Tn-polyagglutinable.[10]

Acquired Nonmicrobial Polyagglutination, (Tn-Polyagglutination, Persistent 'Mixed-Field' Polyagglutination)

Tn is perhaps the most interesting of all categories of erythrocyte polyagglutination, because it is almost certainly due to the appearance in a previously normal person of an abnormal erythropoietic clone as the result of somatic mutation. The work of Cartron et al.[55,56] has established that a single genetic defect is responsible. Tn red cells lack the enzyme β-3-D-galactosyltransferase(T-transferase) so that there is failure of complete synthesis of the carbohydrate moiety of the MN glycoprotein which stops at an intermediate stage, Tn (Fig. 5-1). It is theoretically possible

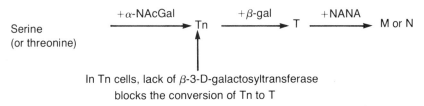

In Tn cells, lack of β-3-D-galactosyltransferase
blocks the conversion of Tn to T

Fig. 5-1. Schematic representation of the MN biosynthetic pathway showing the site of the biochemical defect in Tn-erythrocytes.

that Tn could also occur through the action of both neuraminidase and a microbial T-destroying enzyme; however, no conclusive sample of such a Tn-polyagglutination has yet been detected.

Anti-Tn is present in most adult sera, so that Tn-polyagglutination is associated with blood grouping anomalies. Since Tn is a clonal condition it typically presents as a mixed-field reaction. Rarely, all red cells become Tn-polyagglutinable so that there is no mixed-field appearance. Other forms of polyagglutination are also associated with mixed-fields but they are due to other causes (Table 5-3).

The first example of Tn-polyagglutinability associated with hemolytic anemia was described after a 12-year-long investigation, throughout which the condition persisted, by Dausset et al.[57] Many further examples have been published,[58,59] and there are even more unpublished examples. All the examples of Tn-studied by the author have reacted identically in serological tests.[58] Although Tn is still a rare condition it is commoner than was originally believed. Acquired hemolytic anemia was also associated with the second and

third examples of Tn,[60] but, strangely, not with subsequent examples. Leucopenia and thrombocytopenia however are almost invariably associated with Tn.[61] The Tn-change affects leucocytes and platelets as well as erythrocytes; this supports the view that somatic mutation has occurred at pluripotent stem cell level. Once developed, the condition persists for years, but may eventually disappear[58] presumably by elimination of the abnormal clone. Tn-cells are deficient in NANA and therefore have a reduced electrophoretic mobility. The normal and Tn-cells of a mixed population can be separated by electrophoresis, or by use of polybrene,[56] AB serum,[61] or a suitable lectin.[62] Treatment of red cells with papain destroys the Tn receptor and enables the correct blood group to be established. The rapid identification of Tn cells was made possible by the discovery of the Tn-specific lectin in the seeds of *Salvia sclarea* and other *Salvias*,[4] which can be used to test cells of all ABO groups.

The first clear indication of the chemical basis of Tn-specificity emerged from the studies of Dahr et al[63] who concluded that Tn is a cryptic determinant of the alkali labile tetra-

Table 5-3. Causes of Mixed-Field Agglutination Reactions

Cause	Examples
Artificial	Accidental, blood transfusion, feto-maternal transfer, bone marrow graft
Low antigen site density	Weak A or B—e.g., A_3, Lutheran, Sd^a
Chimeras	Twin chimeras, Dispermic chimeras
Somatic mutation	Old age, malignant blood disorders, inherited erythrocyte "mosaicism"
Erythrocyte polyagglutination	T, Tk, Th, VA, Tn, etc.

saccharide isolated from human glycolipids, and is represented by terminal N-acetyl-D-galactosamine α-glycosidically linked to serine (or threonine) of the peptide backbone. This conclusion has been completely supported.[55,56,64]

It is of interest that there may be an association between Tn-polyagglutination and leukemia. In 1976 Bird et al.[65] described Tn-polyagglutination in an unusual example of acute myelocytic leukemia, and in 1977 Ness et al.[60] described an individual, whose red cells were known to be Tn-polyagglutinable, who subsequently developed acute myelomonocytic leukemia. It is reasonable to suggest therefore that all persons, whose red cells are known to be Tn-polyagglutinable, should be kept under regular hematological surveillance.

It is also interesting to note the remarkable similarity in certain respects of Tn-polyagglutination and paroxysmal nocturnal hemoglobinuria.[4] Both conditions are acquired (somatic mutation), both are associated with more than one population of red cells, both may eventually disappear, presumably by elimination of an abnormal clone of stem cells, and both may be associated with malignant blood disease.

The relationship of Tn to the MN biosynthetic pathway and to breast cancer is described separately below.

Cad-Polyagglutination

Cad may be a very strong form of the blood group antigen Sd[a],[67] or an independent character.[68] If it is a very strong form of Sd[a] it cannot be classified under polyagglutination as defined above. However, since the strongest form of Cad erythrocytes are agglutinated by many sera, Cad is generally classified as a form of polyagglutination.

That the *Dolichos biflorus* lectin could rarely react with group B or O cells was first demonstrated in Japan.[69] The term Cad was however first applied to the red cell antigen involved by Cazal et al.[70] It is generally agreed that the Cad antigen occurs in varying strengths which represent a continuous distribution curve, and that it is therefore difficult precisely to classify the various grades. However, red cells of the strongest form, arbitrarily classified as Cad 1, are polyagglutinable, whereas cells of the lower orders e.g. Cad 2 to Cad 4, although agglutinated by the *Dolichos* lectin, are not polyagglutinable.

Cad cells are readily detected by use of the Cad-specific lectin from *Leonurus cardiaca*[71] or, if papain-treated cells are tested, by the Cad-specific lectins from *Salvia horminium* or *Salvia farinacea*.[3,4] With Wingham, the author has recently shown (unpublished observations) that extracts of the seeds of *Spartium junceum* may be used by the tile method rapidly to detect Cad erythrocytes.

Anti-Sd[a] sera also agglutinate Cad cells much more strongly than ordinary Sd(a+) cells.

Cad-polyagglutination is of little clinical significance. However, a hemolytic transfusion reaction has been attributed to anti-Sd[a].[72] Cad-positive blood would of course be dangerous if transfused in an emergency without prior crossmatching. This is unlikely to happen in a modern transfusion service.

HEMPAS

The acronym HEMPAS stands for hereditary erythroblastic multinuclearity with a positive acidified serum test. It is a congenital dyserythropoietic anemia, type II (CDA II). HEMPAS red cells have an abnormal membrane. The bone marrow is hypercellular, with a predominance (up to 90 percent) of erythroblasts. Intermediate and late normoblasts may have from two to seven nuclei. Electron microscopy of erythroblasts shows an extra linear structure inside and parallel to the cell membrane.

HEMPAS red cells are agglutinated (and lysed in the presence of complement) by an

IgM antibody, anti-HEMPAS, present in many (acidified) sera, but not in the serum of HEMPAS patients. HEMPAS is therefore a polyagglutinable state as defined above. The NANA levels of HEMPAS cells are below normal and their electrophoretic mobility is reduced. HEMPAS erythrocytes are however different to other sialic acid deficient red cells, e.g. the polyagglutinable T- or Tn-erythrocytes or the nonpolyagglutinable En(a−), M^g, M^k and other red cells. HEMPAS red cells are strongly agglutinated by anti-i and readily lysed by anti-I and anti-i. HEMPAS cells are weakly agglutinated by the lectin from *Helix pomatia*.[73]

The H-antigen is deficient in HEMPAS cells.[73,74] Bird and Wingham[73] tested many seed extracts with HEMPAS cells, but failed to find a specific anti-HEMPAS lectin. Useful reviews of various aspects of HEMPAS appear in a book on dyserythropoiesis.[75]

Relationship of Polyagglutination to Blood Group Antigens

ABH   Antigens. Tn-polyagglutination has been described as "A-like."[58] Tn-cells react better with sera which contain anti-A. The basis of the association between Tn and A is simply the fact that both receptors have the same immunodominant sugar, N-acetyl-D-galactosamine in terminal α-linked position.

In both the passively-acquired and enzymic forms of acquired B, the red cells acquire, in each case, a B-like antigen, not completely identical with each other or with human B.

H-receptors are slightly depressed in HEMPAS[73,74] and grossly weakened or destroyed in Tk- or VA-polyagglutination.[37–39] A- or B-receptors are also weakened in Tk-polyagglutination.[37–39]

Ii Antigens. I and i antigens may be weakened in Tk-polyagglutination.[39]

MN Antigens. T and Tn represent intermediate stages in the MN biosynthetic pathway. Although there is general agreement way. Although there is general agreement that, in this pathway, Tn is the precursor of T (figure 5-1), there is controversy as to the final stage or stages of the synthesis of M and N.

According to Springer[76] the addition of NANA residue to T converts it to N and the addition of another NANA to N converts it to M. Others believe that there is no difference between the carbohydrate moieties in M and N, so that the difference between them depends on the configuration imparted to the carbohydrate chain by differences in the amino acid sequence of the protein backbone of the MN glycoprotein. Furthermore the protein itself may form an essential part of the M or N antigen structure. Protein differences therefore, particularly in the NH$_2$ terminus, may solely or in combination with the immunodominant sugar determine the difference between M and N.[77–79]

Whatever the true answer may be makes no difference to the fact that in T- and Tn-erythrocytes the M and N antigens are depressed or absent, and that T- is depressed or absent in Tn.

At one time the N$_{Vg}$ receptor (the receptor for the *Vicia graminea* seeds), and not T, was thought to be the precursor of M and N.[34] If, however, the specificity of the single lectin from *Vicia graminea* lectin is regarded as anti-N+T in that it reacts not only with N but also on its substrate (T) which is exposed after treatment of red cells with neuraminidase, there would be no need to postulate an N$_{Vg}$ receptor; there is serological evidence in support of this view.[4] This interpretation is made without prejudice to the fact that N$_{Vg}$ might form part of a second carbohydrate chain in the MN structure, or that an N$_{Vg}$ receptor may occur, as does T, in other parts of the red cell membrane quite unrelated to the MN glycoprotein.

The hemagglutinins in the hemolymph of the Horseshoe "Crabs", *Limulus polyphemus* and *Tachypleus tridentatus,* which are specific for NANA, understandably fail to agglutinate T-transformed cells. However they agglutinate Tn cells, which are NANA-deficient, as strongly as normal cells. In Tn cells therefore they react with NANA unrelated to the MN biosynthetic pathway.

For reasons which are as yet unclear, the M, N, "N_{Vg}" and T antigens of Cad cells are depressed.[10]

Mixed-Fields

A mixed-field agglutination reaction (firm agglutinates distributed against a background of unagglutinated red cells) is associated with most forms of red cell polyagglutination. There are other causes of mixed-fields (Table 5-3) which should be carefully excluded before a "diagnosis" of erythrocyte polyagglutination is made. There have been errors in interpretation, published and unpublished, of mixed-field reactions. Tn-polyagglutination has been mistaken for an atypical blood group chimera[80]; polyagglutination has been mistaken for weak forms of A or B; and the author's laboratory has received several alleged examples of polyagglutination which were identified as post-transfusion mixtures, or as examples of autoagglutination. Furthermore some alleged paternity exclusions have been based on the erroneous blood grouping of children whose red cells were polyagglutinable.

Positive Antiglobulin Tests in Red Cell Polyagglutination

Antiglobulin sera may contain significant amounts of anti-T, anti-Tn, or other antibodies for polyagglutinable red cells. To avoid error in interpretation, these antibodies must first be absorbed out of the antiglobulin serum.

Lectins in the Elucidation of Erythrocyte Polyagglutination

The rapid proliferation in knowledge which has occurred in recent years is largely due to the application of lectins to the study of polyagglutination, which originated with the demonstration of anti-T in peanuts (*Arachis hypogaea*).[21] Besides *Arachis* several other lectins are essential in the classification of polyagglutination[34] (Tables 5-4, 5-5, 5-6).

Preliminary screening of polyagglutinable red cells with the lectins of *Dolichos biflorus* and *Arachis hypogaea* will divide the possibilities into three categories (Table 5-4), 1) positive with *Dolichos*, negative with *Arachis*: Tn or Cad, 2) negative with *Dolichos*, positive with *Arachis*: T, Tk, or Th, 3) negative with both: other forms of polyagglutination.

In the first of these categories, Tn and Cad can be distinguished by use of the lectins from *Salvia sclarea*, *Salvia horminium* and *Leonurus cardiaca* (Table 5-5), and in the second T, Tk and Th can be distinguished by the use of BS II and the lectin from *Glycine soja*, and by other means (Table 5-6). In the third category the lectin from *Helix pomatia* is useful in the detection of VA polyagglutination in persons of group B or O as described above. Various anti-H lectins, e.g. *Cytisus glabrescens*,[3,73] are useful in the demonstration of depressed H-receptors, but it must be remembered that H-receptors are also depressed in Tk and HEMPAS. Acquired B is detected by ordinary blood grouping. The *Dolichos* lectin reacts relatively more weakly on A_1 cells which have acquired the B-character than on normal A_1 cells. The diagnosis of HEMPAS is usually made during hematological investigation.

The polyagglutinable cells under test should also be compared with known examples of the various forms of polyagglutination. The serum of the person under investigation must also be checked for antibodies to various forms of polyagglutinable erythrocytes because, the absence of an antibody is a diagnostic aid, e.g., in T-polyagglutination, anti-T is absent from the serum, except in the very early or very late stages of the condition.

The fact that lectins react with bacteria or their soluble antigens may be a potential source of error in the elucidation of polyag-

Table 5-4. Preliminary Screening of Polyagglutinable Red Cells with Lectins

Dolichos biflorus	Arachis hypogaea	Polyagglutination
+[a]	−	Tn, Cad
−	+	T, Tk, Th
−	−	Other

[a] group B or O cells

glutination by use of lectins, e.g. the lectin of *Dolichos biflorus* and *Salvia sclarea* react specifically with type C *streptococci* and would therefore agglutinate red cells coated with this organism or its polysaccharide, which might then be mistaken for Tn cells.

T, Tn, and Breast Cancer

It is convenient to deal separately with this important clinicopathological aspect of two antigens, T and Tn, which were originally discovered during studies of polyagglutinable red cells, as discussed above.

Extensive work on the subject by Springer and his associates has recently been reviewed.[81] In malignant cells in breast and other cancers there is loss of NANA with exposure of the T-antigen. Serum anti-T titres are significantly reduced in some cases of breast cancer, but not others. Perhaps in some patients there is enhanced production of anti-T to compensate for the antibody adsorbed by cancer cells. When anti-T levels are depressed they rise again after mastectomy. There is no correlation however between anti-T titres and the severity of the condition.[82,83] The T-antigen of cancer cells in-

duces both humoral as well as cell-mediated responses.[81]

Loss of surface structure may go beyond NANA.[84] The T-antigen itself may be lost, with exposure of Tn, which may also be shed, with exposure of the protein backbone of the MN glycoprotein.

The work of Springer and his colleagues[81] on the exposure of precursor antigens in breast and other cancers may be of value in the diagnosis, prognosis and even immunotherapy of cancer. For immunotherapy anti-T antibodies, or even the anti-T lectin obtained in purified form from the seeds of *Arachis hypogaea*, may be used. A "vaccine" consisting of a combination of T-antigen (extracted from red cells or breast cancer cells) and BCG may be used to raise the patients' anti-T titres. There is of course a fundamental difficulty in using anti-T lectins as an immunotherapeutic agent. Peanut proteins are of course foreign to man, so that they would evoke antibody formation, and therefore have only short-term value. However, it may not be impossible to modify the structure of the lectin to reduce or abolish antigenicity without loss of specificity. Lectins might then be used as a cytotoxic agent, either singly or

Table 5-5. Differentiation of Tn and Cad Polyagglutination with Lectins

Salvia sclarea	Salvia horminum	Leonurus cardiaca	Polyagglutination
+	+	−	Tn
−	+[a]	+	Cad

[a] with red cells treated with papain Tn cells are not agglutinated, and agglutination of Cad cells is enhanced.

Table 5-6. Differentiation of T-, Tk- and Th-Polyagglutination with Lectins

Arachis hypogaea	Glycine soja	BSII	Polyagglutination
+	+	−	T
+	−	+	Tk[a]
+	−	−	Th[b]

[a] enhanced agglutination of protease-treated red cells
[b] depressed agglutination of protease-treated red cells

in conjunction with other forms of treatment. This important subject of immunotherapy of breast cancer has been discussed elsewhere.[84,85]

Polybrene and Other Red Cell Aggregators

Various highly positively charged substances such as polybrene, poly-L-lysine, protamine, DEAE-dextran, methylcellulose, Alcian blue, Ruthenium red and lanthanum nitrate, aggregate erythrocytes, partly by neutralizing their negative charge.[55] Polybrene is the most frequently used aggregator. Whereas it aggregates normal red cells, it fails to aggregate NANA-deficient red cells e.g. T, Tn or protease-treated erythrocytes. In high concentrations (over 5 percent), polybrene fails to aggregate.[55] Very dilute solutions of polybrene (less than 0.003 percent) can detect red cells with only a 10 percent charge reduction. Cartron et al.[55] have successfully used polybrene to separate Tn from normal cells in the bloods of persons with Tn-polyagglutination (persistent mixed-field polyagglutination).

there will be useful developments in the future, which will contribute further to our knowledge of red cell membrane structure and its anomalies.

There is already a probable example of a fourth type of polyagglutination in which the red cells are agglutinated by the peanut lectin, and one of a third inherited form. Both of these new forms of polyagglutination are still under investigation.

If we were to change the generally accepted definition of polyagglutination mentioned above to one the author has used previously[8] i.e. the agglutination of altered, defective or otherwise abnormal erythrocytes by many sera, Cad, probably an abnormally strong form of the human blood group antigen Sd^a, acquired B, in which the red cells are abnormal, and HEMPAS in which there is clearly an abnormal red cell membrane, can all be included as regular members of the polyagglutination clan without question or quibble. The scope of this definition would however theoretically include some forms of drug-dependent hemagglutination e.g. that induced by hemagglutinating antibody to penicillin. Nevertheless, most workers would know where to draw the line.

CONCLUSION

Ever since the first description of in vitro polyagglutination by Hübener in 1925,[14] and of in vivo polyagglutination by Levine and Katzin in 1938,[86] the subject has expanded to become a valuable and interesting facet of Clinical Pathology. The extensive work of Friedenreich[17] on T-transformation really stimulated interest in the subject. His brilliant hypothesis that T-transformation was due to a bacterial enzyme was later confirmed.[87,88] More recently, the discovery of the anti-T lectin of *Arachis hypogaea*[21] provided the basis of the now widespread use of lectins in the study of red cell polyagglutination, and led to a rapid and extensive expansion of knowledge in this field. It is expected that

REFERENCES

1. Gold, E.R. and Balding, P.: Receptor-specific proteins. Plant and animal lectins. Excerpta Medica, Amsterdam, 1975.
2. Cohen, E., ed.: Biomedical perspectives of agglutinins of invertebrate and plant origins. Ann. N.Y. Acad. Sci. Vol 234, 1974.
3. Bird, G.W.G.: The application of lectins to some problems in blood group serology. Rev. Fr. Transf. Immuno-Hematol. 21:103, 1978.
4. Bird, G.W.G.: Significant advances in lectins and polyagglutinable red cells. Plenary Sessions. Main Lectures. XVII Congress of the International Society of Hematology. XV Congress of the International Society of Blood Transfusion. Librairie Arnette, Paris, 1978, p. 87.
5. Bird, G.W.G.: Specific agglutinating activity

for human red blood corpuscles in extracts of *Dolichos biflorus*. Curr. Sci. 20:289, 1951.

6. Prokop, O., Rackwitz, A. and Schlesinger, D.: A "new" human blood group receptor A_{hel} tested with extracts from *Helix hortensis* (garden snail). J. Forens. Med., S. Africa 12:108, 1965.

7. Winzler, R.J.: A glycoprotein in human erythrocyte membranes. In Red Cell Membrane. Structure and Function. Jamieson, G.A. and Greenwalt, T.J., eds. Lippincott, Philadelphia, 1969, p. 157.

8. Bird, G.W.G.: Erythrocyte polyagglutination. Nouv. Rev. Fr. d'Hematol. 11:57, 1971.

9. Bird, G.W.G.: Erythrocyte polyagglutination. In Handbook Series in Clinical Laboratory Science. Section D. Blood Banking. Vol I. Greenwalt, T.J. and Steane, E.A., eds., CRC Press, Cleveland, Ohio, 1977, p. 443.

10. Bird, G.W.G.: Complexity of erythrocyte polyagglutinability. In Human Blood Groups. 5th Int. Convoc. Immunol., Buffalo, N.Y., 1976. Karger, Basel, 1977, p. 335.

11. Neter, E.: Bacterial hemagglutination and hemolysis. Bact. Rev. 201:166, 1956.

12. Chorpenning, F.W. and Dodd, M.C.: Polyagglutinable erythrocytes associated with bacteriogenic transfusion reactions. Vox Sang. 10:460, 1965.

13. Weedon, A.R., Datta, N. and Mollison, P.L.: Adsorption of bacteria on to red cells leading to positive antiglobulin reactions. Vox Sang. 5:523, 1960.

14. Hübener, G.: Untersuchungen Uber Isoagglutination mit besonderer Berücksichtigung scheinbarer Abweichungen vom Gruppenschema. Z. Immunitaetsforsch. Immunobiol. 45:223, 1925.

15. Schiff, F. and Halberstädter, W.: Uber Agglutinationsercheinungen bei gealteren Blutkörperchen. Z. Immunitaetsforsch. Immunobiol. 48:414, 1926.

16. Thomsen, O.: Ein Vermehrungsfahiges Agens als Veranderer des isoagglutinatorischen Verhaltens der roten Blutkörperchen, eine bisher unbekannte Quelle der Fehlbestimmungen. Z. Immunitaetsforsch. Immunobiol. 52:85, 1927.

17. Friedenreich, V.: The Thomsen Haemagglutination Phenomenon. Levin and Munksgaard, Copenhagen, 1930.

18. Vaith, P. and Uhlenbruck, G.: The Thomsen agglutination phenomenon. A discovery revisited 50 years later. Z. Immunitaetsforsch. Immunobiol. 154:1, 1978.

19. Lauf, P.K.: Blood group antigens and membrane permeability in erythrocytes of man and ruminants. In Human Blood Groups. 5th Int. Convoc. Immunol., Buffalo, N.Y., 1976. Karger, Basel, 1977, p. 383.

20. Chorpenning F. and Hayes, J.C.: Occurrence of the Thomsen-Friedenreich phenomenon *in vivo*. Vox Sang. 4:210, 1959.

21. Bird, G.W.G.: Anti-T in peanuts. Vox Sang 9:748, 1964.

22. Rickard, K.A., Robinson, R.J. and Worlledge, S.M.: Acute acquired haemolytic anaemia associated with polyagglutination. Arch. Dis. Child 44:102, 1969.

23. Gray, J.M., Beck, M. and Oberman, H.A.: Clostridial-induced Type I polyagglutinability associated with intravascular hemolysis. Vox Sang. 22:379, 1972.

24. Bird, T. and Stephenson, J.: Acute hemolytic anemia with polyagglutinability of red cells. J. Clin. Pathol. 26:868, 1973.

25. Moores, P., Pudifin, D. and Patel, P.L.: Severe hemolytic anemia in an adult associated with anti-T. Transfusion 15:329, 1975.

26. Tanaka, H., Okubo, Yu, Yamaguchi, H., Matsumoto, T. and Okubo, Y.: Acute acquired hemolytic anemia with T-polyagglutination. Ann. Paed. Japn. 23:48, 1977.

27. Van Loghem, J.J., Jr., van der Hart, M. and Land, M.E.: Polyagglutinability of red cells as a cause of severe hemolytic transfusion reaction. Vox Sang. (Old Series) 5:125, 1955.

28. Klein, P.J., Bulla, M., Newman, R.A., Müller, P., Uhlenbruck, G., Shaefer, H.E., Kruger, G. and Fisher, R.: Thomsen-Friedenreich antigen in hemolytic-uremic syndrome. Lancet ii:1024, 1977.

29. Poulsen, M.P.E.: Polyagglutinabilitet og T-omdannelse. Med. Dissertation, Copenhagen, 1961.

30. Obeid, D., Bird, G.W.G. and Wingham, J.: Prolonged erythrocyte T-polyagglutination in two children with bowel disorders. J. Clin. Pathol. 30:953, 1977.

31. Seger, R., Joller, P., Kenny, A., Hitzig, W., Metaxas, M. and Metaxas-Bühler, M.: Potential hazards of blood transfusion in Clostridia-associated necrotising enterocolitis. Lancet i:48, 1979.

32. Jørgensen, J.R.: Prenatal T-transformation? A

case of polyagglutinable cord blood erythrocytes. Vox Sang. 13:225, 1967.

33. Bird, G.W.G. and Wingham, J.: Tk: a new form of red cell polyagglutination. Br. J. Hematol. 23:759, 1972.

34. Inglis, G., Bird, G.W.G., Mitchell, A.A.B., Milne, G.R. and Wingham, J.: Erythrocyte agglutination showing properties of both T and Tk, probably induced by *Bacteroides fragilis* infection. Vox Sang. 28:314, 1975.

35. Bird, G.W.G., Wingham, J., Inglis, G. and Michell, A.A.B.: Tk polyagglutination in *Bacteroides fragilis* septicaemia. Lancet i:286, 1975.

36. Inglis, G., Bird, G.W.G., Mitchell, A.A.B., Milne, G.R. and Wingham, J.: Effect of *Bacteroides fragilis* in the human erythrocyte membrane: pathogenesis of Tk polyagglutination. J. Clin. Pathol. 28:964, 1975.

37. Inglis, G., Bird, G.W.G., Mitchell, A.A.B., and Wingham, J.: Tk polyagglutination associated with reduced A and H activity. Vox Sang. 35:370, 1978.

38. Beck, M.L., Myers, M.A., Moulds, J., Pierce, S.R., Hardman, J., Wingham, J., and Bird, G.W.G: Co-existent Tk- and VA-polyagglutinability. Transfusion, 18:680, 1978.

39. Andreu, G., Mativet, S., Doinel, C., Cartron, J.P. and Salmon, Ch.: In vitro Tk polyagglutination—relations with acquired B, I and i antigens. Abstracts, XVII Congress of the International Society of Hematology/XV Congress of the International Society of Blood Transfusion, 1978, p. 551.

40. Judd, W.J., Beck, M.L., Hicklin, B.L., Shanker Iyer, P.N. and Goldstein, I.J.: BS II lectin: a second haemagglutinin isolated from *Bandeiraea simplicifolia* seeds with affinity for type III polyagglutinable cells. Vox Sang. 33:246, 1977.

41. Springer, G.F., Williamson, P. and Brandes, W.C.: Blood group activity of Gram-negative bacteria. J. Exp. Med. 113:1077, 1961

42. Pardoe, G.I., Bird, G.W.G. and Uhlenbruck, G.: Structural and serological studies of the lipopolysaccharide of Proteus vulgaris OX 19. Z. Immun. forsch. 136:488, 1968.

43. Pettenkofer, H.J., Maassen, W. and Bickerich, R.: Antigengemenishaften Zwischen menslichen Blutgruppen und Enterobacteriaceen. Z. Immun. forsch. 119:415, 1960.

44. Garratty, G., Willbanks, E. and Petz, L.D.: An acquired B antigen associated with *Proteus vulgaris* infection. Vox Sang. 21:45, 1971.

45. Cameron, C., Graham, F., Dunsford, I., Sickles, G., Macpherson, C.R., Cahan, A., Sanger, R. and Race, R.R.: Acquisition of a B-like antigen by red blood cells. Br. Med. J. 2:29, 1959.

46. Salmon, Ch. and Gerbal, A.: The acquired B antigen. In Handbook Series in Clinical Laboratory Science. Section D. Blood Banking. Vol. I. Greenwalt, T.J. and Steane, E.A., eds. CRC Press, Cleveland, Ohio, p. 193.

47. Gerbal, A., Maslet, C. and Salmon, Ch.: Immunological aspects of the acquired B antigen. Vox Sang. 28:398, 1975.

48. Gerbal, A., Ropars, C., Gerbal, R., Cartron, J.P., Maslet, C. and Salmon, Ch.: Acquired B antigen disappearance by in vitro acetylation associated with A_1 activity restoration. Vox Sang. 31:64, 1976.

49. Andersen, J.: A weak atypical B-like character in the blood cells of 7 group A persons. Acta. Pathol. Microbiol. Scand. 48:289, 1960.

50. Graninger, W., Rameis, H., Fisher, K., Poschmann, A., Bird, G.W.G., Wingham, J. and Neumann, E.: 'VA' a new type of erythrocyte polyagglutination characterized by depressed H receptors and associated with hemolytic anemia. I. Serological and hematological observations. Vox Sang. 32:195, 1977.

51. Graninger, W., Poschmann, A., Fisher, K., Schedl-Giovannoni, I., Hörander, H. and Klaushofer, K.: 'VA' a new type of erythrocyte polyagglutination characterized by depressed H receptors and associated with hemolytic anemia. II. Observations by immunofluorescence, electron microscopy, cell electrophoresis and biochemistry. Vox Sang. 32:201, 1977.

52. Bird, G.W.G., Wingham, J., Beck, M.L., Pierce, S.R., Oates, G.D. and Pollock, A.: Th, a "new" form of erythrocyte polyagglutination. Lancet i:1215, 1978.

53. Veneziano, G., Rasore-Quartino, A. and Sansone, G.: Th erythrocyte polyagglutination. Lancet ii:483, 1978.

54. Stratton, F.: Personal communication, 1978.

55. Cartron, J.P., Cartron, J., Andreu, G., Salmon, Ch. and Bird, G.W.G.: Selective deficiency of 3-β-D-galactosyltransferase (T-transferase) in Tn-polyagglutinable erythrocytes. Lancet i:856, 1978.

56. Cartron, J.P., Andreu, G., Cartron, J., Bird,

G.W.G., Salmon, Ch. and Gerbal, A.: Demonstration of T-transferase deficiency in Tn-polyagglutinable blood samples. Eur. J. Biochem. 92:111, 1978.

57. Dausset, J., Moullec, J. and Bernard, J.: Acquired hemolytic anemia with polyagglutinability of red blood cells due to a new factor present in normal human serum (anti-Tn). Blood 15:1079, 1959.

58. Bird, G.W.G.: Tn-polyagglutination. Rev. Fr. Transf. Immunohématol. 19:231, 1976.

59. Kourteva, B.T., Manolova, V.R. and Mitova, D.K.: Tn-polyagglutinability of red blood cells and acquired A-like specificity. Transfusion 17:272, 1977.

60. Van der Hart, M., Moes, M., Van Loghem, J.J., Enneking, J.H.J. and Leeksma, C.H.W.: A second example of red cell polyagglutinability caused by the Tn antigen. Vox Sang. 6:358, 1961.

61. Bird, G.W.G., Shinton, N.K. and Wingham, J.: Persistent mixed-field polyagglutination. Br. J. Haematol. 21:443, 1971.

62. Bird, G.W.G. and Wingham J.: The M, N and N_{Vg} receptors of Tn-erythrocytes. Vox Sang. 26:171, 1974.

63. Dahr, W., Uhlenbruck, G. and Bird, G.W.G.: Cryptic A-like receptor sites in human erythrocyte glycoproteins: proposed nature of Tn-antigen. Vox Sang. 27:29, 1974.

64. Springer, G.F and Desai, P.R.: Common precursor of blood group M and N specificities. Biochem. Biophys. Res. Comm. 61:470, 1974.

65. Bird, G.W.G., Wingham, J., Pippard, M.J., Hoult, J.G. and Melikian, V.: Erythrocyte membrane modifications in malignant diseases of myeloid and lymphoreticular tissues. Br. J. Haematol. 33:289, 1976.

66. Ness, P.H., Garratty, G. and Morel, P.A.: Tn-polyagglutination preceding acute leukaemia. In Abstracts of Volunteer Papers, 30th Ann. Meeting Am. Assoc. Blood Banks, Atlanta, Georgia, 1977, p. 6.

67. Sanger, R., Gavin, J., Tippett, P., Teesdale, P. and Eldon, K.: Plant agglutinin for another human blood-group. Lancet i:1130, 1971.

68. Gerbal, A., Lopez, M., Chassaigne, M., Genetet, B., Selva, J., Yvart, J. and Salmon, Ch.: L'antigène Cad dans la population française. Rev. Fr. Transf. Immunohématol. 19:415, 1976.

69. Ikuta, S. and Murakami, S.: An example of

group O red cells agglutinable by *Dolichos biflorus* extract (translated from Japanese). J. Japn. Soc. Blood. Transf. 9:37, 1962.

70. Cazal, P., Monis, M., Caubel, J. and Brives, J.: Polyagglutinabilité héréditaire dominante: antigène privé (Cad) correspondant à un anticorps public et à une lectin de *Dolichos biflorus*. Rev. Fr. Transf. Immunohématol., 11:209, 1968.

71. Bird, G.W.G. and Wingham, J.: Anti-Cad lectin from the seeds of *Leonurus cardiaca*. Clin. Lab. Haematol. 1:57, 1979.

72. Peetermans, M.E. and Cole-Dergent, J.: Haemolytic transfusion reaction due to anti-Sd[a]. Vox Sang. 18:67, 1970.

73. Bird, G.W.G. and Wingham, Jr.: The action of seed and other reagents on HEMPAS erythrocytes. Acta. Haematol. 55:174, 1976.

74. Rochant, H., N'go Minh, M., Ton That, H., Henri, A., Basch, A., Sultan, C. and Dreyfus, B.: Un nouveau cas de dyserythropoiese congénitale de type II. Caractères immunologiques et transmission hérédetaire de l'antigène de polyagglutinabilité distinct des antigènes Tn et Cad. Nouv. Rev. Fr. Hématol. 13:649, 1973.

75. Lewis, S.M. and Verwilghen, R.L., eds.: Dyserythropoiesis. Academic Press, London, 1977.

76. Springer, G.F., Tegtmeyer, H. and Huprikar, S.V.: Anti-N reagents in elucidation of the genetical basis of human blood group MN specificities. Vox Sang. 22:325, 1972.

77. Lisowska, E. and Duk, M.: Effect of modification of amino groups of human erythrocytes on M, N and N_{Vg} blood group specificities. Vox Sang. 28:392, 1975.

78. Dahr, W., Uhlenbruck, G. and Knott, H.: Immunochemical aspects of the MNSs blood group system. J. Immunogenet. 2:87, 1975.

79. Springer, G.F., Yang, H.J. and Desai, P.R.: Three-dimensional model of highly M-active NH_2-terminal sialoglycopentapeptide from human blood group MM red cells. Nature 65:547, 1978.

80. Sturgeon, P., McQuiston, D.T., Taswell, H.F. and Allan, C.J. Permanent mixed-field polyagglutinability (PMFP). I. Serological observations. Vox Sang. 25:481, 1973.

81. Springer, G.F., Desai, P.R., Yang, H.J. and Murthy, M.S.: Carcinoma-associated blood group MN precursor antigens against which

all humans possess antibodies. Clin. Immunol. Immunopathol. 7:426, 1977.

82. White, W.L. and Roper, S.: Anti-T microtitres and breast carcinoma. Abstracts of volunteer papers. 31st Ann. Meeting Am. Assoc. Blood Banks, New Orleans, 1978, p. 24.

83. Bird, G.W.G. and Roy, T.C.F.: Hitherto unpublished observations, 1978.

84. Anglin, J.H. Jr., Lerner, M.P. and Nordquist, R.E.: Blood group-like activity released by human mammary carcinoma cells in culture. Nature 269:254, 1977.

85. Bird, G.W.G.: Haematoserology of neoplasms. Rev. Fr. Transf. Immunohematol. 21:57, 1978.

86. Levine, P. and Katzin, E.M.: Temporary agglutinability of red blood cells. Proc. Soc. Exp. Biol. 39:167, N.Y., 1938.

87. Gottschalk, A.: The chemistry and biology of sialic acids and related substances. Cambridge University Press, 1960.

88. Klenk, E.: Chemie und Biochemie der Neuraminosäure. Angew Chem. 68:349, 1956.

6

The HLA System

William V. Miller, M.D.

INTRODUCTION

The HLA genetic complex is a series of closely linked genes located on the short arm of chromosome six. The gene products of the HLA complex were first identified by antisera obtained from polytransfused patients and, later, from multiparous women. The antigens detected by these antisera were initially thought to be genetically determined leukocyte alloantigens analogous to red cell alloantigen systems; but it was soon established that the HLA antigens were actually present on most cells in the body except mature erythrocytes. Although the basic biological function served by these gene products and coded by these loci are still unclear, they are important determinants of allograft rejection—hence, the name, histocompatibility antigens. They are also a major cause of immune destruction of transfused platelets in alloimmunized recipients. Recently, these products have been shown to play a critical role in the regulation of the cellular interactions required for effective immune responses.

All mammalian and avian species studied have a defined major histocompatibility complex (MHC) analogous to the human HLA complex. These genetic factors were first discovered by their ability to serve as transplantation antigens, since allograft survival between inbred strains of mice was significantly prolonged if the strains were genetically matched for the MHC antigens. MHC antigens in all species show marked polymorphism—i.e., many alternative alleles per locus. Initially, the only observed function of MHC gene products was an ability to serve as transplantation antigens; but most investigators believe other functions must also exist, since allograft exchange is an artificial model and could not provide evolutionary pressures to generate the diversity of gene products found at the MHC. Evidence for other functions developed in the late 1960s when McDevitt and his colleagues[1] observed that immune responsiveness of normal inbred animal strains to specific antigens was, in part, determined by genetic factors coded within the MHC. These genes were termed immune response or Ir genes, and the general region of the MHC in coding for these genes was called the I region.[2,3] Ir genes in humans, although not conclusively demonstrated, very likely exist. At least some of the observed HLA associations of certain diseases may be related to genetic control of immune responses.

Thus, the major functions of the HLA complex appear to involve regulation of immune responsiveness. Some gene products are important in the recognition phase of the primary immune response and serve as target antigens for a variety of immune effector mechanisms. These functions help explain why these antigens are important determinants of allograft rejection and immune platelet destruction, and may account for susceptibility to certain diseases associated with specific HLA antigens.

HISTORICAL BACKGROUND

The first evidence of human leukocyte blood groups was advanced in 1954 by Dausset, who observed that patients whose sera contained leukoagglutinins had received a larger number of blood transfusions than other patients; and that these agglutinins were not autoantibodies, as had been thought previously, but rather alloantibodies produced by the infusion of cells carrying alloantigens not present in the recipient.[4] In 1958, several independent investigators provided strong support for this assumption. Dausset observed that sera from seven polytransfused patients agglutinated leukocytes from about 60 percent of the French population, but not the leukocytes of the seven patients.[5] He termed the leukocyte alloantigen MAC, now known to be HLA-2. Family studies showed that the leukocyte antigens were genetically determined. At about the same time, Payne showed that serum from patients with febrile nonhemolytic transfusion reactions often contained leukoagglutinins.[6]

Van Rood developed a computer analysis program to unravel these serologic complexities and discovered several diallelic leukocyte antigen systems, including 4A and 4B (now called Bw4 and Bw6).[7] He also found that leukocyte antigens were present on most human tissues. Because of the complex and often insensitive nature of the leukoagglutination technique, it was of great importance when, in 1964, Terasaki and McClelland introduced the more sensitive microlymphocytotoxicity test which, in various modifications, has maintained its major role in HLA typing until the present time.[8,9]

Following the discovery of the first leuko-

cyte antigens and a suitable test system, the number of defined serologic specificities increased rapidly. By 1967, they were clearly shown to belong to the same genetic system, and the term HL-A was approved by the World Health Organization's Nomenclature Committee.[10] Earlier, it had been suggested that the HLA system was composed of two closely linked loci with genes controlling two segregant series of antigens.[11] The model was substantiated by discovery of a family showing cross-over between the two loci and by analysis of family inheritance patterns, specifically in twins and triplets. In 1970, the existence of a third serologically defined segregant series was suggested, and its value to the HLA system in organ transplantation was clearly established.[12]

Another line of research arose from the discovery that lymphocytes from two different individuals undergo blast transformation and divide when they are mixed and cultured in vitro—the mixed-lymphocyte reaction (MLR) test.[13,14] In 1967, Bach and Amos discovered that the MLR test gave negative results when leukocytes from a pair of HLA identical siblings were mixed together, indicating that a separate locus controlling MLR existed within the HLA complex.[15] In 1973, it became possible to type for MLR determinants by means of MLR homozygous cells, and the polymorphism at the MLR locus, now called the D locus, became clearer.[16] In 1975, investigators found serologically demonstrable gene products closely identified with the D locus.[17] By 1977, it was clear that these D-related (DR) antigens were present on B lymphocytes and monocytes, and that they had very high association with HLA-D locus gene products.[18,19]

Nomenclature

The genetic region encompassing this group of interrelated loci is called HLA. The genetic loci belonging to the HLA system are

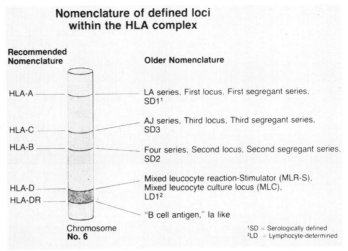

Nomenclature of defined loci within the HLA complex

Recommended Nomenclature

Older Nomenclature

HLA-A —— LA series, First locus, First segregant series, SD1[1]

HLA-C —— AJ series, Third locus, Third segregant series, SD3

HLA-B —— Four series, Second locus, Second segregant series, SD2

HLA-D —— Mixed leucocyte reaction-Stimulator (MLR-S), Mixed leucocyte culture locus (MLC), LD1[2]

HLA-DR —— "B cell antigen," Ia like

Chromosome No. 6

[1]SD = Serologically defined
[2]LD = Lymphocyte-determined

Fig. 6-1. The recommended nomenclature for the HLA complex is compared with older nomenclature, and the relative location of the major loci indicated. The D and DR loci are not yet clearly delineated and are indicated by the shaded region.

designated by one or more letters following the HLA—that is, HLA-A, HLA-B, HLA-C, HLA-D, and HLA-DR. (Figure 6-1) Each locus contains many individual alleles, and the corresponding allelic specificities are designated by numbers following the actual locus symbol—e.g., HLA-A1, HLA-B5, etc. Provisionally identified specificities carry the initial letter w (for workshop) inserted between the locus letter and the allele specificity number. For example, HLA-Bw21 indicates that the Bw21 specificity is not fully agreed upon by the World Health Organization Committee on HLA nomenclature.[20]

Table 6-1 shows many of the currently established HLA specificities and their approximate antigen frequencies in Caucasian Americans. Note that specificities within the A and B locus are not numbered consecutively, as are those within the C, D, and DR locus. This is because many of the A and B specificities were established prior to discovery of the latter loci, and, to avoid renumbering, the existing numbers for A and B locus alleles were used. Note, also, that there is no 4 or 6 within either the A or the B locus, since these numbers were reserved for leukocyte antigen systems under active investigation at the time the nomenclature was established.

During recent years, it has become clear that the antigens previously called 4 and 6 are now properly termed Bw4 and Bw6.[21,22] These antigens migrate with the HLA-B determinants by various protein separation techniques, suggesting that the Bw4 and Bw6 determinants reside on the same polypeptide chain as the other HLA-B locus determinants. It has been suggested that Bw4 and Bw6 are alleles which code for a precursor substance upon which the latter HLA-B alleles operate to form final gene products. Strong associations of Bw4 and Bw6 with their perspective associated alleles is given in Table 6-2.

GENETICS AND BIOCHEMISTRY OF THE HLA COMPLEX

The inheritance of the HLA complex is best understood by comparing it to the classical Fischer/Race hypothesis for the Rh system. Each locus can be thought of as a bead on a string, one bead representing the A locus, another the B locus, a third the C locus, a fourth the D locus, and a fifth the DR locus. Only one bead may occupy a place on the string at any one time, and the string must be handed intact to offspring; that is, the alleles

Table 6-1. HLA Specificities and Approximate Frequencies in American Caucasoids

A Locus		B Locus		C Locus	
A1	29%	B5	12%	Cw1	6%
A2	48%	B7	21%	Cw2	10%
A3	26%	B8	19%	Cw3	21%
A9	18%	B12	26%	Cw4	19%
A10	12%	B13	6%	Cw5	10%
A11	10%	B14	10%	Cw6	——
Aw23(9)*	4%	B15	12%	Cw7	——
Aw24(9)	14%	Bw16	6%	Cw8	——
A25(10)	6%	B17	10%	C Blank*	46%
A26(10)	6%	B18	6%		
A28	8%	Bw21	8%	**D Locus**	
A29	8%	Bw22	4%	Dw1	14%
Aw30	6%	B27	12%	Dw2	23%
Aw31	10%	Bw35	17%	Dw3	17%
Aw32	8%	B37	4%	Dw4	10%
Aw33	2%	Bw38(16)	4%	Dw5	12%
Aw34	1%	Bw39(16)	2%	Dw6	17%
Aw36	1%	Bw40	17%	Dw7	19%
Aw43	1%	Bw41	1%	Dw8	4%
A Blank**	4%	Bw42	1%	Dw9	1%
		Bw44(12)	20%	Dw10	1%
		Bw45(12)	6%	Dw11	1%
		Bw46	1%	Dw12	——
		Bw47	1%	D Blank*	62%
		Bw48	1%		
		Bw49(w21)	4%	**DR Locus**	
		Bw50(w21)	4%	DR1	10%
		Bw51(5)	7%	DR2	26%
		Bw52(5)	5%	DR3	23%
		Bw53	1%	DR4	29%
		Bw54(w22)	1%	DR5	23%
		Bw55(w22)	——	DRw6	21%
		Bw56(w22)	——	DR7	23%
		Bw57(17)	——	DR8	——
		Bw58(17)	——	DR9	——
		Bw59	——	DR10	——
		Bw60(40)	——	DR Blank*	48%
		Bw61(40)	——		
		Bw62(15)	——		
		Bw63(15)	——		
		Bw4	——		
		Bw6	——		
		B Blank*	6%		

* Numbers in parentheses are the "parent alleli" of the preceding "split".
** "Blanks" represent alleles which are undiscovered, or "missing", parts of the locus as calculated by the Hardy-Weinberg calculations.

are inherited en bloc. Since human chromosomes exist in pairs, it is now theoretically possible to demonstrate ten gene products in an individual—five from each chromosome. But amorphs, or absence of a detectable antigen, might occur; and homozygosity is fairly common. Furthermore, detection of D antigens is technically quite complex; and DR sera are not widely available, so that ten antigens may not always be detected.

In the Rh system we speak of the relationship between the alleles in a kind of shorthand; for example, R1, R2, or r, where R1 represents "CDe on the same chromosome." There is no equivalent shorthand notation in the HLA system, but it is important to think of this coupled relation of A, B, C, D, and DR series alleles. The genes on the same chromosome are called a *haplotype*, and, except for the instance of crossing-over, are always

Table 6-2. B Locus Associations with w4 and w6

Bw4 (4a)	Bw6 (4b)
B5	Bw35 (not complete)
B12 (w44)	B12 (w45)
B13	B40
B17	B8
B37	B14
Bw38 (16.1)	Bw39 (16.2)
Bw49 (21.1)	Bw50 (21.2)
B27	B7
15.2 (in caucasians)	15.1
	Bw22
	B18
	Bw41
	Bw42

(Data taken from Oliver and Festenstein, Tissue Antigens 5:395, 1975; and Hunter and Duquesnoy, Transplantation Proceedings, 9:47, 1977 (and workshop discussions.)

found to segregate together. An example of a mating and its four possible offspring is given in Figure 6-2. Note that the father's A chromosome contains an A1 and a B8 together as a haplotype, and that the haplotypes segregate independently, but that the alleles within the haplotype always travel together.

There is a one-in-four chance that children of this mating will share the same two haplotypes, a one-in-two probability that two siblings will share at least one haplotype, and a one-in-four probability that two siblings will share no haplotype. An important corollary is that a parent and child can share only one haplotype—that is, the child must have gotten one haplotype from the other parent, making genotypic identity impossible. However, phenotypic identity can occur as a result of either parental homozygosity or a marriage within the family unit. Indeed, recent reports regarding bone marrow transplantation from donors other than HLA-identical siblings in-

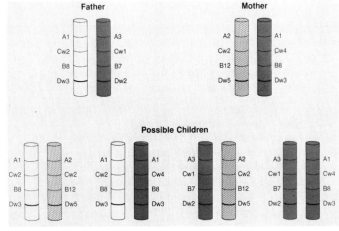

Fig. 6-2. For a given mating, children of only four HLA phenotypes may result, unless there is crossing-over. Implications for donor selection are reviewed in the text.

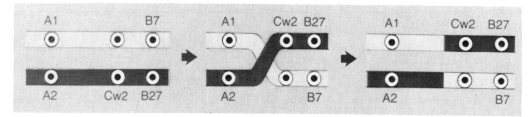

Fig. 6-3. An example of a cross-over during meiotic division. Cross-overs in the HLA complex are unusual (less than 1 percent) but happen frequently enough to have provided considerable information regarding the MHC in man.

dicates that tissue typing of the parents, siblings, and children of patients referred for marrow transplantation may be of value. Experience has indicated that relatives with one haplotype that is genotypically HLA identical are common outside the immediate family unit, and search for fortuitous similarity at the other haplotype could reasonably be extended to aunts, uncles, and cousins.[22a]

Although the genes of the A, B, C, and D series are closely linked, a number of families showing crossing-over between these series have been reported (see Fig. 6-3). One large study of 4,614 meiotic divisions showed 40 crossing-overs, with a recombination frequency of 0.0087, expressed as 0.87 centimorgans, the distance between A and the B locus.[23] The distance between the B and the D locus is about 0.5 centimorgans. The C locus is between A and B, and is estimated to be 0.7 centimorgans from A and 0.2 centimorgans from B (Fig. 6-4).[24] Recently there have been reports of families showing crossing-over between D and DR; but the frequency, while low, is not yet established.[25]

Some HLA genes tend to occur more frequently in the same haplotypes than would be expected on the basis of chance alone. One of the best known examples of this *linkage disequilibrium* occurs with the A1, B8 haplotype, which occurs about five times as frequently as one would expect. This association at the haplotype level is reflected in a strong association between A1 and B8 antigens of the population level as well. About 81 percent of all B8 positives also possess the A1 antigen, al-

though this antigen has a frequency of only 29 percent of the random population. Table 6-3 shows some of the strong linkage disequilibrium associations between HLA alleles.

Because of the phenomenon of linkage disequilibrium, it is not possible to determine the frequency of the given haplotype by simply multiplying frequencies of each constituent allele; instead, actual observed frequencies are necessary. The observed frequencies for Caucasians are given in Table 6-3. It is important to recognize that these frequencies are based on comparatively small numbers of actual observation and that haplotype frequencies for other racial groups have not yet been determined.

As indicated earlier, the association of some alleles of DR with D determinants is very strong. Indeed, typing for DR3 and DR4 gives inferential evidence regarding the individual's HLA-D alleles. Unfortunately, however, the initial promise of a serologic test for DR determinants has not been fulfilled, since

Table 6-3. Linkage Disequilibrium
(Gametic Association)

Haplotype			Frequency %	
A	B	D	observed	expected
A1	B8		9.8	2.1
A3	B7		5.4	2.1
	B8	D3	8.6	1.4
	B7	D2	3.9	1.8

The expected haplotype frequencies were calculated under the assumption of no association.

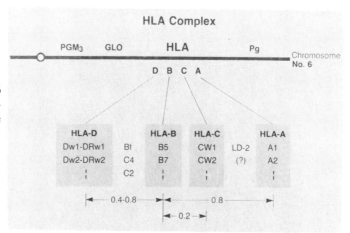

Fig. 6-4. A current map of the C6 chromosome, showing the location and relative distances of the loci of the MHC.

some DR determinants are not correlated with HLA-D determinants with sufficient frequency as to be useful in typing.

Geographic Variation

During the Fifth International Histocompatibility Testing Workshop in 1972, there was an attempt to clarify the genetics of the HLA system in various populations of the world. Many antigens which were apparently well-defined in Caucasians were not in other groups. Several sera, reacting identically with Caucasians' cell panels, failed to react with cells from other populations, and it became clear that some HLA antigens are present only in some populations.

Caucasians are marked by the common occurrence of the A1 and B8 antigens, which are infrequent or absent in most other groups. Another typical Caucasian haplotype is A3, B7, but it is worth noting that these haplotypes are truly European rather than Caucasian and that they decline in frequency from the north to the south of Europe. In contrast, B5 and Bw35 increase from north to south.[26]

Two antigens, Aw36 and Bw42, seem to exist only in African Negroes, in whom B17 is the most frequent antigen. Most well-known Caucasian HLA antigens, including A1, A3,

B7, and B8, are also present in African Negroes.

In Mongoloids, high frequencies of A9, Bw40, and Bw22 are characteristic. A1, A3, B7, and B8 are absent in most Mongoloid populations. The A2 antigen has appreciable frequencies in almost all populations studied and reaches its highest occurrence, about 80 percent, in American Indians. Some HLA antigens—i.e., A1, A11, B15, B17, and Bw22—are recognizable by human alloantisera in chimpanzees while other antigens, including A2, are absent.

HLA Antigen Biochemistry

Biochemical characterization of the HLA antigens has been slow because of the difficulty in procuring sufficient quantities of purified material for analysis, and conflicting results have been reported. It now seems clear that the HLA antigens are glycoprotein in nature and that the allelic antigenic determinants rest in the polypeptide portion of the molecule, not in its carbohydrate side chains. The molecule (Fig. 6-5) is composed of two chains: a heavy chain bearing the antigenic determinant, and a light chain.[27]

The glycopeptides contain about 3 percent carbohydrate and have a molecular weight of

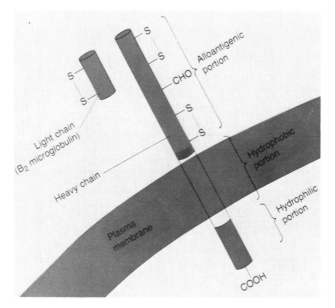

Fig. 6-5. A possible model for the structure of the HLA-A, -B, and -C molecules. The antigenic determinants are located on the heavy chain, beta-2-microglobulin is formed by the light chain.

about 44,000. Enzymatic digestion cleaves the HLA molecule into two parts, one of which (MW 35,000) carries the antigenic determinants as well as the carbohydrates. The other part remains imbedded in the membrane. Detergent procedures release more-or-less intact molecules of larger size (MW 45,000) from the membrane. There is evidence suggesting one or two intrachain disulfide bonds.[28]

Work on the redistribution of surface markers caused by antibodies and shown by fluorescent indicators has given important knowledge about the native configuration of HLA antigens. This technique, known as *cap formation,* is performed by incubating divalent antibodies to form complexes on the surface. The complexes can be induced to aggregate into a single cap by the addition of antimmunoglobulins marked with fluorescent label. The capping process is not entirely passive, as it requires intact energy metabolism; and the cap will be internalized by endocytosis leaving a cell with almost none of the original surface antigens left, a phenomenon called *stripping.* Capping and stripping techniques have shown that two different antigens belonging to the same series—HLA-A1 and A2 for example—will form caps and strip

independently. Two antigens belonging to different series—A1 and B8 for example—also will cap and strip independently, whether or not they are coded by genes in the same haplotype. These studies indicate that the gene products of both allelic genes (A1, A2) and antigenic determinants on the same haplotype (A1, B8) are present on distinct molecules in the cell membrane.[29,30]

Beta-2-microglobulin is a recently discovered protein (MW 11,000 to 12,000) of unknown function. It is present in small amounts in serum and present as a cell surface component of the HLA antigen. Beta-2-microglobulin is believed to be the light chain of the HLA molecule and has some structural similarities to the light chain of immunoglobulin.[31]

HLA-D and DR molecules have more restricted tissue distribution than ABC molecules (Table 6-4). They are found only on macrophages, B lymphocytes, endothelial cells, and spermatozoa. Their structure is less well defined, but they are apparently composed of two noncovalently linked polypeptides of 25,000 and 33,000 MW.[32] They are highly polymorphic and induce strong T-cell proliferation and antibody production. The T-cell activating determinants are named D,

Table 6-4. General Properties of HLA Gene Products

Property	Gene Product	
	HLA-A, B or C	HLA-D or DR
Inheritance	Autosomal codominant	Autosomal codominant
Tissue Distribution	Ubiquitous. On cell membranes of all nucleated cells; platelets; soluble in plasma; occasional remnants on young erythrocytes.	Restricted. On cell membranes of B lymphocytes, monocytes, sperm, some epidermal cells, ? some T cells
Structure	44,000 d glycoprotein noncovalently associated with 12,000 d protein (beta-2-microglobulin)	HLA-DR: a complex of a 33,000 d and a 25,000 d glycoprotein. No beta-2-microglobulin.
Method of Direction	Serologic. using defined HLR antisera.	HLA-DR: Serologic. HLA-D: MLR against a panel of homozygous D locus cells.
Some functions	Targets for a variety of immune effector mechanisms.	Probably important in the afferent, cognitive phase of immune response.

while those producing antibody formation are called DR.

Serologic cross-reactivity is a phenomenon in which an antiserum directed against one HLA antigenic determinant also reacts with other antigenic determinants as well. Anti-A28, for instance, often reacts with A2, and anti-A11 will react with A3. These patterns of cross-reactivity have not been fully explained, but it has been suggested that cross-reactive antigens share important structural elements with one another but retain specific recognizable portions. Examples of some of the more common cross-reactivities within the A and B locus are given in Table 6-5.

HISTOCOMPATIBILITY TESTING TECHNIQUES

Techniques for histocompatibility testing are similar in purpose to those used for erythrocyte compatibility testing. Because the ABO antigens are important histocompatibility antigens in themselves, ABO typing is an important part of histocompatibility testing. The analog of Rh typing is HLA typing, which will be discussed in detail.

The examination of donor and recipient sera for antibodies to HLA antigens is important in that these antibodies may cause significant complications in transplantation or transfusion. Antibody to recipient leukocytes in donor plasma has been associated with severe pulmonary infiltrates and respiratory distress following transfusion.[33,34] If the serum of a potential renal allograft recipient contains cytotoxic antibodies reacting with the lymphocytes of the intended kidney donor, hyperacute rejection of the graft is an almost inevitable result.[34a,34b] Lymphocytotoxic or leukoagglutinating antibody in the recipient is also associated with febrile, nonhemolytic transfusion reactions[35,36] and, less predictably, with poor response to platelet or granulocyte transfusion.

Table 6-5. Some Cross-reactive Associations of Alleles of the HLA-A and HLA-B Loci

HLA-A Locus	HLA-B Locus
A1, A3, A11	B5, B18, B15, B17, Bw21, Bw35
A2, A28	B7, B27, Bw22
A9 (Aw23/Aw24), A1, A2	B7, B13, Bw40
A10 (A25/A26), A11, Aw32, Aw30	B8, B14
Aw30, Aw31, Aw32, Aw33	Bw16 (Bw38, Bw39)

Note: The alleles in parenthesis represent splits of the preceding allele.

Crossmatching in the histocompatibility system may involve examination for both serologically defined and lymphocyte-defined compatibility. Serologic crossmatching is performed by a leukoagglutination technique or by cytotoxicity, either conventional or enhanced by a variety of methods. Lymphocyte-defined compatibility is assessed by the mixed lymphocyte reaction method or one of its modifications.

TECHNIQUES TO DEMONSTRATE ANTIGENS AND ANTIBODIES

Serotyping for A, B, and C Alleles

The agglutination methods used initially to define the HLA complex have given way to a standardized, precise microlymphocytotoxicity test.[9] Cytotoxicity methods require only one to three μl of serum. These methods are sensitive and reproducible and do not require exceptional skill or equipment.

Briefly, a heparinized whole-blood specimen is collected and centrifuged, and the buffy coat is aspirated. A purified lymphocyte suspension is prepared by a wide variety of techniques, the most popular of which involves centrifugation on a ficoll-hypaque gradient. Purified lymphocytes are aspirated from the interface and washed, and 1 μl is added to 1 μl of antiserum in special 72-well microtest plates. The cell-serum mixture is incubated 30 minutes at room temperature, 5 μl of rabbit complement is added, and the incubation is continued for an additional 60 minutes at room temperature. Eosin dye is added to each well to assess the reaction. Injured or dead cells will take up the dye, indicating the presence of antigen on the cell corresponding to the antibody.

Since there is considerable variability even with the best typing reagents, at least two antisera are used to define each specificity whenever possible. Careful attention to methodology and quality control will assure 95 percent reproducibility with the cytotoxicity method.

A number of modifications of the cytotoxicity method have been introduced, including the addition of extra rabbit complement, modified incubation times and temperatures, and the use of fluorescent dyes to measure the end point. Since most antiserums are standardized for the NIH cytotoxicity method, they must be restandardized to the modified method if they are to give accurate results.

Detection of HLA Antibodies

Techniques for the demonstration and identification of HLA antibodies are similar in principle to those for demonstrating unexpected red cell antibodies—i.e., the unknown serum is tested againt a panel of cells whose antigens are established. Unlike red cells, however, cells from a fairly large panel of donors must be selected if antibodies to relatively uncommon specificities are to be demonstrated. A panel of at least 12 to 15 carefully selected cells is required for initial screening, and a panel of at least 40 cells is required for accurate antibody identification. Because the cells can only be preserved for a short period of time, laboratories that do not have a high volume of typing must either rely on a "walking panel" or freeze lymphocytes for subsequent testing. Freezing lymphocytes in trays has the advantage of rapid preparation, enabling serum to be screened within just a few hours.[37]

Crossmatching Techniques for Serologic Incompatibility

Although cytotoxicity is the standard method for HLA typing and the most widely used method for detection of serologic incompatibility, a variety of other methods are in use. Leukoagglutination techniques, usually performed on glass slides, have the advantage of detecting non-HLA antibodies to leukocytes.[38] A number of enhanced cytotoxicity methods using enzymes or antiglobulin serum have been described,[39] but few have found widespread acceptance. A granulocyte cytotoxicity method has been investigated by a number of workers as a crossmatch for granulocyte transfusion.[40] Similarly, crossmatches for platelet transfusions employ special techniques including platelet aggregometry,[41] serotonin release assays,[41d, e] fluorescent platelet antibody tests,[41a] and radioimmunoassays for platelet-bound IgG.[41b,d]

In all the crossmatch techniques, serum from the recipient is mixed with cells from the donor, incubated, and examined for possible antigen antibody reaction. Unfortunately, none of the crossmatch techniques can reliably predict the outcome of a transplant or transfusion because of problems of specificity and sensitivity, a host of unrelated clinical variables, and unknown factors. Indeed, platelet transfusions may result in adequate platelet count increments in patients with HLA antibodies to donor leukocytes,[41c] and the significance of HLA antibodies on the effectiveness of granulocyte transfusions has not yet been defined (see *Granulocyte Transfusion Therapy*). Still, transfusions of granulocytes and platelets in this setting may be ineffective or associated with severe and even fatal febrile reactions, and renal transplantation is not indicated in the presence of a positive crossmatch. Limited experience with marrow transplantation indicates that the presence of lymphocytotoxic antibodies against donor cells does not preclude successful engraftment.[22a] In this instance, plasma exchange was done prior to transplantation to remove detectable antibody.

Typing for HLA-D Alleles

Since rejection of allografted tissue is thought to involve lymphocyte-mediated immune response as well as serologic (antibody) response, a number of tests have been developed which use the biologic responses of lymphocytes to foreign antigens as a measure of histocompatibility. The mixed lymphocyte reaction (MLR) test is especially important, since it provides an in vitro model in which lymphocytes can be used as responders to foreign antigens and as stimulators carrying those antigens. For example, lymphocytes of a potential recipient are mixed with the lymphocytes from a potential donor. They are either activated (responders) or not activated (nonresponders). The response in MLR is measured by the incorporation of radioactive thymidine into the responding cells.

In the MLR test, the responding cells are mixed with the stimulating cells which have been pretreated with irradiation or Mitomycin-C to prevent them from dividing. The mixture is incubated for 5 to 7 days, and radioactive thymidine is added to the mixture. If the responding cells have, indeed, been stimulated, large amounts of labeled thymidine are incorporated into the newly synthesized DNA. This incorporation can be quantitated by placing the washed cell mixture in a liquid scintillation counter. Appropriate controls and duplicate samples must be run, which means that the test is not only time-consuming but expensive.

HLA-D Typing and Other Assays; Cell-Mediated Immunity

Since the cell-surface markers which cause a response in the MLR are genetically determined, assay systems have been developed to differentiate between the HLA-D antigens, as these markers are called. The MLR recognizes antigenic differences on stimulator cells; therefore, it follows that cells that bear the same HLA-D antigens as the responding cell will cause no stimulation.

In D typing, stimulator cells from individuals who are known to be homozygous for all antigens of the HLA haplotype (including the antigens of the D series) are used. Initially, these homozygous D typing cells were ob-

Mitomycin Treated Stimulator Cell Type	Unknown, Untreated Responder Cell	Result of Reaction of Stimulator with Cell XYZ
Dw1/Dw1		No Stimulation
Dw2/Dw2		Stimulation
Dw3/Dw3	Cell X,Y,Z in MLC	No Stimulation
Dw4/Dw4		Stimulation
Dw5/Dw5		Stimulation
Dw6/Dw6		Stimulation

Fig. 6-6. HLA-D typing is performed by one-way stimulation, using homozygous mitomycin-treated stimulator cells. The types are determined by the pattern of response and nonresponse. Since cell xyz is not stimulated by cell homozygous for Dw1 and Dw3 but was stimulated by the others, it must be of the fena type Dw1/Dw3.

tained from HLA-identical children of first-cousin marriages. More recently, similar cells have been found, although infrequently, in the general population.[42] Cells of both types are called homozygous typing cells. In order to type, homozygous typing cells of each type are set up in MLR as stimulators against the test cells. Lack of response in MLR indicates that the test cell bears the same antigen as the homozygous typing cell. So far, there are at least 12 recognized HLA-D phenotypes (See Table 6-1).

D typing is complicated, time-consuming, and expensive; it has not been established outside of a handful of typing laboratories. Serologic demonstration of the D antigens or a simplified culture technique might make the system much more widely available. Sheehy recently described a method for detecting the LD antigen using the primed lymphocyte typing (PLT) test.[43] Cells stimulated in MLR and left for 9 to 14 days (beyond their peak of proliferative activity) will give a very rapid and strong proliferative response if restimulated with cells of the same D type as the original stimulating cell donor. This secondary response can be assayed with radioactive thymidine within 24 hours, and at an even earlier time with radioactive uridine. The PLT test results can be available within a few hours.

If the MLR technique is a measurement of the recognition phase of lymphocyte interaction, the cell-mediated lympholysis (CML) test can be thought of as a test for the effector phase of the process. In the CML assay, the stimulator cells are incubated with the responder cells, just as in MLR. The responder lymphocytes, so generated, are then challenged with ^{51}Cr-labeled target lymphocytes from the original stimulating donor. If the responder cells are capable of effecting a "killer" response, there is lysis of the target cells, releasing ^{51}Cr into the medium.

The CML test is positive when there are HLA-D differences between the sensitizing cell donor and the responding, effector cell donor; the response is substantially greater when there are both D and A, B, and C differences.

Ideally, compatibility testing would involve typing for D antigens by the techniques previously described, evaluation of the effector mechanism by the CML test, and MLRs involving both donor and recipient as stimulator and responder cells. Because MLR testing is technically demanding and requires sophisticated counting equipment, relatively few laboratories are able to do good MLR testing. Still fewer are able to do D typing because of the lack of availability of appropriate lymphocyte test cells.

Recent evidence[22a] suggests that differences within the D region do not preclude successful marrow transplantation. Also, typing for D antigens is of no known significance in transfusion, since D antigens are not present on platelets or on mature granulocytes.[44] D antigens are of little value in the pretransplant evaluation of cadaveric organ donors, since they require 4 to 6 days of incubation before the results can be read.

Typing for DR Alleles

While it is likely that HLA-D and DR are located at separate points along the MHC, the fact that the molecular structure of D and DR alloantigens has not been determined makes it impossible to know the relationship between the D and DR genes themselves. HLA-DR is a newly defined system of serologically detected HLA antigens which are close to, but distinct from, the HLA-D specificity. The D and DR specificities have a much more restricted tissue distribution than the HLA-A, B, D, C antigens; they are readily detectable only on B lymphocytes, monocytes, spermatozoa, Langherhans cells of the skin, and granulocyte precursors. They are not readily detectable by microlymphocytotoxicity testing on mature granulocytes, platelets, red cells, or T-lymphocytes. To test for these specificities by microlymphocytotoxicity, it is necessary to enrich lymphocyte suspension for B cells. There are three techniques in general usage: (1) Sheep RBC rosette depletion of T cells; (2) adherence of B cells to petri dishes coated with antihuman globulin; and (3) differential adherence of B cells on nylon columns.

Erythrocyte rosette depletion provides the purest form of B cells for testing, but, because differential adherence in nylon wall columns is relatively simple, a majority of laboratories have changed to this procedure. Once a purified B lymphocyte preparation has been obtained, antiserum may be used as in a conventional microlymphocytotoxicity system. Antiserum for the DR alleles comes from the same sources as conventional A, B, and C serums—i.e., pregnant or postpartum women, patients with a history of allograft rejection, and cultured cell lines. Typing for DR alleles is difficult —not only because of the scarceness of quality antiserums, but because of the difficulty in preparing B cell suspensions. Because it gives much valuable information about HLA-D alleles, however, and because of its association with immune response gen-

esis in other species, DR typing is likely to grow in importance in coming years.

HISTOCOMPATIBILITY TESTING AND BLOOD TRANSFUSION

As indicated previously, human histocompatibility testing is a science derived from the evaluation of febrile nonhemolytic transfusion reactions in the blood bank. These febrile reactions were found to be due to preformed antibodies reacting with transfused granulocytes. It was soon shown that, if the granulocytes could be removed, the reactions would diminish or disappear. Greenwalt described a method of removing granulocytes by using nylon fiber adhesion, but most of the lymphocytes and platelets were in the transfused product.[45] Frozen deglycerolized blood was found to contain relatively few intact granulocytes, lymphocytes, or platelets; and centrifugal methods have been developed which remove more than 85 percent of these products without the expense and disadvantages of cumbersome washing techniques. These products are of great value in preventing febrile transfusion reactions in patients sensitized to leukocyte antigens by pregnancy or multiple blood transfusions.

There have been several reports of serious reactions to transfused donor plasma which contains potent antibodies to HLA antigens on granulocytes. These "minor side" reactions have become less common as more red blood cell concentrates are used, but plasma products are still commonly used and serious febrile reactions, some of which are associated with severe pulmonary symptoms such as dyspnea and hypoxia, may occur.

Alloimmunization to HLA Antigens by Blood Transfusion

During the last decade, there has been a great deal of interest in the prevention of alloimmunization to HLA antigens by limiting exposure to the antigens in transfusion products. Frozen blood and leukocyte-poor products have been recommended for those patients who will require multiple transfusions or subsequent transplantation, with the hope that alloimmunization may be prevented. Clinical investigations show that recipients of frozen or leukocyte-poor blood do not form cytotoxic or agglutinating antibodies nearly as frequently (5 to 15 percent) as those who receive ordinary packed cells or whole blood (60 to 70 percent).[46] The value of this difference in the patient who is receiving multiple blood transfusions, especially platelets and granulocytes, is under active investigation.

Similarly, it was originally felt that patients requiring renal transplantation might benefit by a lack of HLA antigen exposure. However, Opelz and Terasaki[46a-c, 47] and others[48] have presented evidence to suggest that graft outcome is better among those who have received at least some transfusions, compared to those who have received none. However, extensive transfusion resulting in sensitization to multiple antigens may make the process of finding a compatible organ quite difficult; but, if a compatible kidney can be found, previous exposure to blood products seems to improve graft survival in the recipient (see Ch. 29).

While HLA A, B, D, and C antigens are not present on mature erythrocytes, they seem to be present on erythrocyte precursors and are found in low concentration on young red cells. There has been a strong association between the leukocyte antigen A7 and the erythrocyte antigen Bg[a], and some investigators have proposed that they are controlled by the same gene.[49] Two blood group substances, Chido and Rodgers, have also been shown to be coded for genes within the HLA complex. Recent studies have conclusively shown that Chido and Rodgers are distinct antigenic components of C4. Since it is known that there are receptors for C4 on the surface of erythrocytes, it is postulated that these receptors absorb one or the other of the markers, so that the cells type as Chido or Rodgers positive.[50]

TESTING FOR PLATELET TRANSFUSIONS

The success of combined chemotherapy programs has led to a dramatic increase in platelet transfusions during the past decade. Six to eight platelet concentrates are often pooled and given to a recipient three or five times a week during periods of thrombocytopenia. A patient may be exposed to hundreds of different donors with as many HLA phenotypes. Alloimmunization to platelets has become common and often limits continuing chemotherapy. Yankee et al. found that HLA-matched platelets could sometimes restore satisfactory increments in patients who are alloimmunized and refractory to random-donor platelet transfusion.[51]

Based on Yankee et al.'s findings, a national pool of typed platelet donors was proposed, and efforts to that end are under way in both American Red Cross and the Council of Community Blood Centers blood banks. Initially, it was felt that the pool would of necessity be very large because the chance of finding a perfectly matched donor for a given patient would be quite small. Duquesnoy and his colleagues found it might not be necessary to match perfectly for all HLA antigens, and that it might be possible to substitute a "cross-reactive" antigen at times.[52] For example, an A1, B8, A11, B17 recipient might receive platelets from an A1, B8, A3, B17 donor, since A3 and A11 have been shown to be similar by cross-reactivity studies. By substituting cross-reactive antigens, a much smaller platelet pool can serve a given group of patients. It should be noted that HLA typing for histocompatible platelet transfusion should be performed before induction chemotherapy is initiated, since the peripheral blood lymphocyte count may drop to such low levels that accurate typing may be impossible.

It soon became obvious that even close HLA matching would not assure good platelet responses in all alloimmunized recipients. Third-locus antigens, untyped until recently, might be responsible for some of the discrepancies in the older studies, but non-HLA antigen systems seem to be even more likely candidates, since HLA-D antigens are not represented on platelets. Thus, it is necessary to develop crossmatch techniques which will identify platelet incompatibility in the face of HLA identity. Although a variety of methods have been studied, as discussed earlier in this chapter, current data concerning their clinical value are scanty.

At the present time, a straightforward lymphocyte cytotoxicity test seems to give the best predictive information of any of the available crossmatch techniques, although newer techniques using donor platelets as antigen are promising.

Granulocyte Transfusion Therapy

The data on the importance of histocompatibility testing for granulocyte transfusion are much more tentative. Graw and his co-workers presented evidence suggesting that improved HLA matching was associated with improved granulocyte increments in granulocytopenic recipients, even though those recipients had no evidence of alloimmunization.[53, 54] These data are puzzling and have not been the experience of others in the field. There is no question that, in patients who are alloimmunized as shown by leukoagglutination or granulocyte cytotoxicity assays, histocompatible granulocytes are important to prevent severe febrile reactions, although there are many false negatives and false positives. Lymphocyte cytotoxicity cell matching is of limited value in predicting either febrile reactions or transfusion response.

During recent years, other forms of crossmatching have been evaluated and seem promising. In one test, purified donor granulocytes are spread on a glass slide and incubated with the recipient's serum. After washing, fluorescein-coupled antihuman globulin is used to demonstrate the presence of immunoglobulins bound to the target cells. In preliminary studies, this immunofluorescent antiglobulin crossmatch seems to have a higher correlation with donor safety and granulocyte effectiveness than previous tests,[55] and is capable of detecting granulocyte specific antigens as well as HLA antigens.

Just as there are platelet-specific antigens detected by special techniques, so are there granulocyte-specific antigens which are not detected by lymphocyte cytotoxicity. They are occasionally responsible for febrile transfusion reactions and poor response to granulocyte therapy, but have been implicated more often in neonatal thrombocytopenia, where maternal antibody to granulocytes crosses the placenta to destroy fetal granulocytes.

HLA typing and matching is probably of value in the alloimmunized recipient, but of questionable value in a patient with no evidence of preformed antibodies to granulocytes.

The HLA Complex and Bone Marrow Transplantation

Bone marrow transplantation is comparatively new as a technique to treat patients with various forms of leukemia, severe aplastic anemia, and certain immunodeficiency diseases. Briefly, the immunosuppressed recipient receives 400 to 800 ml of aspirated bone marrow by the intravenous route. Rejection and graft-versus-host disease are two of the major problems associated with marrow transplantation in which histocompatibility plays a major role. There is a high risk of rejection of the marrow if the patient is not HLA-identical as measured by HLA typing.[22a] In contrast, ABO incompatibility does not preclude successful marrow transplantation.[56]

Because many of the patients may require multiple blood transfusions prior to transplantation, it is especially important to consider donor selection for supportive transfusion therapy. Family members (other than children of the proposed recipient) should not be used as blood donors even though they are HLA-identical, since they may immunize the recipient to non-HLA determinants for which it is currently impossible to test.[56]

Usually, HLA-A, B and C-compatible persons can be found in the general population by using large pools of HLA matched individuals such as the national pool described above. Uncommonly, donors who are also identical at the HLA-D locus can be identified in the random population, but, as the size of the national pool grows, the likelihood of identifying compatible donors increases. At present, some success has resulted from marrow transplantation from family-member donors other than HLA-identical siblings,[22a] and some successful transplants have been performed utilizing nonfamily members matched at the HLA-A, B, and C loci but mismatched at the D locus. Marrow donation is associated with substantially more risk than donation of platelets and granulocytes by pherersis, and the ethical issues of using volunteer marrow donors from the random population must be considered. Because of the high risk of graft-versus-host disease, blood products for bone marrow transplant patients should be irradiated to destroy transfused donor lymphocytes unless the product is from the transplant donor.

Since histocompatible bone marrow transplantation offers great promise for the treatment of aplastic anemia, immunodeficiency disease, and acute leukemia,[57, 58] solutions to the clinical and immunologic problems of the transplant procedure are important. It is possible that cadaveric sources could be used, especially if they could be preserved in the frozen state for histocompatibility testing and transportation. Indeed, a bank of preserved marrow from cadaver donors now seems technically feasible.

HLA Serotyping in Cases of Disputed Paternity

As a result of expanding the knowledge of the HLA system, there has been a revolution in paternity testing. Using the available erythrocyte blood groups alone, it is possible to exclude only 60 percent of falsely accused men; but, using the HLA system in addition, it is possible to exclude over 95 percent of falsely accused men and to indicate those men who are highly likely to be the biologic father. Indeed, most men not excluded by HLA typing have a high probability of paternity.[59] The addition of erythrocyte blood grouping to HLA typing makes paternity testing highly accurate and informative.

The HLA system fills a number of important criteria for paternity testing. HLA factors are inherited in a classical Mendelian codominant fashion, with antigen frequencies less than 50 percent, and most less than 15 percent. Since most antigen frequencies are low, calculations for probability of paternity are highly informative. Now that reagents are generally available, this system is practical, and testing is done in several laboratories. The system is reliable and reproducible, with a very low error rate.

Because the commonest haplotypes (HLA A1, B8, and A2, B12) are comparatively rare, the child's HLA factors can be thought to represent two haplotypes—one from each parent—each haplotype rare and distinctive. If the child lacks either of the putative father's possible haplotypes, the man is obviously excluded. Conversely, if the child possesses a rare type which the putative father also possesses, there is presumptive evidence of paternity. An example is given in Figure 6-7. In this case, the putative father A shares only one antigen with the child, A1. A1 in the putative father must be associated with either B17 or B14, but neither is present in the child. The child, in fact, has inherited A1 and B8 from the mother. The putative father is therefore excluded. On the other hand, putative father B possesses the A11, B12 haplo-

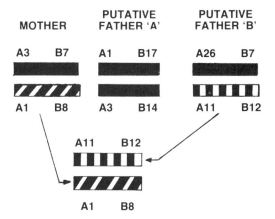

Fig. 6-7. HLA typing in disputed paternity: a case in which only one of two possible fathers could have contributed A11, B12, the required paternal haplotype.

type which is also found in the child. Since the A11, B12 haplotype is rare (frequency about .026) and since it is found in both the putative father and the child, paternity by putative father B seems likely. The actual calculation of probability of paternity can be performed using the haplotype frequency, or, if there is no appreciable linkage disequilibrium, the gene frequencies for A and B.

Disease Associations

The association of HLA antigens with a variety of diseases has opened new vistas into the pathogenesis of these processes. These associations may yield not only clues about the genetics of disease which may be relevant to the diagnosis, prognosis, treatment, and prevention, but they also may give new dimensions to our understanding of the biologic importance of the HLA complex. Mice exhibit genetic susceptibility to a lupus-like syndrome, autoimmune thyroiditis, lymphocytic choroimeningitis, and murine leukemia, as well as experimental viral diabetes.[60] This susceptibility appears to be controlled by genetic factors associated with the mouse H2 complex.

It has long been known that there is an association between certain red blood cell groups and disease, but the strongest association is that found between blood group O and duodenal ulcer with a risk of 1.33 (that is, a 33 percent increment in the risk of developing duodenal ulcer for subjects with the blood group O). The relative risks for HLA in disease are considerably higher, with ankylosing spondylitis being the most notable. Individuals positive for a B27 antigen are 120 times as likely to develop ankylosing spondylitis as individuals who are B27-negative.[61]

These associations point to an important function of HLA and certain red blood cell antigens in natural selection. Since many antigens may be lethal and occur before the age of reproduction, they may have a role in producing differences in blood group and HLA gene frequencies in the world populations. The most appealing aspect of the HLA studies in disease is the promise that the populations at risk for certain disorders will be identified and opportunities for preventive medicine will emerge.

The clinical applications of HLA antigens in daily diagnostic practice are still limited. Rheumatologists are finding tissue typing useful in the diagnosis of ankylosing spondylitis, and the same is true of Reiter's disease, which is also associated with HLA B27. There is a tentative evidence that diabetic microangiopathy may be more severe in B8-positive diabetics; that progression of multiple sclerosis is faster in Dw2-positive patients; that Hodgkin's disease responds more favorably to treatment in B8-positive patients; and that acute lymphocytic leukemia is less severe in patients with A2 and A9.[62]

Despite the broad range of diseases associated with HLA antigens, the diseases tend to share some general features in common: weak familial propensity; chronicity; disease onsets during adulthood; and immunologic aberrations such as autoimmunity.

The mechanism responsible for the association of HLA types and certain diseases is not known. A number of theories have been proposed which are currently being tested. The theories can be divided into two general categories: First, the HLA gene product is directly responsible for increased susceptibility, perhaps through molecular mimicry and cross tolerance. Second, the HLA antigen is not directly involved but is serving as a marker for some other gene product closely linked such as an immune response gene. It seems likely that susceptibility to disease is somehow related to altered immunologic responsiveness, and it is probable that the diseases in question have multifactorial etiologies involving multiple gene interactions and environmental factors.

REFERENCES

1. McDevitt, H.O., Landy, M., Eds.: Genetic Control of the Immune Responsiveness Relationship to Disease Susceptibility. Academic Press, New York, 1972.
2. McDevitt, H.O. and Bodmer, W.F.: HLA, Immune-response Genes and Disease. Lancet 1:1269, 1974.
3. Zinkernagel, R.M.: Major Transplantation Antigens in Host Responses to Injection. Hosp. Pract. 13:83, 1978.
4. Dausset, J.: Leukoagglutinins. IV. Leukoagglutinins and Blood Transfusion Vox Sang. 4:190, 1954.
5. Dausset, J.: Iso-leuco-anticorps. Acta haemat. 20:156, 1958.
6. Payne, R.: The association of febrile transfusion reactive with leukoagglutinins. Vox Sang. 2:233, 1957.
7. van Rood, J.J., vanLeeuwen, A.: Leukocyte Grouping: A method and its application. J. Clin. Invest. 42:1382, 1963.
8. Terasaki, P.I., McClelland, J.P.: Microdroplet assay of human serum cytotoxins. Nature 204:998, 1964.
9. Terasaki, P.I., et al.: Microdroplet Testing for HLA-A, -B, -C and -D Antigens Am. J. Clin. Pathol. 69:103, 1978.
10. WHO: Nomenclature for factors of the HL-A system. Bull. WHO 39:483, 1968.
11. Ceppellini, R., et al.: Genetics of leukocyte antigens. A family study of segregation and linkage. Histocompatibility Testing 1967, p. 149, Munksgaard, Copenhagen.
12. Sandberg, L., et al.: Evidence for a third sublocus within the HLA chromosomal region. Histocompatibility Testing 1970, p. 165. Munksgaard, Copenhagen.
13. Bach, F. H. and Hirshhorn, K: Lymphocyte Interaction: A potential histocompatibility test in vitro. Science 143:813, 1964.
14. Bain, B. and Lowenstein. L.: Genetic studies on the mixed leukocyte reaction. Science 145:1315, 1964.
15. Bach, F.H. and Amos, D.B.: Hu-1: Major histocompatibility locus in man. Science 156:1506, 1967.
16. Dupont, B. et al.: Typing for MLC determinants by means of LD-homozygote and LP-heterozygote test cells. Transplantation Proc. 5:1543, 1973.
17. van Rood, J.J., et al.: The serological recognition of the human MLC determinants using a modified cytotoxicity technique. Tissue Antigens 5:73, 1975.
18. Thorsby, E., et al.: Typing for HLA (LD-1 or MLC) determinants. Histocompatibility Testing 1975, p. 415, Munksgaard, Copenhagen.
19. Albrechtsen, D., Solheim B.G., and Thorsby, E., Serological Identification of Five HLA-D Associated (Ia-Like) Determinants. Tissue Antigens 9:153, 1977.
20. WHO: No nomenclature for factors of the HLA system. Histocompatibility Testing 1975, p. 5, Munksgaard, Copenhagen.
21. D'Amaro, J.: W4 (4a) and W6(4b) in Diverse Human Populations. Demonstrations of their Genetic Identity in Population and Segregation Studies. Tissue Antigens 5:386, 1975.
22. Barnstable, C.J. et al.: The Structure and Evolution of the HLA-Bw 4 and Bw6 Antigens. Tissue Antigens, 13:334, 1979.
22a. Clift, R.A., Hansen, J.A., Thomas, E.D., et al.: Marrow transplantation from donors other than HLA-identical siblings. Transplantation 28:235, 1979.
23. Belvedere, M.C.: et al.: On the heterogenetics of linkage estimations between LA and four loci of the HLA system. Tissue Antigens 5:99, 1975.
24. Nielsen, L. Staub and Svejgaard, A.: The Third (AJ) segregant series. Histocompatibility Testing 1975, p. 324, Munksgaard Copenhagen, 1975.

25. Reinsmoen, N.L., et al.: Anomalous Lymphocyte culture reactivity between HLA-A, -B, -C and -DR Identical siblings. Tissue Antigens 13:19, 1979.

26. Joint Report of the Fifth International Histocompatibility Workshop. Histocompatibility Testing 1972, p. 618. Munkgaard, Copenhagen, 1972.

27. Klein, J.: Biology of the Mouse Histocompatibility 2 Complex; Springer, Berlin, 1975.

28. Hess, M. and Smith, W.: Comparative studies on mouse (H-2) and human (HLA) histocompatibility antigens. Eur. J. Bioch. 43:471, 1974.

29. Bernoco, D. et al.: HLA molecules at the cell surface. Histocompatibility Testing 1972; p. 527, Munksgaard, Copenhagen 1972.

30. Bourguignon, L.Y., et al.: Participation of histocompatibility antigens in capping molecularly independent cell surface components by their specific antibodies. Proc. Nat'l Acad. Sci. 75:2406, 1978.

31. Franklin, E.C.: Beta, Microglobulin—small molecule—Big Role? N. Engl. J. Med. 293:1254, 1975.

32. Thorsby, E., The Human Major Histocompatibility Complex HLA: Some Recent Developments. Transplantation Proc. 11:616, 1979.

33. Thompson, J.S., Severson, C.D., Parmely, M.J., et al.: Pulmonary "hypersensitivity" reactions induced by transfusion of non-HL-A leukoagglutinins. N. Engl. J. Med. 284:1120, 1971.

34. Andrews, A.T., Zmijewski, C.M., Bowman, H.S.: Transfusion reaction with pulmonary infiltration associated with HLA-specific leukocyte antibodies. Am. J. Clin. Path. 66:483–487, 1976.

34a. Kissmeyer-Nielsen, F., Olsen, S., Petersen, V.P., and Fjelborg, O.: Hyperacute rejection of kidney allografts, associated with pre-existing humoral antibodies against donor cells. Lancet 2:662, 1966.

34b. Patel, R. and Terasaki, P.I.: Significance of the positive crossmatch test in kidney transplantation. N. Engl. J. Med. 280:735, 1969.

35. van Rood, J.J., et al.: Leukocyte groups: the normal Leukocyte Transfer test, and homograft sensitivity. In: Histocompatibility Testing 1965. Balner H., Clefton, F.J., Eerniss, J.G., Eds. Willierams & Wilkins, Baltimore, 1966, p. 31–50.

36. Perkins, H.A., Payne, R., Ferguson, J., et al.: Non-hemolytic febrile transfusion reactions; quantitative effects of blood components with emphasis on isoantigenic incompatibility of leukocytes. Vox Sang. 11:578–600, 1966.

37. Shaw, J.F.: Preliminary screening and tentative identification of HL-A lymphocytotoxic antibodies in a hospital blood bank. Transfusion 13:44–49, 1973.

38. Zmijewski, C.M.: EDTA agglutination assay, in Manual of Tissue Typing Technics. DHEW Publication (NIH) 76-545, Washington, D.C., 1974, p. 18.

39. van Rood, J.J. Microagglutination method, in Manual of Tissue Typing Technics. DHEW Publication (NIH) 76-545, Washington, D.C., 1974, p. 17.

40. Hasegawa, T., Graw, R.G., Terasaki, P.I.: A microgranulocyte cytotoxicity test, in Manual of Tissue Typing Technics. DHEW Publication (NIH) 76-545, Washington, D.C., 1974, p. 89.

41. Wu, K.K., Hoak, J.C.: Thompson, J.S., et al.: Use of platelet aggregometry in selection of compatible platelet donors. N. Engl. J. Med. 292:130, 1975.

41a. Brand, A., van Leeuwen, A., Eernisse, J.G., et al.: Platelet transfusion therapy. Optimal donor selection with a combination of lymphocytotoxicity and platelet fluorescence tests. Blood 51:781, 1978.

41b. Slichter, S.J.: Platelet Antibody Detection by Radiolabeled Protein Staph A. Blood 54 (Suppl. 1):115a, 1979.

41c. Tomasulo, P.A.: Management of the alloimmunized patient with HLA-matched platelets. In: Platelet Physiology and Transfusion, Am. Assoc. Blood Banks, 1978.

41d. Slichter, S.J.: Selection of compatible platelet donors. In: Platelet Physiology and Transfusion, Am. Assoc. Blood Banks, 1978, pp. 83–89.

41e. Gockerman, J.P., Bowman R.P., and Conrad, M.E.: Detection of platelet isoantibodies by (^{3}H) serotonin platelet release and its clinical application to the problem of platelet matching. J. Clin. Invest. 55:75, 1975.

42. Thorsby, E. and Piazza, A., eds.: Joint Report from the Sixth International Histocompatibility Conference, II. Typing for HLA-D (LD-1 or MLC) determinants, in Histocompatibility Testing, Munksgaard, Copenhagen, 1975, p. 414.

43. Sheehy, M.J., Sondel, P.H., Bach, M.L., et al.: HL-A LD (lymphocyte defined) typing: a rapid assay with primed lymphocytes. Science 188:1308–1310, 1975.

44. vanLeeuwen, A., Schuit, H.R.E., vanRood, J.J.: Typing for MLC (LD), II. The selection of nonstimulator cells by MLC inhibition tests using SD-identical stimulator cells (MISIS) and fluorescence antibody studies. Transplant. Proc. 5:1539–1542, 1973.

45. Greenwalt, T.J., Gajewski, M., McKenna, J.L.: A new method for preparing buffy coat-poor blood. Transfusion 2:221–229, 1962.

46. Polesky, H.F., McCullough, J., Helgeson, M.A., et al.: Evaluation of methods for the preparation of HL-A antigen-poor blood. Transfusion 13:383–387, 1973.

46a. Opelz, G. and Terasaki, P.I.: Prolongation effect of blood transfusions on kidney graft survival. Transplantation 22:380, 1976.

46b. Opelz, G. and Terasaki, P.I.: Enhancement of kidney graft survival by blood transfusions. Transplant. Proc. 9:121, 1977.

46c. Opelz, G. and Terasaki, P.I.: Improvement of kidney-graft survival with increased numbers of blood transfusions. N. Engl. J. Med. 299:799, 1978.

47. Opelz, G., Sengar, D.P.S., Mickey, M.R., et al.: Effect of blood transfusion on subsequent kidney transplants. Transplant. Proc. 5:253–259, 1973.

48. Van Es, A.A. and Balner, H.: Effect of pre-transplant transfusions on kidney allograft survival. Transplant. Proc. 11:127, 1979.

49. Morton, J.A., Pickles, M.M., Sutton, L.: The correlation of the Bg^a blood group with the HL-A7 leukocyte group: Demonstration of antigenic sites on red cells and leukocytes. Vox. Sang. 17:536–547, 1969.

50. O'Neill, G.J., Yang, S.Y., and Dupont, B.: Chido and Rodgers Blood Groups; Relationship to C4 and HLA, Transplant. Proc. 10:749, 1976.

51. Yankee, R.A., Grumet, F.C., Rogentine, G.N.: Platelet transfusion therapy; the selection of compatible platelet donors for refractory patients by lymphocyte HL-A typing. N. Engl. J. Med. 281:1208, 1969.

52. Duquesnoy, R.J., Filip D.J., and Aster, R.H.: Hemostatic effectiveness of selectively mismatched platelet transfusions in refractory thrombocytopenic patients. Blood 46:1056, 1975.

53. Graw, R.G., Jr., Goldstein, I.M., Eyre, H.J., et al.: Histocompatibility testing for leukocyte transfusion. Lancet 2:77, 1970.

54. Graw, R.G., Jr., Herzig, G., Perry, S., et al.: Normal granulocyte transfusion therapy: treatment of septicemia due to gram-negative bacteria. N. Engl. J. Med. 287:367, 1972.

55. Verheugt, F.W.A., et al.: The detection of granulocyte alloantibodies with indirect immunofluorescence test. Br. J. Haematol. 36:533, 1977.

56. Thomas, E.D., Storb, R., Clift, R.A., et al.: Bone-marrow transplantation. N. Engl. J. Med. 292:832 & 895, 1975.

57. Storb, R., Buckner, C.D., Fefer, A., et al.: Marrow transplantation in aplastic anemia. Transplant. Proc. 6:355, 1974.

58. Blume, K.C., Beutler, E., Bross, K.J., et al.: Bone-marrow ablation and allogeneic marrow transplantation in acute leukemia. N. Engl. J. Med. 302:1041, 1980.

59. Terasaki, P.I.: Resolution for HLA testing of 1000 paternity cases not excluded by ABO testing. J. Family Law 16:543, 1977.

60. Barbosa, J., Yunis, E.J.: HLA and disease, in HLA Typing. Washington, Am. Assoc. Blood Banks, 1976.

61. Brewerton, D., Caffrey, M., Hart, F., et al.: Anklyosing spondylitis and HL-A27. Lancet 1:904–907, 1973.

62. Svejgaard, A., Platz, P., Ryder, L., et al.: HL-A and disease associations—A survey. Transplant. Rev. 22:3–43, 1975.

7

Red Cell Compatibility Testing

Lawrence D. Petz, M.D., Scott N. Swisher, M.D.
Donald R. Branch, M.T. (A.S.C.P.) S.B.B.

The first segment of this chapter concerns aspects of compatibility testing that are of direct concern to clinicians. This section includes a discussion of the principles of compatibility testing, reviews the relationship between in vitro incompatibility and in vivo survival of transfused red cells, and relates this information to clinical decision making.

Other aspects of compatibility testing that are of more immediate interest and concern to blood bankers are considered in the second segment of this chapter, "Techniques of Compatibility Testing." These topics include the origins of the compatibility test, the application of antibody detection techniques to compatibility testing, and recent concepts in compatibility test procedures.

THE CLINICAL SIGNIFICANCE OF COMPATIBILITY TESTING

The Principles of Compatibility Testing

Tests for red cell compatibility have as their purpose the prevention of hemolytic transfusion reactions. In brief, compatibility testing involves typing the donor and recipient red blood cells for ABO and Rho(D) antigens and testing the recipient's serum for the presence of red cell alloantibodies which react in vitro with the red cells of the potential donor.

The Ninth Edition (1978) of *Standards for Blood Banks and Transfusion Services* of the American Association of Blood Banks[1] indicates that testing the recipient's serum for antibodies should be performed by two methods which may be done concurrently. The first of these is usually referred to as the antibody screening test and is performed by testing the patient's serum with samples of red cells containing red cell antigens known to have been implicated in almost all hemolytic transfusion reactions. This requires testing against the red cells of at least two donors; these red cells are readily available from commercial sources.

The second method for antibody detection is the "major crossmatch" test, which is performed by testing the patient's serum against a sample of red cells from each potential donor unit. For antibody screening and for the crossmatch, the American Association of Blood Banks' *Standards* indicates that the tests "shall employ methods which will demonstrate significant coating, hemolyzing, and agglutinating antibodies active at 37° C, and shall include an antiglobulin test."

The definition of "significant" is not given, nor are more details given concerning appropriate methodology. Both of these topics are of intense current interest and continuing investigation. As a result, our present concepts are rapidly evolving and are discussed in some detail in the second segment of this chapter, "Techniques of Compatibility Testing."

The Biological Problem of Donor-Recipient Compatibility for Red Cells

It is fortunate that there is a relatively high correlation between serological evidences of donor-recipient compatibility or incompatibility and the fate of the donor red cells when they are delivered into the recipient's circulation. Faith in this relationship, gained over a long experience, has permitted development of modern blood transfusion and all those medical and surgical procedures which depend upon it.

Yet, it has been known for a long time that there are notable exceptions to the high general correspondence between in vivo and in vitro evidences of donor-recipient compatibility. These exceptions occur in both directions. Red cells thought to be compatible by in vitro tests may be found to be destroyed at a variably accelerated rate, even very rapidly, in the donor's circulation.[2-10] In contrast, some red cell alloantibodies are found not to result in rapid red cell destruction in vivo,[11-15] even though they react in vitro at 37°C in compatibility tests. The existence of these exceptions and the clinical importance of them is poorly understood by physicians who employ transfusion therapy. The biological basis for some of these seeming paradoxes is understood equally poorly even by researchers active in the field.

The ultimate definition of donor-recipient compatibility is based upon what happens when the donor red cells are delivered into the recipient's circulation. It is mandatory to regard the administration of a transfusion as an essential part of the compatibility testing procedure. It is in effect an in vivo crossmatch of donor and recipient. This is particularly true of the early period of a transfusion administered for reasons other than acute blood loss, during which a limited amount of blood—about 25 ml of red cells or 50 ml of whole blood—should be administered over about 30 minutes. The patient should be observed carefully during this period. If any suspicion of incompatibility is observed, the transfusion should be stopped promptly and the matter investigated, as discussed in Chapter 37.

When donor red cell destruction is relatively rapid, it is recognizable clinically, either as an immediate or delayed transfusion reaction. However, red cell survival may even be shortened in the absence of overt indications of an adverse reaction to transfused red cells. At slower rates of red cell destruction, hemolysis may be recognized as an inefficient transfusion as indicated by a suboptimal rise in hemoglobin or by the rapid reappearance of anemia. If hemolysis is still slower, with the donor cells eliminated over 60 days or so, donor-recipient incompatibility will rarely be recognized in the absence of serological evidence of it.

The Fate of Donor Red Cells in the Presence of Alloantibody

The philosophy that has generally prevailed in the past among blood bankers has been that all red cell alloantibodies must be regarded as having the potential for causing shortened survival of transfused red cells that have the corresponding antigen. As indicated above, it has become increasingly evident that this is not true; some antibodies cause rapid hemolysis with associated morbidity and mortality, whereas others have no discernable in vivo effects. This intriguing biologic problem has led to efforts to develop in vitro methods to assess the hemolytic potential of antibodies in vivo.

Many factors may influence whether or not

Table 7-1. Factors Which May Influence the Clinical Significance of Red Cell Antibodies

1. Specificity
2. Thermal Range of Antibody
3. Number of Antigen Sites on Red Cell Membrane
4. Mobility of Antigens Within Membrane
5. Class of Immunoglobulin
6. Subclass of IgG
7. Quantity of Antibody Sensitizing Red Cell
8. Equilibrium Constant of Antibody
9. Presence of Blood Group Antigenic Substances in Donor Plasma
10. Ability of Antibody to Activate Complement
11. Amount of Blood Transfused
12. Activity of Recipient's Reticuloendothelial System

a red cell antibody will cause hemolysis in vivo. These are summarized in Table 7-1. Unfortunately, there is as yet no recognized in vitro characteristic or group of characteristics which can be used to indicate the in vivo significance of all red cell antibodies. Serologic characteristics of an antibody correlated empirically with past clinical experience has provided most of our present fund of knowledge. In addition, red cell survival studies have contributed significantly.

Clinical Significance of Red Cell Alloantibodies

The two serologic characteristics of a red cell antibody that have been found most helpful in predicting its in vivo significance are its specificity and its ability to react at 37° C.

Experience has indicated that antibodies that are reactive only at temperratures below 37° C are clinically benign.[16] Antibodies that react at 37° C and that cause a large majority of hemolytic transfusion reactions are antibodies of the ABO, Rh, Kell, Kidd, Duffy, and SsU blood group systems. The incidence of these antibodies in four large studies is indicated in Table 7-2.

In contrast, numerous blood group antibodies are now considered by most blood bankers to be benign, although, until recently, the transfusion of antigen-negative blood was often considered necessary when these antibodies were present. For example, cold-reactive antibodies such as anti-A_1, -P_1, -M, -N, and -Lu^a can safely be ignored, except when their thermal amplitude is up to 37° C.[16] Even when antibodies of these specificities react at 37° C, their in vivo significance is uncertain.

Other alloantibodies are "benign" even though reacting at 37° C in the compatibility test; examples are anti-Vel, -Ge^a, -Yk^a, -Co^a, -Ch^a, -Rg^a, and -Bg.[11,16,17]

Anti-Lewis antibodies are frequently encountered, but only a small proportion of anti-Le^a antibodies can cause significant red cell destruction.[16] Since criteria have not been established to distinguish by in vitro tests the clinically important Le^a antibodies from those that do not cause in vivo hemolysis, Le(a−) blood is customarily given to patients whose serum contains anti-Le^a reactive at 37° C. In contrast, anti-Le^b is often ignored.

Still other antibodies are inconsistent in regard to their in vivo significance. Published data on the hemolytic potential of anti-Yt^a (Cartwright) is conflicting, and the few reported studies suggest that the hemolytic potential must be individually determined. In the first case of anti-Yt^a to be described, Yt(a+) cells were still detected 64 days after transfusion, and the direct antiglobulin test remained positive for 39 days, suggestive that the antibody was incapable of red cell destruction.[9] Other, apparently benign, examples have been reported with chromium survival studies indicating a strictly normal survival.[11] On the other hand, four cases have been described in which chromium-labeled Yt(a+) red cells were rapidly destroyed by anti-Yt^a in vivo.[9,11,18,19]

Finally, antibodies are occasionally found that react with "high-frequency antigens"— i.e., antigens found on almost all human red cells, such as k, Kp^b, Js^b, Yk^a, Ch^a, Vel, Yt^a, Ge, Jo^a, Jr^a. Although reference laboratories possess red cells lacking such high-frequency antigens, identification of the antibody may

Table 7-2. 37°C Antibodies Detected in Blood Transfusion Recipients in Four Studies

	Grove-Rasmussen and Huggins* [16a] (1973)	Tovey[16b] (1974)	Spielman and Seidl[16c] (1974)	Walker[16d] (1977)	Total	Order of Frequency
AntiD	8,772	3,002	245	778	12,797	1
Anti-E	1,079	231	45	118	1,473	3
Anti-c	619	154	14	53	840	5
Anti-e	86	20	0	2	108	8
Anti-C (together with D)	2,156	28	52	163	2,399	2
Anti-Kell (K, k)	978	174	41	181	1,374	4
Anti-Duffy (Fy^a, Fy^b)	372	72	16	55	515	6
Anti-Kidd (Jk^a, Jk^b)	141	17	12	13	183	7
Anti-Ss	0	9	0	0	9	9
Others (eg, Le^a, Le^b, Wr^a M, N, P_1, unidentified)	1,177	0	72	184	1,433	
	15,758	3,707	497	1,537	21,131	

* Does not include antibodies when detected together with other antibodies (except for Anti-C when present with anti-D)

(Garratty, G.: Clinically Significant Antibodies Reacting Optimally at 37 °C. *In:* Clinically Significant and Insignificant Antibodies, Am. Assoc. of Blood Banks, Wash., D.C., 1979, p. 29.)

be difficult and its in vivo significance uncertain.

It is also true that the severity of hemolysis caused by antibodies that are considered clinically significant varies strikingly. Anti-A and anti-B antibodies usually, but not always, cause immediate symptomatic transfusion reactions which, in a minority of cases, may even be fatal. Some antibodies in the Rh, Kell, and Kidd blood group systems may cause serious degrees of hemolysis, whereas, in other instances, only modest shortening of red cell survival occurs and there are no important clinical sequelae.

Finally, red cell autoantibodies are of varying clinical significance and cause unique problems in compatibility testing. These are discussed in detail in Chapter 31.

Clinical Interpretation of the Compatibility Test

Clinicians, in consultation with the physician director of the blood transfusion service, must determine the appropriate course when in vitro incompatibility exists. In each case of incompatibility, the clinician has a right to expect the director of the blood transfusion service to provide as accurate an assessment as is possible of the risk of tranfusion. The clinician, in turn, should have adequate understanding of compatibility testing to allow for meaningful communication with the blood bank director, and must incorporate information regarding the risks of blood tranfusion into his decision-making process concerning management of the patient.

For example, if a patient has an antibody in his serum which would appear to be clinically significant because of its specificity and temperature of reactivity, the course of least risk to the patient may be to delay a surgical procedure, even if it is urgently needed, for the amount of time necessary to provide compatible blood. Most such incompatibility problems can be resolved within a few hours.

In other instances of serologic incompatibility, it may be inappropriate to delay surgery or to delay the transfusion of an anemic patient not requiring surgery.

Some patients may develop multiple antibodies or a clinically significant antibody against a high-frequency antigen, thus making it extremely difficult to find units of blood lacking the relevant antigen(s). In such situations, the most appropriate course of action must be decided on an individual basis. In some cases, compatible blood may be obtained from a large donor center, from a rare donor file, or from family members. Autologous transfusion would be a safe approach, if feasible (see Ch. 15) and, in the future, blood substitutes may play a significant role (see Ch. 35). In some cases, particularly when antibodies against high-frequency antigens are present, red cell survival studies of an aliquot of cells may be useful in predicting safety of transfusion (see below). Finally, one must recognize that, in life-threatening emergencies, transfusion of red cells that will not survive normally is nevertheless warranted if the only available alternative is to allow the patient to die.

Donor Erythrocyte Destruction in the Absence of Serological Evidence of Alloimmunization

Since 1957, a number of reports have appeared describing rapid destruction of transfused red cells despite apparent in vitro compatibility between the recipient serum and donor erythrocytes.[2-10,20] In spite of increasing sensitivity of serologic techniques, the problem continues to be recognized and reported in the modern literature.[10] Other cases not reported are known in many blood centers and transfusion services.

In the laboratory of one of the authors (SNS) it has been shown that the phenomenon can be evoked quite easily in dogs by following the fate of repeated transfusions from the same donor of ^{51}Cr-labeled red cells which are not recognized as antigenically different by typing with the limited number of sera which detect canine erythrocyte antigen systems.[21] After several such transfusions, shortening of red cell life span in vivo has been observed in about 10 percent of animals so challenged. In about half of these responders, weak serological evidence of alloimmunization has been found, but the specificities of many of these antibodies have been incompletely investigated. They are difficult to work with in the laboratory because of the weak reactions they produce;

they may, in some instances, be parts of already recognized systems.

In the case of man, it was recognized shortly after practical methods for determining the life span of donor red cells in vivo that, in some instances, apparently compatible donor red cells disappeared more rapidly than expected.[9] There may be an initial phase of normal survival testing for 10 days or more, followed by a phase of accelerated destruction, suggesting that the transfusion has induced an immune response; this type of curve has been called a "collapse" curve (Fig. 7-1). In other instances, however, accelerated destruction of transfused red cells begins at the time of transfusion (Figs. 7-2 and 7-3).

Accelerated red cell destruction in the absence of demonstrable antibodies may be a serious clinical problem and may be difficult or impossible to resolve. In some instances, the accelerated destruction occurs as a delayed hemolytic transfusion reaction during the early stages of an immune response.[22] The small amount of antibody initially produced may be absorbed onto red cells but not yet be detectable in the patient's serum (see below, "Significance of the Direct Antiglobulin Test and Autocontrol in Pretransfusion Testing"). In these patients, antibody often becomes detectable in the patient's serum in subsequent days or weeks.

A much more difficult problem is presented by those patients in whom accelerated red cell destruction occurs repeatedly but antibody is never detected. Most commonly, attempts to find a compatible donor fail. For example, a patient described by Heistø et al.[6] developed hemoglobinuria six days after the transfusion of 2800 ml of blood. Tests were subsequently carried out with red cells from eight different donors. The red cell survival as measured by [51]Cr T$\frac{1}{2}$ varied from 14 days to less than 24 hours. Incidentally, the administration of large doses of prednisone did not prevent rapid red cell destruction.

In a patient with sickle-cell disease who had 58 blood transfusions, rapid destruction of transfused red cells occurred repeatedly.[20]

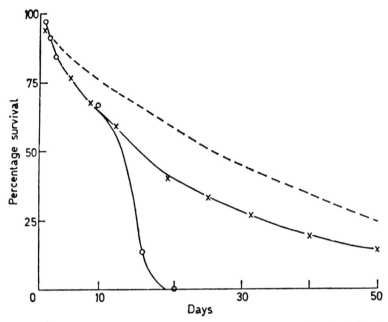

Fig. 7-1. Survival of ^{51}Cr-labeled red cells from two newborn infants following injection into a normal adult. Small samples of blood were taken from two infants, the first aged 35 h and the second aged 50 h. The samples were mixed with ACD and then labeled with ^{51}Cr in the usual way. o-o Cr survival of red cells from the first infant; 2 ml of red cells were labeled. x - x Cr survival of red cells from the second infant; 8 ml of red cells were labeled. The interval between the two injections was 34 d. The dotted line shows the normal Cr survival curve observed when red cells from normal adults are labeled with ^{51}Cr in the same way. (Mollison, P.L.: Blood Transfusion in Clinical Medicine. Blackwell Scientific Publication, London, 1979.)

Seventeen measurements of in vivo red cell survival were performed and all were abnormal except on one occasion when red cells from a sibling survived normally. However, a repeat transfusion from the same donor six months later survived normally for only five to seven days. Subsequently, the donor's cells disappeared rapidly from the circulation. In another case, described by Vullo and Tunioli,[23] red cells from the patient's father survived better than those from another donor. Mollison described a case in which numerous unsuccessful attempts were made to find a compatible donor for a patient who had received many previous transfusions (Fig. 7-4).

More recently, Davey, et al.[10] described a patient in whom anti-c was suspected because transfusion of four units of crossmatch compatible red cells resulted in a severely delayed hemolytic transfusion reaction, and the only common antigen lacking on the patient's cells and present on the donor's cells was c. Anti-c could not be detected in vitro, but ^{51}Cr survival of c-positive red cells was 1 percent at 24 hours, while survival of c-negative red cells was 80 percent at 24 hours. Eight c-negative units were transfused without evidence of a hemolytic reaction.

It is widely assumed that hemolysis of donor red cells in the absence of demonstrable serum antibody has an immunological basis. This viewpoint has been strengthened by observations made in certain patients with what clinically appears to be autoimmune hemolytic anemia, but who have negative direct antiglobulin tests. They may also lack other usual laboratory evidences of red cell-bound autoantibodies. Nevertheless, Gilliland et al.

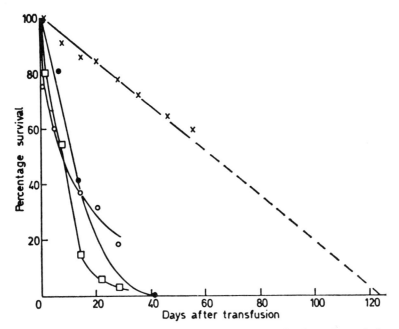

Fig. 7-2. Accelerated destruction of transfused red cells starting at the time of transfusion; no antibody demonstrable in vitro. ●-● Survival of red cells from a particular donor estimated by the method of differential agglutination. □-□ Survival of red cells from the same donor on a subsequent occasion estimated by labeling with ^{51}Cr. o-o Further estimate using ^{51}Cr as a label. x-x Survival of donor's own red cells in her own circulation, estimating with ^{51}Cr. All results corrected for Cr elution. (Mollison, P.L.: Blood Transfusion in Clinical Medicine. Blackwell Scientific Publications, Oxford, 1979.)

Fig. 7-3. Very rapid removal from the circulation of transfused cells, compatible by all the usual serological tests. For comparison, the survival of the patient's own red cells is shown. (Mollison, P.L.: Blood Transfusion in Clinical Medicine. Blackwell Scientific Publications, Oxford, 1979.)

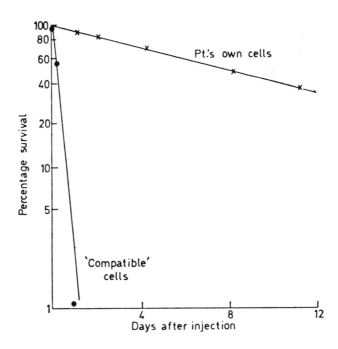

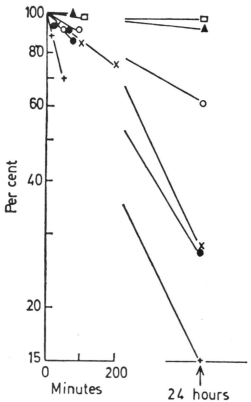

Fig. 7-4. Survival of red cells from six different donors in a patient with paroxysmal nocturnal hemoglobinuria who had received many previous transfusions; in vitro all six samples of red cells appeared to be compatible. (Mollison, P.L.: Blood Transfusion in Clinical Medicine. Blackwell Scientific Publications, Oxford, 1979.)

cules/cell.[24,25] These observations indicate that, under certain circumstances, even very small amounts of bound red cell IgG can be associated with increased red cell destruction in vivo. These methods have not been applied definitively to the problem of incompatibility between donor and recipient without serologically demonstrable antibody. Nevertheless, this seems to be a reasonable research approach. The problem thus becomes one of greatly increasing the sensitivity of antibody detection methods.

Alternatively, red cell destruction by cellular immunity may provide an explanation of this phenomenon. Antibody-mediated cellular immunity is an attractive possible mechanism. In this hypothetical instance, donor red cells minimally "identified" by a small increase in surface-bound IgG interact with reticuloendothelial cells which then hemolyze them by cellular cytotoxicity. Although other hypotheses for the phenomenon can be generated, a biological view of the problem strongly suggests that an immunological explanation ultimately will be found.

In Vivo Compatibility Tests

Transfusion services are occasionally faced with the dilemma of providing safe blood for a patient for whom it is difficult to obtain a negative crossmatch. This may occur when alloantibodies against high-frequency antigens or antibodies of dubious significance are present. In this situation, in vivo compatibility testing has been advocated by some and is based on measuring the survival of an aliquot of red cells. The most sensitive method is the use of a small volume (e.g., 0.5 to 1 ml) of radiolabeled red cells. The details of the methodology are given elsewhere.[9,11,26]

The results of such tests may be of distinct value but must be interpreted appropriately. Mollison points out that when survival at 60 minutes is within normal limits (i.e., 99% ± approximately 5%)[9] the red cells can be regarded as compatible, and it is certain that if

have shown that increased amounts of immunoglobulin (IgG) are bound to the surface of these patients' red cells.[24] This was accomplished by employing a sensitive quantitative method of measurement of red cell-bound IgG. Normal human red cells have fewer than 35 molecules of IgG per cell. Usually, several hundred molecules of IgG antibody per red cell are required for a positive antiglobulin test, the precise number depending on the characteristics of the red cell, the red cell antibody, and the antiglobulin serum.[25] The "Coombs negative" acquired hemolytic anemia patients usually have red cell burdens of IgG in the range of 50 to 400 mole-

the two units from which the samples have been taken are transfused, there will be no danger of an immediate reaction. The data of Silvergleid et al.[11] are in agreement with this conclusion. Twenty-nine of their 42 ^{51}Cr survival studies revealed that the 1-hour survival was 94 percent or greater, and none of these patients who were subsequently transfused had evidence of hemolysis.

However, if survival of the radiolabeled red cells is less than normal, interpretation of the results is less clear. The International Committee for Standardization in Hematology commented that, if survival is at least 70 percent at one hour, the "deduction" is that the concentration of the offending antibody is very low, so the destruction of a large volume of incompatible red cells either will be negligible or will take place only slowly.[26] Indeed, there is a limited body of data supporting such a deduction.[27,28] However, 70 percent survival at 60 minutes represents a T½ of less than 2 hours, and this rate of hemolysis can be dangerous. For example, Silvergleid et al.[11] reported one patient with warm antibody autoimmune hemolytic anemia who had a 1-hour survival of 87 percent, a pretransfusion hematocrit level of 10.5 percent, a posttransfusion hematocrit of 20.6 percent, but a hematocrit of only 10 percent just 16 hours posttransfusion. Another patient, with paroxysmal cold hemoglobinuria, had a 1-hour survival of Tj(a+) red cells of 87 percent and was transfused with 0.5 units of blood; survival at 48 hours was only 53 percent. Other patients reported by Silvergleid in whom 1-hour survival of ^{51}Cr-labeled red cells was between 87 and 94 percent had no evidence of posttransfusion hemolysis. Thus, it is not possible to predict the survival of red cells given in therapeutic amounts after a 1-hour survival that is less than normal but greater than 70 percent.

Some proponents of the use of ^{51}Cr red cell survival studies point out that an "acceptable" in vivo compatibility test, which is variously defined as greater than 70 to 85 percent at one hour,[11,26] will allow one to be quite confident that an *acute life-threatening symptomatic hemolytic transfusion reaction* will not occur. This seems to be true in the cases studied but the number of cases reported is small. However, it is also true that even poorer survival of radiolabeled test cells does not necessarily preclude transfusion. For example, Mayer et al.[29] described 16 patients who had a 24-hour survival of less than 70 percent. Life-threatening conditions necessitated transfusing 11 of these patients, and only one suffered complications directly attributable to the transfusion. Data are not available to determine the rate of destruction of a test dose of red cells that would be predictive of an acute symptomatic hemolytic reaction.

Another factor that seems not to have been taken into account in published reports of survival studies of aliquots of donor units is the duration of storage of the red cells prior to their use in the survival studies. Blood stored for 21 days in CPD anticoagulant will have a 24-hour survival of at least 70 percent when transfused into compatible recipients but survival will not approach 99 percent. Thus, the survival at 24 hours must be compared with the survival that is expected depending on the duration of storage and the anticoagulant used for storage.

Other investigators have performed in vivo compatibility studies using simpler methods. These involve the testing for grossly visible evidence of hemoglobinemia following infusion of 10 to 15 ml of donor red cells (25 to 40 ml of whole blood) over a 30-min period.[30] This is an extension of good routine transfusion practice in which close observation of the patient is made during the administration of the first portion of a unit of blood. In the event of rapid red cell destruction, the patient may exhibit mild-to-moderate symptoms. Since the intravascular lysis of as little as 5 ml of red cells will raise the plasma hemoglobin concentration of an adult recipient by approximately 50 mg per 100 ml, an amount easily detectable by gross visualization, the failure to observe hemoglobinemia suggests that immediate catastrophic hemolysis will not occur with infusion of the entire unit of blood. Although this test is easier to perform, it is less sensitive than the isotope method.[30]

Finally, the problem arises as to the management of patients with poor "in vivo compatibility" tests. Autotransfusion is a safe approach, if feasible. If the patient's serum antibody is against a high-frequency antigen, blood from family members or from a rare donor file or, in an emergency, a blood substitute may be needed. In urgent situations, transfusion can be carried out with the knowledge that an immediate symptomatic hemolytic reaction appears to be unlikely if survival of a small aliquot of cells at one hour is greater than 70 percent. For extreme, life-threatening emergencies, utilization of blood that one knows will be hemolyzed rapidly is nevertheless warranted.

The interpretation of in vivo survival studies in patients who have autoimmune hemolytic anemia is further discussed in Chapter 31.

TECHNIQUES OF COMPATIBILITY TESTING

The Origins of the Compatibility Test

A review of the early twentieth century origins of the compatibility test is fascinating.[31,32] Many blood bankers have the impression that modern concepts of pretransfusion testing followed quickly and logically upon Karl Landsteiner's reports of the discovery of the ABO groups in 1900 and 1901.[33,34] As emphasized by Rosenfield,[32] this was certainly not the case. Indeed, very few persons noticed Landsteiner's reports, and blood transfusion in the early part of this century was developed without blood typing.

Alexis Carrel, a Nobel Prize recipient for the development of end-to-end blood vessel anastomosis, suggested that this surgical technique might be useful for blood transfusions; the method was actually employed successfully until 1913. George Crile, later famous for his thyroid surgery, was trained by Carrel and became the best known transfusionist of the day. He performed hundreds of direct anastomosis transfusions and published a book on the subject in 1909.[34a] However, he never performed ABO typing! Crile did, however, search for hemolysins prior to transfusion, apparently using methods that had been described for blood compatibility between goats.

ABO typing prior to transfusion was first used in 1907, when Richard Weil suggested it to his fellow intern, Reuben Ottenberg. However, as Ottenberg has pointed out,[35] surgeons resented requests for pretransfusion laboratory tests and often proceeded without them—the first recorded instance of a difference of opinion between surgeons and blood transfusionists. The only benefit of this obstinacy was that it allowed Ottenberg to observe that immune hemolysis in vivo often far exceeded anything to be observed in vitro. As indicated in the previous section of this chapter, this is a problem that still occasionally plagues serologists, in spite of the enormous efforts that have been put forth in pretransfusion testing.

In 1914 and 1915 there were several descriptions of the use of sodium citrate as an anticoagulant for human blood.[36-39] The report of Weil[39] was unique among these in that it contained two other very important observations. One was that citrated whole blood could be refrigerated safely for at least several days—the first suggestion for blood banking. The other observation was that serologic tests for compatibility did not require separate serum and erythrocyte samples, but that citrated whole blood of both patient and donor could be mixed. Weil's proportions were 1:1, 9:1, and 1:9. These mixtures were placed in narrow tubes and, after 1 hour of incubation, both agglutination and hemolysis were sought as indications of incompatibility. Rous and Turner[40] improved Weil's compatibility test; the value of pretransfusion testing was further documented in 1921 by Unger,[41] who described five cases of serious reactions to ABO compatible transfusions for which Rous-Turner tests had been positive.

The discovery, in 1940, of the Rhesus (Rh) blood group system[41a] allowed the recognition of the fact that hemolytic transfusion reactions could follow the transfusion of Rh-positive blood cells into Rh-negative recipients. It was subsequently recognized that agglutination methods for demonstration of Rh antibodies in the sera of sensitized individuals were inadequate in that 40 to 50 percent of the subjects in whom sensitization was later confirmed by the birth of an erythroblastotic child or by a hemolytic transfusion reaction showed negative tests for anti-Rh agglutinins.

In 1944, an explanation for such failures was found independently by Wiener and by Race. Race[42] found an additional evidence of Rh sensitization which he called an "incomplete antibody" that did combine with the antigen, the Rh-positive red cell, but failed to cause agglutination in the saline suspension of cells in the test tube. Wiener[43] also recognized failure of agglutination of Rh-positive cells after incubation with the serum of some sensitized individuals. He demonstrated it as follows: To the usual mixture of 2 percent suspension of Rh-positive cells in saline and unknown serum from the sensitized person, he added one drop of an anti-Rh serum known to be capable of agglutinating the test cells. The difference in degree of agglutination of this system, after incubation at 37° C, and centrifugation, from the expected gross or 4 plus agglutination, was the degree of inhibition or "blocking" caused by the unknown serum. Diamond and Abelson[44] showed that the combination of ordinary agglutination plus the "blocking test" was much more satisfactory than agglutination alone, in that the combination demonstrated the presence of Rh antibody in 92 percent of their cases of sensitization.

The year 1945 was notable for the publication by Diamond and Denton[45] pointing out that albumin was a more satisfactory medium for suspending test cells than saline. They reported that some "incomplete" antibodies that reacted with or "sensitized" red cells did not cause them to agglutinate in saline but did cause agglutination of the red cells suspended in albumin-containing media.

Also in 1945, Coombs, Mourant, and Race[45a] reported the use of antiglobulin serum for the detection of weak or "incomplete" Rh antibodies. Dr. Coombs, a veterinarian, later explained[45b] that the antiglobulin test was first described by Carlo Moreschi in 1908 for bacterial agglutination. The antiglobulin test was only very briefly noted by Karl Landsteiner[45c] as evidence that precipitins could also be agglutinins. Coombs and coworkers rediscovered the test while deliberately searching for ways to demonstate "incomplete" red cell antibodies.[32]

In 1947, Morton and Pickles[46] reported that treatment of red cells with the proteolytic enzyme trypsin caused agglutination of cells sensitized with "incomplete" antibody. Subsequently, other proteolytic enzymes were found to react similarly. Kuhns and Bailey (1950)[47] and Löw (1955)[48] worked with the enzyme papain from papayas; Haber and Rosenfield (1957)[49] used an extract from figs called ficin; and Pirofsky and Mangum (1959)[50] used bromelin extracted from pineapples.

In 1964 and 1965, there were several reports[51,52,53] of evaluations of another technique which has gained wider popularity in the United States than the use of enzyme-treated red cells—that is, the addition of bovine serum albumin to the incubation medium prior to antiglobulin testing. These reports pointed out that the use of bovine albumin increased the sensitivity of the antiglobulin test.

In 1955, Jerne and Skovsted[53a] reported that lowering the salt concentration from 1.0M to 0.001M caused a striking increase in the rate of association between antigen and antibody in a bacteriophage neutralization system. This was applied to red cell agglutination tests in 1964,[53b, 53c] but interest in low-ionic-strength solutions (LISS) waned until 1974, when Löw and Messeter reported their experience with the use of LISS in cross-matching more than 100,000 units of blood.[53d]

The Application of Antibody Detection Techniques to Compatibility Testing

Considering the limitations of hemagglutination techniques, an astonishing fund of knowledge concerning blood groups developed, and this information was applied with vigor to compatibility testing. ABO and Rh antibodies in a recipient were, of course, known to cause disastrous results when incompatible blood was transfused. In addition, there was ample documentation of hemolytic transfusion reactions caused by antibodies directed against red cell antigens of blood group systems other than ABO and Rh. Thus, the principle that became firmly established was that, when a patient was found to have a red cell alloantibody against an antigen of any blood group system, antigen-negative blood should be transfused.

Tests were performed which detected antibodies at various temperatures, particularly 37° C, 30° C and room temperature (20 to 25° C). Since various tranfusionists had their own preferences among the antibody detection systems available, there was no uniformity of compatibility test methodology. This fact understandably led to concern among blood bankers and regulatory agencies. Extensive quality control procedures were superimposed on the multitude of tests used to detect donor and recipient antibodies in various media and at various temperatures, and paperwork was added to provide documentation of their performance.[54] Industries developed to supply materials for such a plethora of tests.

In the 1970s, the complexity and extent of pretransfusion testing reached its zenith; as late as 1976, Issitt[55] commented on antibody screening tests as follows: "The object of screening tests is *to detect all antibodies* present so that tests using saline, albumin, enzymes, synthetic potentiating media and antiglobulin serum should all be used." [Emphasis added.]

A nationwide survey of blood bank policies and procedures performed in 1977[56] indicated that 90 percent of responding hospitals used both room temperature incubation in saline (SRT) and incubation in albumin at 37° C with subsequent antiglobulin testing (Alb-AHG) for antibody screening; 80 percent used a two-tube crossmatch technique consisting of both SRT and Alb-AHG. Sixty-two percent used an autocontrol in each phase of the antibody screen. It was also evident that the minor crossmatch was resisting elimination from the battery of tests performed, since it was still used by 34 percent of responding hospitals.

Although not specified in the above survey, it is probable that most blood banks used at least a 30-minute incubation period prior to antiglobulin testing, although other laboratories used incubation times as short as 15 to 20 minutes. In contrast, Mollison[9] suggested a 1-hour incubation period using saline-suspended red cells.

Recent Concepts in Compatibility Test Procedures

Recently, an evolution of blood banking techniques has been taking place which at times has taken on the fervor of a revolution. Gradually, a realization has developed that all of the serologic testing that was being performed was not necessary. As the significance of the various techniques that were commonly utilized in all phases of compatibility testing have been carefully scrutinized, an astonishing number have been deemed overutilized or superfluous. The first technique to be seriously questioned was the minor crossmatch in which the donor serum is incubated with the potential recipient's red cells. Next to be questioned was the necessity of screening donor units for all irregular antibodies. As momentum gained, blood bankers questioned the significance of antibodies other than those reactive at 37° C, and have also suggested that preoperative crossmatching is highly overutilized and should often be replaced by the antibody screening test; this is usually referred to as the "type and screen" procedure. In addition, studies documenting the high degree of safety of the type and screen procedure have led some to suggest that the major crossmatch may be eliminated in instances in which an appropriately performed antibody screening test is negative.

It is of value to examine the evidence relating to each of these aspects of pretransfusion testing.

Minor Crossmatch. The minor or "indirect" crossmatch is a test between the donor serum or plasma and the recipient red cells. Its performance has been the subject of considerable controversy for many years. Although a definitive answer to the question of whether or not a minor crossmatch need be performed now seems obvious, it has taken many years and is still not totally resolved.

As early as 1956,[57] it appeared that the minor crossmatch was losing importance, mainly due to lack of reports in the literature of transfusion problems caused by transfused donor antibody and a beginning desire to eliminate the complexity of pretransfusion tests. In 1958, Jennings et al.,[58] in an attempt to put the minor crossmatch into proper perspective, polled a representative group of blood bank directors concerning the incidence of donor antibody-related transfusion problems as well as whether or not a minor compatibility test was routinely performed. Based on the information obtained, it was concluded that the performance of a minor crossmatch was not essential and that more emphasis should be placed on methods for insuring reliable ABO grouping, antibody detection in the recipient's serum, and "direct matching"—i.e., the major crossmatch. Jen-

nings' sound recommendations apparently fell upon quite deaf ears, and the subject of the performance of the minor crossmatch remained a topic of considerable discussion and debate.

In the very first volume of the scientific journal *Transfusion* in 1961,[59] the question of the performance of the minor crossmatch was addressed by a panel of blood banking experts. Although the panelists' opinions concerning the necessity for performing the minor crossmatch varied from an unqualified "no" to a flat "yes," it became apparent that its major function was to detect errors in ABO grouping. The majority of the panelists felt that, if the patient's and donor's blood groups are determined properly, then the minor crossmatch becomes unnecessary.

Today, the minor crossmatch is considered obsolete and has been replaced by requirements for deliberate screening for the detection of significant blood group antibodies contained in the donor serum. Minor crossmatching is not even mentioned in the current *Standards for Blood Banks and Transfusion Services* of the American Association of Blood Banks,[1] and it is not supported by any recent literature. Even so, it was still performed in a rather astonishing 34 percent of the institutions polled by Waheed.[56]

Donor Antibodies. The above-mentioned panel discussion concerning the minor crossmatch[59] also included data presented by Mohn concerning the significance of screening donor serum for antibodies. He indicated that, of 76,380 units of whole blood transfused over an 18-year period, no transfusion accidents were recorded which could be attributed to transfused donor antibody. During this period, no minor compatibility tests and, apparently, no deliberate screening for donor antibodies were performed. Mohn felt that the additional amount of work and expense required for routine antibody screening for all donor sera was not warranted or was, at least, questionable.

In 1977, Giblett further questioned the necessity of testing the serum of all donors for the presence of irregular antibodies.[16] She pointed out that, because the blood of a small proportion of Group O donors contains high-titered anti-A (or anti-B) hemolysins, it is certainly desirable to avoid giving Group O whole blood to non-Group O recipients except under unusual circumstances. However, she indicated that there is no evidence at all to suggest that other naturally occurring antibodies, such as anti-A_1, -P_1, -Le^a, -Le^b, -M, and -N, have any destructive potential when transfused to incompatible recipients. Therefore, it seemed obvious that laboratory procedures designed for their detection in the screening of donors should be discouraged.

In regard to antibodies of other specificities, screening of Rh-negative donors for anti-D has some merit because anti-D in Rh-negative blood does carry a small risk when given to some Rh-positive patients. Among those few who are at risk are infants with hemolytic disease of the newborn, where appropriate testing of donor plasma is clearly indicated. Another possible risk lies in transfusing Rh-negative women who are subsequently tested for Rh antibodies prior to injecting Rh-immune globulin, since the donor's anti-D might be misinterpreted as the product of the patient's immune system and prevent the proper administration of Rho(D)-immune globulin.

Subtracting the small hazard posed by anti-D and considering only the remaining antibodies found in donor blood, the problem shrinks considerably. In the Puget Sound Blood Center, the serum of only about 1 in 1,000 donors contains incomplete antibodies, other than anti-D, stimulated by previous transfusion or pregnancy. In most instances, the irregular antibodies in donor serum are weakly reactive, and the likelihood of their causing overt red cell destruction in patients with the corresponding antigens is exceedingly small. Indeed, Mollison[9] points out that there does not seem to be a single record in the literature of a hemolytic reaction in the course of a clinical transfusion due to the destruction of the recipient's red cells by a donor antibody other than anti-A and anti-B.

In very rare instances, however, hemolysis has occurred in K-negative patients receiving tandem units of blood containing K-positive red cells and anti-K antibodies.[22, 60, 61] The cost-effectiveness of screening all donor units to prevent such extraordinarily rare hemolytic episodes is highly questionable.

Anti-K and anti-E are by far the most common "immune" antibodies in donors, exclusive of anti-D. Since only about 30 percent of patients have the E antigen and less than 10 percent have the K antigen, the overall likelihood that immune antibodies will be infused into a patient with the corresponding antigen is further reduced to around one in 25,000. Assuming that this unlikely event does take place, and further assuming that the antibody has a high titer, the worst that usually happens is that the patient develops a transiently positive direct antiglobulin test. Even if one makes the assumption that significant red blood cell destruction will occur in one percent of these instances, one can anticipate that the overall likelihood of a hemolytic episode due to donor antibodies will be something like 1 in every 2 or 3 million transfusions. Viewed in this way, the policy of using the antiglobulin test to screen the serum of all blood donors seems overconservative, time-consuming, and unnecessarily expensive.[16]

The 1978 edition of *Standards for Blood Banks and Transfusion Services* of the American Association of Blood Banks[1] indicates only that "blood from donors with a history of prior transfusion or pregnancy should be tested for unexpected antibodies." For the reasons indicated above, this number of tests would appear wasteful except in Rh negative donors, and further refinements in the indications for and techniques of donor antibody screening can be expected in the future.

Cold-Reactive Antibodies. In Giblett's 1977 report,[16] she pointed out, in an essentially parenthetical manner, that her experience indicated that there was no need to be concerned with alloantibodies that do not react at 37°C. This conclusion was thought to be justified by the fact that in vivo hemolysis was not observed in association with cold-reacting alloantibodies, such as anti-A_1, -P_1, -M, -N, -Lu^a, etc., during a 20-year period. During this time, over a million units of blood were transfused. On the rare occasions that antibodies of these specificities are found to react at 37°C (i.e., when cells and serum are warmed to 37°C, then combined and incubated at that temperature), blood lacking the specific antigen is still considered appropriate.

It is evident that Giblett's statements were made as the result of retrospective impressions rather than on the basis of a carefully constructed prospective study. Nonetheless, here conclusions are consistent with the experimental observations of Mollison,[9] and convincing data refuting her statements have not been published.

Many blood bankers expected that conservatism and inertia would prevail and that detection of cold-reactive antibodies would continue to be required by accrediting agencies. However, the Ninth Edition (1978) of the *Standards for Blood Banks and Transfusion Services* of the American Association of Blood Banks[1] indicates that "Tests for incompatibility shall employ methods that demonstrate significant coating, hemolyzing, and agglutinating antibodies *active at 37°C*, and shall include an antiglobulin test." [Emphasis added.]

The Type and Screen Procedure. In 1976, Mintz et al.[62] compiled data on the number of units of blood crossmatched compared to the number of units used for each elective surgical procedure at a university medical center. They pointed out that there were a number of operations for which blood is routinely crossmatched but rarely used. For example, 213 units of blood were crossmatched for 97 patients undergoing cholecystectomy, but only 5 units were actually transfused. This represented a crossmatch-

to-transfusion ratio (C/T) of 42.6. This ratio contrasts strikingly with the ratio of 2.1 to 2.7, which has been considered reasonable.[63]

Since blood crossmatched for surgery is unavailable to other patients for one to two days, an excessive number of preoperative crossmatches results in increased blood wastage or outdating. Further, unnecessary crossmatches result in unnecessary expense to the patient and inefficient utilization of technologists' time. Mintz et al.[62] recommended that, when blood is not likely to be utilized, only blood typing and a preoperative screen for unexpected recipient antibodies should be performed—the "type and screen" procedure. As a guideline, they advocated replacing a preoperative crossmatch with a preoperative type and screen in those surgical procedures shown to have utilized an average of fewer than 0.5 units of blood per patient.

Also in 1976, Friedman et al.[64] introduced the concept of a maximum surgical blood order schedule, or MSBOS, a mnemonic likely to appeal to fans of Al Capp who remember his comic strip character named Joe Btfsplk. The MSBOS represented an attempt to equate more nearly the amount of blood crossmatched with the amount which actually will be transfused. The number of units crossmatched preoperatively for elective surgery was compared to those ultimately transfused. On the basis of these data, a suggested maximum blood order for various surgical procedures was derived and implemented with the cooperation of the medical staff. This was found to be a simple way for a hospital blood bank medical director to reduce the number of units of blood crossmatched daily. Further articles substantiating the advantages of decreasing the number of crossmatches and of performing a type and screen more frequently have been published[65-73] (see also Ch. 18).

Safety of the Type and Screen Procedure. Implementation of policies of more limited crossmatching require assurances that, if more blood were to be needed urgently, it can be provided without undue risk.

Boral and Henry[65] studied this problem by examining 12,848 blood specimens using the type and screen as well as the crossmatch and detected 283 antibodies in 247 patients. The reagent screening cells used were able to detect 96.11 percent of the antibodies. They calculated that if the antigen frequencies corresponding to those antibodies not detected by the screening cells were taken into consideration (i.e., the incompatibility frequencies), the type and screen was 99.99 percent effective in preventing the transfusion of serologically incompatible blood.

Oberman, Barnes, and Friedman[68] reported a retrospective study of 82,647 crossmatches performed on serum from approximately 13,950 patients. In eight instances, antibodies that were considered of potential clinical significance (i.e., Kell, Kidd, or Rh antibodies), were detected in the crossmatch even though the antibody screening test had been negative. All but one of these antibodies, anti-Js[a], would have had the corresponding antigen on the reagent screening cells but were somehow missed. The antibodies undetected by the screening test, but recognized by the crossmatch, were uniformly weakly reactive. Had one of the 13,950 patients in this study required blood on an urgent basis—in which case the blood would have been released after the "immediate spin" phase of the crossmatch (which seems imperative as a final check on ABO compatibility)—there would have been a probability of one in 1,744 that a "clinically significant" but extremely weak recipient antibody would have gone undetected.

Heistø[71] supplied further data by analyzing 73,407 compatibility tests that were performed in association with antibody screening tests for 23,857 patients. The screening test procedure utilized two techniques: (1) an antiglobulin test against two red blood cell samples, and (2) a pre-papainized R_1R_2 (CDe/cDE) red cell, which he used in order to add increased sensitivity in detection of Rh antibodies. The only benefit of the antiglobulin phase of the 73,407 compatibility tests was

the detection of a very weak anti-Le[a] and two possible antibodies, too weak to be identified.

The Value of the Antiglobulin Phase of the Major Crossmatch.   Since the above data suggest that the type and screen procedure is quite safe, the next obvious consideration is whether the crossmatch need be performed at all. This seemingly new concept was actually suggested in 1964 by Grove-Rasmussen, who stated that, if a carefully controlled screening test is negative, it seems unnecessary to carry out the antiglobulin phase of the crossmatch.[74] Further, the Third Edition of the *Standards for a Blood Transfusion Service* of the American Association of Blood Banks, which was published in 1962,[75] was in agreement with this concept because it stated that the antiglobulin test could be performed either as part of the major crossmatch or as part of a screening test for unexpected antibodies provided that the patient's serum lacked such antibodies. Grove-Rasmussen was perhaps ahead of his time, and the Ninth Edition of the *Standards for Blood Banks and Transfusion Services* of the American Association of Blood Banks, published in 1978,[1] clearly mandates the use of the major crossmatch including an antiglobulin test, except for urgent requirements.

Indeed, even the authors cited above regarding the safety of the type and screen procedure still generally recommended that it only be utilized to reduce preoperative crossmatch testing but that, when blood is required, the crossmatch should be performed. Boral and Henry[65] stated that blood volume expanders could be used during the approximately 30 minutes that were considered necessary for performance of an emergency crossmatch. Rouault[67] espoused a somewhat more liberal policy stating that the crossmatch was appropriate when time permits, but that an acceptable alternative was to repeat only ABO and $Rh_o(D)$ typing to assure that the appropriate type-specific unit was sent prior to proceeding with the crossmatch.

In 1977, Walker[16d] strongly recommended establishment of a surgical blood order list for elective surgery but advocated that the cross-match test be used for all patients who have a reasonable chance of using blood during surgery.

The first published recommendation since that of Grove-Rasmussen that disagreed with the policy of using a crossmatch as well as the type and screen was that of Heistø in 1979,[71] who concluded that a careful screening for antibodies, including the use of enzyme-treated red cells, may be preferable to the continued use of the antiglobulin phase of the compatibility test.

A review of the literature regarding clinically significant antibodies coupled with information concerning antigens not usually contained on commercially available screening cells tends to support a position that the antiglobulin phase of the major crossmatch is not justified after an appropriately designed serum screening test proves negative. Table 7-3 lists those antibodies which have been implicated as causes of hemolytic transfusion reactions or hemolytic disease of the newborn and which are reactive with antigens that are not usually contained on commercially supplied antibody detection cells. However, there is no evidence indicating that antibodies that cause hemolytic disease of the newborn will necessarily cause hemolytic transfusion reactions; indeed, only six of these antibodies have been reported to have caused hemolytic

Table 7-3. Antibodies Reported to Have Caused Hemolytic Transfusion Reaction (HTR) or Hemolytic Disease of the Newborn (HDN) and which Recognize Antigens Not Usually Present on Commercially Supplied Antibody Detection Cells

Antibody	Number of Reported Examples Causing:		Reference(s)
	HTR	HDN	
Anti-f (ce); Rh:6	0	2	109, 110
Anti-rh$_i$ (Ce); Rh:7	1*	0	76
Anti-C^w; Rh:8	0	4	111–114
Anti-C^x; Rh:9	0	2	115, 116
Anti-E^w; Rh:11	0	2	117, 118
Anti-Go^a (Gonzales); Rh:30	0	2	113, 119
Anti-Evans	0	1	113
Anti-Zd	0	1	120
Anti-Be^a (Berrens)	0	4	113
Anti-Kp^a (Penny)	1#	1	74, 121
Anti-Js^a (Sutter)	1#	1	74, 122
Anti-Lu^a (Lutheran)	1*	1	76, 123
Anti-Wr^a (Wright)	2	4	77, 78, 113
Anti-Di^a (Diego)	0	5	113, 124
Anti-Kamhuber (Far)	1	0	79
Anti-Rd (Radin)	0	5	125
Anti-V^w (Verweyst)	0	1	113
Anti-Mi^a (Miltenberger)	0	2	113
Anti-Hut (Hutchinson)	0	2	113
Anti-Mur (Murrell)	0	2	113
Anti-Hil (Hill)	0	1	113
Anti-By (Batty)	0	1	126
Anti-Good	0	1	113, 127
Anti-Heibel	0	1	128
Anti-Ht^a (Hunt)	0	1	113
Anti-Becker	0	1	129
Anti-Ven	0	1	130
Anti-Rm	0	1	131
Anti-Do^a (Dombrock)	0	1	132
Anti-Re^a (Reid)	0	1	133

\# Only one example reported to Grove-Rasmussen but no documentation in the literature (see text).

* Reaction was of the delayed type (see text).

transfusion reactions.[74, 76-79] Further, a critical review of these latter reports reveals inadequate documentation in all instances.

For example, Croucher et al.[76] reported an association of anti-rh$_i$(Ce) and anti-Lu^a with delayed type hemolytic transfusion reaction, but it is very unclear to what extent these antibodies contributed, if at all, to the hemolysis. In both cases, other significant antibodies known to cause delayed type hemolytic transfusion reactions were also present. In one case, anti-Fy^a and anti-e antibodies were both found in addition to an anti-rh$_i$(Ce); in the other case, anti-Fy^a was found in addition to an anti-Lu^a. Further, Greendyke et al.[80] have demonstrated that Lu^a-positive blood survives normally in individuals having anti-Lu^a, even though the anti-Lu^a is highly potent and reacts well at 37° C.

Hemolytic transfusion reactions caused by anti-Kp^a or anti-Js^a have not been adequately described. Although one example of each was reported to Grove-Rasmussen,[74] no further information is given.

Anti-Kamhuber (Far) was reported to cause a "severe transfusion reaction" in a multiply transfused patient, but no data are presented to indicate that the reaction was hemolytic in nature.[79]

Anti-Wr^a was demonstrated in the serum of a multiply transfused patient who had repeated transfusion reactions characterized by chills and fever.[77] However, white cell agglutinins were also found in high titer, platelet antibodies were detected, and washed red cells were much better tolerated. The authors point out that there was no proof of abnormal red cell destruction caused by anti-Wr^a. In another report,[78] a patient developed renal insufficiency after a 3½-hour-long surgical procedure for removal of a large ovarian tumor together with both adnexae. Jaundice was also said to develop, although no bilirubin values were reported. The patient's serum contained anti-Wr^a, and the jaundice and renal failure were attributed to a hemolytic transfusion reaction caused by one unit of Wr^a+ blood transfused during surgery. Nei-

ther hemoglobinemia nor hemoglobinuria was noticed on the day of surgery; both were definitely not present the next day, and no other evidence supporting the diagnosis of hemolytic transfusion reaction was reported.

Although the data incriminating the antigens listed in Table 7-3 as being of significance in hemolytic transfusion reactions are inconclusive, red cells containing most of these antigens are obtainable on the screening cells of some commercial suppliers, although this would necessitate the use of an expanded screening cell system using 3 or 4 reagent red cells. However, since their clinical significance is unproven, there is no evident advantage in using screening cells containing these unusual antigens. More importantly, carefully selected screening cells can be homozygous for several important antigens with dosage effects—e.g., c̄, E, Jk^a, and Fy^a. Thus, the screening test is potentially safer than the crossmatch.

Finally, the economic benefits of omitting the crossmatch should be considered. If one combines the data in the studies of Boral and Henry,[65] Oberman et al.[68] and Heistø,[71] 168,302 crossmatches were performed. Considering a charge of $20.00 per crossmatch, this number of crossmatches represents an expenditure of $3,366,040.00. The 99.99 percent safety reported by Boral and Henry, the eight "extremely weak" antibodies detected by Oberman et al., and Heistø's report of the lack of any significant benefit of the crossmatch indicate a lack of justification for continuation of such charges.

All of the above considerations suggest that the antiglobulin phase of the crossmatch test should no longer be utilized, except when the antibody screening test reveals the presence of unexpected antibodies. When no unexpected antibodies are found, only an "immediate spin" saline crossmatch need be performed as a final check on ABO compatibility prior to release of blood from the blood bank for transfusion. Since this is a striking departure from customary compatibility test procedures, the implementation of this policy should await approval by accrediting agencies.

Low-Ionic-Strength Solutions (LISS).
The effect of salt concentration on the rate of association between antigen and antibody was first described by Jerne and Skovsted (1955),[53a] who found that the rate of neutralization of bacteriophage was increased 1000-fold when the salt concentration was reduced from 1.0M to 0.001M. Cann and Clark (1956)[81] and Tsuji, Davis, and Gindler (1962)[82] also found that a reduction in salt concentration increased the rate of association of an antibacteriophage and anti-luciferase antibody, respectively. Both groups interpreted this effect as due to the interaction of oppositely charged ionic groups at the combining sites.

In 1964, two groups of investigators reported on the significance of suspending red cells used for antibody detection in media with salt solution of low ionic strength.[53b,53c,83,84] They indicated that the rate of association of anti-D with D-positive red blood cells can be increased 1000-fold by lowering the salt concentration of the medium in which the reaction takes place from 0.17M to 0.03M. In detecting a wide variety of blood group antibodies by the indirect antiglobulin test, the use of a low-ionic-strength medium allowed the incubation time to be reduced from 1 hour to 5 minutes; moreover, the titer of a wide range of antibodies was increased. However, some false positive results were also noted,[85-86] and low ionic strength media were not applied to routine compatibility testing, even by the blood bankers who authored the original reports.

Interest in this methodology was suddenly awakened in 1974 by the report of Löw and Messeter,[53d] who reported that the LISS method had been routinely used in the blood bank at University Hospital in Lund, Sweden, since 1967. They utilized a 5-minute incubation time and stated that nonspecific reactions were negligible when the salt concentration was at least 0.03M. At lower salt concentrations, both γ-globulin and

complement components were demonstrable on the red cells.[85,86] Although a "scarcity of technicians" did not permit parallel testing with isotonic media, the percentage of samples in which antibodies were detected increased, the reactions were more clear-cut and easier to interpret, and the number of unidentified antibodies remained about the same. Further, more than 100,000 units of blood crossmatched with this method were transfused without any transfusion reaction due to unidentified blood group antibodies.

Further reports followed at a rapidly increasing rate.[87-98] Moore and Mollison's data[87] indicated that a 10-minute incubation time was wiser because there were several instances in which reactions were stronger at 10 minutes than at 5 minutes. Included in their study were data concerning selected Rh antibodies which gave very weak or negative reactions in the saline indirect antiglobulin test but which strongly agglutinated enzyme-treated red cells. When these sera were tested against red cells in LISS, the indirect antiglobulin titer was sometimes almost as high as the titer with enzyme-treated cells. The authors also compared LISS with techniques using albumin-suspended red cells. They concluded that LISS was more sensitive than suspending red cells in albumin and that sensitivity was slightly greater than that achieved by prolonged incubation (90 minutes or more) with saline-suspended cells.

Wicker and Wallas[88] reported that all of more than 50 Rh antibodies and more than 75 non-Rh antibodies were detected in the antiglobulin test after incubation for 15 minutes in low-ionic-strength medium, whereas 30 to 60 minutes were required to detect some of these antibodies using a conventional albumin-fortified isotonic medium.

Garratty, Petz, Webb, et al.[89] evaluated several aspects of LISS for detection of alloantibodies. The effect of preservatives was studied because Moore and Mollison had emphasized that the solution should be discarded after a few days to prevent the growth of microorganisms. Garratty et al. found that

Table 7-4. Reactivity in Antiglobulin Test of 30 Selected Weak Antibodies* Using Red Cells Suspended in Saline (SAL), Albumin (ALB), and Low-Ionic-Strength Solution (LISS)

INCUBATION (37 °C) (Minutes)	SAL	ALB	LISS	ANTIBODIES DETECTED IN LISS ONLY**
	(% DETECTED)			
5	43	47	77	Jk^a(2), Fy^a(3), Fy^b, D, e, k
10	50	63	100	Jk^a(2), Fy^a(3), Fy^b, D(2), C, E, e
15	77	80	100	Jk^a, Fy^a, Fy^b, D, C, E
30	90	90	100	Fy^a, Fy^b, D, C
60	100	100	100	None

* 7 Rh, 7 Kell, 5 Jk, 7 Fy, and 4 Le
** No antibodies were detected in SAL and ALB but not in LISS at any incubation period.

the addition of 0.1 percent sodium azide, 0.01 percent thimerosal, or 0.1 percent chloramphenicol with 0.02 percent neomycin to the LISS did not affect antibody detection but did prevent bacterial and fungal growth at 4°C, 25°C, and 37°C. A later report by Garratty, Petz, Hafleigh et al.[90] indicated that such solutions were stable for at least 6 months. Using 30 *selected* weak antibodies, 100 percent were detected after only 10 minutes incubation in LISS, compared with only 50 percent after incubation in saline or 63 percent after incubation in albumin (Table 7-4). After 15 minutes incubation, 20 percent were still missed in albumin; examples of Rh, Duffy, and Kidd antibodies were not detected.[89] In testing 130 antibodies of various specificities and potency, 44 percent were found to give enhanced reactions in LISS in the antiglobulin test (Table 7-5). In tests with 57 antibodies that reacted by agglutination at room temperature, no important differences were noted among LISS, saline, or albumin-suspending media.

A prospective study[90] of 5009 sera sent for compatibility testing compared results in LISS with albumin and enzyme techniques. Incubation in LISS for 10 to 15 minutes at 37°C detected all antibodies that were detected by nonpapainized red cells, except for three anti-I(IH) antibodies reacting at room temperature only, and one anti-IH, one anti-P$_1$, and one unidentified antibody reacting when room temperature incubation preceded 37°C incubation. Pre-papainized red cells yielded 16 additional positive reactions, but in only three could specificity be determined (weak anti-Le^a).

Further reports confirmed and extended these findings and studied variations of the techniques such as the use of polycation aggregation[99] and the use of albumin in LISS.[100]

In general, there is agreement that the use of low ionic strength media allows for detection of red cell antibodies in the antiglobulin test after only 10 minutes of incubation, with a sensitivity somewhat but not strikingly greater than incubation in albumin media for

Table 7-5. Comparison of the Strength of the Reaction of Antibodies Using Red Cells Suspended in Saline (SAL), Albumin (ALB) or Low-Ionic-Strength Solution (LISS)*

A. 130 ANTIBODIES REACTIVE IN ANTIGLOBULIN TEST (37 °C)
(Rh, Fy, Kell, Lu, S, s, Jk, Kp, Js, Ge, Di, Xg, Yt, Vel, Bg, Le)
   Stronger reactions in LISS than SAL 44%
   Stronger reactions in LISS than ALB 31%
   Strongest reactions in ALB 6%
   Strongest reactions in SAL 0
B. 57 AGGLUTINATING ANTIBODIES (22 °C to 25 °C)
(A, B, M, N, I, H. Le, P$_1$)
   Stronger reactions in LISS than SAL 26.5%
   Stronger reactions in LISS than ALB 19.4%
   Stronger reactions in SAL than LISS 23%
   Stronger reactions in ALB than LISS 23%

* Incubation time = 10 min in LISS; 30 min in SAL or ALB.

15 to 30 minutes. Also, somewhat stronger reactions than with albumin-suspended cells are obtained with a significant percentage of sera. Although "false positive" or nonspecific reactions and the detection of clinically insignificant cold antibodies occur somewhat more frequently with LISS than with saline or albumin techniques, they may not be a significant problem if the room temperature incubation phase of the crossmatch is omitted.[91] Also, the reagent as described by Moore and Mollison[87] is easy and inexpensive to prepare, thus considerably decreasing the expense of reagents required for the performance of the antibody screen and crossmatch. Some large blood transfusion services make their own LISS to take advantage of this considerable savings.[91] Modifications of this reagent have been manufactured, but no published data indicate that they are significantly superior to the Löw and Messeter or Moore and Mollison reagent.

Significance of the Direct Antiglobulin Test and Autocontrol in Pretransfusion Testing. Another aspect of pretransfusion testing where some frequently performed procedures appear superfluous or overutilized is the autocontrol. The Technical Manual of the American Association of Blood Banks[101] advises that an autocontrol be performed when testing pretransfusion blood samples for unexpected antibodies. Also, the College of American Pathologists lists the omission of an autocontrol as a blood bank deficiency.[102] The autocontrol may be accomplished by performing one of the following: a minor crossmatch; an autocontrol (patient's serum mixed with patient's washed red cells) in parallel with either the antibody screen or major crossmatch; or a direct antiglobulin test.

An evaluation of this aspect of pretransfusion testing was performed by Judd et al.[103] who reviewed results of pretransfusion tests on 12,187 blood samples. They performed a detailed serologic evaluation on samples with a positive direct antiglobulin test on the following patients: (1) patients with a hemoglobin of less than 10gm/dl without evident blood loss (i.e., patients with suspected hemolysis); (2) patients who had been transfused within the past 14 days; and (3) patients with serum antibodies detectable by routine pretransfusion studies. They found that, even in these circumstances, a detailed serological evaluation of serum and eluate was fruitless in more than 95 percent of the cases studied. Nevertheless, they did detect six alloantibodies in red cell eluates which were not detectable in concomitantly tested serum samples. They believe that such cases should not go undetected, for further transfusion of unselected blood to these patients may result in antibody-mediated red blood cell destruction.

They also found 64 autoantibodies and three drug-related antibodies but indicated that such findings were clinically insignificant unless associated with evidence of hemolytic anemia. They expressed the opinion that it is the responsibility of the patient's physician to initiate studies aimed at diagnosing anemias and that it is not appropriate or necessary to perform a detailed serologic evaluation on all anemic patients found to have a positive direct antiglobulin test with the hope of uncovering new cases of autoimmune hemolytic anemia.

Based on these findings, the authors concluded that an appropriate and safe approach to the management of blood samples with a positive direct antiglobulin test would be to restrict the preparation of testing of eluates to those samples from patients transfused during the previous 14 days. Thus, the purpose of the direct antiglobulin test in pretransfusion testing should primarily serve to detect alloantibody formation, and should not be used to screen patients for unsuspected autoimmune hemolytic anemia. They also questioned the necessity for the routine performance of an autocontrol and suggested that it could be performed on a more selective basis, dependent on the patient's recent transfusion history.

These recommendations appear to be

sound and are a step in the right direction in eliminating unnecessary work. However, it seems unreasonable for the blood bank to completely abrogate any responsibility in the detection of new cases of autoimmune hemolytic anemia. A practical approach might be to report all positive direct antiglobulin tests to the attending physician so that he may consider whether further workup is indicated.

The Anticomplement Component of Antiglobulin Serum. Prior to 1977, only polyspecific antiglobulin reagents were commercially available in the United States. Anticomplement antibodies in antiglobulin serum are important in the direct antiglobulin test when used for the detection and differential diagnosis of immune hemolytic anemias,[25] but only a very small percentage of antiglobulin serum is used for this purpose. Most of it is used, instead, for compatibility testing. In recent years, an unresolved problem has been the definition of the optimal qualitative and quantitative characteristics of the anticomplement component of antiglobulin sera used for compatibility tests.[104]

The central question in this regard is: "What is the incidence and clinical significance of red blood cell alloantibodies that are detectable, when using standard serologic techniques, only by the antiglobulin test and only by the anticomplement component of the antiglobulin serum?" To be more specific, we are referring to alloantibodies that are not detectable by direct agglutination in saline or albumin or by the anti-IgG component of antiglobulin serum, but that are detected by the anticomplement component of antiglobulin serum. Also of importance are reports of antibodies whose reactivity in the indirect antiglobulin test is significantly enhanced because of the role of complement.

There have been numerous reports of red cell alloantibodies that were not detectable with anti-IgG antiglobulin serum but which were detected with the anticomplement component of antiglobulin serum; this information was reviewed by Petz and Garratty in 1978.[104] Subsequently, additional antibodies with similar characteristics have been reported,[105-107] and evidence has been presented indicating that complement-fixing blood group antibodies are frequently detected at a higher dilution and/or higher titer score when a polyspecific antiglobulin serum containing anticomplement antibodies is used rather than a monospecific anti-IgG.[106] This was true even though the monospecific antiserum contained the same concentration of anti-IgG as the polyspsecific antiserum, as determined by titration tests.

In spite of such evidence indicating the need for anticomplement antibodies for the detection of some clinically significant red cell alloantibodies, there is justification for further study of this point. This is true for two reasons. First, the total number of clinically significant antibodies reported to have been detected only with the anticomplement component of antiglobulin serum in a period of more than 15 years is small. Second, past techniques used in performing the compatibility test were frequently different from those currently utilized. Specifically, many early studies utilized antiglobulin tests performed on tiles rather than techniques involving centrifugation; some investigators did not include albumin in the incubation procedures; some blood transfusion services now utilize low ionic strength solutions; and it is possible that the anti-IgG present in modern reagents is better.

Also, clinically insignificant positive indirect antiglobulin tests may result from complement fixation by cold antibodies. These are often improperly called "false positive" reactions. The incidence of such clinically insignificant reactions varies, depending on the compatibility test procedures used, and can be minimized but certainly not eliminated by omitting the room temperature incubation phase of the crossmatch. The detection and identification of clinically insignificant antibodies wastes time and reagents, and can only be tolerated if balanced by benefit obtained from anticomplement antibodies in antiglobulin serum. Finally, the difference in cost of monospecific anti-IgG reagents and polyspecific reagents, if any, must be considered.

At present, widely divergent conclusions have been expressed in the medical literature. Beck and Marsh[108] stated that antibody screening of more than 5.5 million sera failed to reveal a single example of an alloantibody that was detectable solely because of its complement-binding ability. Their opinion is that anticomplement antibodies in antiglobulin serum are not necessary in compatibility testing. In contrast, Wright and Issitt[106] found 8 of 140 selected antibodies (5.7 percent) which gave positive indirect antiglobulin reactions with a polyspecific reagent but which were nonreactive with anti-IgG. Many additional antibodies reacted stronger with polyspecific antiglobulin serum than with anti-IgG. Wright and Issitt stated that workers who wish to detect all blood group alloantibodies in the sera of patients who are to be transfused and wish to obtain maximal strength reactions in vitro must continue to use a polyspecific antiglobulin reagent that contains potent anti-IgG and anticomplement antibodies.

A prospective study relating to the significance of the anticomplement component of antiglobulin serum is now in progress and will be completed in 1981. Preliminary data have been presented,[105] and it is intended that information gained from the study will allow for a reasonable analysis of both the benefits and disadvantages of polyspecific antiglobulin serum in compatibility testing.

Recommendations for Compatibility Testing. On the basis of the above information, it seems reasonable to make the following recommendations concerning appropriate procedures for compatibility testing, recognizing that not all concepts are in accord with those of some accrediting agencies. Approval should be obtained from accrediting agencies prior to implementation of any policies that are in conflict with current standards.

1. Screening tests for antibodies in donor serum which use an antiglobulin test are not cost effective except on blood from Rh negative donors.

2. A minor crossmatch is superfluous.

3. The room temperature incubation phase of the crossmatch is unnecessary.

4. An autocontrol on all specimens is unnecessary and may be replaced by performance of a direct antiglobulin test on recently transfused patients (although it may be more convenient to perform the direct antiglobulin test routinely if a high percentage of crossmatches are performed on recently transfused patients). A detailed serologic evaluation need be performed when the direct antiglobulin test is positive only when the patient has been transfused recently or when hematologic data are consistent with the possibility of hemolytic anemia.

5. The risk of omitting the antiglobulin phase of the major crossmatch after a negative serum screening test using an antiglobulin test with two reagent screening cells is extremely low. Since screening cells can be homozygous for several antigens with important dosage effects, screening with appropriate cells can be safer than a crossmatch and the continued use of the crossmatch with an antiglobulin test after a negative type and screen procedure is not justified when the type and screen reveals no "unexpected" or "irregular" antibody.

6. A screening test (or crossmatch test) can be performed using an "immediate spin," incubation at 37° C, and an antiglobulin test. Incubation in saline media for 30 to 60 minutes will only rarely miss antibodies, but incubation in the significantly more expensive albumin medium for 15 to 30 minutes is discernably more sensitive. Incubation in low-ionic-strength solutions for 10 minutes is at least as sensitive as incubation in albumin for 15 to 30 minutes and appears somewhat more sensitive.

7. A polyspecific antiglobulin serum should presently be used in the indirect antiglobulin test, although prospective studies

may indicate that this is unnecessary or is not cost-effective.

8. If the antiglobulin phase of the cross-match is omitted after a negative serum screening test, final check on ABO compatibility of donor and recipient using an "immediate spin" saline test should be performed before blood is released from the blood bank.

REFERENCES

1. Standards for Blood Banks and Transfusion Services, Am. Assoc. Blood Banks, Oberman, H., Ed., 9th Ed., 1978.

2. Jandl, J.H. and Greenberg, M.S.: The selective destruction of transfused "compatible" normal red cells in patients with splenomegaly. J. Lab. Clin. Med. 49:233, 1957.

3. Stewart, J.W. and Mollison, P.L.: Rapid destruction of apparently compatible red cells. Br. Med. J. 1:1274, 1959.

4. Heistø, H., Myhre, K., Vogt, E., and Heier, A.M.: Hemolytic transfusion reaction due to incompatibility without demonstrable antibodies. Vox Sang. 5:538, 1960.

5. Kissmeyer-Nielsen, F., Bjorn Jensen, K., and Ersbak, J.: Severe hemolytic transfusion reactions caused by apparently compatible red cells. Br. J. Haematol. 7:36, 1961.

6. Heistø, H., Myhre, K., Borresen, W., Vogt, E., and Heier, A.M.: Another case of hemolytic transfusion reaction due to incompatibility without demonstrable antibodies. Vox Sang. 7:470, 1962.

7. van der Hart, M., Engelfriet, C.P., Prins, H.K., and van Loghem, J.J.: A haemolytic transfusion reaction without demonstrable antibodies *in vitro.* Vox. Sang. 8:363, 1963.

8. van Loghem, J.J., van der Hart, M., Moes, M., and von dem Borne, A.E.G.: Increased red cell destruction in the absence of demonstrable antibodies *in vitro.* Transfusion 5:525, 1965.

9. Mollison, P.L.: Blood Transfusion in Clinical Medicine, 6th Ed. Blackwell Scientific Publications, 1979.

10. Davey, R.J., Gustafson, M., and Holland, P.V.: Accelerated immune red cell destruction in the absence of serologically detectable alloantibodies. Transfusion 20:348, 1980.

11. Silvergleid, A.J., Wells, R.F., Hafleigh, E.B., Korn, G., Kellner, J.J., and Grumet, F.C.: Compatibility test using ^{51}Chromium-labeled red blood cells in crossmatch positive patients. Transfusion 18:8, 1978.

12. Colledge, K.I., Kaplan, H.S., and Marsh, W.L.: Massive transfusion of Sd(a+) blood to a recipient with anti-Sd^a, without clinical complication (abstract). Proceedings of the 26th Annual Meeting, American Association of Blood Banks, 1973.

13. Macvie, S.I., Morton, J.A., and Pickles, M.M.: The reactions and inheritance of a new blood group antigen, Sd^a. Vox. Sang. 13:485, 1967.

14. Wells, R.F., Korn, G., Hafleigh, B., and Grumet, F.C.: Characterization of three new apparently related high frequency antigens. Transfusion 16:427, 1976.

15. Moore, H.C., Issitt, P.D., and Pavone, B.G.: Successful transfusion of Chido-positive blood to two patients with anti-Chido. Transfusion 15:266, 1975.

16. Giblett, E.R.: Blood group alloantibodies: An assessment of some laboratory practices. Transfusion 17:299, 1977.

16a. Grove-Rasmussen, M. and Huggins, C.E.: Selected types of frozen blood for patients with multiple blood group antibodies. Transfusion 13:124, 1973.

16b. Tovey, G.H.: Preventing the incompatible blood transfusion. Haematologia 8:389, 1974.

16c. Spielman, W. and Seidl, S.: Prevalence of irregular red cell antibodies and their significance in blood transfusion and antenatal care. Vox. Sang. 26:551, 1974.

16d. Walker, R.H.: Is a crossmatch utilizing the indirect antiglobulin test necessary for patients with a negative antibody screen? Current Topics in Blood Banking. Ann Arbor, University of Michigan, 1977.

17. Tilley, C.A., Crookston, M.C., Haddad, S.A., and Shumak, K.H.: Red blood cell survival studies in patients with anti-Ch^a, anti-Yk^a, anti-Ge and anti-Vel. Transfusion 17:169, 1977.

18. Bettigole, R., Harris, J.P., Tegoli, J., and Issitt, P.D.: Rapid *in vivo* destruction of Yt(a+) red cells in a patient with anti-Yt^a. Vox. Sang. 14:143, 1968.

19. Gobel, U., Drescher, K.H., Pöttgen, W., and Lehr, H.J.: A second example of anti-Yt^a

with rapid *in vivo* destruction of Yt(a+) red cells. Vox. Sang. 27:171, 1974.

20. Chaplin, H. and Cassell, M.: The occasional fallibility of *in vivo* compatibility tests. Transfusion 2:375, 1962.

21. Swisher, S.N., Young, L.E., and Trabold, H.: *In vitro* and *in vivo* studies of the behavior of canine erythrocyte-isoantibody systems. Annals of the New York Academy of Sciences, 97:15, 1962.

22. Pineda, A.A., Brzica, S.M., and Taswell, H.F.: Hemolytic transfusion reaction. Recent experience in a large blood bank. Mayo Clin. Proc. 53:378, 1978.

23. Vullo, C. and Tunioli, A.M.: The selective destruction of "compatible" red cells transfused in a patient suffering from Thalassaemia major. Vox. Sang. 6:583, 1961.

24. Gilliland, B.C.: Coombs-negative immune hemolytic anemia. Seminars in Hematol. 13:267, 1976.

25. Petz, L.D. and Garratty, G.: Acquired Immune Hemolytic Anemias. Churchill-Livingstone, New York, 1980.

26. International Committee for Standardization in Haematology: Recommended methods for radioisotope red cell survival studies. Br. J. Haematol. 45:659, 1980.

27. Mollison, P.L., Johnson, C.A., and Prior, D.M.: Dose-dependent destruction of A_1 cells by anti-A_1. Vox. Sang. 35:149, 1978.

28. Chaplin, H.: Studies on the survival of incompatible cells in patients with hypogamma-globulinaemia. Blood 14:24, 1959.

29. Mayer, K., Chin, B., Magnes, J., Harris, J.P., and Tegoli, J.: Further experiences with the *in vivo* crossmatch and transfusion of Coombs incompatible red cells. *In:* XVII Congress of International Society of Hematology and XV Congress of International Society Blood Transfusion Book of Abstracts, July 23-29, 1978, p. 49.

30. Chaplin, H.: Special problems in transfusion management of patients with autoimmune hemolytic anemia. *In:* A Seminar on Laboratory Management of Hemolysis. Bell, C.A., Ed. Amer. Assoc. of Blood Banks, Washington, D.C., 1979.

31. Rosenfield, R.E.: Early 20th century origins of modern blood transfusion therapy. Mt. Sinai J. of Med. 41:626, 1974.

32. Rosenfield, R.E.: The past and future of immunohematology. Am. J. Clin. Path. 64:569, 1975.

33. Landsteiner, K.: Zur kenntnis der antifermentativen, lytischen und agglutinierenden wirkungen des blutserums und der lymphe. Zbl. Bakt. 27:375, 1900.

34. Landsteiner, K.: Über agglutinationserscheinungen normalen menschlichen blutes. Wein Klin Wochenschr 14:1132, 1901.

34a. Crile, G.W.: Hemorrhage and Transfusion. London and New York, D. Appleton and Co., 1909.

35. Ottenberg, R.: Reminiscences of the history of blood transfusion. J. Mt. Sinai Hosp. (New York) 4:264, 1937.

36. Agote, L.: Nuevo procediemento para la transfusión del sangre. An. Inst. Mod. Clin. Med. (Buenos Aires) 1:3, 1915.

37. Hustin, A.: Principe d'une nouvelle methode de transfusion. J. Med. Bruxelles 12:436, 1914.

38. Lewisohn, R.: A new and greatly simplified method of blood transfusion. Med. Rec. 87:141, 1915.

39. Weil, R.: Sodium citrate in the transfusion of blood. J.A.M.A. 64:425, 1915.

40. Rous, P. and Turner, J.R.: A rapid and simple method of testing donors for transfusion. J.A.M.A. 64: 1980, 1915.

41. Unger, L.J.: Precautions necessary in selection of a donor for blood transfusion. J.A.M.A. 76:9, 1921.

41a. Landsteiner, K. and Wiener, A.S.: Agglutinable factor in human blood recognized by immune sera for rhesus blood. Proc. Soc. Exper. Biol. & Med. 43:223, 1940.

42. Race, R.R.: An "incomplete" antibody in human serum. Nature (London) 153:771, 1944.

43. Wiener, A.S.: A new test (blocking test) for Rh sensitization. Proc. Soc. Exp. Biol. (New York) 56:173, 1944.

44. Diamond, L.K. and Abelson, N.M.: The demonstration of anti-Rh agglutinins, an accurate and rapid slide test. J. Lab. Clin. Med. 30:204, 1945.

45. Diamond, L.K. and Denton, R.L.: Rh agglutination in various media with particular reference to the value of albumin. J. Lab. Clin. Med. 30:821, 1945.

45a. Coombs, R.R.A., Mourant, A.E., and Race, R.R.: A new test for the detection of weak and "incomplete" Rh agglutinins. Br. J. Exp. Pathol. 26:255, 1945.

45b. Coombs, R.R.A.: History and evaluation of the antiglobulin reaction and its application in clinical and experimental medicine. Am. J. Clin. Pathol. 53:131, 1970.

45c. Landsteiner, K.: The Specificity of Serological Reactions. New York, Dover Publications, Inc., 1962, p. 114.

46. Morton, J.A. and Pickles, M.M.: Use of trypsin in the detection of incomplete anti-Rh antibodies. Nature 159:779, 1947.

47. Kuhns, W.J. and Bailey, A.: Use of red cells modified by papain for detection of Rh antibodies. Am. J. Clin. Pathol. 20:1067, 1950.

48. Löw, B.: A practical method using papain and incomplete Rh-antibodies in routine Rh blood-grouping. Vox. Sang. (series one) 5:94, 1955.

49. Haber, G. and Rosenfield, R.E.: Ficin treated red cells for hemaglutination studies. P.H. Andresen—Papers in dedication of his 60th birthday, p. 45, Munksgaard, Copenhagen, 1957.

50. Pirofsky, B. and Mangum, M.E.J.: Use of bromelin to demonstrate erythrocyte antibodies. Proc. Soc. Exp. Biol. 101:49, 1959.

51. Griffitts, J.J., Frank, S., and Schmidt, R.P.: The influence of albumin in the antiglobulin crossmatch. Transfusion 4:461, 1964.

52. Stroup, M. and MacIlroy, M.: Evaluation of the albumin antiglobulin technique in antibody detection. Transfusion 5:184, 1965.

53. Clayton, E.M., Brown, R.B., and Bove, J.R.: The antiglobulin reaction on albumin enriched cell suspensions. Transfusion 5:344, 1965.

53a. Jerne, N.K. and Skovsted, L.: The rate of inactivation of bacteriophage T4R in specific anti-serum. Ann. Inst. Pasteur 84:73, 1955.

53b. Hughes-Jones, N.C., Polley, M.J., Telford, R., Garndner, B., and Kleinschmidt, G.: Optimal conditions for detecting blood group antibodies by the antiglobulin test. Vox. Sang. 9:385, 1964.

53c. Elliot, M., Bossom, E., Dupuy, M.E., and Masouredis, S.P.: Effect of ionic strength on the serologic behavior of red cell isoantibodies. Vox Sang. 9:396, 1964.

53d. Löw, B. and Messeter, L.: Antiglobulin test in low-ionic strength salt solution for rapid antibody screening and cross-matching. Vox. Sang. 26:53, 1974.

54. Guy, L.R., Neitzer, G.M., and Klein, R.E.: Quality control—How much is enough? Transfusion 17:183, 1977.

55. Issitt, P.D. and Issitt, C.H.: Applied Blood Group Serology. 2nd Ed. Spectra Biologicals, 1975, p. 273.

56. Waheed, A.: A survey about blood bank policies and procedures. Transfusion 18:482, 1978.

57. van Loghem, J.J.: Panel discussion, serologic aspects of blood transfusion. Vox. Sang. 1:207, 1956.

58. Jennings, E.R., Hindmarsh, C., and Renaud, M.: The significance of the minor crossmatch. Am. J. Clin. Path. 30:302, 1958.

59. Dunsford, I., Giblett, E.R., Mohn, J.F., Moore, B.P.L., and Stern, K.: Panel Discussion: The minor crossmatch. Transfusion 1:239, 1961.

60. Zettner, A. and Bove, J.R.: Hemolytic transfusion reaction due to interdonor incompatibility. Transfusion 3:48, 1963.

61. Franciosi, R.A., Awer, E., and Santana, M.: Interdonor incompatibility resulting in anuria. Transfusion 7:297, 1967.

62. Mintz, P.D., Nordine, R.B., Henry, J.B., and Webb, W.R.: Expected hemotherapy in elective surgery. N.Y. State J. Med. 76:532, 1976.

63. Myhre, B.A.: Quality Control in Blood Banking. John Wiley and Sons, 1974.

64. Friedman, B.A.: An analysis of surgical blood use in United States hospitals with application to the maximum surgical blood order schedule. Transfusion 19:268, 1979.

65. Boral, L.I. and Henry, J.B.: The type and screen: A safe alternative and supplement in selected surgical procedures. Transfusion 17:163, 1977.

66. Henry, J.B., Mintz, P.D., and Webb, W.R.: Optimal blood ordering for elective surgery. J.A.M.A. 237:451, 1977.

67. Rouault, C. and Gruenhagen, J.: Reorganization of blood ordering practices. Transfusion 18:448, 1978.

68. Oberman, H.A., Barnes, B.A., and Friedman, B.A.: The risk of abbreviating the major crossmatch in urgent or massive transfusion. Transfusion 18:137, 1978.

69. Boral, L.I., Hill, S.S., Apollon, C.J., and Folland, A.: The type and antibody screen, revisited. Am. J. Clin. Path. 71:578, 1979.

70. Boral, L.I., Dannemiller, F.J., Stanford, W., Sherwood, S.H., and Cornell, T.A.: A guideline for anticipated blood usage during elective surgical procedures. Am. J. Clin. Path. 71:680, 1979.

71. Heistø, H.: Pretransfusion blood group serology: Limited value of the antiglobulin phase of the crossmatch when a careful screening test for unexpected antibodies is performed. Transfusion 19:761, 1979.

72. Boyd, P.R., Sheedy, K.C., and Henry, J.B.: Type and screen: Use and effectiveness in elective surgery. Am. J. Clin. Path. 73:694, 1980.

73. Lee, K. and Lachance, V.: Type and screen for elective surgery—Results of one year's experience in a small community hospital. Transfusion 20:324, 1980.

74. Grove-Rasmussen, M.: Routine compatibility testing: Standards of the AABB as applied to compatibility tests. Transfusion 4:200, 1964.

75. Standards For A Blood Transfusion Service, 3rd Ed., American Association of Blood Banks, Chicago, 1962.

76. Croucher, B.E.E., Crookston, M.C., and Crookston, J.H.: Delayed haemolytic transfusion reactions simulating auto-immune haemolytic anaemia. Vox. Sang. 12:32, 1967.

77. van Loghen, J.J. van der Hart, M., Bok, J., and Brinkerink, P.C.: Two further examples of the antibody anti-Wr[a]. Vox. Sang. (series one) 5:130, 1955.

78. Metaxas, M.N. and Metaxas-Bühler, M.: Studies on the Wright blood group system. Vox. Sang. 8:707, 1963.

79. Speiser, P., Kühböck, J., Mickerts, D., Pausch, V., Reichel, G., Lauer, D., Poremba, I., Doering, I., and Hamacher, H.: "Kamhuber" a new human blood group antigen of familial occurrence, revealed by a severe transfusion reaction. Vox. Sang. 11:113, 1966.

80. Greendyke, R.M. and Chorpenning, F.W.: Normal survival of incompatible red cells in the presence of anti-Lu[a]. Transfusion, 2:52, 1962.

81. Cann, J.R. and Clark, E.W.: Kinetics of the antigen-antibody reaction. Effect of salt concentration and pH on the rate of neutralization of bacteriophage by purified fractions of specific antiserum. J. Am. Chem. Soc. 78:3627, 1956.

82. Tsuji, F.I., Davis, D.L., and Gindler, E.M.: Effect of sodium chloride and pH on the rate of neutralization of Cypridina luciferase by specific antibody. J. Immunol. 88:83, 1962.

83. Atchley, W.A., Bhagavan, N.V., and Masouredis, S.P.: Influence of ionic strength on the reaction between anti-D and D-positive red cells. J. Immunol. 93:701, 1964.

84. Hughes-Jones, N.C., Gardner, B., and Telford, R.: The effect of pH and ionic strength on the reaction between anti-D and erythrocytes. Immun. Lond. 7:72, 1964.

85. Mollison, P.L. and Polley, M.J.: Uptake of γ-globulin and complement by red cells exposed to serum at low ionic strength. Nature 203:535, 1964.

86. Stratton, F. and Rawlinson, V.I.: Interaction between human serum complement and normal human red cells at low ionic strength. Nature (London) 207:305, 1965.

87. Moore, H.C. and Mollison, P.L.: Use of a low-ionic-strength medium in manual tests for antibody detection. Transfusion 16:291, 1976.

88. Wicker, B. and Wallas, C.H.: A comparison of a low ionic strength saline medium with routine methods for antibody detection. Transfusion 16:469, 1976.

89. Garratty, G., Petz, L.D., Webb, M., and Yam, P.: Evaluation of low ionic strength saline (LISS) as a red cell suspending medium for the detection of alloantibodies. Clin. Res. 26:347, 1978.

90. Garratty, G., Petz, L., Hafleigh, E., Howard, J., and Grumet, C.: Evaluation of low ionic strength solution (LISS) for compatibility testing including a prospective study comparing saline, albumin, and enzyme techniques. 31st Annual Meeting of the American Association of Blood Banks. New Orleans, 1978. (Abstract Book p. 41.)

91. Hafleigh, E.B., Svoboda, R.K., and Grumet, F.C.: LISS technique without room temperature phase. Extensive transfusion experience. 31st Annual Meeting of the American Association of Blood Banks. New Orleans, 1978. (Abstract Book p. 41.)

92. Branch, D.: LISS: A revolution in blood banking. Lab. Med. 9:17, 1978.

93. Rock, G., Baxter, A., Charron, M., and Jhaveri, J.: LISS—An effective way to increase blood utilization. Transfusion 18:228, 1978.

94. Herron, R. and Smith, D.S.: Use of low ionic strength salt solution in compatibility testing. J. Clin. Path. 31:1116, 1978. (Correspondence)

95. Fitzsimmons, J.M. and Morel, P.A.: The effects of red blood cell suspending media on hemagglutination and the antiglobulin test. Transfusion 19:81, 1979.

96. Lown, J.A.G., Barr, A.L., and Davis, R.E.: Use of low ionic strength saline for crossmatching and antibody screening. J. Clin. Path. 32:1019, 1979.

97. Greendyke, R.M., Banzhaf, J.C., and Inglis, J.: A comparison of six procedures for compatibility testing. Transfusion 19:782, 1979.

98. Langley, J.W., McMahan, M., and Smith, N.: A nine-month transfusion service experience with low-ionic-strength saline solution (LISS). Am. J. Clin. Path. 73:99, 1980.

99. Rosenfield, R.E.: Low ionic incubation and polycation aggregation ("LIP") to augment hemagglutination in test tubes. American Association of Blood Banks Abstracts of Volunteer Papers. 31st Annual Meeting. New Orleans, 1978, p. 42.

100. Leikola, J. and Perkins, H.A.: Red cell antibodies and low ionic strength: A study with enzyme-linked antiglobulin test. Transfusion 20:224, 1980.

101. American Association of Blood Banks Technical Manual, 7th Ed. Miller, W.V., Ed., Washington, D.C., 1977.

102. College of American Pathologists—Commission on Inspection and Accreditation: Inspection Checklist, Section V, Blood Bank, Chicago, 1976.

103. Judd, W.J., Butch, S.H., Oberman, H.A., Steiner, E.A., and Bauer, R.C.: The evaluation of a positive direct antiglobulin test in pretransfusion testing. Transfusion 20:17, 1980.

104. Petz, L.D. and Garratty, G.: Antiglobulin sera—Past, present and future. Transfusion 18:257, 1978.

105. Howard, J.E., Gottlieb, C.E., Hafleigh, E.B., Grumet, F.C., Petz, L.D., and Garratty, G.: Clinical importance of the anti-complement activity in antiglobulin antisera. American Association of Blood Banks Abstracts of Volunteer Papers. 31st Annual Meeting. New Orleans, 1978, p. 6.

106. Wright, M.S. and Issitt, P.D.: Anticomplement and the indirect antiglobulin test. Transfusion 19:688, 1979.

107. Neppert, J.: Plasma or serum. Transfusion 20:116, 1980. (Correspondence.)

108. Beck, M.L. and Marsh, W.L.: Complement and the antiglobulin test. Transfusion 17:529, 1977.

109. Levine, P., White, J., Stroup, M., Zmijewski, C.M., and Mohn, J.F.: Haemolytic disease of the newborn probably due to anti-f. Nature (London) 185:188, 1960.

110. Spielmann, W., Seidl, S., and von Pawel, J.: Anti-ce(anti-f) in a CDe/cD- mother, as a cause of haemolytic disease of the newborn. Vox. Sang. 27:473, 1974.

111. Lawler, S.D. and van Loghem, J.J.: Rhesus antigen C^w causing haemolytic disease of newborn. Lancet 2:545, 1947.

112. Anderson, G.H. and Fenton, E.: A case of anti-C^w sensitization resulting in hemolytic disease of the newborn. Canad. Med. Assn. J. 89:28, 1963.

113. Race, R.R. and Sanger, R.: Blood Groups in Man. Blackwell Scientific Publications, 6th Ed., 1975.

114. Monaghan, P.W.: Hemolytic disease of the newborn due to anti-C^w (rh^w). Lab. Med. 8:33, 1977.

115. Stratton, F. and Renton, P.H.: Haemolytic disease of the newborn caused by a new rhesus antibody, anti-C^x. Brit. Med. J. i:962, 1954.

116. Finney, R.D., Blue, A.M., and Willoughby, M.L.N.: Haemolytic disease of the newborn caused by the rare rhesus antibody anti-C^x. Vox. Sang. 25:39, 1973.

117. Greenwalt, T.J. and Sanger, R.: The Rh antigen E^w. Br. J. Haematol. 1:52, 1955.

118. Grobel, R.K. and Cardy, J.D.: Hemolytic disease of the newborn due to anti-E^w: A fourth example of the Rh antigen, E^w. Transfusion 11:77, 1971.

119. Alter, A.A., Gelb, A.G., Chown, B., Rosenfield, R.E., and Cleghorn, T.E.: Gonzales (Go^a), a new blood group character. Transfusion 7:88, 1967.

120. Švanda, M., Prochazka, R., Kout, M., and

Giles, C.M.: A case of haemolytic disease of the newborn due to a new red cell antigen, Zd. Vox. Sang. 18:366, 1970.

121. Jensen, K.G.: Haemolytic disease of the newborn caused by anti-Kp[a]. Vox. Sang. 7:476, 1962.

122. Donovan, L.M., Tripp, K.L., Zuckerman, J.E., and Konugres, A.A.: Hemolytic disease of the newborn due to anti-Js[a]. Transfusion 13:153, 1973.

123. Francis, B.J. and Hatcher, D.E.: Hemolytic disease of the newborn apparently caused by anti-Lu[a]. Transfusion 1:248, 1961.

124. Graninger, W.: Anti-Di[a] and the Di[a] blood group-antigen found in an Austrian family. Vox. Sang. 31:131, 1976.

125. Rausen, A.R., Rosenfield, R.E., Alter, A.A., and Hakim, S.: A "new" infrequent red cell antigen, Rd (Radin). Transfusion 7:336, 1967.

126. Simmons, R.T. and Were, S.O.M.: A "new" family blood group antigen and antibody (By) of rare occurrence. Med. J. Aust. ii:55, 1955.

127. Frumin, A.M., Porter, M., and Eichman, M.F.: The Good factor as a possible cause of hemolytic disease of the newborn. Blood 15:681, 1960.

128. Ballowitz, L., Fiedler, H., Hoffmann, Ch., and Pettenkofer, H.: "Heibel" a new rare human blood group antigen, revealed by a haemolytic disease of a newborn. Vox. Sang. 14:307, 1968.

129. Elbel, H. and Prokop, O.: Ein neues erbliches Antigens als Ursache gehaufter Fehlgeburten. Zeitschr. f. Hygiene 132:120, 1951.

130. van Loghem, J.J. and van der Hart, M.: Een zeldzaam voorkomende bloedgroep (Ven.). Bull. Cen. Lab. Bloed transf. Dienst. ned. Rode Kruis 2:225, 1952.

131. van der Hart, M., Bosman, H., and van Loghem, J.J.: Two rare human blood group antigens. Vox. Sang. (series one) 4:108, 1954.

132. Polesky, H.F., Swanson, J., and Smith, R.: Anti-Do[a] stimulated by pregnancy. Vox. Sang. 14:465, 1968.

133. Guévin, R.M., Taliano, V., Fiset, D., Bérubé, P., and Kaita, H.: L'antigène Reid, un nouvel antigène privé. Rev. fr. Transf. 14:455, 1971.

8

Qualifications, Management, and Care of Blood Donors

Dennis Donohue, M.D.

INTRODUCTION

In 1978 there were 11.1 million single units (450 ml) of whole blood and 2.5–3.5 million liters of plasma collected in the United States.[1] Whole blood donors are primarily volunteers in community-oriented, not-for-profit blood programs. Their participation is essential to medical and surgical care.

Plasmapheresis for source plasma is organized mainly as a commercial process including direct monetary payment to the donor and distribution and sale of plasma derivatives by for-profit corporations. The world-wide rapid increase in the use of albumin and Factor VIII has resulted in intense competition for plasma and for albumin markets. In both the voluntary and commercial systems, there is comparable obligation to the donor and the patient. The collection process and the criteria used to select donors should protect both the donor and patient to the extent possible while considering the need for blood and blood products.

This presentation reviews the available information which can be applied to rational selection of donors, defines specific criteria where possible, and discusses the prevention and treatment of acute donor reactions.

MEASURES TO PROTECT THE DONOR

Blood donors are registered and examined by personnel with varying levels of training and experience, including volunteers and registered nurses and physicians. It is frequently convenient to screen donors rapidly in order to decrease waiting time. Efficiency in screening is improved by establishing criteria for donor selection which results in immediate acceptance or rejection of the donor. A third group requires more individual and experienced evaluation in order to maximize the opportunity to donate and minimize the risk of a donor reaction.

SINGLE UNIT (450 ML) WHOLE BLOOD DONATION

Acute Donor Reaction

The donation of blood is frequently associated with intense emotion and physical discomfort. Anxiety, fear, pain, and the effects of an abrupt change in circulating blood volume result in an acute donor reaction in 3 to 5 percent of individuals who give a single unit

Table 8-1. Symptoms in 899 Blood Donor Reactions

	(452) Males	(447) Females
Pallor	86%	83%
Perspiration	72%	60%
Weakness	51%	51%
Dizziness	53%	56%
Nausea	25%	33%
Emesis	4%	3%
Fainting	4%	5%
Clonic Movements	4%	4%
Incontinence	0%	0%

(Tomasulo, P. A., Anderson, A. J., Paluso, M. B., et al.: A study of criteria for blood donor deferral. Transfusion. Accepted for publication.)

of whole blood (450 ml).[1-4] The frequency of disabling or fatal complications is not reported and is presumably very small; however, this potential is obvious. In addition, unpleasant side effects are frequently given as a reason for not again donating.

Donor reactions are characterized by pallor and sweating, followed by a change in pulse pressure and heart rate, and symptoms of coldness, anxiety, nausea, faintness, and, finally, loss of consciousness (Table 8-1). The degree and direction of changes in blood pressure and heart rate are variable. An increase in heart rate is frequently followed by a decrease (30 to 50 beats per minute), and initial compensatory vasoconstriction may be followed by dilation of skeletal muscle arterioles with resulting hypotension due to pooling of blood. These signs and symptoms are the result of activation of the autonomic pressor and depressor regulatory systems—the syndrome of "vasovagal syncope."[5] Hyperventilation is another major cause of signs and symptoms of many donor reactions.

Scientific evaluation of these reactions has included studies of the effects of experimental acute hypovolemia and comparison of the frequency of reactions with physical, physiologic, and environmental variables in different donor groups and donation settings (Table 8-2). These reports are the basis for the commonly accepted criteria of selection designed to protect the healthy donor.[6,7] In addition, certain criteria have intended to exclude donors with preexisting disease which could be aggravated by acute reactions. These have been based upon the potential hazard of activating the autonomic regulatory system in patients with cardiovascular

Table 8-2. Factors Correlating with Donor Reactions

	References Positive Correlation	
	Yes	No
Physical Factors		
Age	1,2,3,4	
Sex	4	1,2,3
Weight	1,2,3,4	
Fatigue		1,4
Temperature (Body)		2
Time Since Eating		1,2,4
Hydration		1
Blood Pressure (<200 mmgh)		3,4
Heart Rate (<50)		3,4
Environmental Factors		
Room Temperature		1,2
Occupation		1,2
Location		4
Season		4
Psychologic Factors		
Prior Donation		3,4
History Fainting	5	
History Nervousness	5	
Expressed Fear	5	

disease or epilepsy. The effect of removing the cellular elements, plasma proteins, and essential nutrients contained in blood has also been considered. Depletion of iron stores, iron deficiency, and anemia are the important factors which limit frequency of donation of whole blood.

The Effect of Acute Hypovolemia

The response of the human body to acute blood loss was reported by Ebert, Stead, and Gibson in 1942.[8] These classic studies of the effects of hypovolemia documented that removal of 15 percent or more of the total blood volume was followed by pallor, sweating, blurred vision, weakness, and nausea. Heart rate increased by 14 to 30 beats per minute, followed by slowing to between 36 to 40 beats per minute in five of six experienced paid blood donors who were used as subjects.

Subsequent reports have confirmed a direct correlation between donor reactions and body weight. A reaction rate which averaged 3.5 percent in all donors increased to 7.6 percent in those weighing between 110 and 119 pounds.[9] The present recommended standards limits donation to those weighing more than 110 pounds, which is equivalent to about 13 percent of the total blood volume. The effects of psychologic factors and hypovolemia appear to be additive, since the reaction rate of first-time donors weighing between 110 and 119 pounds was 12.8 percent, whereas reactions occurred among experienced donors weighing between 100 and 110 pounds.[9]

All donors weighing less than 100 pounds should be rejected. Those weighing 100 to 110 pounds may be accepted if there is a prior history of uncomplicated successful donation. Donors weighing between 110 and 120 pounds should be accepted only if there are no other factors which might increase the risk of an unpleasant reaction. Phlebotomy should be performed by experienced personnel who should use particular caution to prevent postural hypotension, as discussed in the section under donor care.

PHYSIOLOGIC, PSYCHOLOGIC AND ENVIRONMENTAL FACTORS

These factors have not been studied as independent variables in relation to acute, disabling, or fatal donor reactions. Age, sex, prior donation, and fasting are associated with an increased frequency of acute reaction (Table 8-2). At present, donors are required to be between 17 and 65 years of age. The younger age is based largely upon legal considerations and the older age on presumption of increased risk of cardiovascular disease with aging. Screening procedures should routinely accept those in this age range. Donors over 65 years of age who appear to be in good health and who meet other criteria should be considered individually.

Fatigue, time since eating, state of hydration, occupation, ambient temperature, and season are factors which are not associated with an increased frequency of reactions. None should be used to exclude donors. Routine practice has commonly excluded anyone who has not eaten within 2 to 4 hours. However, there is no correlation between donor reactions and eating. Hypoglycemia does not occur, and measured blood sugar levels are normal. Similarly, even moderate dehydration does not increase the frequency of reactions, and administering fluids i.v. at the time blood is collected does not affect the reaction rate.

Preexisting Disease

It has been assumed that preexisting cardiovascular disease such as hypertension, cardiac arrythmias, and coronary insufficiency increase the risk from acute hypovolemia or vasovagal syncope during blood donation. Usual practice is to exclude donors with cardiac arrythmias, symptomatic heart failure, and recurring symptoms of coronary insufficiency. Donors who are free of symptoms for 6 months are usually accepted.

Hypertension greater than 150/100 mmHg has been an absolute criteria for rejection. A recent study indicates donors with a blood pressure up to 200/100 mmHg do not have increased rate of acute donor reactions.[9] However, the relation of hypertension to disabling or lethal reactions is unknown. Donors with a blood pressure between 150–200/90–100 mmHg frequently become normotensive when rested. If hypertension is sustained, a decision to accept the donor should be made only if there are no other factors which would increase the likelihood of an acute reaction—i.e., previous history of fainting, expressed fear, first-time female donor, etc.

Bradycardia (heart rate < 50) is not a contraindication to donating in the absence of other signs of excess vagovagal activity. An increased heart rate (> 100) should primarily be used as an indication of nervousness and anxiety, and not as a reason for rejection.

Donors who have diabetes and require insulin should be permanently deferred. Stable diabetics who meet other criteria should be accepted. Chronic symptomatic renal disease and all forms of hepatic disease prevent blood donation. Epilepsy excludes the donor unless there is no history of unusual nervousness or donor reactions and the donor has had no seizures for 5 years. The ingestion of antiseizure medication such as Dilantin or phenobarbital is not in itself a contraindication.

DRUG THERAPY

Drug therapy is a particular problem in selecting donors. Drugs are frequently prescribed without good reason and are difficult to identify and categorize. Cardiovascular and antihypertensive agents may be particularly important, since their major mode of action involves the regulatory system of the circulation. These agents inhibit or augment adrenergic or cholinergic neuromuscular transfer or block receptor sites.[10] Drugs such as propranolol and guanethedine are an absolute contraindication to donating because they enhance vagal effects by blocking beta-adrenergic receptor sites and adrenergic neurohumeral transmission.[1] Other drugs such as central nervous system depressants seem less likely to increase donor risk, and the donor should be accepted if there are no other factors which would increase the likelihood of acute reactions.

A *Physicians' Desk Reference* (PDR) should be available in each donor checking area to help identify drugs. An updated list of generic and trade names of drugs which contraindicate donation should be posted quarterly.

THE CELLULAR ELEMENTS, PLASMA PROTEINS, AND ESSENTIAL NUTRIENTS

The physiologic adjustment to acute blood loss is initiated while blood is being collected. Within 15 minutes, hemoglobin concentration is decreased by 1.5 percent. It continues to fall for 48 to 72 hours to a level that reflects the portion of total red cell mass that has been removed. Thereafter, red cell regeneration restores the hematocrit to normal over a period of 30 days.[11] An initial decrease in circulating platelet and white cell concentration parallels the change in red cells. The lowest level reached is never pathologic and is rapidly restored to normal.

The decrease in concentration of cellular elements is the result of hemodilution. Total circulating blood volume is restored by movement of water from the extracellular to the intravascular space. Albumin concentration falls initially. The plasma concentration is then restored as albumin also shifts from the extracellular space to the intravascular over about a 12-hour period. Albumin synthesis is increased in about 4 hours, and total body albumin is restored to normal in 3 days.[12] Detailed studies of the responses of other plasma proteins are not available; however, there is no indication that the effect of collecting a single unit of whole blood is significant.

Iron is the only nutrient affected by single unit blood donation. Loss from the body of 1 ml of red cells includes a loss of 1 mg of iron bound to hemoglobin. Each blood donation involves a loss of 250 mgm of iron, an average additional daily requirement of 0.68 mgm for one year. The approximate normal basal requirement of iron for women is 1.3 mgm and for men 1 mgm/day. If one unit of blood is donated per year, the basal requirement thus becomes 1.5 mgm and 1.97 mgm/day respectively. Iron absorption is carefully regulated and does not exceed 3 to 4 mgm/day in normal adults. These facts suggest that the donation of more than 3 units per year in males and 2 in menstruating females would result in iron deficiency, after iron stores (900 mgm average) are depleted. Finch et al. used serum ferritin levels to measure iron stores in 2981 blood donors.[13] Serum ferritin levels were reduced in direct proportion to the number of donations per year. The pathophysiologic significance of depletion of iron stores has not been established. Some evidence suggests iron-containing enzymes may be affected before anemia is measurable, but this is unsettled.

Assay of serum ferritin provides a valuable tool to study the relationship between phlebotomy, iron stores, anemia, and iron intake. Until the relationship between these variables is determined, donation should be limited to 4 units per year for men and 3 per year for menstruating women. Administration of prophylactic iron to blood donors is under investigation at present.

Normal hemoglobin values of 12.5 gm for women and 13.5 gm for men should be used to screen individuals for anemia. Values below these levels should disqualify the donor. Measurement of hemoglobin is the most important procedure performed prior to collecting blood and must be done with great care. Inaccuracy may defer too many donors or too few. Laboratory procedures include the use of copper sulfate to determine specific gravity, and direct measurement of hemoglobin or microhematocrit. All methods should be maintained by a careful quality control program to assure fresh solutions and calibrated machines. The specific gravity of copper sulfate solutions should be measured and recorded daily. Both finger-stick and ear lobe puncture are used to obtain a blood sample. Everyone authorized to perform the test must be carefully trained to collect the sample properly. At the Puget Sound Blood Center 1.8 percent of donors were rejected because of a hemoglobin below 12.5 gm (female) or 13.5 gm (male) measured by the cyanmethemoglobin method.

SUMMARY OF DONOR QUALIFICATION TO PROTECT THE DONOR

Absolute Criteria for Donor Acceptance or Rejection

Procedures to qualify donors of a single unit of whole blood can be organized to accept or reject the majority of donors quickly, safely, and with use of relatively inexperienced personnel. The basic screening procedure should accept individuals who are 17 to 65 years of age, in good health, who have not donated within 8 weeks and not more than 4 times (male) and 3 times (menstruating female) in the past year, who are not under a doctor's care or taking medicine, have not had a major illness, and are not pregnant. Blood pressure should be less than 150/mm/Hg, oral temperature less than 100 °F, weight 110 lb or more, and hemoglobin 12.5 gm female and 13.5 gm male.

Prospective donors who are absolutely excluded are: those who are under 17 years of age; those who have donated within 8 weeks or 4 times (male) and 3 times (female) in the past year; and those who have had a major illness in the past 6 months or are pregnant.

Selective Criteria

The following donors should be separately evaluated by appropriately trained personnel: donors older than 65 years; those who are under a doctor's care or are taking prescribed medicines; those who have had a major illness or surgery in the past 6 months; and those who have measured blood pressure of 150–200/100. Individual evaluation should determine the reason for medical care; identify the type of previous major medical illness; identify and classify the medication; and determine the prospective donor is cardiovascular status. Recurrent vascular insufficiency—including coronary insufficiency, congestive heart failure, or cardiac arrhythmias—is reason for rejection. Donors with recorded blood pressure of 150–200 mmHg should lie down for 15 minutes; if hypertension persists, they should be accepted as donors only after careful historical review to exclude associated cardiovascular disease.

Careful distinction should be made between permanent rejection and temporary deferral because of time sequences of conditions such as pregnancy. Notation of the nature of rejection (temporary or permanent) and the reason should be recorded and become a part of the donor data base where such is used. Permanent rejection should be explained with care by experienced personnel to maintain proper public relations and to decrease the potential of another attempt to donate.

APHERESIS

Apheresis means "taking off" and is applied to the individual components of whole blood, plasma, platelets, and white blood cells. Plasmapheresis is performed by collecting whole blood in a multiple bag system and returning the red cells to the donor after centrifugation. Plateletpheresis and leukopheresis are usually done by connecting disposable plastic bags and tubing vein-to-vein through a centrifuge. Centrifugation may be continuous or interrupted. In either case, the vein-to-vein connection to the donor is not broken. In plasmapheresis and cytopheresis, precision in technique is essential in order to prevent identification errors, circulatory overload, air embolism, etc. None of these are related to donor selection.

Plasmapheresis

Plasmapheresis was used to collect between 2.5 and 3.5 million liters of plasma in 1978 for commercial fractionation to produce albumin and Factor VIII. During World War II, pooled, dried plasma was used extensively to treat hemorrhagic shock. Post transfusion hepatitis was identified as a major hazard of pooling the plasma from very many donors prior to lyophilization. A single unit containing hepatitis virus could contaminate an entire lot.[14] Various techniques were used to inactivate the virus, including room temperature storage of plasma for 6 months and exposure to ultraviolet light. In 1968, Redeker reported that plasma obtained from two commercial sources and presumably so treated transmitted hepatitis to 5 percent of recipients.[15] Subsequently, the Division of Biologic Standards withdrew the licensing of this biologic.

The initial methodology for collecting, lyophilizing, and processing pooled plasma was developed by Cohn and associates.[16] Further investigation of the physical chemistry of plasma proteins resulted in the development of the Cohn method of fractionation, by which albumin could be prepared as a nearly homogeneous protein. Since albumin is stable when heated to 60° for 10 hours, it can be completely pasteurized, eliminating the risk of posttransfusion hepatitis. The availability of a purified, sterile, intravenous protein led to a rapid world-wide increase in its use as an oncotic agent, and, inappropriately in most cases, as a nutritional supplement.

The average adult male has a plasma volume of 3000 ml, containing 130 grams of intravascular albumin. There is an additional 200 gm of extravascular albumin in the interstitial space. The removal of blood is followed by the movement of interstitial fluid into the vascular compartment within minutes. All plasma proteins are thereby diluted, as are the red cells. However, in contrast to red cells, there is an influx of albumin from the extravascular space, and the concentration of albumin returns to normal within 24 hours.

The long-term effects of plasmapheresis were studied in healthy volunteers[17, 18] and in prisoners[19-20] participating in hyperimmunization programs for periods up to three years. Most of the statistically significant alterations in serum proteins and immunoglobulins occur in the initial six months of plasmapheresis. There tends to be a small decrease (0.5% $\pm$) in albumin, a rise in and α_2 globulins, and a decrease in IgG, IgA, and IgM. IgG and IgA values return to normal while IgM may continue to be depressed. These data have been combined with knowledge of the distribution, synthesis, and catabolism of albumin to establish legal donor qualifications for plasmapheresis.[21]

Status of Health

All plasmapheresis donors are required to be in good health and not under the influence of alcohol. The status of health is established at every donation as indicated by normal body temperature, pulse, and blood pressure and hemoglobin determination which is required to be 12.5 gm/100 ml or greater. A blood sample is collected to measure total serum protein, and HbsAg is determined on the collected plasma. Every four months, serum protein electrophoresis or quantitive measurement of immunoglobulin must be

found to be within normal limits of the testing laboratory, and accumulated data are reviewed by a licensed physician who approves the donor. An initial and annual physical examination is also performed by a qualified physician.

These criteria define the status of health of the donor at the time of plasmapheresis. Reliable laboratory results and consistent evaluation of accumulated data should effectively exclude repeating donors who develop measurable plasma protein abnormalities (see Table 8-3).

The Frequency and Volume of Plasmapheresis

The frequency and volume of plasma permitted to be removed by plasmapheresis is in part based upon body weight. Donors weighing less than 175 lb can give 1000 ml of plasma per 48 hr to a total of 2000 ML weekly or 50 l annually. Donors weighing over 175 lbs can give 1200 ml per 48 hr to a total of 2400 ml weekly or 60 l annually. If 1000 ml of plasma is removed, about 45 gm of albumin is lost from a total of 120 gm of intravascular albumin. About 10 percent of the total albumin pool of 300 gm is catabolized daily, and the synthesis rate can be increased to 2 to 3 times normal. Between 30 and 90 gm daily of new albumin is thus potentially available to restore circulating albumin removed in plasmapheresis. These calculations support the reported albumin levels measured in studies of plasmapheresis donors.

Effectiveness of Established Requirements

Many factors affect albumin synthesis including adrenocortical hormone levels, ingestion of alcohol, and the donor's nutritional state, particularly the availability of essential amino acids and total calories ingested. The majority of plasmapheresis donors are from

Table 8-3. Qualifications of Plasmapheresis Donors

To Establish Health Status		
Physical Requirements:	Required	Frequency
*General Good Health	yes	Each Visit
Temperature	< 100 F.	"
Blood Pressure	∠ 150/100mmHg	"
Pulse	∠ 100	"
*Weight	> 120	"
Laboratory:	> 13.5 gm (M)	
Hemoglobin	> 12.5 gm (F)	"
Total Protein	6. gm	"
Quantitative Immunoglobulin	Normal Limits	4 Months
Physician Review of Data		Each Visit

To Maintain Health Status		
Volume and Frequency		
Weight	Volume	Frequency
< 175 lbs.	1000 ml	every 48 hrs.
	2000 ml	every 7 days
	50,000 ml	annually
> 175 lbs.	1200 ml	every 48 hrs.
	2400 ml	every 7 days
	60,000 ml	annually

socially and economically deprived segments of our population. Alcoholism has been a very common phenomenon among them. There are no published data which establish the effectiveness of these regulations of the Bureau of Biologies in protecting the health of the plasma donor. Cited references only include selected donors who could be expected to have[17,18,20] or are defined as having[18] good nutritional status. In addition, there is no regulation which requires an objective evaluation of the donor's nutritional status. Consequently, recording data to permit time-trend analysis of body weight, as well as laboratory measurements, could be used to indicate an adverse change in nutritional status.

Validation of the effectiveness of these regulations in protecting the health of the donor requires information about the frequency and reason for rejection of repeat donors and description of the subject's subsequent health history after rejection. Since only those donors who return are reexamined, a carefully designed study to determine the reasons for dropping out of the plasmapheresis program is needed in order to exclude a change in health status as the cause. The potential long-term pathophysiologic effects of maximum continuous stimulation of cellular and biochemical systems involved in synthesis of albumin or immunoglobulins are unknown. Hyperimmunization programs that use incarcerated donors should permit appropriate studies to assess this question. Present U.S. requirements have been severely criticized by European authors as endangering the health of the donor.[22]

Cytopheresis

Plateletpheresis and leukopheresis most frequently involve a patient's family members or individuals specially selected by HLA matching. Plateletpheresis of healthy, normal adults has not been reported to adversely affect the donor. Daily plateletpheresis using the four-bag technique or six passes in a semicontinuous flow centrifuge result in a decrease in platelet count to 60 percent of normal on the third day, followed by recovery to levels 80 percent of normal over the ensuing 10 days.[23] Changes in bleeding time as a measure of platelet function have not been studied. The levels of circulating leukocytes and B and T lymphocytes are not significantly affected by these procedures.

Leukopheresis has been performed by continuous and semicontinuous centrifugation and by filtration through specially formulated nylon fibers. Collection of a therapeutically adequate number of leukocytes requires administration of adrenocortical hormones to increase blood levels of granulocytes and/or hydroxyethyl starch to sediment these cells. Both substances may cause adverse reactions. The potential effects of the former are well known. The latter may cause allergic reactions, and the long-term effects are unknown. Filtration leukopheresis has been reported to cause respiratory distress and priapism because of circulating nylon fibers (see Ch. 9).

It is difficult for even large cytopheresis laboratories to evaluate the immediate or long-term risks to donors in these programs. Donor selection therefore should be highly individualized and should include informed consent equivalent to that used for clinical human research projects. Accumulation of prospectively collected data in interinstitutional cooperative studies might create a base for long-term follow-up and a reporting system for acute reactions.

Protection of the patient who receives the products of cytopheresis entails rigorous search for potential hepatitis carriers. HbsAg assay and serology should be completed before cytopheresis is started. In addition, SGOT and ALT levels should be normal, and tests should be repeated frequently on continuing donors.

PROTECTION OF THE RECIPIENT

The principal risk to the recipient from the donor of blood is the transmission of infectious disease, particularly the risk of virus-induced hepatitis. In addition to the acute morbidity and mortality, cirrhosis, primary hepatoma, and vertical transmission (mother-to-fetus) among populations heavily infected with hepatitis B virus are major world problem.

Posttransfusion Hepatitis

Posttransfusion hepatitis (PTH) occurs in 7 to 13 percent of patients who receive blood or blood products.[23-25] Intense scientific effort has identified the etiologic agents of infectious hepatitis (HAV) and homologous serum hepatitis (HBV). Antigen and antibody assay of these viruses has identified a third cause of PTH, by exclusion: non-A, non-B (NANB) hepatitis. NANB is now the etiologic agent in 90 percent of cases of PTH.[23] Immunological detection of this agent will certainly be available in the future. Certain facts about HAV, HBV, and NANB hepatitis have been established that are important to selecting donors for blood products.

HAV is not transmitted by parenteral injection, including transfusion. It has been the primary agent in epidemic hepatitis. Its route of transmission is fecal-oral, and the virus is shed only in the prejaundice phase—i.e., in the initial 6 to 8 days of the disease. HAV does not cause chronic liver disease.

HBV is known to be transmitted by parenteral injection or direct contact with blood. HbsAg (antigen) assay has been supplemented by assays for the antigens Core, and "e" and their respective antibodies. All donor blood is now tested by third-generation procedures for HbsAg. About 10 percent of cases of PTH continue to be caused by HBV, but the number of cases has decreased by 50 percent since HbsAg testing has been introduced.[26] HBV causes chronic liver disease on occasion.

NANB hepatitis is transmitted by parenteral injection, including blood transfusion, and in secretions probably only after direct contact. Jaundice is frequently minimal and not observed clinically. However, chronic liver disease, including its progressive form, is most commonly caused by this agent. The frequency with which NANB agent(s) exist concurrently with HBV or HAV is not known.

The Transfusion Transmitted Virus Study Group have reported that an elevated serum alanine aminotransferase (ALT) level correlated most closely with the development of NANB hepatitis in recipients of volunteer blood. Thirty-eight percent of recepients who received blood from donors with an elevated ALT level[24] developed PTH.

Population Screening

The application of epidemiologic data to donor qualifications is the only available method for diminishing the risk of postransfusion hepatitis. Subsets of the population that are identified as having an increased risk of transmitting PTH should not be the target of or donor recruitment programs. Individual prospective donors should be carefully screened by history-taking before blood is collected. All collected blood should be HbsAg tested before components are distributed. The results of HbsAg testing should be incorporated into information about the donor base of the collection facility, along with the names of all donors who are identified to have provided blood to a patient with PTH, so that they can be rejected if they present as donors in the future.

The risk of transmitting hepatitis is increased 5 to 20 times by transfusing blood collected from commercial paid donors;[23] every published, reliable, scientific study confirms this fact. Other determinants of increased risk of hepatitis are: crowded and unsanitary living conditions, low income, institutionalized donors, newly recruited military personnel, and minimum education.[27,28] These characteristics are found among the social and economically disadvantaged. Direct monetary payment to donors, location of donor centers in ghetto or "skid row" areas, and advertisements directed at the needy should be discontinued until laboratory testing or vaccination eliminates the risk of posttransfusion hepatitis (if this ever occurs!).

Occupational hazard of hepatitis has been defined among health care professionals. Physicians and dentists are HbsAg or anti-Hbs positive four times more frequently than comparable controls, and 11 to 30 percent of all hospital workers studied[29] were found to be positive. Soliciting of workers in hospitals as donors should be discontinued until specific tests for NANB carriers are available.

Screening Individuals

Screening of individual donors should identify previous illness presumed to be hepatitis and possible exposure in the preceding 6 months to hepatitis through blood transfusion or needles which are not disposable and not used by health care professionals. The latter includes illicit parenteral drug use, tattooing, acupuncture, and ear piercing.

Specific questions should include a query regarding jaundice. However, a history of jaundice as a newborn or during childhood should not exclude the donor unless it followed blood transfusion or occurred during an epidemic. An isolated instance of jaundice in adolescents is not a reason for exclusion and is frequently due to infectious mononucleosis. Similarly, a demonstrated serologic reaction with any of the three HBV antigens or antibodies excludes the donor; this may change when the relationship between HBV and NANB hepatitis has been established. The increased frequency of HbsAg positivity and observed NANB PTH hepatitis from commercial donors suggests this caution, even if anti-Hbs and anti-Core carriers are proven to be noninfective. The purpose is to decrease the frequency of PTH, 90 percent of which is now NANB.

Donor-Patient Data Base

Data collection used to eliminate potential hepatitis carriers requires linking donors to the patients who develop PTH and methods to access the results of previous laboratory tests performed on donors who have previously donated. Data may be examined before blood is collected by listing suspect donors in printed updated "telephone books," or by on-line data processing terminals. An alternative is to collect and process each donor's blood and then to complete data entry and recall *before* releasing blood or components for transfusion. Regulations require that all individual units of transfused blood or components be traceable to the donor, regardless of where the blood is collected. There is no regulation, however, that requires this connection actually to be made when a patient has PTH. However, the importance of these mechanisms is illustrated by the fact that, in our experience, there were 16 donors identified in one 6-month period who had been implicated previously in PTH transmission or who were known to be HbsAg-positive. Informing donors that they are HbsAg-positive by letter and person-to-person communication has not prevented all of these individuals from again donating.[30] Shaeffer has also emphasized this point.

Malaria

Malaria has been reported following transfusion of whole blood, red cells, and platelets.[32,33] There is a world-wide resurgence of malaria with increased travel to malarious areas and increasing number of immigrants from malarious areas. Of 616 cases of malaria that occurred in the U.S. in 1977, 95 percent were in civilians.[34] Donors are deferred for three years if they have had malaria or have taken prophylatic antimalarial drugs while in a malarious area. This period is based upon the known latent infectivity of *P. falciparum.* The latent period of quartan malaria may be very long, but the infection is much more benign. Donors who have been in malarious areas but who have not used prophylactic medication are accepted six months after their last potential exposure, since 96 percent of *P. falciparum*

infections develop within that period. Of the 616 malaria cases reported in the U.S. in 1978, the largest number were acquired in India, Nigeria, the Philippines, Kenya, and El Salvador.

Other Infectious Diseases

In addition to posttransfusion viral hepatitis and malaria, syphilis and brucellosis have been considered important. The transmission of other infectious diseases or agents such as cytomegalovirus, Epstein-Barr virus, etc. has been presumed to occur; however, they are not relevant to today's transfusion practice.

The spirochete of syphilis does not survive in blood after storage at 4 °C longer than 48 to 72 hours. Freshly drawn blood and platelets which are stored at 22 °C could contain viable spirochetes. The value of performing routine serology on all blood has recently been questioned; a positive serological reaction for syphilis cannot be expected during the spirochetemic phase of the disease, when the donor is infectious.

Brucellosis has largely been controlled by testing cows in the milk-producing industry, and it should ordinarily not be considered in donor selection.

Donors are deferred until 48 hours after having dental procedures to avoid transient bacteremia. Skin rashes or abrasions in the antecubital fossa are likewise reason for rejection because of the potential of bacterial contamination during the venepuncture for a blood donation.

SUMMARY OF DONOR QUALIFICATIONS TO PROTECT THE RECIPIENT

The protection of the recipient of blood products from transfusion-transmitted diseases consists almost entirely of measures to decrease posttransfusion hepatitis, 90 percent of which is caused by Non-A, Non-B virus (es). Protective measures include:

A. Elimination of donor solicitation methods which involve socioeconomically deprived subsets of the population. Monetary and other incentives to donate should not be used.
B. Selection of individual donors only after careful screening for the following:
  1. A history of jaundice or hepatitis is cause for donor deferral, unless it occurred at birth or was an isolated occurrence before age 21 and not transfusion-related.
  2. A history of possible exposure to Non-A, Non-B virus by surgery, needles, tattooing, or transfusion in the preceding 6 months.
C. Laboratory Testing:
  1. Testing of all collected blood for HbsAg before transfusion and discard all HbsAg positive units.
  2. Testing of ALT and SGOT levels of cytopheresis donors (levels should not be elevated).
D. Record Keeping
  Screening of all donors against continuously updated files which show previous HbsAg-positive donors and donors implicated in past cases of PTH.

DONOR MANAGEMENT AND CARE

The Prevention and Treatment of Donor Reactions

The psychological and environmental factors which contribute to donor reactions have been reviewed. Physically attractive facilities for blood collection and cheerful, attentive personnel specially trained in the techniques of interpersonal communication can diminish the effects of stress. Professional, factual, and unemotional interpretation of the steps involved in screening and blood collection is important. The effects of needle sticks and blood collection, including the potential for pain and discomfort, should be recognized. Each donor should be continuously observed for early signs of vasovagal reaction or hyperventilation and predisposing factors—age, first-time donors, minimal weight, history of nervousness or fainting, and donors subjected to individual evaluation prior to acceptance should be identified to personnel collecting blood.

The collection process should be organized to provide a minimum of 15 minutes time for removal of the blood and in-place recovery. Discussion of the reason for each step, including skin preparation, tourniquet application, and the venipuncture itself, is helpful.

The use of an automatic shut-off to limit the amount of blood collected should be mentioned. Many donors appreciate a positive statement that their blood looks normal. The pain of venipuncture may be decreased by the use of an ethyl chloride spray; this has never been documented. Intracutaneous injection of a drop of anticoagulant on the tip of the needle is particularly painful.

At the conclusion of phlebotomy, the donor should be deliberately appraised for signs of hyperventilation or impending vasovagal syncope. Inappropriate perspiring and/or a pulse rate below 60 beats per minute requires retention on the donor bed until these signs have reversed. All predisposed donors, as previously described, should be allowed to sit before standing and should be escorted to the rest area or canteen in order to avoid postural hypotension or to deal with it promptly and safely, should it occur. The reduction of total circulating blood volume by a phlebotomy of 450 ml of blood is intended to be limited to a maximum of about 13 percent. Vasovagal activity has the effect of pooling blood in skeletal muscle. Gravity tends to pool blood in the distal veins. This effect is augmented by sitting erect as at a table, which constricts veins in the legs. Eating or drinking tends to pool blood in the stomach and intestines; the result of pooling of blood may be to further decrease the total circulating blood volume to a level which induces the physiologic response to acute hypovolemia.[8]

Approximately 60 percent of all donor reactions occur in the "canteen" for these reasons. Ideally, the donor would rest in a reclining chair, safe from falling, for a period of at least 30 minutes and would not be overtly encouraged to eat or drink. Even so, certain donors will have a syncopal attack as they leave the premises, with the danger of cuts and bruises or more serious complications. All donors should stand and walk in the presence of trained personnel before they leave the rest area and be unobtrusively observed again for signs of vasomotor collapse.

Treatment of vasovagal syncope should include observing for a potentially obstructed airway or cardiac arrhythmia. Blood pressure will vary, but heart rate will be slow (< 60 beats/minute). An increase will indicate impending recovery. Treatment is limited to maintaining the donor in a reclining position until recovery ensues. Encouraging consumption of liquids, application of cold compresses, etc. are not consistent with the known pathophysiology of this condition and should not be used as an expression of concern.

The potential for disabling or fatal reactions requires that resuscitative equipment such as airways and oxygen be available and that at least one person skilled in cardiorespiratory resuscitation be available at each donor center and mobile operation. Prior arrangements for immediate transportation of severely affected donors to appropriate hospital facilities, including preferred routing, should be made, and details should be included in readily available procedure manuals—particularly when mobile units are set up in outlying communities.

REFERENCES

1. Greenbury, M.B.: An analysis of the incidence of "fainting" in 5897 unselected blood donors. Br. Med. J. 1:253, 1942.
2. Poles, F.C., Boycett, M.: Syncope in blood donors. Lancet 2:531, 1942.
3. Moloney, W.C., Lonergan, L.R., et al.: Syncope in blood donors. N. Engl. J. Med. 234:114, 1946.
4. Graham, D.T.: Prediction of fainting in blood donors. Circulation: 23:901, 1961.
5. Ruetz, P.P., Johnson, S.A. et al.: Fainting: a review of its mechanisms and a study in blood donors. Med. 46:363, 1967.
6. 21 CFR 640.3
7. Standards for Blood Banks and Transfusion Services, American Association of Blood Banks, 1978.
8. Ebert, R.V., Stead, E.A., Gibson, J.G.: Response of normal subjects to acute blood loss. Arch. Intern. Med. 68:578, 1941.
9. Tomasulo, P., Anderson, A. et al.: A study of criteria for blood donor deferral. Transfusion. (Accepted for publication).
10. Goodman, L., Gilman, A.: Pharmacologic basis of therapeutics. MacMillan Publishing Co., Inc. 5th Ed. 404–575 and 653–744.
11. Wadsworth, G.R.: Recovery from acute hemorrhage in normal men and women. J. Physiol. 129:583, 1955.
12. Rothschild, M., Oratz, M., Schreiber, S.S.: Albumin synthesis and albumin degradation. Proceedings of the Workshop on Albumin, DHEW Publication No. (NIH) 76-925, p. 57.
13. Finch, C., Cook, J., et al.: Effect of blood donation on iron stores; an evaluation of serum ferritin. Blood 48:449, 1976.
14. Murray, R.: Viral hepatitis. Bull. N.Y. Acad. Med. 31:341–358, 1955.
15. Redecker, A.G.: Controlled study of the safety of pooled plasma stored in the liquid state at 20–32 °C for six months. Transfusion 8:60, 1968.
16. Cohn, E.J.: History of plasma fractionation. In: Advances in Military Medicine, Vol. 1, Little, Brown & Co., Boston, 1948, pp. 363–364.
17. Kliman, A., Carbone, P.P., et al.: Effects of intensive plasmapheresis on normal blood donors. Blood 23:647, 1964.
18. Friedman, M.A., Schork, M.A., et al.: Short-term and long-term effects of plasmapheresis on serum proteins and immunoglobulins. Transfusion 15:467, 1975.
19. Shanbrom, E., Lundak, R., Walford, R.L.: Long term plasmapheresis effects on specific plasma proteins. Transfusion 12:162, 1972.
20. Salvaggio, J., Arquembourg, P., et al.: Effects of prolonged plasmapheresis on immunoglobulins, other serum proteins, delayed hypersensitivity, and phytohemaglution induced

lymphocyte transformation. Int. Arch. Allergy 41:873, 1971.

21. Proceeding of the Workshop on Albumin, DHEW, Publication No. (NIH) pp. 76–925.

22. Lundsgaard-Hansell, P.: Volume limitations of plasmapheresis. Vox Sang. 32:20, 1977.

23. Alter, H.J., Purcell, R., et al.: Non-A, Non-B hepatitis: a review and interim report. In: Viral Hepatitis, Vyas G, et al. Eds. Franklin Institute Press, Philadelphia, 1978.

24. Aach, R., Lander, J., et al.: Transfusion transmitted virus: interim analysis of hepatitis among transfused and non-transfused patients. In: Viral Hepatitis. Vyas, G., et al., Eds. Franklin Institute Press, Philadelphia, 1978.

25. Seeff, L.B., Wright, E., et al.: Post transfusion hepatitis, 1973–1975, a veterans administration cooperative study. In: Viral Hepatitis. Vyas, G. et al., Eds. Franklin Institute Press, Philadelphia, 1978.

26. Calculations made by the author.

27. Goldfield, M., Bill, J., Colosimo, F.: Control of transfusion—associated hepatitis. In: Viral Hepatitis. Vyas, G., et al., Eds. Franklin Institute Press, Philadelphia, 1978.

28. Szmuness, W. Harley, E., et al.: Sociodemographic aspects of the epidemiology hepatitis B. In: Viral Hepatitis. Vyas, G., et al., Eds. Franklin Institute Press, Philadelphia, 1978.

29. Maynard, J.: Viral hepatitis as an occupational hazard in the health care profession. In: Viral Hepatitis. Vyas, G., et al., Eds. Franklin Institute Press, Philadelphia, 1978.

30. Personal observation by the author.

31. Shaeffer, A.: Hazardous donors. J.A.M.A. 239:2446, 1978.

32. Garfield, M., Ershler, W., Maki, D.: Malaria transmission by platelet concentrate transfusion. J.A.M.A. 240:2285, 1978.

33. Dover, A., Schultz, M.: Transfusion induced malaria. Transfusion 11:353, 1971.

34. Malaria surveillance, parasitic disease. CDC Division, Bureau of Epidemiology, Atlanta, Ga, Weekly Report, Dec. 14, 1979.

35. Personal observation by the author.

9

Preparation of Components and Their Characteristics; Plasmapheresis and Cytapheresis

Cynthia Murray, MT(ASCP)SBB and Garson H. Tishkoff, M.D., Ph.D.

The key to component therapy is the ability of blood centers to isolate specific plasma or cellular products in a concentrated form and make them available to the clinician within a reliable and reasonable time frame. In order to practice component therapy properly and effectively, it is also necessary to be aware of the relevant properties of the available products.

DEFINITIONS

A blood component is a portion of blood which is separable by physical or mechanical means, such as differential centrifugation. A plasma fraction is a derivative of plasma obtained by chemical processes, such as alcohol precipitation. The general term, blood product, is usually interpreted to include both blood components and plasma fractions.

Most hospital technologists and physicians are unaware of the effort required to produce even one platelet concentrate, fresh frozen plasma, or cryoprecipitate. Many small hospital and community blood banks have chosen to merge their resources with larger blood collection centers where the production of these components is dealt with on a routine basis. Notwithstanding, even large centers at times have difficulty interfacing the logistics involved in adequate and proper collection, processing, and distribution of these specific components of human blood. This chapter will attempt to outline some of the major considerations that are involved in the preparation, storage, shipment, and pretransfusion care of platelet concentrates, cryoprecipitate, and the various types of single donor plasma. Red cell products are considered in Chapter 12. We will also address these same issues with reference to the several products of pheresis now in vogue. In the latter instance, diligent care of the donor and rapid delivery of the product to the transfusion facility are of prime importance.

GENERAL REQUIREMENTS FOR COMPONENT PRODUCTION

There are several general considerations that are relevant to the activities of the Regional Blood Center as it attempts to fully meet component needs in a given geographic area. Whole blood collections must be predictable and uniform. This means that annual collections must be smoothly distributed throughout each collection day of the entire 12-month calendar year. Appropriate arrangements must be made for holidays occurring on Mondays and Fridays, as a Center which provides platelets cannot restrict drawing of whole blood donors for a period of more than 72 hours. A predetermined percentage of each day's collection must occur within a two-hour transportation radius of the processing center. Units intended for component preparation should have a normal distribution of blood groups. Drivers must be made available for continuous "shuttling" of freshly drawn whole blood units from the collection site to the component preparation site. Generally, component preparation will occur at the Blood Center or at a fixed subcenter. Mobile laboratory vehicles have been used with variable degrees of success. In general, donors respond positively to the fact that their blood is being drawn in specialized containers and then "whisked off" to a centralized location where it will be "divided" into different parts, each having different uses. This appeal is in fact heavily used in the recruitment of whole blood donors.

Physical aspects of blood collection are very important in the quality control of blood components. Venipuncture must be nontraumatic and should result in a smooth, uninterrupted blood flow for 8 to 12 minutes. Frequent mixing of the whole blood and the anticoagulant contained in the collection bag is important when coagulation factors are to be isolated from the plasma. Blood from which platelets are prepared is maintained at room temperature (20° to 24° C) from the time of collection until after the platelet-rich plasma has been removed. If this is not to be done, blood must be packed in insulated boxes under generous amounts of wet ice until it can be transported back to the Blood Center.

Component preparation is by its nature a program with exaggerated peaks and valleys of activity. When fresh blood is delivered to the center for separation, several trained technologists must be available immediately to perform the several steps involved in the preparation of the products derived from the plasma. Collection and preparation of these components from adequate numbers of fresh bloods is the major factor in assuring their availability for transfusion. Also inherent in availability is the concept of projection of need and inventory management. These variables must be calculated several times daily for each product. They generally strongly reflect the assigned blood component shelf life. The fact that component hemotherapy may or may not be limited to ABO and Rh identical products for a given recipient will bear directly on the type-specific donor recruitment goals of the blood center. Reasonable regional outdate rates will vary greatly depending on the blood component in question.

Quality control standards exist for almost all plasma products as established by federal regulatory agencies or by individual blood collection institutions. Further standards cover the shipment and storage of plasma products. For these and other reasons, component production has become a program that most hospital transfusion services would rather delegate to large blood-collecting facilities, and appropriately so. Our experience as a blood center serving a large geographic area has also shown that patients requiring specific component replacement, particularly platelets, are probably better cared for in the larger tertiary care facility where hospital staff is familiar with the proper storage and administration techniques for these products.

PREPARATION OF COMPONENTS

The specifics of preparation and storage of each of the major plasma components are considered below:

Platelet Concentrate Preparation

Transfusion of platelet concentrates has increased dramatically because of improved means of isolating and concentrating platelets, more intense use of chemotherapy and cytostatic immunosuppression, and an increasing awareness by physicians of the therapeutic usefulness of platelets in these situations.

Platelet production requirements largely dictate the pattern of whole blood collection in a regional blood service. Platelets survive poorly in stored blood so that platelet concentrates must be obtained from individual donations of fresh whole blood. Federal regulations require that the platelet-rich plasma be separated from the red cell concentrate within 4 hours of collection. A blood center may typically produce 30 to 50 percent more platelets than it anticipates distributing to hospitals in its region. This strategy insures, or attempts to insure, that adequate numbers of platelet concentrate will be available to meet emergency therapeutic demands as well as planned prophylactic platelet therapy.

Effects of Drug Ingestion

The drug ingestion history of the donor may have a significant impact on platelet component production. Ingestion of acetylsalicylic acid (ASA) has been shown to interfere irreversibly with the platelet's functional ability to adhere to collagen.[1] Studies by aggregometry of ASA "paralyzed" platelets demonstrate that the secondary release reaction, normally seen following stimulation with adenosine diphosphate (ADP) or epinephrine, does not occur. The once advocated practice of not drawing units of blood from donors who have ingested aspirin in a 7-day period prior to donation had a disastrous impact on the realities of platelet production.[2] Fortunately, current in vivo and in vitro studies suggest that the mixing of 20 percent or more normal platelets with the platelets of donors who have ingested aspirin corrects the functional defects caused by ASA[3,4] although contradictory studies have been reported.[5] Platelet concentrates are nearly always

transfused in pools of six units or more; therefore, it is no longer necessary to screen whole blood donors for aspirin ingestion. This is true unless a patient—for example, an infant—is to receive platelets derived from a single donor; or, in the case of plateletpheresis, when multiple units of platelets are collected from a single donor. In these latter instances, the donor should not have ingested aspirin-containing drugs for at least 48 hours prior to the donation.[6]

Platelet Isolation

Platelets must be isolated in such a way as to make them suitable for storage. Traditionally, platelet concentrates are prepared by performing two separate centrifugations on whole blood in a large four- or six-place rotor, constant temperature (20 to 24° C) centrifuge. The initial spin under low gravitational force results in the separation of the red cell concentrate from the platelet-rich plasma (PRP). Ninety percent of the donor platelets are retained in the PRP, which is then centrifuged at a higher gravitational level to effect the separation of the platelet concentrate from the platelet-poor supernatant. Federal regulations require that these two centrifugations result "in an unclumped product, without visible hemolysis, that yields a count of not less than 5.5×10^{10} platelets per unit in at least 75 percent of the units tested." A minimum of four platelet concentrates must be assayed per month by any facility "manufacturing" this product, although most larger facilities conduct quality control procedures on many more units per month.

While no published data exist that indicate that the initial centrifugation can affect viability of the platelet concentrate, it has been shown that the second centrifugation step can be critical and can result in reduced viability after 72-hour storage at room temperature.[7]

The problem of platelet "clumping" refers to the formation of reversible aggregates caused by ADP release from platelets colliding during centrifugation and from increased foreign surface contact. If platelet concentrates are allowed to repose for 60 to 90 minutes following separation from the platelet-poor supernatant plasma, gentle manipulation may then be used to resuspend the platelet pellet.[8] It is, therefore, only after this "resting" period that platelet concentrates may be labeled and distributed, even under emergency situations. This tactic avoids irreversible aggregation and loss of viability.

Storage Conditions

Federal regulations permit continual storage of platelet concentrate at a temperature of 1 to 6°C for 48 hours or at a temperature of 20 to 24°C for up to 72 hours. Whichever temperature is chosen for storage, the pH of the concentrate must be maintained within defined limits. The production of lactic acid by platelet glycolysis and the accumulation of CO_2 from oxidative phosphorylation may cause the pH to drop from its initial value of between 7.0 and 7.2,[9] particularly during storage at ambient temperatures.

As pH decreases, platelets progressively change from their typical discoid shape into spheres. This shape change is reversible in vivo if pH of the concentrate is maintained above 6.0. Below this point, irreversible damage occurs as evidenced by platelet lysis and fragmentation. The pH fluctuation can be stabilized to some degree by the retention of an adequate volume of autologous plasma in the platelet concentrate and by storing the platelets in an environmental chamber that accurately maintains a temperature of 20 to 24°C. Continual gentle agitation and adequate spacing of the plastic bags containing the platelet concentrates will allow CO_2 diffusion across the polyvinylchloride (PVC) membrane of the storage container.[10] The pH will also be more reliably controlled if the number of platelets per bag is held at approximately 7.7×10^{10}.[11] These measures will influence directly the oxygen supply to the platelets within the storage container. Figure 9-1 illustrates schematically the effect of these variables on the pH of platelet concentrates stored at room temperature.

Hemostatic Effectiveness

Platelets prepared at room temperature and stored at 1 to 6°C are thought to be initially hemostatically more effective as compared with platelets stored at ambient temperatures. However, platelets stored at 1 to 6°C have reduced survival time in the circulation after only 18 hours in the cold as compared with platelets stored at 20 to 24°C.[12,13] That platelets stored at room temperature may have suboptimal hemostatic effectiveness is suggested from studies showing that posttransfusion circulation of up to 24 hours may be required for normalization of certain intrinsic metabolic characteristics.[14] In contrast, bleeding times were significantly corrected within 2½ hours posttransfusion when carefully prepared platelets that had been stored at room temperature were transfused to aplastic thrombocytopenic patients.[15]

While no single in vitro test adequately documents the viability of stored platelets, several measurements may serve as indicators of the platelets' tolerance to different forms of storage as well as provide clues to explain the functional defects which occur when platelets are stored. Table 9-1 compares cold- and ambient-temperature-stored platelets with respect to a number of properties.

Proponents of ambient-temperature storage of platelets agree that five key factors are involved in the maintenance of platelet viability:

(1) pH, (2) concentration of platelets, (3) continual gentle agitation during storage, (4) temperature of storage, and (5) plastic composition of storage container.[16] When vigilant attention is paid to these variables, it is possible to recover 86 ± 1 percent of the platelets available in whole blood in the platelet concentrate. Approximately 50 percent of these platelets are recovered in the circulation after transfusion when stored for 24 hours at 20 to

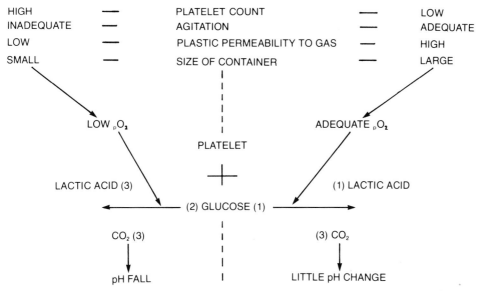

Fig. 9-1. Interaction of factors influencing pH of platelet concentrates during storage. Four factors interact to determine the pO_2 in the stored PC. When the pO_2 is low, glucose consumption per platelet is accelerated twofold with production of lactic acid, which lowers the pH of platelet concentrates. In addition to this effect, the higher the platelet count, the greater will be the production of lactic acid. Finally, if gas diffusion through the bag is impaired, pCO_2 will be higher for a given rate of CO_2 production. This will also lower the pH. (Murphy, S.N.: Harvesting of platelets and problems of storage. Greenwalt, T.J. and Jamieson, G.A., eds. The Blood Platelet in Transfusion Therapy. Alan R. Liss, Inc., New York, 1978.)

Table 9-1. Comparison of Physical Characteristics Between Platelets Stored at Ambient and Cold Temperatures

Parameter	Storage Temperature	
	1–6 °C	20–24 °C
Sterility[80, 81]	Bacterial growth not reported	Potential for contamination
Platelet survival in vivo[82]	4 days	1½ days
Adenine nucleotide metabolism impaired[83–85]	yes	yes—greater than that noted at 1–6 °C
Irreversible loss of discoid shape[86, 87] due to loss of microtuble	yes—rapid	no
Response to aggregating agents (ADP, Epinephrine, Collagen)[88–92]	increased	lost after 18 hours at 20–24 °C
Response to hypotonic stress[93–95]	severely depressed	depressed to 70% of normal
Electrophoretic mobility[96]	reduced	reduced
Proteolysis of platelet myosin[97]	yes	yes
Sensitivity to thrombin[98]	greater than normal	less than 1–6 ° storage
Alteration of membrane glycoproteins[99]	noted	noted—significant loss of sialic acid which may contribute to increased aggregability
Membrane lipid[100]	no change	10% of total lost after 72 hours

24°C. Further loss of viability as measured by platelet survival occurs with longer periods of storage. After 48 and 72 hours of room-temperature storage, approximately 40 percent and 30 percent of the transfused platelets are recovered in vivo, respectively.[17]

Agitation

Continual gentle agitation of stored platelet concentrates prior to transfusion may be achieved in a number of ways. Platelets stored on a horizontal shaker evidence post-transfusion yields superior to those stored on a ferris-wheel type of apparatus, and these findings can be correlated with specific morphologic changes in the platelets. Collisions with the plastic walls of the storage bag with release of platelet constituents may be responsible in part for these observations.[18]

Plastic Formulation

Plastics used in the production of the storage bag vary in suitability for preservation of platelet function. Fenwal PL 146 is clearly superior, and this fact has created a virtual monopoly in the blood bag industry for its manufacturers.[19] It has also been proposed that the use of thinner plastic than the standard PVC sheet used in the construction of the storage bag would allow greater gas permeability across the plastic membrane and may result in improved platelet viability.[20] Platelet concentrates prepared from blood of female donors appear to tolerate storage less well than those derived from male donors, presumably due to a lower initial pH which may be related to the lower hematocrits of female donors.[21]

Practical Considerations of Storage

Out of this morass of information have developed some suggestions for the practical management of the patient who requires transfusion of platelet concentrates. As graphically depicted in Figure 9-2, 1 to 6°C stored platelets are superior in hemostatic effectiveness for the first 4 hours. Between 4 and 24 hours of storage, cold and ambient stored platelets are comparable in hemostatic effectiveness; however, beyond 24 hours of storage, the quality of cold-stored platelets clearly declines in comparison to the room temperature stored platelet.[22]

One possible logistic strategy for a blood center would be to provide 1 to 6°C-stored platelets to control active bleeding and 20 to 24°C-stored platelets for prophylactic treatment of thrombocytopenia secondary to chemotherapy, etc.[23,24] This, of course, seriously increases the general logistic problem of platelet supply.

With in vitro function better preserved at 1 to 6°C and in vivo viability superiorly maintained at 20 to 24°C, a recent novel approach to the platelet storage problem proposes 30-minute "pulses" of 37°C storage after every 12 hours of 1 to 6°C storage.[25] Temperature "cycling" appears to improve the response of cold stored platelet to hypotonic stress and acts to prevent the irreversible disassembly of platelet microtubules which is observed during continuous storage at 1 to 6°C. The loss of discoid shape which is associated with the disassembly of microtubules appears to be the major cause of loss of viability during cold storage.[26] Platelets stored under temperature cycling conditions maintain normal aggregometry responses up to 96 hours following isolation. Presumably, this measure of in vitro function may correlate with improved in vivo viability for the temperature cycled cold stored platelet.

Immunologic Considerations

Survival of the transfused platelet may be dependent on specific immunologic factors as well. ABO incompatibility has been known to reduce the effectiveness of transfused plate-

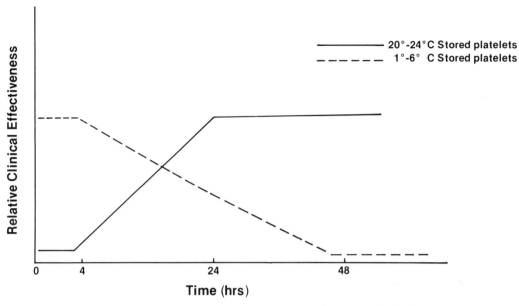

Fig. 9-2. Comparison of the hemostatic quality of cold and ambient stored platelets over a storage period of 0 to 48 hours.

lets[27] in some recipients; however, subsequent studies have not supported this phenomenon.[28,29]

Although platelet concentrates are derived from the plasma compartment of whole blood, they will inevitably contain small quantities of red cells which are capable of immunizing the recipient to red cell antigens, particularly $Rh_o(D)$. If $Rh_o(D)$ negative platelets are not available for $Rh_o(D)$ negative recipients, immunization can be prevented when necessary by administration of Rh immunoglobulin. Blood centers attempt to prepare platelets from all blood groups in order to supply compatible, if not identical, platelets in most instances. With understanding of the logistics of platelet preparation and supply, it should not be difficult to accept the occasional inability of the blood center to provide every patient with platelets of a specific blood group and type. In light of an immediate clinical platelet need, this point should be considered of minor importance.

Presence of lymphocytotoxic antibodies in the serum of patients receiving multiple random-donor platelet transfusions is correlated with poor platelet survival in this group.[30] This "refractory" condition is credited to alloimmunization to tissue antigens present on the platelet surface. A 24-hour posttransfusion platelet recovery of less than 20 percent indicates the development of the "refractory" state and may result in a failure of the platelets to support hemostasis. While it is recognized that matching donors and patients for histocompatibility antigens does not reliably predict platelet transfusion responses,[31] alloimmunized patients frequently respond successfully to platelets from donors who are matched or "selectively mismatched" for HLA antigens.[32] (This subject will be returned to in the discussion of Single Donor Platelets, and is also discussed in Chapters 26 and 27.)

Cryopreservation of Platelets

Cryopreservation of platelets has been under investigation for a number of years.[33,34,35] The advantage of frozen-stored viable platelets would be to increase acceptable storage periods to permit stockpiling of matched platelets and to preserve autologous platelets. At the present time, the methodology for cryopreservation of platelets employs 5 percent dimethylsulfoxide (DMSO) or 5 percent glycerol. Platelets have been shown to be stable for up to 8 months stored at −80° C when protected in DMSO. Recovered platelets up to 6 hours post-thaw have been reported to yield satisfactory results. When 5 percent glycerol with 4 percent glucose is used as the cryoprotective agent, storage should be in the vapor phase of liquid nitrogen. These recovered platelets are known to be stable 4 to 6 hours post-thaw. A significant role for autologous platelets may be found in the support of alloimmunized patients undergoing maintenance chemotherapy. As much as 40 percent of a patient's platelet needs may be able to be met by means of intensive platelet-pheresis and cryopreservation when it can be tolerated, followed by the subsequent thawing and reinfusion of autologous platelets.[36] Further clinical investigations are now underway to determine the in vitro and in vivo effectiveness of cryopreserved platelets by both methods.

Summary

Platelets must be prepared and stored in such a way as to effect the desired hemostatic response in the thrombocytopenic recipient. Every step of preparation and the specific conditions of storage, in addition to numerous immunologic and physical conditions in the recipient, will influence the success of the platelet transfusion.

OTHER PRODUCTS FROM PLASMA

Several unique plasma products are generally available from regional blood centers. Of prime importance are those prepared to preserve labile coagulation factors, notably Cryoprecipitate and Single Donor Plasma, Fresh Frozen.

Cryoprecipitated Antihemophilic Factor

Cryoprecipitated Antihemophilic Factor, which provides a major source of Factor VIII procoagulant for treatment of hemophiliacs in the U.S., has been produced by blood collection centers by the method first described by the late Dr. Judith Pool.[37] This relatively simple method, which resulted in isolation of cryoprecipitate rich in Factor VIII from donor plasma virtually revolutionized the treatment of classical hemophilia. Once prepared, cryoprecipitate may be stored for one year at −18° C or below (preferably −30° C). Cryoprecipitate is a labile product that must not be allowed to thaw at any point during storage because a dramatic loss of Factor VIII procoagulant activity will result. The source plasma, from which cryoprecipitate is isolated, must be frozen within 6 hours of collection (21 CFR 640.54), necessitating a transportation network similar to that required for platelet concentrate production. Platelets and cryoprecipitate may be prepared from a single unit of whole blood that has been drawn into a quadruple blood collection bag, if there is at least 200 ml of cell-free plasma remaining after the platelet concentrate has been removed. Bureau of Biologics quality control regulations require a minimum yield of 80 units of antihemophilic factor (AHF) per final container. At least four representative units must be assayed and reported monthly by each blood center that prepares cryoprecipitate to insure conformity to these potency requirements.

Technique of Preparation

While storage of cryoprecipitate at −18° C poses no problem, step-by-step preparation of this material rivals, indeed surpasses, that of platelet preparation in difficulty and the need for vigilant attention to detail. Investigators have identified as many as 90 variables which might conceivably affect the final cryoprecipitate quality and potency. As with platelet preparation, the whole blood from which cryoprecipitate is to be isolated must be collected in a smooth and uninterrupted manner. The donor unit should be mixed frequently with the anticoagulant contained in the collection bag during the phlebotomy. If platelets are not to be harvested in addition to cryoprecipitate, the whole blood should be refrigerated immediately after collection. It has been shown, however, that the amount of Factor VIII activity in a unit of whole blood stored at 22°C or 4°C after collection was virtually identical and that equal amounts of Factor VIII can be cryoprecipitated from blood maintained at either of the two temperatures.[38]

If platelets are not to be harvested, red cells and plasma should be separated by means of a relatively hard initial spin in a refrigerated centrifuge. As much cell-free plasma as possible should be expressed into an attached container. The major clinical disadvantage of cryoprecipitate is the individual variation in Factor VIII levels from bag to bag. This variation is at least as great as the range of Factor VIII activity in normal human plasma which is 50 to 200 percent. (Factor VIII content may be expressed either as a percent or as units per ml, with reference to a normal pooled plasma standard containing 100 percent activity or 1 unit per ml.) Additionally, a multitude of other variables of preparation will affect Factor VIII potency in cryoprecipitate, beginning with the relative amounts of plasma available after the first centrifugation. This variability results in some unpredictability of the required therapeutic dose.

Of utmost importance to blood center logistics is the fact that the source of plasma intended for cryoprecipitation must be frozen within 6 hours of collection. Extension of this time interval can result in a loss of as much as 25 percent of the original AHF activity.[39]

Plasma should be frozen quickly at temperatures of −40°C or below;[40] it can be held in the frozen state for 2 to 3 months without significant loss of AHF.[41] Perhaps the most critical step in cryoprecipitate preparation involves the means by which the frozen plasma is thawed and the cryoprecipitate is "captured." Source plasma may be thawed at 4°C in air or aqueous medium. The thawed plasma should be centrifuged promptly at 0°C at the point where a small amount of ice slush remains.[42] This will occur after approximately 90 minutes in a 4°C waterbath or 12 hours in a 4°C refrigerator.[43] All but 10 to 15 ml of autologous plasma is expressed from the cryoprecipitate after centrifugation, and the bag containing the AHF-poor plasma is clamped and separated. The cryoprecipitate should be promptly refrozen at a temperature of −30°C or below for optimal Factor VIII recovery and storage.

Preparation of Cryoprecipitate for Infusion

Certain precautions also must be taken in preparing cryoprecipitate for infusion. Cryoprecipitated AHF should be thawed and dissolved in the residual plasma in a circulating constant temperature waterbath maintained at 37°C. Use in hospitals usually includes pooling several cryoprecipitates into a single transfusion unit. Care must be taken during pooling, since each drop of thawed concentrate lost represents a significant loss in the amount of transfusible AHF. Containers can be rinsed with small volumes of normal saline after removal of the thawed cryoprecipitate and plasma in order to minimize this loss.

Cryoprecipitate must be administered through a filter. A significant amount of "insoluble debris" consisting of immunoglobulin, fibrinoprotein and cold-insoluble globulin remains after thawing. These may be responsible for some of the adverse reactions reported after infusion such as bronchospasm and hypotension.[44]

The final preparation of cryoprecipitate prepared under optimal conditions contains 35 to 50 percent of the original Factor VIII content of the plasma from which it was obtained in approximately 5 percent of the original plasma volume. It also contains 20 to 25 percent of the plasma fibrinogen, a point of equal importance.

Therapeutic Fibrinogen

For many years, fibrinogen—which precipitates in the first step of the Cohn cold ethanol plasma fractionation procedure—was made available for treatment of various fibrinogenopenic states. Fibrinogen always carried an alarmingly high risk of hepatitis due to the pooling of large volumes of plasma in the fractionation procedure and because fibrinogen, unlike albumin, cannot be pasteurized to inactivate the hepatitis virius.[45] Each unit of cryoprecipitate contains approximately 250 mg of fibrinogen and carries a hepatitis risk equal to that of a single unit of whole blood.[46] Since pooled plasma fibrinogen prepared by cold ethanol fractionation is no longer marketed, cryoprecipitate is the material of choice for fibrinogen replacement.

Single-Donor Plasma, Fresh Frozen

Other than antihemophilic factor and fibrinogen, cryoprecipitate does not contain appreciable amounts of other clotting factors. Single Donor Plasma, Fresh Frozen, contains 0.7 to 1.0 unit per ml of each clotting factor. Its use is indicated in the following conditions:

1. when deficiencies of multiple clotting factors exist as in liver disease,

2. at times in disseminated intravascular coagulation, or

3. when a specific factor deficiency has not yet been established.

Fresh Frozen Plasma (FFP) must be separated from the red cell concentrate and frozen within 6 hours of collection at $-18°C$ or below. It may be stored in the frozen state for one year. Both Cryoprecipitated Antihemophilic Factor and Single Donor Plasma, Fresh Frozen, may alternatively be prepared from plasma collected by pheresis. The presence of an appreciable amount of anti-A and anti-B isoagglutinins in FFP necessitates ABO compatibility between patient and donor plasma; therefore, blood centers must inventory all types for transfusion. In that plasma is virtually cell-free, it is not necessary to be concerned about the $Rh_o(D)$ type of the plasma donor, except possibly in the transfusion of neonates.[47]

Other Products

Single Donor Plasma. Several other specialized therapeutic plasma products may be available from the regional blood center. Single Donor Plasma, in which no attempt has been made to preserve the labile coagulation factors, is generally available in all blood types. This plasma is used clinically in much the same manner as albumin, and each unit carries a risk of hepatitis transmission equal to a unit of whole blood. It may also be employed in the maintenance of normal immunoglobulin concentrations in hypogammaglobulinemia. If frozen at $-18°C$, single-donor plasma may be stored for 5 years.

IgA Deficient Plasma. Larger centers will stock or have access to plasma collected from donors who lack IgA immunoglobulin. Transfusion of this plasma is indicated in the treatment of patients sensitized to either class specific or allotype specific IgA antigens or those known to be congenitally deficient in IgA immunoglobulin. Severe anaphylactic transfusion reactions have been reported in association with these antibodies.[48]

Source Plasma. Blood centers may serve to collect Source Plasma for the production of specific immunoglobulins. For example, Zoster Immune Globulin (ZIG) is produced from the plasma of donors exhibiting high-titered antibody during the recovery phase of herpes zoster or chicken pox. Donor centers have worked closely with clinicians for many years in collecting zoster immune plasma from these otherwise healthy donors. ZIG appears to be effective in attenuating or preventing herpes or chicken pox infection in immunosuppressed patients.

Blood centers may also become involved with the collectin of Source Plasma for hyperimmune gammaglobulin preparations from a donor population selectively immunized to rabies or tetanus—e.g., Veterinary Medicine students.

Recovered Plasma. A large proportion of the national supply of Recovered Plasma used by commercial or state-operated plasma fractionators is collected by donor centers. Recovered Plasma removed from outdated blood or plasma not needed for other purposes is primarily fractionated into albumin and immunoglobulin products. If Recovered Plasma is frozen within 6 hours of collection, it may serve as a source of lyophilized AHF concentrate as well.

CYTAPHERESIS

Iatrogenic bone marrow hypocellularity secondary to the administration of radiation, cytotoxic drugs, and chemotherapy encountered in modern oncology practice, has provided a new challenge to the facilities responsible for blood collection and component preparation. In order to provide significant numbers of granulocytes for hemotherapy, it is necessary to process large volumes of blood from a single donor in a relatively short period of time. While platelets can be effectively harvested from a single whole blood donation as described earlier, there are both theoretical and immunologic advantages and some disadvantages to providing the equivalent of 8 to 10 units of platelet concentrate to the thrombocytopenic patient from a single donor. This strategy may be very useful after a recipient has become

alloimmunized. (For further discussion of this topic, see Chapters 26 and 27.) In response to this need, the technology of component production by cytapheresis from a single donor has accelerated over the last 18 years and, with it, a progression of supportive instrumentation has appeared on the market (see Ch. 10).

With this technology has come new concerns for donor safety as well as controversy concerning in vitro and in vivo function of the collected platelets and granulocytes. In the first instance, the plateletpheresis/leukapheresis donor, unlike the whole blood donor, is subject to the potential of several mechanical and biochemical hazards. In an attempt to monitor the frequency and characteristics of these adverse reactions, the American Red Cross Blood Service has formed a committee charged with the collection and analysis of data pertinent to the safety of the donor undergoing pheresis procedures.

Adverse reactions have been reported in 4 to 6 percent of all donors undergoing cytapheresis procedures.[49] As in whole blood donation, anxiety is the most common manifestation. Some specific reactions are related to hypervolemia as well as to the drugs administered to the donor. These include sodium citrate, colloid volume substitutes (hydroxyethyl starch), corticosteroids, and heparin. Drug administration may be dictated by the particular theory upon which the collection method is based.

Techniques of Cytapheresis

There are two major leukapheresis formats: centrifugation and filtration (CFFL). Platelets are harvested exclusively by centrifugation. Centrifugation methods may be intermittent flow (IFC) or continuous flow (CFC). The essential features of the major equipment currently in use in most centers are shown in Figures 9–3, 9–4, and 9–5. The Haemonetics Model 30 (Haemonetics Cor-

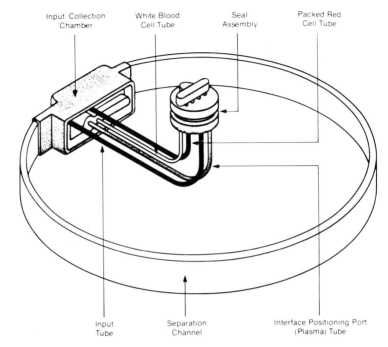

The IBM 2997
Blood Cell Separator

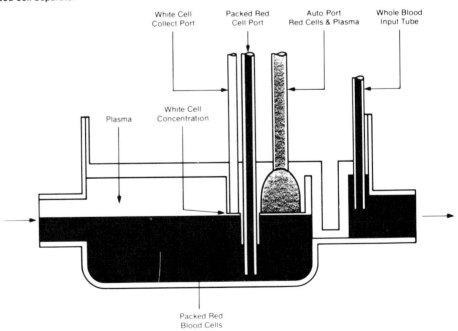

Fig. 9-3. IBM 2997 Blood Cell Separator Single Stage Separation Channel (IBM 2997 Blood Cell Separator Brochure, No. G570 1488-0). (Courtesy of International Business Machines Corporation.)

poration, Natick, MA) operates on the principle of intermittent flow centrifugation, while the IBM 2997 (International Business Machine Corporation, Princeton, NJ) is a continuous flow centrifuge. The Fenwal Filtration Set (Fenwal Laboratories, Deerfield, IL) which is used only for leukocyte collection, operates also as a continuous flow system with filtration (CFFL). It is comprised of a preassembled, closed sterile tubing set with two in-line nylon filters coupled with a compact peristaltic pump.

In both CFC and IFC, donor blood enters a reservoir where red cells, leukocytes, platelets, and plasma are separated centrifugally by virtue of their different specific gravities. The leukocytes and/or platelets are harvested, and the rest of the blood is returned to the donor. CFFL exploits the specific adhesion of phagocytic cells to nylon fiber of the filter in the presence of divalent cations. Citrate anticoagulation is therefore inappropriate, and the donor must be anticoagulated with heparin, administered either as a continuous infusion or as a bolus just prior to the start of the procedure. The usual heparin dose is 17,500 u. Donors may be given protamine (50 mg) at the end of the procedure to neutralize the heparin effect. CFFL donors must not have a history of bleeding tendency or allergy to beef, pork, or fish, hypersensitivity to heparin or protamine, or be women in menses. A unique reaction has been described in approximately 1.0 percent of CFFL donors.[50] Almost all the reactions occur in female donors and are characterized by severe lower abdominal, perineal, and upper thigh cramping resembling menstrual pain. Donors pretreated with corticosteroids to induce leukocytosis have a statistically significant reduction in the incidence of this pain syndrome. The incidence of the abdominal pain reaction has decreased recently and may have been associated with certain lots of nylon used in the filters. A more alarming adverse reaction associated with CFFL has occurred twice to date and has prompted the American Red Cross Blood Service to suspend CFFL in males. In these two instances, irreversible priapism occurred during the CFFL procedure, which required surgical intervention. In neither case had steroid pretreatment been given.

Most techniques require two venipunctures, which are necessary for effluent and return blood flow respectively. Eight to ten liters of whole blood are processed in approximately two hours. While undergoing leukapheresis, the donor is continuosly mobilizing granulocytes from the marginal pool and tissues reserve to replace those removed; postpheresis white cell count is usually not significantly altered. A peripheral platelet decrement in the range of 70,000/mm^3 to 90,000/mm^3 may occur in donors during plateletpheresis. A prepheresis platelet count is needed to establish normal levels of circulating platelets on prospective donors. Similarly, hematocrit values may decrease 2 to 4 percent during the cytapheresis procedure. These hematologic changes are thought to be due in part to physical removal and in part to hemodilution from the slight net excess of I.V. fluid administered during the procedures.[51] While the red cell loss is predictable in consecutive cytapheresis procedures, prepheresis hemoglobin levels do not return to initial values within a 24-hour period. Some evidence exists to support the notion that procedures utilizing hydroxyethyl starch (HES) as a rouleaux-inducing agent may result in the removal of 60 to 80 percent of the circulating reticulocytes causing a sustained mild anemia in donors undergoing repeated leukapheresis.[52]

Use of Hydroxyethyl Starch

Hydroxyethyl starch (HES), a high-molecular-weight colloid plasma volume expander, is employed in granulocyte collection as a rouleaux-inducing agent. Because separation of the cellular constituents depends upon dif-

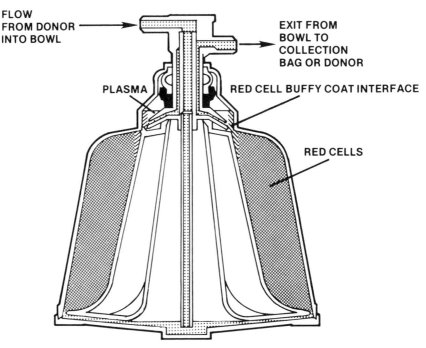

Fig. 9-4. (*A*) Cross-section diagram of the disposable centrifuge bowl used in the Haemonetics Model 30. (Haemonetics Corporation Owner's Manual, Natick, Mass., 1975.)

ferential centrifugation, the extracorporeal addition of a red cell sedimenting agent is necessary to obtain significant numbers of granulocytes.[53] When HES is used, hypervolemia may occur due to its oncotic effect which favors fluid retention, causing mild donor discomfort which generally abates in the first 24-hour postpheresis period. HES had been reported to be free of adverse in vivo reactions in man.[54] However, the authors have observed that, while the incidence of adverse reactions is admittedly low, acute hypersensitivity reactions have been experienced in as many as 0.3 percent of a leukapheresis donor population.

Tissue retention of HES has been well documented. Enhanced tissue storage appears to be related in part to the formation of HES-protein complexes. A high-molecular-weight HES-amylase complex retained by the reticuloendothelial system has been reported, and some preliminary reports in animal studies have indicated that this retention may result in impaired phagocytosis.[55] It has been recommended that the total HES burden per donor be limited. In our American Red Cross Center, that limit has been established as 200 grams of HES or seven leukapheresis donations.

Corticosteroid Administration to Donors

The number of granulocytes collected by any leukapheresis technique may be increased by inducing an elevation in the donor's preleukapheresis granulocyte count. The discovery that leukocytosis occurs following the administration of steroids,[56] and that the increase is composed entirely of young and mature neutrophilic granulocytes, formed the basis for the premedication of normal donors with corticosteroids. The steroids most commonly used are prednisone (60 mg. p.o.), etiocholanolone (i.m. 12 hours before), and dexamethasone (4 to 8 mg i.v. immediately before[57]). Recently, very im-

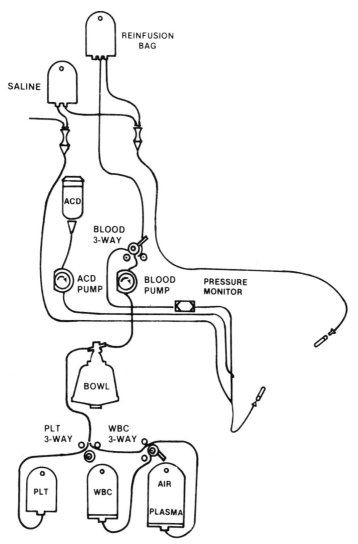

Fig. 9-4. (*B*) Disposable harness utilized with Haemonetics Model 30. (Haemonetics Corporation Owners Manual, Natick, Mass., 1975.)

pressive granulocyte yields (30×10^9) have been obtained using a double-dose dexamethasone protocol 12 hours prepheresis and again 3 hours prepheresis.[58] Steroid administration has been reported to cause adverse donor effects such as flushing, tingling of the scalp and perianal area, mild euphoria or depression, insomnia, indigestion, and headache. Donors with a history of peptic ulcer, cataracts, glaucoma, or hypersensitivity to steroids must not be premedicated.

Citrate Reactions

Citrate reactions in donors have also been reported. As whole blood leaves the donor's arm, it is immediately admixed with an anticoagulant, generally Acid Citrate Dextrose (Formula B). Donors may exhibit symptoms suggestive of citrate-induced hypocalcemia characterized by paresthesias, cooling sensations, and a quivering sensation of the diaphragm. A severe reaction may progress to

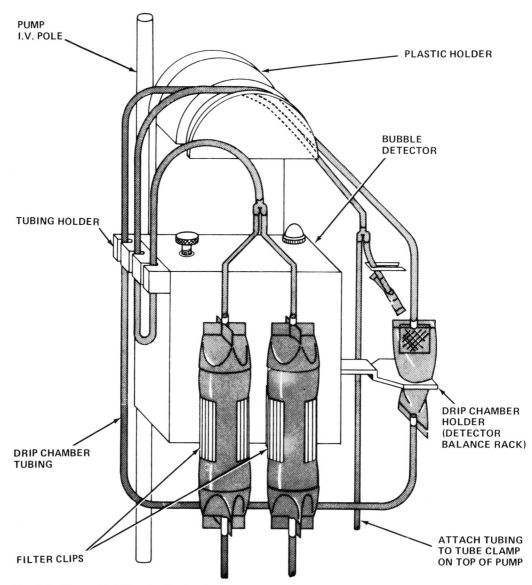

PUMP
I.V. POLE

PLASTIC HOLDER

BUBBLE
DETECTOR

TUBING HOLDER

DRIP CHAMBER
HOLDER
(DETECTOR
BALANCE RACK)

DRIP CHAMBER
TUBING

FILTER CLIPS

ATTACH TUBING
TO TUBE CLAMP
ON TOP OF PUMP

Fig. 9-5. Disposable Filtration Leukopheresis Set utilized in Fenwal system. (Fenwal Laboratories Operators Manual, Division of Travenol Laboratories, Deerfield, Illinois, 1977.)

the sensation of severe chest pressure and shortness of breath.[59] The reaction appears to be dependent upon the concentration of citrate used, the accumulation of the citrate load, and the rate of citrate administration. Massive extracorporeal clotting has been observed when citrate added to HES was not continuously mixed throughout a procedure and was apparently delivered in too low a concentration to provide anticoagulation. In this instance, fibrin monomer was present in the donor plasma indicating in vivo coagulation.[60]

Procedure Induced Hemolysis

Marked intravascular hemolysis has been observed following cytapheresis procedures on the Haemonetics Model 30.[61,62] In neither case could a specific mechanism for the red cell destruction be found. Both donors exhibited gross hemoglobinemia and hemoglobinuria, but without renal impairment. Neither donor had abnormal red cell fragility. Mild hemolysis in the range of 40 to 100 mg percent free hemoglobin continues to be seen in the supernatant plasma of whole blood that has been processed through the Haemonetics Model 30 prior to reinfusion. The mechanism of hemolysis presumably is mechanical, and in many instances the donor has had a slightly elevated prepheresis hematocrit in the range of 49 to 51 percent.

Safety

Despite these rather disconcerting reactions, pheresis procedures are regarded as safe and carry only minimal risk to the donor population. When cytapheresis procedures are conducted by qualified medical personnel who can anticipate and recognize adverse donor reactions, serious sequelae very rarely occur. A physician need not be present during these procedures but should be available within a reasonably few minutes for consultation.

Written informed consent of the donor is obligatory. The donor must be properly informed of the nature of the procedure and the recognized side effects or risks associated with it. Any potentially harmful side effect associated with drugs that might be administered also must be explained to the donor. The donor should understand that he is clearly free to refuse to participate in the procedure. A sample donor consent form is shown in Figure 9-6 (p. 231).

Cytapheresis Schedules

The most commonly used clinical schedule of leukocyte administration used in practice is three or four consecutive daily transfu-

sions.[63] Thus, these products must be available on a seven-day-a-week basis. The support of a highly cooperative and committed group of donors is therefore indispensable to a successful program. Cytapheresis donors seem to be strongly motivated by feelings of self-worth; participating in such a program supplies a high degree of emotional gratification.[64] Family members and acquaintances of particular patients often serve as cytapheresis donors but the frequency of repetitive procedures on an individual donor should be dictated by local policy and hematologic parameters such as platelet count and hematocrit.

Single Donor Platelets prepared by IFC and CFC may only be stored for 24 hours because of the open system used for collection. The platelets are most generally stored at ambient temperature (20 to 24°C) and should be continually agitated during storage. There is some suggestion that, due to increased numbers of platelets contained in the storage bag, pH and morphology are better maintained when very large plastic bags (2000 ml capacity) are used.[65]

Leukocyte Function

While absolute numbers of granulocytes infused have a direct relationship to clinical response,[66] it is of prime importance to establish whether the collection method has altered the cellular function of the transfused granulocyte. For the most part, current evidence supports the theory that the abnormal morphology observed in granulocytes collected by CFFL (vacuoles, degranulation) is correlated with abnormal function in vivo, particularly in poor migration to sites of infection.[67] Cells eluting from the filters prior to tapping of the filter casings seem to show less morphologic abnormalities and appear to perform better in functional analysis.[68] The number of normally functioning granulocytes obtained by CFFL can be increased by employing a combination of the following strategies:

1. pretreatment of the donor with steroids (4 mg/sq M dexamethasone I.V. or 30 to 50 mg p.o. of prednisone),

2. pretreatment of the donor with colchicine (2.4 mg by mouth to prevent neutrophil degranulation),

3. use of a carefully prepared solution for recovery of the granulocytes, and

4. control of the centrifuge speed used to pack the cells.[69]

White cells collected by CFC and IFC fare much better in both in vitro[70] and in vivo[71] functional studies including chemotaxis, NBT reduction, bactericidal function, post-transfusion recovery, and half-life measurement.

The duration and temperature of storage of granulocyte concentrates can also have a profound effect on the functional competence of the cells. Granulocytes collected by IFC and CFC are best preserved at 20 to 24 °C and may be stored for 24 hours prior to transfusion. They should not be agitated during storage.[72] Storage at 1 to 6 °C results in a greatly decreased chemotactic response within the first 24-hour period. Granulocytes collected by CFFL perform so poorly following storage that they must not be stored at all.

Yields

CFFL yields approximately 2.0 to 4.0×10^{10} leukocytes in a 3-hour collection period, the majority of which are granulocytes. The relative benefit of the superior yields obtained by CFFL is somewhat compromised by the abnormal function of many of these cells.

In order to achieve a therapeutic dosage of granulocytes by CFC or IFC, the donor must be exposed to either HES, steroid pretreatment, or both. Table 9-2 contrasts results obtained by IFC and CFC when both steroid pretreatment and HES is employed. The enhancement of granulocyte yields utilizing HES and corticosteroids is cumulative, and as much as four times as many granulocytes as

can be harvested when both additives are employed.[73] Using HES alone in our Center, we have experienced average leukocyte yields of 1.3×10^{10} (72 percent granulocytes) using the IFC method and 1.8×10^{10} (53 percent granulocytes) using the CFC method. When both HES and steroid pretreatment are used in conjunction with the IBM 2997, very impressive yields in the range obtained by CFFL have been reported. Further, granulocyte yield can be reliably predicted, with donor precount and blood volume being the most significant variables.[74]

Leukocyte Platelet Collection

Simultaneous Single Donor Platelet and granulocyte collection is possible when IFC is used. In our hands, an average of 5.0×10^{11} platelets or the equivalent of 9 to 10 single units of platelet concentrate can be harvested along with granulocytes. Tandem collection of leukocytes and platelets is possible by CFC although again, in our experience, platelet collection has not been as efficient as by IFC. This feature of leukocyte and platelet collection deserves serious consideration because many patients requiring platelets also need granulocytes during the course of their treatment. Approximately 50 percent of the procedures performed in our Center provide for the combination of platelets and granulocytes.

It is desirable that the ABO type of the leukocyte/platelet donor be compatible with the plasma of the recipient, as the red blood cell contamination of these products may be very high. If necessary, the incompatible red blood cells can be removed by a second differential centrifugation prior to transfusion; however, this maneuver will be accompanied by a significant loss of leukocytes. As in the case of the transfusion of platelet concentrate, Rh incompatibility is of minor consequence although usually avoided, and immunization can be avoided by the administration of Rh

LEUKAPHERESIS DONOR CONSENT FORM

I. I hereby volunteer and consent to serve as a donor for granulocyte and platelet transfusion with the collection of granulocytes and platelets by centrifugation of my blood.

II. The procedure has been explained to me by _____. I also understand that I have the opportunity to request further description and explanation of this procedure from a physician. I understand the nature of the leukapheresis procedure to be the removal of blood from a vein in one arm, passage of the blood through the centrifuge instrument where white cells, platelets and some plasma will be removed, the remainder of my blood being returned to my other arm or the same arm. I understand that the cycle of filling the centrifuge bowl with my blood, removing white cells, platelets and some plasma and returning the remaining blood to me will be repeated several times and require 2-3 hours. I may be asked to take a dose of steroid medication to raise my white cell count prior to donation. I also understand that an agent which helps to separate white cells, hydroxyethyl starch, will be mixed with my blood during the collection and that some of it will be returned to me. During the course of the procedure I will receive the anticoagulant citrate.

III. I have been made aware that the risks are similar to those involved in whole blood donation and include nausea, vomiting, fainting or dizziness, hematoma (accumulation of blood at the needle puncture site), seizures, blood loss, and infection. Potential problems of leukapheresis with hydroxyethyl starch and citrate include air embolus (collection of air in the circulation), muscle cramping, numbness, chilliness, tingling sensations, feelings of anxiety, heart rhythm disturbances, headache, ankle swelling, fluid overload, low blood pressure and allergic reactions to hydroxyethyl starch.

IV. It has been explained to me that after leukapheresis my platelet count may be decreased temporarily. The lost platelets will be replaced by my body so that the platelet count should be back to normal within 1 to 2 days after donation.

V. I am aware that the practice of medicine is not an exact science and I acknowledge that no guarantees have been made to me concerning the results of this procedure. I desire to participate of my own free will. I understand that I may withdraw from this procedure at any time.

It is clear to me that there is no advantage or benefit to me accompanying this procedure, but that I am volunteering to donate sufficient normal granulocytes to be useful for transfusion, and to aid in the developing of this new process. I understand that if the granulocytes and/or platelets which I have donated for any reason are not used in all or part for transfusion, the remainder can be used for laboratory purposes. I also agree to have small samples of my blood drawn for research related to pheresis and for quality control procedures.

I understand that if I have any questions about the theory behind this work, the need for the program, the benefits or hazards involved or any other related questions, I am free to ask them at any time.

_____   _____
(Witness)   (Signature of Donor)

_____
(Date)

Fig. 9-6. Leukapheresis Donor Consent Form. (American Red Cross Blood Services, Great Lakes Region, Lansing, Michigan.)

Table 9-2. Granulocyte Yield from Currently Available Leukapheresis Technique

Method	Instrument	Donor Treatment	Granulo-cytes $\times 10^9$
CFCL	IBM Blood Cell Separator or Aminco Celltrifuge	None	6
		HES*	10
		Steroids and HES*	16–22
IFCL	Haemonetics Model 30	HES*	6–13
		Steroids and HES*	—
FL	Fenwal pump	None	25
Gravity leukapheresis	Plastic bags	Steroids and HES*	17.9
NEW CFCL	IBM 2997 Blood Cell Separator	HES*	11
		Steroids and HES*	20–27

*HES = Hydroxyethyl Starch. Yields for CFCL, IFCL, and FL are summarized from many reports.

(Twenty second Annual Meeting American Society of Hematology Education Program Pg. 59)

immunoglobulin. Stimulation of anti-$Rh_{o(D)}$ in these situations is rare, probably due to the immunosuppressed state of most recipients.

HLA Donor/Recipient Matching

Appreciable controversy revolves around the role of HLA matching and granulocyte transfusion.[75] In spite of varying opinions regarding the clinical effectiveness of mismatched or incompatible leukocytes, most clinical evidence sustains the view that posttransfusion granulocyte increments are greater when HLA matching has been done.[76]

At this point in time, no pretransfusion method stands out as a good predictive tool for determining which patients might respond poorly to granulocyte transfusion due to immunologic incompatibility.[77] Most patients currently do not receive HLA-matched granulocytes due to logistical restraints, but for the sensitized patient this strategy may be of major importance.

The case for HLA matching for Single Donor Platelets is clearer, particularly in patients who have become refractory to random platelets. While matched platelet transfusions are not always successful, and mismatched platelets in refractory patients are not always unsuccessful, response to matched or "selectively mismatched" platelets (as measured by posttransfusion recovery in the peripheral blood) is significantly higher.[78] Platelets are highly immunogenic. Recognizing that 70 percent of patients who receive repeated platelet transfusions will develop lymphocytotoxic antibody,[79] many clinicians subscribe to the concept of "limited antigen exposure" when treating patients destined to receive multiple platelet transfusion. The patient is thus exposed to only one HLA phenotype per transfusion episode, and the onset of the refractory state is *possibly* delayed. This approach, however, places a high demand on the donor, without assurance that a refractory state will be delayed (see Ch. 27).

Cytapheresis for the procurement of platelets and granulocytes is now a recognized strategy of hemotherapy. While possible effects on the donor should not be overplayed, they must be dealt with in a responsible manner. Effective therapeutic yields, proper patient selection and transfusion schedules, and in vivo evaluation of transfusions are essential areas that must be examined.

PLASMAPHERESIS

Plasmapheresis is the only pheresis procedure currently regulated by the Bureau of Biologics. Plasma is harvested by pheresis methods for a variety of uses including fractionation into albumin and immunoglobulins, production of platelets and cryoprecipitates, and use as Single Donor Plasma, Fresh Frozen.

The largest collectors of plasma by pheresis for fractionation are the commercial plasma collectors located throughout the country, who offer between $7 and $10 per 500 ml donation of plasma. These are primarily manual operations where the whole blood is withdrawn, plasma is separated from the red cells by centrifugation, and the red cells are returned to the donor. The process is then repeated. The maximum whole blood removed in a 48-hour period must not exceed 1,000 ml (or 1,200 ml if the donor weighs over 175 pounds). A donor identification system must be developed to insure proper return of the red cells to the donor. Chances of a mix-up can be decreased by the use of a portable refrigerated centrifuge that is placed at the bedside, keeping the donor close to his withdrawn red cells.

In addition, the donor must be examined by a physician upon entry into the plasmapheresis program and every four months thereafter. Serum protein levels and protein electrophoresis or quantitative immunodiffusion measurements must be performed and reviewed at regular intervals.

Manual plasmapheresis has advantages over automated collection in that it can be performed away from the main location. Automated plasma collection can be accomplished by use of the Haemonetics Model 50. This apparatus operates on the same principle as the Haemonetics Model 30 used for platelet and leukapheresis. A major advantage in safety is that the donor and his red cells are never separated.

The issue of commercial versus volunteer plasma for fractionation purposes is one of local and national interest. Still unsettled is the effect of long-term repetitive plasmapheresis on donor health. Since much of the plasma collected by commercial concerns in the United States is marketed outside the country, this issue has sociological significance as well.

REFERENCES

1. Moroff, G. and Jamieson, G. A.: Biochemical aspects of platelet function. In: The Blood Platelet in Transfusion Therapy. Greenwalt, T. J., and Jamieson, G.. A., eds. Alan R. Liss, Inc., New York, 1978, p. 25.
2. Mielke, C.H., Dr., and Britton, A. F.: Aspirin: A new nightmare for blood bankers. N. Engl. J. Med., 286:268, 1972.
3. O'Brien, J.R.: Effects of salycylates on human platelets. Lancet 1:1431, 1968.
4. Stuart, M.J., Murphy, S., Oski, F.A., Evans, A.E., Donaldson, M.H., and Gardner, F.H.: Platelet function in recipients of platelets from donors ingesting aspirin. N. Engl. J. Med., 287:1105, 1972.
5. Rock, G. and Trepanier, J.: The effect of aspirin on the hypotonic shock response. Transfusion, 18:423, 1978.
6. Aster, R.H.: Clinical use of platelet concentrates. In: Transfusion and Immunology. Skkola, E. and Nykanen, A., eds. International Society of Blood Transfusion, 1975 p. 223.
7. Slichter, S.J, and Harker, L.A.: Preparation and storage of platelet concentrates. Transfusion 16:8, 1976.
8. Mourad, N.: A simple method for obtaining platelet concentrates free of aggregates. Transfusion 8:48, 1968.
9. Murphy, S.N. and Gardner, F.H.: Platelet storage at 22 °C: Role of gas transport across plastic containers in maintenance of viability. Blood 46:209, 1975.
10. Murphy, S.N.: Harvesting of platelets and problems of storage. In: The Blood Platelet in Transfusion Therapy. Greenwalt, T.J., and Jamieson, G.A. eds. Alan R. Liss, Inc., New York, 1978, p. 101.
11. Kunikci, T.J., Tuccelli, M., Becker, G.A., and Aster, R.H. A study of variables af-

fecting the quality of platelets stored at room temperature. Transfusion 15:414, 1975.

12. Becker, G.A., Tuccelli, M., Kunicki, T., Chalos, M.K., and Aster, R.H.: Studies on platelets stored at 22 °C and 4 °C. Transfusion 13:61, 1973.

13. Aster, R.H., Becker, G.A., Hamid, M., and Calvert, D.N. Storage of platelet concentrates at 4 °C; Use of refrigerated platelet concentrates in the treatment of hemorrhage in thrombocytopenic patients. Baldini, M.G. and Ebbe, S. eds. Platelets: Production, Function, Transfusion, and Storage. New York: Grune and Stratton, Inc., 1974, p. 631.

14. Murphy S.N. and Gardner, F.H.: Platelet storage at 22 °C; metabolic, morphologic and functional studies. J. Clin. Invest. 50:370, 1971.

15. Slichter, S.J. and Harker, L.A.: Preparation and storage of platelet concentrates. Br. J. Haematol. 34:403, 1976.

16. Slichter, S.J. and Harker, L.A.: Preparation and storage of platelet concentrates. Transfusion 16:8, 1976.

17. Valeri, C.R.: Circulation and hemostatic effectiveness of platelets stored at 4 °C or 22 °C. Transfusion 16:20, 1976.

18. Holme, S., Vaidja, K., and Murphy, S.: Platelet storage at 22 °C: effect of type of agitation on morphology, viability, and function in vitro. Blood 52:425, 1978.

19. Aster, R.H., Becker, G.A., and Filip, D.J.: Studies to improve methods of short term platelet preservation. Transfusion 16:4, 1976.

20. Murphy, S.N.: Harvesting of platelets and problems of storage. Greenwalt, T.J., and Jamieson, G.A., eds. The Blood Platelet in Transfusion Therapy. Alan R. Liss, Inc., New York, 1978, p. 101.

21. Kunikci, T.J., Tuccelli, M., Becker, G.A., and Aster, R.H.: A study of variables affecting the quality of platelets stored at room temperature. Transfusion 15:414, 1975.

22. Aster, R.H., Becker, G.A., and Filip, D.J.: Studies to improve methods of short term platelet preservation. Transfusion 16:4, 1976.

23. Kattlove, H.E.: Platelet preservation—what temperature? A rationale for strategy. Transfusion 14:328, 1974.

24. Valeri, C.R.: Circulation and hemostatic effectiveness of platelets stored at 4 °C or 22 °C. Transfusion 16:20, 1976.

25. McGill, M.: Platelet storage by temperature cycling. Greenwalt, T.J. and Jamieson, G.A., eds. The Blood Platelet in Transfusion Therapy. Alan R. Liss, Inc., New York, 1978, p. 119.

26. Behnke, O.: Some possible practical implications of the lability of blood platelet microtubules. Vox Sang. 13:502, 1967.

27. Aster, R.H.: Effect of anticoagulation and ABO compatibility on recovery of transfused human platelets. Blood 26:732, 1965.

28. Lohrmann, H., Bull, M.I., Decter, J.A., Yankee, R.A., and Graw, R.G.: Platelet transfusions from HLA compatible unrelated donors of alloimmunized patients. Ann. Intern. Med. 80:9, 1974.

29. Duquesnoy, R., Anderson, A., Tomasulo, P., and Aster, R. ABO compatibility and platelet transfusions of alloimmunized thrombocytopenic patients. Blood 54:595, 1979.

30. Howard, J. and Perkins, H.A.: The natural history of alloimmunization to platelets. Transfusion, 18:496, 1978.

31. Tosato, G., Appelbaum, F.R., and Deisseroth, A.B.: HLA matched platelet transfusion therapy of severe aplastic anemia. Blood 52:846, 1978.

32. Duquesnoy, R.: Donor selection in platelet transfusion therapy of alloimmunized thrombocytopenic patients. Greenwalt, T.J. and Jamieson, G.A., eds. The Blood Platelet in Transfusion Therapy. Alan R. Liss, Inc., New York, 1978, p. 229.

33. Klein, E., Toch, R., Farber, S., Freeman, G., and Florentino, R.: Hemostasis in thrombocytopenic bleeding following infusion of stored frozen platelets. Blood 11:693, 1956.

34. Cohen, P. and Gardner, F.H.: Platelet preservation II. Preservation of canine platelet concentrate by freezing in solutions of glycerol plasma. J. Clin. Invest. 41:10, 1962.

35. Djerrasi, I., Farber, A.R., and Cavens, J.: Preparation and in vivo circulation of human platelets preserved with combined demethylsulfoxide and dextrose. Transfusion 6:572, 1966.

36. Shiffer, C.A., Aisner, J., and Wiernik, P.H.: Platelet transfusion therapy for patients with leukemia. Greenwalt, T.J. and Jamieson, G.A., eds. The Blood Platelet in Transfusion Therapy. Alan R. Liss, Inc., New York, 1978, p. 267.

37. Pool, J. and Shannon, A.E.: Production of high potency concentrate of antihemophilic globulin in a closed bag system. N.E.J.M. 273:1443, 1965.

38. Rock, G. and Tittley, P.: The effect of temperature variation on cryoprecipitate. Transfusion 19:86, 1979.

39. Slichter, S.J., Counts, R.B., Henderson, R., and Harker, L.A.: Preparation of cryoprecipitated Factor VIII concentrate. Transfusion 16:616, 1976.

40. Rock, G. and Tittley, P.: The effect of temperature variation on cryoprecipitate. Transfusion 19:86, 1979.

41. Kasper, C., Myre, B.A., McDonald, J.D., Nakasako, Y., and Feinstein, D.I.: Determinants of Factor VIII recovery in cryoprecipitate. Transfusion 15:312, 1975.

42. Burka, E., Harker, L.A., Kasper, C., Kevy, S.V., and Ness, P.N.: A protocol for cryoprecipitate production. Transfusion 15:327, 1975.

43. Kasper, C., Myre, B.A., McDonald, J.D., Nakasako, Y., and Feinstein, D.I.: Determinants of Factor VIII recovery in cryoprecipitate. Transfusion 15:312, 1975.

44. Eyster, M. and Nau, ME.: Particulate material in antihemophilic factor (AHF) concentrates. Transfusion 18:576, 1978.

45. Barker, L.: Transmission of Viral Hepatitis, Type B, by plasma derivatives. Div. Biol. Stand. 27:128, 1974.

46. Bove, J.: Fibrinogen—is the benefit worth the risk? Transfusion 18:129, 1978.

47. Konungres, A.: Transfusion therapy for the neonate. Bell, C., ed. A seminar on Perinatal Blood Banking. American Association of Blood Banks, 1978, p. 93.

48. Vyas, G.N., Holmdahl, L., and Perkins, H.A.: Serologic specificity of human anti-IgA and its significance in transfusion. Blood 34:573, 1969.

49. Haddy, T.B. and Fratantoni, J.C.: Reactions in leukocyte donors. N.E.J.M. 299:833, 1975.

50. Wiltbank T.B., Nusbacher, J., Higby, D.J., and MacPherson, J.L.: Abdominal pain in donors during filtration leukapheresis. Transfusion 17:159, 1977.

51. McCullough, J.: Leukapheresis and granulocyte transfusion. CRC Crit. Rev. Clin. Lab. Sci. 10:275, 1979.

52. Woods, A.H., Gibbs, R., and Holmberg, A.: The anemia associated with repeated leukapheresis. Gold, J.M. and Lowenthal, R.M., eds. Leukbcytes: Separation, Collection and Transfusion. Academic Press, London, 1975, p. 106.

53. Sussman, L.N., Colli, W., and Pichetshote, C.: Harvesting of granulocytes using a hydroxyethyl starch solution. Transfusion 15:461, 1975.

54. Mishler, J.M.: Hydroxyethyl starch as an experimental adjunct to leukocyte separation by centrifugal means: Review of safety and efficacy. Transfusion 15:449, 1975.

55. Kohler, H., Kirch, W., and Horstmann, J.J.: J. Clin. Pharmacol. Biopharm. 15:428, 1977.

56. Bishop, C.R., Athens, J.W., Boggs, D.R., and Cartwright, G.E.: The mechanism of cortisol induced granulocytosis. Clin. Res. 15:130, 1967.

57. McCullough, J.: Leukapheresis and granulocyte transfusion. Critical Reviews in Clinical Laboratory Sciences 10:275, 1979.

58. Winton, E.F. and Vogler, W.R.: Development of a practical oral dexamethasone premedication schedule leading to improved granulocyte yields with the continuous flow blood cell separator. Blood 52:249, 1978.

59. Olson, P.R., Cox, C., and McCullough, J.: Laboratory and clinical effects on the reinfusion of ACD solution during plateletpheresis. Vox. Sang. 33:79, 1977.

60. Drescher, W.P., Shih, N., Hess, K., and Tishkoff, G.H.: Massive extracorporeal blood clotting during discontinuous flow leukapheresis. Transfusion 18:89, 1978.

61. Howard, J.E. and Perkins, H.A.: Lysis of donor RBC during plateletpheresis with a blood processor. J.A.M.A. 236:289, 1976.

62. Personal observation of authors.

63. Graw, R.G., Herzig, G., Perry, S., and Henderson, E.S.: Normal granulocyte transfusion therapy. N. Engl. J. Med. 287:367, 1972.

64. Szymanski, L.S., Cushna, B., Jackson, B.C.H., and Szymanski, I.O.: Motivation of platelet pheresis donors. Transfusion 18:64, 1978.

65. Katz, A., Houx, J., and Ewald, L.: Storage of platelets prepared by discontinuous flow centrifugation. Transfusion 18:220, 1978.

66. Mathé, G., Amiel, J.L., and Schwarzenberg, L.: Leukocyte transfusion. In: Bone Marrow Transplantation and Leukocyte Transfusion.

Charles C. Thomas, Springfield, Ill., 1971, p. 104.

67. Wright, D.G., Kauffmann, J.C., Chused, M.J., Herzig, G.P., and Gallin, J.L.: Functional abnormalities of human neutrophils collected by continuous flow filtration leukapheresis. Blood 46:901, 1975.

68. *ibid.*

69. Higby, D. and Burnett, D.: Granulocyte transfusion: current status. Blood 55:2, 1980.

70. Strauss, R.G., Koepke, J.A., and Maguire, L.C.: Properties of neutrophils (PMN) prepared for transfusion by the Haemonetics Cell Separator. Blood 50 (suppl. 1):310, 1977.

71. Prince, T.H. and Dale, D.C.: Neutrophil and collection method on neutrophil blood kinetics. Blood 51:789, 1978.

72. McCullough, J., Weiblen, B.J., Peterson, P.K., and Quie, P.G.: Effects of temperature on granulocyte preservation. Blood 52:301, 1978.

73. McCredie, K.B., Freireich, E.J., Hester, J.P., and Vallejos, C.: Increased granulocyte collection with the blood cell separator and the addition of etiocholanolone and hydroxyethyl starch. Transfusion 14:357, 1974.

74. Hester, J.P., Kellogg, R.M., Mulzet, A.P., Kruger, V.R., McCredie, K.B., and Freireich, E.J.: Principles of blood separation and component extraction in a disposable continuous-flow single stage channel. Blood 54:254, 1979.

75. McCredie, K.B., Hester, J.P., Freireich, E.J., Brittin, G.M., and Vallejos, C.: Platelet and leukocyte transfusions in acute leukemia. Hum. Pathol. 5:699, 1974.

76. Graw, R.G., Jr., Eyre, H.J., Goldstein, I.M., and Terasaki, P.J.: Histocompatibility testing for leukocyte transfusion. Lancet 2:77, 1970.

77. Ungerleider, R.S., Appelbaum, F.R., Trapani, R.J., and Deisseroth, A.B.: Lack of predictive value of anti-leukocyte antibody screening in granulocyte transfusion therapy. Transfusion 19:90, 1979.

78. Duquesnoy, R.: Donor selection in platelet transfusion therapy of alloimmunized thrombocytopenic patients. Greenwalt, T.J. and Jamieson, G.A. eds. The Blood Platelet in Transfusion Therapy. Alan R. Liss, Inc., New York, 1978, p. 229.

79. Howard, J. and Perkins, H.A.: The natural history of alloimmunization to platelets. Transfusion 18:496, 1978.

80. Buckholtz, D.H., Youngh, V.M., Friedman, N.R., Reilly, J.A., and Mardinez, M.K.: Bacterial proliferation in platelet products stored at room temperature. N.E.J.M. 285:429, 1971.

81. Kahn, R.A. and Flinton, L.J.: The relationship between platelets and bacteria. Blood 44:715, 1974.

82. Valeri, C.R.: Circulation and hemostatic effectiveness of platelets stored at 4 °C or 22 °C. Transfusion 16:20, 1976.

83. Filip, D.J., Eckstein, J.D., and Sibley, C.A.: The effect of platelet concentrate storage temperature on adenine nucleotide metabolism. Blood 45:749, 1975.

84. Kim, B.K. and Baldini, M.G.: Glycolytic intermediates and adenine nucleotides of human platelets. Transfusion 12:1, 1972.

85. Kotelba-Witkowska, B., Holmsen, H., and Murer, E.H.: Storage of human platelets: Effects on metabolically active ATP and the release reaction. Br. J. Haematol. 22:429, 1972.

86. White, J.G. and Krivit, W.: An ultrastructural basis for the shape changes induced in platelets by chilling. Blood 30:625, 1967.

87. Zucker, M.B. and Borrelli, J.: Reversible alterations in platelet morphology produced by anticoagulants and by cold. Blood 9:602, 1954.

88. Kattlove, H.E. and Alexander, B.: The effect of cold on platelets. I. Cold induced platelet aggregation. Blood 38:39, 1971.

89. Shively, J.A., Gott, C.L., and DeJengh, D.S.: The effect of storage on adhesion and aggregation of platelets. Vox Sang. 18:204, 1970.

90. Silva, V.A. and Miller, W.V.: Platelet transfusion survey in a regional blood program. Transfusion 17:255, 1977.

91. Aster, R.H., Becker, G.A., Hamid, M., and Calvert, D.N.: Storage of platelet concentrates at 4 °C: Use of refrigerated platelet concentrates in the treatment of hemmorrhage in thrombocytopenic patients. Baldini, M.G. and Ebbe, S. eds. Platelets: Production, Function, Transfusion, and Storage. Grune and Stratton, Inc., New York, 1974, p. 631.

92. Murphy, S.N. and Gardner, F.H.: Platelet storage at 22 °C; metabolic, morphologic and

functional studies. J. Clin. Invest. 50:370, 1971.

93. Rock, G. and Figueredo, A.: Metabolic changes during platelet storage. Transfusion 16:571, 1976.

94. Kim, B.K. and Baldini, M.G.: The platelet response to hypotonic shock. Its value as an indicator of platelet viability after storage. Transfusion 14:130, 1974.

95. Valeri, C.R., Feingold, H., and Marchionni, L.D.: The relation between response to hypotonic stress and the ^{51}Cr recovery of preserved platelets. Transfusion 14:331, 1974.

96. Ando, Y., Steiner, M., and Baldini, M.G.: Effect of chilling on membrane related functions of platelets. Transfusion 14:453, 1974.

97. Abramowitz, J., Stracher, B., and Detweler, T.C.: Proteolysis of myosin during platelet storage. J. Clin. Invest. 53:1493, 1974.

98. Robblee, L.S., Shepro, D., Vecchione, J.J., and Valeri, C.R.: Increased thrombin sensitivity of human platelets after storage at 4°C. Transfusion 18:45, 1978.

99. George, J.N.: Platelet membrane glycoproteins: alteration during storage of human platelet concentration. Thromb. Res. 8:719, 1976.

100. Aster, R.H., Becker, G.A., Hamid, M., and Calvert, D.N.: Storage of platelet concentrates at 4°C; Use of refrigerated platelet concentrates in the treatment of hemorrhage in thrombocytopenic patients. Baldini, M.G., and Ebbe, S., eds. Platelets: Production, Function, Transfusion, and Storage. Grune and Stratton, Inc., New York, 1974, p. 631.

10

Equipment, Devices, and Instruments Associated with Transfusion

William C. Sherwood, M.D.

INTRODUCTION

Blood banking and its related disciplines have not suffered from a lack of human ingenuity in a search to develop instruments and applications to assist with their many functions and responsibilities. From the ultra-simple bladder of a dog and quill of goose, the first syringe, attributed to Christopher Wren, to the highly complex Groupamatic System, with its microswitches, laser beam, and thousands of integrated circuits, developed by Claude Matte for automated blood grouping,[1] a plethora of equipment and utensils have come and gone. Come, to satisfy the exigencies of a situation, and gone, to be replaced by a better tool. Throughout most of this time, the equipment was designed and developed by the user. Only in recent years have many other disciplines applied themselves to this task. Today, the development of such equipment is supported by mechanical and electrical engineers, computer specialists, chemists, industrial designers and, more recently, bioengineers and biomaterials specialists. An important incentive has been the competition of the "marketplace." Often, a number of manufacturers' products are available that essentially carry out similar functions.

Today, the equipment used in blood banking and blood transfusion therapy includes items utilized for: the collection of blood, the production of individual blood components; the processing of blood into components and fractions; the diagnostic testing of blood to characterize its group and type and determine its safety; the storage of blood and components in temperature controlled environments; the transfusion or administration of the blood product to the patient; and the removal of certain blood elements for therapeutic reasons.

This chapter is intended to provide basic information on the types of equipment in use. All manufacturers' products could not be exhibited, and the reader should be aware that, for many items discussed, a number of manufacturers' products are often available that are at least as satisfactory as those depicted or described.

BLOOD COLLECTION EQUIPMENT

Fortunately, the equipment required to collect units of whole blood for transfusion purposes is quite simple, although attempts have been made to complicate the process. The simplicity of this equipment contributes to the high degree of mobility of blood collection teams. Blood donors can be handled in stable, fixed units that may accommodate as few as one donor at a time to large mobile extravaganzas that, given the space, may collect blood from hundreds of donors in a single session. Today, this mobility is essential to procure the large number of blood products required by our health care system.

The early equipment used in the collection of blood, although functional, had little appeal to the sensitivities of anxious blood donors. In some cases, the equipment was fearsome. However, in recent years, there have been attempts to develop blood collection equipment which, in addition to being functional, is pleasing in appearance and comfortable to the donor. If the donor has a pleasant blood donation experience, he will be more likely to return. Contoured donor lounges, such as the one depicted in Figure 10-1, have been developed for fixed donor facilities. The American Red Cross, in conjunction with the Rhode Island School of Design, developed an integrated "system" of mobile blood collection equipment (Figs. 10-2, 10-3) which is lightweight, compact, provides comfort and ease for both donor and staff, and is pleasing to the eye.

Given the flexibility of mobile unit sys-

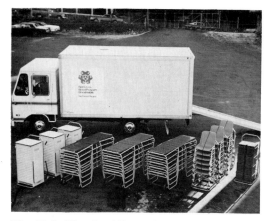

Fig. 10-2. Bloodmobile equipment, modern and compact, developed for the American Red Cross by the Rhode Island School of Design. (Courtesy American Red Cross, Washington, D.C.).

tems, blood can be collected in even the most unexpected locations. For special situations, self-contained mobile vans have been designed in which the entire blood donation process is carried out within the van, under environmental control (Fig. 10-4).

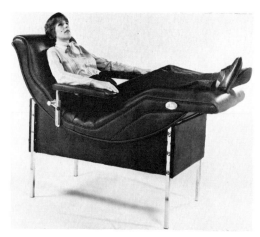

Fig. 10-1. Blood donation lounge. For fixed blood donor locations. By sliding action, lounge allows the rapid and convenient change to a Trendelenberg position. (Courtesy Fenwal Laboratories, Deerfield, Illinois).

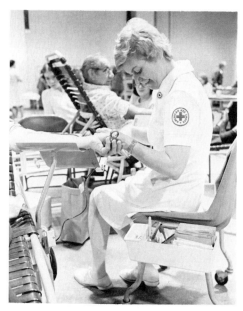

Fig. 10-3. Bloodmobile equipment, in use by the American Red Cross. Comfort and ease of use for both donor and phlebotomist. (Courtesy American Red Cross, Washington, D.C.).

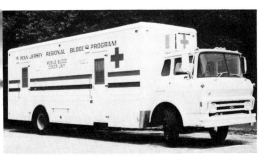

Fig. 10-4. Blood donor van. Self-contained. Accommodates three donors, recovery bed, work bench, refrigerator, and canteen area. (Courtesy Penn-Jersey Regional Red Cross Blood Service.)

For donor areas, federal regulations[2] require adequate space, lighting, and ventilation. In addition, they specify handwashing and toilet facilities, and privacy of the donor during interview. Given the almost universal presence of pleasant, comfortable blood collection sites and equipment, there are not many excuses for not being a regular blood donor.

Blood Collection Containers

For the past 10 years, the predominant containers used for the collection of donor blood have been pliable, sterile, prepackaged, disposable plastic containers that have multiple compartments with sealed, in-line connections (Fig. 10-5). The use of these containers has made possible the extensive practice of blood component therapy. The pliability of the containers allows easy component transfer following differential centrifugation. The sterile, sealed connections make blood component production possible without opening the system to risk from bacterial contamination. The shelf life of the components is based upon component viability rather than the limited 24 hours required for components produced in "open" systems. Current federal regulations require that some blood components be prepared in closed systems.[2]

The majority of plastic films in use for

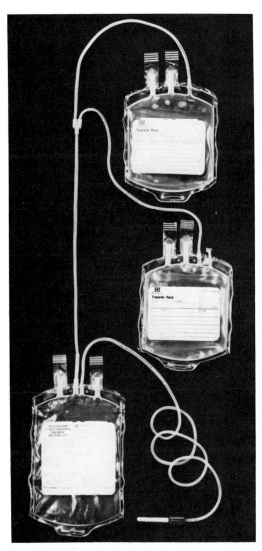

Fig. 10-5. Blood collection set. Primary blood collection container with anticoagulant storage media and two satellite containers attached with sealed, sterile in-line tubing. Prepackaged, nonreusable. (Courtesy Fenwal Laboratories, Deerfield, Ill.).

blood containers are variants of polyvinyl chloride. However, other plastics, such as polyolefin, have been used for special circumstances such as storage of frozen red cells. Although plastic blood containers have many important advantages over the glass vacuum bottles used previously, there are disadvantages which cannot be disregarded. One of the more disquieting features is the leaching of the plasticizer di-2-ethylhexylphthalate (DEHP) from the polyvinylchloride (PVC) plastic film into the blood or component during the period of storage.[3,4] The leaching of this material from the container into the product appears to increase with time, temperature, and the lipid concentration of the contents.[5]

There is no clear evidence of deleterious effects of the infusion of DEHP into humans in the concentrations found in blood products.[6] However, there is an accumulation of its metabolite, mono-2-ethylhexylphalate, in fat tissue,[7] and any long-term effects of this have yet to be recognized. Although it has been suggested that the leaching of DEHP into blood may be associated with microaggregate formation during blood storage, this could not be proven.[8]

Unlike red cells, which metabolize glucose via the anerobic Emden-Meyerhof pathway, platelets and leukocytes require oxygen for the tricarboxylic acid (Krebs) cycle. The current plastic films used as blood and component containers effect gas transport very poorly. Murphy[9] has shown that platelet viability is much improved when platelet concentrates are stored in containers that allow improved oxygen and CO_2 transport across the container wall.

Currently there is a major effort to develop plastic films that possess the strength, pliability, and transparency of PVC yet do not contain leachable ingredients and allow a high degree of gas diffusion.

Pheresis Equipment

Pheresis equipment was developed primarily to harvest granulocytes and single donor platelets in large numbers from normal donors in order to provide replacement therapy to patients with granulocytopenia and/or thrombocytopenia. This development was stimulated by the more aggressive chemotherapy applied to patients with malignant disease and the prolonged pancytopenia that followed. The majority of equipment in current use utilizes either continuous or discontinuous centrifugation cell separation principles.

There was early evidence that granulocytes, which could be collected in large numbers from patients with chronic myelogenous leukemia, were useful in the support of some patients with severe granulocytopenia.[10-12] In 1965, The National Cancer Institute along with the IBM Corporation developed a cell separator for the main purpose of collecting granulocytes for transfusion.[13] Although this initial instrument functioned well, it was cumbersome to operate and after each use required sterilization of a number of reusable parts.

Expansion in the preparation and use of granulocytes occurred when more simple and operator-oriented equipment became available. The earliest method to experience widespread use, filtration leukapheresis, adopted a principle recognized by Greenwalt in 1962.[14] Granulocytes, in the presence of calcium (heparinized blood), will adhere to scrubbed nylon wool fibers. The granulocytes collected on the nylon wool filters can be eluted with citrated plasma and be further concentrated by centrifugation. The equipment for filtration leukapheresis consists only of a calibrated roller pump used to pump blood continuously from the vein of a heparinized donor, through two or more disposable nylon wool filter cartridges,[15-18] and back to the donor. Although more granulocytes can be harvested per liter of blood processed by this method than by centrifugation methods, granulocyte concentrates prepared in this manner are associated with a higher incidence of febrile reactions.[17-19] There is evidence that this phenomenon is a result of membrane changes caused by the adherence-elution process. This method went into a rapid decline when two male donors, while undergoing filtration leukapheresis, developed severe priapism requiring surgical decompression.[20] Although a direct cause-and-effect relationship has not been established, this same unusual complication has been noted in patients undergoing renal hemodialysis.[21-23]

The pheresis cell separation equipment currently in widespread use utilizes centrifugation principles. This equipment includes: the Model 30 (Haemonetics Corporation) (Fig. 10-6), the Celltrifuge Blood Cell Separator (Fenwal Laboratories), and the IBM 2997 Blood Cell Separator (IBM Corporation) (Fig. 10-7).

The Celltrifuge is a continuous flow system employing the same operating principle as the NCI-IBM apparatus. Blood is citrated as it is removed from the donor and is pumped to a spinning reusable centrifuge bowl. Exit ports within the bowl provide for the removal of various layers which develop as centrifugation proceeds. As the rate of blood flow is adjusted against centrifugation speed, the position of layers within the bowl can be adjusted to collect the desired fraction.

The Haemonetics Model 30 (or 30S) (Fig. 10-6) is a discontinuous flow system which also uses a unique centrifugation bowl that is disposable after use. Citrated blood is pumped to the bottom of the spinning bowl.

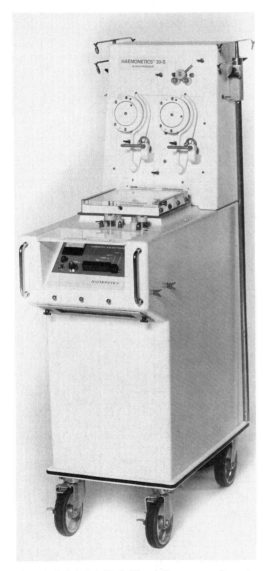

Fig. 10-6. Model 30-S Blood Processor. A portable cell separator used for the collection of leukocyte and/or platelet concentrates from normal donors and for therapeutic plasma and cytopheresis. Utilizes a discontinuous flow centrifugation principle. (Courtesy Haemonetics Corporation, Braintree, Mass.)

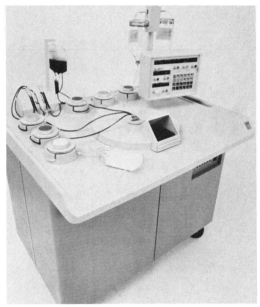

Fig. 10-7. Model 2997 Blood Cell Separator. Used for the collection of leukocyte and/or platelet concentrates and for therapeutic plasma and cytopheresis. Utilizes a continuous flow principle. Cell separation is achieved as blood from the donor is pumped into a disposable plastic, belt-like separation chamber (Fig. 10-8). (Courtesy International Business Machines Corporation.)

Plasma, platelets, and leukocytes layer above the red cells. As additional blood is added from the bottom, separation continues. The various layers which reach the top port can be separately collected as they are sequentially pumped upward and out of the bowl. The centrifugation is then discontinued, the bowl is emptied of the remaining red cells, and the red cells and plasma are returned to the donor while the process is repeated.

The IBM 2997 Blood Cell Separator utilizes a spinning centrifuge chamber in the configuration of a loop, or belt (Fig. 10-8). The "buckle" of the belt is an area of enlargement of the chamber designed for anticoagulated whole blood entry and separated cell plasma exit ports.

Each of the centrifugation devices described requires a rotating seal through which must pass the blood as it is pumped into the

bowl and the various blood fractions as they are removed. Each of these seals is a unique device designed to be "leakproof" and maintain sterility of the contents passing through, while rotating at high speed.

A new cell separation system has been developed (CS3000 Blood Cell Separator, Fenwal Laboratories) (Fig. 10-9), which provides continuous flow cell separation, using centrifugation principles, without a rotating seal. Centrifugation without twisting of efferent and afferent lines is accomplished with an ingenious design of rotating loops.[24,25]

All of the systems described also provide for the collection of platelets from the pheresis donor. However, platelets are of a lighter density than leukocytes. When collecting granulocytes by the centrifugation methods described, large numbers of platelets

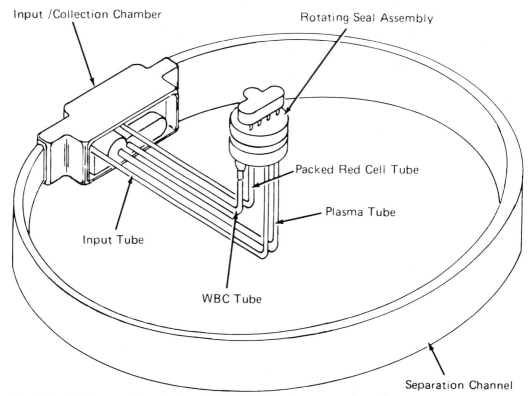

Fig. 10-8. Belt-like centrifugation chamber used by the IBM Model 2997 Cell Separator. Citrated blood from the donor is continually pumped into the chamber during centrifugation. Leukocyte and/or platelet collection occurs in the "buckle" of the spinning belt. Plasma and red cells are reunited and continually returned to the donor. (Courtesy International Business Machines Corporation.)

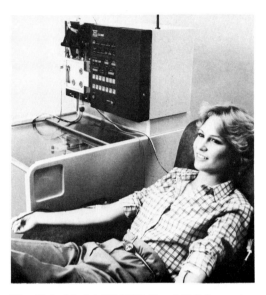

Fig. 10-9. Model CS-3000 Blood Cell Separator. Used for the collection of platelet concentrates and possible leukocyte concentrates (protocol in development). Cell separation achieved by a continuous-flow separation principle. The absence of rotating seals provide for a "closed" sterile system to reduce leaks and contamination. (Courtesy Fenwal Laboratories, Deerfield, Ill.).

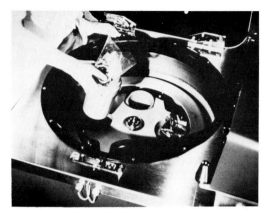

Fig. 10-10. Refrigerated centrifuge. Capable of centrifuging 6 units of blood at 4500 RPM. A "work-horse" for most blood centers and large blood banks engaged in blood component production. Sorvall RC-3 (Courtesy E.I. du Pont de Nemours and Co., Wilmington, Del.)

are concentrated in the white cell product. Depending upon the method used, granulocyte concentrates can also provide treatment doses of platelets with the same product.

Currently, the majority of plasmaphereses, in order to provide plasma for fractionation into blood derivatives (serum albumin, AHF concentrate, gamma globulin), does not utilize special equipment; rather, plasmapheresis is conducted by the sequential collection of whole blood into sodium citrate containing blood collection bags and attached satellite containers specifically designed for this purpose. The units of blood collected, along with appropriate satellite bags, are removed from the plastic harness and needle, which remains in place in the vein of the donor. The units are placed in a large refrigerated centrifuge (Fig. 10-10), the plasma and/or platelets are removed, and the red cells returned to the donor. The procedure may then be repeated.

However, all of the centrifugation devices, continuous and discontinuous, used for cell separation and collection can also be used for therapeutic plasmapheresis as well as for plasma collection from normal donors intended for production of blood derivatives or reagents.

Although cell separators were originally developed for harvesting granulocytes (and later for platelets), in recent years they have been used extensively for therapeutic plasma and cytapheresis. Such equipment, now available in many community hospitals as well as major medical centers and blood centers, is being used to treat empirically a number of heterogeneous and unrelated disorders. Although for some disorders there is a clear rationale for the use of therapeutic pheresis, for many patients the procedure is just one more modality to be used in desperate situations for which little else is helpful. Until there is more information from controlled studies, cell separators will continue to carry the epithet of "machines in search of a disease."

The Haemonetics Model 50 Plasmapheresis System, using principles similar to cell separators, was developed exclusively for plasmapheresis. Although the Model 50 may be used for therapeutic plasmapheresis, it has been developed for use by blood banks in collecting plasma from normal donors for blood derivative or reagent production.

A most innovative yet highly experimental method of plasmapheresis has been developed by the American Red Cross and is undergoing clinical trials. The method, "continuous flow filtration plasmapheresis," utilizes a transmembrane filtration process.[26] Blood is citrated as it is removed from the donor, pumped through a membrane filtration chamber, and returned to the donor in a continuous fashion (Fig. 10-11). In the filtration chamber (Fig. 10-12), plasma and red cells are separated as a feature of membrane pore characteristics, and the plasma is removed. Considerable refinement will be necessary in order for such a system to be cost-effective in comparison to current techniques.

Red Cell Washing Equipment

Parallel to the development of plasma and cytapheresis equipment has been the use of

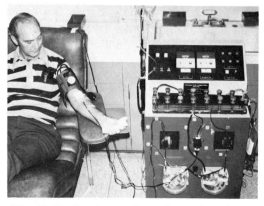

Fig. 10-11. Continuous flow plasmapheresis system which uses membrane filtration as the operating principle for plasma separation. In its prototype form, citrated donor plasma is pumped through a membrane filtration chamber (Fig. 10-12) and concentrated blood cells returned to the donor (ref. 26). (Courtesy Dr. Leonard I. Friedman, Bethesda, Md.)

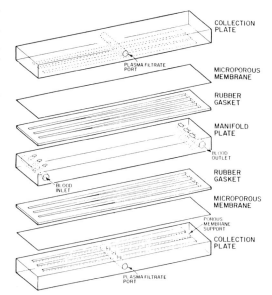

Fig. 10-12. Diagram of the filtration chamber for a continuous flow plasmapheresis system using membrane filtration (prototype). The membrane (Nucleopore, Pleasonton, California) has a pore diameter of 0.6 microns and allows the passage of the largest plasma proteins yet retains the blood cellular elements. (Courtesy Dr. Leonard I. Friedman, Bethesda, Md.)

equipment, similar in principle, to wash red cells. These are either continuous or discontinuous flow centrifugation devices used for the "washing out" of plasma, white cells, and platelets from packed red cells, the deglycerolization of previously glycerolized-frozen-thawed red cells, or the washing of red cells aspirated during major surgical procedures for return infusion to the patient. Examples of this equipment are demonstrated in Figures 10-13, 14, 15, and 16. For the most part, they may be used interchangeably for the function required, with variations in operating protocol. As an exception, "spark-proof" equipment will be required for operating suites.

Depending upon the operating protocol used, the extent to which white cells, platelets, and plasma may be removed from units of blood is generally not significantly different among the various devices. Using standard

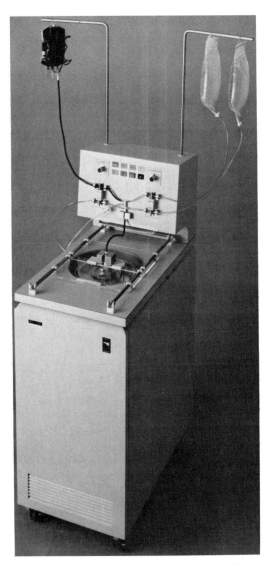

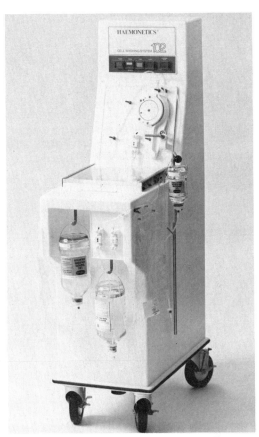

Fig. 10-14. Model 102 cell washing system for continuous flow cell washing and deglycerolization using the Haemonetics disposable plastic centrifugation bowl. "Hard-wire" programming provides for automated protocols. (Courtesy Haemonetics Corporation, Braintree, Mass.)

Fig. 10-13. Model 2991 cell washing device. Principle use is for the washing and deglycerolization of red cells. A batch-wash system that uses a disposable "donut" shaped washing container which may also be used as the final container for transfusion. (Courtesy International Business Machines Corporation.)

protocols, the operator can depend upon removing at least 85 percent of the white blood cells[27-30] and diluting plasma albumin to 1:1200 from starting values.[28,31]

The IBM 2991 cell washer (Fig. 10-13) uti-

lizes a unique rotating soft plastic "donut" in which the cells are washed. Since the donut is disposable, it may also serve as the final container from which the red cells are transfused to the patient. The Haemonetics Systems utilize their standard plastic disposable bowl similar to that used for their pheresis devices. Most pheresis devices can be used by the blood bank as cell washers; however, it is an expensive alternative when compared to the cheaper and simpler cell washing devices.

The earliest devices utilized in the operating room to salvage blood from the wound for reinfusion to the patient served mainly as res-

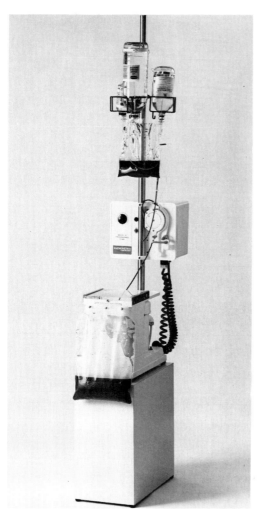

Fig. 10-15. Model 15 centrifuge coupled with Model 16 programmed pump. A simple, less expensive system for cell washing and deglycerolization using the Haemonetics plastic disposable centrifuge bowl. (Courtesy Haemonetics Corporation, Braintree, Mass.)

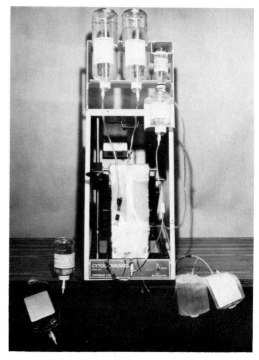

Fig. 10-16. Cytoagglomerator. For frozen-thawed red cell deglycerolization. Utilizes red cell agglomeration and rapid sedimentation in low-ionic-strength (fructose) solutions as a batch wash principle. Used in some large hospital transfusion services. (Courtesy Cryosan, Inc., Hyde Park, Mass.)

ervoirs to anticoagulate and "debubble" the blood collected. Little attention was directed to the hemolyzed plasma containing activated coagulation factors and free-floating fat, which were reinfused. The Haemonetics "Cell Saver," intended for operating room use, provides for the removal of plasma from aspirated blood by centrifugal batch washing prior to the return of red cells to the patient.

With some imaginative adjustments, cell washers have been used as pheresis devices. However, they lack the appropriate safety devices, and these practices should be discouraged.

The first practical red cell washing system developed for the deglycerolization of red cells, the cytoagglomerator (Fig. 10-16), is still in use today.[32,33] This device makes use of the agglomeration and rapid sedimentation of red cells which occur when low-ionic-strength solutions such as 5 percent fructose are added. Glycerolized-frozen-thawed red cells are batch washed using such solutions; the supernate is rapidly removed from the agglomerates, and the agglomeration is reversed by the addition of isotonic electrolyte solutions. Although this method of deglycerolizing red cells may have some advantages for large hospital blood banks,[34] there is some evidence that there is a slight increase in red cell loss when compared to centrifugation methods.[35]

BLOOD STORAGE EQUIPMENT

The objectives of blood storage equipment go further than the mere provision of appropriate storage temperature. Depending on the product in storage, there are often physical-mechanical characteristics to be considered, monitoring and alarm components, reliability and back-up power features, and compartment design, all of which play major roles.

Refrigerators

Federal regulations require that whole blood and red cells be maintained at a temperature between 1 and 6° C.[2] In addition to the reliable maintenance of this temperature range, equipment in which blood is stored must also be equipped with a constant recording device which provides an historical log of temperature throughout the period of storage. The sensor for this monitor should be placed in a container inside the refrigerator which contains a liquid simulating a unit of packed red cells (200 ml of 10 percent glycerol). Suitable alarms must be incorporated which provide an adequate alert for either high or low variances in temperature. Since power failure may be a cause for refrigerator failure, it is necessary that such alarms be connected to independent circuits or operated by battery power. Quality control steps, which calibrate temperature recording devices, alarm threshold settings, and alarm reliability on all storage equipment, are very important procedures. Where emergency generators provide for backup power, scheduled periodic testing of the generator is essential.

Freezers

Fresh-frozen plasma and cryoprecipitated antihemophilic factor must be stored at −18° C or colder. Similar temperature monitoring and alarm devices are required for such freezer equipment. The temperature-monitoring sensor may be placed in a 200 ml solution containing 6 parts automobile antifreeze to 4 parts water. Only a high-temperature alarm threshold is required. It is useful for freezers to incorporate a "defrost" cycle to prevent buildup of ice in the compartment and on the coils and diffuser. For freezers used in the storage of blood products, the defrost cycles are designed to provide a short burst of warm air within the compartment which will not raise the product temperature or monitor sensor above −18° C.

Frozen red cells may be maintained at either −85° C (the temperature of mechanical freezers) or −120° C (the temperature of the vapor phase of liquid nitrogen). Maintenance of glycerolized red cells at −85° C require higher glycerol concentrations (40 percent w/v) than those maintained at −120° C (20 percent w/v). Selection of frozen red cell storage equipment will determine the red cell freezing and thawing protocol to be used. Although mechanical freezers have a high initial capital cost, the operational cost can be expected to be significantly lower than liquid nitrogen freezers. The high w/v glycerol technic provides the added advantage of short-term red cell storage (several days) at higher temperatures, such as those maintained by dry ice (−70° C). This feature allows the shipment of red cells maintained in the frozen state and the ability to endure mechanical freezer failures by temporarily storing the frozen blood inventory in dry ice. Mechanical freezers that maintain these low temperatures usually require a "dual-cascade" refrigeration system. One compresser system, using conventional refrigerant, is utilized to precool the refrigerant (ethane) of the second system. Given an adequate supply of liquid nitrogen, liquid nitrogen freezers enjoy a freedom from breakdown, are highly reliable, and are virtually noiseless.

Room Temperature Storage

Surprisingly, the maintenance of room temperature (20-24° C) conditions for platelet concentrate storage provides special problems. Most rooms, including laboratories, are not continuously maintained at 20-24° C. Environmental chambers (Fig. 10-17) for platelet concentrate storage have been developed in order to maintain this range. Since ambient room temperatures often fluctuate above and below 20 to 24° C, such equipment requires both heating and cooling elements. And, since platelets should be stored with a continual rotary motion (vide infra), these chambers provide or accommodate platelet rotator devices.

Platelet Agitators

Of the many variables associated with optimum platelet concentrate storage, continuous gentle platelet agitation appears to play a critical role.[36,37] Platelet concentrates stored at room temperature without agitation will lose their normal discoid shape and some of their ultrastructural characteristics more rapidly and will fail to provide adequate in vivo survivals as compared with platelet concentrates stored with gentle agitation.[37,38] However, it appears that not all methods of agitation are equivalent.

The majority of commercial platelet agitators provide for a vertical rotational movement of the platelet concentrate unit (Fig. 10-18). Although this motion and configuration may be the most efficient for storage and engineering design, there is information that horizontal gentle rotation is superior, as evidenced by improved viability, maintenance of normal morphology, and aggregation function.[39] However, Lee, et al.,[40] to the contrary, have provided evidence to indicate that platelet morphology is better preserved by agitation when rotated through a vertical 90° arc. Until this issue is resolved, gentle agitation of platelet concentrates regardless of the geometrics, is far superior to no agitation at all.

DIAGNOSTIC EQUIPMENT

Given the necessary reagents, antiserum, and red cells, uncomplicated ABO grouping is the simplest of all laboratory tests. If necessary (and it has been necessary) the admix-

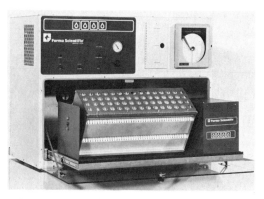

Fig. 10-17. Model 3605 Platelet Incubator housing a Model 4715 Platelet Rotator. This "environmental" chamber contains both heating and cooling elements in order to maintain a temperature of 20 to 24 °C. (Courtesy Forma Scientific, Marietta, Oh.)

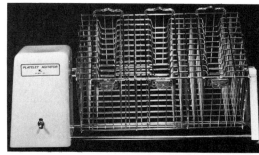

Fig. 10-18. Platelet Agitator. Providing gentle platelet agitation by vertical motion through a 90° arc. (Courtesy Helmer Labs., Somerset, Pa.)

ture of reagents and the interpretation can be performed in the palm of the hand. Under normal clinical circumstances this simplicity fades since more complex issues regarding hemagglutination reactions arise. These include: weak variants of A and B antigens, weak anti-A and anti-B isoagglutinins, variations in the quality of commercial reagents, and "coating" antibodies which require antiglobulin testing for the recognition of the many red cell antigens other than A and B.

Since Karl Landsteiner first recognized the variation of blood groups among his colleagues in 1900,[41,42] hemagglutination has been the standard tool for the recognition of red cell antigen-antibody reactions. In addition, the red cell has served as a convenient vehicle in test systems for the recognition of antigen-antibody reactions other than those associated with red cells.[43,44] As a fundamental procedure, hemagglutination has sustained the trials of time. However, the interpretation has remained highly subjective and, at best, only "semi-quantitative." Detecting weak reactions requires skill, long experience, and good eyesight. As a further problem, the clinical significance of such reactions is often beclouded—a status that seems unusual in an era of such a high degree of clinical laboratory instrumentation and objective results.

For the most part, automated equipment that provides objective interpretations of hemagglutination reactions is confined to large blood centers where large numbers of donor samples are tested daily and to those few laboratories that maintain a special interest in hemagglutination reactions. Most hospital transfusion services and smaller blood centers rely exclusively on subjectively interpreted manual techniques. For these laboratories the equipment is simple: water bath, refrigerator, magnifying glass, centrifuge, possibly a microscope, and a strong light.

The quality of work produced by immunohematology laboratories is much less a function of the equipment on hand than of the reagents available and the skill of the personnel. One of the most respected reference laboratories in the United States—the Pearson C. Cummin Memorial Laboratory in Villanova, Pennsylvania—is in the basement of a private home and was equipped for only a few hundred dollars.

Curiously, instruments for blood grouping and typing arose as labor-saving devices rather than to fulfill a need for objective results. The initial instruments for practical use were developed by the Technicon Corporation (Fig. 10-19). These instruments have adapted the basic principles found to be successful for automated clinical chemistry devices: automated sampling and sample changing followed by a continuous flow of reagents and sequential samples. The design of the flow-through coils of the Technicon Blood Grouping Autoanalyzer provides for appropriate red cell antiserum admixture and the concentration and siphoning of red cell agglutinates. As many as 15 separate reaction channels are available. As a final step, the red cell agglutinates (or the red cell suspension of negative reactions) are deposited on a moving filter paper. The technologist interprets each reaction from the appearance of the blot and summarizes a group and type from the results of each channel for the sample tested. The filter paper may be retained as a permanent record of the reactions. Recently, this basic system has been upgraded extensively (Fig. 10-20) to provide for electronic optical interpretation and grading of the hemagglutination reactions of each channel and data processing of the results of these reactions to develop a group and type summary.

For a number of years the "ultimate" in automated blood grouping has been the Groupamatic 360 System (Fig. 10-21), manufactured in France and distributed by Roche Medical Electronics. Unlike the Technicon Autoanalyzer, this system is an automated replication of the grouping and typing procedure like that carried out in a hand-held test tube. It provides a fully automated sequence of events which begins with the preparation of a cell suspension and deposits

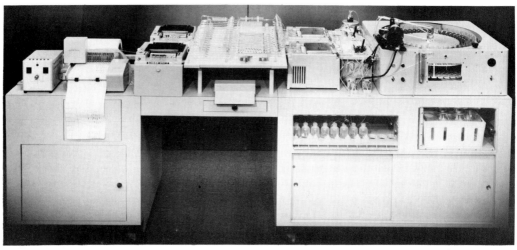

Fig. 10-19. Blood Grouping Autoanalyzer-15 channel. An automated blood grouping and typing instrument. Can provide ABO and Rh results for 120 samples per hour. Red cell agglutinates are deposited on a moving filter paper and a manual interpretation is necessary. (Courtesy Technicon Corporation, Tarrytown, N.Y.).

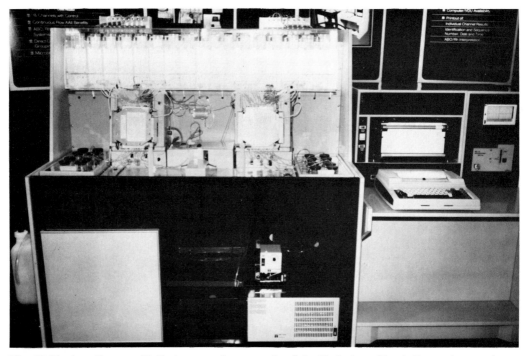

Fig. 10-20. AutoGrouper 16-C. An extensive upgrade of the Technicon Blood Group Autoanalyzer. The continuous-flow serologic principle is retained, however photo-optic interpretation of reactions and a data processor are added to fully automate the system. (Courtesy Technicon Corporation, Tarrytown, N.Y.)

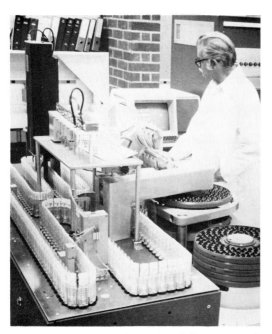

Fig. 10-21. Groupamatic 360C. A fully automated blood grouping system which can provide comprehensive serologic results of 360 blood samples per hour. A programmable computer component provides for a variety of data permutations. (Courtesy Roche Medical Electronics, Cranbury, N.J.)

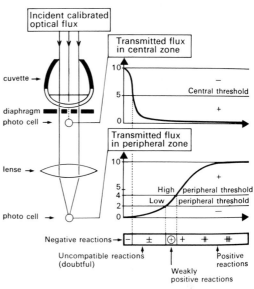

Fig. 10-22. Optical principle of reaction interpretation by the Groupamatic 360 C System. The presence of red cell agglutinates (positive reaction), which localize to the central area of the reaction cuvette cause an increased extinction of light to the photocells recording the central zone and an increased transmission of light to the photocells recording the peripheral zone. The reactions may be graded (in millivolts), and the computer will monitor the complementarity of results from the two zones. As many as 12 reactions are available for each sample; the computer receives all results, develops the interpretation, and provides the logic for a final group and type summary. (Courtesy Roche Medical Electronics, Cranbury, N.J.)

donor serum or cells in a reaction cuvette along with appropriate reagents.[1] Following a period of incubation at room temperature, the cuvettes are centrifuged, then agitated in such a manner as to swirl any red cell agglutinates to the center of the cuvette. A series of photocells respond to light passed through the central and peripheral portions of the cuvette (Fig. 10-22). The presence and degree of hemagglutination are determined by the photocell-voltmeter responses. The graded reactions are provided to the data processing element of the system, which carries the logic for interpretation and summary results. The software and data storage capability of this system provide for a number of sorting features and data permutations. One of these features is the ability to use the data base maintained by the Groupamatic as a data source for labeling blood and components utilizing bar code or other optical characters and hand-held light wands. Although a major advantage of this system is speed (360 samples per hour), its distinct benefits are accuracy, variations of data permutation, and serologic flexibility. Hemagglutination reactions can be accurately quantitated, antisera can be standardized,[45] and weak reactions such as weak D(D^u) reactions can be reliably detected.[46,47] A smaller and less versatile version of the Groupamatic (Fig. 10-23) is also available. This model utilizes similar operating principles and provides results for 75 samples per hour.

Both the newly upgraded Technicon Sys-

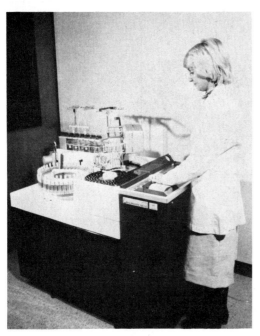

Fig. 10-23. Groupamatic MG 50. An automated blood grouping system. Smaller and less versatile than the Groupamatic 360; but, operating by similar serologic, optical and data processing methods. Provides readings for 75 samples per hour. (Courtesy Roche Medical Electronics, Cranbury, N.J.)

tem and the Groupamatic utilize an optical character recognition system (Fig. 10-24) for pilot sample identification. With automated sample identification, grouping and typing, data storage; and finally, automated blood product labeling using optical characters, such as bar code labels on blood containers, a "closed-loop" free from human error in blood processing is at hand. Such systems will provide a basis for the development of electronic safeguards for donor unit-patient matching to be conducted in the hospital blood bank and at the bedside of the patient.

BLOOD ADMINISTRATION EQUIPMENT

Plastic blood containers in current use provide for easy and rapid access to sterile entry ports in which a variety of blood administration devices may be inserted. Blood administration sets are available, with in-line filters (vide infra), which have attached "Y" arms for the convenient administration of saline through the same set (Fig. 10-25). This is the most appropriate method to introduce saline, by retrograde flow, into a unit of packed red cells in order to reduce viscosity and speed the administration rate.

Some blood administration equipment and supplies are manufactured for pediatric use. These include administration sets with mini-drip chambers and filters. Scales are available to monitor accurately the amount infused to infants and children. Primary blood containers may have attached as many as four satellite containers in order that sterile, in-line division of a single donor unit into multiple dosages may be accomplished for pediatric use.

Blood Filters

It is important that blood and certain blood components be administered through a filter. Filters have been utilized for blood transfusion for two basic reasons: 1) the removal of blood clots, which may occur in any blood product which contains plasma 2) the removal of microaggregates, which occur in all units of whole blood and packed red cells and which accumulate in proportion to the duration of blood storage.

The rationale for a filter to prevent the inadvertent infusion of clots of donor blood is clear. Under normal circumstances, the amount of citrate used to anticoagulate donor blood is in excess of physiologic requirements; however, blood clots of various sizes occasionally are observed in donor units. Although the reason for such clot formation is often not apparent, it is known that inadequate mixing during collection or "over-collection" of a standard volume will promote clot formation.

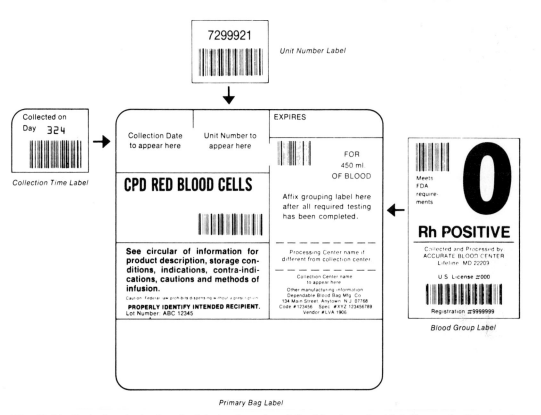

Fig. 10-24. Optical code (code-a-bar) being introduced for blood product labeling and pilot sample identification. May be read with laser devices or hand held "wands." (Courtesy American Blood Commission, Washington, D.C.)

In the earliest days of transfusion therapy, donor blood was merely poured through several layers of cheese cloth to remove clots prior to transfusion. However, in more recent years standard blood filters of the type depicted in Fig. 10-26 have been universally used. Usually these are constructed of polyvinyl chloride and contain a simple one-layer filter screen of 170 micron pore size. Such filters usually allow the rapid transfusion of blood and components, including platelet and white cell concentrates, without deleterious effects on the quality of the product, yet effectively prevent fibrin clots from entering the circulation. Usually, two to four units of blood may be sequentially administered to a patient through the same filter, depending upon the degree of filter obstruction that may

occur. Single donor plasma, platelet concentrates, white cell concentrates, and cryoprecipitate are also capable of clot formation and should be administered through filter sets as well.

From the first day of storage, microaggregates composed of platelets, leukocytes, and fibrin will accumulate in units of whole blood and packed red cells.[48] Such aggregates will range in size from 10 to 200 microns.[49] The majority will pass through a standard 170-micron filter but will be retained by a 25 to 40 micron micropore filter. As microaggregates increase in concentration in a unit of blood, the pressure required to maintain a constant flow rate through a micropore filter screen will also increase.[48] The "screen filtration pressure" has been used as an indirect mea-

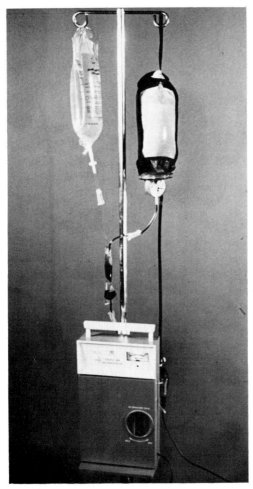

Fig. 10-25. Blood administration set. One arm of the "Y" allows for the introduction of saline, retrograde into a unit of packed red cells. This procedure reduces the viscosity of red cells with high hematocrit and increases the administration rate. (Courtesy Fenwal Laboratories, Deerfield, Ill.)

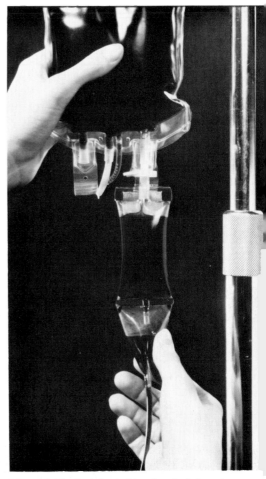

Fig. 10-26. Standard blood administration set with 170 micron filter. (Courtesy Fenwal Laboratories, Deerfield, Ill.)

surement of the degree of microaggregate formation.[48,50] Figures 10-27, 28, and 29 demonstrate a 40-micron mesh filter and the detritus retained following the passage of one unit of CPD blood 14 days of age.

Theoretically, the transfusion of large volumes of blood containing microaggregates, as may occur in the resuscitation of patients with massive hemorrhage, would result in extensive accumulation of these particles in the pulmonary capillary bed with resultant clinical effects. The occurrence of the adult respiratory distress syndrome (ARDS) during massive transfusion has been attributed, at least in part, to the accumulation in the pulmonary circulation of transfused microaggregates.[51-53] However, many events may lead to respiratory distress in the traumatized patient, and there is contrasting evidence on the significance of microaggregates. Studies in transfused casualties in Vietnam,[54] in patients undergoing abdominal aortic surgery,[55] and a carefully controlled study in baboons[56] have revealed little evidence that the transfusion of

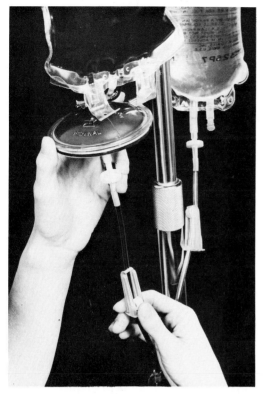

Fig. 10-27. Microaggregate filter, during blood administration 40 micron mesh. (Courtesy Fenwal Laboratories, Deerfield, Ill.)

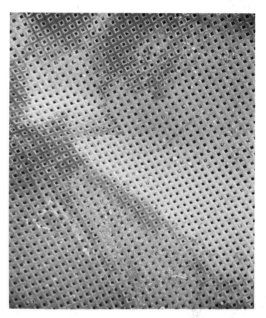

Fig. 10-28. Microaggregate filter. Scanning electron photomicrograph (× 500). (Courtesy Dr. Brian Marshall, Philadelphia, Pa.)

microaggregates is deleterious. Many investigators that have followed this issue closely, for the massively transfused patient, either do not use microfilters or recommended their use only after the first four or five units of blood have been administered.[57] A major drawback of most microaggregate filters is the relatively slow maximum infusion rate that can be attained. As one surgeon has stated ". . . it must be remembered that most bleeding patients who die, die of the blood they did not receive, not from the blood they were given."[57]

A new use for microaggregate blood filters has been introduced by Wentz et al.[58] These workers have shown that the degree of leukocyte removal by microfilters may be sufficient to prevent febrile reactions in sensitized patients. Used in this manner, the filter removed an average of 60 percent of the total

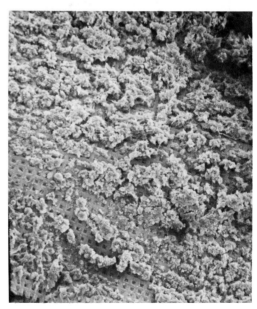

Fig. 10-29. Microaggregate filter following the passage of one unit of CPD blood 14 days of age. Scanning electron photomicrograph (× 500). (Courtesy Dr. Brian Marshall, Philadelphia, Pa.)

leukocytes and virtually all of the granulocytes from CPD blood stored for 14 days. As expected, the efficiency of leukocyte removal improves as the duration of storage increases. This method will not remove leukocytes to the degree achieved by the usual red cell washing methods and will not remove plasma proteins which may be associated with sensitization and febrile reactions; however, it may be a useful expedient when the clinical situation cannot wait for the delay required for washed red cell preparations.

Blood Warmers

There is good evidence that the rapid transfusion of large amounts of refrigerated blood, without prewarming, may have serious cardiotoxic effects.[59–61] Boyan[59] has described two patients who, during massive transfusion with nonwarmed blood, devel-

oped cardiac arrest. Esophageal temperatures behind the heart fell to 27.5 °C and 32 °C, respectively, during transfusion, and premonitory EKG signs gave warning of these episodes. In Boyan's controlled study, cardiac arrest occurred much less frequently in patients receiving massive transfusion with prewarmed blood than in those who received blood transfusions that were not warmed.

Warming of red cells and whole blood for transfusion should be performed at the time of administration and, preferably, intercurrent with the infusion. Three general techniques of blood warming have been used:

1. Coils of blood administration tubing placed in warm water during the infusion. This is a satisfactory method and has the advantage of constant temperature monitoring of the water bath. Although commercial devices are available (Du Pa Co.) a number of

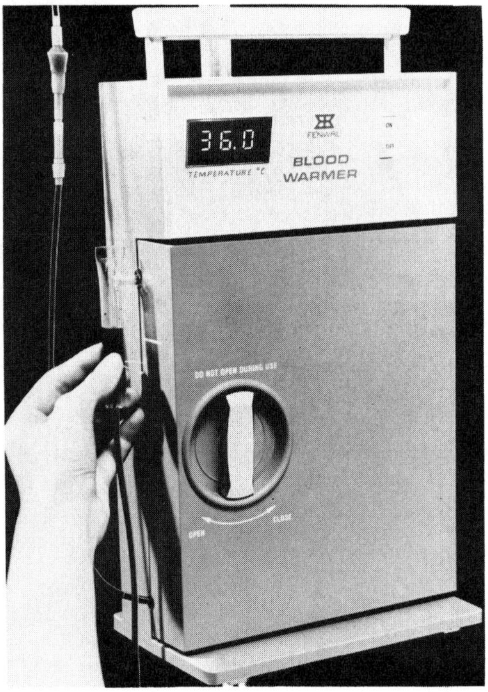

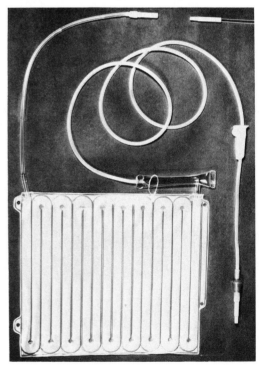

Fig. 10-30. Blood warmer. Electric heating plates warm the blood intercurrent with transfusion. Unit contains constant temperature monitor. (Courtesy Fenwal Laboratories, Deerfield, Ill.)

Fig. 10-31. In-line coil, used in the Fenwal blood warmer depicted in Figure 10-30. (Courtesy Fenwal Laboratories, Deerfield, Ill.)

"self-made" devices are in use. The routine blood administration set usually does not provide an adequate length of tubing for optimal warming during rapid infusion. Particular care must be taken to maintain the water bath that warms the coils at a temperature below 40 °C.

2. Coils of administration tubing warmed by electric heating plates (Figs. 10-30, 31). Because of simplicity, prepackaged heating coils, and relative safety, these are the most widely used blood warmers. Calibration of the temperature measuring and controlling device should be performed for each use.

Table 10-1. Equipment Quality Control for Blood Banks and Blood Centers

Equipment	Performance Check
Aneroid sphygmomanometers	Standardize against mercury manometer monthly
Blood container scales and dietary scales	Standardize against calibrated weights each day of use
Copper sulfate solution	Check specific gravity for each lot number used
Emergency power supply	Check at least once monthly
Freezers and refrigerators used for storage of blood and blood products	Monitored by a constant temperature recording device to be read and recorded twice daily. In addition, monitored by at least one standard thermometer to be read and recorded twice daily. Alarm system to be checked monthly.
Gamma counters	Background and known source standards counted daily. Empty tube holders counted weekly.
HB^{s}Ag RIA Test washing devices	Check volume delivered each day of use.
Mercury thermometers	Check with a National Bureau of Standards certified thermometer on receipt.
Microhematocrit centrifuges	Standardize with control sample each day of use. Check with tachometer and stopwatch every 6 months.
Plasma pooling areas	Place a nutrient agar plate on work surface for one-half hour during pooling (colony count should not exceed 5).
Recording constant temperature devices	Calibrate semiannually.
Refrigerated blood centrifuges	Observe and record temperature and speed each day of use. Check with tachometer and stop watch every 6 months.
Resuscitation equipment	Test flowmeter and pressure gauge of O_2 tank, self-filling resuscitator bag weekly.
Rotators for serologic test for syphilis	Calibrate oscillations per minute daily.
Shipping containers	Monitor temperature of shipments, in transit, quarterly.
Storage environment-20–24 °C	Temperature monitored by a 24 hour continuous recorder. Inspected and recorded twice daily.
Vacuum blood agitators	Standardize against blood container filled with 513 ml each day of use.
Laboratory waterbaths	Read and record temperature on laboratory record for each series of tests performed. Secure temperature adjustment knobs.
Waterbaths for thawing frozen red cells	Read and record temperature on laboratory record for each unit thawed. Change water each day of use. Temperature adjustment knobs secured.

(Condensed from: Technical Manual: American Association of Blood Banks, Washington, D.C., 7th. edition, 1977; Blood Services Directives: Technical, Nursing and Distribution Sections; The American Red Cross Blood Services, Washington, D.C., and Quality Control in Blood Banking: A Technical Workshop Manual, American Association of Blood Banks, Washington, D.C., 1973.)

3. Microwave (2450 mHz) and radio wave (27 mHz) "Ovens." These devices cannot be recommended. Although they are appealing because of the simplicity and rapid warming a full unit prior to transfusion, microwave ovens have been associated with hemolysis of red cells, presumed to be a result of excessive and uneven heating.[62, 63] As an additional problem, units warmed in this manner occasionally may not be transfused as intended and erroneously returned to the blood bank for storage and reissue.

The warming of a unit of blood, manually, under a warm water faucet, in a basin or sink should be prohibited. Temperature control and even warming of the full volume are usually inadequate.

QUALITY CONTROL

For laboratories associated with health care, where life and health are final outcomes, the concepts associated with quality control procedures are undisputed. However, there is not uniform agreement on the extent to which quality control procedures should be applied in a blood bank setting.

Where products are produced, such as in the pharmaceutical industry, it is appropriate to concentrate quality control procedures upon the product, during manufacture and at the finish. Often, as in the blood bank, this is not possible, and only a small number of random samples may be evaluated. To assist in the control of product quality, quality control procedures for the equipment utilized in blood collection, processing, testing, and storage are essential and may be the only practical procedures to assure some quality characteristics.

In order for quality control procedures of equipment to be effective, they must: (1) have a meaningful purpose; (2) have a clear and measurable endpoint; (3) be established as a nonvarying routine, and (4) produce results which are recorded and brought to periodic attention of the laboratory director. When improperly functioning or miscalibrated equipment is recognized, it is occasionally found that quality control methods signaled the problem much earlier but that the results were ignored.

Guy et al.[64] provide an excellent, well-balanced series of recommendations of quality control procedures for both reagents and equipment used in blood banks. As they indicate, quality control procedures should be applied (1) on receipt, (2) if in doubt, (3) after adjustment or repairs, and (4) at regular, scheduled intervals. Table 10-1 outlines the quality control procedures for equipment that are carried out in most blood banks and regional blood centers. This information is a composite of the procedures used by the American Red Cross Blood Centers and those recommended by the American Association of Blood Banks.[65-67] Some equipment quality control procedures indicated are required by the Code of Federal Regulations of the Food and Drug Administration and have the force of federal law.

REFERENCES

1. Matte, G.: Le Groupamatic, appareil pour la determination automatique des groups sanguins. 12th. Congress Inter. Soc. Blood Trans., (Moscow, 1969). Part II, p. 123. S. Karger, Basel, 1971.
2. Code of Federal Regulations, Food and Drug Administration, Volume 21, part 606.40, revised April 1, 1979.
3. Guess, W.L. and Haberman, S.: Toxicity profiles of vinyl and polyolefinic plastics and their additives. J. Biomed. Mater. Res. 2:313, 1968.
4. Jaeger, R.J. and Rubin, R.J.: Migration of phthalate ester plasticizer from polyvinyl chloride blood bags into stored human blood and its localization in human tissues. N. Engl. J. Med. 287:1114, 1972.
5. Jaeger, R.J. and Rubin, R.J.: Plasticizers from plastic devices: Extraction, metabolism, and accumulation by biological systems. Science 170:460, 1970.
6. Petersen, R.V.: Toxicology of plastic devices

having contact with blood. Final Report NIH Contract NIH-NHLI-73-2908-B, 1975.

7. Rock, G., Secours, V.E., Franklin, C.A., Chu, I., and Villenueve, D.C.: The accumulation of mono-2-ethylhexylphthalate (MEHP) during storage of whole blood and plasma. Transfusion 18:553, 1978.

8. Contreras, T.J., Sheibley, R.H., and Valeri, C.R.: Accumulation of di-2-ethylhexyl-phthalate (DEHP) in whole blood, platelet concentrates, and platelet-poor plasma. Transfusion 14:34, 1974.

9. Murphy, S. and Gardner, F.H.: Platelet storage at 22 °C: Role of gas transport across plastic containers in maintenance of viability. Blood 46:209, 1975.

10. Freireich, E.J., Levin, R.H., Whang, J., Carbone, P.P., Bronson, W., and Morse, E.E.: The function and fate of leukocytes from donors with chronic myelocytic leukemia in leukemic recipients. Ann. N.Y. Acad. Sci. 113:1081, 1964.

11. Freireich, E.J., Judson, G., and Levin R.H.: Separation and collection of leukocytes. Cancer Res. 25:1516, 1965.

12. Morse, E.E., Freireich, E.J., Carbone, P.P., Bronson, W., and Frei, E.: The transfusion of leukocytes from donors with chronic myelocytic leukemia to patients with leukopenia. Transfusion 6:183, 1966.

13. Jones, A.L.: Continuous-flow blood cell separation. Transfusion 8:94, 1968.

14. Greenwalt, T.J., Gajewski, M., and McKenna, J.L.: A new method for preparing buffy coat-poor blood. Transfusion 2:221, 1962.

15. Djerassi, I., Kim, J.S., Mitrakul, C., Suvansri, V., and Ciesielka, W.: Filtration leukopheresis for separation and concentration of transfusable amounts of normal human granulocytes. J. Med. (Basel) 1:358, 1970.

16. Herzig, G.P., Root, R.K., and Graw, R.G.: Granulocyte collection by continuous-flow filtration leukopheresis. Blood 39:554, 1972.

17. Buchholz, D.H., Schiffer, C.A., Wiernik, P.H., Betts, S.W., and Reilly, J.A.: Granulocyte transfusion: A low cost method for filtration leucapheresis. In: Leucocytes, Separation Collection and Transfusion. Academic Press, London, 1975, pp. 137–144.

18. Schiffer, C.A., Buchholz, D.H., Aihser, J., and Wiernik, P.H.: Transfusion of granulocytes obtained by filtration leucapheresis. In: Leu-cocytes, Separation Collection and Transfusion, Academic Press. London, 1975, pp. 316–323.

19. Ruder, E.A. and Hartz, W.H.: Transfusion reactions in patients receiving leucocyte concentrates collected from normal donors by filtration leucapheresis. In: Leucocytes, Separation Collection and Transfusion, Academic Press, London, 1975, pp. 332–339.

20. Dahlke, M.B., Shah, S.L., Sherwood, W.C., Shafer, A.W., and Brownstein, P.K.: Priapism during filtration leukapheresis. Transfusion 19:482, 1979.

21. Port, F.K., Hecking, E., Fiegel, P., Kohler, H., and Distler, A.: Priapism during regular haemodialysis. Lancet 2:1287, 1974.

22. Sale, D. and Cameron, J.S.: Priapism during regular dialysis. Lancet 2:1567, 1974.

23. Fassbinder, W., Frei, V., Issantier, R., Koch, K.M., Mion, C., Shaldon, S., and Slingeneyer, A.: Factors predisposing to priapism in haemodialysis patients. Proc. Eur. Dial. Transplant. Assoc. 12:380, 1976.

24. Ito, Y., Suaudeau, J., and Bowman, R.L.: New flow-through centrifuge without rotating seals applied to plasmapheresis. Science 189:999, 1975.

25. Suaudeau, J., Kolobow, T., Vaillancourt, R., Carvalho, A., and Ito, Y.: The Ito "flow-through" centrifuge: A new device for long-term (24 hours) plasmapheresis without platelet deterioration. Transfusion 18:312, 1978.

26. Friedman, L.I., Castino, F., Lysaght, M.J., Solomon, B.A., Sanderson, J.E., and Wiltbank, T.B.: A continuous flow plasmapheresis system. Final Report: NIH-NHLBI Contract No. 1-HB-6-2928 June 1976-April 1979.

27. Crowley, J.P. and Valeri, C.R.: The purification of red cells for transfusion by freeze preservation and washing. I. The mechanism of leukocyte removal from washed, freeze-preserved red cells. Transfusion 14:188, 1974.

28. Crowley, J.P. and Valeri, C.R.: The purification of red cells for transfusion by freeze preservation and washing. II. The residual leukocytes, platelets and plasma in washed, freeze-preserved red cells. Transfusion 14:196, 1974.

29. Crowley, J.P. and Valeri, C.R.: The purification of red cells for transfusion by freeze preservation and washing. III. Leukocyte removal and red cell recovery after red cell preserva-

tion by the high or low glycerol concentration method. Transfusion 14:590, 1974.

30. Contreras, T.J. and Valeri, C.R.: A comparison of methods to wash liquid-stored red blood cells and red blood cells frozen with high or low concentrations of glycerol. Transfusion 16:539, 1976.

31. Sherwood, W.G.: Unpublished observation.

32. Huggins, C.E.: Reversible agglomeration used to remove dimethylsulfoxide from large volumes of frozen blood. Science 139:504, 1963.

33. Huggins, C.E.: A general system for the preservation of blood by freezing. In: "Long-Term Preservation of Red Blood Cells". National Academy of Sciences-National Research Council Bulletin 1965, pp. 160–180.

34. Grove-Rasmussen, M.: Selection of donors for frozen blood based on specific blood group combination. J.A.M.A. 193:48, 1965.

35. Hornblower, M. and Meryman, H.T.: Relative efficiency and interchangeability of Huggins and American Red Cross red cell freezing procedures. Transfusion 17:417, 1977.

36. Murphy, S. and Gardner, F.H.: Platelet preservation: effect of storage temperature on maintenance of platelet viability, deleterious effect of refrigerated storage. N. Engl. J. Med. 280:1094, 1969.

37. Slichter, S.J. and Harker, L.A.: Preparation and storage of platelet concentrates. II. Storage variables influencing platelet viability and function. Br. J. Haematol. 34:403, 1976.

38. Kunicki, T.J., Tuccelli, M., Becker, G.A., and Aster, R.A.: A study of variables affecting the quality of platelets stored at room temperature. Transfusion 15:414, 1975.

39. Holme, S., Vaidja, K., and Murphy, S.: Platelet storage at 22 °C: Effect of type of agitation on morphology, viability, and function in vitro. Blood 52(2):425, 1978.

40. Lee, E.L., Azar, H.A., and Kasnic, G.: Ultrastructure of human platelets processed for transfusion under standard blood bank conditions. Transfusion 19:732, 1979.

41. Landsteiner, K.: Zur Kenntnis der Antifermentativen, lytischen und agglutinierenden Werkungen des Blutserums und der Lymphe. Zbl. Bakt. 27:357, 1900.

42. Landsteiner, K.: Uber Agglutinationserscheinungen normalen menschlichen Blutes Wien. Klin. Wschr. 14:1132, 1901.

43. Nelson, D.S.: Immune adherence. Adv. in Immunol. 3:131, 1963.

44. Gold, E.R. and Fudenberg, H.H.: Chromic chloride coupling reagent for passive hemagglutination reactions. J. Immunol. 99:859, 1967.

45. Sherwood, W.C., Glackin, K., Busch, S., and Dahlke, M.: The standardization of blood bank antisera with the Groupamatic 360C System. Rev. Fr. Transfus. Immunohematol. 21:311, 1978.

46. Garretta, M., Muller, A., and Gener, J.: Determination of the D^u factor with the Groupamatic System. Rev. Fr. Transfus. Immunohematol. 17:121, 1974.

47. Glackin, K., McIntyre, K., and Sherwood, W.C.: Weak $D(D^u)$ antigen testing—the Groupamatic 360 System. (To be published.)

48. Swank, R.L.: Alteration of blood on storage: Measurement of adhesiveness of "aging" platelets and leukocytes and their removal by filtration. N. Engl. J. Med. 265:728, 1961.

49. Solis, R.T. and Gibbs, M.B.: Filtration of microaggregates in stored blood. Transfusion 4:245, 1972.

50. Hisson, W. and Swank, R.L.: Screen filtration pressure and pulmonary hypertension. Am. J. Physiol. 209:715, 1965.

51. Reul, G.J., Greenberg, S.D., Lefrak, E.A., McCollum, W.B., Beall, A.C., and Jordan, G.L.: Prevention of post-transfusion pulmonary insufficiency. Arch. Surg. 106:386, 1973.

52. Connell, R.S. and Swank, R.L.: Pulmonary microembolism after blood transfusions. Ann. Surg. 177:40, 1973.

53. Jenevein, E.P. and Weiss, D.L.: Platelet microemboli associated with massive blood transfusion. Am. J. Pathol. 45:313, 1964.

54. McNamara, J.J., Molot, M.D., and Stremple, J.F.: Screen filtration pressure in combat casualties. Ann. Surg. 172:334, 1970.

55. McDanal, J.T., Wickline, S. Suehiro, G.T., Thomas, V.E., and McNamara, J.J.: Further studies on the significance of microaggregates in stored blood. Surg. Forum. 26:213, 1975.

56. Tobey, R.E., Kopriva, C.J., Homer, L.D., Solis, R.T., Dickson, L.G., and Herman, C.M.: Pulmonary gas exchange following hemorrhagic shock and massive blood transfusion in the baboon. Ann. Sug. 179:316, 1974.

57. Bredenberg, C.E., Collins, J.A., Fulton, R.L., McNamara, J.J., Solis, R.T., and Walker, B.D.: International Forum: Does a relationship exist between massive blood transfusions

and the adult respiratory distress syndrome? If so, what are the best preventive measures? Vox Sang. 32:311, 1977.

58. Wenz, B., Gurtlinger, K., O'Toole, A., and Dugan, E.: Leukocyte poor red blood cells prepared by microaggregate blood filtration. 32nd. Annual Meeting, American Association of Blood Banks, Las Vegas, Nov. 3–8, 1979.

59. Boyan, C.P. and Howland, W.S.: Cardiac arrest and temperature of blood bank: J.A.M.A. 183:58, 1963.

60. Boyan, C.P.: Cold or warmed blood for massive transfusions. Ann. Surg. 160:282, 1964.

61. Wilner, R.D., Fekete, M., and Hodge, J.S.: Influence of donor blood temperature on metabolic and hormonal changes during exchange transfusion. Arch. Dis. Child. 47:933, 1972.

62. Arens, J.F. and Leonard, G.L.: Danger of overwarming blood by microwave. J.A.M.A. 218:045, 1971.

63. Dalili, H. and Adriani, J.: Effects of various blood warmers on the components of bank blood. Anesth. Analg. 53:125, 1974.

64. Guy, L.R., Neitzer, G.M., and Klein, R.E.: Quality Control—How much is enough? Transfusion 17:183, 1977.

65. Technical Manual: American Association of Blood Banks, Washington, D.C., 7th. edition, 1977, p. 279.

66. Blood Services Directives: Technical, Nursing and Distribution Sections; The American Red Cross Blood Services, Washington, D.C.

67. Quality Control in Blood Banking: A Technical Workshop Manual, American Association of Blood Banks, Washington, D.C., 1973.

11

Erythrocyte Metabolism and Its Relation to the Liquid Preservation of Human Blood

Ernst R. Jaffé, M.D.

The mature human erythrocyte is a disadvantaged cell.[1] It lacks a nucleus and mitochondria; the ability to synthesize proteins, heme, and lipids; a complete cytochrome system; and an intact tricarboxylic acid cycle. The erythrocyte can neither divide nor carry out many of the commonly accepted biochemical activities with which nucleated cells are endowed. During its maturation from a nucleated precursor, the erythroblast or normoblast, through the stage of being a reticulocyte, it progressively loses its ability to synthesize nucleic acids, loses its deoxyribonucleic and ribonucleic acids, its ribosomes and mitochondria, and a number of enzymatic activities critical for other cells. The activities of several of the remaining enzymes also decline sharply as the cell gradually changes from being a reticulocyte, which can still carry out many but not all of the metabolic reactions that characterize nucleated cells, to become a mature, circulating erythrocyte. Further decreases in the activities of certain enzymes continue throughout the aging of the cell and may play important roles in the ultimate death and destruction of the erythrocyte.

For its modest metabolic needs, the erythrocyte is left dependent upon the anerobic Embden-Meyerhof glycolytic pathway and its associated shunts (see Table 11-1).

This least efficient pathway for the metabolism of the only substrate normally available to the erythrocyte, glucose, is essential for the cell to survive in vivo during its normal lifespan of about 120 days. It is not surprising, therefore, that deficiencies in the activities of glycolytic enzymes are associated with hemolytic disorders and that impaired metabolic activity consequent to storage in vitro results in shortened survival of erythrocytes upon reinfusion beyond limited periods of time.

THE METABOLISM OF THE MATURE NORMAL HUMAN ERYTHROCYTE

Glucose Metabolism

Glucose is the normal energy source for the erythrocyte. This sugar is metabolized by the cell through the direct anaerobic glycolytic pathway and, to a lesser degree, through the hexose monophosphate shunt. The enzymatic reactions in these pathways are essentially the same as those in other tissues and organisms. Before glucose can be utilized, it must cross the cell membrane. Glucose transport into erythrocytes is believed to require an insulin-independent carrier which reversibly combines with glucose and other sugars at the

Table 11-1. Metabolic Characteristics of Erythroid Cells, Reticulocytes, and Mature Human Erythrocytes

	Erythroid precursor cell	Reticulocyte	Erythrocyte
Replication	+	−	−
Synthesis of DNA	+	−	−
DNA present	+	−	−
Synthesis of RNA	+	−	−
Completion of -CCA terminus, tRNA	+	+	−
RNA present	+	+	−?
Biosynthesis of cofactors:			
Purine nucleotides de novo	+	+	−
Purine nucleotides by salvage	+	+	+
Pyridine nucleotides de novo	+	+	+
Pyridine nucleotides, salvage	+	+?	+?
Flavin nucleotides de novo	+	+	+
Pyrimidine nucleotides de novo	+	+	−
Pyrimidine nucleotides, salvage	+	+?	+?
Synthesis of new protein	+	+	−
Synthesis of new heme	+	+	−
Synthesis of new lipid	+	+	−
Metabolic pathways:			
Tricarboxylic acid cycle	+	+	−
Complete electron transport chain	+	+	−
Anaerobic (Embden-Meyerhof) glycolysis	+	+	+
Hexose monophosphate shunt	+	+	+
Diphosphoglycerate shunt	+	+	+

+ = present, − = absent, ? = uncertain

cell surface and at the interior surface of the membrane.[2]

Once inside the erythrocyte, glucose is phosphorylated by hexokinase with adenosine triphosphate (ATP) in the first reaction of the Embden-Meyerhof pathway (Fig. 11-1).[3,4] A second molecule of ATP is used by phosphofructokinase to phosphorylate fructose-6-phosphate to fructose-1,6-diphosphate. The rate of glucose utilization is limited largely by the activities of hexokinase and phosphofructokinase, which both have relatively high (about 8.2) pH optima and exhibit very little activity below pH 7. Aldolase cleaves the six-carbon fructose diphosphate into two three-carbon phosphorylated fragments. One of the three-carbon compounds, dihydroxyacetone phosphate, can be isomerized to glyceraldehyde-3-phosphate, and both halves of the glucose molecule can then continue to traverse the glycolytic pathway with the potential of generating ATP at the phosphoglycerate kinase and pyruvate kinase steps. The end product of glycolysis is pyruvate or lactate, both of which can diffuse out of the cell and be metabolized by other tissues. The final result of this glycolytic pathway, then, is the potential generation of four molecules of ATP for every two molecules utilized, with a net gain of two molecules of ATP. The high-energy ATP that is generated by this series of reactions is utilized for the various energy needs of the erythrocyte (vide infra).

Since the erythrocyte apparently does not require the large potential energy pool of

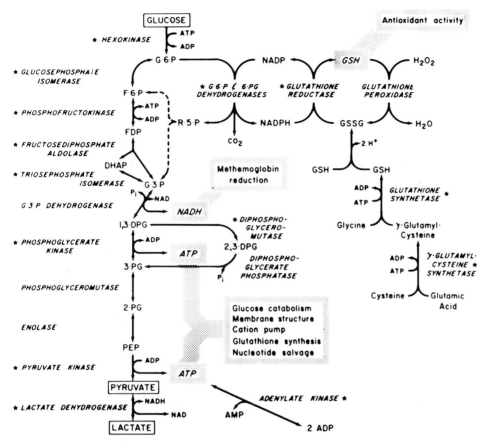

Fig. 11-1. The anaerobic glycolytic pathway and its associated shunts in human erythrocytes, and their relationship to the functions of the erythrocyte. (Valentine, W. N.: Hemolytic anemia and inborn errors of metabolism. Blood 54:549, 1979. With permission.)

ATP that would be generated by the uninterrupted metabolic flow of glucose to lactate, the branching of the metabolic reaction chain at the 1,3-diphosphoglycerate step provides for an "energy clutch." The Rapoport-Luebering diphosphoglycerate bypass permits the generation of 2,3-diphosphoglycerate (2,3-DPG), avoiding the first ATP-generating reaction catalyzed by phosphoglycerate kinase. The 2,3-DPG is dephosphorylated by a phosphatase that has the lowest activity of any enzyme in glycolysis to form 3-phosphoglycerate, which then reenters the mainstream of glycolysis. Regulation of glucose catabolism at this branch point determines not only the rate of adenosine diphosphate (ADP) phosphorylation to ATP, but also the

concentration of intracellular 2,3-DPG, an important regulator of oxygen binding by hemoglobin.

Nicotinamide adenine dinucleotide (NAD) is reduced to reduced nicotinamide adenine dinucleotide (NADH) at the glyceraldehyde-3-phosphate dehydrogenase step. Normally, the NADH generated here is used to reduce pyruvate to lactate at the lactate dehydrogenase step with the regeneration of NAD. Alternatively, the NADH can be utilized for the reduction of methemoglobin to hemoglobin through the activity of NADH-methemoglobin reductase, an enzyme that appears to be a cytochrome b_5 reductase. If significant methemoglobin reduction has occurred, pyruvate is the end product of glycolysis. Normally, however, little methemoglobin reduction is required, and lactate is the terminal product of the flexible Embden-Meyerhof pathway.

Shunt Pathway

In the absence of "oxidant" stress by a drug or chemical, about 10 to 15 percent of the glucose phosphorylated by hexokinase flows through the hexose monophosphate (pentose phosphate, Horecker) shunt pathway. In this series of enzymatic reactions, glucose-6-phosphate is first converted to 6-phosphogluconolactone and then to ribulose-5-phosphate with the loss of a molecule of carbon dioxide. In the reactions catalyzed by glucose-6-phosphate dehydrogenase and 6-phosphogluconolactone dehydrogenase, nicotinamide adenine dinucleotide phosphate (NADP) is reduced to reduced nicotinamide adenine dinucleotide phosphate (NADPH). The NADPH generated appears to function primarily in the reduction of oxidized glutathione (GSSG) to reduced glutathione (GSH) and the reduction of mixed disulfides of hemoglobin with GSH through the intervention of oxidized glutathione reductase. GSH is oxidized to GSSG in the process of the conversion of potentially deleterious peroxides to innocuous water, catalyzed by glutathione peroxidase. The percentage of glucose flowing through the hexose monophosphate shunt pathway is normally directly related to the rate of oxidation of GSH; this process, in turn, varies widely depending upon the "oxidant" stress to which the erythrocyte is exposed. The hereditary deficiency of glucose-6-phosphate dehydrogenase activity is the most common known enzymatic deficiency of human erythrocytes, and the gene controlling this enzyme has been demonstrated to reside on the sex (X) chromosome. The pentose phosphate formed when glucose traverses the hexose monophosphate shunt undergoes a series of molecular rearrangements leading to the formation of glyceraldehyde-3-phosphate and fructose-6-phosphate, which rejoin the anaerobic glycolytic mainstream.

Regulation of Glycolysis

The regulation of glycolysis in erythrocytes, while simpler than that in other cells, is still complex. It depends upon the temperature, the surrounding pH, the inherent activity of the enzymes involved, and especially on the effects of substrates and metabolic products that serve to control the enzymatic reactions by feedback or product inhibition or stimulation.[3] The actual activity of any enzyme in the glycolytic chain is usually determined by the concentration of one or more substrates. Under normal steady-state conditions, all of the enzymes function below their maximum capacities and below saturation. *Hexokinase* has the lowest activity of the main pathway glycolytic enzymes, and it has been called the "conductor of the enzyme orchestra." Hexokinase activity is inhibited at a pH above or below its optimum (8.1 to 8.3), and by glucose-6-phosphate, ADP, and 2,3-DPG. *Phosphofructokinase,* the second and perhaps most important control enzyme, is also very sensitive to changes in pH. Regulation of its activity is effected by the reciprocal interaction of its substrates, fructose-6-phosphate and ATP, by the property of ATP to be both substrate and an inhibitor, and by the inhibitory effect of 2,3-DPG. It is stimulated by AMP, fructose-1,6-diphosphate, ADP, inorganic phosphate, and ammonium ion. The other enzymes in the pathway are also influenced by their substrates, products, and environmental factors, but hexokinase and phosphofructokinase appear to be the most critical. At the midpoint and end of the glycolytic pathway, the NAD/NADH ratio, reflected in the pyruvate/lactate ratio, is an important regulator of metabolic activity.

Other Metabolic Substrates

The human erythrocyte has the ability to utilize several other substrates, in addition to glucose, as a source of energy.[5] Erythrocytes in the circulation normally either are denied access to these compounds or use them much less effectively than glucose; however, their utilization is of interest and potential importance during blood storage and in certain experimental situations. Adenosine is readily deaminated to inosine by adenosine deaminase. Inosine, formed from adenosine or added directly, can enter the erythrocyte and undergo phosphorylation without the use of ATP to form hypoxanthine and ribose-1-phosphate. The ribose-1-phosphate may then be metabolized further to yield high-energy phosphate compounds. Other purine nucleosides can also be metabolized by human erythrocytes, provided that they can enter the cell and are either substrates for purine nucleoside phosphorylase or can be converted to suitable forms. Fructose is readily utilized, although at a rate somewhat slower than glucose. It is phosphorylated by hexokinase with ATP to yield fructose-6-phosphate that can then proceed down the normal anaerobic glycolytic pathway. Mannose is also phosphorylated by hexokinase, and the mannose-6-phosphate is converted to fructose-6-phosphate by phosphomannose isomerase (which, however, has a very low activity in mature erythrocytes). Galactose utilization by erythrocytes is more complex; it involves the activities of galactokinase, galactose-1-phosphate uridyl transferase, phosphoglucomutase, and phosphoglucose isomerase to form fructose-6-phosphate. Glyceraldehyde and dihydroxyacetone can both be phosphorylated by triokinase with ATP. Since the products, glyceraldehyde-3-phosphate and dihydroxyacetone phosphate, are normal metabolic intermediates, they can be utilized further for the formation of 2,3-DPG and the regeneration of ATP.

FUNCTIONS OF THE MATURE NORMAL HUMAN ERYTHROCYTE

Despite its serious metabolic handicap, the human erythrocyte must carry out a number of activities required to preserve its *raison d'être*—the transport of oxygen from the lungs to the tissues and of carbon dioxide from the tissues to the lungs. The human erythrocyte must really be looked upon as a metabolically moderately active, flexible, biconcave, discoid container, limited by a plasma membrane composed of lipids and specific proteins arranged in a lipid-globular protein mosaic. The functions of the erythrocyte and their relationships to the cell's metabolism are listed in Table 11-2 and are discussed briefly below.

Gas Transport

The transportation of oxygen is almost totally dependent upon the heme moiety of hemoglobin, which is able to bind oxygen in a stable but reversible complex without the iron undergoing oxidation from the ferrous state of deoxyhemoglobin to the ferric state of methemoglobin. Mechanisms exist within erythrocytes to protect the heme iron against oxidation to methemoglobin and to reduce any methemoglobin formed in the high-oxygen environment that exists within the cell to functional hemoglobin.[6] Although a small amount of carbon dioxide produced in the tissues is transported in simple solution in plasma, most of the carbon dioxide diffuses into the erythrocytes. Inside these cells, about 5 percent remains in solution, while about 25 percent combines with the alpha amino groups of hemoglobin to form carbaminohemoglobin and 70 percent is hydrated to carbonic acid by carbonic anhydrase.[7] When hydrogen ion is bound by deoxyhemoglobin, carbonate ion diffuses out of the erythrocyte

Table 11-2. Functions of the Erythrocyte and Their Relation to Metabolism

1. Transport oxygen to the tissues, carbon dioxide to the lungs
   A. Dependent upon functional hemoglobin (ferroprotoporphyrin IX-globin)
   B. Oxygen affinity influenced by concentrations of organic phosphate esters, especially 2,3-diphosphoglycerate

2. Maintain intracellular cation concentrations against electrochemical gradients
   A. High intracellular potassium, low intracellular sodium
   B. Maintained by ATPase system, coupled to glycolysis

3. Maintain intracellular concentrations of nucleotides and cofactors
   A. Adenine nucleotides via glycolysis; and salvage pathway*
   B. Pyridine nucleotides via glycolysis; and synthesis de novo from nicotinic acid*
   C. Flavin nucleotides via synthesis de novo from riboflavin*
   D. Pyrimidine nucleotides via salvage pathway*
   E. Pyridoxal- and thiamine-containing cofactors*

4. Maintain lipids of the erythrocyte membrane
   A. Turnover of cholesterol and phospholipids by exchange from plasma
   B. Exchange of fatty acids dependent upon glycolysis*

5. Maintain hemoglobin in a functional state
   A. Protect hemoglobin against oxidation to methemoglobin and/or denaturation
   B. Reduce methemoglobin to hemoglobin via reductase coupled to glycolysis

6. Maintain intracellular concentration of reduced glutathione
   A. Reduce oxidized to reduced glutathione via reductase coupled to hexose monophosphate shunt pathway activity
   B. Synthesis de novo from glutamine, cysteine, and glycine

7. Maintain intracellular organization, structure, and biconcave disc shape
   A. Maintenance of shape and flexibility related to glycolysis
   B. Maintain membrane structural proteins; spectrin phosphorylation

* Although these synthetic activities can be demonstrated with erythrocytes in vitro and the processes may occur in mature cells in vivo under certain conditions, their physiologic significance is unclear.

into the plasma; chloride and water enter the cell, and the erythrocyte swells (the "Hamburger shift"). In the lungs, all these processes are reversed. The reversible binding of oxygen to hemoglobin and the transportation of carbon dioxide do not require appreciable energy in and of themselves.

Human erythrocytes contain very significant concentrations of organic phosphate esters, especially ATP and 2,3-DPG. Many studies have demonstrated the influence of these compounds on the binding of oxygen by hemoglobin. Since 2,3-DPG is present at the higher concentration and the level approaches that of intracellular hemoglobin (about 4mM versus 5mM), most attention has been directed to the effects of this compound. The preferential binding of 2,3-DPG to deoxyhemoglobin changes the configuration of the molecule and decreases its affinity for oxygen. Increased concentrations of 2,3-DPG, therefore, favor the release of oxygen

to tissues at low-oxygen tensions, leading to a "shift to the right" of the oxygen dissociation curve (Fig. 11-2).[8] Conversely, low concentrations of 2,3-DPG enhance the binding of oxygen to hemoglobin and induce a "shift to the left" of the oxygen dissociation curve. Enzymatic activities are involved in the generation and degradation of 2,3-DPG and thereby influence this vital function of the erythrocyte. It has been estimated that as much as 20 percent of the glucose metabolized by human erythrocytes may flow through the 2,3-DPG bypass.[9] The relationships between metabolic activity and the regulation of the affinity of hemoglobin for oxygen have been reviewed in great detail.[9,10]

Cation Transport

Human erythrocytes are characterized by high concentrations of intracellular potas-

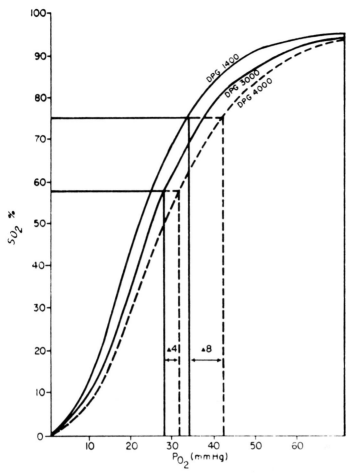

Fig. 11-2. The relationship between oxyhemoglobin dissociation and the concentration of 2,3-DPG in erythrocytes. Dashed curve = normal 2,3-DPG concentration of 4/umoles/ml erythrocytes and P_{50} of 27.5 ml of mercury. Solid curves = 2,3-DPG concentration of 3/umoles/ml erythrocytes and P_{50} of 24 ml of mercury, and 2,3-DPG concentration of 1.4/umoles/ml erythrocytes and P_{50} of 21 ml of mercury. Solid vertical lines drawn from measured central venous pO_2 to corresponding curve. Central venous pO_2 (dashed vertical lines) and increment in central venous pO_2 (delta) predicted if a normal dissociation curve was present and central venous saturation ($SO_2\%$) remained constant (horizontal solid lines). (Sugarman, H. J. et al.: The basis of effective oxygen delivery from stored blood. Surgery, Gynecology & Obstetrics 131:733, 1970. With permission.)

sium (90 to 100 meq/1 of cells) and low concentrations of intracellular sodium (5 to 15 meq/1 of cells). These levels must be maintained against the electrochemical gradients that result from the approximately inverse concentrations of sodium and potassium in the plasma. The ATPase system involved in this process is magnesium-dependent and is probably membrane-bound.[11] The ATPase system is activated by sodium and potassium and is coupled to glycolysis and the generation of ATP. The relationship between the need to pump cations and the metabolic activity of human erythrocytes has been the subject of extensive investigations. It has been estimated that only about 8.5 calories per liter of cells per hour are required for active cation pumping.[12] Since erythrocytes theoretically can produce about 84 calories per liter of cells per hour by glycolysis, cation transport can account for only approximately 10 percent of the potential energy production of the cell, although other estimates have ranged between 7 and 30 percent. Cations other than sodium and potassium, such as calcium, are transported across the membrane of the erythrocyte by mechanisms probably different from this ATPase pump.

Adenine Nucleotides

Adenine nucleotides are essential cofactors for glycolysis, and their maintenance is dependent upon metabolic activity. Although the mature erythrocyte preserves its ATP levels by phosphorylating ADP in the course of the conversion of glucose to lactate (see Fig. 11-1), it has no mechanism for the net synthesis of adenine nucleotides from small molecule precursors other than adenine itself (Fig. 11-3).[13] Lacking adenylsuccinate synthetase, it is unable to convert inosine monophosphate (IMP) to adenosine monophosphate (AMP). Purine nucleotides can, however, be formed by the salvage pathway in which preformed purines react with phosphoribosyl pyrophosphate (PRPP) in the presence of the appropriate phosphoribosyl transferase. Adenine, hypoxanthine, xanthine, and guanine can be incorporated into AMP, IMP, xanthine monophosphate (XMP), and guanine monophosphate (GMP), respectively; however, the roles of the last three purine nucleotides in human erythrocytes have not been definitively elucidated. The PRPP required is derived from the metabolism of glucose (or purine nucleosides) and involves the utilization of ATP. Adenylate kinase activity can convert one mole of AMP plus one mole of ATP to two moles of ADP and can thereby serve to prevent the irreversible loss of AMP from the cell's metabolic pool which might otherwise result from the activity of adenylate deaminase. Although adenosine kinase can form AMP from adenosine and ATP, this reaction apparently is significant only at high concentrations of adenosine and may not occur under physiologic conditions. Thus, the reactions of the anaerobic glycolytic pathway, the purine nucleotide salvage pathway, adenylate kinase, and adenosine kinase can serve to preserve the pool of adenine nucleotides for mature erythrocytes.

Pyridine Nucleotides

The pyridine nucleotides, NAD and NADP, are also essential cofactors for the glycolytic activity of erythrocytes (see Fig. 11-1). Mature and immature erythrocytes have the capacity to synthesize large amounts of NAD upon incubation in vitro with nicotinic acid, glutamine, glucose, and inorganic phosphate.[14] Glycolytic activity is required for the generation of the PRPP and ATP that are substrates for the enzymes involved in the nicotinic acid pathway for the biosynthesis of pyridine nucleotides (Fig. 11-4). The only known pathway for the synthesis of NADP involves the activity of NAD-kinase, which catalyzes the formation of NADP from NAD plus ATP in the presence of magnesium; this reaction appears to take place in human erythrocytes. Nicotinamide can be incorporated into NAD and NADP by exchange reactions catalyzed by NADase(s) that play major roles in the degradation of pyridine nucleotides, but that might also participate in a salvage pathway. It is uncertain whether or not synthesis of pyridine nucleotides occurs in human erythrocytes under physiologic conditions.

Flavin Nucleotides

The content of flavin nucleotides in human erythrocytes is very low: flavin adenine dinucleotide (FAD) about 0.5 μM. FAD, however, appears to be an important component of oxidized glutathione reductase and the

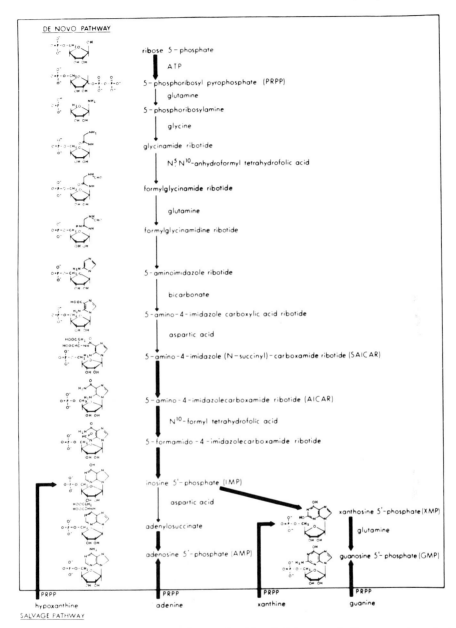

Fig. 11-3. Pathways for the synthesis of purine nucleotides. Bold arrows indicate reactions that can occur in human erythrocytes. (Lowy, B. A.: Synthesis and metabolism of nucleic acids and nucleotides. In: Hematology, 2nd ed., Williams, W. J. et al., eds. McGraw-Hill Book Company, New York, 1977. With permission.)

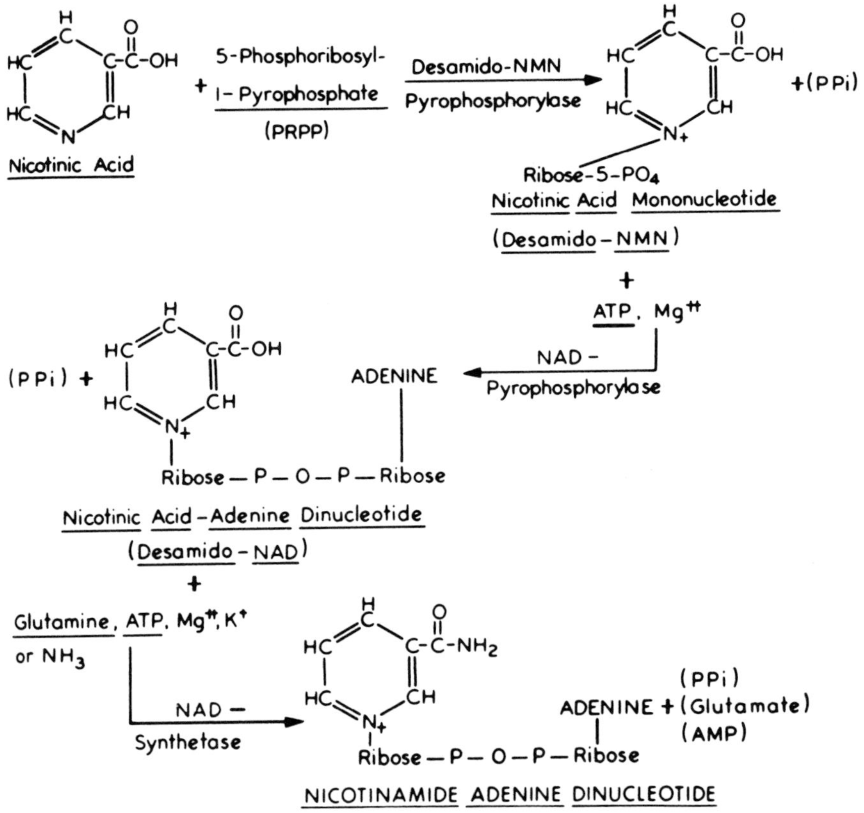

Fig. 11-4. The nicotinic acid pathway for the biosynthesis of NAD. (Jaffé, E. R.: Synthesis and metabolism of pyridine nucleotides. In: Hematology, 2nd ed. Williams, W. J. et al., eds. McGraw-Hill Book Company, New York, 1977. With permission.)

NADH-dependent methemoglobin reductase. Mature human erythrocytes are able to incorporate riboflavin into FAD and flavin mononucleotide (FMN) in vitro and to carry out the net synthesis of FAD in vivo and in vitro.[15] ATP is required by both flavokinase activity, which converts riboflavin into FMN, and flavin nucleotide phosphorylase activity, which converts FMN to FAD.

Pyrimidine Nucleotides

The mature human erythrocyte can synthesize some precursors of pyrimidine nucleotides, but it is incapable of complete synthesis de novo because of the absence of dihydroorotate dehydrogenase activity.[13] The function of the pyrimidine nucleotides in the metabolic activity of erythrocytes is uncertain. Their biosynthetic pathways require ATP and PRPP. The salvage pathway for pyrimidine nucleotides may be present in mature human erythrocytes. In the presence of a severe deficiency of the degradative enzyme, pyrimidine-5'-nucleotidase, pyrimidines accumulate in the erythrocytes. The deficiency of this enzyme is associated with a hereditary hemolytic disorder that is being recognized with increasing frequency.[16]

Pyridoxal Phosphate

Pyridoxal phosphate can be synthesized from pyridoxine by erythrocytes in vivo and in vitro through the activity of pyridoxal kinase, which utilizes ATP.[17] The role of pyridoxal phosphate in the metabolism of mature human erythrocytes is unclear, but an increase in the activities of erythrocyte transaminases has been observed after pyridoxine administration. Similarly, the administration of thiamine to patients whose erythrocytes have been shown to have decreased transketolase activities results in apparent correction of this defect.

Summary

All of these metabolic pathways that are involved in the formation or regeneration of the various cofactors present in human erythrocytes are dependent upon the generation of ATP and/or PRPP; however, data are lacking about how much of the cells' energy is normally devoted to these activities.

Membrane Lipids

The lipids of mature human erythrocytes, composed primarily of cholesterol and phospholipids, are confined to the membrane of the cell. The mature erythrocyte probably cannot synthesize these components de novo. The cholesterol, however, can be shown to undergo an equilibrium exchange reaction with the free cholesterol that is bound to lipoproteins in plasma, both in vitro and in vivo. The exchange of cholesterol is not dependent upon temperature and does not appear to require energy. Although mature erythrocytes are unable to synthesize fatty acids de novo, they are able to bring about chain lengthening.[18] Plasma free fatty acids exchange rapidly with those of the erythrocyte membrane, and the free fatty acids are incorporated into lysophosphatides by reactions requiring ATP and coenzyme A. From data obtained in experiments in vitro, it has been estimated that about 10 percent of the ATP production of human erythrocytes may be utilized for the incorporation of plasma free fatty acids into membrane lipids. The acylation mechanism provides a means for repairing damaged membrane phospholipids. Nonenergy requiring renewal of phospholipids may also occur through dismutation reactions and by direct exchange of intact phospholipid molecules between cells and plasma. Conflicting observations have been reported about the turnover of the phosphate group of phospholipids, but there is consistent evidence that the phosphate of phosphatidic acid, which is present in trace amounts, can be derived from ATP. Although perhaps of limited importance under ordinary circumstances, the restoration of erythrocyte lipids is dependent upon the presence of an intact glycolytic pathway. The accelerated destruction of glucose-6-phosphate dehydrogenase-deficient erythrocytes upon exposure to "oxidant" drugs may, in part, be the result of lipid peroxidation in the absence of the normal protective mechanisms.

Resistance to Oxidation

Conversion of hemoglobin to methemoglobin and further oxidative denaturation destroy the ability of hemoglobin to bind oxygen reversibly. The inherent structure of normal human hemoglobin with the heme moieties located in intensely hydrophobic pockets tends to shield the iron against oxidation. Protective mechanisms, related to metabolic activity, exist within erythrocytes to remove hydrogen peroxide or equivalent free radicals that may be involved in the formation of methemoglobin and in the oxidative denaturation of hemoglobin. Destruction of hydrogen peroxide is facilitated by glutathione peroxidase activity (see Fig. 11-1), but catalase appears to play an insignificant role in the presence of low concentrations of hydrogen peroxide. Direct protective effects of such reducing agents as GSH, NADPH, ergothioneine, and cysteine have been postulated but not proved. When methemoglobin is formed in normal human erythrocytes, it can be reduced to hemoglobin through reactions dependent upon the generation of reduced pyridine nucleotides. The major, most significant pathway involves a NADH-dependent methemoglobin reductase ("diaphorase," NADH dehydrogenase, cytochrome b_5 reductase). Human erythrocytes also contain a NADPH-dependent dehydrogenase that can act as a methemoglobin reductase, but that appears to be effective only in the presence of certain dyes (such as methylene blue) that can serve as artificial electron carriers. Ascorbic acid and GSH can reduce methemoglobin directly, but only at slow rates. Their roles in this process are probably not physiologically important.

In patients with an inherited deficiency of NADH-methemoglobin reductase activity, methemoglobin reappears at a linear rate of 0.5 to 3 percent of the total hemoglobin per day, after all of the methemoglobin has been reduced to hemoglobin by appropriate therapy. Since the normal concentration of methemoglobin in human erythrocytes is less than one percent, no more than about 0.5 to one percent of the metabolic activity of these cells may be required to maintain this concentration. The metabolism of methemoglobin and its relationship to erythrocyte metabolism have been reviewed in detail elsewhere.[6,19]

The normal human erythrocyte contains about half as many molecules of GSH as of hemoglobin, 2.0 to 2.5 μmoles of the tripeptide per milliliter. Almost all of the nonprotein sulfhydryl groups of erythrocytes are present as glutathione, 99.8 percent of which is in the form of GSH in the steady state.[20] This GSH turns over with a half-life of about four days in vivo,[21] suggesting that it may be continuously resynthesized from its component amino acids, especially since an active transport system capable of removing GSSG from erythrocytes exists. Erythrocytes possess the enzymatic machinery necessary for the synthesis de novo of GSH (see Fig. 11-1). Gamma-glutamyl cysteine synthetase uses ATP to catalyze the formation of gamma-

glutamyl cysteine from glutamate and cysteine. Glutathione synthetase makes GSH from gamma-glutamyl cysteine and glycine, again requiring ATP. The amount of ATP required for the synthesis of new GSH, however, cannot account for more than about 1 percent of the total potential ATP production of the erythrocytes. Erythrocytes also contain the enzymes necessary for the oxidation of GSH to GSSG (glutathione peroxidase) and the reduction of GSSG to GSH (oxidized glutathione reductase). Despite many investigations and numerous hypotheses, the fundamental role of GSH has defied definition.[22] However, GSH appears to provide "reducing power" for erythrocytes because it contains a reduced sulfhydryl group in the cysteine moiety. It may be involved in shielding essential enzymes against inactivation—especially hexokinase, glyceraldehyde-3-phosphate dehydrogenase, and oxidized glutathione reductase that contain active sulfhydryl groups. It may guard membrane lipids against peroxidation. It probably protects hemoglobin against irreversible oxidative denaturation, for hemoglobin has an exposed sulfhydryl group at the beta-93 position. Its most important function appears to be the detoxification of hydrogen peroxide, formed spontaneously or as the consequence of drug administration. The superoxide radical may be formed first, being converted to hydrogen peroxide by superoxide dismutase and then to water by glutathione peroxidase. Oxidized glutathione reductase not only reduces GSSG to GSH, but can also reduce mixed disulfides of GSH and proteins, such as hemoglobin A_3.[5,20] Conjugation of GSH with drugs and chemicals or their metabolites may serve to detoxify these agents and permit their excretion,[22] but such a function for GSH in erythrocytes has not been reported.

Maintenance of Shape

Finally, metabolic activity and the maintenance of an adequate supply of ATP appear to be essential for the preservation of the characteristic biconcave disc shape and deformability of human erythrocytes.[23] This characteristic shape results in an advantageous surface area-to-volume relationship. As long as the membrane is deformable and the cell contents are liquid, the erythrocyte can traverse the very small (about 2.8 micra) passages provided by the microcirculation, especially in the reticulo-endothelial system as exemplified by the spleen. When the ATP levels fall below about 5 to 15 percent of normal, the erythrocytes leak cations and become rigid, echinocytic (spiculated, crenated), and, finally, spherical. These changes result, in part, from alterations in the membrane skeletal structure, especially in the protein spectrin, which accounts for 76 percent of the skeletal protein.[24] Spectrin phosphorylation is accomplished by membrane-bound and cytoplasmic cyclic AMP-independent protein kinases. Cyclic AMP-dependent protein kinases, which do not phosphorylate spectrin, may also be involved in protecting the membrane skeleton against alterations that can lead to sphering of the cells.

A decrease in the content of ATP, associated with a decrease in deformability and the development of a spherical shape, is also associated with an increase in the calcium content of the membrane.[25] It has been postulated that small local alterations in the membrane ATP/calcium ratios may lead to changes in deformability before total cell ATP and calcium concentrations have changed markedly. Calcium appears to be 90 percent bound to the lipid and integral membrane proteins, but not to spectrin or actin. However, the widely accepted view that calcium makes erythrocyte membranes rigid has recently been challenged.[26] Although the exact details remain unknown, the shape, volume, and deformability characteristics of human erythrocytes all appear to depend upon the preservation of normal metabolic activity. The fraction of glycolytic activity required for these important properties has not been established.

Summary

This overview of the metabolic capacities of normal human erythrocytes has made it clear that this cell can no longer be considered to be an "inert bag of hemoglobin" designed simply to serve as a neat package for its essential gas transport functions. The observation that only about 20 percent to at most 50 percent of the ATP-generating capacity of the erythrocytes can be accounted for by the known functions of this cell emphasizes the importance of the glycolytic regulatory processes inherent in the enzymes of the Embden-Meyerhof pathway. Despite being metabolically disadvantaged, the erythrocyte must carry out a number of reactions, related directly or indirectly to the generation and utilization of the high-energy compound, ATP, to withstand the "slings and arrows of outrageous fortune" as it is buffeted about in the circulation during its 300-mile, 120-day journey.

METABOLIC ALTERATIONS OF ERYTHROCYTES DURING LIQUID STORAGE IN VITRO

With the background of information about the metabolic activities and functions of erythrocytes, it is possible to explain and understand the changes that occur when blood is removed for storage prior to transfusion and the attempts that have been made to extend the useful "shelf life" of human blood. The history of the progress made in these efforts has been reviewed elsewhere[27,28] and in this volume (Ch. 1 and 12). When whole blood is collected into the standard preservative solutions—acid-citrate-dextrose (ACD) or citrate-phosphate-dextrose (CPD)—and stored at 4 °C, the erythrocytes gradually lose their viability so that after about 21 to 28 days only approximately 70 percent of the cells survive in the recipient's circulation for more than a few hours upon reinfusion. The fraction of erythrocytes that fails to survive is rapidly removed, most likely by the reticulo-endothelial system and because of irreversible changes in the membrane, perhaps as a consequence of increased rigidity with loss of deformability. Since the erythrocytes at the very end of their life span cannot readily be isolated and examined, the precise mechanisms leading to the death of the cells, either in vivo as the result of normal aging, or after storage in vitro, remain unidentified.

Preservative Solutions

The basic ingredients of the preservative solutions have their specific useful purposes, although they may at times have counterproductive effects. The sodium citrate-citric acid mixture prevents coagulation by binding calcium ions and lowers the pH. The pH of ACD solution is about 5.0. Glucose (dextrose) provides the essential substrate for the erythrocytes' energy metabolism and thus their viability. Inorganic phosphate in CPD raises the mixture's pH somewhat and aids the formation of organic phosphate esters. The pH of CPD solution is about 5.6. Storage at 4 °C lowers the metabolic rate of the erythrocytes and thereby retards loss of viability. Because temperature exerts a profound effect on the pH of blood, the initial extracellular pH of ACD-preserved blood at 4 °C is actually approximately 7.5 and the intracellular pH about 7.6, while in CPD-preserved blood at 4 °C the extracellular pH is about 7.7 and the intracellular pH approximately 7.8.[29]

Storage Lesion

When whole blood or packed erythrocytes are stored in either ACD or CPD, a series of well-defined biochemical alterations, designated the storage lesion,[30] takes place. The modifications of erythrocytes and their metabolism that occur in vitro, however, should not be confused with the changes that occur with aging in vivo. They are quite different,

for the latter are associated with a progressive decline in the activities of certain glycolytic enzymes, while the former are not. A common denominator, however, appears to be a decrease in the concentration of ATP, the compound that has received so much attention because of its central role in glycolysis. The gradual fall in the concentration of ATP, therefore, has been the focus of many studies on the metabolic phenomena that occur during storage (Fig. 11-5).[31] Although a relationship exists between ATP levels and erythrocyte viability, the effect of ATP is clearly significant only when its levels are very low, below about 1.5 μmol/g of hemoglobin (normal: 4 μmol/g hemoglobin or 1.35 μmol per ml erythrocytes).[32] When the ATP level declines to about 30 percent of normal, the erythrocytes' ability to phosphorylate glucose is impaired, but not lost. Even lower levels of ATP may still permit satisfactory survival of the erythrocytes upon transfusion. Conversely, maintenance of high ATP concentrations in itself is no guarantee that the cells will be viable when reinfused. Thus, all media, even those that maintain ATP concentrations very well, must be subjected to evaluation by survival studies in vivo.

With the loss of ATP, the concentrations of ADP and AMP increase, but then decrease as the AMP is irreversibly deaminated to IMP.[33] When the pool of adenine nucleotides is so depleted, survival is seriously impaired and only the addition of exogenous adenine can restore the blood's usefulness (vide infra).

2,3-DPG Maintenance

More recent attention has been directed to the changes in the 2,3-DPG concentrations in stored blood.[32] At the end of one week of storage in ACD and two weeks in CPD, most of the 2,3-DPG has been lost. Correlated with this loss of 2,3-DPG is a rapid increase in the oxygen affinity (binding) of the blood, raising concern about the usefulness of such depleted blood for transfusion in situations where ox-

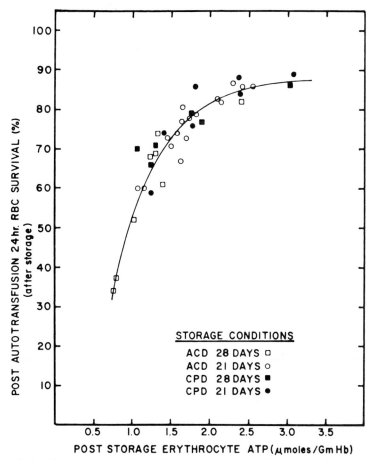

Fig. 11-5. The relationship between ATP levels in erythrocytes and post-transfusion viability in blood stored in ACD or CPD solutions for 21 or 28 days. (Dern, R. J., et al.: Studies on the preservation of human blood. II. The relationship of erythrocyte adenosine triphosphate levels and other in vitro measures to red cell storageability. J. Lab. Clin. Med. 69:968, 1967. With permission.)

ygen transport may be critical. There is a body of opinion that blood with nearly normal hemoglobin-oxygen affinity should be utilized for massive transfusions, especially in older patients and those with pulmonary or cardiovascular disease, and infants; however, this has not been adequately documented. Fortunately, regeneration of 2,3-DPG occurs relatively rapidly after reinfusion of depleted blood so that about half of the original amount may be resynthesized within 4 to 12 hours. It should be recalled that the low pH of ACD-preserved blood at 37 °C or after prolonged storage shifts the oxygen dissociation curve to the right, favoring the release of oxygen, as does an elevated concentration of 2,-3-DPG. At the same time, however, the low pH tends to inhibit the activity of the two most important glycolytic control enzymes, hexokinase and phosphofructokinase, which utilize ATP. A higher pH, induced by the addition of inorganic phosphate in CPD, enhances glycolytic activity by decreasing this inhibition and favors the synthesis of 2,3-DPG, but shifts the oxygen dissociation curve to the left. These opposing actions of pH and 2,3-DPG on the oxygen affinity of hemoglobin are complex and have been considered extensively.[3,9,34] The effect of pH, however, appears to be the most important factor in regulating the oxygen binding by hemoglobin in vivo, and it can usually be rapidly altered upon reinfusion of stored blood.

The effects of different preservative media on the maintenance of ATP and 2,3-DPG levels and erythrocyte viability are summarized in Table 11-3.[35] It should be noted, however, that these data are from selected experiments, and somewhat different values have been reported, due to unexplained donor variation and unidentified alterations in storage conditions.

Fragility and Membrane Changes

Because the sodium-potassium pump (ATPase) is exquisitely sensitive to changes in temperature, potassium rapidly leaks out of stored erythrocytes, and sodium seeps in.[36] The cells' osmotic fragility gradually increases, and some hemolyze spontaneously, giving rise to an increased plasma hemoglobin. Similarly, erythrocytes stored in ACD undergo a progressive loss of both cholesterol and phospholipid amounting to about 25 percent after seven weeks.[18] The loss of phospholipids affects all of the major phosphatides, and no change in their relative amounts is evident after eight weeks of storage. A decrease in critical hemolytic volume accompanies this lipid loss. Some controversy exists about whether or not membrane proteins are lost during the budding or fragmentation loss of membrane which accompanies ATP depletion during storage.[37] These changes, however, are paralleled by the well-known alterations in shape—i.e., the conversion of the biconcave disc to a crenated echinocyte and then to a spherocyte or echinospherocyte.

As a consequence of the decreased ability to metabolize glucose that occurs during storage in ACD solution, the concentrations of inorganic phosphate esters other than ATP and 2,3-DPG also decline significantly.[38,39]

Relatively little attention, however, has been paid to the fate of other compounds in erythrocytes during storage, including the various cofactors. Contradictory data have been reported about the stability of pyridine nucleotides. Trace amounts are still present after 18 weeks of storage,[39] and the steady-state levels of NAD, NADH, NADP, and NADPH and the activities of pyridine nucleotide-dependent enzymes appear to be maintained at nearly normal levels after storage for 48 days.[14] There is a decline in the capacity of human erythrocytes that have survived prolonged storage to synthesize NAD from small molecule precursors and to incorporate nicotinic acid into NAD.

Associated with all of the metabolic alterations that occur during storage is a progressive increase in the rigidity of the erythrocyte membrane, as measured by the rate-of-flow of erythrocytes through fine paper filters and their viscosity as determined with a cone-plate viscometer.[40] The decrease in posttransfusion survival of the cells correlates with the disc-to-sphere transformation, the loss of ATP and lipid, and a decrease in the critical hemolytic volume. These changes may be related to the increase in calcium binding to the erythrocyte membrane. The degree of calcium binding in erythrocytes stored in ACD or CPD, however, may not be extensive because it is firmly chelated by the citrate in the preservative solutions. Regardless of the mechanisms involved, the stored erythrocytes are less deformable than freshly collected cells.[41] They can be expected to encounter difficulty in passing through the microcirculation and to be more susceptible to destruction.

Currently, there is little doubt that satisfactory posttransfusion survival of stored human erythrocytes is dependent on the maintenance of a sufficiently high ATP content and the preservation of a flexible, deformable membrane. It is conceivable, however, that these two properties may be dissociated in such a manner that the erythrocyte membrane will have been damaged by fragmen-

Table 11-3. ATP, Post-transfusion Viability, and 2,3-DPG Levels During Storage of Blood in Various Preservatives at 4°C

Preservative	Storage period (weeks)																	
	1			2			3			4			5			6		
	ATP	Vi-ability	DPG	ATP	Vi-ability	DPG	ATP	Vi-ability	DPG	ATP	Vi-ability	DPG	ATP	Vi-ability	DPG	ATP	Vi-ability	DPG
ACD	90	>90	60	80	85	10	60	80	5	40	65–70	5	30	60	—	25	45	—
ACD-Adenine 0.50 mM	110	>90	40	>90	90	10	80	85	5	70	85	5	60	75–80	5	40	70	—
CPD	75	—	120	70	—	85	65	80	40	40	70	40	30	55	5	25	—	—
CPD-Adenine 0.25 mM	85	—	110	85	—	70	80	85	70	65	75–80	30	50	70	5	40	—	—
CPD-Adenine 0.50 mM	95	—	100	90	—	40	85	—	10	70	75–80	10	60	75–80	—	—	70	—
ACD-IAG Inosine 10 mM Adenine 0.5 mM Guanosine 0.5 mM	—	—	—	80	—	85	75	85	85	70	85	30	60	85	—	60	75–80	20
ACD-AG Adenine 0.5 mM Guanosine 0.5 mM	—	—	—	—	—	—	100	—	—	—	—	—	65	80	—	55	70	—
ACD-AI Adenine 0.25 mM Inosine 2.5 mM	—	>90	—	—	90	—	—	80	—	—	80	—	—	80	—	—	65	—
CPD-ad-DHA-pH7 Adenine 0.5 mM Dihydroxy-acetone 20 mM	95	—	110	75	—	130	65	—	115	75	—	100	—	—	65	—	—	—

Values are percent of initial values or percent survival.
(Högman, C.F., Åkerblom, O., Arturson, G., de Verdier, C.H., Kreuger, A., and Westman, M.: Experience with new preservatives: summary of the experiences in Sweden. In: The Human Red Cell in Vitro. Greenwalt, T.J., and Jamieson, G.A., eds. Grune & Stratton, New York, 1974. By permission.)

tation or other alterations so that survival in the circulation will be jeopardized even with a high ATP content. It is not ATP alone which is important, but also the various systems that use it to preserve and protect the delicate functional and structural elements of this effete cell. Therefore, efforts to devise tests in vitro to predict the viability of stored erythrocytes on reinfusion have met with only limited success. ATP determinations are only a good screening technique. There are no substitutes for survival studies in vivo.

REJUVENATION OF LIQUID STORED HUMAN ERYTHROCYTES

Extending the useful "shelf life" of blood by even a few weeks would increase flexibility in blood banking by improving the logistics of supply and reducing wastage due to outdating of a product for which demand not infrequently exceeds supply. Efforts to develop better blood preservative solutions began in the early 1950s. A series of classic studies initiated by Finch, Gabrio, Huennekens, Donohue, and their associates, as well as by other investigators, demonstrated that the addition of purine nucleosides at the beginning of storage or their incubation at 37° C with blood after several weeks of storage would either delay the breakdown of organic phosphate esters or permit their resynthesis, and would improve the posttransfusion survival of the erythrocytes.[28,30,41,42] Added adenosine was shown to be deaminated to inosine by adenosine deaminase. Inosine was then cleaved to hypoxanthine and ribose-1-phosphate by purine nucleoside phosphorylase, which could metabolize either inosine or guanosine but not other nucleosides. Because of the known hypotensive effect of adenosine, most attention was directed to inosine as an additive. Ultimately, it was shown that both adenosine and inosine supplementation would foster the maintenance or resynthesis of ATP

and 2,3-DPG to different degrees, depending upon the length of the preceding storage period. Inosine provided a means for the formation of organic phosphate esters without the expenditure of ATP, and permitted the regeneration of adenine nucleotides, provided a minimal essential amount was still present. Adenosine, on the other hand, could serve both as a source of organic phosphate esters after conversion to inosine and for the synthesis of new ATP through the adenosine kinase and adenylate kinase reactions with a trace residual amount of ATP (vide supra). The decline in the ability of erythrocytes to synthesize pyridine nucleotides from nicotinic acid was also prevented, in part, by including inosine in the incubation medium after the cells had been stored for about five weeks.[14]

The studies of Simon and his associates[43] demonstrated that the addition of small amounts of adenine (0.25 to 0.5 μmol per ml of ACD blood) retarded the decline in ATP concentration by being continually incorporated into adenine nucleotides in the reaction between adenine and PRPP (formed from glucose or inosine) catalyzed by adenine phosphoribosyl transferase (see Fig. 11-3). Addition of adenine extended the storage period in vitro with satisfactory posttransfusion survival of the erythrocytes from 21 to at least 35 days. Unfortunately, the addition of adenine did not prevent the loss of 2,3-DPG; actually, it appeared to accelerate it slightly. This effect was found to be dose-dependent: the higher the adenine concentration, the more rapid the fall in 2,3-DPG. With adenine added to CPD solution, adequate levels of 2,3-DPG were maintained for 12 to 14 days—only slightly less than with CPD alone and definitely longer than with ACD alone.

Maintenance of satisfactory ATP and 2,3-DPG levels with these various additives also promoted the maintenance of the normal biconcave disc shape of the erythrocytes and their deformability. Incubation with purine nucleosides and especially with added adenine after prolonged storage resulted in the restoration of the normal shape, filterability, and viscosity of the erythrocytes, but not their lipid content.[40,44]

Concern about the use of adenine or inosine in human blood preservation was voiced in terms of the ultimate metabolic fate of the purine moieties. About 5 percent of infused adenine was found to be converted to 2,8-dihydroxyadenine (DOA), a compound insoluble in neutral aqueous solutions, including plasma and urine.[43] Fear was expressed that DOA would be precipitated in the renal tubules and cause nephrotoxicity. Several studies, however, have demonstrated that adenine could probably be administered safely to animals or man in single doses up to 20 mg per kg, well above the amount needed to bestow the beneficial effects of this purine on several units of stored blood.[41]

The hypoxanthine formed upon the phosphorolytic cleavage of inosine would be converted to poorly soluble xanthine and uric acid and might lead to dangerous hyperuricemia. Hypoxanthine was also found to arise from the breakdown of the purine portion of adenine nucleotides (ATP→ADP→AMP-→IMP) that occurred during prolonged storage. It must be noted, however, that large numbers of blood transfusions with added inosine have been administered in Germany without difficulty, although increases in uric acid were observed when three or more units of blood were administered over a short time period, especially to patients with impaired renal function.[45] Although the formation of urate could be effectively lowered by the prior administration of allopurinal, it was observed that the effect of this xanthine oxidase inhibitor extended beyond the desired one and decreased the utilization of inosine.[35]

Some caution, therefore, in the use of purine or purine nucleoside supplemented blood would appear to be indicated when massive or exchange transfusions are required, especially in elderly or chronically ill subjects. Extensive European experience with these preservative solutions documents their general safety. The infusion of undesired metabolites may be minimized when necessary if packed erythrocytes are used with most of the supernatant plasma removed, or with washed, resuspended erythrocytes.

Efforts to maintain satisfactory concentrations of 2,3-DPG and, therefore, the normal oxygen affinity of blood, led to other studies of the metabolism of stored erythrocytes with added compounds.[35,41,42,45] A very successful mixture was found to consist of inosine (10 μmol per ml of anticoagulated blood), pyruvate (4 μmol per ml), and phosphate (4 μmol per ml) ("PIP cocktail"). The inorganic phosphate facilitated the metabolism of inosine by purine nucleoside phosphorylase. The pyruvate increased the reoxidation of NADH to NAD by lactate dehydrogenase to stimulate the metabolism of glyceraldehyde-3-phosphate and to relieve the block that resulted from the accumulation of fructose-1,-6-diphosphate and triose phosphate that followed upon incubation with inosine alone. Supernormal 2,3-DPG concentrations and an extremely right shifted oxygen dissociation curve could be effected by incubating human erythrocytes, either fresh or after storage, with the PIP cocktail (Fig. 11-6).[46] The clinical importance of the oxygen affinity of transfused blood and the effectiveness of its delivery of oxygen to the tissues, especially in a hypoxic patient, have turned out to be difficult questions to answer. Because of the potential toxic effects of the metabolites of inosine, it was suggested that, if a supernormal 2,3-DPG concentration in the erythrocytes were desired, it would be preferable to incubate blood with the nucleosides in vitro and to wash the erythrocytes prior to transfusion.

An almost infinite number of variations in the composition and pH of the standard preservative solutions, in the ratios of preservative solution to blood, and in the size and composition of the containers used for blood storage have been examined. Their detailed consideration is beyond the scope of this discussion. Note should be taken, however, of the effects of some other additives on the preservation of human erythrocytes in vitro.[32] Al-

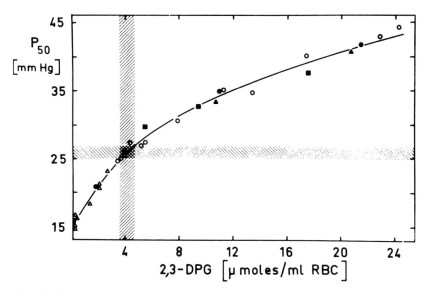

Fig. 11-6. The relationship between 2,3-DPG levels and oxygen affinity (P_{50}) of blood depleted of 2,3-DPG, with normal 2,3-DPG content, and with enhanced 2,3-DPG levels after incubation with PIP. Normal ranges indicated by shaded areas. (Duhm, J. et al.: Complete restoration of oxygen transport and 2,3-diphosphoglycerate concentration in stored blood. Transfusion 11:147, 1971. With permission.)

though glucose, mannose, and fructose can be metabolized by human erythrocytes via its hexokinase and all have approximately the same ability to maintain ATP levels, no advantage to the use of the latter two sugars has been demonstrated. Galactose, which can also be metabolized by human erythrocytes, but at a much slower rate, has very little ATP-sustaining ability.

Dihydroxyacetone, which is phosphorylated by triokinase and not hexokinase with a pH optimum of about 6.7, is a promising substrate for the maintenance of 2,3-DPG levels, but not ATP. Its apparent lack of toxicity also commends it for further evaluation. The addition of as little as 1.4 μmol per ml to ACD- or CPD-preserved blood of ascorbic acid, but not dehydroascorbic acid, significantly improves the maintenance of 2,3-DPG levels, albeit at the expense of ATP. The effect of ascorbate is additive to that of dihydroxyacetone. Ascorbate's mechanism of action remains unknown. The addition of methylene blue in a concentration of 10 μM to CPD solution improves the maintenance of 2,3-DPG levels, especially with the addition

of inosine. Methylene blue probably exerts its effect by stimulating the hexose monophosphate shunt pathway by reoxidizing NADPH to NADP, removing the inhibition of hexokinase by glucose-6-phosphate, and providing more substrate for 2,3-DPG synthesis. It may also facilitate the conversion of glyceraldehyde-3-phosphate to 1,3-diphosphoglycerate by directly oxidizing NADH to NAD. Methylene blue, however, will probably not gain wide acceptance for blood preservation because it is an unphysiologic substance and because its stimulation of the hexose monophosphate shunt pathway will be minimal and may be harmful in glucose-6-phosphate dehydrogenase-deficient erythrocytes. Finally, it should be pointed out that 2,3-DPG preservation is greater in bags of stored blood that are repeatedly mixed, and that glucose consumption and the fall in pH are greater in unmixed samples. This phenomenon has been attributed to the rapid fall in pH that occurs in the vicinity of the packed erythrocytes in the lower part of the container, leading to depletion of the 2,3-DPG, relief of the 2,3-DPG-induced inhibition of hexokinase and phosphofructokinase, increased glucose utilization, and further decrease in the pH as more lactic acid accumulates.

As suggested by Bartlett,[41] one approach to improve the preservation of human blood in vitro could involve the initial storage of blood in the usual manner in ACD or CPD solution. Just before administration, a mixture of the minimal necessary amounts of inosine, adenine, pyruvate, and inorganic phosphate, or other additives, could be added from an attached satellite container under sterile conditions. The blood-additive mixture could then be incubated at body temperature for approximately one hour or less to restore the ATP and 2,3-DPG levels to normal. In the event that large volumes of blood were required, the undesired excess metabolites could be removed by packing the erythrocytes or washing and resuspending them in a suitable medium.

CONCLUSION

The exquisitely designed human erythrocyte, despite its relatively simple structure and limited metabolic machinery, is eminently suited for the transport of oxygen and carbon dioxide and is capable of maintaining its structural integrity for about 120 days in vivo. Knowledge about its metabolic needs and functions has permitted the development of preservative solutions and containers that maximize the usefulness of stored blood upon transfusion. Future progress in enhancing the capacity to store human blood, therefore, will require even more information about the subtleties of the erythrocyte's structure, function, and metabolism to permit their exploitation in accordance with the requirements of a national blood policy.

REFERENCES

1. London, I.M.: The metabolism of the erythrocyte. Harvey Lectures 56:151, 1961.

2. Widdas, W.F.: Membrane transport of sugars. p. 1. In: Carbohydrate Metabolism and Its Disorders, vol. 1. Randle, P.J. and Whelan, W.J., Eds. Academic Press, New York, 1968, p. 1.

3. Rapoport, S.: Control mechanisms of red cell glycolysis. In: The Human Red Cell in Vitro. Greenwalt, T.J., and Jamieson, G.A., Eds. Grune & Stratton, New York, 1974, p. 153.

4. Valentine, W.N.: Hemolytic anemia and inborn errors of metabolism. Blood 54:549, 1979.

5. Beutler, E.: Energy metabolism and maintenance of erythrocytes. In: Hematology, 2nd Ed. Williams, W.J., Beutler, E., Erslev, A.J., and Rundles, R.W., Eds. McGraw-Hill Book Company, New York, 1977, p. 171.

6. Hsieh, H.-S. and Jaffé, E.R.: The metabolism of methemoglobin in human erythrocytes. In: The Red Blood Cell, 2nd Ed., Vol. 2. Surgenor, D.Mac.N., Ed. Academic Press, New York, 1975, p. 799.

7. Tyuma, I.: Gas transport. In: Cellular and Molecular Biology of Erythrocytes. Yoshikawa, H., and Rapoport, S.M., Eds. University of Tokyo Press, Tokyo, 1974.

8. Sugarman, H.J., Davidson, D.T., Vibul, S., Delivoria-Papadopoulos, M., Miller, L.D., and Oski, F.A.: The basis of defective oxygen delivery from stored blood. Surg. Gynecol. Obstet. 131:733, 1970.

9. Duhm, J. and Gerlach, E.: Metabolism and function of 2,3-diphosphoglycerate in red blood cells. In: The Human Red Cell in Vitro. Greenwalt, T.J., and Jamieson, G.A., Eds. Grune & Stratton, New York, 1974, p. 111.

10. Brewer, G.J. and Eaton, J.W.: Erythrocyte metabolism: interaction with oxygen transport. Science 171:1205, 1971.

11. Post, R.L., Merritt, G.R., Kinsolving, C.R., and Albright, C.D.: Membrane adenosine triphosphatase as a participant in the active transport of sodium and potassium in the human erythrocyte. J. Biol. Chem. 235:1796, 1960.

12. Nathan, D.G. and Shohet, S.B.: Erythrocyte ion transport defects and hemolytic anemia: "hydrocytosis" and "desiccytosis." Seminars in Hematology 7:381, 1970.

13. Lowy, B.A.: Synthesis and metabolism of nucleic acids and nucleotides. In: Hematology, 2nd Ed. Williams, W.J., Beutler, E., Erslev, A.J., and Rundles, R.W., Eds. McGraw-Hill Book Company, New York, 1977, p. 142.

14. Jaffé, E.R.: Synthesis and metabolism of pyridine nucleotides. In: Hematology, 2nd Ed. Williams, W.J., Beutler, E., Erslev, A.J., and Rundles, R.W., Eds. McGraw-Hill Book Company, New York, 1977, p. 146.

15. Mandula, B. and Beutler, E.: Synthesis of riboflavin nucleotides by mature human erythrocytes. Blood 36:491, 1970.

16. Valentine, W.N., Fink, K., Paglia, D.E., Harris, S.R., and Adams, W.S.: Hereditary hemolytic anemia with human erythrocyte pyrimidine 5'-nucleotidase deficiency. J. Clin. Invest. 54:866, 1974.

17. Anderson, B.B., Fulford-Jones, C.E. Child, J.A., Beard, M.E.J., and Bateman, C.J.T.: Conversion of vitamin B_6 compounds to active forms in the red blood cell. J. Clin. Invest. 50:1901, 1971.

18. Cooper, R.A.: Lipids of human red cell membrane: normal composition and variability in disease. Seminars in Hematology 7:296, 1970.

19. Schwartz, J.M. and Jaffé, E.R.: Hereditary methemoglobinemia with deficiency of NADH dehydrogenase. In: The Metabolic Basis of Inherited Disease, 4th Ed. Stanbury, J.B., Wyngaarden, J.B., and Fredrickson, D.S., Eds. McGraw-Hill Book Company, New York, 1978, p. 1452.

20. Beutler, E.: Glucose-6-phosphate dehydrogenase deficiency. In: The Metabolic Basis of Inherited Disease, 4th Ed. Stanbury, J.B., Wyngaarden, J.B., and Fredrickson, D.S., Eds. McGraw-Hill Book Company, New York, 1978, p. 1430.

21. Dimant, E., Landsberg, E., and London, I.M.: The metabolic behavior of reduced glutathione in human and avian erythrocytes. J. Biol. Chem. 213:769, 1955.

22. Arias, I.M. and Jakoby, W.B., Eds.: Glutathione: Metabolism and Function. Raven Press, New York, 1976.

23. Weed, R.I.: Disorders of the red cell membrane: history and perspectives. Semin. Hematol. 7:249, 1970.

24. Lux, S.E.: Spectrin-actin membrane skeleton of normal and abnormal red blood cells. Semin. Hematol. 16:21, 1979.

25. Palek, J. and Liu, S.-C.: Dependence of spectrin organization in red blood cell membranes on cell metabolism: implications for control of red cell shape, deformability, and surface area. Semin. Hematol. 16:75, 1979.

26. Clark, M.R., Mohandas, N., Jacobs, M.S., and Shohet, S.B.: Calcium does not rigidify red blood cell membranes. Blood (suppl.1) 54:25a, 1979.

27. Chaplin, H., Jaffé, E.R., Lenfant, C., and Valeri, C.R., Eds.: Preservation of Red Blood Cells. National Academy of Sciences, Washington, 1973.

28. Swisher, S.N.: The introduction of adenine fortified blood preservatives: introduction and an interpretation of its history. Transfusion 17:309, 1977.

29. Tsuda, S., Kakinuma, K., and Minakami, S.: Intracellular pH of red cells stored in acid citrate dextrose medium. Experientia 28:1481, 1972.

30 Gabrio, B.W., Finch, C.A., and Huennekens, F.M.: Erythrocyte preservation: a topic in molecular biochemistry. Blood 11:103, 1956.

31. Dern, R.J., Brewer, G.J., and Wiorkowski, J.J.: Studies on the preservation of human blood. II. The relationship of erythrocyte adenosine triphosphate levels and other in vitro measures to red cell storageability. J. Lab. Clin. Med. 69:968, 1967.

32. Beutler, E.: Experimental blood preservatives for liquid storage. In: The Human Red Cell in Vitro. Greenwalt, T.J. and Jamieson, G.A., Eds. Grune & Stratton, New York, 1974, p. 189.

33. Bishop, C.: Changes in the nucleotides of stored or incubated human blood. Transfusion 1:349, 1961.

34. Caldwell, P.R.B., Nagel, R.L., and Jaffé, E.R.: The effect of oxygen, carbon dioxide, pH and cyanate on the binding of 2,3-diphosphoglycerate to human hemoglobin. Biochem. Biophys. Res. Commun. 44:1504, 1971.

35. Högman, C.F., Åkerblom, O., Arturson, G., de Verdier, C.H., Kreuger, A., and Westman, M.: Experience with new preservatives: summary of the experiences in Sweden. In: The Human Red Cell in Vitro. Greenwalt, T.J., and Jamieson, G.A., Eds. Grune & Stratton, New York, 1974, p. 217.

36. Wood, I. and Beutler, E.: Temperature dependence of sodiuim-potassium activated erythrocyte adenosine triphosphatase. J. Lab. Clin. Med. 70:287, 1967.

37. Weed, R.I., LaCelle, P.L., and Udkow, M.: Structure and function of the red cell membrane: changes during storage. In: The

Human Red Cell in Vitro. Greenwalt, T.J. and Jamieson, G.A., Eds. Grune & Stratton, New York, 1974, p. 65.

38. Bartlett, G.R. and Barnet, H.N.: Changes in the phosphate compounds of the human red blood cell during blood bank storage. J. Clin. Invest. 39:56, 1960.

39. Shafer, A.W. and Bartlett, G.R.: Phosphorylated carbohydrate intermediates of the human erythrocyte during storage in acid citrate dextrose. III. Effect of incubation at 37°C with inosine, inosine plus adenine, and adenosine after storage for 6, 10, 14, and 18 weeks. J. Clin. Invest. 41:690, 1962.

40. Haradin, A.R., Weed, R.I., and Reed, C.F.: Changes in physical properties of stored erythrocytes: relationship to survival in vivo. Transfusion, 9:229, 1969.

41. Bartlett, G.R.: Red cell metabolism: review highlighting changes during storage. In: The Human Red Cell in Vitro. Greenwalt, T.J. and Jamieson, G.A., Eds. Grune & Stratton, New York, 1974, p. 5.

42. Valeri, C.R.: Metabolic regeneration of depleted erythrocytes and their frozen storage. In: The Human Red Cell in Vitro. Greenwalt, T.J. and Jamieson, G.A., Eds. Grune & Stratton, New York, 1974, p. 281.

43. Simon, E.R.: Adenine in blood banking. Transfusion 17:317, 1977.

44. Nakao, M.: ATP-requiring phenomena in red-cell membranes. In: Cellular and Molecular Biology of Erythrocytes. Yoshikawa, H. and Rapoport, S.M., Eds. University of Tokyo Press, Tokyo, 1974, p. 35.

45. Spielmann, W. and Seidl, S.: Summary of clinical experiences in Germany with preservative-anticoagulant solutions with newer additives. In: The Human Red Cell in Vitro. Greenwalt, T.J. and Jamieson, G.A., Eds. Grune & Stratton, New York, 1974, p. 255.

46. Duhm, J., Deuticke, B., and Gerlach, E.: Complete restoration of oxygen transport and 2,3-diphosphoglycerate concentration in stored blood. Transfusion 11:147, 1971.

12

Transfusion of Red Blood Cell Products

Jacob Nusbacher, M.D.

The transfusion of red blood cell products is a major medical therapy; the magnitude and significance of this form of therapy are not generally appreciated. Approximately 10 million units of blood are now being transfused annually in the United States, and this activity is increasing at a rate of 3 to 5 percent per year. It would not be an overstatement to assert that medical practice as we know it could not exist without hemotherapeutic support. Open heart surgery and other major surgical procedures, the support of patients with neoplastic diseases, and the maintenance of patients with chronic anemias, are but examples of therapies that would be impossible without the ready availability of red cell products for transfusion. Thus, reliance on transfusion support has become routine and perhaps casual; often, insufficient attention is paid to the hazards in transfusing red cell products, to choosing from among the different products available for transfusion, and to their specific indications for clinical use. This chapter will deal primarily with identifying the available red blood cell products, the approach to the patient needing transfusion of red cell products, the clinical circumstances that mandate red cell transfusion, and the determination of efficacy after transfusion.

HISTORY

The history of blood transfusion is covered in detail in Chapter 2. However, it seems worthwhile to highlight some of the important historical developments that relate specifically to the transfusion of red cell products, and particularly to some of the issues to be discussed in this chapter.

The establishment of blood banking and blood transfusion practice could not occur until two major problems had been solved: immunological donor-recipient incompatibility and blood storage without clotting. In 1900, the discovery by Landsteiner[1] of what we now designate as the ABO groups was of fundamental importance; but it was not until much later in the early 1940s with the discovery of the Rh system by Landsteiner and Weiner[2] and Levine and Stetson[3] that immunologically safe blood transfusion could be practiced. Equally important at this time was the development of the antiglobulin test by Coombs et al.[4] for the detection of nonagglutinating red cell antibodies which set the stage for sophisticated donor-recipient compatibility testing.

After the discovery of the ABO blood group, direct donor-recipient transfusion became the standard practice for many years.

289

Storage was not possible because a safe anticoagulant for intravenous use was not available. The safety of citrate for intravenous administration was demonstrated by Hustin in 1914[5] and by others.[6,7] Rous and Turner[8] in 1916 showed the beneficial effect of added dextrose on red blood cell preservation, thereby making red cell storage possible. Many years later, Maizels[9] demonstrated that dextrose exerted its favorable effect by providing a source of energy for the synthesis of organic phosphate compounds. The acidification of the anticoagulant-preservative solution was introduced by Loutit et al.[10] in 1943 to prevent caramelization of the dextrose solution during sterilization. Fortunately, it was found that acidification also gave better red cell preservation as judged by posttransfusion survival. The original Acid-Citrate-Dextrose (ACD) solution for preservation of red cells was suggested by Loutit and Mollison in 1943.[11] This solution has been modified through the years, but the essential constituents have remained little altered. A further comparison of different anticoagulant-preservative solutions will be considered later.

A major development in blood bank practice occurred in the mid-1960s with the introduction of plastic collection containers which have replaced glass bottles as the standard blood container. This made possible the separation of whole blood into its various constituents in an integral, closed sterile system and opened the way for the practice of blood component therapy. An inevitable result of component production from whole blood has been the ready availability of red blood cells (human) ("packed cells") as well as other red cell products that are more easily manipulated and altered in plastic storage containers.

RED BLOOD CELL PRODUCTS

The modern blood transfusion service can provide a variety of red blood cell products. When faced with a patient needing transfusion, the physician must choose from among these the one that is "best" for the particular clinical situation. It is important, therefore, that the physician know how these red cell products are prepared, the cellular and liquid composition of the final products, the advantages and drawbacks of each, and their relative costs before arriving at a choice for transfusion. Table 12-1 lists the red blood cell

Table 12-1. Red Blood Cell Products and Their Important Characteristics

Product	Shelf Life (Days)	Characteristics	Clinical Use
1. Whole Blood, ACD or CPD	21	510 ml	massive bleeding
2. Whole blood, CPD-A1	35	510 ml	massive bleeding
3. Whole blood, heparin	2	450 ml	a. exchange transfusions b. extracorporeal pump
4. Red blood cells, ACD or CPD	21	200 ml RBC/ 100 ml plasma	general transfusion
5. Red blood cells, CPD-A1	35	same	same
6. Leukocyte-poor red blood cells	1	few WBC or platelets	a. febrile transfusion reactions b. prevention of leukocyte alloimmunization
7. Washed red blood cells	1	same	a. same as leukocyte-poor RBC b. allergic reactions c. IgA deficiency
8. Frozen-deglycerolized red blood cells	1	same	a. same as leukocyte-poor or washed red blood cells b. long-term storage for rare phenotypes

products that are currently available for transfusion and some of their important characteristics.

Whole Blood—The Citrate Anticoagulants

The standard "unit" of whole blood consists of 450 ml of blood collected in one of three different anticoagulant solutions: ACD, CPD, and CPD-adenine (CPD-A1). These also function as red blood cell preservatives because they contain dextrose and other metabolites that help maintain cell viability and function during the storage period. The three anticoagulant-preservatives are quite similar to each other. Their formulas are given in Table 12-2.

All red blood cell products stored in the liquid state must be refrigerated continuously at 1 to 6°C prior to transfusion. Cold storage serves to slow glycolytic enzyme activity in the cells so that the energy source, glucose, is not depleted rapidly[12,13] from the anticoagulant-preservative solution and the accumulation rate of acidic metabolic by-products, principally lactic acid, is minimized. Cold storage also serves to inhibit effectively the proliferation of bacteria that may have contaminated the blood during donor venipuncture.[14] The permissible duration of storage depends on the anticoagulant-preservative used and is based on the arbitrary standard that requires that, on the last day of storage, at least 70 percent of red cells transfused must be recovered in the circulation of the recipient after 24 hours; these red cells will then survive normally.

For many years, ACD was the only anticoagulant-preservative suitable for red blood cell storage. Blood collected in ACD met the viability criteria for up to 21 days storage. In 1957, Gibson et al.[15] published studies on modified ACD solutions buffered by phosphate to higher pH levels. This anticoagulant-preservative, citrate-phosphate-dextrose (CPD), was found to be superior to ACD in that 80 percent of the red blood cells were reported to have retained viability after 32 days storage. However, while other studies[16,17] confirmed that CPD-stored erythrocytes have better survival than those stored in ACD, the improvement was not as great as originally thought. Thus, as with ACD, storage in CPD was permitted for only 21 days in the United States although, with CPD, posttransfusion red blood cell recovery often exceeded considerably the 70 percent standard. In some European countries, however, 28 days of storage in CPD was instituted. CPD became the major anticoagulant-preservative in general use, having supplanted ACD soon after its introduction in 1971.

The preservation of red blood cell viability in vitro is thought to correlate with levels of intracellular ATP.[18,19] Depletion of erythrocyte ATP leads to a cell that is less deformable and therefore prone to sequestration and removal in the microcirculation after transfusion. Although the role of erythrocyte ATP as the critical erythrocyte survival determinant has been questioned recently,[20] the better viability of CDP-stored erythrocytes when compared with those stored in ACD has been attributed to better maintenance of cellular ATP levels resulting from the higher pH of the former anticoagulant-preservative. The

Table 12-2. Formulations for ACD, CPD, and CPD-A1

	ACD	CPD	CPD-A1
trisodium citrate (dihydrate)	1.485 g	1.656 g	1.656 g
citric acid (monohydrate)	0.540 g	0.206 g	0.206 g
sodium dihydrogen phosphate (monohydrate)	—	0.139 g	0.139 g
dextrose	1.687 g	1.606 g	2.0 g
adenine	—	—	.017 g
water to	67.5 ml	63 ml	63 ml

addition of adenine to the CPD formulation (CPD-A1) further improves ATP maintenance during storage by providing adenine as a precursor for continued nucleotide synthesis. Studies of blood stored in CPD-A1 have shown that red blood cell viability is well-maintained so that 35 days of storage is permissible.[21,22] CPD-A1 has been licensed recently in the United States, and its use for red blood cell storage is becoming widespread.

Ideally, preservation of red blood cell viability during storage should be accompanied by preservation of optimal cellular function. The major erythrocyte function, delivery of oxygen to tissues, is related to many factors that play interdependent roles during blood transfusion, particularly when transfusion is massive. At the cellular level, erythrocyte function is related to the level of intracellular 2,3-diphosphoglycerate (2,3-DPG).[23-25] This organic phosphate compound facilitates unloading of oxygen from red blood cells to tissues. Thus immediately after transfusion, red blood cells depleted of 2,3-DPG release oxygen to tissues less readily than those that have normal levels and the oxygen dissociation curve is shifted to the left. However, 2,3-DPG levels and normal oxygen delivery are replenished within 6-24 hours after transfusion.[26]

During the first five to seven days of storage of red blood cells in ACD, there is a rapid fall in red blood 2,3-DPG levels which is associated with a rapid fall in pH when this anticoagulant-preservative is used.[27,28] In contrast, CPD solution, with its higher initial pH level and slower fall in pH, serves to preserve 2,3-DPG levels at normal or increased levels for about seven to ten days, and levels are considered adequate for about two weeks—i.e., about 0.6 μmol/μmol Hgb. With storage in CPD-A1, DPG levels fall slightly more rapidly when compared with CPD but are still much better preserved than with ACD storage.[29]

When blood is collected in one of the citrate anticoagulant-preservatives, a number of changes occur immediately or soon after storage in the refrigerator. Frequently ignored is the fact that whole blood is diluted by the anticoagulant-preservative by about 12 percent and that the hematocrit of the final product, which varies with the original hematocrit of the donor, is usually between 35 to 40 percent. Other immediate changes include a drop in pH reflecting the acidity of the anticoagulant-preservative and the disappearance of all ionized calcium because of chelation with citrate. In addition, there is an excess of "free" citrate present to assure anticoagulation, but which is available to bind further the recipient's ionized calcium after transfusion.

Within the first 12 to 24 hours of storage, the viability of platelets[30] and phagocytic leukocytes progressively decrease,[31] but at least some lymphocytes seem to survive the rigors of regular blood storage.[32] Among the plasma coagulation factors, factor VIII (antihemophilic factor, AHF) levels fall by about one-third during the first 24 hours of storage.[33] However, even after storage for 21 days, a small amount of factor VIII activity remains.

Continued storage of whole blood leads to further changes in its composition.[34] These are summarized in Table 12-3. As discussed above, red blood cell metabolic waste in the form of lactic acid contributes to a falling pH; red blood cell senescence and death result in leakage of potassium and hemoglobin from the cell and accumulation in the plasma. Levels of labile clotting factors, Factors VIII and V, also fall during storage. The clinical significance of these and other alterations that occur during blood storage will be discussed briefly below and in greater detail in Chapter 11.

Indications for Whole Blood Transfusion. Whole blood transfusion is indicated whenever a patient needs red blood cells and plasma simultaneously. Specifically, whole blood is the transfusion product of choice for the actively bleeding patient where both oxygen-carrying capacity and plasma volume support can be administered together con-

Table 12-3. Some Changes That Occur in Blood During Storage (CPD)
(% of initial value)

	Days of Storage			
	1	7	21	35*
RBC viability	95	90	80	80
**Functional platelets	? few	probably 0	0	0
ATP	100	96	86	56
DPG	100	99	44	
Factor VIII	60	30	15	
Factor V	100	70	35	
Factor IX	100	100	100	
Prothrombin	100	100	95	
Plasma K^+ (mEq/1)	3.9	12	21	
pH	7.1	7.0	6.9	

* CPD-A1
** Available data in the literature is very limited on platelet function vs viability.

veniently. Other red blood cell products may be substituted effectively for whole blood and used in combination with one of the following: (1) crystalloid solutions such as normal saline or Ringer's lactate solution; (2) volume expanders such as hydroxyethyl starch or dextran; (3) plasma derivatives such as normal serum albumin or plasma protein fraction; and, on occasion, (4) plasma. Artificial plasma expanders are used infrequently today. However, whole blood has the advantages of convenience and, in some cases, lower cost when compared with some of the red cell-volume expander combinations and should be used whenever possible in the proper clinical setting.

Whole Blood—Heparinized

Heparin anticoagulant is used infrequently as the medium for whole blood collection. Heparin is not a suitable anticoagulant for long-term storage of blood because with time its anticoagulant effects are neutralized by normal constituents of blood. It also has no red blood cell preservative properties.[35] Thus, blood storage in heparin may be for no longer than 48 hours. However, even within this short storage period, there are few studies documenting adequate red blood cell viability with this anticoagulant.

Heparinized whole blood has been used in cardiovascular surgery, particularly for priming the extracorporeal pump, and in exchange transfusion for hemolytic disease of the newborn. With the development of small-volume extracorporeal pumps that do not require blood at all, the use of this product has diminished greatly. The use of heparinized blood for neonatal exchange transfusion was based on the desire to obviate the citrate toxicity that may occur with the standard citrate anticoagulants. However, citrate toxicity is minimized by the use of packed red cells rather than whole blood[36] and, alternatively, is easily treated by periodic administration of calcium gluconate to the infant. Heparinized blood for neonatal exchange also has disadvantages. The infant becomes anticoagulated and there is an associated rise in plasma-free fatty acids which may increase the plasma levels of unconjugated bilirubin after exchange.[37] For these reasons, heparinized whole blood is rarely used now.

Red Blood Cells ("Packed Cells," Red Cell Concentrates)

Red blood cells are simply concentrates of whole blood prepared by removing from whole blood about two-thirds of the plasma after sedimentation or centrifugation. This product may be prepared either soon after collection or at any time during the storage period. When red blood cell concentration is performed in a closed, sterile system—the usual case with current plastic collection equipment—the final product may be stored for as long as whole blood, depending on the anticoagulant-preservative used. With storage, changes occur in red blood cell concentrates that are similar to those seen with whole blood.

The final hematocrit of red blood cell concentrates depends on the blood donor's hematocrit and the amount of plasma removed in the concentration process. Hematocrits of 65 to 70 percent are usual, but there are wide variations among laboratories.

Indications for Red Blood Cell Transfusion. Red blood cells have become accepted as the standard transfusion unit for the correction of a red blood cell deficit. When compared with whole blood, more erythrocytes can be delivered to the recipient for each volume of blood transfused. Hypervolemia is thereby minimized. This product is indicated in the transfusion of patients with chronic anemia, slow hemorrhage, and other conditions where the threat of acute hypovolemic hypotension is not present. The increased use of red blood cells has also permitted increased use of other blood components such as platelet concentrates and plasma derivatives which are obtained as by-products during the process of red blood cell concentration.

An important advantage of red blood cell concentrates is their use in situations where donor blood identical with the recipient's ABO type is unavailable. This may occur during blood inventory shortages or when the recipient has multiple alloantibodies that make it difficult to find compatible blood. In these circumstances, group O blood is often used as universal donor blood for all recipients, while group A or B may be used for AB recipients. In exercising such alternatives, using whole blood has the attendant risk of

infusion of a large amount of donor plasma containing alloantibodies directed against recipient red blood cells (so-called "minor" incompatibility). Severe hemolytic transfusion reactions have been reported under those circumstances.[38] In contrast, the use of red blood cells in this setting reduces this risk considerably.

Leukocyte-Poor Red Blood Cells

Leukocytes may be removed from blood by a variety of processes; these include differential centrifugation (either manual or automated), filtration, and washing, either alone or in various combinations.[39-42] Intact platelets, or platelet fragments are often removed concomitantly. Thus, the term "leukocyte-poor" red blood cells is generic, describing red blood cell transfusion products of differing characteristics prepared by a variety of techniques.

The degree of leukocyte removal achieved depends largely on the technique used and varies between 70 and 90 percent. Thus, many leukocytes—primarily viable lymphocytes but also some granulocytes—often remain in the final product. A significant number of red blood cells also are lost during these maneuvers (10 to 30 percent). This must be taken into account when assessing the efficacy of this product after transfusion, especially if the recipient does not demonstrate the expected rise in red blood cell count after transfusion. Leukocyte-poor red blood cell products can be prepared only by entering the collection bag. Thus, such products are considered "open," and only a 24-hour shelf life is permitted because of possible bacterial contamination.

Indications for Leukocyte-Poor Red Blood Cell Transfusion. Patients receiving many transfusions of whole blood or red blood cells will often develop nonhemolytic, "febrile" transfusion reactions. In one large series, febrile reactions occurred in about 4 percent of all blood recipients.[43] Other studies show rates of about 0.5 percent. Since the studies by Payne in 1957,[44] it has been clear that these reactions result from the presence of antileukocyte antibodies in the recipient. Payne showed a direct correlation between the quantity of blood previously transfused and the presence of leukoagglutinins.[45] She also demonstrated the presence of leukoagglutinins in 65 percent of patients with a history of febrile transfusion reactions and correlated the earliest detection of leukoagglutinins with their onset.[44] Studies by Brittingham and Chaplin[46] firmly established the pathogenicity of leukocyte antibodies in producing febrile transfusion reactions and demonstrated clearly the effectiveness of leukocyte-poor blood in preventing them. Finally, Perkins et al.[47] showed that the severity of the febrile reaction was related to the number of leukocytes transfused.

Clear immunological definition of the precise pathogenesis of febrile reactions is not yet at hand. It is thought that granulocytes play a greater role than lymphocytes in producing these reactions; but, antibodies directed against platelets—particularly those of the Pl antigen system—may also play a role on occasion.[48,49] The specificity of leukocyte antibodies causing febrile symptoms is thought to be most frequently related to the granulocyte-specific antigen system, which is at present poorly defined; but there is evidence that HLA antibodies—which are directed against antigenic determinants best expressed on lymphocytes but also present on granulocytes and platelets—are also related to febrile reactions.

Leukocyte-poor red blood cells are indicated when transfusing patients with a history of febrile, nonhemolytic transfusion reactions. As noted above, these patients have almost always received many previous blood transfusions. Therefore, in some institutions, it is a common practice to use leukocyte-poor red blood cells prophylactically—that is, prior to the occurrence of febrile reactions— for patients who have a life-long transfusion requirement such as those with thalassemia or sickle cell anemia.

The decision to treat patients with leukocyte-poor blood is usually made empirically. A history of febrile reactions is enough, and few laboratories try to demonstrate leukoagglutinins or other possible pathogenetic antibodies before commencing use of this product. In patients with large amounts of leukocyte antibody, multiple separations and washings may be required before febrile reactions are eliminated. In some cases, frozen red blood cells may be useful (see below).

Leukocyte-poor red blood cells also have been used *prophylactically* in two other clinical settings: to prevent HLA immunization in patients expected to need platelet or granulocyte transfusions, and in prospective renal allograft recipients. The studies of Yankee et al.[50] and others have demonstrated the detrimental role of HLA alloimmunization on increments of platelet count after platelet concentrate transfusion. Studies on human recipients of granulocyte concentrates are less clear, but experiments in dogs show the deleterious effects of prior blood transfusion on the efficacy of granulocyte transfusion.[51] It would thus seem logical to use leukocyte-poor blood in these patients, but the value of this approach remains to be demonstrated. With current technology, it is impossible to make red blood cell products totally devoid of leukocytes, and it is therefore questionable whether the possible benefit of delay or mitigation of alloimmunization is possible or, in practical terms, worth the effort and expense. The use of leukocyte-poor red blood cells for potential renal allograft recipients will be discussed below in the section on frozen red blood cells (see also Ch. 29).

Washed Red Blood Cells

Red blood cell products may be washed with isotonic NaCl solutions to remove almost all of the plasma and most nonerythrocytic constituents. Both manual and automated wash methods may be used, although mechanical systems seem to be more efficient and effective. The final product is largely one of red blood cells suspended in saline, but the degree of leukocyte, platelet, and plasma "contamination" varies considerably with the technique and the volume of wash solution used. As with leukocyte-poor blood, significant erythrocyte loss attends such manipulations. Also, because the collection pack must be entered for the introduction of wash solution, storage is permitted for only 24 hours after washing.

Indications for Washed Red Blood Cell Transfusion. Allergic reactions to plasma constituents occur in about 1 to 3 percent of all blood recipients.[43,52] The severity of allergic manifestations varies from the appearance of a few hives to generalized urticaria. Systemic symptoms such as asthma or anaphylaxis may occur occasionally. The pathogenesis of allergic reactions is not known in most cases, but it is generally believed to be attributable to IgE antibody directed against a donor plasma constituent or against an exogenous material such as a drug present in the donor plasma.

Anaphylactoid reactions have been reported to occur in patients with IgA deficiency. The incidence of complete IgA deficiency in the general population is about 0.1 percent,[53,54] and class-specific IgA antibodies may occur in these patients in the absence of previous transfusion or pregnancy.[54] Transfusion of blood into these patients has resulted in severe anaphylactoid reactions including dyspnea, laryngeal edema, and vascular collapse. The occurrence of antibodies to IgA in the general population is quite frequent, however, having been observed in 2 to 15 percent of all patients.[55] These antibodies have been shown to have specificity to some IgA subclass proteins. Anaphylactoid reactions in such patients may occur if the patient has been previously transfused or pregnant.

Washed red blood cell transfusions are in-

dicated for patients with a history of allergic transfusion reactions and in IgA-deficient recipients. Severely sensitized patients may have reactions even with red blood cells that have been washed once, and repeated washings may be necessary to remove completely the immunogen. In rare cases, only transfusion of frozen-deglycerolized red blood cells are tolerated.[55] As indicated above, washed red blood cells also have few leukocytes and platelets and are used often when leukocyte-poor transfusions are indicated.

Frozen-Deglycerolized Red Blood Cells

This subject is dealt with in greater detail in Chapter 14. Red blood cells may be stored in the frozen state in either mechanical freezers at −30 °C or less,[57] or in liquid nitrogen[58] but only after the prior addition of a cryoprotective agent which maintains red blood cell viability during the freeze-thaw cycle. Glycerol is the usually used cryoprotective agent. Conditions for the cryopreservation of erythrocytes are not appropriate for other blood cells, although some lymphocytes survive the rigors of the red cell freezing process. After thawing of a previously frozen red blood cell unit, the glycerol is removed by one of a variety of washing techniques. Also removed with the washing are most nonerythrocyte cells, red cell stroma, and plasma. Thus, the final product—red blood cells, deglycerolized—consists of erythrocytes suspended in an isotonic electrolyte solution. Depending on the freeze-thaw technique used, about 7 to 30 percent of the initial red blood cell mass is lost during these manipulations. In terms of the properties of the final product, frozen deglycerolized red blood cells are similar to washed red blood cells.

Red blood cells may be stored for many years in the frozen state. After thawing and washing, however, only a 24-hour shelf life is permitted because of possible bacterial contamination during processing in an open system.

Indications for Frozen-Deglycerolized Red Blood Cell Transfusions. The development of cryopreservation of red blood cells was based primarily on the desire to prolong the shelf life of donated blood. Prolonged storage could be advantageous in three areas: maintenance of a ready resource of phenotyped or rare bloods, autologous transfusion, and blood inventory balancing.

Prospective blood recipients who have alloantibodies require blood that has been found to be negative for those antigenic specificities. Occasionally such blood may be difficult to find because of the rarity of the required phenotype. Cryopreserved blood that has been phenotyped previously or obtained from donors known to have the same rare red blood cell types provides a ready resource in these situations. This important use of frozen-deglycerolized blood accounts for only a small percentage of all blood transfused. Cryopreservation also has been used for autologous transfusion, either for patients with unusual red blood cell phenotypes or on a routine basis (see Ch. 15 for a discussion of autologous transfusion). This application is also used infrequently.

Of greater potential is the use of frozen-deglycerolized blood as an inventory balancing strategy. Blood collected during periods of oversupply can be frozen for use when there are blood shortages. Unfortunately, the cost associated with freezing and deglycerolization, and the one hour's time required to process each unit prior to transfusion, make this use unattractive at present. Future improvements in the technology of the processing may make this a useful application, however.

Previously frozen blood was also thought to be free of the risk of hepatitis transmission. In a retrospective study, Tullis et al.[59] noted a complete absence of hepatitis among recipients of frozen-deglycerolized blood. How-ever, studies by Alter et al.[60] in chimpanzees have demonstrated that units of frozen-deglycerolized red blood cells infected with hepatitis B virus and transfused could transmit the disease to recipients. A recent analysis by Haugen[61] of more than 31,000 blood transfusions, in which 78 percent used only frozen or washed red blood cells, revealed 56 cases of posttransfusion hepatitis. In 37 of these, only frozen or washed red blood cells were transfused and non-A, non-B hepatitis accounted for 95 percent of the cases. Thus, it is clear that frozen-deglycerolized blood may transmit hepatitis.

The most common use of frozen-deglycerolized blood is in situations where immunization to leukocyte or platelet antigens is undesirable or where previous immunization has led to febrile, nonhemolytic transfusion reactions. This blood product is as effective as washed red blood cells and may be used in these cases, but the cost is much greater. The relative efficiency of leukocyte removal in frozen-deglycerolized blood as compared with washed red blood cells depends largely on the particulars of the processing techniques used. Frozen-deglycerolized red blood cells may also be used in lieu of washed red blood cells for patients with a history of allergic transfusion reactions and in recipients with IgA deficiency (see discusison above).

Until recently, most frozen-deglycerolized red blood cell transfusions were given to patients with chronic renal disease awaiting the availability of a kidney graft. The rationale for this practice was based on the desire to avoid alloimmunization to HLA antigens which might compromise the survival of the future renal graft. Recent evidence has accumulated that this practice may be undesirable. Opelz and Terasaki,[62] in a study of 1360 cadaver-donor kidney transplants, found a striking correlation between increased numbers of pretransplant blood transfusions and improved transplant survival. They also noted that frozen blood was less effective than nonfrozen blood in producing this effect. Other studies tend to confirm these observations.[63] While the mechanism by which prior blood transfusion appears to protect against renal graft rejection is far from clear, it does seem likely that eliminating or mitigating HLA alloimmunization by using frozen-deglycerolized blood is an undesirable practice. Thus, in recent years, many blood centers have noticed a sharp drop in frozen blood transfusions for this purpose. (See Ch. 29 for further discussion of this subject.)

HAZARDS OF TRANSFUSION

It is not surprising that undesirable effects resulting from transfusion—those that are immediately apparent as well as those that are long-term, more subtle, but of no less significance—occur quite frequently. Blood is a heterogeneous mixture of diverse cellular elements and plasma constituents that is transfused from one immunologically distinct individual to another. Diseases that are present in donor blood may also be transmitted to susceptible recipients. The metabolic products that are inherent in the artificial anticoagulant-preservative and those which are further generated by cells during the storage period may present additional risks for the recipient.

The potential hazards of blood transfusion can be categorized as those that result from:

1. the depletion of coagulation factors and accumulation of undesirable by-products during storage in vitro ("storage lesions").

2. immunological differences between donor and recipient.

3. diseases present in the donor that may be transmitted to the recipient.

4. recipient circulatory and iron overload. A complete discussion of the potential hazards of blood transfusion is given in Chapters 37 and 38.

As Collins[64] has pointed out so perceptively, transfusion hazards may be related either to the total cumulative quantity of blood transfused, regardless of the rate of transfusion, or to the volume of blood trans-

fused only when combined with a rapid rate of infusion. Hazards of immunological origin and those related to disease transmission (categories 2 and 3, above) increase with each transfusion regardless of rate of blood administration, while problems related to blood storage (category 1) exist primarily when large quantities of blood are given rapidly—i.e., in the massive transfusion setting. In the latter case, the effect is one of an exchange transfusion wherein the patient's own blood is replaced with previously stored blood which has somewhat different metabolic and other characteristics as a result of storage. The extent of risk to the recipient in this circumstance depends, therefore, on the rate and magnitude of the transfusion, the age of the blood transfused, and also on the integrity of the recipient's homeostatic mechanisms in dealing with these exogenous materials. Table 12-4 shows the different levels of exchange achieved at various levels of massive transfusion, assuming that the transfused material is "inert" and that no new cell release or synthesis occurs in the recipient. It can be seen, even in this obviously hypothetical situation, that exchange transfusion per se, which is only dilution of the patient's own blood with donor blood, would not lead to dangerous depletion of vital recipient blood constituents until approximately two blood volumes, about 20 units of blood in the average adult, are transfused.

Stored blood, of course, is not metabolically inert; the rate of decline in viability and function of the different cellular and plasma

Table 12-4. Percent of Original Blood Volume Remaining After Massive Hemorrhage and Transfusion (Exchange Transfusion)*

Blood Volume Exchanged**	Percent Original Volume Remaining
1 (10 units whole blood)	34.9
2 (20 units whole blood)	12.2
3 (30 units whole blood)	4.2

* after Collins, J.A.: Problems associated with the massive transfusion of stored blood. Surgery 75:274, 1974.

** approximate for adult recipient

constituents varies. Some are unaltered with storage. Some of the changes that do occur in blood during storage have been listed in Table 12-3.[65] It can be seen that, in the usual massive transfusion setting wherein the recipient receives blood stored for various times, it is unlikely for dilutional depletion to result unless the amount of blood transfused has been extraordinarily large. (See Ch. 24.) Other factors, then, must play a significant role. Of particular importance with regard to coagulation factor depletion is the presence of a consumption coagulopathy during massive transfusion. This complication may occur when there is extensive tissue necrosis in the recipient or when an incompatible blood transfusion has been given.

The accumulation of "toxic" metabolites during blood storage—potassium, and lactic acid, and the added citrate—has often been cited as hazardous for the massively transfused blood recipient. However, it seems clear that the recipient's own homeostatic mechanisms can compensate adequately for these metabolic "toxins" in most cases, as long as tissue perfusion is maintained by timely and adequate blood volume support.[63] Conversely, when tissue perfusion has been inadequate, the transfusion of stored blood may present the recipient with an additional undesirable metabolic load that he is incapable of handling effectively.

Immunological Differences Between Donor and Recipient

Blood transfusion is, of necessity, associated with the injection of many antigens into a recipient lacking these antigens. Because of the extreme complexity of the red cell blood group systems, the HLA and other antigens of white blood cells and platelets, and the polymorphisms of plasma proteins, it is impossible to give transfusions in which the donor and the recipient are antigenically identical, or even similar. Therefore, each blood transfusion has a potential for immunizing the recipient to any cellular or plasma antigen that he may lack. In the previously nonimmunized blood recipient, the immunizing transfusion is not compromised because it usually takes many weeks for the recipient to mount an antibody response.

The red blood cell antigens A, B, and $Rh_o(D)$ are of sufficient immunizing potential that all donors and recipients are tested for these antigens routinely so that incompatibilities can be eliminated. Transfusion to recipients who lack these antigens should be from donors who are also negative for the antigen in question. No such routine testing is required or desirable for other red blood cell antigens because antigenic heterogeneity would make selection of blood virtually impossible. As a consequence of this practice, the risk of alloimmunization in recipients to red cell antigens other than ABO and $Rh_o(D)$ is about 1 percent per unit of blood transfused.[66] Once immunized, recipients are at increased risk if additional transfusions are required, especially if multiple alloantibodies have developed. The alloantibody, if directed against a high frequency red blood cell antigen, makes it difficult or impossible to find compatible blood. Fortunately, this is infrequent. In addition, the antibody may not be detectable at the time of pretransfusion testing, so that apparently compatible blood will lead to an anamnestic response in the recipient and a delayed hemolytic transfusion reaction.

Most *fatal* hemolytic transfusion reactions are characterized by rapid intravascular hemolysis associated with complement activation. In nearly all cases, ABO incompatibility is responsible. Furthermore, it is rare for this to occur because of inadequate serologic technique in the laboratory. ABO incompatible transfusions result from clerical errors or other failings in the system of documentation prior to transfusion, such as giving the patient the wrong unit of blood or mislabeling of a specimen. This most serious complication of transfusion can be eliminated only by strict adherence to proper "paperwork" procedures in identifying specimens and patients, in avoiding data transciption errors, and in careful attention to labeling.

Alloimmunization to white cell and platelet antigens present in red cell products may occur.[45,46] These antibodies are directed primarily against antigens in the HLA system. HLA immunized recipients may have transfusion reactions; or, if they are candidates for granulocyte or platelet transfusions, they may show decreased effectiveness of these transfusions. Alloimmunization to plasma protein antigens is seen in the IgG, IgM, IgA, and lipoprotein systems. Anaphylactic transfusion reactions in such alloimmunized patients have been reported.[54,56]

Diseases That May Be Transmitted to the Recipient

A number of infectious agents may be transmitted by blood transfusion. These include viral hepatitis, malaria, cytomegalovirus, Epstein-Barr (EB) viral infection, and syphilis. Other diseases such as brucellosis, toxoplasmosis, filariasis, trypanosomiasis, and kala azar may also be transmitted in those countries where they are endemic. Chapter 37 discusses the hazard of disease transmission in detail.

Cytomegalovirus (CMV), a leukocyte-borne virus, is perhaps the most common pathogenic microorganism known to be transmitted by blood transfusion.[67,68] One large study[69] found serological evidence of CMV infection in 35 percent of recipients of fresh blood. Clinical manifestations of CMV infection such as fever, atypical lymphocytosis, splenomegaly, and mild hepatic dysfunction occurring two to six weeks after transfusion, are uncommon.

The most important disease transmitted by blood transfusion is viral hepatitis. Infection with hepatitis B was thought to be the most common type of posttransfusion hepatitis but, with the advent of hepatitis B surface an-

tigen (HBsAg) testing of all donors and a shift to volunteer blood donors, infection with this virus now accounts for less than 10 percent of all cases.[70] Hepatitis A has been found to be rarely, if ever, transmitted by blood transfusion. Thus, the most common type of posttransfusion hepatitis is now designated as non-A, non-B hepatitis, a syndrome of moderate severity with an incubation period intermediate between hepatitis A and B. Non-A non-B infections may account for 90 percent of all posttransfusion hepatitis at present. Control of this complication will require serological detection and identification of the causative agent(s).

Recipient Volume Overload

Volume overload may occur in the massively transfused patient when insufficient attention is paid to the quantity of fluid replacement relative to the amount of blood loss. In patients with chronic anemia and stable blood volumes, overload may occur even after one transfusion, particularly in the elderly recipient with diminished cardiovascular reserve. Often, these patients have expanded plasma volumes, which magnifies the apparent degree of anemia present. This hazard can be minimized with the use of red blood cell concentrates, and by a proper rate of transfusion administration (see Ch. 30 and 32).

Recipient Iron Overload

Iron overload is a major cause of morbidity in patients with large, chronic transfusion requirements. Because each unit of transfused blood contains about 250 mg of iron, this complication is difficult to avoid; however, new approaches with the use of iron-chelating agents are helpful. The problem is most severe in cases of thalassemia major and sickle cell anemia (see Ch. 32).

THE PHYSIOLOGY OF BLOOD TRANSFUSION

Anemia

The correction of a red cell deficit is probably the commonest reason for transfusing blood, but the benefits of transfusions are not as clear as they may seem. The red cell mass in any patient represents a dynamic equilibrium between production and loss. Disorders with decreased production or increased loss that can be corrected, should be. This will be more effective than the temporary benefit of transfusing red cells. If the hematocrit remains elevated for a long time after transfusion, it is because the balance between production and loss has changed favorably, not because the transfused cells are somehow persisting indefinitely.

Given that transfusion brings about only a temporary increase in red cell mass accompanied by significant risk, there are situations where such temporary benefits outweigh the risks. Increasing the hematocrit increases oxygen *availability* by increasing the oxygen content of blood, while at the same time may decrease oxygen *delivery* by increasing the intrinsic resistance to blood flow. In order to predict the optimal hematocrit under varying conditions, detailed and accurate quantitative data on blood viscosity are required. The few studies in vivo that have been attempted indicate that the resistance of blood to flow is probably an exponential function of hematocrit, but with different relative changes in different vascular beds.[71,72] Factors other than hematocrit are also demonstrably important.[73-75]

Most authors agree that, under the conditions that apply in the normal state, there is maximal oxygen delivery at normal hematocrits.[76-78] As flow rate decreases, there may be an advantage in moderate hemodilution, but more studies of this question are needed under conditions that more nearly approximate those in vivo.

The hemodynamic changes in acutely anemic patients and animals have been reviewed recently.[79,80] Perhaps the most fundamental observation is that, when other variables are kept constant, increased cardiac output is a most important compensatory mechanism to maintain nearly normal oxygen delivery. There are probably elements of both increased left ventricular work and decreased viscosity in the compensatory increase in cardiac output. Such changes in cardiac output can occur only if blood volume is maintained near normal. Therefore, it is mandatory that hypovolemia be avoided in the acutely anemic patient. Indeed, loss of blood volume is more detrimental to oxygen delivery than is loss of blood oxygen-carrying capacity, except at extreme levels of anemia. The primacy in importance of blood volume over red cell mass is a well-recognized principle of resuscitation from hemorrhage.

In studies of patients with chronic anemias, it has been difficult to detect a deficit in work capacity with hemoglobin concentrations as low as 7 grams per dl.[81-87] Other investigators have found evidence of only moderately impaired function.[88-90] This correlates with the failure to detect much increase in cardiac output at rest with similar hemoglobin levels.[91] Unfortunately, many of these studies were carried out before there was awareness of the lability and responses of oxyhemoglobin affinity in vivo to stresses on oxygen delivery. By changing levels of 2,3-DPG in red cells, these shifts can compensate to some degree for losses of red cell mass by proportionally increasing the efficiency of hemoglobin as an oxygen-delivering agent at physiologic gas tensions. In view of the seeming importance of the affinity of hemoglobin for oxygen in the oxygen delivery system, it is surprising how little has been done to investigate the interaction between hemoglobin function and hemoglobin concentration in the response to stress. These experiments will be difficult to define and carry out in man, particularly in ill patients where they are of greatest importance.

The heart occupies a unique position in the

oxygen-delivering system apart from its central role as pump. With loss of blood volume and/or loss of red cell mass as well as with most other acute stresses to the oxygen-delivering system, the heart works harder to increase total flow or to minimize any decrease in flow at lower filling pressures. The oxygen requirements of the heart increase, either absolutely or relatively, at a time when systemic oxygen delivery is decreasing. Most other organs can greatly increase oxygen extraction by working at the lower partial pressure of oxygen, but this important mechanism is almost completely unavailable to the heart, which works at all times near the minimum functional pO_2. This unusual constellation of circumstances—increased oxygen requirements, a tendency to decreased blood supply from purely physical factors, and inability to extract more oxygen from available blood—places extraordinary importance on the ability to the coronary vessels to dilate in order for the heart to perform satisfactorily and the patient to survive during hemorrhage. Against this background, factors such as hemoglobin function and hematocrit could conceivably become survival-limiting variables in patients with coronary artery disease.[92]

With respect to oxygen delivery as an integrated system, the body has regulatory mechanisms controlling a number of important components: cardiac output, blood volume, hematocrit, and red cell 2,3-DPG levels. Presumably, other variables are manipulated to give high efficiency to the cardiac mechanism—that is, maximum peripheral oxygen delivery per unit of energy consumed in pumping.

For the clinician faced with the problem of what is best for the anemic patient, it is important to keep in mind the risks of transfusion and the transitory nature of the improvement that results from transfusion. Chronic anemia down to hemoglobin concentrations that are one-half normal is tolerated even by patients who must perform physical work. Even acute anemia can be well tolerated at similar hemoglobin levels if demands on the

oxygen-delivering system are minimal. On the other hand, factors such as coronary insufficiency, fever, hypovolemia, and likely further acute loss of blood greatly increase the risks of acute or chronic anemia. There are no simple guidelines or rules for establishing the need for transfusion to correct anemia. Need will vary with circumstances, and the decision to transfuse must be made on an individual basis after considering both the current status and the projected future course of the patient and the risks of all other courses of action.

Hemorrhage

Hemorrhage is a clear and logical indication for transfusion when a significant percentage of the patient's blood volume has been lost. Limited hemorrhage can be treated with simple salt solutions or natural or artificial colloidal solutions. The use of such solutions results in hemodilutional anemia, and the considerations discussed in the previous section on anemia apply. These solutions can be used as the sole replacement for limited hemorrhages to keep the patient alive until blood is available, or in combination with blood to lessen the total amount needed.

The important consideration in the management of hemorrhage is that blood volume must be maintained. Most patients can tolerate acute loss of half their red cell mass, but acute untreated loss of half of the blood volume is usually fatal. Therefore, volume replacement, not necessarily in the form of blood alone, must be begun as soon as possible.

Replacement Solutions. Simple electrolyte solutions are effective, safe, and practical for initial resuscitation from hemorrhage. Experience in Vietnam[93, 94] and detailed studies in the U.S.[91,95] indicate that blood volume can be restored by electrolyte solutions after hemorrhage. With electrolyte solutions alone, however, each volume of lost blood must be replaced by three volumes of solution. The disadvantages of replacement with electrolyte solutions are: (1) overexpansion of extracellular fluid which must be excreted subsequently by the patient; (2) failure of the central venous pressure to reflect dangerous degrees of volume overloading; (3) loss of efficacy of the solution in terms of the fraction retained in the vascular space as hemorrhage progresses; and (4) lowering of plasma colloid osmotic pressure. The advantages are: (1) administration of electrolyte solutions can be begun quickly and safely even outside the hospital; (2) no adverse reactions except for overloading; (3) reduced risk of posthemorrhagic renal failure; and (4) sequestration loss can be treated as it occurs. Artificial colloids given I.V. preserve plasma osmotic activity, but those now available in the U.S.—dextran and hydroxyethyl starch—may interfere with clotting and are used infrequently.[96] The natural colloids, albumin or albumin with other plasma proteins, do not interfere with clotting and carry almost no risk of hepatitis, but they are expensive. They should be used in the presence of continued active bleeding after replacing 15 to 20 percent of the blood volume with electrolyte solutions.

Whatever is used initially, as the hemorrhage approaches half the blood volume, replacement with red cells and/or whole blood will be necessary. The more rapid the rate of bleeding and the more significant the associated diseases or disorders, the sooner blood must be used. Nonblood replacement of blood loss should be continued only if the anticipated loss is limited, the patient is doing well, and there are no associated conditions that make acute anemia less tolerable.

Uncrossmatched Blood. In severe situations in which exsanguination is imminent, it may be necessary to use uncrossmatched blood in order to save the patient's life. If possible, this should be ABO and Rh specific. The military experience with the use of uncrossmatched

blood has been excellent,[97] but few of those recipients had been transfused or pregnant previously, and donor blood with high titer anti-A and anti-B was eliminated. In extensive bleeding, the cause of hemorrhage must be identified and corrected as soon as possible. Evaluation of the clotting system early in the course of severe hemorrhage occasionally yields evidence of a clotting defect that can be corrected. Some patients with rapid exsanguination must be operated on to control bleeding before resuscitation is complete because the maximum possible rate of administration of fluid and blood may not equal the rate of loss.

Monitoring central venous pressure can be helpful in the extensively hemorrhaging patient, but may not reflect overloading with simple salt solutions or, occasionally, acute left ventricular failure. Pulmonary capillary wedge pressure measurement is more informative but carries added risks and should be reserved for difficult situations. Blood pressure, pulse rate, respiratory rate, state of consciousness, urinary output, and skin temperature and color all can be valuable indicators of the adequacy of perfusion, but any one of them alone can be misleading. Hematocrit is a measure of red cell concentration and reflects changes in whole blood volume only over a longer span of time than is appropriate for resuscitation. Hematocrit, therefore, does not reflect acute blood loss accurately. Similarly, the central venous pressure (CVP) does not always bear a linear relationship to blood volume. The rate of change of CVP with fluid administration is often more informative than the absolute level itself. CVP monitoring is most valuable as an aid to the early detection of fluid overload when administering blood or other fluids with colloid osmotic activity.

Clotting System Abnormalities Associated with Massive Transfusion. Component therapy guided by appropriate laboratory studies is the rational way to manage clotting system abnormalities. The use of platelet concentrates, fresh frozen plasma, cryoprecipitate, and cryoprecipitate-poor plasma are indicated in the various clinical abnormalities. The use of clotting factor concentrates, which are prepared from large plasma pools, is not indicated in the usual situation of massive transfusion because of the high risk of hepatitis and other hazards.

The use of blood transfusions to correct coagulation abnormalities may be thought to imply the use of fresh whole blood. This becomes rational only when: (1) multiple clotting deficiencies are to be treated simultaneously; (2) appropriate components are not on hand; (3) there is a concomitant need for red blood cells; and (4) fresh blood is easily available. Such circumstances are most likely to occur in a small hospital when the need arises for platelet replacement in an actively bleeding patient. Even here, the use of fresh whole blood should be considered a temporary measure until platelet concentrates can be obtained. For replacement of plasma clotting factors, except for Factor VIII, blood that is 24 to 48 hours old is quite adequate (see Ch. 24 and 25).

Exchange Transfusion

Exchange transfusion is an established therapeutic procedure for hemolytic disease of the newborn. Special precautions are necessary for this particular version of massive transfusion because the metabolic compensations of these sick newborn infants are not as efficient as those of adults, especially if the infant is premature. The blood must be warmed and should be less than five days old. Also, adjunct therapy with calcium chloride and sodium bicarbonate may be necessary. The exchange rate must be carefully controlled, input and removal must be balanced against cardiovascular function, and the infant must be monitored closely. Mortality rates of 1 to 5 percent have been reported, although most deaths were probably due to an underlying disease and not to the exchange procedure.

In performing exchange transfusion in the neonatal period, whole blood, heparinized whole blood, and frozen red cells reconstituted with fresh frozen plasma are used, each having a number of real and theoretical advantages. It has been suggested, when using citrate anticoagulated blood, that half the plasma should be removed.[98] This will reduce the risk of citrate toxicity and leave the infant with a higher hematocrit at the end of the procedure (see Ch. 33).

Exchange transfusion has been extended to several other conditions, usually various forms of poisonings. Recently, exchange transfusion has been used in the treatment of disseminated intravascular coagulation in infants, but there are no controlled clinical studies. Exchange transfusion is being evaluated in high-risk infants and in infants with respiratory distress syndrome.[99] Preliminary results are encouraging. A modification of exchange transfusion has been used experimentally for hepatic coma in adults. Total body blood washout is achieved by rapid exchange with cold asanguineous fluid followed by a short run on cardiopulmonary bypass to support the circulation, restore temperature, and restore red cell mass. The most notable successes have been in patients with Reye's syndrome but not in those with hepatitis A or B. Again, proof of benefit by controlled clinical trials is needed.

Extracorporeal Circulation

Some blood is necessary for cardiopulmonary bypass, but most such operations are now done using very little blood in the priming solution. Instead, hemodilution occurs during bypass, and slow replacement of the red cell mass occurs after bypass is completed. It is difficult to justify the persistent use of large amounts of blood in the priming solution in some cardiovascular surgical programs or to understand the marked interinstitutional discrepancies in utilization of blood for similar bypass procedures.

Some Misconceptions about Blood Transfusion

Whole blood is occasionally given to provide a "general support," or to treat hypoproteinemia with some degree of concomitant anemia, or even to prepare a nutritionally depleted patient for some form of stressful treatment. All of these approaches and concepts represent serious misconceptions about the efficacy of blood transfusion, the dynamics of blood cell protein turnover in disease and malnutrition, the optimal management of the undernourished patient, and even more serious misconceptions about the risks of transfusion. General support and the correction of malnutrition are not legitimate indications for transfusion. Wound healing is impaired by protein deficiency and hypoproteinemia, but it is not impaired by anemia. Transfusion to promote wound healing is not indicated; quite the contrary, this is usually a florid example of poor medical practice.

INDICATIONS FOR TRANSFUSION

Despite a large and long-standing experience, the indications for transfusion of red blood cell products are not always easy to delineate. This is to be expected because of the wide variety of available transfusion products, wide variations in the homeostatic capabilities of patients, and the multiplicity of clinical situations that may be encountered. Thus, rules of thumb about when to tranfuse, optimal hematocrit levels, and other such notions are unrealistic. Despite this, there are a few general principles that are useful in selecting patients to be transfused and determining how much blood to give.

The transfusion of red blood cell products is indicated when there is a red cell deficit, chronic or acute, and when the deficit is se-

vere enough to cause signs or symptoms resulting from tissue oxygen deprivation. Transfusion is also indicated when such signs and symptoms are anticipated if the patient's red blood cell deficit is not corrected. Patients vary considerably in their tolerance of anemia. For example, patients with cardiovascular insufficiency, pulmonary insufficiency, or cerebrovascular disease may not be able to tolerate low hemoglobin levels as well as healthier patients. Anemias of insidious onset may be better tolerated than those that occurred more rapidly. Active patients may require higher hemoglobin levels than those who lead more sedentary lives. Thus, the decision as to when to transfuse must be individualized, taking into account these specific patient variables. Some patients, especially those with chronic anemia, may have to decrease their level of activity as do other patients with chronic diseases.

In considering blood transfusion, the physician must keep in mind that transfusion is never definitive therapy; in all cases the underlying cause of the red blood cell deficit must be corrected or the patient will either succumb or require further transfusion indefinitely, with all its attendant hazards. It follows, therefore, that the quantity of blood given should be kept at a minimum consistent with the goals of the transfusion. It is the general opinion of most transfusion therapists that much blood is given inappropriately. In some situations where blood transfusion has had to be restricted, as in certain types of surgery on Jehovah's Witnesses, patient outcome has not been affected adversely. Lessons can be learned for management of all patients from these experiences.

Impaired Red Blood Cell Production

Patients may become anemic because of a deficiency in metabolic precursors necessary for normal erythropoiesis. In this group are patients with iron deficiency, pernicious anemia, folate deficiency, and endocrine disorders. In such patients the necessity for transfusion is infrequent because response to specific therapy is usually effective. Often, such patients can tolerate severe degrees of anemia without manifesting major symptoms.

Impaired red blood cell production is diagnosed easily: The patient demonstrates anemia without adequate reticulocytosis. In some cases, the pathogenesis of these anemias is complex; there may be concomitant elements of increased red blood cell destruction as in pernicious anemia or increased loss, as in iron deficiency anemia secondary to slow hemorrhage. In these cases, there may be some reticulocytosis reflecting these complicating factors, but its magnitude will be inappropriate to the degree of red blood cell deficit.

Inadequate red blood cell production is also seen in patients with bone marrow failure. While in rare instances marrow failure may be restricted to the erythrocyte series, pure red cell aplasia, it is usually seen in combination with decreased production of other blood cell elements. This group of disorders includes patients witih aplastic anemia, myelofibrosis, leukemia, and metastatic carcinoma. The ultimate outcome is invariably related to the underlying conditions rather than to the anemia. As these conditions are chronic; however, frequent blood transfusion is often necessary. In all cases of impaired red blood cell production, red blood cell concentrate is the product of choice for transfusion. After a while, many of these patients will require leukocyte-poor or washed red cell products. These issues have been discussed previously (see Ch. 30).

Increased Red Blood Cell Destruction—Intracorpuscular Defects

When red blood cell destruction occurs at a rate greater than six times the compensatory ability of the bone marrow, anemia will occur. Patients with a variety of red blood cell enzymatic defects, hereditary spherocytosis, hemoglobinopathies, and thalassemia are in this category. The presence of mild or moderate anemia, however, is usually not an indication for transfusion. These patients may have to limit their activities because of the anemia. Since these hereditary conditions and the concomitant anemia are lifelong, blood transfusion, because of its attendant risks, should be used judiciously. Where effective therapy can be instituted—such as splenectomy in patients with hereditary spherocytosis—this should be done, certainly in preference to transfusion.

In children, but also occasionally in adults, aplastic crises may develop in patients with inherited hemolytic disorders. These events are manifested by an acute, severe decrease in hemoglobin level. They require treatment with red blood cell tranfusions until the episode, often the result of infection or folate deficiency, remits spontaneously or by treatment.

Transfusion therapy is most frequent in patients with thalassemia major. These patients are often transfused vigorously in childhood to increase the peripheral hemoglobin levels so that marrow erythroid hyperplasia, which leads to bone expansion and serious disfigurement, can be suppressed. As a result of this chronic transfusion program, severe iron overload with tissue deposition and destruction is frequent and is a significant cause or morbidity in later years. Treatment with the iron chelation compound, deferoxamine, has been used to increase iron excretion and serves to mitigate the occurrence of this serious complication. Recently, Propper et al. have shown that collection by mechanical means of a donor's youngest cell population, the "neocytes," can reduce the requirement for transfusion in thalassemia major.[99a] (See Ch. 32.)

PNH

The red blood cells of patients with paroxysmal nocturnal hemoglobinuria have increased sensitivity to complement-mediated lysis. When transfusion is necessary in these patients, it has been the general practice to use only washed or frozen-deglycerolized red blood cells.[99b, c, d] This was done to avoid transfusion of additional complement components present in plasma which might provide a replenished source of mediators for continued hemolysis. This practice has been questioned recently by Sherman and Taswell[100] who found no difference in the reaction rate between whole blood/red cell transfusions and washed red cell transfusions. This issue requires further study, but most investigators still rely on washed red blood cells for transfusion in patients with paroxysmal nocturnal hemoglobinuria.

Jenkins has recently reviewed this problem.[100a] He agrees that transfusion of plasma components per se does not seem responsible for exacerbations of hemolysis in PNH patients posttransfusion. The observations of Sirchia et al. regarding a mechanism in which donor leukocytes and corresponding alloantibodies interact with resultant complement activation and injury of the hypersensitive PNH erythrocyte seem convincing.[100b] Jenkins has adopted frozen-deglycerolized red cells as the principal transfusion product for his large group of PNH patients. This policy has been adopted as a practical, fail-safe measure, with full recognition that other methods of removing leukocytes from donor blood will be adequate for many patients most of the time.

Increased Red Blood Cell Destruction—Extracorpuscular Defects

Increased red blood cell destruction may result from both nonimmune and immune extracellular factors. Hemolysis resulting from a prosthetic heart valve or microangiopathic processes may require treatment with blood transfusion. Unfortunately, the effectiveness of transfusion in these cases is limited and short-lived because the transfused cells will have the same shortened survival as the patient's own red blood cells.

Immune mediated extracorpuscular hemolytic phenomena present special problems in transfusion. In these cases, an autoantibody which is present on the patient's red blood cells, and which usually can also be found in the plasma, causes the premature destruction of the cells. The autoimmune hemolytic anemias are usually categorized as either the warm or cold type, based on the serologic thermal optima of the autoantibodies involved in the process. In occasional cases of the warm type of autoimmune hemolytic anemia, the antibody is directed against a well-defined antigenic specificity, and compatible blood transfusion is possible.[101] The transfused cells will then have a normal survival. Much more frequently, however, the autoantibody has a "broader" specificity, and it is virtually impossible to find compatible blood.[102] Survival of transfused red cells in these cases will be similar to the shortened survival of the patient's own cells, and transfusion is usually avoided if possible. Exceptions to this practice are made if the patient is in dire straits because of the severity of the anemia and severe complications appear imminent. Transfusion in these circumstances must be considered dangerous but may prolong life long enough for the institution of and response to more definitive therapy.

The serologic evaluation and, by extension, the selection of blood prior to transfusion in patients with warm type autoimmune hemolytic anemia are complicated further by the possible presence in the serum of a red cell alloantibody which is masked by the autopanagglutinin. Newer serological techniques are now available which use the patient's own red blood cells after partial elution from the cells of existing autoantibody.[103] This technique "uncovers" erythrocyte alloantibodies that might be present in the patient's serum.

Alphamethyldopa. The technique of autoabsorption after partial elution is most valuable in the pretransfusion evaluation of patients with a positive direct antiglobulin test due to alphamethyldopa therapy. Approximately 25 percent of all patients taking alpha-methyldopa have a positive direct antiglobulin test and usually a serum panagglutinin as well.[104] Only 2 to 3 percent of these patients have evidence of hemolysis, however, Serologically, even in the absence of hemolysis, these cases are indistinguishable from the usual case of autoimmune hemolytic anemia and serologically compatible blood is impossible to find. If transfusion is not urgent, the drug should be stopped, but it may take months for the serological phenomena to disappear. If transfusion is required promptly, perhaps because of the immediate necessity for cardiovascular surgery, then autoimmune *hemolysis* should be ruled out by appropriate laboratory tests. In some cases, a ^{51}Cr-red cell survival measurement may be necessary, although a reticulocyte count usually suffices. The absence of evidence for hemolysis indicates that the drug-induced serological phenomena are not detrimental to the patient's own cells and are likely not to affect transfused cells. Autoabsorption following partial elution, as described above, helps assure the absence of any significant red cell alloantibodies. A history of no previous blood transfusion or pregnancy also aids in assuring that dangerous alloantibodies are not present. After such an evaluation, necessary blood transfusion may be instituted even though the transfused cells are "incompatible" in vitro.

In autoimmune hemolytic anemia of the cold agglutinin type, the specificity of the antibody is usually anti-I. Transfusion is usually avoided because the I antigen is present on all adult red blood cells except for the rare I-negative individual. Woll et al.[105] reported a patient with cold agglutinin disease who did not require transfusion until her hematocrit fell to 9 percent. Successful transfusion with previously frozen I-negative blood was accomplished and a ^{51}Chromium-labeled red cell survival study showed a normal survival curve. (See Ch. 31 for further discussion.)

Hemorrhage

The physiology and transfusion management of the hemorrhaging patient has been discussed earlier in this chapter. The rate or anticipated rate of bleeding determines which blood product should be selected. Slow hemorrhages are best managed with red blood cell concentrates; rapid bleeding requires the simultaneous replacement of volume and red blood cells, and is best accomplished with whole blood. Red cell concentrates given in combination with volume expanders, electrolyte solutions, or albumin preparations are suitable alternatives to whole blood.

REFERENCES

1. Landsteiner, K.: Zur kenntnis der antifermentativen, lytischen und agglutinierenden wirkungen des blutserums und der lymphe. Zbl. Bakt. 27:357, 1900.
2. Landsteiner K. and Wiener, A.S.: An agglutinable factor in human blood recognizable by immune sera for Rhesus blood. Proc. Soc. Exper. Biol. Med. 43:223, 1940.
3. Levine P. and Stetson, R.: An unusual case of intra-group agglutination. J.A.M.A. 113:126, 1939.
4. Coombs, R.R.A., Mourant, A.E., and Race, R.R.: A new test for the detection of weak and "incomplete" Rh agglutinins. Br. J. Exp. Pathol. 26:255, 1945.
5. Hustin, A.: Principe d'une nouvelle methode de transfusion muqueuse. J. Med. Brux. 2:246, 1914.
6. Agote, L.: Nuevo procidimiento para la transfusion de sangre. Ann. Inst. Modelo. Clin. Med. (B. Aires) 1, 1915.
7. Lewisohn, R.: Blood transfusion by the citrate method. Surg. Gynecol. Obstet. 21:37, 1915.
8. Rous, P. and Turner, J.R.: Preservation of living red blood corpuscles in vitro. II. The transfusion of kept cells. J. Exper. Med. 23:219, 1916.
9. Maizels, M.: Preservation of organic phosphorus compounds in stored blood by glucose. Lancet 1:722, 1941.
10. Loutit, J.F., Mollison, P.L., and Young, M.I.:

Citric acid-sodium citrate-glucose mixtures for blood storage. Quart. J. Exper. Physiol. 32:183, 1943.

11. Loutit, J.F. and Mollison, P.L.: Advantages of a disodium-citrate-glucose mixture as a blood preservative. Br. Med. J. 2:744, 1943.

12. Strumia, M.M.: Methods of blood preservation in general and preparation and use of red cell suspension. Am. J. Clin. Pathol. 24:260, 1954.

13. Chaplin, H., Crawford, J., and Cutbush, M., et al.: Post-transfusion survival of red cells stored at −20°C. Lancet 1:852, 1954.

14. Chaplin, H., Chang, E., and Kolb, R.W.: Report of routine tests for psychrophilic and mesophilic contaminants in banked blood. Appl. Microbiol. 3:213, 1955.

15. Gibson, J.G., Rees, S.B., and McManus, T.J., et al.: A citrate-phosphate-dextrose solution for the preservation of human blood. Am. J. Clin. Pathol. 28:569, 1957.

16. Dern, R.J., Brewer, G.J., and Wiorkowski, J.J.: Studies on the preservation of human blood. II. The relationship of erythrocyte adenosine triphosphate levels and other *in vitro* measures of red cell storageability. J. Lab. Clin. Med. 69:968, 1967.

17. Orlina, A. and Josephson, A.: Comparative viability of blood stored in ACD and CPD. Transfusion 9:62, 1969.

18. Haradin, A.R., Weed, R.I., and Reed, C.F.: Changes in physical properties of stored erythrocytes: relationship to survival *in vivo*. Transfusion 9:229, 1969.

19. Weed, R.I. and LaCelle, P.L.: ATP dependence of erythrocyte membrane deformability. In Jamieson, G.A. and Greenwalt, T.J.: Red Cell Membrane Structure and Function. P. 318, 1969, Lippincott, Philadelphia.

20. Kirkpatrick, F.H., Muhs, A.G., and Kostuk, R.K., et al.: Dense (aged) circulating red cells contain normal concentrations of adenosine triphosphate (ATP). Blood 54:946, 1979.

21. Simon, E.R., Chapman, R.G., and Finch, C.A.: Adenine in red cell preservation. J. Clin. Invest. 41:351, 1962.

22. Simon, E.R.: Adenine and purine nucleosides in human red cell preservation: a review. Transfusion 7:395, 1967.

23. Benesch, R. and Benesch, R.E.: The effect of organic phosphates from the human erythrocyte on the allosteric properties of hemoglobin. Biochem. Biophys. Res. Commun. 26:162, 1967.

24. Benesch, R.E. and Benesch, R.: The mechanism of interaction of red cell organic phosphates with hemoglobin. Adv. Protein Chem. 28:211, 1974.

25. Chanutin, A. and Curnish, R.R.: Effect of organic and inorganic phosphates on the oxygen equilibrium of human erythrocytes. Arch. Biochem. Biophys. 121:96, 1967.

26. Beutler E. and Wood, L.: The *in vivo* regeneration of red cell 2,3-diphosphoglyceric acid (DPG) after transfusion of stored blood. J. Lab. Clin. Med. 74:300, 1969.

27. Chanutin, A.: The effect of the addition of adenine and nucleosides at the beginning of storage on the concentrations of phosphates of human erythrocytes during storage in acid-citrate-dextrose and citrate-phosphate-dextrose. Transfusion 7:120, 1967.

28. Dawson, R. B., Kocholaty, W.F., and Gray, J.L.: Hemoglobin function and 2,3-DPG levels of blood stored at 4C in ACD and CPD: pH effect. Transfusion 10:299, 1970.

29. Akerblom, O.C. and Kreuger, A.: Studies on citrate-phosphate-dextrose (CPD) blood supplemented with adenine. Vox Sang. 29:90, 1975.

30. Slichter, S.J. and Harker, L.A.: Preparation and storage of platelet concentrates. II. Storage variables influencing platelet viability and function. Br. J. Haematol. 34:403, 1976.

31. McCullough, J., Carter, S.J., and Quie, P.G.: Effects of anticoagulants and storage on granulocyte function in bank blood. Blood 43:207, 1974.

32. McCullough, J., Benson, S.J., and Yunis, E.J., et al.: Effect of blood-bank storage on leukocyte function. Lancet 2:1333, 1969.

33. Slichter, S.J., Counts, R.B., and Henderson, R., et al.: Preparation of cryoprecipitated factor VIII concentrates. Transfusion 16:616, 1976.

34. Bailey, D.N. and Bove, J.R.: Chemical and hematological changes in stored CPD blood. Transfusion, 15:244, 1975.

35. Perkins, H.A., Rolfs, M.R., and Acra, D.J.: Studies on bank blood collected and stored under various conditions with particular reference to its use in open heart surgery. Transfusion 1:157, 1961.

36. Veall, N. and Mollison, P.L.: The rate of red-cell exchange in replacement transfusions. Lancet 2:792, 1950.

37. Johnson, L., Garcia, M.L., and Figueroa, E., et al.: Kernicterus in rats lacking glucuronyl transferase. Am. J. Dis. Child. 101:322, 1961.

38. Ervin, D.M., Christian, R.M., and Young, L.E.: Dangerous universal donors. II. Further observations on the in vivo and in vitro behaviour of isoantibodies of immune type present in group O blood. Blood 5:553, 1950.

39. Miller, W.V., Wilson, M.J., and Kalb, H.J.: Simple methods for production of HL-A antigen poor red blood cells. Transfusion 13:189, 1973.

40. Tenzcar, F.J.: Comparison of inverted centrifugation, saline washing, and dextran sedimentation in the preparation of leukocyte-poor red cells. Transfusion 13:183, 1973.

41. Perkins, H.A., Senecal, I., and Howell, E.: Leukocyte contamination of red cells in leukocyte-poor and frozen deglycerolized units. Transfusion 13:194, 1973.

42. Greenwalt, T.J., Gajewski, M., and McKenna, J.L.: A new method for preparing buffy coat-poor blood. Transfusion 2:221, 1962.

43. Walker, R.H.: cited in Mollison, P.L.: Blood Transfusion in Clinical Medicine. p. 617, 1979, Blackwell Scientific, Oxford.

44. Payne, R.: The association of febrile transfusion reactions with leukoagglutinins. Vox Sang. 2:233, 1957.

45. Payne, R.: Leukocyte agglutinins in human sera. Arch. Intern. Med. 99:587, 1957.

46. Brittingham, T.E. and Chaplin, H.: Febrile transfusion reactions caused by sensitivity to donor leukocytes and platelets. J.A.M.A. 165:819, 1957.

47. Perkins, H.A., Payne, R., and Ferguson, J., et al.: Nonhemolytic febrile transfusion reactions. Quantitative effects of blood components with emphasis on isoantigenic incompatibility of leukocytes. Vox Sang. 11:578, 1966.

48. Perkins, H.A., Payne, R., and Vyas, G., et al.: Nonhemolytic reactions to blood transfusion and organ transplantation. Proc. 12th Congr. Int. Soc. Blood Transf. Moscow, 1969.

49. Heinrich, D., Muller-Eckhardt, C., and Steir, W.: The specificity of leukocyte and platelet alloantibodies in sera of patients with non-hemolytic transfusion reactions. Absorptions and elution studies. Vox Sang. 25:442, 1973.

50. Yankee, R.A., Graff, K.S., and Dowling, R., et al.: Selection of unrelated platelet donors by lymphocyte HL-A matching. N. Engl. J. Med. 288:760, 1973.

51. Westrick, M.A., Debelak-Fehir, K.M., and Epstein, R.B.: The effect of prior whole blood transfusion on subsequent granulocyte support in leukopenic dogs. Transfusion 17:611, 1977.

52. Huestis, D.W., Bove, J.R., and Busch, S.: Practical blood transfusion (2nd Ed.). P. 261, Little Brown, Boston.

53. Bachman, R.: Studies on serum gamma A globulin level: III. Frequency of a-gamma A globulinemia. Scand. J. Clin. Lab. Invest. 17:316, 1965.

54. Vyas, G.N., Perkins, H.A., and Yang, Y.M., et al.: Healthy blood donors with selective absence of immunoglobulin A: prevention of anaphylactic transfusion reactions caused by antibodies to IgA. J. Lab. Clin. Med. 85:838, 1975.

55. Vyas, G.N., Levin, A.S., and Fudenberg, H.H.: Intrauterine isoimmunization caused by maternal IgA crossing the placenta. Nature 225:275, 1970.

56. Miller, W.V., Holland, P.V., and Sugarbroker, E., et al.: Anaphylactic reactions to IgA: a difficult transfusion problem. Am. J. Clin. Path. 54:618, 1970.

57. Meryman, H.T. and Hornblower, M.: A method for freezing and washing red blood cells using a high glycerol concentration. Transfusion 12:145, 1972.

58. Rowe, A.W., Eyster, E., and Kellner, A.: Liquid nitrogen preservation of red blood cells for transfusion: a low glycerol-rapid freeze procedure. Cryobiology 5:119, 1968.

59. Tullis, J.L., Hinman, J., and Sproul, M.T., et al.: Incidence of post-transfusion hepatitis in previously frozen blood. J.A.M.A. 214:719, 1970.

60. Alter, H.J., Tabor, E., and Meryman, H.T., et al.: Transmission of hepatitis B virus infection by transfusion of frozen-deglycerolized red blood cells. N. Engl. J. Med. 298:637, 1978.

61. Haugen, R.K.: Hepatitis after the transfusion of frozen red cells and washed red cells. N. Engl. J. Med. 301:393, 1979.

62. Opelz, G. and Terasaki, P.I.: Improvement of kidney-graft survival with increased numbers of blood transfusions. N. Engl. J. Med. 299:799, 1978.

63. Vincenti, F., Duca, R.M., and Amend, W. et al.: Immunologic factors determining survival of cadaver-kidney transplants. The effect of HLA serotyping, cytotoxic antibodies and blood transfusions on graft survival. N. Engl. J. Med. 299:799, 1978.

64. Collins, J.A.: Problems associated with the massive transfusion of stored blood. Surgery 75:274, 1974.

65. Simon, T.L. and Henderson, R.: personal communication.

66. Lostumbo, M.M., Holland, P.V., and Schmidt, P.J.: Isoimmunization after multiple transfusions. N. Engl. J. Med. 275:141, 1966.

67. Kaarianen, L., Klemola, E., and Palokeimo, J.: Rise of cytomegalovirus antibodies in an infectious-mononucleosis-like syndrome after transfusion. Br. Med. J. 1:1270, 1966.

68. Lang, D.J. and Henshaw, J.B.: Cytomegalovirus infection and the post perfusion syndrome: recognition of primary infection in four patients. N. Engl. J. Med. 280:1145, 1969.

69. Henle, W., Henle, G., and Scriba, M., et al.: Antibody responses to the Epstein-Barr virus and cytomegalovirus after open-heart surgery and other surgery. N. Engl. J. Med. 282:1068, 1970.

70. Tabor, E. and Gerety, R.J.: Non-A, non-B hepatitis: New findings and prospects for prevention. Transfusion 19:669, 1979.

71. Agarwal, J.B., Paltoo, B.R., and Palmer, W.H.: Relative viscosity of blood at varying hematocrits in pulmonary circulation. J. Appl. Physiol. 29:866, 1970.

72. Djojosugito, A.M., Folkow, B., and Oberg, B., et al.: A comparison of blood viscosity measured in vitro and in a vascular bed. Acta. Physiol. Scand. 78:70, 1970.

73. Braasch, D.: Red cell deformability and capillary blood flow. Physiol. Rev. 51:679, 1971.

74. Rowlands, S. and Skibo, L.: Erythrocyte flow in tubes of capillary size. Can. J. Physiol. Pharmacol. 49:373, 1971.

75. Greene, R., Hughes, J.M., and Iliff, L.D., et al.: Red cell flexibility and pressure-flow relations in isolated lungs. J. Appl. Physiol. 34:169, 1973.

76. Chien, S.: Present state of blood rheology. In: Hemodilution, Theoretical Basics and Clinical Application. Messmer, K., Schmid-Schonbein, eds. Karger, Basil, 1972, p. 1.

77. Crowell, J.W., Bounds, S.H., and Johnson, W.W.: Effect of varying the hematocrit ratio on the susceptibility to hemorrhagic shock. Amer. J. Physiol. 192:171, 1958.

78. Gordon, R.J., Snyder, G.K., and Tritel, H., et al.: Potential significance of plasma viscosity and hematocrit variations in myocardial ischemia. Am. Heart. J. 87:175, 1974.

79. Carey, J.S.: Cardiovascular response to acute hemodilution. J. Thoracic. Cardiovasc. Surg. 62:103, 1971.

80. Varat, M.A., Adolph, R.J., and Fowler, N.O.: Cardiovascular effects of anemia. Amer. Heart. J. 83:415, 1972.

81. Beutler, E., Larsh, S., and Tanzi, F.: Iron enzymes in iron deficiency. VII. Oxygen consumption measurements in iron deficient subjects. Am. J. Med. Sci. 239:759, 1960.

82. Rowell, L.B., Taylor, H.L., and Wang, Y.: Limitations to prediction of maximal oxygen intake. J. Appl. Physiol. 19:919, 1964.

83. Cotes, J.E., Dabbs, J.M., and Elwood, P.C., et al.: The response to submaximal exercise in adult females; relation to haemoglobin concentration. J. Physiol. 203:79P, 1969.

84. Elwood, P.C. and Hughes, D.: Clinical trial of iron therapy on psychomotor function in anaemic women. Br. Med. J. 3:254, 1970.

85. Ericsson, P.: Total haemoglobin and physical work capacity in elderly people. Acta. Med. Scand. 188:15, 1970.

86. Elwood, P.C.: Evaluation of the clinical importance of anemia. Am. J. Clin. Nutrit. 26:958, 1973.

87. Hermansen, L.: Oxygen transport during exercise in human subjects. Acta. Physiol. Scand. suppl. 399, 1973.

88. Sproule, B.J., Mitchell, J.H., and Miller, W.F.: Cardiopulmonary physiological responses to heavy exercise in patients with anemia. J. Clin. Invest. 39:378, 1960.

89. Davies, C.T.M. and VanHaaren, J.P.M.: Anemia: affect of therapy on responses to exercise. J. Physiol. 227:36P, 1972.

90. Ekblom, B., Goldbarg, A.N., and Gullbring,

B.: Response to exercise after blood loss and reinfusion. J. Appl. Physiol. 33:175, 1972.

91. Sharpey-Schafer, E.P.: Cardiac output in severe anaemia. Clin. Sci. 5:125, 1944.

92. Case, R.B., Berglund, E., and Sarnoff, S.J.: Ventricular function. VII. Changes in coronary resistance and ventricular function resulting from acutely induced anemia and the effect thereon of coronary stenosis. Am. J. Med. 18:397, 1955.

93. Carey, L.C., Lowery, B.D., and Cloutier, C.T.: Hemorrhagic shock. Current Problems in Surgery, Jan. 1971.

94. Collins, J.A.: The causes of progressive pulmonary insufficiency in surgical patients. J. Surg. Res. 9:685, 1969.

95. Shires, T., Coln, D., and Carrico, J., et al.: Fluid therapy in hemorrhagic shock. Arch. Surg. 88:688, 1964.

96. Alexander, B.: Recent studies on plasma colloid substitutes: Their effects on coagulation and hemostasis. In: Fox, C.L., and Nahas, G.G.: Body Fluid Replacement in the Surgical Patient. Grune and Stratton, New York, 1970, p. 157.

97. Barnes, A.: Status of the use of universal donor blood transfusion. CRC Critical Reviews in Clinical Laboratory Sciences. 4:147, 1973.

98. Veall, N. and Mollison, P.L.: The rate of red-cell exchange in replacement transfusions. Lancet 2:792, 1950.

99. Delivoria-Papadopoulos, M., Miller, L.D., and Forster, R.E., et al.: The role of exchange transfusion in the management of low-birth-weight infants with and without severe respiratory distress syndrome. I. initial observations. J. Peds. 89:273, 1976.

99a. Propper, R.O., Button, L.H., and Nathan, D.G.: New approaches to the transfusion management of thalassemia. Blood 55:55, 1980.

99b. Dacie, J.V. and Lewis, S.M.: Paroxysmal nocturnal hemoglobinuria: clinical manifestations. Haematology and nature of the disease. Ser. Haematol. V:3, 1972.

99c. Dacie, J.V. and Firth, D.: Blood transfusion in nocturnal hemoglobinuria. Br. Med. J. 1:626, 1943.

99d. Gockerman, F.P. and Brouillard, R.P.: RBC transfusions in paroxysmal nocturnal hemoglobinuria. Arch. Intern. Med. 137:536, 1977.

100. Sherman, S.P. and Taswell, H.F.: The need for transfusion of saline-washed red blood cells to patients with paroxysmal nocturnal hemoglobinuria: A myth. Transfusion 17:683, 1977 (Abstr.)

100a. Jenkins, D.E.: Paroxysmal nocturnal hemoglobinuria hemolytic systems, In: A Seminar on Laboratory Management of Hemolysis. American Assoc. Blood Banks, C. Bell, Ed., Washington, D.C., 1979, p. 45.

100b. Sirchia, G., Ferrone, S., and Mercuriali, F.: Leukocyte antigen-antibody reaction and lysis of paroxysmal nocturnal hemoglobinuria erythrocytes. Blood 36:334, 1970.

101. Weiner, W. and Vos, G.H.: Serology of acquired anemias. Blood 22:206, 1963.

102. Leddy, J.P., Peterson, P., and Yeaw, M.A., et al.: Patterns of serologic specificity of human gamma G autoantibodies: Correlation of antibody specificity with complement fixing behavior. J. Immunol. 105:677, 1970.

103. Technical Manual, American Assoc. Blood Banks, 1977, p. 204.

104. Worlledge, S.: Immune drug-induced hemolytic anemias. Semin. Hemat. 10:327, 1973.

105. Woll, J.E., Smith, C.M., and Nusbacher, J.: Treatment of acute cold agglutinin hemolytic anemia with transfusion of adult i rbc's. J.A.M.A. 229:1779, 1974.

13

Cryopreservation of Blood and Marrow Cells; Basic Biological and Biophysical Considerations

Harold T. Meryman, M.D.

Investigators early in this century, observing freezing in tissues and cell suspensions under the microscope, were impressed by the extent to which tissue cells appeared to be crushed between ice crystals (Fig. 13-1B) or in jeopardy from rapidly advancing spears of ice (Fig. 13-2). They tended to conclude, with some justification, that freezing injury was probably the result of the mechanical destruction of cells. Much of the early research therefore centered about the formation and growth of ice in biological systems and ways of influencing its development through the manipulation of the solute environment and the freezing rate.[1]

Of particular significance was the observation that cells that were uniformly destroyed at low cooling rates often showed some survival at higher rates. Since elevated cooling rates also resulted in smaller and more uniformly distributed ice crystals (Fig. 13-1C), this reinforced the hypothesis that freezing injury was somehow related to the formation of ice. These observations also suggested that, if the frreezing and thawing rate could be sufficiently rapid, the formation and growth of ice might be prevented altogether, permitting cell survival. Although theoretically probably correct, freezing and thawing rates sufficiently rapid to achieve this end are not

attainable in practice because of the physical limitations of heat transfer. In fact, contrary to expectation, ultrarapid cooling rates often resulted in the same total destruction that was seen at very slow rates of freezing.[2] Figure 13-3 illustrates this schematically. At low rates of cooling (A), no recovery is seen, but as the cooling rate is accelerated there is a progressive increase in survival (B). However, there is almost inevitably an optimum cooling rate above which survival again falls off (C), ultimately to zero. Much of the cryobiological research of the last three decades has been directed at an explanation of this relationship between cooling rate and cell survival.

Probably the single most significant milestone in cryobiology was the report by Polge, Smith, and Parkes in 1949 that glycerol could prevent freezing injury in bovine spermatozoa[3] and human red cells.[4] Of particular importance were the subsequent classic papers by Lovelock,[5,6] who showed that injury to red cells was always proportional to the concentration of salt produced by the freezing out of water, regardless of the temperature of freezing or the presence or absence of glycerol. Lovelock's experiments effectively contradicted the mechanical injury theory, since they demonstrated that injury resulted not from the physical presence of the ice but from

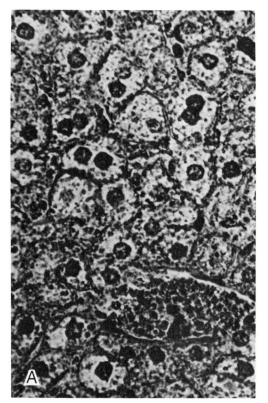

Fig. 13-1*A*. Control section of rabbit liver, formalin fixed, H & E stain. Magnification approximately 1000 ×. (Meryman, H.T.: Ice crystal formation in frozen tissues. NMRI Rept. Lect. and Rev. Series No. 53-3, 1953.)

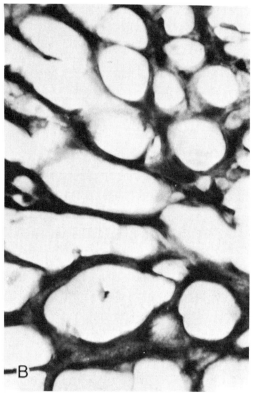

Fig. 13-1*B*. Section of rabbit liver frozen to −30° C at a rate of approximately 1°/min, then lyophilized at −60° C, transferred to anhydrous alcohol-ether, and embedded in hard collodian for sectioning. The white spaces represent the areas originally occupied by ice. (Meryman, H.T.: Ice crystal formation in frozen tissues. NMRI Rept. Lect. and Rev. Series No. 53-3, 1953.)

the concentration of solutes which Lovelock presumed caused injury on a biochemical basis. The biochemical theory of injury was also consistent with the fact that cell survival could be seen at accelerated cooling rates, presumably because insufficient time was then available for processes of degradation to take place.

The biochemical injury theory failed, however, to explain the cell injury at excessive rates of cooling. It was not until the mid-1960s that it became apparent that the decline in survival with increasing cooling velocity appeared to coincide with the appearance of intracellular ice.[7,8] On this basis, Mazur[9] proposed that two independent processes were involved in freezing injury: one at slower cooling rates, resulting from solute concentration which he termed "solute effects"; the other at high cooling rates, resulting from intracellular ice which caused mechanical damage. Although there is some evidence that cells with minimal intracellular ice may survive very rapid thawing, in general the proposal that the descending portion of the survival curve of Figure 13-3 is associated with intracellular ice remains unchallenged.

The emphasis in our laboratory over the

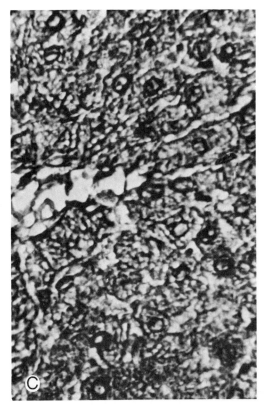

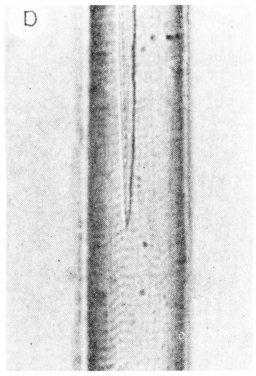

Fig. 13-1C. This section was obtained after freezing by direct immersion of a one half inch diameter sample of rabbit liver into a liquid bath at −30° C, producing a freezing rate in excess of 20° per minute. The gross anatomy of the tissue is well preserved, and ice appears to be predominantly intracellular. (Meryman, H.T.: Ice crystal formation in frozen tissues. NMRI Rept. Lect. and Rev. Series No. 53-3, 1953.)

Fig. 13-2. This photograph shows a spear of ice advancing down the interior of a muscle fiber. (Rapatz, G. and Luyet, B.: On the mechanism of ice formation and propagation in muscle. Biodynamica 8:121-144, 1959.)

last two decades has been on the mechanism of slow freezing injury, corresponding to that portion of Figure 13-3 labeled "A." It is tempting to recount our studies as an historical narrative, with each new discovery building on the previous one and driving us progressively toward an unexpected answer to the mechanism of freezing injury. Such an account, however, is probably more satisfying to the author than to the reader who is more interested in the conclusion than in the steps that led to its formulation. In fact, it is now possible to present a unified theory of freez-

ing injury which can account for the entire curve of Figure 13-3 on what is essentially a physical basis.

INJURY AT SLOW RATES OF COOLING

As suggested above, at least for cell suspensions, extracellular ice crystals do not appear to be damaging on the basis of their physical presence. They do not crush or pierce the cells; in fact, there is evidence that ice does not grow through the intact cell membrane nor can extracellular ice stimulate the development of intracellular ice across an intact membrane.[10] Furthermore, it appears that intact cells do not contain the mysterious

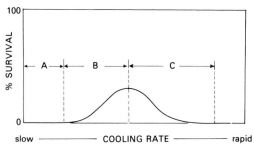

Fig. 13-3. Schematic illustration of the general effects of cooling rate on cell survival. At very slow rates of cooling (*A*), injury is generally complete for those cells that lack any natural resistance to freezing. As the cooling rate increases, some survival may be seen (*B*). But, as the cooling rate is still further increased, survival falls, ultimately to zero (*C*).

"motes" that nucleate ice crystal growth (heterogeneous nucleation), presumably by hydrogen bonding water in a crystalline array to form a template for continued crystal growth. This means that a cell with an intact membrane will not spontaneously freeze internally at ordinary subfreezing temperature. Only when the temperature falls to the vicinity of −40° C, at which random aggregations of water molecules can nucleate ice (homozygous nucleation), does spontaneous intracellular freezing occur. In other words, as the temperature of a cell suspension falls below the melting point, ice will first appear only in the extracellular solution. Cells remain suspended in the remaining unfrozen solution. The removal of extracellular water to form ice concentrates extracellular solutes. The increased osmotic pressure of the extracellular solution causes a movement of water out of the cell, with the result that the intracellular solution is also concentrated and the cell volume is reduced.

Lovelock assumed that it was the concentration of solutes, particularly of salts, that was responsible for cell injury. Although entirely reasonable, this theory became increasingly untenable as cells from a wider variety of species were studied. For example, red cells frozen in isotonic sucrose were injured to the same extent at the same temperatures as when frozen in isotonic sodium chloride, demonstrating that denaturation from extracellular electrolytes was clearly not responsible for lysis. Furthermore, red cells depleted of intracellular electrolytes were lysed at a higher freezing temperature than normal cells but at approximately the same volume.[11] Still more compelling is the kind of data shown in Fig-

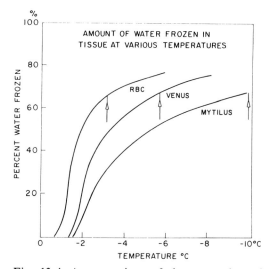

Fig. 13-4. A comparison of the proportion of water frozen as a function of temperature for three different tissues. The arrows indicate the point at which freezing injury is first seen. Red blood cells (RBC) are isotonic at 300 mOsm, with a freezing temperature of −5.5° C. Hemolysis first appears at approximately −3° C when the salt concentration is approximately 1600 mOsm. *Venus mercernaria* is isotonic at 1000 mOsm, has a freezing temperature of −1.9° C; tissue damage is seen at −6° C, where the solution osmolality is approximately 3200 mOsm. *Mytilus edulis,* which has some natural tolerance to freezing, is also isotonic at 1000 mOsm, but tissue injury is not seen until the temperature has reached −10° C at an osmolality of approximately 5400 mOsm. The only common denominator in these three systems is the observation that approximately the same proportion of water has been frozen out at the point of injury in each system. (Meryman, H.T.: The exceeding of a tolerable cell volume in hypertonic suspension as a cause of freezing injury. In: The Frozen Cell. G.E.W. Wolstenholme and M. O'Connor, eds., J. & A. Churchill, London, 1970.)

ure 13-4. Human red cells, isotonic at 300 mOsm, first show lysis at about $-3°C$, where the salt has been concentrated to nearly 5 percent with an osmolality of about 1500 mOsm. Tissues from *Venus mercernaria,* a marine clam isotonic at 1000 mOsm, are first injured by freezing at around $-6°C$, which produces a salt concentration of nearly 12 percent with an osmolality of approximately 6000 mOsm. *Mytilus edulis,* the common mussel of the shoreline, has developed a modest resistance to freezing, apparently by rendering some of its water unfreezeable. *Mytilus* is not injured until frozen to $-10°C$, where the sodium chloride concentration is nearly 16 percent with an osmolality of over 6000 mOsm. As shown in Figure 13-4, whereas the killing temperatures, and therefore the salt concentrations and water activities vary widely, the proportion of water frozen out is virtually identical. These experiments suggest that it is the loss of intracellular water and the associated reduction in cell volume rather than the absolute concentration of solutes that is directly responsible for cell injury. The next question is, then, how can volume reduction cause cell damage?

In plant cells, as cell volume is reduced by freezing, there is no observable event as the cell volume passes the point of no return. It is only on deplasmolysis with return of the cell to its original volume that injury is observed. Shortly before the cell regains its original volume, it bursts, as though the membrane were no longer of sufficient area to permit achieving the original volume.[12] Studies of cell phospholipids in monolayer have shown that compression of the monolayer does result in the loss of membrane constituents.[13] One particularly frost-resistant wheat has been found to possess a mechanism whereby lipids lost from the membrane are stored in intracellular liposomes and returned to the membrane during thawing.[12] These cells are able to survive plasmolysis to a substantially smaller volume when this adaptive mechanism is functioning than during the summer, when they possess no frost resistance.

These observations suggest that it is volume reduction rather than salt concentration that is the basis of freezing injury and that the injury itself is basically mechanical or physical-chemical rather than biochemical.

We have therefore proposed[11] that there is a resistance to cell volume reduction on the part of the plasma membrane. Indirect support of this hypothesis has been found in a number of experiments, although difficult to demonstrate directly. If the cell membrane does resist cell volume reduction, this implies that the cell is incrementally larger than it would be if there were no resistance to volume change. This in turn means that the intracellular osmolality must be slightly lower than the extracellular. The unrelieved osmotic pressure gradient across the membrane would therefore result in a difference in hydrostatic pressure between the cell's interior and exterior. This was directly tested by measuring the internal pressure in the giant algal cell, *Nitella,* during plasmolysis in hyperosmotic calcium chloride solutions. As the cell was reduced in volume, the intracellular pressure was found to fall below atmospheric.[15]

Another implication of membrane resistance to volume reduction is that some energy is being stored in the membrane just as is true when a spring resists compression. This in turn implies an increase in surface energy and, therefore, a decrease in surface tension. Measurements of the surface tension of the sea urghin egg using the contact angle method, showed that the surface tension of the egg did decrease as the cell decreased in volume in hyperosmotic suspension.[16] Of particular interest was the observation that when the contact angle between the egg and the substrate reached $90°$, which implies equality between the surface tension of the egg surface and the suspending medium, the egg lysed. This suggests first that the integrity of the cell membrane depends on interfacial energies rather than only on membrane "structure" and, second, that injury from osmotic water loss and volume reduction may also produce a decrease in cell surface tension with a resulting loss of interfacial stability.

FREEZING AT ELEVATED COOLING RATES

Mazur[17] showed that it was possible to formulate and to some extent to predict the cooling rate that would result in spontaneous intracellular freezing. He argues that, since intracellular water must diffuse out of the cell to the ice crystal in response to the osmotic gradient created when extracellular water is frozen, one can clearly attach a time constant to this process by considering the diffusion constant of the cell interior, the surface to volume ratio, and the water permeability of the cell membrane. If the cooling rate is sufficiently rapid, there may be insufficient time for water to leave the cell before very physically stabilizing temperatures are reached. In other words, the intracellular solution will remain dilute and its melting point will be substantially higher than the actual temperature. If this discrepancy is large enough and the temperature low enough, spontaneous intracellular crystallization will occur.

It should now be apparent that both intracellular freezing and dehydration injury are the result of the diffusion of water from the cell: in the first case too little, in the second case too much. This observation leads readily to an explanation of cell recovery at intermediate cooling rates, that portion of the recovery curve in Figure 13-3 designated as "B."

A UNIFIED HYPOTHESIS FOR FREEZING INJURY

Figure 13-5 illustrates schematically the results of freezing at slow, intermediate, and rapid rates corresponding to sections A, B, and C of Figure 13-3. At a slow rate of cooling, there is ample time for water to diffuse from the cell in response to the osmotic gradi-

ent created when extracellular water freezes. The cell is dehydrated and reduced in volume and, regardless of the precise mechanism involved, is injured as a result. However, as the cooling rate is increased, less time is available for the movement of water from the cell before a stabilizing temperature is reached. As a result, less dehydration and less volume reduction result. If the cooling rate is fast enough, some cells may not be dehydrated to the point of injury, and survival can be expected. On the other hand, further increasing the cooling rate and decreasing cell dehydration may render the cell interior sufficiently dilute so that spontaneous crystallization takes place and recovery again falls. The optimum cooling rate will presumably be just short of that rapid enough to cause intracellular freezing. As Leibo and Mazur have shown,[18] the optimum cooling rate varies widely from cell to cell depending on the surface to volume ratio and the permeability of the membrane to water.

CRYOPROTECTION

Historically, there has been the same lack of consistency to the theories of cryoprotection as was true of theories of freezing injury. Some cryoprotectants, such as glycerol, penetrate the cells and protect against slow freezing. Other agents such as sugars and polymers are nominally extracellular and protect only at elevated cooling rates. The variety in the character of cryoprotectants—which includes alcohols, glycols, sugars, and sugar alcohols, polymers, and even some electrolytes—provided no clue to any common mechanism. However, starting with the unified mechanism of injury summarized above, it should be evident that, to be effective, a cryoprotectant for slow freezing must either increase the resistance of the cell to dehydration injury or reduce the extent of dehydration. To be effective at accelerated cooling rates, a cryoprotectant might in addition inhibit intracellular freezing or in-

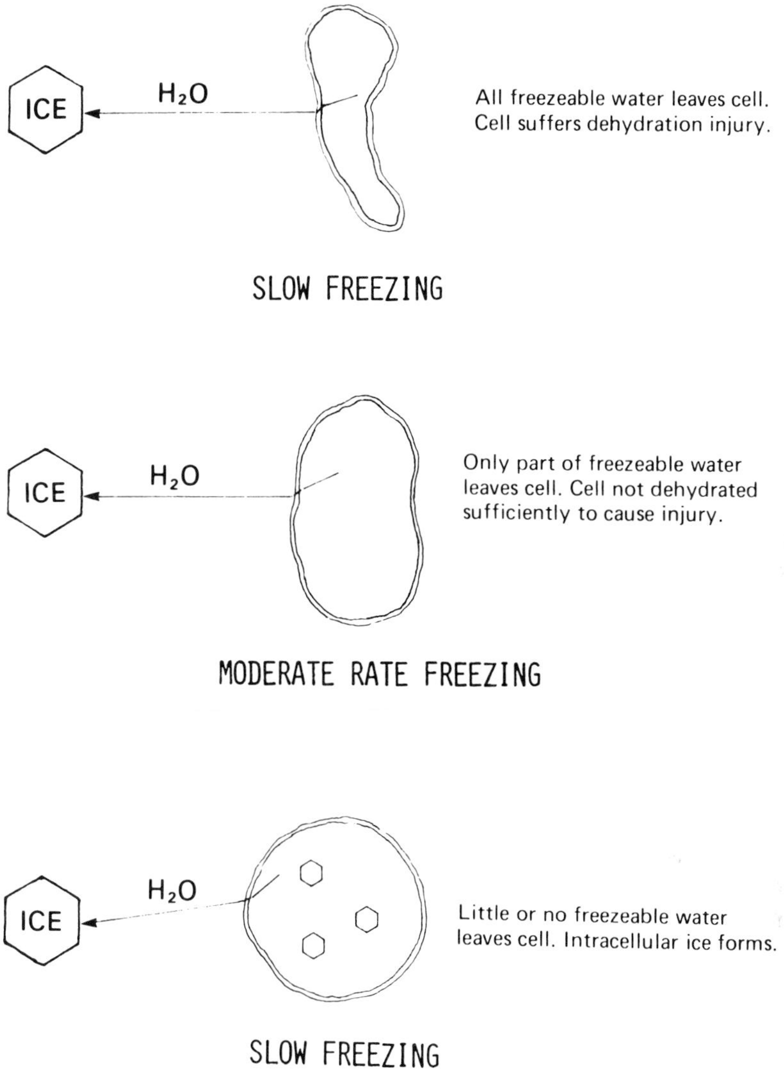

All freezeable water leaves cell.
Cell suffers dehydration injury.

SLOW FREEZING

Only part of freezeable water
leaves cell. Cell not dehydrated
sufficiently to cause injury.

MODERATE RATE FREEZING

Little or no freezeable water
leaves cell. Intracellular ice forms.

SLOW FREEZING

Fig. 13-5. Schematic illustration of the effects on the cell of varying the rate of freezing.

crease the resistance of the cell to damage from that source.

CRYOPROTECTION AGAINST SLOW COOLING

Lovelock's original analysis of the mechanism of glycerol protection for red cells[6] remains essentially unchallengeable. Lovelock showed that red cell injury was proportional to the concentration of extracellular salt and that the function of glycerol was simply that of an antifreeze: to reduce the amount of ice formed at any temperature and, therefore, to reduce the salt concentration. If the glycerol concentration is sufficiently high, insufficient ice will be formed at any temperature to cause cell injury. Obviously, to function as a cryoprotectant on this antifreeze basis, a compound must possess two critical characteristics: First, it must penetrate the cell membrane; otherwise, it will osmotically dehydrate the cell and cause the very injury that it is intended to prevent. Second, the compound must be nontoxic at the relatively high concentrations that are necessary to produce a useful antifreeze effect.

Our own studies have not only confirmed Lovelock's observations regarding glycerol but have shown that a variety of other compounds are equally cryoprotective for slowly frozen red cells, provided the two criteria of permeation and nontoxicity are met.[19] We have shown that ethanol, methanol, dimethyl sulfoxide (DMSO), and ammonium acetate are as effective as glycerol at equiosmolal concentrations as long as the concentrations are less than toxic. These experiments also indicated that none of these compounds increase the resistance of the cell to dehydration since, in every case, hemolysis was proportional to the osmolality of extracellular salt regardless of the cryoprotectant used, its concentration, or the temperature of freezing. Nonpenetrating solutes such as sucrose and polyvinylpyrrolidone (PVP), although possessing cryoprotective properties at accelerated cooling rates, were wholly ineffectual when the cooling was very slow. In fact, they contributed to the cell injury by increasing the extracellular osmolality and the consequent cell dehydration. These experiments support the contention that, at slow cooling rates, known cryoprotectants do not alter the susceptibility of the cell to dehydration but function purely on an antifreeze basis.

CRYOPROTECTION AT ACCELERATED COOLING RATES

As implied in earlier paragraphs, the goal of accelerated rate freezing, generally referred to as controlled rate freezing, is to find a cooling rate that will dehydrate most of the cells sufficiently to prevent intracellular crystallization but not so much as to result in dehydration injury. There are probably three ways by which cryoprotectants can assist in this objective.

The antifreeze properties of penetrating cryoprotectants continue to be useful under kinetic conditions. The higher the concentration of a penetrating cryoprotectant, the less ice will be formed at any temperature, the less dehydration will result, and the greater the possibility of reaching a stabilizing temperature before a damaging extent of dehydration has developed.

Second, the presence of an intracellular solute can reduce the temperature for spontaneous intracellular ice formation. DMSO, when used as a cryoprotectant during controlled rate freezing, is generally used in concentrations betwen 5 and 10 percent (.7 to 1.4 m). Most cells will easily tolerate an extracellular salt osmolality 4 to 5 times isotonic. This means that, with a starting concentration of 1 m DMSO, the cell will tolerate at least a quadrupling of intracellular solute concentration. A 4 m concentration of DMSO will substantially reduce the temperature of spontaneous crystallization and, more importantly, will markedly increase the viscosity of the unfrozen solution, particularly at low temperature. Since crystal growth requires the diffusion of water, an increase in viscosity can inhibit or even prevent crystal growth—even though, in theory, nucleation still can occur. Penetrating compounds like DMSO and glycerol may, therefore, substantially widen the window between too much and too little dehydration by both reducing the extent of dehydration and decreasing the rate of crystal growth.

Yet another effect of cryoprotectants during kinetic freezing is that they shift optimum recovery to a lower cooling velocity. One of the best examples is in red cell freezing. The original rapid freezing procedure reported by Meryman and Kafig[20] in 1954 required that cell suspensions be sprayed in small droplets onto the surface of liquid nitrogen to achieve the optimum cooling rate of approximately 100° C/sec. This impractical procedure was improved upon by Strumia,[21] who was able to reduce the optimum cooling rate by the addition of sugars to one that could be achieved in thin-walled, envelope-shaped metal containers. Unfortunately, the transfusion of sugars at concentrations of the order of 10 to 15 percent caused pulmonary edema, and the technique proved unsatisfactory. Doebbler et al.[22] then showed that PVP still further reduced the optimum cooling velocity but without the problems of excessive osmolality. Rapatz and Luyet[2] have shown that glycerol also reduces the optimum cooling rate for red cells.

All of the compounds that have been reported effective during kinetic freezing substantially increase the viscosity of the unfrozen solution as concentration is increased and temperature decreased. Compounds such as ethanol and methanol, which do not increase solution viscosity, do not affect the optimum cooling velocity. It is probable that the former compounds influence cooling velocity simply by increasing the resistance to water diffusion from the cell to the ice crystal. Clearly, any reduction in the overall diffusion rate of water from the cell to ice will increase the time required to achieve optimum dehydration.

The major advantage in reducing the cooling rate is convenience, but it is also probable that some increase in recovery may result. The higher the cooling velocity, the more difficult it will be to achieve uniformity within the specimen and the more likely it is that portions of the specimen will be cooling too rapidly or too slowly. At a lower cooling rate there is more opportunity for the diffusion of heat through the specimen, and temperature gradients will be lessened.

It is also probable that some compounds, particularly DMSO, may alter the permeability of the cell membrane to water. Such an effect is implied by experience in freezing platelets. The optimum cooling rate for platelets cryoprotected with 5 percent DMSO is between 1° C and 4° C/min.[23] With glycerol at an equimolal concentration, the optimum cooling rate is 30° C/min.[24] The implied difference in water diffusion rates is far greater than can be attributed to any difference in the viscosity of glycerol and DMSO solutions; the most probable interpretation is that the DMSO is increasing the permeability of the membrane to water.

No experiments have been reported which were designed to determine whether cryoprotectants could modify the damaging effects of intracellular ice, and there is no evidence that intracellular ice can be rendered innocuous by the addition of any protective agent.

CRYOPRESERVATION IN PRACTICE

Colligative Cryoprotection

As defined in prior paragraphs, colligative cryoprotection demands the use of a solute which will penetrate the cell membrane and which is not toxic in concentrations sufficiently high to prevent excessive cell dehydration as ice forms. For all practical purposes, glycerol is the only compound that fully meets the toxicity requirement but its use is seriously limited by its relatively low rate of permeation into many cell types. Even when the penetration rate is high, as in red cells, its flux rate will be several orders of magnitude slower than that of water. Because of this, an isotonic salt solution containing added glycerol will transiently appear to a cell as a nonpenetrating solution, and water will leave the cell in response to the total osmotic gradient. As the glycerol slowly comes to equilibrium across the cell membrane, its osmotic effect will diminish. Ultimately, only the nonpenetrating solutes exert long-term osmotic effects and determine the volume of the cell.

It is because of the transient osmotic effects of glycerol, or any other penetrating cryoprotectant, that careful attention must be paid to the process of addition and removal of the agent before and after freezing. To design a glycerolizing and deglycerolizing protocol, two critical parameters must be known: the rate of permeation of the compound and the osmotic tolerance of the cell.

The kinetics of glycerol permeation can be determined using ^{14}C glycerol[25] or, more easily, by observing cell volume change. Knowledge of the kinetics of cryoprotective permeation is essential in order to determine the equilibration times that are necessary during addition and removal of the agent.

It is also essential to explore the response of the cell to hyper- and hypotonic solutions of nonpenetrating solutes in order to establish the limits of cell volume which the cell will tolerate. Most animal cells appear to be able to tolerate hyperosmotic exposure of at least 4 times isotonic. Human platelets have been found to withstand osmolalities 6 times isotonic when held at $-5°C$ supercooled,[26] and Chinese hamster ovary cells can survive suspension in solutions of as much as 10 times isotonic.[27] Human granulocytes, on the other hand, are sensitive to even moderate increases in osmolality.[28]

Figure 13-6 illustrates a glycerolizing protocol for red cells based on the assumption that the cell is tolerant to solutions ranging in osmolality from half isotonic to 4 times isotonic. As this figure indicates, each glycerolizing step can increase the total osmolality of the solution by a factor of 4. With each change of suspending solution, the cell is abruptly decreased in volume; but, as the glycerol slowly penetrates the cell, its volume returns to that dictated by the salt concentration of the suspending medium.

Figure 13-7 illustrates a similar stepwise prodedure for deglycerolizing. Each time the glycerol concentration is reduced, the cell will swell in response to the reduction in total osmolality, and return to isotonicity as the glycerol equilibrates. Since the cell can only tolerate a hypotonic osmolality of half isotonic, each step can reduce the total osmolality by only a factor of two. It is clear that this can be a tedious process. In fact, it was this obstacle[29] that prevented the prompt clinical application of frozen red cells following the publications by Smith[4] and by Lovelock[5, 6] in the 1950s.

It is, however, possible to accelerate substantially the glycerolizing and deglycerolizing process by taking advantage of the full capacity of the cell to swell and shrink. As illustrated in Figure 13-8, if the first resuspension of the cells is into a glycerol solution containing salt at only one-half isotonic, the cells will then subsequently equilibrate at their maximum volume rather than at isotonic volume. The next increase in total osmolality can then be by a factor of 8 rather than 4, and the number of resuspension steps required to achieve full glycerolization can be reduced.

In practice, for the glycerolization of red

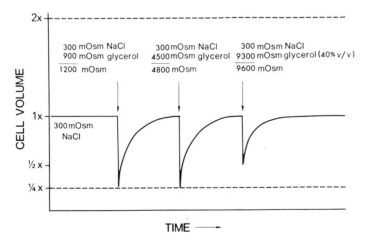

300 mOsm NaCl
900 mOsm glycerol
1200 mOsm

300 mOsm NaCl
4500 mOsm glycerol
4800 mOsm

300 mOsm NaCl
9300 mOsm glycerol (40% v/v)
9600 mOsm

300 mOsm NaCl

Fig. 13-6. Glycerolizing: This figure illustrates the effect on cell volume of transferring the cells into a succession of glycerol solutions, each solution having a total osmolality four times the previous.

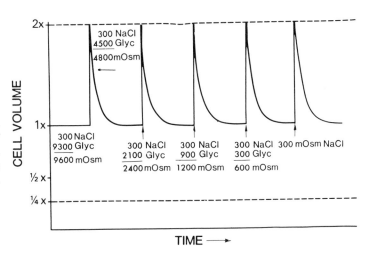

Fig. 13-7. Deglycerolizing: This figure illustrates the effect on cell volume of transferring the cell through a series of glycerol solutions, each one of which has a total osmolality one half of the previous solution. It is necessary to go through five solution changes to deglycerolize cells using this program.

cells, it is inconvenient to use more than one glycerolizing solution. The standard procedure[30] therefore requires that, to glycerolize a unit of red cells, 100 ml of a 6.2 M glycerol solution in isotonic lactate solution be added slowly with vigorous mixing. This is a sufficient quantity of glycerol to raise the extracellular concentration to approximately 1500 mOsm, shrinking the cells but not beyond their limit of tolerance. The suspension is then allowed to equilibrate for several minutes until the cells have reestablished their normal volume. Since the osmolality of the 6.2 M glycerol solution does not now exceed 4 times that of the cell suspension, the remain-

der of the glycerol solution can be added without danger of lysis.

The use of hypertonic salt to simplify deglycerolization yields even more dramatic results. As shown in Figure 13-9, if the first resuspending solution contains salt at a 4 times isotonic osmolality, the cells will come to equilibrium at their minimum safe volume and the next resuspension can then be in a solution of one-eighth the osmolality. In the standard deglycerolizing procedure for red cells, the actual steps are different but the principle remains the same. Thawed cells in equilibrium with approximately 4.5 M glycerol in isotonic lactate solution are diluted

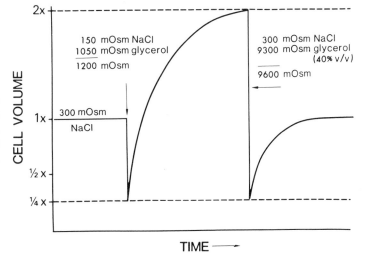

Fig. 13-8. This figure illustrates the fact that adjusting the salt concentration in order to take advantage of the full range of tolerated volume of the cell can reduce the number of steps required for glycerolizing from three (Fig. 13-6) to two.

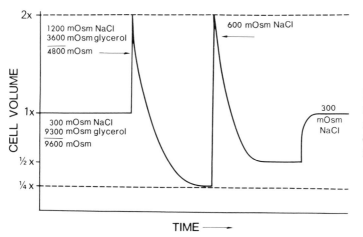

Fig. 13-9. Utilizing the entire range of tolerated volume can reduce the number of steps required for deglycerolization from five (Fig. 13-7) to three.

with 150 ml of 12 percent NaCl. The osmolality of the salt solution is approximately one-half that of the cell suspension so that cells coming into transient contact with this solution will not suffer hypotonic lysis. The quantity of the hypertonic salt solution added is such that after mixing with the cell suspension the total osmolality of the nonpenetrating sodium salts approaches 4 times isotonic. The cell volume is then sufficiently small so that the cells can be washed directly with the 1.6 percent NaCl (500 mOsm) solution—or even, in more recent protocols, directly with isotonic saline.[31] It is the development of this concept of deglycerolizing with a hyperosmotic salt that has transformed the processing of red cells from the several-hour procedure of the 1950s[29] to the 30-minute procedure in general use today.

Kinetic Cryoprotection

One of the great virtues of kinetic cryoprotection is that the concentration of cryoprotectant need not be high and the osmotic obstacles of addition and removal do not approach those experienced in the colligative system. However, even a 5 percent (0.7 M) glycerol solution in isotonic saline cannot be dealt with in cavalier fashion. Since the total osmolality of such a solution will be approximately 1000 mOsm, most cells will easily tolerate transfer to such a solution. However, subsequent resuspension of the cell in isotonic medium can cause it to swell by a factor of more than 3, a stress which many cells will not tolerate. There is no question but that many of the reported failures of cryopreservation may in fact be no more than failures to appreciate the transient osmotic stresses associated with glycerolization and deglycerolization.

There are several cryoprotectants that are valuable in kinetic freezing; the most ubiquitous of these is DMSO, which contributes some colligative protection, increases solution viscosity, and probably reduces the hydraulic permeability of the cell membrane. Concentrations around 5 percent are commonly used. DMSO has the important value of penetrating most cells rapidly at room temperature or above. In the cold, permeation may be very slow. At $0°C$, DMSO penetrates human red cells more slowly than glycerol (unpublished observation). Concentrations above 10 percent (1.4 M) may be toxic.[27]

Glycerol can also be used in the kinetic mode. Its rate of penetration is slow in most cells, and care must be taken in its introduction and removal. Certain extracellular agents are also useful, although probably only to reduce the cooling rate for optimum recovery. Commonly used are PVP, HES,

Dextran, and albumin. Sugars and sugar alcohols can serve a similar function, but the concentrations at which they can be used are limited by their osmotic effects.

One potential drawback to the kinetic approach is the requirement for a controlled rate of cooling. Where the optimum rate of cooling is of the order of 1°/min, freezing does not pose a major obstacle. In fact, it is often possible by trial and error to find a combination of container geometry and insulation that will result in the desired freezing rate when the specimen is simply placed into a freezer. On the other hand, when freezing rates are more demanding, controlled rate freezing devices may be required. Another problem encountered at accelerated cooling rates will be the lack of uniformity throughout the specimen. This will be particularly true of a large specimen, where cooling rates throughout the interior may differ widely.[32] It may be impossible to cool all of the specimen at anything close to the optimum rate.

An alternate and in some ways preferable procedure is the two-step freezing method. This was described first by Sakai,[33] then rediscovered and exploited by McGann and Farrant.[34] In the two-step procedure, the specimen is rapidly cooled, usually by direct immersion in a cold bath, to some intermediate temperature of the order of −10°C to −30°C. As long as the temperature is above the homogeneous nucleation temperature of around −40°C, no intracellular freezing will take place. Because the cooling is rapid, ice will be well distributed throughout the extracellular spaces. The specimen is then held at the intermediate temperature while cell dehydration proceeds. At the critical moment, presumably just before cell dehydration is sufficient to cause injury, the specimen is transferred to liquid nitrogen temperature. By empirically optimizing the intermediate temperature and the holding time, survival at least equivalent to controlled rate freezing can be obtained. The procedure has the advantage that controlled-rate freezing apparatus is not required and, more important, better uniformity in thermal history throughout the specimen can often be attained.

Choice of Method

The nature of the specimen very frequently dictates whether the colligative or the kinetic approach should be used. The colligative requires either successive transfers of the cells from one solution to another as the cryoprotectant concentration is increased or decreased, or else some means of restraining the cells while the suspending solution is changed. In many situations this is impractical. With platelets, for example, progressive dilution of the suspension to alter the glycerol concentration results in sample volumes that become unmanageable. Centrifugation, on the other hand, to remove excess suspending solution leads to the loss of cells so that only the kinetic approach appears to be feasible for platelets.

It is fortunate that red cells are relatively tolerant to centrifugation. For red cells, the optimum cooling rate for kinetic freezing is of the order of 100°C per second, a rate that could only be achieved with bulk blood by spraying it onto the surface of liquid nitrogen.[20] To reduce the cooling velocity to a feasible rate permitting the use of closed containers, the addition of quite high concentrations of sugars[21] or of polymers such as PVP[22] or HES[35] is necessary. These agents however, create problems in transfusion, as is true of virtually every other known cryoprotectant with the exception of glycerol. Red cells represent one of the few systems frozen as a cell suspension in which colligative freezing with a high concentration of glycerol is superior to a kinetic approach. A "low glycerol" red cell freezing procedure, using approximately 20 percent glycerol, has been reported.[34a] However, this reduction in glycerol concentration is not sufficient to permit much simplification in the deglycerolizing procedure.

Kidney cryopreservation is an example of a situation where colligative cryoprotection is almost obligatory. The large mass of the organ makes it difficult to achieve a uniform cooling rate throughout unless the rate is extremely low. Rapid thawing is equally difficult. This then means that high concentrations of glycerol must be built up in the organ by perfusion before freezing can be contemplated. However, although concentrations of 3 to 4 M glycerol may prevent cell damage from dehydration, ice formation is not prevented. While extracellular ice may be innocuous for a cell suspension, interstitial or intravascular ice may not be for an organized tissue, and the cryopreservation of organs represents a particularly difficult challenge.

CRYOPRESERVATION OF BLOOD CELLS

Red Cells

Three different approaches to red cell cryopreservation are currently available for clinical use. One of these,[36] used by the American Red Cross, is based on the original procedure of Smith,[4] using approximately 40 percent glycerol in isotonic salt. Because of the high concentration of glycerol, cells frozen by this method are stable at any temperature and even rather prolonged freezer failure can be tolerated.[25] The rates of freezing and of thawing are not critical, storage at -65° C or below provides very long term stability and shipping in dry ice is feasible. The principal disadvantages of this method lie in the introduction and removal of the high concentration of glycerol, although recent developments in deglycerolizing apparatus have made it possible to deglycerolize in less than 30 minutes using only two wash solutions.[31]

Because of the magnitude of the obstacles of glycerolization and deglycerolization during the late 1950s and 1960s, two other approaches were developed in an attempt to circumvent some of the problems. One of these, the so-called low glycerol procedure,

achieves cryoprotection with 20 percent glycerol in isotonic salt instead of 40 percent.[33] However, since this is an insufficient concentration to afford complete protection during slow freezing, an accelerated freezing rate is necessary. The principal disadvantage of this method is that both freezing and storage in liquid nitrogen are mandatory.

The second method is the ingenious agglomeration procedure devised by Huggins.[37] This method uses a high concentration of glycerol but in glucose-fructose rather than salt. After thawing, the cells are diluted with hypertonic glucose followed by isotonic fructose solution. In the presence of this low-ionic, low-pH solution, the cells agglomerate into large clumps and sink spontaneously to the bottom of the container. The supernatant solution can be expelled and the cells rediluted to repeat the process. Following the agglomeration procedure, the cells are resuspended in isotonic saline, which reverses the clumping. The cells are then sedimented in a centrifuge, and the excess solution is discarded. Like the Red Cross method, this procedure has the advantage of not requiring liquid nitrogen. However, the cells are not as stable at higher temperatures, and freezer failures are not well tolerated.[35a]

The clinical quality of red cells processed by all three methods is equally good. The recovery of cells processed by agglomeration is slightly less than with the other systems because of the loss of cells that fail to agglomerate.[35a] The agglomeration procedure takes substantially longer to complete than with the other methods. On the other hand, a technician with multiple stations can process more units by agglomeration than by the other methods. Detailed protocols of all three methods have been published.[33, 36, 37]

It is unlikely that there will be any radical new developments in red cell freezing during the next several years. We have reported a modification of the freezing technique that permits the freezing of the cells as packed cells.[31] This reduces storage volume, somewhat simplifies the deglycerolizing procedure, and permits manual deglycerolization in a clinical centrifuge. Valeri has recently described a similar procedure.[38] We have also reported[39] a modification of the technique used by Chaplin and Mollison in 1955 which permits storage at −20° C to −30° C.[40] Our modification consists in adding adenine, isosine, and pyruvate to the glycerol solution to support cell metabolism during storage rather than attempt to rejuvenate the cells following thawing as originally reported by Chaplin et al.[29] We are also aware of preliminary experiments in the application of ultrafiltration[41] and of electroosmosis[42] as novel approaches to deglycerolization. However, neither of these techniques has yet been proven effective and it cannot be predicted whether, even if effective, they would offer significant advantages in either cost or speed of processing.

The possibility of using a kinetic freezing approach with a sufficiently low concentration of clinically acceptable protectant so that the thawed cells can be infused without further processing continues to be an elusive goal. The original procedure which we reported in the 1950s[20] required that the cell suspension be sprayed onto the surface of liquid nitrogen in order to achieve the very high rate of cooling necessary for acceptable recovery. The procedure was clearly impractical for routine clinical use. Subsequent improvements consisted primarily in changes in cryoprotectant in order to reduce the optimum cooling rate to one that could be achieved within a closed container. As mentioned earlier, the use by Strumia[21] of higher sugar concentrations led to osmotic problems. The substitution of PVP by Doebbler et al.[22] gave good recoveries at feasible cooling rates; however, the demonstration that PVP accumulated in the reticular endothelial system and was neither completely excreted nor metabolized led to concern regarding its long term safety. Hydroxyethyl starch was subsequently substituted for PVP, yielding equally good recoveries.[35]

Freezing methods using either of these polymers have been plagued by intravascular hemolysis of the order of 5 to 15 percent. This was recently explained by Williams,[43] who showed that PVP, HES, and dextran in cryoprotective concentrations could prevent the loss of hemoglobin through membrane defects by modifying the interfacial tensions between the hemoglobin and the suspending medium. However, this is a temporary bandaid; although damaged cells may fail to lose all of their hemoglobin in the presence of the polymers, when the polymer is diluted by transfusion, lysis goes to completion.[19] Another problem with the one-step method using HES is the viscosity of the cell suspension which makes transfusion a lengthy process. It is probable that the one-step approach will not be competitive with existing methods, barring some radical new development.

Platelets

For more than a decade, platelets have been cryopreserved using the kinetic approach with DMSO.[23] The procedures used have all been empirical and differ one from another only in minor details. In general, the concentration of DMSO ranges from 4 to 6 percent with a cooling rate between 1° C and 4° C/min. Recoveries of circulating platelets range from 40 to 70 percent of control. The principal problems with this procedure are related to the DMSO itself. Questions regarding its toxicity have never been fully resolved. Following the infusion of DMSO, patients produce an unpleasant odor. If quantities much in excess of a gram are administered, patients display symptoms of dizziness, nausea, and vomiting. For this reason, it is necessary to reduce the DMSO concentration to a minimum following thawing, and all protocols currently in use require a sedimentation and resuspension step, which can be a major cause of cell loss. The final quantity of DMSO remaining in the infused sample is of the order of 15 mg/unit, and recipient odor is reported not to be a problem with the usual platelet transfusion. Platelets cryopreserved by such a method are reported to be clinically effective.[44]

In 1976, Dayian and Rowe reported promising results with a preservation method using glycerol.[24] The original method reported by Dayian and Rowe suffered from a high degree of variability in recovery. However, a more recent report by Dayian and Pert,[45] who introduced modifications of the freezing bag and freezing procedure, suggests that the unreliability of the earlier method has been overcome and that there is some reason for optimism that a usable procedure will be available shortly. The glycerol procedure has the disadvantage of requiring liquid nitrogen for freezing and storage; but, it has the very considerable advantage of using a clinically acceptable cryoprotectant that need not be removed prior to administration. Cells frozen with glycerol can be directly administered after dilution and a brief period of incubation following thawing.

Granulocytes

Granulocytes have so far proven to be particularly refractory to cryopreservation. One contributing factor is probably the relative intolerance of the cell to osmotic stress. Luyet and Menz[28] reported the destruction of granulocytes in plasma concentrated by freezing to only twice isotonic, and we have confirmed this observation. Since hypertonic suspension is an unavoidable consequence of freezing, it is not surprising that the conventional empirical approaches have been unsuccessful. The literature is a litany of promising reports based on in vitro assays followed by either silence or retractions when more sophisticated assays were employed.[46] Most recently, Lionetti and colleagues have reported excellent recoveries of baboon granulocytes.[47] The cells are frozen in the presence of DMSO, HES, and albumin and a variety of quite demanding in vitro assays suggest a recovery of

the order of 70 percent. In vivo studies have yet to be reported.

Bone Marrow

So far, the freezing of bone marrow has been restricted to material destined for autologous transplantation, since a period of preservation is unnecessary when allogeneic transplants from a living donor are employed. The cryopreservation of bone marrow appears to be an example of a purely empirical approach that worked the first time. Several investigators have reported cryopreservation protocols, all of which use DMSO at concentrations between 5 and 10 percent with freezing at a rate of around $1°C/min$.[48, 49] The frozen marrow is stored in liquid nitrogen, rapidly thawed in warm water and infused without further processing. It is interesting that none of the methods makes any serious attempt to minimize osmotic stresses during the addition of DMSO nor, in some of the protocols, is there any attempt made to reduce the concentration of DMSO prior to infusion in order to minimize the hypotonic stresses attending sudden dilution. This implies a particular tolerance on the part of the stem cells to osmotic stresses, an adequate explanation for the apparent ease with which they are frozen. On the other hand, excessive cooling rates are still destructive. In unpublished experiments of our own conducted at Yale Medical School in 1955, mouse marrow which was droplet-frozen in liquid nitrogen failed to protect lethally irradiated litter mates.

One interesting application of cryopreservation may well be the freezing of allogeneic marrow with the intent of exercising some selection over the types of cells that are preserved. On the assumption that graft-versus-host disease is the result of the transplantation of partially or completely differentiated cells of the lymphocytic series, the goal of selectively destroying these cells while preserving the pluripotent stem cell could possibly be achieved by manipulating the conditions of freezing. Since the cooling rate for optimum recovery has been shown to vary from one cell type to another, this raises the possibility that careful adjustment and control of cooling rate might be a mechanism of selection. In the past, freezing was generally used either to obtain total destructin of all cells, as in cryosurgery, or to preserve a single cell type, with the preservation or destruction of other accompanying cells left to chance. Deliberate attempts to exploit the differences between cells as a means of cell selection could be a new and potentially useful application of cryobiology.

ACKNOWLEDGMENT

Contribution No. 483 from the American Red Cross Blood Services–Bethesda. Supported in part by NIH Grant No. GM 17959.

REFERENCES

1. Luyet, B.J. and Gehenio, P.M.: Life and death at low temperatures. Normancy, Mo:Biodynamica, 1940.
2. Rapatz, G. and Luyet, B.: Effects of cooling rates on the preservation of erythrocytes in frozen glycerolated blood. Biodynamica 9:125, 1963.
3. Polge, C., Smith, A.U., and Parkes, A.S.: Revival of spermatozoa after vitrification and dehydration at low temperatures. Nature (Lond.) 164:666, 1949.
4. Smith, A.U.: Prevention of haemolysis during freezing and thawing of red blood cells. Lancet 2:910, 1950.
5. Lovelock, J.E.: The haemolysis of human red blood cells by freezing and thawing. Biochim. Biophys. Acta 10:414, 1953.
6. Lovelock, J.E.: The mechanism of the protective action of glycerol against haemolysis by freezing and thawing. Biochim. biophys. Acta. 11:28, 1953.
7. Mazur, P. and Schmidt, J.: Interactions of cooling velocity, temperature, and warming

velocity on the survival of frozen and thawed yeast. Cryobiology 5:1, 1968.
8. Rapatz, G., Sullivan, J.J., and Luyet, B.: Preservation of erythrocytes in blood containing various cryoprotective agents, frozen at various rates and brought to a given final temperature. Cryobiology 5:18, 1968.
9. Mazur, P., Leibo, S.P., and Chu, E.H.Y.: A two-factor hypothesis of freezing injury. Exp. Cell. Res. 71:345, 1972.
10. Mazur, P.: The role of cell membranes in the freezing of yeast and other single cells. Ann. N.Y. Acad. Sci. 125:658, 1965.
11. Meryman, H.T.: Osmotic stress as a mechanism of freezing injury. Cryobiology 8:489, 1971.
12. Williams, R.J. and Hope, H.J.: The relationship betwen cell injury and osmotic volume reduction: III. Freezing injury and frost resistance in winter wheat. Cryobiology. (In Press.)
13. Williams, R.J. and Willemot, C.: The relationship between cell injury and osmotic volume reduction: IV. The behavior of hardy wheat membrane lipids in monolayer. Cryobiology. (In Press.)
14. Meryman, H.T.: A modified model for the mechanism of freezing injury in erythrocytes. Nature 218:333, 1968.
15. Baker, H.: The intracellular pressure of *Nitella* in hypertonic solutions and its relationship to freezing injury. Cryobiology 9:283, 1972.
16. Williams, R.J. and Takahashi, T.: Evidence for injurious surface pressures developing in the membranes of osmotically stressed sea urchin eggs. Cryobiology 15:688, 1978.
17. Mazur, P.: Kinetics of water loss from cells at subzero temperatures and the likelihood of intracellular freezing. J. Gen. Physiol. 47:347, 1963.
18. Leibo, S.P. and Mazur, P.: The role of cooling rates in low-temperature preservation. Cryobiology 8:447, 1971.
19. Meryman, H.T., Williams, R.J., and Douglas, M.: Freezing injury from "solution effects" and its prevention by natural or artificial cryoprotection. Cryobiology 14:287, 1977.
20. Meryman, H.T. and Kafig, E.: Rapid freezing and thawing of whole blood. Proc. Soc. Exp. Biol. and Med. 90:587, 1955.
21. Strumia, M.M., Colwell, L.S., and Strumia, P.V.: In vitro recovery after freezing and

thawing of red cells modified with sugars. J. Lab. Clln. Med. 56:576, 1960.

22. Doebbler, G.F., Rowe, A.W., and Rinfret, A.P.: Freezing of mammaliana blood and its constituents. In: Cryobiology. Meryman, H.T., Ed. Academic Press, London, 1966, p. 407.

23. Meryman, H.T. and Burton, J.L.: Cryopreservation of platelets. In: The Blood Platelet in Transfusion Therapy. Greenwalt, T.J. and Jamieson, G.A., Eds. Alan R. Liss, New York, 1978, p. 153.

24. Dayian, G. and Rowe, A.W.: Cryopreservation of human platelets for transfusion. A glycerol-glucose, moderate rate cooling procedure. Cryobiology 13:1, 1976.

25. Meryman, H.T.: The cryopreservation of blood cells for clinical use. In: Progress in Hematology. Brown, E.B., Ed. Grune & Stratton, New York, 1979, p. 193.

26. Kahn, R.A. and Meryman, H.T.: The effects of various solutes on platelets exposed to hypertonic stress. Am. J. Physiol. 225:77, 1973.

27. Mironescu, S.: Hyperosmotic injury in mammalian cells. III. Volume and alkali cation alterations of CHO cells in unprotected and DMSO-treated cultures. Cryobiology 15:178, 1978.

28. Luyet, B. and Menz, L.: Effects of freezing on peripheral leukocytes. Biodynamica 10:241, 1969.

29. Chaplin, H., Crawford, H., and Cutbush, M., et al.: Post-transfusion survival of red cells stored at −20°C. Lancet 1:852, 1954.

30. Meryman, H.T. and Hornblower, M.: A method for freezing and washing red blood cells using a high glycerol concentration. Transfusion 12:145, 1972.

31. Meryman, H.T. and Hornblower, M.: A simplified procedure for deglycerolizing red cells frozen in a high glycerol concentration. Transfusion 17:438, 1977.

32. Meryman, H.T.: Review of biological freezing. In: Cryobiology. Meryman, H.T., Ed. Academic Press, London, 1966, pp. 25–48.

33. Sakai, A.: Survival of plant tissue at super-low temperatures by rapid cooling and rewarming. Proc. Int. Conf. Low Temp Sci., Univ. Hokkaido 2:119, 1967.

34. McGann, L.E. and Farrant, J.: Survival of tissue culture cells frozen by a two-step procedure to −196°C. I. Holding temperature and time. Cryobiology 13:261, 1976.

34a. Rowe, A.W.: Preservation of blood by the low glycerol-rapid freeze process. In: Red Cell Freezing: A Technical Workshop. Valeri, C.R., Ed. American Association of Blood Banks, Washington, D.C., 1973, p. 55.

35. Knorpp, C.T., Merchant, W.R., and Gikas, P.W. et al.: Hydroxyethyl starch: Extracellular cryophylactic agent for erythrocytes. Science 157:1312, 1967.

35a. Hornblower, M. and Meryman, H.T.: Relative efficiency and interchangeability of Huggins and American Red Cross red cell freezing procedures. Transfusion 17:417–425, 1977.

36. Meryman, H.T.: A high glycerol red cell freezing method. In: Red Cell Freezing: A Technical Workshop. Valeri, C.R., et al., Ed. Washington, D.C., 1973, p. 73.

37. Huggins, C.E.: Practical preservation of blood by freezing. In: Red Cell Freezing: A Technical Workshop. Valeri, C.R., et al., Ed. American Association of Blood Banks, Washington, D.C., 1973, p. 31.

38. Valeri, C.R., Valeri, D.A. and Anastasi, J., et al.: A new system for freezing red blood cells: Higher quality at lower cost. Transfusion 18:633, 1978.

39. Meryman, H.T.: Advances in red cell freezing. Transfusion 18:632, 1978.

40. Chaplin, H. and Mollison, P.L.: Improved storage of red cells at −20°C. Lancet 1:215, 1953.

41. Castino, F., Van Reis, R., and Daniels, J., et al.: The deglycerolization of frozen, thawed RBC by filtration. Transfusion 19:651, 1979.

42. Zellman, A. (personal communication)

43. Williams, R.J.: A proposed mechanism for PVP cryoprotection. Cryobiology 13:653, 1976.

44. Schiffer, C.A., Aisner, J., and Wiernik, P.H.: Frozen autologous platelet transfusion for patients with leukemia. N. Engl. J. Med. 299:7, 1978.

45. Dayian, G. and Pert, J.H.: A simplified method for freezing human blood platelets in glycerol-glucose using a statically controlled cooling rate device. Transfusion 19:255, 1979.

46. Meryman, H.T. and Howard, J.: Cryopreservation of granulocytes. In: The Granulocyte. Greenwalt, T.J. and Jamieson, G.A., Eds. Alan R. Liss, New York, 1976, p. 193.

47. Lionetti, F.J., Hunt, S.M., and Mattaliano, R.J.: In vitro studies of cryopreserved baboon granulocytes. Transfusion 18:685, 1978.

48. Adamson, J.W. and Storb, R.: The proliferative potential of frozen stored human marrow cells. Transplantation 14:490, 1972.

49. Lewis, P.L., Passovoy, M., and Conti, A., et al.: The effect of cooling regimens on the transplantation potential of marrow. Transfusion 7:17, 1967.

14

Clinical Uses of Frozen-Stored Red Blood Cells

Hugh Chaplin, Jr., M.D.

INTRODUCTION

The term "frozen blood" is a misnomer commonly applied to packed red blood cells (RBC) that have been mixed with a cryopreservative solution, stored frozen, then thawed and washed free of the cryopreservative. Thus, "frozen-stored RBC" is a preferable term and will be used throughout this chapter. Similar techniques (with important modifications) have been applied to the frozen storage of platelets (see Ch. 27), bone marrow cells, and various populations of peripheral blood leukocytes; these will be referred to only briefly, since their application is largely investigative at the present time.

The possibility for more-or-less indefinite preservation of living tissue, long a preoccupation of science fiction, became a reality with respect to human RBC largely as the result of studies in the late 1940s on the frozen preservation of vinegar eels and fowl spermatozoa.[1,2] Cryobiologists hypothesized that the usually fatal effects of freezing were in some way related to damage by intracellular ice crystal formation, denaturation of proteins by high-solute concentrations, and osmotic stresses during the freezing and thawing processes. While the precise nature of freeze-thaw damage is still not completely understood, it became clear that various penetrating and nonpenetrating solvents could protect single cells from irreversible freeze-thaw damage if careful attention were given to the concentration of the solvent and of the accompanying buffer salts, as well as to rates of freezing and thawing and the ultimate temperature at which the cells were stored.

The solvent almost universally employed for RBC cryopreservation is glycerol, chosen from among a variety of polyhydric alcohols because of its effectiveness in preventing freeze-thaw damage and because of its established low toxicity following parenteral administration to humans. "High glycerol" concentrations (about 40 percent w/v) are employed when freezing is relatively slow and the storage temperature relatively high—e.g., $-80°C$ in a mechanical freezer. "Low glycerol" concentrations (about 20 percent w/v) may be employed when RBC are quick-frozen by direct immersion in liquid nitrogen ($-192°C$) and stored at relatively low temperatures—e.g., in the gas phase of liquid nitrogen at $-150°C$. After thawing, the intracellular glycerol must be reduced to <1 to 2 percent to prevent osmotic lysis of the RBC on introduction into the recipient's circulation. Glycerol removal is accomplished by a variety of dilutional washing procedures employing a series of progressively less hypertonic buffered crystalloid and sugar solutions. Deglycerolization utilizes one or another specially designed machines for introduction and removal of the wash solutions—e.g., serial batch centrifugation, continuous flow centrifugation, cytoagglomeration. The above details are mentioned briefly to emphasize that *"frozen-stored RBC" cannot be considered a uniform product and can be expected to vary in a number of essential characteristics depending on particulars of the cryopreservative conditions employed for its production.*

CHARACTERISTICS OF FROZEN-STORED RBC

As indicated in the preceding paragraph, products designated as frozen-stored RBC will differ depending on preparative methods employed for their production. However, certain generalizations are useful in comparing frozen-stored RBC to whole blood or packed RBC derived from whole blood.

Viable RBC Content

Incident to the numerous procedures outlined above, 10 to 15 percent of the RBC present in the original donor unit is lost en route to the final product. Freeze-thaw lysis accounts for less than ⅓ of the loss; mechanical losses in the numerous transfers from original container to freezing container, then to the washing device, then to the final container, plus additional osmotic lysis and overflow of RBC during washing account for most of the loss. The 24-hour in vivo survival of RBC transfused within 24 hours of thawing has been extensively documented and is within 85 to 90 percent. The extremely important concept of "index of therapeutic effectiveness"[3] combines the in vitro and in vivo losses to indicate that the content of *viable* RBC in a unit of frozen-stored RBC is equivalent to approximately 75 percent of the RBC present in the original fresh whole blood unit.

Platelet and Leukocyte Content

Conditions optimal for preservation and recovery of nonnucleated RBC are not optimal for nucleated cells (leukocytes) and for platelets. The numbers of intact leukocytes and platelets remaining in frozen-stored RBC will vary from 1 to 5 percent of those present in the original donor unit[4]; a small amount of leukocyte and platelet "debris" can also be identified but is impossible to quantify in terms of the intact components from which it is derived. Most of the recovered leukocytes and platelets are believed to be nonviable; but the presence of a proportion of viable leukocytes (principally lymphocytes) has been definitely established.[5]

Plasma Content

Studies employing radiolabeled serum proteins added to the original donor unit have demonstrated approximately 0.025 percent of residual plasma in the final product.[6] It must be emphasized that residual plasma will depend importantly on the amount of plasma present in the mixture originally frozen (i.e., the amount present with the RBC to which the cryopreservative solution was added) and on the volume of wash solutions and dilutional kinetics of the washing procedure employed for deglycerolization. If future modifications in deglycerolization employ smaller volumes of wash solutions (with attendant reductions in cost and time required for washing), it may be expected that the percent of residual donor plasma will increase.

Supernatant Hemoglobin

Within 4 hours of deglycerolization, supernatant hemoglobin concentrations are in the range of 50 to 100 mg per dl—i.e., 2 to 4 times that present in liquid stored blood; by 24 hours postdeglycerolization, supernatant hemoglobin concentrations have increased a further 2- to 6-fold.[6]

Residual Glycerol

Glycerol concentrations in the final product are <2 percent w/v, and generally <1 percent w/v.[6]

RBC 2,3-DPG and ATP

These will vary depending on their concentration in the RBC immediately prior to freezing. If absolutely fresh donor blood has been employed, 2,3-DPG and ATP concentrations in the frozen-stored RBC will be at least 90 percent of normal.[7] If the donor units have been stored for several days prior to processing for frozen storage, 2,3-DPG and ATP concentrations will have declined by predictable amounts, depending on the preservative solution originally employed (e.g., ACD, CPD, CPD-adenine). A further loss of up to 10 percent of the prefreeze values may be expected in the frozen-stored RBC product. Concentrations of 2,3-DPG and ATP are essentially stable during refrigerated storage for 24 hours following deglycerolization. It should be noted that RBC severely depleted of 2,3-DPG and ATP by prolonged liquid storage of whole blood or packed RBC may be restored to near normal concentrations by incubation with "rejuvenating" solutions (containing pyruvate, inosine, glucose, phosphate, and adenine) prior to glycerolization.[8] In current RBC freezing practice, use of relatively fresh donor blood has precluded the necessity for prefreeze "rejuvenation."

Sterility and Shelf Life

Under existing U.S. Bureau of Biologics requirements, once a product under liquid storage at 4 to 10° C has been entered (i.e., the bacteriological seal has been broken), the product must be transfused within 24 hours. Since current cryopreservation procedures involve multiple entries and transfers, a 24-hour shelf life has been imposed, and units not transfused within that period must be discarded. Numerous bacteriological studies on frozen-stored RBC have revealed a very low incidence of contamination.[9,10] However, in any center processing a large number of frozen units, occasional units demonstrate a crack in the plastic storage container, presumably due to its brittle state at extreme low temperatures; such units are discarded and are generally not cultured. Several manufacturers are working on designs for "sterile docking devices"[11]; if these devices prove reliable in prohibiting bacterial contamination associated with container entries, it should be possible to extend the shelf life beyond 24 hours, with attendant major logistic advantages.

Cost

It is evident that frozen storage incurs substantial additional costs related to technician salaries, plastic softwares, cryoprotective and washing solutions, refrigerants, special refrigerators, and mechanical washing devices, plus the increased space required if this technology is utilized on a large scale. Current estimates place the cost to the patient of one unit of frozen-stored RBC at 2 to 3 times the cost of a unit of whole blood or packed RBC.

Recapitulation

Frozen-stored RBC have an "index of therapeutic effectiveness" equivalent to approximately 75 percent of the RBC present in the original fresh donor unit. The final product generally contains less than 5 percent of the original donor platelets and leukocytes, most of which are nonviable; residual donor plasma is generally <0.025 percent of that present originally. Supernatant hemoglobin is in the range of 50 to 200 mg/dl and glycerol is generally <1 percent w/v. RBC 2,3-DPG and ATP concentrations are near normal. One unit of frozen-stored RBC costs the patient 2 to 3 times the cost of one unit of whole blood or packed RBC. Because of multiple entries during processing, the shelf life is currently restricted to 24 hours. Because cryopreservation techniques are not standardized, frozen-stored RBC cannot be considered a uniform product; variations and modifications in details of processing may result in significant alterations in one or more of the product characteristics outlined above.

COMMON ARGUMENTS FAVORING EXPANDED USE OF FROZEN-STORED RBC

Those who enthusiastically support expanded use of frozen-stored RBC usually stress the following points.

1. Frozen storage assures the availability of rare bloods to supply the transfusion needs of patients who are sensitized to high-incidence blood group antigens. Frozen storage also permits such patients, when they are not anemic, to donate their own blood for subsequent autotransfusion should they need it in the future.

2. Because of the near-normal RBC 2,3-DPG and ATP, frozen-stored RBC are superior for oxygen transport and delivery compared to liquid stored RBC units that have been stored more than 1 week prior to transfusion.

3. Frozen-stored RBC constitute the "purest" RBC product available in relation to their low contents of residual donor platelets, leukocytes and plasma, thereby fulfilling the cardinal principle of component therapy—namely, to transfuse only the blood product(s) that the patient definitively needs.

4. Posttransfusion hepatitis is reported to be significantly less frequent following transfusions of frozen-stored RBC, presumably because of their markedly reduced content of residual donor plasma.

5. For the same reason, frozen-stored RBC is the component of choice for administration to those rare patients who experience transfusion-associated anaphylactic reactions secondary to antibodies directed against donor IgA gobulin.

6. Sensitization to histocompatibility and other leukocyte and platelet antigens occurs less frequently following transfusions of frozen-stored RBC, which may be important in relation to subsequent kidney and bone marrow graft survival. Furthermore, patients who are already sensitized to leukocyte and platelet antigens and who experience distressing febrile reactions following transfusions of whole blood or packed RBC will tolerate transfusions of frozen-stored RBC with little or no fever and associated symptoms.

7. Frozen-stored red cells are a practical, albeit expensive, means of inventory control as a safeguard during periods of severe blood shortages.

UNDESIRABLE CHARACTERISTICS OF FROZEN-STORED RBC

Frozen-stored RBC compare unfavorably with whole blood or packed RBC in the following respects.

1. They are cumbersome to prepare and therefore cannot be made available as quickly as liquid stored blood.

2. Their unit cost to the patient is 2 to 3 times that of whole blood or packed RBC, for the reasons outlined previously.

3. Their index of therapeutic effectiveness is only 75 percent that of fresh blood—i.e., they compare with liquid stored blood that is nearing its storage expiration date.

4. The 24-hour shelf life limits flexibility in assignment to other patients in the event a frozen-stored RBC unit is not transfused to the originally designated patient. The short shelf life also limits possibilities for interhospital and intercity shipment.

5. Because of the multiple container transfers required during processing, there is enhanced danger of inaccurate donor identifi-

cation compared to liquid-stored blood which is transfused from the original container into which blood was drawn from the donor.

6. A number of minor drawbacks include the occasional coating of RBC by the fourth component of complement (and to a lesser extent the third) during glycerolization of RBC from donors with modestly elevated cold agglutinin titers; the bound C4 may cause problems in the major indirect antiglobulin test crossmatch when polyspecific antiglobulin-sera are employed.[12] Furthermore, unsatisfactory RBC recovery has sometimes been noted when RBC from donors with G-6-PD deficiency or with sickle cell trait are subjected to frozen storage procedures. It is therefore probably wise to prescreen donor units for these erythrocyte abnormalities so as to exclude them from frozen storage.

FURTHER CONSIDERATION OF ALLEGED ADVANTAGES OF FROZEN-STORED RBC

Rare Donor Red Cells

The capability of frozen storage to assure the availability of rare donor RBC cannot be questioned and is universally accepted as a uniquely valuable feature of cryopreservation technology. Rare donor RBC frozen storage depots have been established in major centers throughout the United States. When rare donor RBC are required for transfusion, the depot responds by providing the frozen-stored RBC directly if the patient is within a few hours driving distance; otherwise the frozen unit is shipped under refrigeration to the deglycerolization facility nearest the patient. The technology is ideally suited to permitting such a sensitized patient, during periods when his hemoglobin is normal, to establish a frozen storage "bank account" of his own blood which can be used for autotransfusion should a subsequent need arise. A good example would be the sensitized patient suffering from recurrent massive gastrointes-

tinal or urinary tract hemorrhage, or a sensitized patient for whom major surgery is a likely future possibility. Blood drawn into standard donor anticoagulant solution is transported promptly (at $4°$ C) to the nearest RBC freezing facility, where plasma and RBC are frozen separately and stored until one or both are needed. Recently, this procedure has also been utilized for some patients with autoimmune hemolytic anemia in remission for reinfusion should relapse occur[13] (see Ch. 31).

2,3-DPG and ATP

The importance of the near-normal 2,3-DPG and ATP of frozen RBC is less clear. It is known that low 2,3-DPG levels are restored to near normal within 6 to 24 hours of transfusion.[14] The Vietnam War provided the opportunity for a vast experience using 2,3-DPG and ATP depleted liquid-stored RBC for massive transfusion to seriously wounded service men.[15] Collins was unable to demonstrate any deficiency in oxygen delivery to the tissues in young battle casualties who received 2 or 3 blood volume exchanges of low 2,3-DPG red cells.[16] Additional mechanisms almost certainly helped to improve oxygen delivery in this young male population; for example, increased cardiac output and a right shift of the oxygen dissociation curve associated with commonly concurrent acidosis. Chronically ill and older patients with impaired pulmonary function and/or heart failure would certainly be more susceptible to impaired oxygen delivery than otherwise healthy servicemen. Frozen-stored RBC, with their normal oxygen affinity, would seem preferable to 2,3-DPG depleted liquid-stored RBC for massive transfusion to such patients. Nevertheless, Weisel[17] found no evidence of impairment of oxygen transport in the first 24-hour period postoperatively in high-risk, elderly patients (average age 70 years) despite the stress of major surgery. It msut be remembered that there is nothing uniquely superior about frozen-stored RBC in the circumstances under discussion; if there is an indication for blood with near-normal 2,3-DPG and ATP, reasonably fresh liquid-stored RBC will be equally suitable and will generally be available.

Hepatitis

The claim of a reduced incidence of posttransfusion hepatitis after frozen-stored RBC is based largely on retrospective and uncontrolled studies[18] and is difficult to evaluate. Remarkably, there has been only a single prospective study reported.[19] Evidence for hepatitis was found in 4 of 104 recipients of 442 units of whole blood or packed RBC, as compared to none of 110 recipients of 623 units of frozen-stored RBC. The numbers are small, and the study employed only one of the various deglycerolization washing procedures (continuous-flow centrifugation). A retrospective review of approximately 3000 frozen-stored RBC transfusions to 88 patients on a renal dialysis unit supports a reduced risk of hepatitis,[20] but conditions of the study do not permit definite conclusions. More recently, Haugen[21] reported on a series of 31,-125 transfusions (excluding platelets and plasma), 78 percent of which were given in the form of frozen or washed red cells. These transfusions were associated with 56 cases of hepatitis, almost all of which were overt. In 37 cases, the recipients had received only frozen or washed red cells (or both). As others have emphasized,[22,23] this is certain to be an underestimate of the total number of cases of hepatitis, since the number of subclinical cases exceeds the number of overt cases by at least five to one.

It is clear from the chimpanzee experiments of Alter et al.[24] that known infected units of whole blood are not rendered noninfectious by frozen storage; four of four animals developed unequivocal hepatitis B infection following transfusion with frozen-stored RBC prepared from experimentally infected human blood, of which two units were deglycerolized by serial batch centrifugation and two by continuous flow centrifugation. The authors wisely emphasize that implications from their results must be drawn with caution. The concentration of virus was in the range to be expected in human hepatitis carriers; however, only a single strain of hepatitis B virus was employed, and it is not known whether similar results would be obtained for other strains of B, A, or non-A, non-B viruses. Furthermore, the susceptibility of chimpanzees to infection may not be strictly analogous to susceptibility in humans.

The severity of human hepatitis B infection is known to be dose-related[25]; after exposure to high doses of virus, clinically evident hepatitis develops after a relatively short incubation period, with frank jaundice and systemic symptoms, whereas low doses of virus more often produce an attenuated illness following a long incubation period and manifested only by mildly abnormal liver function tests and persistent HB-antigenemia (carrier state). Because of its markedly reduced content of donor plasma, frozen-stored RBC derived from hepatitis carrier donors would be expected to deliver a low dose of hepatitis virus to the transfusion recipient, and any resultant disease would likely be of the attenuated variety. It is essential, therefore, that much-needed prospective studies be designed to detect modest chemical alterations and employ sensitive serological methods for detection of hepatitis viral antigens and antibodies. This is particularly important because Barker et al.[26] have clearly shown that the attenuated illness has definite potential for causing chronic liver impairment (persistent antigenemia and abnormalities in thymol turbidity tests and BSP retention) for at least 6 to 36 months following initial infection. It will also be important that prospective studies be applied to frozen-stored RBC deglycerolized by *each* of the commonly employed methods (and any modified methods that are introduced), since it cannot be assumed that the incidence of posttransfusion hepatitis is not affected by differences among the methods.

Reactions to Donor IgA

Frozen-stored RBC as the RBC component of choice for transfusions to patients suffering anaphylactic reactions to donor IgA is justified only because it is the currently available product containing the lowest concentration of donor IgA globulin. However, it should be possible to prepare IgA-depleted RBC suspensions by serial batch washing or continuous flow washing with isotonic saline to achieve equivalent dilutional removal of donor IgA. Six wash steps in one commercial cell washing apparatus is said to dilute the plasma from a unit of whole blood 3-million-fold.[27] Glycerolization and frozen storage are irrelevant to IgA depletion. Frozen-stored RBC used for this purpose represent an unnecessarily costly product and one with a lower index of therapeutic effectiveness than suitably washed fresh donor RBC. (See also Ch. 37.)

Sensitization to Leukocyte and Platelet Antigens

The virtues of frozen-stored RBC for minimizing sensitization to HLA and other leukocyte and platelet antigens are generally cited in relation to two clinical circumstances: patients who are likely to receive multiple transfusions over prolonged periods of time (e.g., congenital hemolytic anemias, aplastic anemia) and patients who may be candidates for organ allografts (e.g., kidney, bone marrow).

The objectives in chronic transfusion therapy are:

1. to delay the development of broadly reactive antileukocyte antibodies which are responsible for severe febrile reactions associated with whole blood and packed RBC transfusions, and

2. to delay the development of broadly reactive antiplatelet antibodies which could preclude functionally effective platelet transfusions should they become necessary in the future. There are few prospective data on platelet antibodies; limited prospective data on antileukocyte antibodies confirm a reduced incidence of sensitization to isologous leukocytes after frozen-stored RBC transfusions compared to transfusions of whole blood or packed RBC.[28] Unfortunately, even less data are available for transfusions of leukocyte-poor RBC prepared by less cumbersome and less expensive methods,[29] including washed red cells prepared by a mechanical cell washer. Unless it can be shown that some essential feature of cryopreservation technology is required to delay antileukocyte sensitization, it would appear reasonable to employ the more economical leukocyte-poor RBC suspensions for this purpose.

The indications for the use of a leukocyte-poor preparation as a prophylactic measure against development of leukocyte and platelet antibodies in chronic anemias are not clearly defined. The use of leukocyte-poor red cell preparations are generally appropriate in patients with severe congenital hemolytic anemia who will require frequent transfusions throughout their lives—e.g.,patients with Thalassemia major being managed with hypertransfusion (see Ch. 32). In most adults who have acquired anemias and who are not candidates for transplantation, it is probably more reasonable to reserve the use of leukocyte-poor red cells for those individuals who become sensitized as manifest by the development of febrile nonhemolytic transfusion reactions (see Ch. 37). Experience in the use of frozen-stored RBC and liquid-stored leukocyte-depleted RBC for prevention of febrile transfusion reactions in already sensitized recipients has demonstrated equally good responses to both products.[30]

The relation of allograft survival to prior antileukocyte sensitization is complex and controversial. This is discussed in detail in

Chapters 28 and 29. In brief, patients with aplastic anemia who are candidates for bone marrow transplantation should not be transfused with any blood product if at all possible.[31] A transplant center should be contacted immediately. If transfusions are absolutely necessary, a leukocyte-poor preparation such as frozen-stored RBC should be used. In contrast, there is at present no indication to restrict the transfusion support for leukemic patients in the pretransplant period, except that transfusions from family members should be avoided (see Ch. 28).

The situation with regard to long-term cadaver kidney allograft survival is much less clear, and continues to evolve as more data become available. On the assumption that kidney graft survival would be maximized by minimizing exposure to donor leukocytes, it became nearly universal practice to transfuse only frozen-stored RBC to candidates for renal transplantation. In fact, renal dialysis units have become the principal users of frozen-stored RBC. The original expectation was that long-term graft survival would be maximum in never-transfused recipients and, in transfused recipients, would correlate inversely with the number of prior transfusions. Opelz and Terasaki were among the first to present convincing data indicating that this is not true.[32] In a study of 1360 cadaver-donor kidney transplants, four-year graft survival in never-transfused recipients was 30 ± 3 percent in contrast to 65 ± 5 percent in patients with >20 pretransplant whole blood or packed RBC transfusions. Indeed, prior exposure to donor leukocytes appears to enhance graft survival, and this rationale for use of frozen-stored RBC has been dealt a severe blow. Nevertheless, it is also clear that when a potential recipient has multiple antileukocyte antibodies as a result of numerous whole blood transfusions, the task of finding a compatible cadaver donor may be formidable, resulting in delayed transplantation and, conceivably, in occasional failure ever to find a compatible donor. Development of nationwide computerized HLA registries will help

to alleviate this problem. On the other hand, it is not yet clear how many prior whole blood transfusions are optimal for enhanced long-term graft survival. Nor is it clear how favorably the few leukocytes present in frozen-stored RBC (and other leukocyte-poor RBC products) compare with whole blood leukocytes in providing the enhanced graft survival effect. The role for frozen-stored RBC will be determined by the results of such studies currently under way, and will reflect a balance between the advantage of restricted sensitization in minimizing the difficulty of finding a compatible donor and the disadvantage of reducing the enhanced graft survival effect (see Ch. 29).

The appropriate role for frozen-stored RBC in candidates for renal transplantation is not currently determined solely on its effect on antileukocyte sensitization. A high incidence of hepatitis has been a serious problem among patients and personnel in large renal dialysis centers.[33]

To the extent that various frozen-stored RBC products can be established to carry a reduced risk of transmitting serum hepatitis (B, A, and non-A, non-B), there will continue to be strong motivation for their use to supply most of the transfusion needs of dialysis center patients. Only when a washed RBC product prepared from liquid-stored blood can be shown to confer equivalent protection against posttransfusion hepatitis will the matter of antileukocyte sensitization become the principal determinant of frozen-stored RBC usage in dialysis center populations.

CLINICAL INDICATIONS FOR TRANSFUSING FROZEN-STORED RBC

Based on considerations put forward in the preceding sections of this chapter, it is possible to summarize guidelines for the transfusion of frozen-stored RBC (Table 14-1). Because of their satisfactory viability and near-normal oxygen-binding characteristics, fro-

Table 14-1. Guidelines for the Transfusion of Frozen-Stored Red Blood Cells

Patient Category	RBC Products in Order of Choice	Comments
Patients with alloantibodies to high incidence blood group antigens	1. Rare donor frozen-stored (F-S) RBC 2. Patient's own F-S RBC for autotransfusion 3. Rare donor liquid-stored blood*	*Likely to be unavailable because of rarity
Patients with febrile transfusion reactions due to antileukocyte sensitization	1. Leukocyte-poor RBC prepared from liquid stored blood* 2. F-S RBC$^\Delta$	*Such RBC have an index of therapeutic effectiveness of 85–90%. $^\Delta$Index of therapeutic effectiveness is approximately 75%, and cost is higher
Patients with demonstrated anti-IgA anaphylaxis	1. F-S RBC 2. Saline-washed reduction of donor IgA* 3. IgA-deficient donor blood$^\Delta$	*RBC extensively washed in commercial cell washer are adequate for most patients who have reactions to donor IgA. $^\Delta$Reported incidence 1/886 normal donors[41]
Candidates for cadaver kidney transplantation	1. Packed RBC—limited number (1 to 5 units)* 2. F-S RBC therafter 3. ? suitably washed "buffy coat-poor" RBC$^\Delta$	Aim to achieve enhanced long-term graft survival yet minimize difficulty in finding compatible donor kidneys and reduce incidence of hepatitis *Absolute number of packed RBC units and schedule in relation to transplant surgery awaits definition $^\Delta$May be substituted for F-S RBC if comparable reduced incidence of antileukocyte sensitization and of hepatitis can be demonstrated
Patients with Cooley's anemia, who will require recurrent transfusions over a long period	1. F-S RBC* 2. Leukocyte-poor RBC prepared from liquid-stored blood*	*Order of preference awaits additional prospective data on incidence of antileukocyte sensitization following leukocyte-poor RBC
Patients with aplastic anemia who are candidates for bone marrow transplantation	1. *Avoid all transfusions,* if possible 2. F-S RBC* 3. Leukocyte-poor RBC*	*Same as immediately above
Patients with hypoxia, respiratory distress syndrome, chronic pulmonary disease or congestive heart failure	1. Freshest available liquid-preserved RBC* 2. F-S RBC	*The importance of RBC 2,3-DPG concentrations in this setting is not well documented; RBC stored in CPD preservative for 14 days will have 50% of original 2,3-DPG concentration

zen-stored RBC can theoretically be used alone or in concert with appropriate plasma products in any circumstances in which a patient requires RBC. However, because of their high cost, difficult preparative requirements, 24-hour shelf life, and somewhat diminished index of therapeutic effectiveness, the use of frozen-stored RBC should probably be considered primarily in relation to the special circumstances listed in Table 14-1 under "Patient Category." Note that frozen-stored RBC is not always the product of choice; whenever liquid-stored RBC is documented to have equivalent pertinent properties, it is shown as the product of choice. Furthermore, Table 14-1 points out, under "Comments," a number of prospective studies, either in progress or greatly needed, whose outcome may modify the relative ranking of liquid-stored and frozen-stored RBC in the future. The need for careful documentation of the hepatitis-transmitting properties of thoroughly washed liquid-stored RBC as well as of frozen-stored RBC prepared by each of the commonly used technologies cannot be overemphasized. This information, plus detailed follow-up for chronic liver damage among recipients who develop attenuated hepatitis viral infection, will help to put the use of frozen-stored RBC into broad rational perspective.

FROZEN STORAGE OF LEUKOCYTES, PLATELETS AND BONE MARROW

Conditions for maximizing the recovery of viable and functionally unimpaired leukocytes,[34] platelets,[35] and hematopoietic bone marrow cells[36] are under intensive study. Compared to the yields of viable functioning RBC, recoveries of the nonerythrocytic elements have been considerably less good, and specific functions are sometimes impaired. Glycerol has not proved to be an optimal cryopreservative; dimethyl sulfoxide (DMSO) is much more effective but is somewhat more toxic than glycerol on parenteral administration to humans. Therapeutic application of frozen-stored platelets[37] and frozen-stored bone marrow[38,39] is in the clinical investigative stage and shows distinct promise. The use of cryopreservation technology in maintaining animal and human tissue culture cell lines for laboratory use is already a common practice.[40]

REFERENCES

1. Luyet, B.J. and Hartung, M.C.: Survival of *Anguillula Aceti* after solidification in liquid air. Biodynamica 3:353, 1941.
2. Polge, C., Smith, A.U., and Parkes, A.S.: Revival of spermatozoa after vitrification and dehydration at low temperatures. Nature (Lond.) 164:666, 1949.
3. Valeri, C.R.: Recent advances in techniques for freezing red cells. Clin. Lab. Sci. 1:381, 1970.
4. Crowley, J. P., Wade, P.H., Wish, C., and Valeri, C.R.: The purification of red cells for transfusion by freeze-preservation and washing. V. Red cell recovery and residual leukocytes after freeze-preservation with high concentrations of glycerol and washing in various systems. Transfusion 17:1, 1977.
5. Kurtz, S.R., Van Deinse, W.H., and Valerie, C.R.: Immunocompetence of residual lymphocytes at various stages of red cell cryopreservation with 40% w/v glycerol in an ionic medium at $-80°$ C. Transfusion 18:441, 1978.
6. Contreras, T.J. and Valeri, C.R.: A comparison of methods to wash liquid-stored red blood cells and red blood cells frozen with high or low concentrations of glycerol. Transfusion 16:539, 1976.
7. Zemp, J.W. and O'Brien, T.G.: In vitro characteristics of glycerolized and frozen human red blood cells. Proceedings of the VIIth International Congress of Hematology, Tokyo, Sept. 4-10, 1960. Vol. 2, Hemocytology and Anemia. Pan-Pacific Press, Tokyo, 1962.
8. Valeri, C.R. and Zarvulis, C.G.: Rejuvenation and freezing of outdated stored human red cells. N. Engl. J. Med. 287:1307, 1972.
9. Myhre, B.A., Nakasado, Y.Y., and Schott, R.: Studies on 4C stored frozen-reconstituted red

cells. I. Bacterial growth. Transfusion 17:454, 1977.

10. Radcliffe, J.H., Denham, M.A., Gaydos, C., and Simpson, M.B.: Bacteriological sterility of washed deglycerolized red blood cells after 72 hours storage. Transfusion 18:365, 1978.

11. Myhre, B.A., Nakasado, Y.Y., Schott, R., Johnson, D., Berkman, R.M., and Cleland, E.L.: An aseptic fluid transfer system for blood and blood components. Tranfusion 18:546, 1978.

12. Moore, J.A., Dorner, I., and Chaplin, H.: Positive antiglobulin reactions with thawed deglycerolized red blood cells. Vox Sang. 27:385, 1974.

13. Goldfinger, D., Connelly, M., Kellum, S., and Rosenbaum, D.: Transfusion of frozen autologous red blood cells in patients with positive direct antiglobulin tests. Blood 54(suppl):124a, 1979.

14. Valeri, C.R. and Hirsch, N.M.: Restoration in vivo of erythrocyte adenosine triphosphate, 2,3-diphosphoglycerate, potassium ion, and sodium ion concentrations following the transfusion of acid-citrate-dextrose-stored human red blood cells. J. Lab. Clin. Med. 73:722, 1968.

15. Collins, J.A., Simmons, R.L., James, P.M., Bredenberg, C.E., Anderson, R.W., and Heisterkamp, C.A.: Acid-base status of seriously wounded combat casualties. II. Resuscitation with stored blood. Ann. Surg. 173:6, 1971.

16. Collins, J.A.: Massive Blood Transfusion: Clinics in Hematology 5:216, 1976.

17. Weisel, R.D., Dennis, R., Manny, J., et al.: Adverse effects of transfusion therapy during abdominal aortic aneurysectomy. Surgery 83:682, 1978.

18. Meryman, H.T.: Red cell freezing: a major factor in the future of blood banking. In: Clinical and Practical Aspects of the Use of Frozen Blood: A technical workshop. Dawson, R.B. and Barnes, A., Jr., Eds. Am. Assoc. Blood Banks, Atlanta, 1977, pp. 1-21.

19. Tullis, J.L., Hinman, J., Sproul, M.T., and Nickerson, R.J.: Incidence of post-transfusion hepatitis in previously frozen blood. J.A.M.A. 214:719, 1970.

20. Huggins, C.E., Russell, P.S., Winn, H.J., Fuller, T.C., and Beck, C.H., Jr.: Frozen blood in transplant patients: hepatitis and HL-A isosensitization. Transplant. Proc. 5:809, 1973.

21. Haugen, R.K.: Hepatitis after the transfusion of frozen red cells and washed red cells. N. Engl. J. Med. 301:393, 1979.

22. Goldfinger, D.: Hepatitis after frozen or washed red cells (correspondence). N. Engl. J. Med. 302:581, 1980.

23. Valeri, C.R.: Blood Banking and the Use of Frozen Blood Products. CRC Press, Cleveland, 1976.

24. Alter, H.J., Tabor, E., Meryman, H.T., Hoofnagle, J.H., Kahn, R.A., Holland, P.V., Gerety, R.J., and Barker, L.F.: Failure of frozen-deglycerolized red blood cells to prevent the transmission of hepatitis B virus infection. N. Engl. J. Med. 298:637, 1978.

25. Barker, L.F. and Murray, R.: Relationship of virus dose to incubation time of clinical disease and time of appearance of hepatitis-associated antigen. Am. J. Med. Sci. 263:27, 1972.

26. Barker, L.F. and Murray, R.: Acquisition of hepatitis-associated antigen: clinical features in young adults. J.A.M.A. 216:1970, 1971.

27. Jones, A.L., Judson, G.T., Kellog, R.M., and Kruger, V.R.: The IBM blood cell processor. IBM Technical Report 01. Nov. 3, 1964.

28. Fuller, T.C., Delmonico, F.L., Cosimi, A.B., Huggins, C.E., King, M., and Russell, P.S.: Effects of various types of RBC transfusions on HLA alloimmunization and renal allograft survival. Transplant. Proc. 9:117, 1977.

29. Miller, W.V., Schmidt, R.D., Luke, R.G., and Caywood, B.E.: Effect on cytotoxicity antibodies in potential transplant recipients of leukocyte-poor blood transfusions. Lancet i:893, 1975.

30. Dorner, I., Moore, J.A., Collins, J.A., Sherman, L.A., and Chaplin, H.: Efficacy of leukocyte-poor red blood cell suspensions prepared by sedimentation in hydroxyethyl starch. Transfusion 15:439, 1975.

31. Storb, R.: Marrow transplantation in thirty "untransfused" patients with severe aplastic anemia. Ann. Intern. Med. 92:30, 1980.

32. Opelz, G. and Terasaki, P.I.: Improvement of kidney-graft survival with increased numbers of blood transfusions. N. Engl. J. Med. 299:799, 1978.

33. Control of hepatitis on hemodialysis units (Editorial). N. Engl. J. Med. 282:1488, 1970.

34. Lionetti, F.J., Hunt, S.M., Mattaliano, R.J., and Valeri, C.R.: *In vitro* studies of cryopre-

served baboon granulocytes. Transfusion 18:685, 1978.

35. Spector, J.I., Yarmola, J.A., Marchionni, L.D., Emerson, C.P., and Valeri, C.R.: Viability and function of platelets frozen at 2 and 3°C per minute with 4 or 5 percent DMSO and stored at −80°C for 8 months. Transfusion 17:8, 1977.

36. Lewis, J.P.: Bone Marrow. In: Organ Preservation for Transplantation. Karow, A.M., Jr., Abouna, G.J.M., and Humphries, A.L., eds. Little Brown, Boston, 1974, pp. 167–184.

37. Schiffer, C.A., Aisner, J., and Wiernik, P.H.: Frozen autologous platelet transfusions for patients with leukemia. N. Engl. J. Med. 299:7, 1978.

38. Applebaum, F.R., Herzig, G.P., Ziegler, J.L., Graw, R.G., Levine, A.S., and Deisseroth, A.B.: Successful engraftment of cryopreserved autologous bone marrow in patients with malignant lymphoma. Blood 52:85, 1978.

39. Tobias, J.S. and Tattersall, M.H.R.: Perspectives in cancer research. Autologous marrow support and intensive chemotherapy in cancer patients. Eur. J. Cancer 12:1, 1976.

40. Roundtable Conference on the Cryogenic Preservation of Cell Cultures. Rinfret, A.P. and La Salle, B., editors. Nat. Acad. Sci., Washington, D.C., 1975.

41. Vyas, G.N., Perkins, H.A., Yang, Y.M., and Basantani, G.K.: Healthy blood donors with selective absence of immunoglobulin A: Prevention of anaphylactic transfusion reactions caused by antibodies to IgA. J. Lab. Clin. Med. 85:838, 1975.

15

Autologous Blood Transfusion and Blood Salvage

Scott N. Swisher, M.D., and Lawrence D. Petz, M.D.

AUTOLOGOUS TRANSFUSION

In this chapter, the term autologous transfusion will refer to procedures in which blood is removed from an individual for later transfusion to that same individual after a period of in vitro storage. Blood salvage will refer to recovery of blood already shed either into a closed body cavity or during or shortly after a surgical procedure, with return of the blood to the same patient. These terms are used in various ways in the literature on this topic.

The idea of employing a patient as his own blood donor is of long standing. The earliest attempts involved intraoperative autologous transfusion, first in the late 19th century and again at about the time of World War I. Theis' and Appleby's cases involved recovery of large hemorrhages in the closed space of the peritoneal cavity caused by ruptured ectopic pregnancies.[1,2] In spite of these relatively successful early efforts, the technique did not develop in the face of the growing effectiveness of the practice of donor-recipient transfusion made possible by development of a successful system of blood anticoagulation.

It was not until true blood banking was made possible by the development of the Acid Citrate Dextrose (ACD) system of 21-day preservation of blood in the liquid state after World War II and very long-term cryopreservation of blood still later that effective autologous transfusion was possible. Autotransfusion and blood salvage were then reinvestigated intensively following the work of Milles, et al. in the early 1960s.[3,4] Shortly afterwards, Wilson, Taswell, and colleagues reexamined the feasibility and utility of intraoperative blood salvage.[5,6] Miller et al. published a monography on this topic in 1971.[7] Since then, the use of autologous transfusion has grown slowly, and intraoperative and postoperative blood salvage have become established procedures with development of new equipment. A monograph published by the American Association of Blood Banks in 1976 on this topic summarizes much of the recent development in this field.[8] Parallel development of these techniques has occurred in other countries.

REASONS FOR AUTOLOGOUS TRANSFUSION AND BLOOD SALVAGE

There are a number of apparent reasons for the present patterns of utilization of these two general techniques. Three general reasons have been proposed in support of both procedures. These are:

1. Improvement of the blood supply or reduction of the need for recruited blood donors.

2. Reduction of the risk of transmission of hepatitis.

3. Reduction of the incidence of recipient alloimmunization, and other adverse effects upon recipients which depend upon immunological mechanisms.

If a recipient's need for transfusion could be satisfied completely by autotransfusions, theoretically the risks due to hepatitis and immune reactions could be eliminated completely. In practice, it has been found that a significant proportion of patients who have been entered into autologous transfusion programs for elective surgery require supplementation with variable amounts of donor blood. The amount of donor blood required will vary with the nature of the surgical procedure. The risks to these patients are reduced by autotransfusion, but not eliminated.

The Rare Compatible Donor Problem

Autotransfusion may be of crucial importance to a small group of patients who lack very high-incidence blood group antigens such as Kp_B of the Kell system and $P + P_1$ of the P system and who have been alloimmunized by previous transfusions. If only one of ten thousand random donors in the United States will be found to be compatible, long-term preservation of the patient's own blood in the frozen state may be life-saving. A patient with the so-called Bombay blood group, O_h, and a group of related very rare, genetically determined abnormalities of expression of the antigens of the ABH(O) system provides an even more urgent problem. These individuals usually have preformed antibodies against the A, B, and H antigens. They are thus incompatible with all other donors except those rare individuals like themselves. Known examples of these blood group abnormalities are widely scattered around the world; only a few such cases have been identified since 1952, when the problem was first identified by Bhende et al.[8]

Predeposit of autologous blood for later autotransfusion is very wise for most patients known to lack a very high-incidence blood group antigen, a so-called "public antigen," or who are already alloimmunized to multiple red cell antigens. Storage of blood in the frozen state is, of course, necessary for this purpose. If elective surgery is contemplated, a more intensive presurgical program of blood collection and storage in the liquid or frozen state can be undertaken, as described later in this chapter. If all the blood is not transfused during surgery, as is frequently the case, the remaining units can be converted to frozen storage and placed in inventory for that particular patient or others like him.

The patient lacking a high-incidence blood group antigen can, of course, be transfused safely the first time blood is needed, unless an antibody to this antigen has appeared for other reasons such as a pregnancy. Most patients with this situation will be identified first when crossmatches are found to be incompatible at the time of subsequent transfusions. They will have become alloimmunized by the first transfusion. Previously undiscovered patients of blood group O_h will be identified at the time they are first cross-matched and found to be incompatible with all available donors. Others may be found by studies of family members. It is for these patients and for alloimmunized individuals who have been unable or unwilling to enter into an autologous transfusion program and who need blood that the national and international registries of rare donors are of great value, and not infrequently life-saving.

Information about the location and availability of rare donor bloods—either as frozen blood or as liquid-preserved blood from a donor who can be called in at the time of need—is widely accessible in all regional blood centers and in most large, hospital-based blood banks. Time is required to obtain these bloods, but, with modern communications and transportation systems, this can be accomplished in many cases with surprising rapidity. It will always be necessary to undertake a period of support of the patient without availability of red cells for transfusion. This period should be devoted to intensive efforts to control blood loss, to recover lost blood if possible, and to maintain the patient's intravascular volume and circulatory perfusion. The potential utility of oxygen-carrying blood substitutes in these critical circumstances may be a consideration in the future (see Ch. 35).

It is very important to enlist all rare donors into a national registry, and to convince the appropriate ones to participate in an autologous transfusion program, even located at some distance from their homes and involving considerable inconvenience. Equally important is the need for them to release their own blood deposits for urgent use by other patients who need them. This requires the blood bank to take responsibility for obtaining additional units from the rare donor whenever the individual donor's blood inventory on deposit has been invaded. In this way, patients with needs for rare donor bloods can form a subsystem of a national, indeed international, blood transfusion system and jointly provide for the needs of others like themselves while providing for their own.

Importance of Communication

It is crucial that the responsible senior clinician in charge of a patient with a rare donor problem be available for early and frequent consultation with the blood bank responsible for supporting his patient. It is not enough to "order blood." The patient's management must be planned in relation to the availability of blood in terms of both amount and timing. The clinician can be helped most by a competent medical blood bank director, but he should not hesitate to communicate directly with technical or other laboratory management personnel if he feels this will be more effective. The blood banks of many hospitals are directed by general or clinical patholo-

gists whose principal interests are in areas other than blood banking. Senior blood bank technologists can be of great help, for they very frequently have an excellent grasp of many clinical problems which involve the need for blood and blood products. They frequently understand the logistics of the local blood supply as well or better than the nominal blood bank director. It is surprising and disheartening to see how infrequently clinicians take optimum advantage of the resources of the blood bank, even in the management of difficult transfusion problems. Status is not lost by discussing a problem with anyone who can help in the management of a patient.

Similarly, it is important that hospital blood banks contact their supplying regional blood centers or support networks early in the course of managing any transfusion problem, particularly a rare donor problem. Time, effort, expense, and patient risk are all minimized by early notification about even a potential problem. It is always a better strategy to inform the regional blood center about a potential problem rather than to await its arrival, even though the actual occurrence of these problems may be infrequent. In the authors' experience, instances of poor performance of either a hospital blood bank or a regional blood center are most often due to lack of adequate exchange of information rather than to true technical or logistic failure. For this reason, most such failures are preventable. The responsibility rests primarily on the clinician in charge of the patient to initiate this chain of information and to assure himself that it is being acted upon appropriately.

The Practice of Autologous Transfusion

It has been demonstrated that autologous transfusion is a safe and practical procedure in many patients. The technology needed is all state of the art. It requires little more than special identification and segregation of the autologous donor blood units to insure that they are appropriately and safely redirected to the person from whom they came. This is not a trivial requirement for blood bank management, but it can be done. It gives rise to the first of two questions which the clinician who is considering employment of autologous transfusion must consider.

1. *Is there an established and functioning autologous transfusion service available?* It is the experience of the authors, shared by many clinicians and blood bankers, that a more reliable, effective, and safe service is rendered by a formally established and experienced autologous transfusion service. Casual or infrequent performance of autologous transfusions is possible, but at the cost of extra effort in personnel education and increased possibilities for error or failure in storage and identification procedures.

A survey in 1974 by the American Association of Blood Banks revealed that, of 800 responding hospitals, 35 percent had established programs of autologous transfusion. Of 50 blood centers which served over 700 hospitals, 64 percent had this capability.[8] These estimates are difficult to generalize to the United States as a whole. Undoubtedly, there has been some slow growth of these programs since 1974, but the data suggest that this service is still not universally available. When it is needed, it is more likely to be available on an organized basis at a regional blood center than at a hospital blood bank.

2. *Does the patient's medical condition permit him to act as his own donor with reasonable safety?* This is the most difficult question to answer. Physicians and surgeons both tend to be extremely conservative on this matter; even clinical situations which have been shown by experience to be quite safe are regarded uncritically as *contraindications* for autologous transfusion. Physicians and surgeons also tend to underevaluate the risks of the usual donor-based transfusions. These attitudes seem to account for much of the low

utilization and slow growth of autologous transfusion.

Medical Evaluation of Patients for Autologous Transfusion

The principal absolute contraindication for autologous transfusion of a patient is the coexistence of any disorder which significantly limits erythrocyte production. Chronic anemic states of even mild degree usually disqualify a patient for autologous transfusion. An exception might be iron deficiency anemia, which can be rapidly repaired by iron administration under circumstances when adequate time is available to do so. Unfortunately, many such patients also have chronic blood loss and cannot be treated effectively enough with iron therapy to permit them to sustain the additional blood loss incurred in autologous transfusion. Patients with the anemia of chronic disease, such as chronic renal insufficiency, a disseminated tumor, or chronic inflammation are also largely excluded from participation in autologous transfusion.

Obviously, the chronically ill patient who is limited in mobility, the patient with multiple significant illness, the very elderly patient, patients suffering from impaired tissue oxygen delivery of any cause, and children and adults of very small body size can in most instances be excluded as autologous donors on the grounds of reasonability and good medical judgment. But there remains a large population of patients facing elective surgery who can safely undergo autologous blood donation in spite of a significant deviation from good health. It has been said that, if a patient cannot donate blood, he may not be a candidate for elective surgery.[10] This clearly overstates the matter, but it does emphasize that a very large proportion of candidates for elective surgery are in fact qualified. The risks to be balanced are those of donation versus receiving blood from another donor.

Autotransfusion in Cardiac Surgery

The modern practice of cardiac surgery employing cardiopulmonary bypass procedures involves a type of autologous transfusion. The patient's own red cell mass is initially diluted to fill the bypass machine, at times with supplementation with donor blood. Most of this blood can be returned to the patient at the termination of surgery or in the immediate postoperative period. If a relatively small amount of the patient's own blood obtained prior to surgery is available, the entire prime of the machine can be made up of the patient's own blood.

Goldfinger et al. have studied the problem of autologous transfusion in cardiac surgery. In over 100 cases, they noted no adverse effects.[10,11] In an earlier series of 44 patients, autologous transfusion accounted for about one-third of the total blood needs of the group. Their practice was to exclude from the program only patients who required emergency surgery. Milles et al. have evaluated by electrocardiography a variety of elective surgery candidates undergoing autologous blood donation.[7] In the group were a number of patients with a variety of EKG abnormalities including arrhythmias, conduction defects, and evidences of old myocardial infarction. Abnormalities attributable to blood donation were not found. Although this study supports the clinical observation that autologous blood donation is well tolerated, it must be remembered that electrocardiography does not reflect a wide variety of significant hemodynamic and pathophysiological changes in the circulatory system. Other authors also support the safety of autologous blood donation in cardiopulmonary surgical patients.[11,12,13,14]

Disadvantages of Autologous Transfusion

In spite of all the seeming advantages of autologous transfusions, programs of this type have not developed in the United States to a point where they have as yet had a significant impact on the total national blood supply. The limitations on this technique have become apparent in a number of ways, based upon experience with it. These limitations are largely logistical in nature.

1. Autologous blood donations incur all of the costs of regular blood collection and distribution, plus the cost of providing special arrangements for collection, storage, and direction of the units to the donor now as recipient. Even associated blood typing and cross-matching procedures cannot be avoided safely; these tests provide significant protection against clerical errors which might result from misidentification of donor as recipient.

2. If an elective surgical procedure is delayed significantly by some relatively common but unpredictable event such as a respiratory infection, the blood will be lost to its donor. The blood may be used for other recipients in some cases if the donor is otherwise qualified, but, in a significant number of instances, this is not the case. The purpose of autotransfusion will have been lost in any event.

3. Many elective surgical patients will require more blood for transfusion than can be reasonably collected from them. These patients will have some reduction in the hazards of isologous transfusion, but will not avoid them totally.

4. Surgeons who attempt to recruit patients to these programs find that a significant proportion refuse or are reluctant to participate. This may reflect a public awareness of an attitude which many physicians have— i.e., it just does not seem "reasonable" to lose blood before a planned operation. They do not believe that the potential benefits outweigh the presumed risks.

5. Some surgeons feel obligated to give back autologous blood if it has been obtained, even though it is not needed by the patient. It should be noted that autologous

transfusion is *not* risk-free. The possibility of clerical error resulting in a hemolytic reaction is always present, as is the remote possibility of the unit becoming infected.

Recent publications and personal discussions of the practice of autologous transfusion confirm the low level of this activity in the United States at this time. For example, Silvergleid reported on the experience of a blood center in which on 178 units of autologous transfusion in 103 patients between 1974 and 1978.[15] This blood center distributes about 45,000 units of blood annually; the autologous transfusion program thus accounted for about 0.1 percent of blood distributed, in the face of systematic efforts to promote the program. Coggiano reported about 1 percent of 55,000 annual units to be autologous.[16] Increasing this program to much over 3 percent of annual activity would incur a significant disproportionate increase in costs of the total program. Aster has expressed similar opinions and has pointed out that an equivalent effort directed toward development of the total blood supply would be more effective on behalf of all the patients who rely on a blood program.[17] These considerations would seem to apply regardless of whether the autotransfusion program is sponsored by a regional blood center or by a hospital blood bank.

Blood Depository

It has been suggested that anyone with any significant chance of needing a transfusion should deposit blood for personal use in a frozen blood repository. However, the costs of cryopreservation in terms of space requirements, energy, and capital, as well as costs of processing make this concept totally unfeasible for any large scale application. Addition of the costs of freezing can raise the total cost of an autologous transfusion by at least a factor of three or more compared to liquid blood storage—i.e., to over $150.00 per unit transfused. This added cost is clearly a limitation on the use of cryopreservation in any routine program in anticipation of elective surgery.

Collection and Storage of Autologous Blood

After a patient has been found to be medically eligible for autologous tranfusion, he should be fully informed of the requirements and risks of the procedure and should sign a specific consent form for this purpose.[18] If blood storage in the frozen state is to be used, the collection schedule usually can be extended, sometimes over several months. If liquid storage is employed, the schedule must encompass the time limits of the blood preservation system employed. This is 21 days when ACD or CPD are used, and 35 days with adenine-supplemented CPD. Although special identification and isolation are needed for these bloods, all other conditions of storage are standard.[19]

The rate of blood donation is limited primarily by the donor patient's ability to regenerate red cells and maintain a reasonable, functionally adequate red cell mass. The rate of tolerable bleeding varies greatly from patient to patient, as does the fall in hematocrit following a standard 500 ml phlebotomy. An average fall of about 4 percent in hematocrit can be expected following each phlebotomy in an average adult male, with a range of 1 to 8 percent. Persons of small body size and, thus, lower blood volume can be expected to show the larger decreases.

An hematocrit of 34 percent or a hemoglobin level of 11 gm/100 ml are generally accepted standards for the lowest acceptable limit for further donation.[19] Initially, it may be possible to bleed the patient every 72 hours; more frequent phlebotomies are probably unwise in virtually all instances. Later, the patient may be able to donate only every 5 to 10 days. Under certain very urgent conditions, it may be possible to bleed patients with lower hematocrits, but this decision should be made only after most careful evaluation of the patient and the overall clinical situation. In all instances, the patient on an intensive bleeding schedule should be carefully evaluated by a physician prior to each donation for any of the following evidences of physiological deterioration: decreased exercise tolerance; increasing cardiovascular abnormalities such as angina, tachycardia, or arrhythmia; postural hypotension; edema; or orthopnea. If adverse effects are encountered, they can usually be reversed promptly by reinfusion of one or more units of the patient's stored red cells.

"Leap Frogging"

A technique called "leap frog" has been proposed to permit a more intensive and larger collection of donor blood from patients. It also may provide blood with somewhat longer periods before outdating.[20] The technique involves a schedule such as the following: Several units of blood might be obtained over a period of several weeks. Following the next phlebotomy, the oldest stored unit is reinfused. this largely restores the patient's blood volume and red cell mass, minus those reinfused cells which are nonviable. A second unit of blood is then removed. Multiple units could be so recycled in a short period of time. This procedure can be employed when there has been short notice of a delay in surgery for a week or so. The system has been found to be workable, although it is time-consuming for the patient and the blood bank, increases costs substantially, and requires exceptionally good access to the patient's veins. However, it has other shortcomings as well.

This procedure results in three significant effects upon the reinfused stored red cells, some of which are removed a second time and stored again. The nonviable cells are removed; the surviving stored cells are diluted in the remainder of the patient's normal red cell mass; and the reinfused stored red cells

are, to varying degrees, rejuvenated in vivo. For the latter effect to occur, some time is required. Significant levels of 2,3-DPG will probably be regenerated within about 12 hours after reinfusion, although complete recovery will take longer.[21] Less is known about recovery of the membrane and other kinds of possible damage induced by blood storage, but it is generally agreed that red cells remaining in the recipient's circulation 24 hours after infusion have a nearly normal life span.[22] This would suggest that the "leap frog" technique might be most effective if 24 hours were to intervene between an infusion of stored cells and removal of the next donation. This adds to the inconvenience for the patient, and apparently it is not common practice. Nevertheless, a convincing argument can be made in support of delay of further bleeding after stored red cell reinfusion. With the availability of CPD-adenine blood preservation, leap-frogging is now rarely justifiable.

Iron Therapy

Availability of iron in the body stores is frequently a significant limitation on the patient donor's ability to regenerate red cells. If iron stores are depleted, even in the presence of an essentially normal red cell mass, only a few units of blood can be expected to be collected before the hematocrit drops to an unacceptable level. Oral iron therapy may promptly correct this situation.[23,24] Oral iron in standard doses, equivalent to at least 150 mg of elemental iron, should be given to all autologous donors unless specifically contraindicated. All of the precautions taken normally to insure adequate iron absorption and tolerance should be taken. These include administration of the drug in a bioavailable formulation, an hour before meals. Enteric-coated or slow absorption preparations should be avoided. Ferrous sulfate USP, if the tablets are fresh and easily crushed, is certainly the cheapest and probably the best absorbed preparation. Although the addition of ascorbic acid, succinate, or fructose is theoretically able to enhance iron absorption, these offer little practical benefit.

Parenteral iron therapy may be indicated in the management of a small number of autologous donors. Parenteral iron treatment will not improve the situation of patients in whom the limit on red cell regeneration is not likely to be due to iron lack—including patients who do not have hypochromic red cells, are normoferremic, or have not responded to oral iron therapy with significant reticulocytosis after phlebotomy. The principal indication for parenteral iron treatment of the autologous donor is preexistent iron deficiency, where not enough time is available to replenish iron stores orally before starting blood collection. Iron malabsorption and true intolerance to oral iron therapy are infrequent and rarely justify parenteral iron administration. Parenteral iron therapy still carries higher risks than does oral iron treatment.[25] All of the usual precautions involved in parenteral iron therapy should be observed carefully in the very few patients who may require it. Even though parenteral iron therapy involves certain risks, they are probably less than the total risks of transfusion.

In spite of iron therapy, one is frequently limited to one or two units of autologous blood for use during surgery. Poor patient acceptance, scheduling problems, and unexpected limitations on the patient's capacity to regenerate red cells contribute to this limitation. In all cases, plans should be made at the outset to supplement the supply of blood for these patients. Under optimal circumstances, up to six or seven units of autologous blood might be available, employing liquid storage in CPD-adenine. If frozen storage is elected and there has been a long period for accumulation, still larger amounts might be obtained; this would be an unusual situation, however. As a practical limit, most programs will accumulate up to a maximum of about ten units for any one patient. Rarely is more blood predictably needed.

Other Considerations

Patients known to be positive for hepatitis B surface antigen, or suspected carriers of non-A, non-B hepatitis should probably not be considered for autologous transfusion or blood salvage programs because of the hazard to exposed personnel. Frozen blood storage is particularly hazardous because of the frequency of bag rupture caused by embrittlement at low temperatures.

The amount of medication carried over in autologous blood is rarely of importance, except in those cases where a significant allergic response to a drug has developed between the time of donation and readministration. Nevertheless, it is probably advisable for the patient to receive as few medications as possible while blood is being collected.[20]

Autologous blood can be collected and stored as whole blood or as sedimented red cells with the plasma returned to the patient. Although rarely indicated, other components can be prepared from these units by standard procedures.

Presurgical Blood Donation

In certain areas of the United States, patients scheduled for elective surgery who are otherwise qualified as blood donors are encouraged to donate blood prior to surgery. Although this is done to increase the blood supply of the area and without specific plans for autologous transfusion, many donors are unclear about the matter and arrive at the blood bank with the expectation that they are donating for their own use. Presurgical blood donation is laudable only if there is a significant amount of time between the blood donation and the surgery (at least two weeks), if the donor is otherwise qualified, and if the patient and surgeon fully understand what will happen to the donated unit in the general blood supply. On the other hand, the practice cannot be strongly encouraged because it does require one more physiological adaptation in a patient who will soon be stressed by surgery—and without the offsetting advantages of autologous transfusion.

BLOOD SALVAGE

Blood salvage techniques provide another type of autologous transfusion. Their use appears to be increasing more rapidly than predeposit autologous transfusion. Shed blood is collected from a wound or body cavity at the time of surgery, or postoperatively, processed in various ways, and reinfused into the bleeding patient. This approach is, in most instances, not fully autologous tranfusion in the sense that it avoids recipient exposure to donor blood. Most of these patients receive donor blood in addition to salvaged blood. It has been estimated that 50 percent of that lost in general surgery and about 75 percent of that lost in cardiovascular surgery can be salvaged.[26] Thus, the aim of blood salvage in most instances is to minimize the amount of donor blood used for what benefits this may have for the patient and for the blood supply.

As has been noted previously, the first efforts to autotransfuse blood occurred in the era 1914 to 1925. Patients with hemorrhage into a closed, sterile serosal cavity were reinfused with the recovered blood. Wilson and Taswell, in the mid 1960s, used a centrifugal washing procedure to prepare the red cells for reinfusion.[5] Since then, a number of systems have been developed and tested. Two are now commercially available.[27] Properly employed, they may be applied to the elective or emergency salvage of shed blood in a wide variety of situations. Their use appears to be increasing, particularly in major surgical centers with cardiovascular surgical programs.

Available Blood Salvage Systems

It is beyond the scope of this chapter to discuss in detail the characteristics and operation of the several systems available for in-

traoperative blood salvage. The technology is still evolving as more experience is gained and as various industrial organizations enter this market. The first available systems required anticoagulation of the patient and did not concentrate the reinfused red cells. They also reinfused plasma containing activated coagulation factors and were thought to be responsible for induction of disseminated intravascular coagulation. It is also probable that microemboli of fat, platelets, and leukocytes and tissue products, and possibly activated complement and kinin systems products were reinfused, leading to an unacceptable level of patient reactions. Air embolism was also a hazard. The red cells were not concentrated before return in some systems; only a limited volume of salvaged blood, five to six units, could be returned to the bleeding patient when there was significant hemodilution by anticoagulant or wound irrigants or where intravascular volume loss was replaced with crystalloid or colloid solutions in large volume. This limited the utility of these systems in just the circumstances where they might be most useful, massive bleeding, in addition to considerations of the hazards involved.

A more recently introduced system avoids these difficulties to a large degree. It is properly an intraoperative or postoperative salvaging system for red blood cells rather than a "whole blood" salvaging system, a distinction that must be kept in mind with respect to need for possible replacement of other blood components in the program of total management of the bleeding patient.[27] All of the systems available or in prospect require trained operators and frequently require addition of a person to the operating room or recovery room team. This is particularly true of the most highly developed system. A significant capital cost is involved as well as costs of operation and disposable supplies. On the other hand, in cases of massive bleeding, blood salvage clearly reduces the work load in the hospital blood bank and in the entire logistic chain of blood supply. Donor blood is undoubtedly conserved in direct proportion to the efficiency of salvage. Only one patient can be served at one time for each unit installed. Some time is required to prepare the system between patients. A comprehensive cost-effectiveness study has not been carried out to evaluate these systems; until this is done, it will be difficult to determine the optimum role of this approach in a transfusion program.

At present, only two systems of blood salvage apparatus are commercially available in the U.S. The Sorenson system provides for collection under controlled vacuum, filtration, and reinfusion under closed system conditions at low capital cost. The system marketed by Haemonetics Corporation provides for red cell washing and concentration before the return to the patient.[27] At least one more such system is under development. The Bentley system, the first to be available, and the Pall system are not currently marketed.

Institutions which decide to undertake blood salvage should examine their needs carefully before selecting a system. Costs, maintenance, operator training, and flexibility are all important considerations.

Contraindications for Blood Salvage

Two virtually absolute contraindications exist for intraoperative blood salvage by any available technique. These are: 1) recovery of blood exposed to a source of bacteria, as in patients with infected wounds or with fecal contamination,[28,29] and 2) procedures in which the shed blood could be contaminated with tumor cells.[30] Since these transfusion systems are in effect open, all intraoperatively salvaged blood should be reinfused as soon as possible, and within a few hours at most, even with refrigeration.

Safety and Efficacy of Blood Salvage

Experience gained during the early years of development of these systems emphasized the

hazards and reactions encountered with their use. More recent reports document their safety when carefully managed.[31,32,33,34,35] Schaff et al. were able to reduce the requirement for postoperative homologous (donor) transfusion by 50 percent by the use of blood salvage in 271 adult and 36 pediatric cardiac surgical patients who received autologous blood collected and reinfused postoperatively.[36] These patients were drawn from a larger series of 592 adults and 108 pediatric patients. Thus, about half of the adults and a third of the children in the total group received salvaged blood. The impact of this program was a reduction in the use of donor blood from an average 8.4 ± 0.7 units of donor blood per adult patient to 4.2 ± 0.3 units after the introduction of routine blood salvage. Thurer et al. confirmed the safety of this procedure but found, in a program already designed to minimize the use of donor blood in cardiovascular surgery, that the impact on further reduction of donor blood was not significant.[36] It seems clear that, in this context, efforts at blood conservation are more important than blood salvage.

Comment

In spite of a number of theoretically attractive aspects, the practices of autotransfusion and blood salvage have grown slowly but substantially in the United States since their introduction as technological possibilities. They have, at present, little total impact upon the national blood supply. Some slow growth of predeposit autologous transfusion can be anticipated, at least in the near future. Practical problems of cost and logistic complexity seem responsible for the present low rate of utilization. Poor physician and patient acceptance and weak public support of programs of autotransfusion are impediments to further development, although these factors might be influenced by education if the program were otherwise cost-effective.

On the other hand, for a very limited number of patients with serious problems of compatibility with random donors, autologous transfusion programs, along with rare donor registries and rapid blood shipment, may be life-saving. The costs of cryopreservation of these autologous blood units clearly can be justified.

In spite of relatively lower cost-effectiveness, it should be possible for at least regional blood centers to accept autologous donors who are strongly motivated, and to accommodate physicians who feel strongly about the medical issues of safety involved in autotransfusion. Autotransfusion should not be carried out casually. A well thought out and standardized program should be employed wherever autotransfusion is practiced, regardless of the scale of the program.

Further growth of blood salvage will probably be more rapid, particularly with development of still better, simpler, and cheaper apparatus. Demonstration of a favorable cost-benefit relationship would no doubt accelerate this use of technology. A recent increase in publications dealing with this technique is evidence of more widespread interest in and application of this technology.[37,38,39,40,41] If this trend continues, it will certainly result in a significant saving of donor bloods. This may be of greatest impact on regional blood supplies in areas of chronic shortage of blood donors. Many such areas in the United States are in large cities which are also major medical centers. It is in just such medical centers that the practice of blood salvage is currently increasing, a trend that seems appropriate to support.

REFERENCES

1. Thies, J.: Zur Behandlung der Extrauterinegraviditat, Zbl. Gynaek. 38:1191, 1914.
2. Appleby, L.H.: Autotransfusion, Can. Med. Assoc. J. 15:36, 1925.
3. Milles, G., Langston, H., and Dalessandro, W.: Experiences with autotransfusions. Surg. Gynecol. Obstet. 115:689, 1962.
4. Milles, G., Langston, H., and Dalessandro, W.: Studies show a patient may be his own best donor. Mod. Hosp. 102:104, 1964.
5. Wilson, J.D. and Taswell, H.F.: Autotransfusion: Historical Review and Preliminary Report on a New Method. Mayo Clinic Proc. 43:26, 1968.
6. Wilson, J.D., Taswell, H.F. and Utz, D.C.: Autotransfusion: Urologic Applications and the Development of a Modified Irrigating Fluid. J. Urol. 105:873, 1971.
7. Milles, G., Langston, H.T., and Dalessandro, W.: Autologous Transfusion. John Alexander Monograph Series, Charles C. Thomas, Springfield, Ill., U.S.A., 1971.
8. Autologous Transfusion, A Tech)ical Workshop. American Association of Blood Banks, R. B. Dawson, Ed., Washington, D.C., 1976.
9. Bhende, H.M., Despande, C.K., Bhatia, H.M., Sanger, R., Race, R.R., Morgan, W.T.J., and Watkins, W.M.: A "New" Blood-group Character Related to the ABO System, Lancet i:903, 1952.
10. Goldfinger, D.: Use of Autologous Transfusion in Elective Surgery. In: Autologous Transfusion, A Technical Workshop. Dawson, B.R., Ed., American Association of Blood Banks, Washington, D.C., 1976, p. 115.
11. Cove, H., Matloff, J., Sacks, H.J., Sherbecoe, R., and Goldfinger, D.: Autologous Blood Transfusion in Coronary Artery Bypass Surgery. Transfusion 16:245, 1976.
12. Silver, H.: Banked and Fresh Autologous Blood in Cardiopulmonary Bypass Surgery. Transfusion 15:600, 1975.
13. Cuello, L., Vazquez, E., Perez, V., and Raffucci, F.L.: Autologous Blood Transfusion in Cardiovascular Surgery. Transfusion 7:309, 1967.
14. Daggett, W.M., Gada, P.H., Leape, L.L., Scannel, J.G., and Taratkoff, J.: Autologous Blood Transfusion in Pulmonary Surgery. J. Thorac. Cardiovasc. Surg. 59:546, 1970.
15. Silvergleid, A.J.: Autologous Transfusions. Experience in a Community Blood Center, J.A.M.A. 241:2724, 1979.
16. Caggiano, V.: Sacramento Medical Foundation Blood Bank, Personal communication, 1980.
17. Aster, R.: Blood Center of Southeastern Wisconsin, Communication to Council of Community Blood Centers, 1979.
18. Basequin, P.P.: Implementation of an autologous blood program in a community blood bank. In: Autologous Transfusion, A Technical Workshop. Dawson, B.R., Ed., Am.

Assoc. Blood Banks, Washington, D.C., 1976, p. 103.

19. American Association of Blood Banks, Standards for Blood Banks and Transfusion Services, 7th Ed., Washington, D.C., 1976.

20. Silver, H.: Liquid Storage of Autologous Blood. In: Autologous Transfusion, A Technical Workshop. Dawson, B.R., Ed., Am. Assoc. Blood Banks, Washington, D.C., 1976, p. 37.

21. Beutler, E. and Wood, L.: The *in vivo* regeneration of red cell 2,3-diphosphoglycerics acid (DPG) after transfusion of stored blood. J. Lab. Clin. Med. 74:300, 1969.

22. Mollison, P.L.: Blood Transfusion in Clinical Medicine, 6th Ed., Blackwell, London, 1979.

23. Hamstra, R.D. and Block, M.H.: Erythropoiesis in response to blood loss in man. J. Appl. Physiol. 27:503, 1969.

24. Zuck, T.F.: Donor response to Predeposit Autologous Transfusion Phlebotomy. In: Autologous Transfusion, A Technical Workshop. Dawson, B.R., Ed., Am. Assoc. Blood Banks, Washington, D.C., 1976, p. 51.

25. Becker, C.E., MacGregor, R.R., and Walker, K.S.: Fatal Anaphylaxis After Intramuscular Iron Dextran. Ann. Intern. Med. 65:745, 1966.

26. Gilcher, R.O.: Autologous Transfusion Blood Salvage. In: Autologous Transfusion, A Technical Workshop. Dawson, B.R., Ed., Am. Assoc. Blood Banks, Washington, D.C., 1976, p. 95.

27. Gilcher, R.O. and Orr, M.: Intraoperative blood salvage, In: Hemotherapy in Trauma Surgery, Barnes, A., Ed., American Association of Blood Banks, Washington, D.C., 1979.

28. Glover, J.L., Smith, R., Yaw, P.B., Radigan, L.R., Benedick, R., and Plawecki, R.: Autotransfusion of blood contaminated by intestinal contents. JACEP 7:142, 1978.

29. Youner, H.J. and Samuelson, P.: Bacteriologic examination of autologous blood. South Med. J. 71:1232, 1978.

30. Yaw, P.B.: Tumor cells carried through autotransfusion. Contraindications to intraoperative blood recovery? J.A.M.A. 231:490, 1975.

31. McKenzie, F.N., Heimbecker, R.D., Wall, W., Robert, A., Black, L., and Barr, R.: Intraoperative autotransfusion in elective and emergency vascular surgery. Surgery 83:470, 1978.

32. Orr, M.: Autotransfusion: The use of washed red cells as an adjunct to component therapy. Surgery 84:728, 1978.

33. Noon, G.: Intraoperative autotransfusion. Surgery 84:722, 1978.

34. Davidson, S.J.: Emergency unit autotransfusion. Surgery 84:703, 1978.

35. Bell, W.: The hematology of autotransfusion. Surgery 84:695, 1978.

36. Schaff, H.V., Houer, J., Gardner, T.J., Donahoo, J.S., Watkins, L., Gott, V., and Brawley, R.K.: Routine use of autotranfusion following cardiac surgery: Experience in 700 patients. Ann. Thorac. Surg. 27:493, 1979.

37. Thurer, R.L., Lytle, B.W., Cosgrove, D.M., and Loop, F.D.: Autotransfusion following cardiac operations: A randomized, prospective study. Ann. Thorac. Surg. 27:500, 1979.

38. Annexton, M.: Autotransfusion for surgery: A comeback? J.A.M.A. 240:2710, 1978.

39. Brzica, S.M., Pineda, A.A., and Taswell, H.F.: Autologous Blood Transfusions, CRC Crit. Rev. Clin. Lab. Sci. 10:31, 1978.

40. Brewster, D.C., Ambrosino, J.J., Darling, R.C., Davison, J.K., and Warnock, D.F.: Intraoperative autotransfusion in major vascular surgery. Am. J. Surg. 137:507, 1979.

41. Lockhart, C., Mattox, K.L., and Philley, C.: A Review of Autotransfusion. J.E.N. 5:38, 1979.

16

The Regional Blood Center: Organization, Management, and Integration into National Systems

Johanna Pindyck, M.D., and Aaron Kellner, M.D.

INTRODUCTION

Within the span of some 40 years since the first blood banks were created in the mid 1930s, these simple structures—originally little more than hospital-based repositories for blood—have evolved into free-standing, multifaceted regional and community blood centers. A recent study by the National Blood Data Center revealed that 80 percent of the blood transfused annually in the United States is collected by such centers,[1] of which there are about 200. The typical center supplies a group of hospitals, usually within a defined geographic area, with blood, blood components, and derivatives, as well as various specialized services tailored to meet the patient care requirements within the service area. The blood center interacts directly and intimately with the hospital blood banks and transfusion services; through them, it interacts with the clinicians in the community. The blood center must also relate to the community at large for the regular supply of blood so essential to its mission.

The National Blood Policy, enunciated for the first time in 1973, called for an all-volunteer donor base for the nation's blood supply.[2] Blood centers, in cooperation with those hospitals which have blood collection capability, have been working toward this goal. It is estimated that in 1979 approximately 5 to 10 percent of the nation's blood supply still came from paid donors.

The blood service complex's greatest challenge for the next five to ten years will be the full development and subsequent stabilization of an adequate all-volunteer blood supply.

In this chapter, we will explore the development, goals, and operational characteristics of blood centers. Their importance to the communities they serve will be examined, as will the mechanisms which they have employed to communicate with the several publics with which they interact—lay, medical, scientific, technical, and administrative. Individual blood centers vary in size from those that collect less than 20,000 units of blood per year to others that collect more than 700,000, and the number of the hospitals served varies from less than 30 to more than 250. The distance of hospitals from the supplying center may vary from a few hundred feet to several hundred miles, requiring the development of unique strategies to cope with logistic problems. We will make no effort to examine exhaustively the many approaches which centers have devised to meet such unusual and highly specialized demands of a particular service area. Instead, we will delineate those features which most centers share regardless of their size and location, and dwell on those activities which have been integrated into the function of typical centers. In addition, we will describe the complex interactions which have evolved betwen blood centers both in this country and abroad and which serve to assure the availability of resources, both ordinary and rare, to all patients throughout the United States.

FUNCTIONS AND SERVICES PROVIDED BY A REGIONAL BLOOD CENTER

Products Provided by the Regional Blood Center

The primary objective of a blood center is the provision of a safe, stable, cost-effective supply of blood and blood products to meet the needs of patients and to assist hospitals in the appropriate use of these materials. In addition to meeting the ordinary requirements for blood, clotting factors, and platelets, special arrangements exist to meet extraordinary blood needs. The center provides a resource of blood from selected donors to meet the requirements of patients sensitized to blood group antigens and also serves as a reservoir from which the unexpected demands of emergencies can be met. The clinical needs of patients can best be met by close cooperation and coordinated planning between the center and the hospitals it serves; the hospital blood bank director and technical staff should form the link between the center staff and the bedside.

The center asesses the usual daily needs of its hospitals, reviewing past usage, projected requirements, and national trends. Preparations are then made to recruit, collect, and process a sufficient number of units of blood each day from essentially unselected donors to meet these constant demands from the hospitals. This must be done in a planned and coordinated manner that provides an ample but not excessive supply in order to optimize usage, minimize outdating and provide sufficient numbers of each blood component. The four functions—recruitment, collection, processing, and distribution—form the backbone operations of the blood center in accomplishing its primary mission. The blood components that are prepared and distributed by the regional blood center are listed in Table 16-1. In addition to these items, plasma derivatives such as albumin, plasma protein solution, clotting factors, and specialized materials necessary to hospital blood bank operations may also be available from the center, as noted in Table 16-2.

Services Available through the Blood Center

In addition to providing the materials noted above, certain specialized laboratory and clinical services are available through the blood center which augment the ability of the hospital blood banks to provide optimal patient care.

The services provided by the blood center vary from place to place and may include: antibody reference facilities; histocompatibility testing, including HLA typing; screening tests for hepatitis antigen or antibodies; and coagulation studies. In addition, procedures may be performed on patients referred to the center, such as collection and storage of blood for autologous transfusion, outpatient transfusion, therapeutic phlebotomy, and, most recently, a wide range of therapeutic pheresis procedures, including plasmapheresis and cytopheresis.

A staff of medical and technical experts is generally available in the larger centers to provide consultation services to the hospitals on transfusion or transfusion-related problems, both serologic and epidemiologic in nature.

Table 16-1. Blood Components Prepared and Distributed by a Regional Blood Center to the Hospitals in Its Service Area

Component	Description
Cryoprecipitate	Contains Factor VIII $\cong$ 130 units; Fibrinogen $\cong$ 200 mg.
Frozen Red Cells	Frozen, thawed red cells from one unit whole blood.
Leukocyte — Single unit	Buffy coat from 1 unit whole blood.
Single donor (pheresis)	Filtration leukopheresis or centrifugation derived leukocytes from 6–8 cycles of leukapheresis.
Leukocyte Poor Packed Red Cells	Buffy coat removed from 1 unit packed cells.
Packed Red Cells	Red cells from one unit whole blood.
Plasma — Fresh frozen plasma	Plasma from one unit whole blood.
Factor VIII depleted plasma, frozen	Plasma from one unit of whole blood, cryoprecipitate removed.
IgA deficient plasma	Plasma from IgA deficient donors.
Platelet rich plasma	Plasma with platelets from one unit whole blood.
Single donor plasma (non-frozen)	Deficient in labile clotting factors.
Zoster immune plasma	Plasma from donors recently recovered from Herpes Zoster.
Platelets — Single unit	Platelets from one unit of whole blood.
Single donor (pheresis)— HLA matched or non-matched	Platelets from 6–8 cycles of plateletpheresis.
Washed Red Cells	Washed red cells from unit of whole blood.
Whole Blood	Blood from which no components have been removed.

In order to provide all the above-noted services to the hospitals 24 hours a day, 7 days a week, most centers have on-call programs and round-the-clock coverage by their medical and technical staff, in keeping with other major health care institutions which face unpredictable emergency demands. Thus, patients with difficult antibody problems, patients requiring rare blood, or victims of accidents may be cared for appropriately and without undue delay, with the blood center providing those resources on a timely basis to all the hospitals in its service area.

Education and Research

As the name implies, a blood center has other functions in addition to provision of products and service; it is also a focus for education and research. This commitment to the improvement of blood services has been well expressed in the Statement of Purpose of the Blood Services of the American National Red Cross,[3] the largest group of affiliated blood centers in the United States.

Education. Educational efforts are aimed at several groups, both within and outside of the blood bank specialty. These groups include laboratory technicians, undergraduate or graduate students, and physicians wishing to enter the field. Continuing education for people already in blood banking as a specialty is also undertaken by the centers.

Blood centers also have responsibilities for educational efforts directed toward two other groups—physicians who utilize blood and its components, and the public, who must be the informed volunteer donors of today and tomorrow. It is with these latter two areas that much work still needs to be done, and in which the practicing physician can play a

Table 16-2. Plasma Derivatives and Other Materials Often Available from the Regional Blood Center for the Hospitals in Its Service Area

Plasma Derivatives
  Albumin 5% Normal Serum Albumin
             25% Normal Serum Albumin
  Factor VIII Concen-
    trate   (Antihemophilic Factor)
  Factor IX Concentrate (Factor IX Complex)
  Gamma Globulin   (Immune Serum Globulin)
  Gamma Globulin, Hyperimmune
    Hepatitis B Immune Globulin
    Tetanus Immune Globulin
    Pertussis Immune Globulin
    Mumps Immune Globulin
    Vaccinia Immune Globulin
  Plasma Protein Solution 5% Solution

Other Materials
  Bags, for blood collection
  Equipment—via joint purchasing arrangements
  Reagent Red Cells for laboratory use
  Reagent Sera for laboratory use

role. It is reasonable to expect that the physician responsible for prescribing blood has an understanding of how it is provided and when and how to use it. The physician audience which needs to be reached is very large and heterogeneous and, for the message to be delivered, the collaborative effort of many groups is required. The several clinical departments within a hospital which utilize blood, as well as the various organized medical groups within an area, such as state or county medical societies, offer the most effective means for accomplishing this. The blood center staff, in cooperation with the medical community, shoulder the responsibility for disseminating information in this increasingly important and rapidly advancing field.[4]

The largest and most unwieldy of all publics, the community at large, is a prime and critically essential target for education by the blood center. Blood donors represent only 4 to 5 percent of the population. They form a natural focus for continuing education because it is the group which has already elected to join the donor ranks. The major thrust of the communication effort directed to influence them usually involves gripping accounts of past or future needs with a "Madison Ave-

nue" slant rather than being truly educational. Future efforts should be directed toward improving the information base presented to these already committed individuals. Attracting new donors in the future will require a broader educational effort that must emphasize not only the need for blood but also the simplicity, safety, and relative painlessness of donation. This educational effort must also stress the risks to the individual and society in general of an insufficient blood supply—that is, that a community's blood supply, for those who need it, is as important as its water supply. Overcoming the natural fears of the first-time donor requires patience, understanding, and the development of sufficient motivation to outweigh fear or apathy. The clinician can play an important role in the education of present and future donors by seeing to it that the friends and family of patients in their care are aware of the activities of the blood service complex within their community and of the responsibility of healthy members of society to sustain the blood supply for all patients. A stable, all-volunteer donor base requires a sensitized donor public which responds promptly and consistently to requests for blood donation.

Broad educational efforts beamed to the general public take place at many locations, through varying channels, and are directed at several age groups in the population. Schools have begun to include information in their curricula on the biology and importance to the health field of blood donation, some beginning even in the primary grades. Provision of educational material through organized industrial and community groups disseminates information to the audience of donor age (17 through 65 in most states). In addition, increased public awareness of blood needs can be stimulated by the news media as a public service. Since the time for such programs is donated to the community's blood program, as to other nonprofit endeavors, this exposure is sharply limited by the availability of free time or space and the competition among public agencies. Each of these avenues needs to be carefully exploited in the increasingly difficult effort to develop a sense of community commitment on the part of the public to donate blood.

Research. The research efforts of a blood center can span the range from basic to applied; they are vital because they are the engine of progress and serve to assure improvements and innovation. These activities may, for example, focus on the biochemistry of blood cells and their preservation, transplantation biology, genetics, the technologies of fail-safe donor-patient identification, or the development of sophisticated, computerized systems for inventory management. As a focal point for long-term contact with many thousands of healthy individuals within the community, the blood center can serve as the locus for extensive epidemiologic investigations in other fields, such as cancer and heart disease, as well as blood-related problems. The dynamic and research-oriented blood center can make a significant contribution to health care in many fields.

ORGANIZATION, GOVERNANCE, AND FINANCING

Hospital blood banks are not usually legal entities unto themselves, but are an integral part of the larger hospital complex in which they function. By contrast, a blood center is a free-standing, separately incorporated, non-profit institution, governed by its own board of directors, or other similarly titled body, which has the responsibility to establish the policies and objectives of the center and provide for its continuity and fiscal health. Depending upon the mode of origin and the affiliation of a blood center, its board may be more or less representative of the total community served. It is usual for the boards of centers within the Red Cross system to have broad representation from the lay community as well as the medical community. Some blood centers that origunated under the sponsorship of a group of concerned physi-

cians or an area's medical society have boards which are largely, and in some cases even totally, comprised of physicians. The trend today is for broader community representation on the boards of directors.

The board has the responsibility to determine policy and to select staff leadership for the center, and then to delegate to it the responsibility of its day-to-day operations. Center management must develop the plans, acquire and train staff at all levels, and prepare the operating documents and protocols which are required for the effective functioning of the enterprise. These activities must be in keeping with the expectations, goals, and policies established by the board and consistent with the medical needs of the community.

The designated leader of a blood center may be either a lay administrator or a physician. In either case, a high level of both administrative competence and medical knowledge are essential in the center's top staff echelons. It is clear that, as independent non-profit corporations, centers must be financially self-sustaining. This is best achieved not by subsidies but by the development of appropriate fees for the products and services provided to the patients in the community. These fees are charged to the hospitals; they are then usually passed along to the individual patient who received the product or service or to the third-party payer involved (i.e., the appropriate insurance company, Medicaid, or Medicare). The fees attached to blood products, the "processing fees" are generally set at a level to permit recovery of the cost of donor recruitment, collection, laboratory processing, and delivery of the products to hospitals. Specialized consulting services, such as for rare blood, are usually not charged specifically to the individual patient but are incorporated into the operating expenses of the center and form part of this "processing fee."

Today, most recipients of blood transfusions have third-party payment available to cover the costs of the "processing fees"—the

Federal Government (Medicare and Medicaid), Blue Cross/Blue Shield, and other forms of health insurance. The increased utilization of blood for patient care has made third-party payment for these charges, which can mount to hundreds or thousands of dollars, an essential part of the health insurance package. As the NBDC report states, "An average of one unit of blood (whole blood and red cells) was transfused for every five hospital admissions."[1] The nation's annual blood bill has been estimated to be in excess of $500,000,000.

ORGANIZATION AND STAFFING OF THE REGIONAL BLOOD CENTER (INTERNAL ORGANIZATION)

The configuration of the regional center's staff will reflect the functions performed. In this section we will not attempt to detail the specialized staff who serve as members of educational or research sections within a center because these functions are similar to those carried out in other institutions and their activities are therefore familiar to the reader. On the other hand, the operating functions of the blood center which are dedicated to fulfillment of its primary mission, the provision of the blood supply, are unique and unfamiliar and thus warrant brief comment.

Medical Staff

Every aspect of the blood center's activities has medical implications insofar as the health of the donor or the recipient may be affected. In view of this, all blood centers have at least one and sometimes several physicians who are charged with establishing policies and procedures directed toward assuring the health and safety of donors and the eventual recipients. Blood donations must by regulation be carried out under the direct supervision of a licensed physician, or by those

trained to carry out the procedures according to protocols designated by him.

Physicians may enter center blood banking via several paths—usually from backgrounds in clinical pathology or internal medicine, the latter often after special training in hematology. The American Board of Pathology has established blood banking as an accepted subspecialty, and many blood center physicians with the requisite training have passed their examination and been so recognized. The physician may serve the center full-time or part-time, depending upon the size and scope of its activities. More and more centers have found it necessary to have at least one full-time physician due to the increasing medical supervision needed during pheresis procedures and to the recognized need for the center to serve as consultant to its area hospitals in the use of blood and components.

Whether a physician is the director of the blood center or works closely with an administrator who has overall responsibilities for directing the center's functions, the ultimate success of the operation will be determined by the ability of the staff within the center to perceive the medical needs of the community it serves and translate these effectively into responsive action, and in a timely fashion. The operating staff is organized to perform the four major blood center functions which are essential to the provision of the blood supply: recruitment, collection, laboratory processing, and distribution.

Recruitment

The recruitment staff may be either paid or volunteer, in varying proportions, depending upon the particular affiliation (Red Cross or non-Red Cross) and the characteristics of the center. This staff has the responsibility to plan, recruit, and schedule the collection of blood from sufficient numbers of volunteer donors to provide the necessary blood and blood components to meet patient needs.

Since the storage life of some blood products is short, 3 days or even less, blood usually must be obtained daily, including weekends. the number of units needed each day by a center may range from 100 to more than 2,-000, depending upon the demands of the hospitals served. The collection of these units requires scheduling of predictable numbers of donors on a regular basis. To achieve this efficiently, centers employ the basic strategy of collecting blood from organized groups of individuals within the community which can be approached in large numbers. Such groups may be businesses, industrial organizations, governmental offices, schools, churches, or fraternal organizations. Frequently, the groups are scheduled a year in advance, in order to build a calendar of collections to provide continuity in meeting patient needs. Group donations, to be cost-effective, are generally scheduled to yield at least 50 units of blood.

An organization's agreement to sponsor donations by its members is a solemn pledge to work with its community blood center to achieve the promised number of donors; it is a serious commitment of interest and support.

Donor recruitment, with its attendant public relations activities, provides the cornerstone on which the rest of the blood center's operations rest. As the need for blood components increases, the demands upon the recruitment department to provide the starting material increase in parallel. No other field depends so heavily each day on the good will and altruistic attitudes of a substantial segment of the population.

Collection

Location. Collections must be undertaken at sites which are convenient to the donor[5] and safe for the performance of the collection procedure. They must also be so located so as to permit the requisite number of components to be prepared within the time

constraint dictated by the regulatory agencies to which the center is subject. To provide convenient donor locations, blood centers have tended to bring the collection site to the donor in the form of a bloodmobile—essentially a traveling collection team, including staff and equipment. This may be set up entirely on the premises of a facility (Fig. 16-1) or may take place in a self-contained mobile unit van (Figs. 16-2*A*, *B*). More than 80 percent of the blood collected daily throughout the country by the American Red Cross and other blood centers is collected on mobile units.

In addition, centers maintain fixed collection stations in convenient locations in the community to which donors may come; some of these are in hospitals which have donor programs affiliated with the local blood center. Whether donating at fixed sites or on a bloodmobile, most donors have been enlisted through the participation of the organized groups referred to above, on whose regular support the center's donor program depends.

Staff and Procedures. Blood collections are carried out under the supervision of the center physician. The guiding principle of the donor screening is that the donation should be safe for the donor and the blood which is collected should be safe for the intended recipient. The guidelines for screening have been detailed in Chapter 8. Collections are performed either by nurses and/or by trained phlebotomists. A team of other individuals, both paid and volunteer, works closely with the phlebotomy staff to offer donor care and service. Each blood collection experience, regardless of where it is carried out, is a medical encounter for the donor and must be undertaken with the professionalism expected in a doctor's office or in a clinic of a hospital.

With the acceptance of a donation, the center establishes a complex relationship to assure the welfare of the donor, the proper utilization of the gift which he has given to society, and the privacy of information which has been obtained during donor processing, whether this is demographic or medical. Each

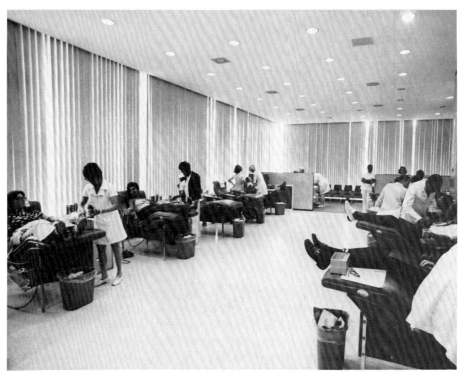

Fig. 16-1. Blood being collected at Center West, one of three Red Cross blood donor stations in Manhattan.

of these aspects must find its proper place in the center's functioning while it performs its task of providing for the community's blood supply.

One mechanism which has been used by blood centers to aid them in providing an adequate supply of blood from volunteer donors has been by developing inventory sharing mechanisms of varying kinds between centers in different communities. The Clearing House of the AABB and the Compass System of Red Cross are examples of such sharing, dealing mostly with acute shortages and overages. A more recent approach to the problem is resource sharing, in which centers that have successfully developed a donor base greater than that required to fill their own needs have entered into long-term, preplanned commitments to serve as regular supplementary suppliers to centers in other areas with insufficient donor support. All cen-

ters participate in resource sharing of rare blood to assure that such special and unusual red cells will be available to all patients according to need regardless of their location.[12]

The most far-reaching of these resource sharing programs is one which was developed by the New York Blood Center soon after its inception and referred to by the code name Euroblood. In 1973, in order to counteract the excessive dependence on commercial blood which had reached more than 60 percent of the blood transfused in the New York area, the New York Blood Center launched a unique international program of cooperation between blood centers. Following World War II, the Swiss, German, French, and other European Red Cross organizations had maintained a strong commitment to Red Cross blood programs. They also entered into the production of blood derivatives from plasma obtained from volunteer blood donors, which

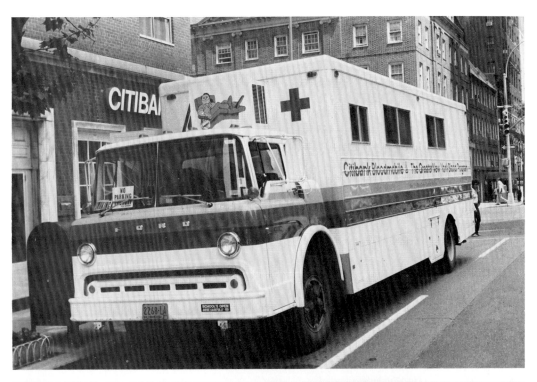

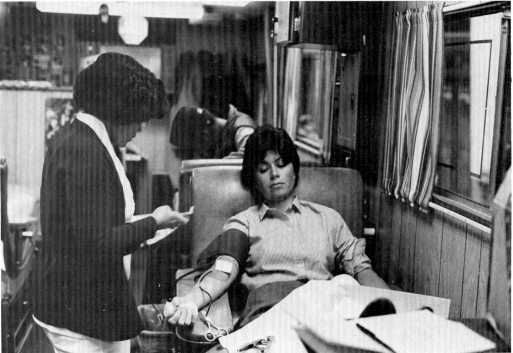

Fig. 16-2 A. Exterior of self-contained mobile collection vehicle of the Greater New York Blood Program. B. Interior view of same vehicle, during a mobile drive.

they accomplished by collecting more blood than was needed in their communities, drawing off the plasma, and discarding the surplus red cells. With the approval of the BOB, the New York Blood Center extended its license to collection activities in Europe. By so doing, blood was collected from voluntary donors, the plasma was separated and left in the country of origin, and the red cells which would otherwise have been wasted were shipped to New York where all the required laboratory tests were performed and the red cells utilized for transfusion. The Euroblood program has also provided support for other cities in the United States and is now aiding other nations which are in the formative stages of their volunteer donor blood programs (e.g., Greece, Portugal, and some of the Mid-Eastern countries). The Euroblood program highlights a difference between the volunteer blood donor programs of the Western European countries and those in the United States—the availability and sustained commitment of the donors. These countries appear to have large cadres of volunteer donors who consider it their responsibility to support their nation's blood supply.

Efforts at planned resource sharing have begun in the United States, but the full development and utilization of this approach is still in its infancy.

Problems in Interagency Interactions

On the surface, the approach of organizing centralized regional systems to provide for a hospital's needs for blood and derivatives would appear to interface optimally with hospital goals, since the hospital's primary concern is the provision of the needed material for the hospitalized patient. That this was not to be the case is one of the unfortunate realities of the blood bank field, and one which has hampered progress. It is important, therefore, to examine briefly the problem in order to be able to understand the situation which confronts the U.S. blood service complex.

Laboratory Processing

Blood is collected into one of several types of plastic containers, depending on the ultimate component production for which it is intended (see Ch. 9). It is then returned to the center for processing prior to entering the inventory. Unlike most materials which can be pooled and tested in batches, each unit of blood must be individually tested to determine ABO group, Rh type, and the presence of any unexpected anti-red cell antibodies in the plasma. Serological tests for syphilis and for hepatitis-B antigen are also performed routinely. If the unit is intended for component production, this is accomplished in parallel with the performance of the above serological tests in another section of the laboratory. After all the studies have been concluded, appropriate labels must be applied to each unit found acceptable for transfusion and to the components produced from it. Those found positive for syphilis or hepatitis are removed and appropriately discarded. The center's responsibility to the public health authorities and the blood donor do not cease when a unit has been found unsuitable for transfusion; mechanisms exist within each center to notify the donor and the responsible agency of such abnormalities, as well as to restrict future donations of persons found to have hepatitis-B surface antigen in the serum or to be implicated in the transmission of posttransfusion hepatitis.

Processing of individual blood units creates a major problem, not only because of the work load involved but also because of the enormous amount of record keeping required. Since each unit, or the components prepared from it, is a therapeutic agent, rigorous attention to detail at every step must be a part of the laboratory's protocol. Written records are required from the time the unit of blood is volunteered by the donor until a product label is applied. Additional records accompany the storage and shipping of the unit to an individual hospital. The unit's subsequent history in the blood bank is reviewed in Chapter 17, and it is clear that record keeping is a concern of equal magnitude in that location. Introduction of automated methods for testing and record keeping has been a major step forward in the safe and efficient handling of the unit of blood.

Automated serological testing can be performed on such instruments as Technicon's Autoanalyzer or Roche's Groupamatic. New technologies in blood labeling have recently been developed with the introduction of machine readable bar code labels for unit and product identification. Combining automated laboratory testing and specimen identification yields a powerful approach to solving the major problems presented by the need to handle each individual unit separately throughout its history, and promises with its gradual introduction throughout the field of blood banking to afford improved levels of performance previously unattainable by manual techniques.[6] As noted in Chapter 17, the clinician can also expect to see extension of this approach within the hospital to minimize the single largest source of serious transfusion reactions—human clerical error.

Distribution (Product Management)

Once the blood and its components have been processed, they must be stored in a fashion appropriate to the product. Storage conditions and durations range from low temperature storage of frozen blood in liquid nitrogen at $-196°$ C for 3 years to brief room temperature storage of platelets at $22°$ C for days. An even shorter storage life—24 hours—is required for any product prepared in an open system because of concern about possible bacterial contamination—e.g., single donor pheresis products or frozen red cells

which have been thawed and washed to remove the cryoprotective agent. A blood center offers the hospitals it serves a broad range of products, each with special characteristics for storage, expiration date, and shipping. In addition, since many of the products are needed only episodically by an individual hospital, the center serves both as a supplier of the hospital's routine inventory and as the backup reserve supply. Thus, an inventory of each product must be developed and maintained consistent with the anticipated demand of all the hospitals served. Management of the blood inventory has become a complex demanding exercise that requires development of procedures to assure availability of products at all times. Several types of approach have been utilized to manage the blood inventory rationally, but regardless of the method chosen, the aim is to make the product available to patients as needed in an efficient and cost-effective manner.

Red cells, either as packed cells or whole blood, are the major product supplied by the centers, and inventory management strategies focus primarily on the provision of this material. The prolonged storage life of red cells (21 to 35 days) permits hospitals to maintain stock inventories of red cells which are obtained on a regular basis from available supplies at the regional center. Fresh-frozen plasma, which may be stored for several months, is also kept on hand in the hospital. Other materials, with shorter life spans or infrequent use, are usually ordered and delivered as needed for individual patients. Inventory management protocols between the center and the hospitals may vary from a simple demand system, in which the hospital places all its blood requests daily, to sophisticated computer-coordinated preplanned shipments based on thorough review of the hospital's past blood use experience.[7] Nevertheless, all centers, regardless of basic inventory management strategy, maintain a regular telephone communication link with the hospitals served. This link acts as an operations center for vital information relay and reactive response between the hospital blood bank and the blood center, permitting rapid adjustment in the case of emergencies or other unusual situations.

Protocols and Procedures Dedicated to Assure Product Quality

Blood centers are strictly regulated by federal, state, and, at times, municipal health agencies. All blood banks in the United States are required to *register* with the Food and Drug Administration (FDA), which exercises federal regulatory authority over them through its Bureau of Biologics (BOB). Blood banks engaging in shipments across state lines (which includes essentially all blood centers) are required to be *licensed* by the FDA. For licensure by the BOB, FDA requires submission of an application that details the protocols and procedures used in the preparation of the licensable products produced by the center as well as the physical plant in which this will be accomplished; it also involves inspection prior to licensure followed by at least annual inspections to ascertain compliance with the licensed protocols and with the regulations promulgated by the FDA for blood banks.[8]

These regulations establish minimum standards for product quality to which all licensed establishments must adhere. In addition, there are state and local regulations which may in some instances be more rigid than the federal standards, but which must not be in conflict with them. Since they are administered by a different agency, they usually involve additional record keeping, reporting, and inspections.

In parallel with these external regulatory requirements, virtually all blood centers have developed quality assurance procedures to assess regularly the performance of staff and equipment in the preparation of blood products. There are also voluntary inspection and accreditation programs in which the center

may participate, such as those operated by the American Association of Blood Banks and the College of American Pathologists. It is important to recognize that every activity involved in handling blood from the initial donor interview to eventual transfusion to the patient can effect the quality of the product. The degree of control which the center and its partner, the hospital blood bank, exert at every step in the path from donor to recipient is motivated by recognition of this critically important fact. No other laboratory with which the clinician deals, and no other therapeutic agent which is regularly administered to patients, is as fragile as the transplantable tissues prepared from blood donations.

BLOOD CENTER—COMMUNITY INTERFACES

The National Level

From an historical viewpoint, blood centers were a natural outgrowth of the recognition of the clinical importance of a stable, coordinated blood supply which first arose during the nation's need to provide blood to the Armed Forces during World War II. Most of the blood collected for the troops during World War II and the Korean War was processed into pooled liquid or dried plasma. Responsibility for the acquisition of more than 20 million units of blood for this purpose fell to the American Red Cross, which responded rapidly and effectively by mobilizing to accomplish this task and establishing 65 collection centers throughout the United States. The success of the endeavor can be appreciated by realizing that in 1944 alone more than 5 million units of blood were collected, about the same number that was collected by all Red Cross blood centers in 1978. Following World War II, many of the European nations continued their Red Cross blood programs, often with government support. By contrast, all centers in the United States ceased to operate following World War II.

It very quickly became clear that, just as a reliable, predictable, centralized supply of blood and derivatives was of great supportive value to military medicine in wartime, a similar advantage would accrue to civilian practice from such blood availability during peacetime. In 1947, American Red Cross leadership decided to endorse the development of a National Blood Program under the aegis of the Red Cross. Blood centers began to arise in communities across the country, sponsored by Red Cross or by independent local civic groups, in response to a need perceived by the medical or lay leadership of the area for a steadily available blood supply for their hospitals.

American Red Cross Blood Services currently include 57 centers across the nation. These function under one Bureau of Biologics license with respect to their production methods; they are strongly linked by common ties within the Red Cross system, and are dedicated to providing for the unique and individual needs of their service areas. Many hospitals in the United States are served by approximately 140 blood centers which are independent of the American Red Cross. Most of those are members of the American Association of Blood Banks (AABB) and/or the Council of Community Blood Centers (CCBC). The former organization was founded in 1947 by physicians, technologists, and administrators, drawn largely from hospital blood banks but also community blood centers who were interested in sharing information and know-how in their specialty. The CCBC was founded in the 1960s to represent the needs and interests of blood centers which were not within the Red Cross system.

The Need for Resource Sharing

Many of the blood centers, particularly those serving the more rural sections of the United States, have succeeded in achieving the goal of providing a stable blood supply for their hospitals from local donors. Those located in urban settings have had more difficulty in attaining this goal. Several factors have contributed to this difficulty. These include (1) changes in the demography of the population in the urban setting, and (2) increased mobility of this population, leading to a decreased sense of community and decreased participation in community activities including blood donation. In addition, the less advantaged population within urban areas, although requiring as much blood per capita in terms of usage, fails to make as substantial a contribution to the supply. Many factors have been identified as playing a role in this phenomenon, including fear, ignorance, and cultural beliefs related to the effects of donation.[9]

Urban blood centers tend to serve the larger and more sophisticated medical complexes which offer advanced medical and surgical therapies and frequently serve as referral centers from other hospitals both near and far. Since these advanced procedures often require the most extensive use of blood and blood components, the demands for these products are frequently greatest on those centers least able to meet them fully from local sources. On the other hand, such centers have tended to develop the most sophisticated reference laboratories, the most complete supplies of rare products, and the most extensive lists of special donors to meet the needs of their hospitals.

Difficulty in receiving total supply from the local blood center has led some hospitals to provide part of their own supply from in-hospital collections. It has also led to the development of for-profit suppliers of blood who use paid blood donors as their source. The reliance on commercial blood donors in the past reached more than 60 percent of the total supply in some parts of the country.

The unacceptability of dependence on commercial blood suppliers for the whole blood and components needed for transfusion was appreciated by leaders in blood banking and related fields[10] long before it became clear that such paid donors were the largest single source of posttransfusion hepatitis in the country.[1] Several approaches have been used to decrease the dependence on paid donors in different areas, and the demise of commercial blood centers has been hastened by the introduction in May, 1978 by the BOB, of a requirement that all blood be conspicuously labeled as to its source from a volunteer or paid donor.

In essence, the early post-World War II organization of blood services in the United States into a coordinated, integrated whole foundered on the rocks of conflict between two opposed philosophies of donor recruitment. One was based on altruism and "community responsibility" espoused by the American Red Cross and many other community blood centers in which blood donations made by the public are available to all according to medical need; the other was that of "individual responsibility," in which persons receiving blood were required to replace it. The conflict revolved around the method used to enlist donors. Since hospitals are the location at which blood is transfused, the replacement concept received its support primarily by hospitals. Compelx schemes to encourage replacement were developed, all revolving essentially around varying degrees of reduction in hospital charges if blood donations were made in the name of a patient. This led to a polarization within the blood service complex which was further complicated by a perception on the part of some hospital blood bankers that this individual responsibility approach to donation was essential for their survival. To complicate the picture further, certain financial advantages were available from the penalty fees which hospitals attached for units of blood which were not replaced. These conflicts have led to less than optimal development of strong regional centers in many areas because the benefits of the regional approach requires compromise from all participants—a degree of cooperation which has been difficult to achieve. The volunteer donor has been trapped in this conflict, and his confusion has contributed to his failure to support fully the needs of the blood service complex.

The American Blood Commission

In 1973, the federal government, which had previously remained aloof from the ethical and social problems confronting blood banking and had concerned itself only with the safety and efficacy of blood products, modified its position and proclaimed its interest in the integrity of the country's blood supply by announcing for the first time a National Blood Policy.[2] The four principles of that policy state that all Americans are entitled to be assured of an adequate blood supply, which should be high-quality, readily accessible, independent of ability to pay, and efficiently managed.

Implementation of the National Blood Policy was then turned back to the private sector, and members of the blood service complex as well as other concerned health professionals were charged with the responsibility of developing a workable plan. Representatives from the American Medical Association, American Association of Blood Banks, American National Red Cross, Council of Community Blood Centers, American Hospital Association, American Society of Clinical Pathologists, and College of American Pathologists worked together in this planning effort, which in due course led to the creation of the American Blood Commission in 1975. The central purpose of the Commission was to serve as a national public forum in which to examine and resolve the major policy issues relating to the provision of optimal blood services for the country.

Membership in and sponsorship for the American Blood Commission (ABC) was sought from those organized groups which have a prime interest in the nation's blood services: the providers of blood services, the donor population, and the patient or consumer. More than 40 organized national groups rallied to join and give their support, contributing both finances and personnel to work with the ABC. ABC member groups are listed alphabetically in Table 16-3. Since 1975, the ABC has concentrated on several areas which are of key importance in the implementation of the National Blood Policy.

Table 16-3. Membership of the American Blood Commission.

American Association for Clinical Histocompatibility Testing
American Association of Blood Banks
American Association of Tissue Banks
American Cancer Society
American College of Emergency Physicians
American College of Physicians
American College of Surgeons
American Federation of Labor-Congress of Industrial Organizations (AFL-CIO)
American Heart Association
American Hospital Association
American Legion
American Medical Association
American Nurse's Association
American Osteopathic Association
American Osteopathic College of Pathologists
American Red Cross
American Society for Medical Technology
American Society of Anesthesiologists
American Society of Clinical Pathologists
American Society of Hematology
American Surgical Association
Association of American Cancer Institutes
Blue Cross Association
College of American Pathologists
Communications Workers of America
Cooley's Anemia Foundation
Council of Community Blood Centers
Health Insurance Association of America
United Automobile Workers
Aerospace & Agricultural Implement Workers of America
Leukemia Society of America
National Association of Manufacturers
National Association of Patients on Hemodialysis and Transplantation
National Association for Sickle Cell Disease
National Hemophilia Foundation
National Kidney Foundation
National Medical Association
National Retired Teachers Association
American Association of Retired Persons
Pharmaceutical Manufacturers Association
Society for Cryobiology
United Way of America
Veterans Administration

(Henry, J.B. and Hubbell, R.C.: Blood resource management. J.A.M.A. 242:261, 1979.)

These include a program for defining and recognizing blood service regions throughout the country;[13] establishment of a National Blood Data Center for the gathering and analysis of essential information on blood collection and utilization;[1] designation of common systems for labeling blood and blood products; and development of ways to address the problem of donor recruitment. Significant progress has been made by the private sector in response to the challenge with which it was presented, although several thorny problems still remain to be resolved.

As indicated throughout this chapter, the critical unresolved problem is donor resource development. Although efforts at resource sharing have been begun, it is clear that the overriding problem is not so much the sharing as it is the obtaining of sufficient resources to share. The American Blood Commission can be of material assistance in this undertaking because of its broad representation and because it is national rather than local in scope. Widespread dissemination of information concerning the importance of voluntary blood donation to the health and well-being of the nation's population by lending support to local efforts at donor recruitment can be a major contribution of the ABC to the successful implementation of the National Blood Policy.

In 1978, the ABC took a much needed step toward resolving the existing confusion and moving the country to a single philosophy of donor recruitment when it endorsed the concept of altruism and community responsibility as the preferred message for delivery to the American public.

Donor resource development will present a continuing challenge to the blood service complex and to the medical and lay community because the need for blood and its products is increasing at a rate estimated to be about 5 percent per year. New products such as interferon derived from human leukocytes and new surgical procedures and cancer therapies can be expected to increase further the need for blood and require even greater responsiveness of the public to become blood donors.

Blood Center—Community Relations—The Local Level

A basic responsibility of the regional blood center is the establishment of effective communication with its diverse publics. The strategies involved in accomplishing this should ensure not only an informed citizenry and a stable blood supply but the continuing responsiveness of the center to its community obligations and methods to permit assessment of this responsiveness. In effect, each blood center must implement the National Blood Policy within its area. The ABC has provided the criteria to assist blood centers and their communities in this effort through its Task Force on Regionalization which has developed the guidelines and bench marks to define a regional association of blood service units.[13] The Task Force has designated broad principles for the governance of such regional associations of blood service units; however, because of the sensitivity of this matter, considerable latitude is provided to permit innovation and responsiveness to local conditions.

Regardless of the governance mechanism, the regional association should permit appropriate input from the following concerned groups:

1. the blood center—which may serve as the focal point for the association;
2. the hospital—which should have a voice for its blood banks, administrators, and transfusionists;
3. the patient—who may be represented by one or more of the organized groups for special hematologic disorders (e.g., thalassemia or hemophilia);
4. the donor—represented by labor, management, and social or religious groups within the community;
5. the medical society;
6. the public health agency.

Having been charged with implementing the National Blood Policy, the blood center, the hospitals, and the local public must work together to accomplish this task. During 1979, the first 14 regions representing approximately 7 percent of the blood collected in the country were recognized as regional associations by the ABC.

Toward a National Blood System

The principles embodied in the ABC's Regionalization Program hold promise for eventual development of an integrated national blood system based on strong local programs, each reflecting the unique characteristics of the region in which it exists. The resource sharing activities which have been developed may provide the beginning for a larger and more integrated network. When achieved, a coordinated national system will assure that the whole country will have equal access to the full range of services needed for modern patient care. It will, in addition, permit the development of a full set of contingency plans to meet local and national disasters. The blood banking community has the challenging opportunity to provide a model for the health care field to demonstrate the effectiveness of the private sector in planning and implementing a coordinated, shared, interdependent national program.

REFERENCES

1. Special Report of the National Blood Data Center, June 1979, American Blood Commission.
2. National Blood Policy, Few Register 39(47):9329, 1974.
3. Statement of American Red Cross Blood Services Purposes, American Red Cross National Headquarters, June, 1979.
4. Hillman, R.S., Helbig, S., Howes, S., Hayes, J., Meyer, D.M., and McArthur, S.R.: The effect of an educational program on transfusion practices in a regional blood program. Transfusion 19:153, 1979.

5. Drake, A.W.: Public Attitudes and Decision Processes with Regard to Blood Donation. Technical Report #138. Operations Research Center, Massachusetts Institute of Technology, 1978.

6. Allen, F.H., Jr., Brodheim, E., Hirsch, R.L., Steele, D.R., and Ying, W.: Regional blood center automation: computer surveillance of donor blood processing. Transfusion 18:716, 1978.

7. Brodheim, E., Hirsch, R., and Prastacos, G.: Setting Inventory Levels for Hospital Blood Banks. Transfusion 16:63, 1976.

8. Code of Federal Regulations, Food and Drugs, U.S. Government Printing Office, Washington, D.C., 1979.

9. Oswalt, R.M.: A Review of Blood Donor Motivation and Recruitment. Transfusion 17:123, 1977.

10. National Heart, Blood Vessel, Lung and Blood Program. Vol. IV Panel Reports. Part IV Report of the Blood Resources Panel. 1.2.1. Voluntarism 1-5, April 6, 1973, U.S. Department of Health, Education and Welfare.

11. Alter, H.J., Holland, P.V., Purcell, R.H., Lander, J.J., Feinstone, S.M., Morrow, A.G., and Schmidt, P.S.: Post-transfusion hepatitis after exclusion of commercial and hepatitis-B antigen-positive donors. Am. Intern. Med. 77:691, 1972.

12. Technical Methods and Procedures of the American Association of Blood Banks, Seventh Edition, Washington, D.C., 1978.

13. Report of the Task Force on Regional Associations of Blood Service Units. American Blood Commission, 1976.

17

Organization and Functions of a Hospital Blood Bank and Transfusion Service

Carl F. W. Wolf, M.D.

INTRODUCTION

As indicated by the title of this chapter, the blood bank laboratory of the past has outgrown its name and now often has the added or substitute designation of tranfusion service. Historically, the simplest hospital blood bank was a place for refrigerated storage of blood and a laboratory to determine blood types and perform compatibility tests. The bank was logically a part of the hospital's clinical laboratory service. The analytical methods used focused on the interactions of cells and immunoglobulins and continue to rely mainly on the phenomena of immune agglutination, lysis, or cytotoxicity; but they have improved in specificity and sensitivity over the years as reagents and methods have improved. At the same time, new knowledge of the genetic and immunologic basis for the results obtained has helped in their application to diagnosis. The blood bank thus continues to have an important role as a diagnostic laboratory not unlike that of any other clinical laboratory. In this role, the blood bank shares the same organizational and managerial problems common to all clinical laboratories and all too familiar to physicians—such as prompt and accurate reporting of results, reliability of assays, establishment of equitable charge schedules, and

accurate billing practices. These functions of the blood bank should pose no unusual problems to the practitioner who is well versed in the use of other laboratory services. Indeed, if wholly new analytical methods such as radioimmunoassay or enzyme-linked immunosorbent assay were to be proved superior, the diagnostic work now done in blood banks might then be better performed in other laboratories, completing the scission in blood bank activities now only apparent functionally.

Unlike other clinical laboratories, however, the blood bank provides a parenteral therapeutic agent. Unlike the pharmacy's primarily synthetic parenterals, blood and its components resemble tissue or organ transplants. They require individual patient-donor matching. The unique aspects of transfusion practice are attributable to the complexity and "impurity" of the biological agent administered, the resultant sequelae, its perishability, and the vagaries of a supply that is dependent on a complex technology of collection and the good will and cooperation of physicians, patients, and the general public. It is these factors which increasingly determine the activities of the hospital blood bank and explain its evolution toward a transfusion service quite unlike its sister laboratories, and not entirely similar to the pharmacy or the organ transplant service, yet sharing with them important similarities.

Hospital blood banks and the products for transfusion are closely regulated by accrediting and governmental agencies. The specialist staffs of blood banks are similarly subject to various proficiency testing, licensing, and credentialing systems. But there is no guarantee that a blood bank and staff which meet all those standards will be able to provide an adequate supply of top-quality donor blood or that the transfusion service will operate well and meet the needs of patients and clinicians for blood products and relevant guidance and information about their use. Because performance is uncertain, even when product and personnel standards are met, the best assurance that a hospital blood bank's services are adequate comes from the interest and participation of the clinician using them. To be most effective, he should be a knowledgeable and demanding consumer and an active participant in the proper functioning of both the hospital transfusion service and the donor blood collecting system which supports it. In the discussion which follows, the basic elements of the organization and function of the hospital transfusion service will be described with the intention of making the clinician's participation in the operation of the service both easier and more effective.

THE OBJECTIVES OF THE HOSPITAL BLOOD BANK AND TRANSFUSION SERVICE

Fundamental Roles

Blood Inventory. The fundamental objectives of a hospital blood bank include the provision of blood for transfusion—in adequate amount, safely, soon enough, and in good condition so that it is efficacious. By studying historical patterns of blood use within the hospital, the size of the inventory which must be on hand to accommodate probable needs for blood can be calculated.[1]

Obviously, if the bank were to keep enough blood on hand to be always prepared even for the rare massive transfusion of uncommon group blood, the inventory would be excessive, and wastage due to outdating would increase. This problem is most troublesome in those hospitals where there is no regional supplier to supplement local supplies or no donors prepared to respond quickly to an emergency need. A wasteful inventory policy may be unavoidable in such unusual circumstances. In practice, it is usually possible to decide that most but not all needs will be met with local inventory and that a backup supply will be arranged for to take care of the unpredictable special need. When applied to the hospitals of a region served by a blood center, this principle can permit the scheduling of blood deliveries and donor blood collection activities in a rational and economic way. Programmed blood distribution[2] can be made to cover an arbitrary percentage of anticipated needs, usually 90 to 95 percent. A similar approach can be used if blood must be collected locally and the donations can be scheduled in advance. Since the program is based upon historical data on blood use, it is important that changes in the circumstances of use be noted and that the program be changed to accommodate them. Addition of a new clinical service, expansion of an existing service, and new knowledge or other factors leading to altered use patterns for a blood product may all make it necessary to adjust the program. Otherwise, the insidious or abrupt appearance of new needs will, in effect, reduce the percentage of needs which the programmed distribution or collection will cover, and more and more shortage situations will develop. The foresight and vigilance of the clinician and blood bank staff and frequent communication with each other and the supplier are needed to keep the assumptions on which blood distribution or collection is based up to date.

Compatibility Testing.   In each hospital, the need to assure compatibility of the blood transfused must be met. Which techniques should be used in crossmatching so as to detect clinically significant incompatibilities continues to be a question of interest to serologists, but acceptable methods are readily identified and implemented, and the risk of abbreviating or omitting them can be quantitated.[3] The latter is of importance in devising a system for coping with the rare extreme emergency need, as is discussed more fully in several other chapters of this book. If emergency needs can occur, some such protocol must be in operation to assure the prompt response of the blood bank to an order by the clinician in a mutually agreed-upon format and terminology. In that way, the risk of not transfusing immediately can better be compared with the risks of a potential incompatibility due to use of abbreviated techniques of typing and matching.

In the routine preparation of blood for transfusion, unexpected patient antibodies can cause red blood cell incompatibility. It is prudent in such cases to identify the antigenic specificity of the antibody so that absence of the antigen on the red cells of the potential donor can be assured. If all such identification were to be referred to a distant reference laboratory, frequent delays in transfusion would result. Since the way in which this common problem is handled bears directly on the convenience of the patient and the physician, the policy followed is of more than passing interest to the clinician.

Each hospital bank must decide how extensively it will analyze patient specimens which pose problems in atypical antibody identification or unusual red cell types. The decision depends on the probable urgency of transfusion needs as dictated by the kinds of patients seen, the availability of a more sophisticated reference laboratory to serve as backup on such cases, and the level of expertise available—either in the blood bank technical and professional staff or through consultation with the reference laboratory.

Commercial serologic blood grouping reagents of high quality are now universally available in the United States. Similarly, the

basic analytical procedures requiring a modest investment in simple equipment are well described in print, such as in the *Technical Manual of the American Association of Blood Banks* (AABB).[4] Necessary technical expertise can be readily acquired and maintained by the professional medical laboratory technologist. With the ready availability of antibody identification red cell panels as laboratory reagents, the majority of antibodies can be promptly and reliably identified by the skilled technologist. Proficiency can be assured by regular participation in one or more of the several available governmental, commercial, or professional proficiency testing programs.

It is not reasonable for most hospital laboratories to aspire to the solution of *all* such antibody identification problems without the occasional need for outside assistance. Regional blood centers and some commercial laboratories, independent or sponsored by suppliers of blood bank reagents, can be consulted on those problems requiring rare red cell types or specialized knowledge and techniques for their solution. It is reasonable to require that any hospital transfusing blood be no more than minutes away from a laboratory able to identify common antibodies by testing against a panel of known red cells. Arrangements should exist for prompt interpretive assistance within the hospital or from a reference center. A mechanism for the explanation of such technical problems directly to the transfusing clinician should also be available.

Blood Components. The technology of blood collection and processing has developed so that whole blood is now used more for the preparation of blood components and derivatives than it is for direct transfusion. The resultant products are increasingly numerous and vary in their indications for use, associated hazards, and cost. A new basic role for the hospital blood bank and transfusion service which has thus emerged is that of an information resource, consultation, and teaching service on the proper clinical use of blood products. The various common approaches to providing for the consultative and teaching role are discussed more fully below. The depth and breadth of local educational resources should parallel the complexity of the transfusion therapy practiced.

Optional Roles

In addition to the most fundamental roles of the hospital blood bank mentioned above, a variety of optional roles have emerged which vary with local circumstances.

Blood Collection and Processing. Frequently, the hospital blood bank is responsible for the collection of donor blood in sufficient quantity to meet all or a significant part of its needs. Even in hospitals where a regional collecting center bears most of the burden for collection, the ability to collect donor blood locally for special needs is often helpful. In either case, the clinician is in a unique position to contribute to the smooth operation of the transfusion service by encouraging the voluntary replacement or altruistic donation of blood by the friends and relatives of patients, directing them to the hospital or regional donor program as local circumstances dictate. Simply having a candidate execute a written pledge and register to be called as a donor may serve the needs of the collecting agency even more effectively than an unsolicited donation. Because blood outdates in a few weeks, a constant stream of a few donors each day is better than an occasional dramatic appeal for donors to meet an acute shortage. The physician-to-patient's family relationship is often qualitatively and temporally well suited to developing the continuous source of donations which constitutes the most helpful and efficient blood supply. The shorter life (3 days) of components such as platelets makes it necessary to have some donor collections every day of the week if a supply is to be available whenever needed. Encouraging donations on weekends and holidays is therefore especially meaningful. The psychology of donor recruitment and the use of various persuasive media to that end are topics of great current interest as the nation attempts to implement the national blood policy's requirement of an adequate volunteer donor blood supply. Success may one day allow those engaged in the transfusion of blood to be unconcerned about its procurement, but that day has not arrived. In the interim, it is difficult to conceive of a more capable and persuasive person to identify the healthy individual willing to volunteer as a blood donor than the physician who knows the value of blood to his patients and can speak with conviction.

Component Preparation and Therapeutic Plasmapheresis. Continuous or intermittent flow centrifuges able to separate blood into its components and return part of the blood to the donor have found growing acceptance in hospital blood banks and blood collection centers. They are used to collect large numbers of platelets or granulocytes from a single donor without depleting his red cells or plasma (plateletpheresis or leukapheresis), and in some cases for collecting plasma (plasmapheresis). Subsequently, interest in the use of such machines for the treatment of patients with a variety of diseases by plasmapheresis has grown rapidly,[5] and the availability of the machinery in the blood bank has led in some hospitals to the blood bank's assuming the role of therapist, presumably to avoid the expense of duplicating the capability elsewhere in the hospital. However, if the therapeutic procedure is viewed as a form of extracorporeal blood processing similar to hemodialysis, it becomes less certain that it is always reasonable to assign the therapeutic plasmapheresis role to the blood bank. The management of acutely ill patients undergoing plasmapheresis contrasts sharply with that of normal blood donors. Furthermore, the development of alternative, less costly means for accomplishing plasmapheresis, such as continuous ultrafiltration,[6] would further divorce the most common therapeutic procedure from the fundamental roles and capabilities of the hospital blood bank.

Less tenuous is the relationship between cytopheresis (leukapheresis and plateletpheresis) and the hospital blood bank. As platelet transfusion has developed, the value to the transfusion service of single donor platelets harvested by plateletpheresis in circumventing refractoriness due to alloimmunization has been clearly demonstrated. Provision for such a service or other means of access to a source of single donor platelets has become necessary if prolonged support of thrombocytopenic patients by platelet transfusion is planned. Similarly, the use of neutrophils for the temporary support of neutropenic infected patients, still a somewhat controversial modality as to efficacy and indications for use,[7] would make a cytopheresis capability necessary.

Rational blood component therapy cannot be practiced without basic hematologic laboratory determinations to assess the indications for transfusion and efficacy of the products after transfusion. The access to hematologic data must match in sophistication the blood products transfused. If not otherwise available, such determinations are sometimes performed and interpreted by the hospital blood bank to directly guide and monitor component therapy.

Histocompatibility Testing. Knowledge of the system of transplantation (HLA) and neutrophil-specific antigens has increased rapidly in recent years. The principal techniques used in their study (such as leukoagglutination and lymphocytotoxicity assays), as well as the basic principles common to inherited antigenic systems expressed on blood cells, have in some cases caused the hospital blood bank to become involved when their study was deemed necessary, usually in connection with organ transplantation. The need for analytical capabilities in the leukocyte antigen systems within the hospital blood bank

organization in relation to basic transfusion therapy has not become clear. In the patient who has become refractory to platelet transfusions from unrelated, randomly selected donors, HLA-matched donors are clearly superior; but discovery of suitably matched donors form a limited random population by the hospital blood bank is unlikely to be rewarding, due to the many alleles at the HLA loci. Related (family) donors, more likely to share HLA antigens with a patient, can be readily evaluated as to compatibility by a trial transfusion. The importance of HLA compatibility in neutrophil transfusion currently is unclear, and similarly cannot at this stage provide justification for developing local analytical capabilities in the leukocyte antigen systems.

In selected patients, it would thus appear that homage to HLA is best paid by reliance on HLA typing capabilities and the fully typed donor rosters of major referral centers. As knowledge increases, however, the need for these analytical tools to guide therapy will have to be frequently reassessed, especially in connection with neutrophil transfusion therapy. In any case, a means for obtaining HLA typing services should be available, since prompt initiation of transfusion or chemotherapy in leukemia patients can make subsequent typing more difficult and analysis of the pretreatment specimen is often preferable.

Preparation of Reagents. Many hospital transfusion services attempt to identify patients having anti-red cell antibodies which are serologically suitably reactive so they can be used, often greatly diluted, as typing reagents. Once identified, solicitation of a donation of serum from a cooperative individual can result in sufficient reagent so that hundreds or thousands of typings can be done to solve antibody identification problems and make transfusions safer for many patients. Although the few common typing reagents are readily purchased, many of the less common specificities are unavailable at any price and are therefore rightly prized by tranfusionists. The help of the understanding clinician in the enterprise can be invaluable in obtaining such antisera.

Medicolegal Blood Typing. The analysis of blood specimens to establish paternity or nonpaternity is a specialized area of blood group serology undertaken by some hospital blood banks. Because of the legal implications of the findings and the recent addition of HLA typing and study of protein polymorphisms to enhance the certainty of results obtained with red cells alone, the work is increasingly referred to specialized forensic laboratories.

Subsidiary Roles

Diagnostic Functions. The sensitivity and specificity of immune agglutination of red cells in saline suspension is so extraordinary that the procedure has successfully stood the test of time, continuing in use since Landsteiner identified the major blood groups by using the principle in 1900. With the advent of antihuman globulin or Coombs serum in 1945, new dimensions of sensitivity and specificity were opened up and the visual detection of immune agglutination was given a new lease on life, continuing to be useful to this day. Further increases in sensitivity have been achieved by use of automated systems,[8] but manual methods suffice for diagnosis in routine transfusion practice and in most patients with the autoimmune hemolytic anemias. As a result, the hospital blood bank, skilled in the art and science of immune agglutination, provides the analytical means for the study of hemolytic disease of the newborn and the antibody-mediated anemias. It is in the diagnostic role that a case might also be made for development in the blood bank of the capability for study of transplantation (HLA), and leukocyte and platelet-specific antigens, since their role in hematologic and other disorders is well established, and many of them require transfusion therapy as well.

COMMON ORGANIZATIONAL ARRANGEMENTS AND TECHNIQUES

Frequent communication between the using physician and his suppliers is essential at every level throughout the blood service complex—from the national level, where physician organizations such as the American Medical Association, American College of Physicians, American Society of Clinical Pathologists, and many others are formally represented on the American Blood Commission, to the individual hospital, where the staff physician knows and deals directly with the transfusion service medical director, supervisors, and technical staff.

The Medical Director

In each hospital, a qualified, licensed physician should be made responsible for the operation of the blood bank laboratory and the transfusion service as required by the Joint Commission for the Accreditation of Hospitals (JCAH)[9] and the American Association of Blood Banks (AABB).[10] That director, recognized by the administrative and professional governing organizations of the hospital, should be charged with overall responsibility for transfusion practice within the institution. The role of blood bank-transfusion service medical director has become increasingly well defined in recent years,[11,12] and training programs for physicians preparing for the position have been developed in several academic centers.[12] The American Board of Pathology began a program for specialty board certification of physicians in the subspeciality of blood banking in 1973. In most hospitals, the director is a clinical pathologist or, less often, an internist, and is usually devoting less than full time to the task.[13,14] Simultaneously, governmental licensing agencies in some jurisdictions have tended to establish separate, additional criteria for physician licensing in blood banking as compared with other clinical laboratory disciplines. This is done in recognition of the increased complexity of immunohematology and transfusion therapy and the unique dependence of patient safety on a well-run transfusion service.

The principal functions of the medical director are: (1) consultant on clinical transfusion problems; (2) director of the laboratory's technical functions; (3) administrator of the transfusion service; and (4) educator for professional and technical hospital staff members. The medical director is responsible for transfusion of all patients in the institution, and the limited blood supply must be used with that in mind. For this reason, it is an important operating principle that blood is not ordered but is requested from the transfusion service, and that it is provided with the approval of the medical director. A corollary must be that no one patient has exclusive rights to a unit of blood, but that it must go to the patient in greatest need.

The blood bank laboratory technical staff traditionally carried much of the burden for translating their findings into clinical decisions, perhaps because of the arcane terminology of blood group genetics and serology. While the technologist frequently became skilled at the task of offering direct consultation to the clinician, the shortcomings encountered were cited by Rosenfield in 1966[15] as an argument for the development of transfusion therapy as a medical specialty—a development which subsequently occurred. Because hospital blood banks differ in scale from a single generalist technician within a small general laboratory to a large blood bank staffed by specialists at all levels, including the medical director, the best means for translating the blood bank's perception of a serologic problem into a proper clinical decision or action will vary. For example, consider the question of whether to transfuse an anemic patient having autoimmune hemolytic disease, an incompatible crossmatch, a history of prior transfusion or pregnancy, and severe cardiovascular disease. Since the labo-

ratory specialist can best describe the serologic situation and the potential hazards of transfusion while the responsible clinician can best appreciate the hazards of the anemia, the problem is how to organize matters even within the smallest hospital so as to facilitate such decision making. Clearly, education of the practitioner in blood bank serology and the laboratorian in clinical matters is an ideal objective and should be vigorously pursued. Practically, however, assured access to an experienced local or distant consultant able to comprehend both areas of knowledge needs to be part of each hospital transfusion system. When available local expertise does not cover the many areas of responsibility described for the director, it may be necessary to arrange that consultation with specialists be available in some areas of practice. Whenever possible, reliance on qualified local staff is preferable, since prompt attention is frequently needed and staff education will be facilitated. Regional blood center medical staff can often provide a necessary consultant; that resource should be explored if needed, and procedures for consultation should be defined in advance.

The Transfusion Committee

The most important single organizational entity in the establishment and smooth operation of a hospital transfusion service is the transfusion committee. The committee should be the primary means for individual clinicians, directly or through their representatives, to influence the local practice of transfusion therapy in all its aspects. The committee should be appointed according to institutional procedures as a permanent professional committee of the medical board or other appropriate body. Representation should reflect local conditions but should include the medical director of the transfusion service and blood bank and could also include the director of laboratories, a general practitioner, a surgeon, an internist, perhaps a hematologist, an anesthesiologist, a pediatrician (perhaps with an interest in neonatal care), an obstetrician, representatives of the hospital administration, the nursing department, and other groups especially concerned with transfusion, such as dialysis or hepatitis surveillance staff.

The transfusion committee should serve as the forum for review of all transfusion practices and services within the institution and its recommendations, and reports of surveillance should be made periodically to its parent organization. Its activities should include advising on the appointment and role definition of the transfusion service director, frequent review of transfusion and blood wastage statistics, adverse reactions, blood bank laboratory proficiency and accreditation surveys, adequacy of transfusion service personnel, facilities and equipment, and generally of transfusion practices, policies, and procedures in the institution. The committee can establish guidelines for the reservation (crossmatch) of blood for elective surgical procedures (e.g., a maximum surgical blood order schedule as discussed in detail in Chapter 18), and decide how to minimize safely the time during which blood will be held in a reserved status. The committee, working with the transfusion service medical director, can serve a vital role in education of clinical staff, identification of problem areas, and promotion of optimum transfusion practices. Formal audits of transfusion practices can be made using criteria such as the clinical indications for use of blood products, the proper reporting and treatment of reactions, and acceptable charting practices established by the transfusion committee.[16]

The Regional Blood Center

Provision for clinician participation in operation and governance of regional blood collection and distribution programs and regional blood centers varies widely among regions throughout the country. It seems self evident that such participation is essential in some form if quality and appropriateness of the services provided to hospitals is to be assured, just as it is essential within each hospital. Whether the individual clinician relates to the regional system through representatives of his professional organizations, through his hospital transfusion service director or other hospital staff representatives, or as a direct participant in regional program management, it is a relationship of great importance at the present early stage of development of the national blood service complex. Adequate feedback to the regional agency from clinicians is needed to insure relevant applications of resources, to promote accurate forecasting of needs as clinical practices change and constantly to provide reports on the quality of the products and services provided. Opportunities for clinician input of this type should be seized and responsibly carried out whenever possible; if not offered, they should be developed. Conversely, the regional center should provide the served hospitals and physicians with frequent information on the needs and activities of the regional program, and serve as an educational and consultative resource as necessary. The roles of the regional center are discussed more fully in Chapter 16.

The hospital transfusion service should usually serve in routine matters as the interface between the practitioner and the regional center, especially in those hospitals where the transfusion service is fully developed and is more or less autonomous. Even in the smaller hospital, the system should, if possible, routinely interpose the medical director and transfusion service between clinician and regional center so as to utilize local resources when possible and minimize unnecessary demands on the center, to keep the hospital service fully informed as to the needs of its staff, and to coordinate better regional center participation in therapy within the hospital. Bypassing the hospital transfusion service with blood products or advice, and direct dealings between the clinician and a regional center can subvert local hospital record keeping, transfusion safety, and billing practices and introduce therapeutic practices at variance with local guidelines. The cooperation of the regional center staff in implementing such a policy is essential.

THE BLOOD BANK AND TRANSFUSION SERVICE LABORATORY

The laboratory staff is usually organized to perform serologic work fundamental to transfusion, similar work needed in diagnosis, and management of the blood inventory and collection or ordering functions so as to minimize blood outdating.

Record Keeping

Because of the great potential for harm to the patient in the event of errors in techniques, clerical procedures, or record keeping, the proper design of blood bank procedures emphasizes accuracy. To date, the development of reliable and economical automated instruments for the performance of routine serologic tests and recording of results on the scale encountered in hospitals has not been successful; manual methods remain superior. Consequently, eliminating human errors in the performance of tests, and the recording and transcribing of results is a persistent challenge. Careful attention to the design of mundane procedures and data recording forms and practices so as to eliminate unnecessary recopying of vital data and avoid obscuring essential facts or procedures with unessential trivia is the key to simplicity, and simplicity begets transfusion safety. Similar opportunities for error arise in manipulation of blood donor and patient identification data, and the same principle applies.

Preventing Errors

Analysis of the causes of fatal transfusion reactions has shown that the vast majority are related to clerical errors in identifying patients when beginning a transfusion or drawing a blood specimen, or in such activities as recopying data or recording blood types in the laboratory. In recognition of human fallibility, accrediting agencies have specified in detail the minimum information which must appear on the label of a blood specimen intended for crossmatching and with the blood bag dispensed for transfusion. Incomplete or incorrectly completed forms and labels which cause doubt about the correctness of the contents must be discarded. Often the experienced laboratory staff, at the crossroads of such communications, sees the potential for harm which is not apparent to the clinician in errors such as mislabeled blood specimens. The need to discard specimens and begin anew to assure patient safety in such cases is difficult to accept and explain unless one has seen the myriad permutations of error which occur. The safest system of specimen collection and blood infusion is probably that based upon a full-time team of nurse-technician specialists assigned to the transfusion service. A system of patient wrist bands and matching labels can be purchased for use solely with transfusion recipients to improve their safety when matching blood specimen, blood bag, and patient. Alternatively, systems have been proposed which would automate the process at the bedside of patient/donor bag matching and patient/crossmatch specimen matching.[17] By using a machine-readable bar code symbol identifying the donor blood on the bag label and similar symbols on patient identification wrist bands and specimen labels, the human factor in matching them up correctly may some day be eliminated.

The blood bank staff, unlike most other clinical laboratorians, produces test results which cannot be seen in the perspective of the clinical picture and accepted or rejected as relevant, irrelevant, or perhaps incorrect by the clinician. The blood type or crossmatch result can rarely be questioned clinically until after the transfusion has gone awry, which is of course too late. Blood bankers consequently can be expected to be concerned about maintaining a high standard of accuracy, adhering to prescribed procedures for testing and data recording; in general, they may seem overly fussy and rigid to the clinician using their services. If viewed in proper relation to patient safety, perhaps the clinician should see those traits as assets rather than liabilities, and encourage their continuation.

Staff Education

The blood bank staff also is unique, as mentioned above, in frequently being called upon to assess the clinical importance of its findings. That role as it persists is aided by experience and formal training, such as the specialist in blood bank technology programs (SBB) developed by the AABB and the American Society of Clinical Pathologists (ASCP) to provide advanced training to qualified medical technologists [MT (ASCP)]. Suitable in-service education programs for the technical staff are also an important aspect of clinical laboratory operation in general and blood banking in particular, where an appreciation of clinical problems is especially helpful.

Need for Clinical Information

In order for the blood bank staff to select donor units for a particular patient, basic demographic data such as age and sex can be invaluable. The need for Rh-negative blood in a young female trauma victim is more urgent than in the elderly male GI bleeder. Similarly, in elective surgery cases, clear communications of the name of the planned procedure and any anticipated unusual blood loss are essential if the blood bank is to provide optimum blood coverage. If the benefits of a maximum surgical blood order schedule are to be realized (Vide Supra), that information is especially important.

The Blood Bank Staff

It should be apparent from the preceding comments that a blood bank laboratory needs to be staffed by responsible, slightly worried people who are reluctant to stray from proven methods despite the pressures of emergencies, very meticulous about clerical and technical work, intolerant of seemingly small omissions or errors in patient identification data, and surprisingly demanding of the kind of information needed such as diagnosis, age, sex, and surgical procedure on forms used to request blood. By seeing those traits not as obstacles or nuisances but rather as virtues which protect the patient from error and exploit the blood supply to the full, the clinician can do much to encourage good transfusion practice.

MAJOR AREAS OF CONCERN, INTEREST, AND RESPONSIBILITY FOR THE CLINICIAN

By definition, peer review of transfusion practice in the hospital must be primarily the responsibility of the clinical staff. The transfusion committee and blood bank director can establish the criteria or standards against which practices should be measured. The maximum surgical blood order schedule can, for example, be used to study surgical blood use practices. More difficult than collecting data and comparing it with standards is how to proceed to alter aberrant or substandard clinical practices when they are discovered, a problem best handled by the local auditors in keeping with local wisdom and custom. Shortcomings can provide the basis for design of educational programs for the clinical staff.

The several aspects of the blood supply are all of direct interest to the clinician. As mentioned above, the recruiting of donors and promotion of voluntarism are worthy activities. Is the blood supplied from healthy volunteers rather than paid donors? As is well known, paid donors are often disadvantaged and in poor health and at greater risk of transmitting hepatitis. Do collection, storage, and shipping practices, equipment, and facilities insure that a sterile, well-preserved product is supplied? Even though increasingly rigid standards cover such matters, the alert clinician might spot unsuspected failures. Surprisingly little is known about the in vivo efficacy of blood products in general, but even less is known about how day-to-day variations in collection and storage practices effect efficacy. Does the patient's hemoglobin rise as expected after transfusion of red cells? Does the platelet count or coagulation factor level rise as expected? Obtaining the answers to these questions on a continuing basis has been described as the new frontier of blood banking: the definition and monitoring of efficacy.[18] Is the supply adequate in amount? Decreased use can do almost as much for the supply as increased collections. Similarly, the use of blood components instead of whole blood can stretch a limited supply to serve more patients. Are the desirable safety features a part of the hospital's transfusion system? The blood bank should maintain patient blood type and transfusion problem records in an accessible form. A cumulative patient data file is readily set up using card files in small hospitals or microfiche, electromechanical card-retrieval systems, or on-line computer files in large ones. The patient/donor identification system should be as simple and convenient to use as possible while providing proven protection against errors when used properly.

Is blood provided when needed? An approach to providing blood in emergencies is described in other chapters of this book. By anticipating blood needs and giving the blood bank advance warning and an opportunity to detect atypical antibodies which could delay successful crossmatches, the clinician can avoid unpleasant and dangerous delays as urgent situations develop with a hard-to-crossmatch patient. Sometimes simply providing a specimen for group, Rh, and anti-

body screen or previous data from another institution well in advance can smooth the way if a less common blood type is involved. A recent specimen is of course always needed for confirmation and actual crossmatching. Are the correct blood products available when needed? Despite valuable general rules, circumstances sometimes dictate special needs. Freshly drawn blood is rarely indicated, but in surgery on neonates it is often the transfusion product of choice. Autotransfusion may currently be impractical for most of our blood needs; but, in defined populations such as healthy, young adults undergoing elective cosmetic or corrective surgery, the only transfusions they are likely to need in their lifetime might better be autologous.

These situations are examples of recurrent special blood needs which are best solved for the transfusion service once and for all by the preparation of a written blood transfusion protocol. Close collaboration between the clinician needing the product and the transfusion service director familiar with the local blood supply should yield a protocol specifying in advance what will be provided, when and to whom, and a common language to be used in dealing with the problem. Each formerly special event then becomes routine, and all concerned are freed to devote their attention to the truly unusual case where they are better employed. The written protocol has the further advantage that it can be used to prevent deterioration of practice as time goes by, it can be used to train new staff, and it serves as a starting point when or if changes become necessary.

Reporting of Adverse Reactions

Adverse reactions to tranfusion due to immunologic mechanisms range in severity from trivial urticaria to anaphylaxis or intractable shock and a hemorrhagic diathesis. The blood bank should be notified promptly of all reactions before proceeding with the transfusion, since even a cursory check may reveal important errors in the case in question. Local practices differ as to how extensive the investigation should be for particular signs or symptoms; but, when specimens of blood are required, it is important that they be drawn so as to avoid hemolyzing red cells, either with high-shear stresses by forcing the blood through a fine needle or by inadvertently mixing blood with nonphysiologic intravenous solutions. The hemolysis artefact would represent hemoglobinemia to the analyst and imply occurrence of a major incompatibility until proven otherwise. Each transfusion service should have a protocol and means for providing emergency therapy in the event of intravascular hemolysis, anaphylaxis, or other serious reactions. Since some reactions can continue to evolve over a period of hours or days, it is prudent to await the outcome of the laboratory study of the reaction before proceeding with patient care decisions such as discharge from the hospital. All significant findings should be reported promptly by the blood bank to the clinician as a matter of course. When a disease is known or suspected to have been transmitted to the patient by a transfusion, notification of the transfusion service by the clinician may prevent repeated donations by a dangerous donor. Records are kept so that each donor unit can be traced to its source. Conversely, when a donor subsequently develops an illness which may have been contagious at the time of donation, notification of the clinician by the blood bank may make prophylaxis in the recipient possible, or at least it may clarify the appearance of new symptomatology.

Continuing Education

Teaching and learning about blood transfusion theory and practice should logically be planned around transfusion service and regional blood center staff, transfusion committee staff, and available local clinicians such as hematologists, anesthesiologists, or surgeons with special interest in and knowledge of the topic. The specific objectives of educational programs should be guided by the results of audits or other evaluations of transfusion practices conducted by the transfusion committee. Teaching materials directed at clinicians on general principles of blood transfusion[19] or specifically on component therapy are available from professional organizations[20-22] in a variety of media including books, slides, cassette tapes, and videotapes, and new materials are undoubtedly in preparation, suitable for use in hospital staff education programs.

New Developments

Few of the many new developments in blood transfusion practice now underway or planned can proceed without the collaboration and eventual acceptance of the practicing clinician. Studies of transfusion-transmitted viruses have revealed that hepatitis B is no longer the major cause of posttransfusion hepatitis, that hepatitis A is not a transfusion-related disease, and that a new agent or agents designated "non-A,non-B" causes most of the posttransfusion hepatitis now encountered. The cooperation of clinicians in granting access to their patients has been essential to the success of those studies. If new methods for automated patient identification are to make transfusion safer, the clinician will have to accept and use the systems provided. Clinical research on the use of newly developed blood products such as cryogenically stored platelets is needed at all stages of development. New uses proposed for existing blood components or derivatives, such as cold insoluble globulin (fibronectin) in cryoprecipitate for treatment of overwhelming sepsis or multiple organ failure in trauma, need to be evaluated.

Such studies need approval of the local institutional review committee for the protection of human rights in research, since no blood product is entirely without hazard to the recipient. In some circumstances, new products and uses will need the approval of the Bureau of Biologics of the Food and Drug Administration (FDA) when studies with human recipients are involved, since blood and its parts are now legally regulated in the same way as drugs. Devices to be used on patients, such as centrifuge-washers to reclaim and prepare shed blood in the operating room for reinfusion, blood warmers, blood microaggregate filters, even the labels on blood products, all now come under the jurisdiction of the FDA as medical devices and cannot be arbitrarily introduced, changed, or employed in novel ways without formal review and approval.

REFERENCES

1. Brodheim, E., Hirsch, R., and Prastacos, G.: Setting inventory levels for hospital blood banks. Transfusion 16:63, 1976.
2. Brodheim, E. and Prastacos, G.P.: The Long Island blood distribution system as a prototype for regional blood management. Interfaces 9:3, 1979.
3. Boral, L.I. and Henry, J.B.: The type and screen: A safe alternative and supplement in selected surgical procedures. Transfusion 17:163, 1977.
4. Technical Manual of the American Association of Blood Banks, 7th Ed., American Association of Blood Banks, Washington, D.C., 1977.
5. Lockwood, C.M.: Plasma exchange: An overview. Plasma Therapy 1:1, 1979.
6. Solomon, B.A., Castino, F., Lysaght, M.J., Colton, C.K., and Friedman, L.I.: Continuous flow membrane filtration of plasma from whole blood. Trans. Am. Soc. Artif. Intern. Organs 24:21, 1978.
7. Higby, D.J. and Burnett, D.: Granulocyte transfusions: Current status. Blood 55:2, 1980.
8. Penwalt, R. and Hogman, C.: Automated red cell antibody analysis. A parallel study. II. Identification of serologic specificity. Vox Sang. 20:356, 1971.
9. Blood Transfusion Service, Pathology and Medical Laboratory Services, Accreditation Manual for Hospitals, p. 124; The Joint Commission for Accreditation of Hospitals, 1979.
10. Standards for Blood Banks and Transfusion Services, 9th Ed., Committee on Standards, American Association of Blood Banks, Washington, D.C., 1978.
11. Grove-Rasmussen, M., Hammer, G.J., Kellner, A., Muirhead, E.E., Swisher, S.N., and Shively, J.A.: Blood bank physician-role and education. Transfusion 12:66, 1972.
12. Kuhns, W.J., Allen, F.H., Jr., and Kellner, A.: Blood banking as a professional discipline in medicine. Transfusion 15:152, 1975.
13. Shively, J.A., Grove-Rasmussen, M., Hammer, G.J., Kellner, A., Muirhead, E.E., and Perkins, H.A.: Survey of blood bank physicians and medical directors. J.A.M.A. 217:1085, 1971.
14. Wallas, C.H. and Grindon, A.J.: Physician involvement in blood banking. Transfusion 18:367, 1978.
15. Rosenfield, R.E.: Transfusion Service Management (Letter). N. Engl. J. Med. 274:580, 1966.
16. Sabatino, F.G., Ed.: Special section on blood utilization. Quality Review Bulletin 3 (entire issue), 1977.
17. Wolf, C.F.W. and Muirhead, E.E.: Blood Banking Automation. J.A.M.A. 240:853, 1978.
18. Zuck, T.F.: In vivo performance evaluation of blood bank components. In: A Seminar on Blood Components: E Unium Pluribus, p. 1, American Association of Blood Banks, Washington, D.C., 1977.
19. Greenwalt, T.J., Ed.: General Principles of Blood Transfusion. American Medical Association, Monroe, Wisconsin, 1977.
20. Blood Component Therapy. Health Sciences Learning Resources Center, SB-56, University of Washington, Seattle, WA.
21. Component Therapy. American Association of Blood Banks, Washington, D.C., 1978.
22. NCME Cassette #297. Blood Components and Their Applications. Network for Continuing Medical Education, N.Y., 1978.

Appendix: Transfusion Committee Procedures

Scott N. Swisher, M.D., and Lawrence D. Petz, M.D.

Transfusion Committees can and should be an important force in developing and monitoring effective and safe transfusion practices in a hospital. There are a number of approaches that can be employed to discharge this responsibility. The procedures of a transfusion committee should be compatible with the general pattern of staff governance of the institution. It is important, however, that the Transfusion Committee have strong and sensitive leadership and that it approach its task actively.

The general procedure described here is one that has been found to be effective in a number of institutions. A number of variations and modifications are obviously possible. The procedure is based upon a method of identifying selected charts of transfused patients for review by record room personnel, and review of these charts by the professional members of the committee for appropriateness of the transfusion therapy and follow-up investigations with corrective action where necessary. The initial chart review by the record room selects for professional review only those in which the transfusion therapy appears to fall outside guidelines established by the Transfusion Committee. Thus, in most institutions, only a relatively small proportion of the charts of transfused patients needs to be reviewed.

Selection of Charts of Transfused Patients for Review

A Transfusion Committee may need to develop an algorithm which may be used by record room personnel to identify records in need of review by the Committee. This algorithm should describe a set of indications for transfusion commonly encountered in the hospital and a set of criteria which *probably* justify a particular transfusion and exempt it from specific review and evaluation of the transfusion committee. If the particular criteria are not met when the record is examined by the record room, the case is referred for review by the professional committee for its judgment in the matter, and appropriate action. It should be emphasized that record room personnel do not exercise the professional judgments of a physician; they are only responsible for examination of the record to see if the criteria established by the medical staff have or have not been met in an individual case where a transfusion has been administered.

Examples

Algorithm #1 is in use in a hospital where large numbers of patients with malignant disorders are treated. The second example shown is from a hospital with large programs in cardiovascular surgery and end-stage renal disease. By comparing them, one can appreciate how an algorithm can be developed or adjusted from time to time to fit the programs of the hospital or to investigate a particular problem which has come to the attention of the blood bank or transfusion committee. The first column contains common indications for transfusion, and the second contains the criteria. The criteria used are not exactly the same. Note that all transfusions in certain categories are reviewed. Also, it is useful to review a sample of "accepted" records in a given category from time to time to "fine-tune" the criteria and to make sure nothing of importance is being missed. For example, Hospital #2 might review records of component replacement or end-stage renal disease.

HOSPITAL #1

BLOOD TRANSFUSION REVIEW ALGORITHM

NUMBER OF TRANSFUSIONS REVIEWED: _____   DATE: _____

NUMBER OF PATIENTS STILL IN HOSPITAL: _____

START

WAS BLOOD GIVEN TO PT. ON CHEMOTHERAPY FOR MALIGNANCY?
  YES ——→ WAS HGB < 10gm?   NO ————————→ REVIEW
  NO
                    YES
                    ↓
                  ACCEPT

WAS BLOOD GIVEN TO COMPENSATE FOR ACTIVE BLEEDING? INTRAOPERATIVE, ETC.
  YES ——→ WAS ESTIMATED BLOOD LOSS > 500ml? DID BP DROP TO < 100? DID PULSE RISE TO > 100?   NO ——→ REVIEW
  NO
                    YES
                    ↓
                  ACCEPT

WAS BLOOD GIVEN IN PREPARATION FOR SURGERY?
  YES ——→ WAS HGB < 10gm?   NO ————————→ REVIEW
  NO   YES
                    ↓
                  ACCEPT

                  IF PLATELETS, WAS PLATELET COUNT < 30,000?   NO ————————→ REVIEW
                    YES
                    ↓
                  ACCEPT

WAS BLOOD COMPONENT GIVEN FOR REPLACEMENT OF SPECIFIC DEFICIENCY, E.G. PLATELETS OR WBC?
  YES
                  IF WBC, WAS GRANULOCYTE COUNT [WBC × (POLYS & BANDS)] < 600?   NO ————————→ REVIEW
  NO
                    YES
                  ACCEPT

WAS BLOOD GIVEN FOR CHRONIC ANEMIA NOT RESPONSIVE TO SPECIFIC THERAPY?
  YES ——→ WAS Hb < 10gm?   NO ————————→ REVIEW
  NO
                    YES
                    ↓
                  ACCEPT

                                                        ————→ REVIEW

HOSPITAL #2

BLOOD TRANSFUSION REVIEW ALGORITHM

NUMBER OF TRANSFUSIONS REVIEWED:_____ DATE: _____

START

WAS BLOOD USED FOR EXTRACOR-
PORAL CIRCULATION? OPEN HEART   YES──────────┐
SURGERY, HEMODIALYSIS.
                                                  ↓
         NO   ACCEPT
         ↓

WAS BLOOD GIVEN FOR REPLACE-   ┌─ WAS DEFICIENCY DOCU-
MENT OF SPECIFIC COMPONENT?   YES──── MENTED ON CHART?   NO────────→REVIEW
PLATELETS, CLOTTING FACTORS,
WBC, ETC.   YES
                                               ↓
         NO   ACCEPT
         ↓

DID PATIENT HAVE END STAGE   YES──────── WAS HCT < 25%?   NO────────→REVIEW
RENAL DISEASE?   YES
                                               ↓
         NO   ACCEPT
         ↓

WAS BLOOD GIVEN TO COMPEN-   ┌ WAS ESTIMATED BLOOD LOSS
SATE FOR ACTIVE BLEEDING?   YES──── > 500 ml? DID BP DROP TO   NO────────→REVIEW
INTRAOPERATIVE, ETC.   < 100 SYSTOL.? DID PULSE
                                      RISE TO > 100?
                                              YES
         NO   ACCEPT
         ↓

WAS BLOOD GIVEN IN PREPARA-   YES──────── WAS HGB < 10 gm?   NO────────→REVIEW
TION FOR SURGERY?   YES
                                               ↓
         NO   ACCEPT
         ↓

WAS BLOOD GIVEN TO PATIENT   YES──────── WAS HGB <9 gm?   NO────────→REVIEW
ON CHEMOTHERAPY FOR MALIG-
NANCY?   YES
                                               ↓
         NO   ACCEPT
         ↓

WAS ONLY ONE UNIT OF BLOOD   YES──────────────────────────────────────→REVIEW
ADMINISTERED?

         NO
         ↓

WAS A TRANSFUSION REACTION   YES──────────────────────────────────────→REVIEW
RECORDED?

REVIEW REMAINDER

Selection of Records for Examination

Ideally, records of all patients receiving a transfusion of any blood product should be examined by the record room. If this is impossible, a carefully selected stratified sample should be selected by a predetermined program for analysis. This should cover records from all services which have employed transfusions during the review interval, and all staff members who have ordered blood. Outpatient transfusion clinics should be included. It is usually preferable to conduct the review monthly to keep its findings in step with current practice in the institution. This also permits questionable cases to be fresh in the memory of those involved where discussions of the appropriateness of a transfusion are required.

Both of the algorithms shown here are designed primarily to detect overutilization of transfusion. Similar algorithms can be developed to identify records of patients where other blood products such as albumin have been used. There is reasonable evidence that, in the U.S. as a whole, red cell products and platelets are overutilized to a significant degree. For this reason, a Transfusion Committee might wish to start with an evaluation of these matters.

In some instances, undertransfusion of patients may be a problem of significance. The Joint Committee on Accreditation of Hospitals recommends review of records of transfusion for this purpose as well. It is more difficult to develop this algorithm for use in the record room. More kinds of data must be examined; knowledgeable intercorrelation of these data are required so that an inordinate number of charts are not presented for review by the committee. For example, a record search for significant hypotension would identify many patients with myocardial infarction or vasodepressor reactions. On the other hand, a search for surgery, trauma and/or bleeding, *and* hypotension would reveal a large number of cases in which transfusion and fluid management was entirely appropriate; but it is much more difficult to establish criteria for this judgment that can be employed by nonphysician personnel. Nevertheless, it is appropriate for a transfusion committee to examine periodically a group of records in this category. The performance of the emergency room, surgical suites, postoperative and intensive care wards, as well as those caring for bleeding medical and pediatric patients, should be evaluated. Transfusion of more blood than was needed is also difficult to define by criteria. This can occur in situations where the use of some blood was clearly required. This question can be evaluated by the same procedures suggested for evaluation of possible undertransfusion of patients.

Actions Taken by Transfusion Committees

If, upon review of the record, the transfusion therapy of a patient is judged to be appropriate, the record is returned to files and nothing further need be done. The fact that the record was reviewed and the findings of the committee should be recorded only in the minutes of the committee.

If a judgment cannot be made from the record alone, and a significant question exists, further information may be sought, formally or informally, from the physician ordering the blood. A final judgment can then be made later in view of this new information.

If a transfusion has been found probably to be inappropriate, the responsible physician should be so notified, and requested to respond formally to the finding. The option to appear at a Committee meeting for discussion of the matter should usually be offered. In most instances, the matter can be closed at this point.

If the inappropriate transfusion has resulted in an unfavorable outcome for the patient, or if the same physician is repeatedly cited for inappropriate practices, an appearance before the Committee should be required. If an agreement about the matter cannot be reached, or if the same issue again arises in the future, the responsible head of the service and/or Chief of Staff should be informed so that the staff as a whole may take up its responsibility in the matter. Staff discipline may then be exercised, if required. It rarely is needed if these proceedings are handled in a nonadversarial, educational way.

In these situations, it is possible that the criteria or procedures employed by the transfusion committee are inappropriate in some areas, and that honest differences of opinion exist among informed physicians about what constitutes good practice. This should be resolved by open discussion, reference to the literature, and, possibly, consultation with outside experts. The transfusion committee may need to revise its procedures and criteria to be in accord with the consensus of the best-informed staff members. It is important that differences of opinion which arise be resolved on the basis of scientifically derived information, informed opinion, and good judgment, not staff or hospital politics. Where an issue is not resolvable scientifically, it is possible to recognize more than one practice as acceptable until further clinical investigation can resolve the matter. Several issues of this type have been identified in the preparation of this book (see Ch. 1).

18

Surgical Blood Ordering, Blood Shortage Situations, and Emergency Transfusion

Harold A. Oberman, M.D.

The primary function of a hospital transfusion service is the efficient provision of safe and effective blood and blood products. Since approximately 70 percent of the blood provided by such a laboratory will be for patients undergoing surgical procedures or for patients with acute unexpected blood loss, it is appropriate to devote a chapter of this text to a consideration of the problems which beset the blood bank director and the laboratory in attempting to meet this obligation. In so doing, it is also appropriate to dwell upon the relatively common problem of providing blood at times of shortage in the institution or in the regional system.

We will first focus on the optimal processing of blood before its issuance for transfusion, and the temporal requirements which pertain. This will be followed by a discussion of preoperative provision of blood, emphasizing issuance of only that amount appropriate for the corresponding surgical procedures. By this mechanism there is resultant conservation of the blood resource and mitigation of the third problem discussed—namely, blood shortage situations. Finally, we will dwell on the provision of blood at times of emergency. Such emergency transfusion pertains both to the patient brought to the hospital who has not previously been evaluated in its blood bank and to the patient suffering acute unexpected blood loss in the course of hospitalization.

PREOPERATIVE PROCESSING OF BLOOD

Donor Blood

Most blood and blood products issued by hospital blood banks are drawn by a regional collection agency. This blood is shipped to the hospital, either on consignment or through some form of purchase by the hospital. This purchase reflects reimbursement of the collection agency for the expenses of collection and processing. Hospital blood banks also may have active donor facilities for collection of special products, provision of supplemental blood needs, or performance of therapeutic procedures.

The hospital must assume that the central collection agency has vigorously applied all appropriate standards of practice to the collection of blood.[1] Specifically, the prospective donor must have been screened through history-taking and physical examination to mitigate the possibility of transmitting disease to the recipient. It is also assumed that the collection agency has performed appropriate red cell typing, including ABO and Rh, and has screened the serum of the donor unit for unexpected antibodies. Finally, it must be assumed that the blood has been collected under aseptic conditions and labeled accurately so that the identification of the unit is not in question, and that a test for hepatitis-B surface antigen has been performed and is negative.

Upon receipt of the blood by the hospital blood bank, it is placed in the hospital's inventory. The hospital verifies the ABO type and, if appropriate, the Rh type of the unit. It is not necessary for the hospital to repeat either the screening test for unexpected antibodies or the test for hepatitis-B surface antigen.

Patient Sample

Upon receiving an order for blood, the blood bank must process a specimen from the patient. Before the request for blood arrives in the blood bank, the patient's specimen must be collected, with scrupulous attention paid to the identity of the donor and to the labeling of the collection tube. There must be verification of identity of the patient by comparing identifying information on the patient's wristband (at least first and last names and patient's identification number) with the same information on the blood bank requisition. This is true not only for hospitalized patients but also for out-patients, who should also have a wristband in place prior to being bled.

Serologic Testing

After receipt in the blood bank, the specimen is typed for ABO and Rh, and a test for unexpected antibodies is performed. The ABO type of the patient is determined by typing the red blood cells with appropriate reagents, and it is confirmed by reacting the patient's serum against red blood cells of known ABO type. Similarly, the Rh type of the patient must be determined with appropriate controls.

The patient's serum is "screened" for unexpected antibodies by reacting the serum against red blood cells which contain the antigenic specificities corresponding to the majority of clinically significant antibodies. Should the antibody screening test be positive, it is necessary to identify the offending antibody so that compatible blood can be located. This necessitates reacting the serum against a panel of cells of known antigenic specificity and determining the presence of an antibody, or a combination of antibodies, by excluding those specificities on red blood cells not reactive with the patient's serum.

The total time required for performance of the ABO and Rh typing and the screening test for unexpected antibodies is usually 20 to 60 minutes. This variation is related to the incubation times necessary for differing methods. However, should the antibody screening test be positive, additional time will be required for antibody identification. In some instances this may be only one or two hours; however, considerably more time may be required when multiple antibody specificities are present in a serum or when the antibody is directed against an antigen of relatively high incidence.

The typing and screening procedures all can be performed well in advance of the transfusion. A negative screening test for unexpected antibodies largely precludes the possibility of a positive crossmatch. If the patient has not been transfused or pregnant during the preceding three months, the antibody screening may be performed days or even weeks in advance of the transfusion, so that if any antibodies are found, adequate time will be available for the blood bank to locate compatible blood. On the other hand, if a patient has been transfused recently or is pregnant, there is greater likelihood of the presence or appearance of unexpected antibodies. In this case, if screening tests are performed several days or more prior to transfusion, they should be repeated using a specimen obtained within 48 hours of the transfusion.

The final test performed before transfusion is the major crossmatch. This involves reaction of the patient's serum with donor red blood cells. The minor crossmatch, which tests the reaction of donor serum with patient's red blood cells, is unnecessary. The crossmatch attempts, in an in vitro setting, to anticipate the survival of red blood cells upon transfusion. If the antibody screening test is negative or if blood has been located which lacks antigens corresponding to antibodies in the patient's serum, the major crossmatch should be compatible. The time required for the crossmatch, depending upon the method employed and the incubation time, as well as the paper work involved, may vary from 15 minutes to an hour. The latter would reflect longer incubation times, while the former would reflect a more abbreviated crossmatch using methods for augmentation of the agglutination reaction. The major crossmatch must be performed in proximity to the time of transfusion, and within 48 hours of the transfusion if the patient either has been pregnant, transfused within the past three months, or such information is uncertain or unavailable.[1]

In some laboratories a direct antiglobulin test is included as part of pretransfusion testing. This permits diagnosis of unsuspected autoimmune hemolytic anemia and, in recently transfused patients, allows detection of unexpected antibodies attached to transfused red cells before such antibodies are evident in the plasma. Although we perform a direct antiglobulin test on all prospective transfusion blood samples, we do not feel it cost-effective or appropriate to perform a detailed serologic evaluation on all samples yielding a positive result. Instead, we evaluate only those samples from patients with a positive test who have been recently transfused or who have clinical evidence of hemolytic anemia.[2] In institutions not dealing with as high a proportion of recently transfused patients as ours, it may be appropriate to perform the direct antiglobulin test on a more selective basis, dependent upon the patient's recent transfusion history (see Ch. 7).

BLOOD ORDER SCHEDULES

Most of the blood crossmatched in a hospital blood bank is for patients undergoing operative procedures. However, most of this blood is not transfused. Once a unit of blood is crossmatched for a patient, it remains out of inventory and is not available for use by other patients, usually for at least 24 hours. When an excessive number of crossmatched units of blood are held for patients, a blood shortage and/or wastage due to outdating may result.

In an effort to maximize the availability of this limited resource, it behooves the hospital blood bank to adopt a mechanism that will improve the chances that the crossmatched units of blood will be transfused. In this way the hospital reduces the time blood is spent in an assigned or crossmatched status, and thereby increases the effective shelf life of the blood. Since this enhances the opportunity for every unit of blood to be transfused, it also results in a greater availability of blood for all patients—not only in the hospital, but also, if a similar practice is implemented by neighboring hospitals, in an entire region.

In assessing the effectiveness of a hospital's transfusion program, a crossmatch-transfusion ratio often is utilized. This relates the number of units of blood crossmatched for all patients to the number of units of blood actually transfused. It is generally acknowledged that this ratio should not exceed 2.5.[3] A ratio of 1.0 might seem optimal; however, this is not reasonable, for it would result in an excessive number of acute blood shortage situations, especially in surgical patients where precise needs are more often unpredictable.

An effective way for a hospital blood bank to reduce the number of units of blood crossmatched each day is to implement guidelines for provision of blood for common surgical procedures. This implies correlating the number of units of blood crossmatched for an operation with the number of units, based on past local experience, which have been transfused to comparable patients having comparable procedures. Such a system need not cover all operations. However, it is most important that it cover elective surgery, and especially those surgical procedures which usually result in tranfusion of three, or less, units of blood. It is this group of operations which prove most wasteful of blood through excess preoperative orders. It must be emphasized that effective inventory control in a hospital blood bank is centered on such guidelines for surgical patients, since blood usage is far less predictable in surgical patients than in medical patients.[4]

Implementation of a maximum surgical blood order schedule (MSBOS) requires close cooperation between the blood bank and the surgical staff. To be most effective, this schedule should be based primarily on blood utilization experience in transfusion of patients with comparable procedures in the respective hospital. Regional and national transfusion practices also may be taken into consideration.[4a] A surgeon's readiness to accept a MSBOS is in direct proportion to his confidence in the hospital blood bank's ability to supply blood and blood components rapidly in the event that unexpected bleeding occurs during a surgical procedure.

An indication of the efficiency of a MSBOS was presented in an article by Devitt, who noted that only 1.4 percent of patients undergoing cholecystectomy were transfused with even a single unit of blood in the operating room.[5] Yet, it is common practice to crossmatch two units of blood for each such surgical procedure. In University of Michigan Hospital, only 3 of 432 patients having cholecystectomy required blood during 1974. If two units of blood had been crossmatched for each of these patients, 858 units of blood would needlessly have been out of inventory for 24 hours and unavailable for other patients. Further, unnecessary cross-match tests result in excessive expense to the patient.

It is essential that any MSBOS be provided with an override mechanism. The clinical situation may indicate that the specified usage guideline for a specific surgical procedure is inappropriate. For example, only one unit of blood may be an appropriate guideline for a routine above-knee amputation. However, such a procedure planned for a patient with hemophilia-A unquestionably should result in provision of considerably more blood for the operation.

When a MSBOS is implemented, only the indicated amount of blood on the schedule is crossmatched for a surgical procedure, regardless of the number of units of blood ordered by the surgeon or house officer. Therefore, if there are mitigating circumstances, these must be specified to the blood bank, either verbally or in writing, by the surgeon, to permit temporary overriding of the schedule.

There are many surgical procedures which usually do not result in intraoperative transfusion. For example, procedures such as appendectomy, thyroidectomy, breast biopsy, hemorrhoidectomy, and many others are unlikely to have sufficient blood loss to occasion transfusion. In such instances the patient's preoperative blood specimen should be typed for ABO and Rh, and a screening test for unexpected antibodies should be performed, but no blood should be crossmatched for the operation. This practice often is referred to as "type and screen," with the connotation that it is a singular form of inventory management.[6] Actually, this is only one part of a MSBOS, providing for those procedures which usually do not result in transfusion of blood. It must be emphasized, however, that ABO compatible blood must be available in the hospital blood bank for such patients should unexpected hemorrhage result.

An example of a portion of a surgical blood order schedule is indicated in Table 18-1. It must be stressed that this schedule was prepared in cooperation with the surgical staff performing these procedures. Moreover, it is

Table 18-1. Maximum Blood Orders Provided for Surgical Procedures (partial list)*
(University of Michigan Hospital)

General Surgery

Procedure	No. Units	Procedure	No. Units
Amputation (A/K or B/K)	1	Hemorrhoidectomy	T&S
Aortic aneurysm resection	5	Hiatal hernia repair	1
Aorto-iliac bypass	5	Hodgkin's staging operation	1
Breast biopsy	T&S	Inguinal hernia repair	T&S
Breast-mastectomy	1	Laparotomy, exploratory	1
Carotid endarterectomy	1	Pancreatectomy	6
Cholecystectomy	T&S	Parathyroidectomy	T&S
Colectomy, subtotal resection	2	Pilonidal cyst or sinus excision	T&S
Colectomy, total or A/P resection	3	Porto-caval shunt	5
Colostomy, revision	T&S	Renal transplant	2
Common bile duct exploration	2	Splenectomy	1
Femoral-popliteal bypass	3	Split thickness skin graft	T&S
Fistula-in-ano repair	T&S	Thyroidectomy	T&S
Gastrectomy, subtotal or total	2	Vagotomy and pyloroplasty	1
Gastrostomy	T&S	Varicose vein stripping	T&S

Gynecology

Procedure	No. Units	Procedure	No. Units
Abortion, therapeutic	2	Radium implant	T&S
Cervical circlage	T&S	Salpingo-oophorectomy	T&S
Cervical conization (non-pregnant)	T&S	Tubal ligation	T&S
Cesarean Section	1	Tuboplasty	T&S
Dilatation and Curettage	T&S	Vaginal (A/P) repair	1
Hysterectomy, abdominal or vaginal	1	Vaginectomy	2
Hysterectomy, radical	3	Vesico-vaginal or rectal-vaginal	
Laparoscopy	T&S	fistula repair	T&S
Oophorectomy	T&S	Uterine suspension	T&S
Ovarian wedge resection	T&S	Vulvectomy, total	1
Pelvic lymph node dissection	3	Vulvectomy, radical	2

* The above schedule of maximum blood provision for common operations *on adults* has been confirmed by the appropriate departmental chairmen and section heads. The Blood Bank will provide no more than the designated amount of blood, although orders for fewer units will be followed. The provision of blood for procedures not on this list will be based, as in the past, on the order of the surgeon scheduling the case in the O.R. The first two units of blood transfused to all such patients will be in the form of "packed cells."

Should the patient's clinical condition indicate that the volume of blood designated on this list is inadequate, the Blood Bank will provide additional units if notified through consultation with the technologist in charge or with the Medical Staff of the laboratory. Additional blood also will be provided if the excess order on the posting schedule is countersigned by the staff surgeon responsible for the patient.

(T & S = Type and Screen)

revised every several years, based upon current blood usage. Therefore, this should not necessarily be transposed for use into another hospital but should merely serve as a model of such a plan.

BLOOD SHORTAGE SITUATIONS

Inability of a hospital blood bank to meet the needs of its patients for blood and blood products may result either from a shortage of blood within the regional system or from de-pletion of a hospital's blood inventory in the face of adequate regional blood resources.

The first situation usually is far more serious, and results from sudden and unexpected depletion of the regional blood resource due to: (1) increased demand, as from a major disaster; (2) poor management of the regional inventory, reflected by excessive outdating of blood, or (3) inadequate blood collections. Inadequate blood collections might arise because of breakdown of the recruitment effort or seasonal variation in willingness of volunteers to donate blood and blood products. In contrast, isolated blood shortage in a hospital blood bank results from a sudden and unanticipated increase in demand, often for a particular blood type. It also may be due to poor management of the blood resource from such practices as holding an excessive number of crossmatched units of blood for specific patients in anticipation of possible transfusion, from reluctance to use blood that is near its time of outdating, or from inappropriate use of freshly drawn blood. Such practices will yield a high outdate rate.

When a hospital blood bank experiences blood shortage, yet there is adequate blood within the region or system, correction can be achieved through manipulation of the regional resource. Depending upon the size of the region, blood can be moved from hospital to hospital, or from central blood bank to hospital, thereby correcting the temporary blood shortage. In an effort to optimize the blood resource within a region, it is desirable to reduce outdating of blood to a minimum. This may be achieved by elimination of hoarding of blood by hospitals and by reduction of the number of older units of blood on the shelves of hospitals which have little likelihood of transfusing such blood. Units of blood can be transferred to larger hospitals, where transfusion is more predictable, at the mid-point of their dating interval. Such a recycling system has been used effectively, especially when units of blood are provided to hospitals on a consignment basis rather than purchased by the hospitals.[7]

In the event of a regional blood shortage, it is often possible to bring blood into the area from neighboring regions in the country. Unfortunately, this may take considerable time and effort, and it must be appreciated that regional shortages often coexist in more than one location.

At times of regional blood shortage, outdating of blood should be held to a minimum. The dating interval of units of blood is based on a requirement that the recovery of transfused red cells 24 hours after transfusion shall be at least 70 percent. In an emergency, however, this requirement may be modified, since transfusion of somewhat older blood is preferable to lack of availability of any blood. Such extension of the dating interval must always be done with the full knowledge of the patient's physician.

The most common type of hospital blood shortage is the temporary depletion of the inventory of one or more types of blood at a hospital within a region. Prevention of such a situation mandates implementation of a strong inventory control program. Use of the above-described MSBOS should reduce outdating of blood and promote effective utilization of a hospital's inventory. It must be appreciated that assignment of a unit of blood to a patient in whom transfusion is unlikely proportionately reduces the number of effective days such a unit of blood is available for transfusion of other patients.

A hospital blood bank should maximize its ability to transfuse all of the blood on its shelves through increasing the flexibility of its blood issuance policies. For example, the usual practice is to maintain eight different inventories of blood; that is, A, B, AB, and O, both Rh-negative and Rh-positive.

Some hospitals also type units of blood for hr′(c) and issue red cells containing this antigen only to patients who test positively for the antigen. This practice is inappropriate—not only from a logistic standpoint, but from a medical standpoint as well, for the incidence of sensitization to hr′ is not of sufficient magnitude to warrant this practice. Furthermore, it results in maintenance of 16 different inventories and thereby accentuates the likelihood of outdating units of blood.

At times of blood shortage, the hospital blood transfusion service director and the patient's physician should not feel constrained to transfusion of blood corresponding only to a patient's ABO and Rh type. As a strategy in overcoming such a situation, switching a patient's transfusion product to that of a different, yet compatible, ABO or Rh type is an effective means of overcoming such a shortage. When this is done, the transfused

Table 18-2. Principles to Be Followed When Switching Blood Groups and Types due to Shortages

Patient's Group and Type	Principles to Follow
O-negative	1. Use only O, Rh-negative if patient is sensitized to D. 2. Use group O, D and Du-negative, C- and/or E-positive in preference to Rh(D)-positive. 3. Avoid transfusing anything but O, Rh-negative to patients (ESPECIALLY FEMALES) under age 45. 4. Restrict the use of O, Rh-positive blood for O, Rh-negative patients to acute emergency situations, and then use only if the patient either has a negative antibody screen, or definitely lacks Rh antibodies. 5. If massive volumes of blood are required, and switching to Rh-positive is inevitable, avoid wasting O, Rh-negative blood by switching as early as possible.
A-negative or B-negative	1. Use only Rh-negative if patient is sensitized to D i.e., Group-specific Rh-negative or O, Rh-negative (as packed cells if possible) 2. Use D and Du negative, C and/or E positive in preference to Rh (D) positive. 3. Avoid transfusing anything but Rh-negative blood to patients (ESPECIALLY FEMALES) under age 45. 4. Restrict use of Rh-positive blood to acute emergency situations; then, use only if the patient has a negative antibody screen or definitely lacks Rh antibodies. 5. If massive volumes of blood are required, and switching to Rh-positive is inevitable, avoid wasting Rh-negative blood by switching as early as possible. 6. Conserve group O blood. Only group O can be given to a group O recipient.
AB-negative	1. Use only Rh-negative if patient is sensitized to D. 2. Use D and Du-negative, C and/or E-positive in preference to Rh(D)-positive. 3. Group A blood may be used (as packed cells if possible) unless the patient has anti A_1. The patient initially should be switched to group A, then, secondarily, may be switched to O. *Always do this before switching Rh types* (see text). 4. Avoid transfusing anything but Rh-negative to patients (ESPECIALLY FEMALES) under age 45. 5. Restrict the use of Rh-positive to acute emergency situations and then use only if the patient has a negative antibody screen, or definitely lacks Rh antibodies. 6. If massive volumes of blood are required, and switching to Rh-positive is inevitable, avoid wasting Rh-negative by switching as early as possible. 7. Conserve group O blood. Only group O can be given to a group O recipient.
O-positive	1. A group O patient may receive only group O blood. 2. Rh-negative may be used, but this should be avoided due to supply problems.
A-positive or B-positive	1. Group O blood may be given (as packed cells if possible). 2. Rh negative may be used but this should be avoided due to supply problems.
AB-positive	1. Group A blood may be used (as packed cells, if possible) unless the patient has anti-A_1. The patient initially should be switched to group A, then, secondarily, to group O. 2. Conserve group O Blood. Only group O can be given to a group O recipient. 3. Rh-negative may be used but this should be avoided due to supply problems.

red blood cells always should be in the form of Red Blood Cells (packed cells), rather than whole blood, thereby avoiding the transfusion of significant amounts of ABO alloantibodies. A plan for the provision of compatible blood in blood shortage situations is presented in Table 18-2.

When deciding as to the appropriateness of switching the blood type of red blood cells being transfused, it is important that the pa-tient's clinical condition be assessed to anticipate the extent of the prospective blood requirement. For example, it would be well to avoid transfusion of Rh positive blood to an Rh negative patient, especially a female in the childbearing years of life, except in life-threatening situations.

It is always wise to plan for a pattern of blood switching that will maintain the greatest flexibility in meeting the patient's requirements. If the blood requirements of an AB, Rh-negative, patient exceed the number of AB-negative units in the blood bank, it would be inadvisable to provide the patient initially with O-negative whole blood.[8] If at least several units of group O cells were to be given, it would not be possible to switch the patient subsequently to type A products because of the anti-A antibody that had been transfused. In contrast, this patient initially could be transfused with A, Rh-negative, Red Blood Cells; should additional units be required beyond the capacity of the A-negative inventory, O-negative (packed) Red Blood Cells could be given. The anti-A antibody present in the small volumes of supernatant plasma will be diluted in the patient and will not cause hemolysis.

Furthermore, if an AB-negative patient is an elderly male, who has an urgent large anticipated blood requirement because of unexpected bleeding during a surgical procedure, and the patient lacks anti-D, it might be well to switch the patient immediately to A-positive Red Blood Cells and have O-positive Red Blood Cells available in reserve. Parenthetically, a shortage of type AB blood should rarely be a significant problem, for such patients always can be transfused with type A Red Blood Cells.

Frozen Red Blood Cells usually are of little help in overcoming a major blood shortage situation. When there is a regional shortage, it is unlikely that there are sufficient units of frozen Red Blood Cells available in the system to provide more than minimally transient relief. Similarly, when there is a shortage of blood of a given ABO or Rh type in a hospital, the patient's needs usually are most easily met through switching to Red Blood Cells of another compatible type. Further, the use of frozen-stored red cells adds considerable expense.

Another example of a blood shortage occurs when it is not possible to obtain sufficient blood for a patient who has an antibody to a high-incidence antigen. In this situation there is really not a shortage within the system, but only a shortage of blood for a specific patient. If the blood requirement is for an elective surgical procedure and the patient's state of health permits, the blood need may be met through predeposit autologous transfusion. Several units of blood can be collected over a period of a few weeks; or, if more protracted accumulation of units of blood is feasible, units of autologous blood can be stored frozen for utilization at the time of the operation.

Another consideration for patients who have an antibody to a high-incidence antigen is to obtain blood from compatible donors. Such donors are most likely to be found among siblings of the patient. A registry of rare donors may be consulted, either at a regional blood center or in a central national location, such as the Rare Donor File of the American Association of Blood Banks. Using such a registry, a donor whose blood lacks the antigen can be identified quickly, blood can be donated and can be transported to the respective hospital, or blood from such donors can be labeled and stored frozen, either regionally or nationally, for future needs.

EMERGENCY TRANSFUSION

While routine processing of blood for transfusion was described previously in this chapter, there are clinical situations wherein delay in provision of blood through routine processing may unduly jeopardize the patient. In these circumstances it may be necessary to issue incompletely processed blood and perhaps to compromise other standard practices of the transfusion service. Nevertheless, an overriding concern is that the blood bank not do anything which may increase the morbidity of the patient.

Orderly management of the patient who requires urgent transfusion of blood necessitates definition of the severity and extent of the emergency. This evaluation must enable the blood bank to determine the appropriate blood product to be issued and the extent of pretransfusion testing that can be completed before transfusion. Furthermore, the approach to management of a single patient who has an urgent requirement for blood is quite different from the approach to a mass casualty situation. The ability of the laboratory to cope with the latter situation is greatly enhanced by development of a plan for management of mass casualties. This should encompass a mechanism for accurate identification of casualties, obtaining blood specimens and accurately labeling such specimens, a notification mechanism for members of the blood bank staff, and a system for assuring proper identification of units of blood with prospective recipients.

When dealing with emergency transfusion, it is appropriate to separate conceptually acute and unanticipated blood loss in a previously unhospitalized patient from such blood loss occurring in a patient in the course of hospitalization. Particular attention should be paid to identification of any blood specimens obtained from a previously unhospitalized patient. Auto accidents often result in patients being brought to emergency rooms who have the same last name. A system must be developed whereby confusion of patient identification can be precluded.

PROVISION OF UNCROSSMATCHED TYPE-SPECIFIC OR O, Rh-NEGATIVE, BLOOD

It is axiomatic that reliance must not be placed on blood typing results performed at other institutions but only on blood typing results performed by the transfusing facility. Determination of the ABO and Rh type should take less than 5 minutes. Most patients brought to the hospital emergency room can receive volume support, as with lactated Ringer's solution, during this brief interval so

that type-specific blood can be administered. If the patient must be transfused immediately, and the patient's ABO and Rh types have not been determined, O, Rh-negative Red Blood Cells can be administered. However, even in times of extreme urgency, a sample from the patient must be obtained for the blood bank before any blood is administered. In well-administered emergency rooms, only rarely is any type O blood used for this purpose, and it is extremely rare for more than one such unit to be required before type-specific blood can be made available. Indeed, even in military combat, transfusion of more than 2,890 severely injured patients required the use of only 157 units of group O, Rh-negative red blood cells because extreme emergency did not allow the obtaining of type-specific blood.[9] Recipients whose ABO and Rh types have been determined by the transfusing facility may receive type-specific blood before tests for compatibility have been completed.

The term "universal donor" often has been applied to O, Rh-negative blood products. It should be evident that there are many blood group antigen systems other than ABO and Rh. The O-negative red cells may be positive for Rh antigens other than Rh_o (D) as well as other antigens such as Kell, Duffy, and Kidd, while the plasma of the prospective recipient may contain antibodies against such antigens. Therefore, the serum from a patient with anti-Jk^a would react with O, Rh-negative, Red Blood Cells containing the Jk^a antigen. Nevertheless, since most of the population lacks unexpected antibodies, and since the most common such unexpected antibody is anti-Rh_o (D), O, Rh-negative, Red Blood Cells are the safest product to transfuse in such a situation.

As indicated, the O, Rh-negative, blood should be given in the form of Red Blood Cells. This will avoid the transfusion of a significant amount of anti-A and anti-B. In the past, such alloantibodies were minimized by providing blood with low titers of anti-A and anti-B. However, only a small fraction of O, Rh-negative, units were then available for such emergency purposes. The policy of using Red Blood Cells greatly increases the utilization of the O, Rh-negative, resource in such situations, and also allows transfusion of type-specific blood for the patient after typing has been completed. Use of O, Rh-negative whole blood might result in transfusion of anti-A or anti-B, which would preclude such return to transfusion of blood of the patient's own type.

Administration of Red Blood Cells may not be as acceptable as whole blood to the physician dealing with the patient requiring emergency transfusion because of the flow characteristics of Red Blood Cells. Most units of red blood cells will have a hematocrit of approximately 80 percent. Transfusion can be accelerated by means of an external pressure cuff around the unit of packed cells. Similarly, the flow rate of the unit can be increased by diluting the unit with a small volume (50 to 100 ml) of isotonic saline. This can readily be accomplished through use of a Y-type administration set.

Ordinarily, lactated Ringer's solution should not be mixed with blood because of the possibility of neutralization of the citrate anticoagulant and the resultant possibility of development of clots in the unit of blood.[10] Under usual circumstances, only isotonic saline solution should be mixed with blood. However, in an emergency this becomes more of a theoretical than a real possibility. It has been demonstrated that, when the ratio of blood to lactated Ringer's solution is greater than 1.0, there is little possibility of clot formation. Clot formation with such mixtures is enhanced by an increased ratio of solution to blood, and also through prolonged contact of the solution with blood at a temperature of 37°C. In emergency situations, necessitating use of O, Rh-negative red blood cells, it is most unlikely that the blood would have time to warm toward 37°C; because of the urgency of the situation, the blood would be administered rapidly, thereby avoiding prolonged contact of the solution with blood.

COMPATIBILITY TESTING IN EMERGENCY SITUATIONS

When there is urgent need for blood transfusion, it may be possible to begin pretransfusion compatibility testing, yet it is often necessary to issue type-specific blood before completion of the major crossmatch or the screening test for unexpected antibodies. Since this creates an increased degree of risk for the transfusion recipient, it is imperative that the patient's records contain a statement indicating that the clinical situation was of sufficient urgency to require release of blood before completion of such testing.[1] This statement must be signed by the requesting physician, although this may be done after the transfusion has been given. Such physician may be either the physician primarily responsible for the care of the patient or the physician responsible for the blood bank. Usually the former is most appropriate. Similarly, when incompletely crossmatched blood is released for transfusion, the tag or label attached to the unit of blood must indicate in a conspicuous fashion that the crossmatch was incomplete at the time of issuance of the blood.[1]

As noted above, even with the use of methods that enhance agglutination and thereby somewhat expedite the crossmatch and antibody screening procedures, 20 to 60 minutes generally are required for completion of all phases of a major crossmatch and antibody screening test. This includes the various centrifugations, incubations, and paper work. When blood must be issued before completion of these procedures, it is imperative that the laboratory continue with the processing and complete the tests promptly. If an unexpected antibody is discovered, or if incompatibility is noted in the major crossmatch, previously issued units must be retrieved and compatible blood should be provided as soon as possible. As stated above, such abbreviation of the major crossmatch in a patient whose serum has not been screened for unexpected antibodies bears an element of risk. The blood bank director and patient's physician must balance this risk against the risk to the patient of postponing transfusion.

When an urgent requirement for blood occurs for a patient in the course of a hospitalization, and the patient's serum previously has been screened for unexpected antibodies, what is the risk of abbreviating the major crossmatch? The most important function of the major crossmatch is the confirmation of ABO compatibility. Life-threatening transfusion reactions usually are due to such incompatibility and most often are a result of human error. Since the haste and disruption of routine procedure associated with an emergency accentuates the possibility of such an error, it is important that this function of the crossmatch be retained. This can be accomplished by an abbreviated procedure involving reaction of recipient serum and donor red cells by immediate centrifugation. The complete crossmatch with antiglobulin serum permits detection of IgG antibodies. In general, such antibodies reacting with incompatible red cells result in decreased posttransfusion survival of the transfused cells but usually do not result in life-threatening intravascular hemolysis of incompatible blood. The "immediate spin" phase of the crossmatch, performed at room temperature, should detect IgM antibodies in the ABO system which might result in life-threatening intravascular hemolysis. This topic is discussed in more detail in Chapter 7.

A hospital blood bank often is requested to transfuse blood on an urgent basis during operative procedures to patients whose blood previously has been typed for ABO and Rh and screened for unexpected antibodies. In such a situation it may be assumed that the screening test for unexpected antibodies has detected most clinically significant antibodies; therefore, abbreviation of the major crossmatch to the "immediate spin" phase may be quite safe. In a recent study of 83,000 crossmatches performed on approximately 14,000 patients at the University of Michigan Hospital, it was shown that only eight weakly reactive, yet clinically significant, antibodies were not detected by the screening test for such antibodies but were detected by the major crossmatch.[11]

Therefore, issuance of blood in urgent situations after an "immediate spin" phase of the major crossmatch for patients whose red cells have been typed for ABO and Rh and whose serum has been screened for unexpected antibodies carries a very low level of risk. Such processing should require less than five minutes. Of course, this would not apply to patients whose serum has not previously been screened for unexpected antibodies.

Parenthetically, it should be noted that the use of such an abbreviated crossmatch, coupled with the demonstrated safety of this procedure when the patient's blood previously has been typed for ABO and Rh and screened for unexpected antibodies, enhances the acceptability of a MSBOS in a hospital since safe blood can be provided at relatively short notice for unexpected operative hemorrhage.

Of necessity, the subject of emergency transfusion often blends into the subject of massive transfusion. This is discussed elsewhere in this text. Nevertheless, it should be appreciated that in a massive transfusion the blood bank may be called upon to perform complete major crossmatches for all issued units of blood. This is inappropriate, for there seems little reason to expend the effort and expense of performing a major crossmatch through the antiglobulin phase after a patient has received a single volume replacement transfusion. In such a situation the patient's welfare can be protected by merely performing an "immediate spin" crossmatch, thereby assuring ABO compatibility.[1] Furthermore, in such a situation it is not necessary for the laboratory to complete the crossmatch after issuance of the blood. It should also be noted that, in some patients, both the blood supply problems and the compatibility testing problems associated with massive transfusion can be circumvented by use of intraoperative autologous transfusion (see Ch. 15).

REFERENCES

1. Standards for blood banks and transfusion services. Ninth edition. Oberman, H., ed. Washington, D.C., 1978.
2. Judd, W.J., Butch, S.H., Oberman, H.A., Steiner, E.A., and Bauer, R.D.: The evaluation of a positive direct antiglobulin test in pretransfusion testing. Transfusion 20:17, 1980.
3. Myhre, B.A.: Quality control in blood banking. John Wiley and Sons, New York, 1974.
4. Friedman, B.A., Oberman, H.A., Chadwick, A.R., and Kingdon, K.I.: The maximum surgical blood order schedule and surgical blood use in the United States. Transfusion 16:380, 1976.
4a. Friedman, B.A.: An analysis of surgical blood use in United States hospitals with application to the maximum surgical blood order schedule. Transfusion 19:3, 1979.
5. Devitt, J.E.: Blood wastage and cholecystectomy: Spin-off from a peer review. Can. Med. Assoc. J. 109:120, 1973.
6. Boral, L.I. and Henry, J.B.: The type and screen: a safe alternative and supplement in selected surgical procedures. Transfusion 17:163, 1977.
7. Brodheim, E. and Hirsch, R.: Effect of adenine on blood usage strategies, shortages and outdating. Transfusion 19:105, 1979.
8. Technical Manual. Seventh edition. Miller, W., ed. American Association of Blood Banks, Washington, D.C., 1977, p. 190.
9. Monaghan, W.P., Levan, D.R., and Camp, F.R., Jr.: Blood transfusion aboard a naval hospital ship receiving multiple casualties in a combat zone, a controlled medical environment. Transfusion 17:473, 1977.
10. Ryden, S.E. and Oberman, H.A.: Compatibility of common intravenous solutions with CPD blood. Transfusion 15:250, 1975.
11. Oberman, H.A., Barnes, B.A., and Friedman, B.A.: The risk of abbreviating the major crossmatch in urgent or massive transfusion. Transfusion 18:137, 1978.

19

Medicolegal Considerations in Blood Transfusion

Harold L. Engel, M.D., J.D.

INTRODUCTION

The use of blood transfusions in the clinical practice of medicine has brought untold benefits to countless individuals. At the same time, as with any medical procedure, it has resulted in numerous injuries and deaths. That the benefits have far outnumbered the harmful incidents cannot be denied. Nonetheless, continuing efforts must be directed toward reducing the dangers of the use of blood and blood products. It is certainly too much to expect that transfusions will ever become 100 percent safe, and so injured persons and their relatives will undoubtedly continue to seek compensation for their injuries. Whenever a bad result follows a blood transfusion and it appears to have been the result of the transfusion, one may anticipate a law suit. Individuals always have the right to bring a suit. Fortunately for the medical profession and for those untold millions who will benefit from transfusions in the future, they do not always succeed. If they did, it might bring an end to this most useful procedure, for the cost of assuming responsibility for every bad result of a transfusion would probably put the price of its use beyond reach. But, where the injury was due to wrongful act, the injured party may be entitled to compensation which is best borne through widespread cost distribution by means of insurance.

The constant threat of malpractice suits in modern medical practice may be turned to the advantage of both physicians and patients if the medical profession will use it as a stimulus continually to seek safer methods and techniques in the utilization of blood transfusions. The following discussion of the legal avenues available to a person seeking compensation, as well as mention of some legal considerations peculiar to blood transfusions, may aid in reducing the number of injuries and thus the number of lawsuits involved with this treatment method. It may also help in the defense of a suit if it is brought.

THEORIES OF LIABILITY

Negligence

In order for a plaintiff to succeed in a suit for negligence, he must prove that the defendant owed him a duty, that the defendant breached that duty, that the breach caused the plaintiff an injury, and that it is an injury that can be compensated in monetary damages. Failure to prove any one of these four will result in a verdict in favor of the defendant.

Duty. A duty arises when a physician-patient relationship is established. There is usually no difficulty in finding such a duty when a doctor undertakes the treatment of a patient or when a patient enters a hospital or when a blood bank obtains and provides blood or a pathologist tests it. Every individual or legal entity which has anything to do with any part of the process which starts with getting the blood from the donor and ends with the receiving of the blood by the recipient has a duty to act in such a manner as not to injure him. It is not uncommon to find as defendants the owners and operators of both commercial and voluntary blood banks or their workers who may be volunteers, employees, or independent contractors. Even those who have provided defective or contaminated equipment or supplies to blood banks, laboratories, or hospitals have been held to have had a duty to the ultimate consumer of the blood. Clearly, any physician, nurse, or technician who has had a direct or indirect role in any part of the blood transfusion has a duty not to injure the patient. The donor himself may have a duty not to injure the recipient by, for example, denying a past history of hepatitis.

A more difficult question is whether a duty is owed to anyone other than the individual who actually receives the transfusion. Certainly a duty is owed to the prospective heirs not to bring about the death of the recipient. Similarly, a duty may be owed to a spouse not to cause a loss of consortium by injuring the recipient. But let us assume that a patient who had developed serum hepatitis following a negligent transfusion had in turn transmitted the disease to another who came in contact with his now infected blood. Did the original negligent actor have a duty to the last injured person? Presumably there was no doctor-patient relationship between the two, and no transmission of blood was ever intended. However, there may definitely be such a duty if it can be shown that injuries to others than the actual recipient of the transfusion are

reasonably foreseeable. Such a decision would probably be left to a jury. One may owe a duty, not only to the recipient but to all others who may be injured as a consequence of a negligent act.

It has been held that one may owe a duty to a person who was not even conceived at the time of the wrongful act.[1] In 1965 a girl thirteen years old who was Rh-negative was given a transfusion of Rh-positive blood. She had no adverse reaction and did not learn of the error at the time. But she must have been sensitized since, in 1974, she delivered a jaundiced baby who required a complete exchange transfusion and suffered damage to her brain and various other organs. The court held that the child could maintain an action against the doctor and the hospital who were allegedly responsible for the incorrect transfusion of her mother "even though the transfusion occurred several years prior to the infant's conception." It was specifically stated that the defendants could have foreseen that a thirteen-year-old girl would probably grow up, marry, and become pregnant. It is not known whether other jurisdictions besides Illinois will adopt this theory, but it indicates that there may be a trend to hold that a physician has a duty to anyone who may foreseeably be injured by his action.

Breach of Duty. The "standard of practice" is used to determine whether a breach of duty has occurred. This term really means that the defendant, such as a physician, is required to practice in a manner consistent with the practice of other physicians of the same or similar qualifications under similar conditions in the same locality at the same time. Plaintiffs usually attempt to show that there is only one standard of practice under a given circumstance, while defendants claim there are several acceptable ways to handle a specific case. This does not mean that one must conform to the majority, but one should conform to at least a substantial minority. Being the only one or two physicians in a community to practice in a given manner may expose one to a charge of not being within "the standard." In recent years there has also been an expansion of the meaning of "locality" so that standards have tended to become national.

What the standard is in any given lawsuit must usually be established in one of two ways. Expert witnesses will be called by each side to give testimony as to that standard. The plaintiff will present an expert who will claim to know what the standard was at the time of the act; he will testify as to what the standard was and to the fact that the defendant did not conform to it. The defendant's expert may agree or disagree as to the actual standard but will insist that the defendant either conformed to or exceeded it. The jury will then weigh the evidence and decide.

If the plaintiff is unable to obtain an expert to testify in his behalf, his case is almost always dismissed. Physicians who are asked to testify on behalf of plaintiffs should consider the fact that without such testimony the plaintiff may be unable to recover. But, if he should decide to undertake giving his opinions, he should keep the definition of "standard of practice" in mind at all times and not hold up as the standard what he himself would have done, or what was done at universities, or what would have been ideal; rather, he should hold the defendant only to what a reasonable number of others would have done under the circumstances at that time. Testimony by an expert that he would like to have had an SGOT test performed on donor blood in 1966 was held to be of no value in the face of proof that no other laboratory used the test then.[2]

Sometimes the standards are established by law or by various organizations. There are many statutes—federal, state, and local—relating to the obtaining, processing, and transportation of blood for transfusion. If these laws are not conformed to and if a person is injured as a result thereof, it may be held that there was a breach of duty. If a laboratory is a member of an organization such as the American Association of Blood Banks, or a hospital has voluntarily obtained accreditation by the Joint Committee on Accreditation of Hospitals, it must conform to all of their regulations. Similarly, if a hospital staff or department has established its own rules, they must be followed even if they call for higher standards than required by law, for any failure to conform to them may be considered a breach. Since the word "standard" has such a specific legal meaning, many organizations have preferred to substitute the word "guidelines" so as to permit the argument that if one did not comply with them exactly he was not falling below the standard of practice but only not following suggestions.

Courts have also consistently held that complete conformity to a set of standards or guidelines promulgated by a hospital or a society does not in and of itself prove that the standard of practice was met and that no breach of duty took place. They have ruled that these regulations themselves may be inadequate to protect the public and that, in effect, the entire "industry" was negligent. But, if the regulations are adequate, compliance has been held to indicate the use of due care.[3] If one doesn't follow the rules, he will surely be held to have fallen below the requisite standards; if one does follow them, he may still be held to have been below if those standards are themselves inadequate.

Expert testimony may, in some instances, not be necessary if the facts are such as to involve the rule of "res ipsa loquitor." In such a situation, the average layperson will know of his own knowledge and experience that the given injury would not have happened unless someone along the line was negligent. Cases involving incorrect labeling of blood, errors in recording results of tests, and giving the blood to the wrong patient are examples in which res ipsa loquitor has been applied.[4] But, where the only evidence of alleged negligence is the bare fact that the patient contracted hepatitis following a blood transfusion, the doctrine has not been allowed.[5] This is based upon the fact that hepatitis may occur even though no one has done anything wrong.

Causation. If a duty to act in a certain way or to refrain from acting has been established and a breach of that duty has occurred, the plaintiff will not prevail unless he can prove that it was the breach that caused the injury. It should be kept in mind that legal proof is not equivalent to scientific proof. One need only convince a jury by a preponderance of the evidence—i.e., it is more likely than not that the injury was caused by the breach of the defendant's duty. Here, too, it is usually necessary to present expert testimony, since what caused the injury is almost always beyond the knowledge of the average person who would be a member of the jury.

A defendant may have fallen below the standard of practice in several areas, and the patient may have been injured without the one following from the other. For instance, a technician may have negligently mistyped blood, resulting in a type-A patient receiving type-O blood. The patient may subsequently develop hepatitis, but since that was caused by a virus in the blood and not by the mismatch, there would be no liability. But, if an immediate transfusion reaction had taken place, there probably would be a decision in favor of the patient-plaintiff.

Lawsuits have been brought alleging negligence caused by almost every conceivable act. Only a few need be mentioned to show that whenever a patient is injured he is likely to look for a cause that was due to someone's error. A blood bank has been accused of negligence in drawing blood too frequently from a donor, in not asking if the donor was tatooed, in not having a medical doctor present to examine or supervise others in examining the donor, and in not testing "to determine whether there were signs of his ever having had hepatitis." A hospital was sued for not inquiring as to the background of the blood bank from which it obtained its blood or as to the conditions under which it obtained blood from its donors. The blood bank

was in New York, but its license to operate a branch was in the process of being revoked in New Jersey.[6] A hospital was sued on the claim that an intravenous needle was contaminated;[7] another was sued for improperly taking, typing, and matching blood as well as failure to provide careful observation during a transfusion to observe for indications of an adverse reaction.[8] The use of paid donors as opposed to volunteers is not negligent in and of itself unless there is a statute against it.[2,3] Any error from the very start of the process up to and including the recognition and treatment of any complication may bring on litigation.

Damages. If a defendant is found guilty of negligence, he will be liable for all reasonable damages suffered by the plaintiff as a result of that negligence. This may vary from state to state but usually includes all past and future medical costs and all past and future loss of earnings as well as pain and suffering. This may well add up to several millions of dollars in a given case. Attempts to limit the amount recoverable for a wrongful death have been more successful than those to limit recovery for pain and suffering. It therefore is wise for anyone who might be exposed to such a judgment to protect himself with insurance.

If the negligence has been so willful and wanton as to constitute an utter disregard for the welfare of the plaintiff, it may be possible to recover punitive damages. These are assessed as a punishment of the wrongdoer and as a warning to others. In most cases one cannot purchase insurance against such damages.

Strict Liability

The theory of strict liability is usually considered to have entered American law through two nonmedical cases in 1944 and 1963.[9,10] These cases held that a defendant may be held liable for damages to a plaintiff even if he was not negligent in any way. Any person who manufactures, sells, distributes, or in any other way places in the stream of commerce a product which proves to have a defect that causes injury to a human being may be held liable, even if he did nothing wrong. It is not difficult to see that it can be argued that this theory would be applicable in relation to patients who developed hepatitis due to transfusion with blood contaminated with a pathogenic virus. If the securing and processing of the blood is considered "manufacturing," the blood could be a product. The charges made in conjunction with administering it in a transfusion could be considered a sale, and the presence of the virus could be the defect.

Arguments made by the plaintiff along these lines were rejected by a New York court in 1954.[11] This court held that a blood transfusion was a service and not a sale, and thus there would be no liability upon the defendant unless it could be shown that he was negligent. This ruling has been followed almost unanimously by other states.[12,13] However, the Illinois Supreme Court (1970)[14] and the Colorado Supreme Court (1978)[15] held just the opposite, namely that a blood transfusion was a sale, not a service, and that it was not necessary for the plaintiff to prove that the defendant did something wrong in order to recover. If this had remained the law, it would have meant that the mere fact that a patient developed hepatitis following a transfusion would have permitted him to recover. In order to prevent such an outcome, more than 40 State Legislatures have passed statutes codifying the rule that a transfusion is a service and not a sale. The California law[16] is a representative example:

"Health and Safety Code § 1606

"The procurement, processing, distribution, or use of whole blood, plasma, blood products, and blood derivatives for the purpose of injecting or transfusing the same, or any of them, into the human body shall be construed to be, and is declared to be, for all purposes whatsoever, the rendition of a service by each and every person, firm, or corporation participating therein, and shall not be construed to be, and is declared not to be, a sale of such whole blood, plasma, blood products, or blood derivatives, for any purpose or purposes whatsoever."

This statute was upheld as being constitutional by the California Supreme Court in 1976.[17]

But it should be kept in mind that the reasoning behind these statutes and decisions holding that a transfusion is a service and not a sale and that the theory of strict liability would therefore not be applied has been that "there was no scientific method available for testing blood for hepatitis."[17] With the development of such tests, it is possible that courts may begin to reverse themselves and that legislatures may repeal statutes so as to make a transfusion a sale and bring hepatitis cases into the area of strict liability. Where such tests for hepatitis virus are available, it would be wise to use them, for a failure to do so could lead to a case of hepatitis which in turn could result in a lawsuit which might lead to holding such statutes unconstitutional.

Breach of Warranty

A cause of action for breach of warranty is sometimes used when the injured party feels that he has been given a guarantee that no harm will come to him. The warranty may be implied or expressed. The implied warranty is usually restricted to cases in which a sale takes place. Courts have almost always refused to allow this cause of action in relation to blood transfusions for reasons similar to their refusal to allow strict liability. They have held that the administration of blood is a service and not a sale. Moneys received by a hospital or laboratory are considered service fees and not receipts from a sale even though they are taxable.[18]

But, where the warranty has been expressed, either by a writing or an oral statement, this cause of action has been allowed.[19] If the patient has been told that the blood transfusion will definitely cause no harm and then it does injure him, he may recover damages even though the defendants were not negligent. The mere happening of what was guaranteed not to happen is enough to render the guarantor liable.

CONSENT TO TRANSFUSION

Informed Consent

Before any transfusion is administered, an informed consent must be obtained. The law as to what constitutes such a consent varies widely throughout the United States and is presently in a constant state of change. Except in cases of emergency, it is probably advisable to obtain a written consent separate from the general hospital treatment consent. This should be obtained after a physician has explained the risks of such a transfusion. Some jurisdictions require as an explanation only that which other physicians in a similar circumstance would give the patient—i.e., what the standard of practice is.[20] Other jurisdictions do not allow the explanation to be based upon such standards; rather, they set their own requirements, including giving the patient information as to the alternative procedures and risks of serious bodily harm and death.[21] If a patient is injured by a transfusion given without his valid consent, he may recover damages even though the defendants did everything else properly.

Jehovah's Witnesses

The official legal reports of appellate cases published throughout the country contain an inordinate number referable to Jehovah's Witnesses. Members of this small religious group usually refuse to consent to receiving transfusions of blood or blood products. Some members will accept plasma expanders and many will agree to autotransfusions. Some hold that their religious beliefs prevent them from giving their consent and that, if they are compelled to accept a transfusion under a court order, they will suffer no religious penalties. But others fear eternal damnation if transfused voluntarily or involuntarily.[22] It is not possible to obtain from these cases any definite set of rules which can be used to attempt to determine whether a physician should order a transfusion for a Jehovah's Witness in a given case. It all depends upon the facts that exist at the time the doctor must make the decision. In general, the greater the emergency, the greater the risk to the patient of withholding the blood; and, the less the competency of the patient to give consent, the less likely the doctor will be held liable if he proceeds. But, where time permits, a court order should be sought. The hospital's attorney is usually helpful in attempting to obtain one.

A court refused to order a transfusion where the patient was a competent, 23-year-old woman who had no children and was not pregnant. It found no compelling state interest which would make it override her refusal.[23] Similarly, another court refused to order the transfusion of a 34-year-old man with two children when it was convinced that provision had been made for the future well-being of the children, both financially and in regard to care by relatives.[24] A 17-year-old was held not to be a neglected child for agreeing with his mother and refusing a blood transfusion for surgery to correct his spine.[25] But a court did order a transfusion to preserve the life of the mother of an infant.[26] A similar ruling could be expected from some courts to preserve the life of a pregnant mother in the interest of the unborn child, but other courts might decide upon the basis of which trimester the pregnancy was.

In one case an adult father refused a

transfusion. His separated wife, mother of his child, and the man's two brothers petitioned the court for an order to force a transfusion. The judge issued the order, the transfusion was given, and the patient recovered. He then appealed against the order, but it was held to be moot since he had already received the blood. He next sued the judge to prevent him from issuing such orders in the future, but his case was dismissed.[27]

Where an automobile accident killed the parents and injured three minors, the court gave temporary guardianship to the Welfare Department when relatives refused transfusions.[28] In another case, when a divorced mother became a Jehovah's Witness, the custody of minor children was transferred from her to the children's father in order to protect them from any danger resulting from the mother's possible refusal to allow them blood transfusions.[29] And in another case, a court ordered the transfusion of a minor because society had an overriding interest to prevent brain damage or death.[30]

If a patient is unconscious and cannot make his wishes known, a court may order a transfusion.[31] One adult who was "in extremis" was held "non compos mentis" and an order was issued.[22] But it is very much uncertain what a court would do when asked for an order for an unconscious patient who had adamantly refused blood when in full possession of his faculties.

It can be seen that every possible situation may arise and that no general rules can be established. Each case must be handled individually. The rights of the patient, the rights of his relatives, the rights of society, and certainly the rights of the physician are all entitled to great consideration. For what it is worth, my personal advice is to follow the law of your own state but, if an error in judgment is made, let it be on the side of preserving life. If a lawsuit follows, it will be rigorously defended, and a verdict favorable to the defendant is much more likely if the patient survived than if, on the other hand, he died and his heirs sued alleging that blood should have been given.

INFREQUENT LEGAL PROBLEMS

Injuries to the Donor

The donor, whether a volunteer or paid, has a right not to be injured. If taking blood from him causes him injury, he may be entitled to recover. Bleeding a donor who does not meet the physical requirements, who may be anemic or hypertensive, or who may have given blood too recently may lead to liability if he has a subsequent myocardial infarction, cerebrovascular accident, or other complication. One donor fainted, fell, and suffered injuries when not observed carefully.[32] Others have developed local infections and even septicemia from improperly sterilized needles and other equipment.

Liability of Donor to Recipient

When a patient developed hepatitis after a blood transfusion, he sued the donor for contaminating him. He was unable to recover against the donor because he was unable to present any evidence that she knew or should have known that she had had hepatitis.[33] Presumably, if a donor knows he has had hepatitis or syphilis or any other disease which can be transmitted by a transfusion and conceals this fact or denies it, he may be liable to a recipient whom he infects.

Charges for Transfusions

A patient refused to pay the charges for a transfusion because the blood was replaced free by a relative. The court held that a charge could be made as compensation for the time and labor involved.[34]

Criminal Case

A blood transfusion has been involved in at least one criminal case. The defendant had inflicted a gunshot wound on the victim. It was definitely not lethal, but he required a blood transfusion. He developed serum hepatitis and died. The defendant was convicted of first-degree murder. The transfusion was not considered to be a sufficient intervening act to break the chain of events and reduce the criminal charge, since it was not a "gross error."[37]

Paid or Voluntary Donors

It is generally held that the incidence of complications is less when voluntary rather than paid donors are used. However, the mere use of paid donors does not constitute negligence if all other precautions have been used.[3] However, at least one state now has a law against the use of paid donors.[35]

OTHER CAUSES OF COMPLICATIONS

All complications which follow blood transfusions are not the result of the transfusion. In many instances, lawsuits may be successfully defended by presenting expert testimony to show that the injury was due to or that it was just as likely to be due to another cause. An example is a Texas case in which a woman suffered a postpartum hemorrhage and was given two units of whole blood. She developed a lower nephron nephrosis and died. Suit was brought alleging that the cause of the nephrosis was incompatible blood. The court found for the defendant, holding that the death could have been caused by shock.[36]

A certain number of individuals who develop jaundice and hepatitis following transfusions would certainly have developed them without the transfusions if they were in the incubation stage of infectious hepatitis. Others may have been exposed to various hepatotoxins such as carbon tetrachloride, halothane, or chlorpromazine. A physician who is called to testify as an expert witness should be extremely careful that he has examined all the available material on the case and that he has ruled out all other possible causes of the injury before condemning the blood transfusion.

REFERENCES

1. *Renslow v. Mennonite Hospital.* 367 NE 2d 1250; 67 Ill. 2d 348 (1977).
2. *Hutchins v. Blood Services.* 506 P 2d 449.
3. *Hines v. St. Joseph Hosp.'* 527 P 2d 1075; 86 N.M. 763.
4. *Redding v. U.S.* 196 F. Supp. 871.
5. *Morse v. Riverside Hosp.* 339 NE 2d 846; 44 Ohio App. 2d 422.
6. *Samuels v. Health & Hosp. Corp.* 591 F 2d 195.
7. *Sommers v. Sisters of Charity.* 561 P 2d 603; 277 Or 549.
8. *Joseph v. W. H. Grove L.D.S. Hosp.* 10 Utah 2d 94; 348 P 2d 935.
9. *Escola v. Coca Cola.* 24 Cal. 2d 453; 150 P 2d 436.
10. *Greenman v. Yuba Power Products.* 50 Cal. 2d 57; 377 P 2d 897.
11. *Perlmutter v. Beth David Hosp.* 308 NY 100; 123 N.E. 2d 792.
12. 45 Amer. Law Review 3d 1353, 1389 (1972).
13. 24 Stanford Law Review 439; 476.
14. *Cunningham v. MacNeal Memorial Hosp.* 47 Ill. 2d 443; 266 NE 2d 987.
15. *Belle Bonfils Blood Bank v. Hansen.* 579 P 2d 1158.
16. Calif. Health and Safety Code § 1606.
17. *McDonald v. Sacramento Medical Foundation Blood Bank.* 62 CA 3d 866; 133 Cal. Rpt. 444.
18. *U.S. v. Garber.* 589 F 2d 843 (1979).
19. *Napoli v. St. Peter's Hosp.* 213 N.Y.S. 2d 6.
20. *Moore v. Underwood Memorial Hosp.* 371 A 2d 105; 147 N.J. Super. 252.
21. *Cobbs v. Grant.* 8 Cal. 3d 229; 104 Cal. Rpt. 505; 502 P 2d 1.
22. "Power of Court to Order Blood Transfusion for Adult." 9 ALR 3d 1391.
23. *In re MELIDED.* 390 N.Y.S. 2d 523.

24. *In re OSBORNE.* 294 A 2d 372.
25. *In re GREEN.* 307 A 2d 279; 452 Pa. 373.
26. Application of Georgetown College. 118 DC 80; 331 F 2d 1000.
27. *Hamilton v. McAuliffe.* 353 A 2d 634; 277 Md. 336.
28. *Guardianship of RANDALL.* 569 P 2d 549.
29. *Stapley v. Stapley.* 485 P 2d 1181; 15 Ariz. App. 64.
30. *Muhlenberg Hosp. v. Patterson.* 320 A 2d 518; 128 N.J. Sup. 498.
31. *Kennedy Hosp. v. Heston.* 279A 2d 670; 58 N.J. 576.
32. *Boll v. Sharp and Dohme.* 121 N.Y.S. 2d 20.
33. *Hubbell v. So. Nassau Comm. Hosp.* 260 N.Y.S. 2d 539.
34. *Local 1140 v. Mass. Mutual Life.* 165 N.W. 2d 234.
35. Calif. Health & Safety Code § 1626.
36. *Billen v. U.S.* 281 F 2d 425.
37. *People v. Fleenan.* 202 N.W. 2d 471; 42 Mich. App. 457.

20

The Role of Government in Blood Services

Scott N. Swisher, M.D.

During the early years of the modern practice of blood transfusion, it was carried out strictly within hospitals and was regarded as essentially a surgical procedure. Each hospital had its own blood bank. In this era, transfusion practice was largely free of regulatory control or other governmental intervention. The growth of transfusion practice and the need for blood and serological reagents to move in interstate commerce soon brought the field under regulatory control of the federal government for safety and efficacy and, in some instances, parallel regulation by state and local governments as well. The growth and influence of regulatory processes has been steadily increasing in recent years.[1]

Recently, the federal and some state governments also have become interested in the overall management of blood as a national resource for health care. This has been implemented in a number of ways. A major study of U.S. blood resources was undertaken.[2] A research program has been established within the National Heart, Lung and Blood Institute of the National Institutes of Health, the Blood Resources Branch, directed to blood resource research and development. A second approach was through the enunciation of a National Blood Policy, announced by the Secretary of Health, Education and Welfare in 1974 after the report by the broadly based national study (previously noted) of the problems which had developed during the period of very rapid growth of blood services in the U.S.[3] The National Blood Policy has led to efforts to unify blood services of the country, based upon formation of a broad coalition of blood service organizations, blood service users, and public members, under the aegis of a new organization the American Blood Commission.

A variety of national and state legislative initiatives have been taken over the last ten years, some now pending, which speak to the organization and operation of blood services. This chapter discussed these several roles of government in the provision of blood services in the United States. It should be recognized that the topics discussed here are all undergoing rapid change. Therefore, only a general discussion of these matters can be given here.

FEDERAL REGULATION

The legal basis for the regulation of blood and blood products along with related reagents and equipment arises from the Biologics Control Act of 1902, now multiply amended. This authority over biologics was initially separate from the law which established the Food and Drug Administration (FDA), the Food and Drug Act of 1906, and, later, the Food, Drug and Cosmetics Act of 1938; again, this act has been amended frequently. The Kefauver-Harris amendments of 1962 provided the most important major recent revisions. The Division of Biologics Standards (DBS), on the campus of the National Institutes of Health, was ultimately established to carry out regulatory function for biologics and some of the necessary related research activities. These responsibilities had rested in several different places before the DBS was founded. Although this agency was responsible for the regulation and standardization of all biological materials, particularly the classical vaccines and antisera, its blood-related activities were at a relatively low level until the early 1960s.

The Bureau of Biologics

A number of problems arose from having two agencies regulating therapeutic materials. These included overlapping jurisdiction with the FDA in the regulation of blood, its products, related reagents, preservatives, equipment and procedures, as well as an increasing requirement for field investigations and enforcement actions. The Division of Biologics Standards was then merged with the FDA, where it became the Bureau of Biologics (BOB) in 1972 in an effort to resolve these issues. Within the BOB, a Division of Blood and Blood Products was established. This organization has grown in size and professional and scientific competence until it is now able to discharge its regulatory function to a very high standard.

The BOB not only establishes standards for blood and blood products which are acceptable for their safety and efficacy, but also establishes good manufacturing practices, inspects manufacturing facilities, and evaluates products for compliance with required standards. It also inspects and licenses blood banks which regularly ship blood or blood products in interstate commerce. More recently, the BOB developed a program of reg-

istration and inspection of all blood banks, including those not formally licensed. This program is designed to insure that all blood services meet minimum standards of good practice.

A number of organizations in the private sector also offer voluntary inspections of blood banks in an effort to upgrade the quality of blood services. For example, the standards and inspection program of the American Association of Blood Banks long antedated the BOB program and was of major importance in calling attention to this important aspect of safe transfusion therapy.

STANDARDS FOR U.S. BIOLOGICALS

The standards now employed in the U.S. for approval of new blood products or changes in the production of old products by new methods are stringent when compared with those employed by much of the rest of the world. A relatively large amount of comprehensive data derived from critically designed and executed investigations by reputable investigators is required for these approvals. Acquisition of these data is often a slow process. Ambiguous results of one study require further investigations.[7] The BOB, like the FDA in the matter of new drug approvals, has been criticized for the slowness of this process, its costs, and the resultant delayed availability of products in this country which are seemingly successful and safe in other countries. Without categorically defending these agencies against well-publicized charges of this type of failure, it should be recognized that the growing public opinion about safety of drugs which has developed during the past decade or more has created a climate in which fully reasonable and responsive regulation has been virtually impossible. The consumerist philosophy of "complete safety" for all therapeutic products has created impossible public expectations by virtue of the very nature of the safety problem. Opportunist politicians from the U.S. Congress and so-called "consumer advocates" have compounded these problems by initiating politically motivated and uninformed interventions. Given these circumstances, it appears remarkable to at least some observers, the author included, that the regulatory process has worked at all in recent years.[4,5,6]

The regulatory process within the BOB which controls blood and blood products is at present in the hands of a group of dedicated, professional, and capable scientists who operate within reasonable, if conservative, guidelines. Prolonged delays encountered in new product approval are more often due to serious inadequacies of the data presented in support of the request than to what is categorically termed "bureaucratic delay." These opinions have been formed during a review by a consultant panel of physicians over a three-year period of all blood and blood products approved prior to 1973 for their safety and efficacy. Clinicians and, more importantly, patients, can be quite confident of the safety and efficacy of the blood and blood products they receive, if they will only recognize that these terms are always relative. Safety, and thus risk, must always be judged in relation to expected benefits, and the risks and benefits to be expected of any available alternatives.*

The report of this consultant panel is to be published in the Federal Register.[8] It should be of value to clinicians and blood banks alike, as well as to commercial organizations in the field; it is a concensus document covering issues of safety, efficacy, therapeutic indications, and adverse reactions of the major-

ity of blood products available for clinical use today. Only a few of the products available in the past were removed from the market for reasons of inadequate safety or unproved efficacy. A few products were identified which required additional information to permit these judgments to be made in the near future.

The panel on Safety and Efficacy of Blood and Blood Products completed its work in 1979. A standing consultant panel of experts outside governmental agencies has been appointed to provide ongoing advice and evaluations to the BOB. This panel will serve, as did the initial panel, as a link between the regulatory agency, clinical and basic science investigators, blood banks, and industry to assist in the expedient and scientifically valid operation of the regulatory process.

STATE AND LOCAL REGULATIONS

A variety of state and in some cases municipal regulations also affect blood services in some areas of the U.S. In a few instances, these appear to be justified by local situations. In most cases, they reflect another layer of burdensome, redundant, expensive, and unnecessary regulation. In some instances, these kinds of regulations are designed to be of specific advantage to various special interest groups. All such regulations should be reexamined, and those that serve no valid purpose should be repealed. This is a move that government itself could make to help control health care costs.

THE IMPACT OF THE NATIONAL BLOOD POLICY

Adoption of the National Blood Policy was the first major federal governmental intervention into the supply and economics of U.S. civilian blood services.[3] The policy speaks to four interrelated goals:

---

* The author of this chapter served as Chairman of Panel 6 on Safety and Efficacy of Blood and Blood Products, BOB, FDA. The opinions expressed here about the functions of the BOB and the Panel's report are his own and do not reflect an official action of the Panel. It is also the author's perception that the opinions expressed here were, in general, also held by his colleagues in that group, but he does not presume to speak for them.

1. Quality of Service.
2. Adequacy of Supply.
3. Accessibility to All Citizens.
4. Efficiency of the System.

The policy was formed in response to a number of perceived defects in U.S. blood services at that time.[2,9-11] Some areas of the country were underserved for reasons of an economic or demographic nature. A still significant proportion of whole blood and the blood bank products prepared from it was derived from commercial, for-profit sources which employed paid donors. Elimination of paid donors became a major goal when it was shown unequivocally that these donors, in all but a few instances, posed a much greater threat for transmission of hepatitis-B than did volunteer donors[12] (see also Ch. 36).

A wide range of conflicts also existed among various blood service agencies and individual blood banks at the time the National Blood policy was promulgated. The issues involved ranged from the philosophical to the financial. These conflicts were deemed to have an adverse effect upon the blood services of the nation. Establishment of a National Blood Policy was regarded as a way to provide guidelines for the resolution of a variety of dysfunctional arrangements within and among the operating agencies and to provide them with a set of measurable goals against which their performance ultimately could be judged. Although not clearly stated by the Congress, it has been widely understood that the alternative to improved performance by the private sector would be, in essence, federal management of blood services.[13]

THE AMERICAN BLOOD COMMISSION

The National Blood Policy has to some extent appeared to stimulate or accelerate a number of reforms and long needed developments in the field. The American Blood Commission (ABC), founded in 1975, was to be one of the principal vehicles for carrying out these public policies.[13] Its multiple constituencies include the major blood service organizations, professional and hospital organizations, user groups, and public representatives including industry and major labor groups. Its authority is limited to that provided by its role as a public forum and focus for organizational and coordinating activities.

The ABC got off to a slow and uncertain start. The deep divisions of philosophy, conflicting interests, and poor communication which have a long history in the field have continued to some degree in the forum of the ABC. ABC funding has been inadequate, since it must now rely largely on funds derived from its own constituents. Much of its activities revolve about issues that are fundamentally political in nature among its various constituent groups. At one time, its early demise was freely predicted.

In spite of these difficulties, the ABC has slowly established itself as a significant force in the field. It has begun a process of regional organization of blood services. A National Blood Service Data Center is being developed. The ABC has undertaken a number of research studies, policy studies, and communicational activities of importance. It has proposed a revised and much improved system of labeling blood and blood products which will be compatible with modern data processing and automated equipment available now and in the future. Recently, it has undertaken to develop on a national basis a program of blood resource sharing based upon a similar program developed jointly by the American Red Cross Blood Program and the Council of Community Blood Banks. Although many of its original roster of inherited problems remain to be resolved, there are now good grounds for the hope that the private section, through the ABC, will be able to accomplish enough of the reforms required by government to forestall federalization of the management of the national blood resources. In doing this, blood services should also improve.

CONFLICTS AMONG BLOOD SERVICE ORGANIZATIONS

During the period since World War II, a number of conflicts have developed among the several agencies providing blood services in the U.S.[14] The basis for these conflicts, their history, and their present status are not relevant to the purposes of this book, and they will not be discussed further here. It is notable, however, that a number of the major differences of position are slowly being resolved, largely under the sponsorship of the ABC. The articulation of public policy reflected in the formal statement of the National Blood Policy is slowly coming into being. The wisdom of these public policy positions can be evaluated only in the future.

RESOURCE SHARING

Another major philosophical difference among blood banks, regardless of their primary affiliation, involves the degree to which a regional blood program is willing to take responsibility for assisting where it can with blood supplies in areas of shortage outside its local region. Few hospital blood banks can be expected to be concerned about the adequacy of blood supplies beyond their own or a few closely related institutions. Similarly, programs in some communities are concerned mainly about their own needs and find it difficult or unreasonable to try to help meet needs in distant places. The trend, however, is clearly in the other direction, and this kind of provincialism is on the wane. Self-sufficiency is a reasonable goal for all areas of the country; but, where this cannot be attained promptly for one reason or another, patient needs should be met by resource sharing. We

have strong social traditions of this type in other areas of our national life. The greatest security of the blood supply in any area, even in those that are now self-sufficient, will come from a well-organized, efficiently managed pattern of strong mutual interdependence; this seems to be developing.

COST CONTROLS

Modern blood transfusion practice developed in an era of expanding fiscal resources for health care in the U.S. Control of costs, until recently, has been a secondary consideration to improvement of service. Because of the highly distributed nature of blood services of all sorts and the lack of required reports of activities and finances, the overall cost of blood services in the U.S. is only roughly known. These costs have risen under the pressure of inflation, as have all costs of health care. This has led to a number of efforts to control costs with direct impact upon the resources available to blood services. It is no longer possible in many areas of the country to "pass through" to third-party payers cost increases which may reflect both inflationary factors and service improvements. Rather, these now must be negotiated within specified "cost caps" allowed by third parties and governmental agencies in many instances.

The U.S. health care community has had little past experience in dealing with problems imposed by limited resources. Indeed, an argument can be made that health care workers should not be responsible for decisions of this nature. Rather, the public, through its various agencies which support health care, should be responsible for resource allocation decisions. The problem inherent in this approach is that the decisions may be made without full knowledge of their impact and the cost/benefit relationships of the possible alternatives. Professional advice will certainly be required in these circumstances, but it will be difficult to remove the element of advocacy from such advice. There is also the hazard, which in reality approaches certainty, that these decisions will become political in nature, with special interest groups exerting influence beyond their equitable involvement.

Unfortunately, there is little information which helps in rational decision making in this area. The typical cost/benefit analysis can be attacked in that it is frequently entirely economic in nature and ignores the "human values" involved. Translation between these two domains still is elusive. Nevertheless, this type of analysis, which is increasingly being applied to laboratory and radiological studies, may well develop in blood services in the near future.[15,16] For example, a recent paper examining the cost/benefit of leukocyte transfusions in acute leukemia received great attention following its publication in a prestigious journal.[17,18]

Uncomfortable as it will be, the blood services community will have to begin a searching analysis of its services and their value and costs, and exert a major effort to increase efficacy of operation. Only through increased efficiency can the adverse impact of reduced service levels, quantitative and qualitative, be minimized. This certainly is the major challenge facing blood services in the U.S. today.

THE ROLE OF GOVERNMENT IN BLOOD SERVICES OF OTHER COUNTRIES

It can be safely said that the quality and availability of blood services throughout the world are related primarily to the economic resources of a country which are available for health care. In those countries of the developed world which have highly managed economies, as in the Eastern Bloc of Europe, governmental economic allocation decisions, which are based largely on international politics, have a powerful effect upon the quality of blood services. Factors such as these seem much more significant in the development of health care services of all sorts than does the availability of knowledge. Adequate numbers of trained personnel are, of course, not available in the absence of adequate economic resources with which to employ them gainfully. Limitations imposed by lack of knowledge of the results of scientific investigation or of development of products and equipment are certainly of secondary importance in the developed countries and in many underdeveloped countries as well. Knowledge travels rapidly, world-wide today.

Beyond their role in control of the economy, governments exert widely different influences on the financing and management of blood services throughout the world. Many nations of Europe, including England, have had "national blood programs" for many years, although this term may mean quite different things in the several countries. For example, in the U.S.S.R., blood services are governmentally financed and managed by a governmental bureaucracy. In England, blood services are financed as a part of the National Health Service, but their organization and management is much more regional in character. In a number of Western European countries—The Netherlands, West Germany and Switzerland, for example—the National Red Cross Societies are the operating agencies of the national blood programs, with a variety of financial and administrative relationships with their respective governments.

In Canada, an arrangement similar to that found in Western Europe exists. The Canadian Red Cross Society Blood Transfusion Service is the designated operating agency. It serves over 900 hospitals from 17 established regional Transfusion Centres. Its annual budget of nearly $42 million in 1979 is negotiated with the Canadian government as part of the national health care program. In that same year, this program collected over 1 million units of blood and served about 250,000 patients.[19] The Canadian Red Cross Blood Transfusion service maintains a wide range of relationships with public groups, industry, universities, and research organizations through which the program is indirectly supported and blood service activities are coordinated. The Canadian national blood program is probably about 10 percent of the size of blood service activities in the U.S., for which comprehensive cost figures are not known.

SUMMARY

By contrast with much of the rest of the developed world, blood services in the U.S. remain distinctly pluralistic. It can be argued that pluralism with its inherent competition has been, and could be in the future, a source of great strength for maximum development and efficiency of national blood services. Others argue, with equal vehemence, that pluralism has been wasteful and divisive. It is already clear that public policy in the U.S. has reduced the boundaries of the pluralism of the past.

From this brief and necessarily incomplete discussion, it can be seen that government at many levels and by many mechanisms affects the operation of blood services in the U.S. and other countries as well. This role of government is similar and parallel to that which it exercises in the health care system as a whole, a role that is rapidly deepening and broadening. Although this is regarded as regrettable by many, it appears to be inevitable now in the present political climate of the U.S. Complex moral, social, and political issues remain intertwined in this arena.[20] There are no prospectively universally "right" answers to most such questions. There is only decision (however inchoate), trial, and retrospective evaluation.

REFERENCES

1. NHLI's Blood Resource Studies: Vol. 2, Federal and State Regulation of the Nation's Blood Resource (DHEW Publication No. (NIH) 73-418), Bethesda, MD, 1972.
2. NHLI's Blood Resource Studies: Supply and Use of the Nation's Blood Resource, Vol. 1 (DHEW Publication No. (NIH) 73-417), Bethesda, MD, 1972.
3. National Blood Policy, Federal Register, 39 (47) 9326, 1974.
4. Swisher, S.N.: The National Research Council Report on Blood Transfusion Services in the United States. Vox Sang. 23:10, 1972.
5. Roll, G.F.: Of Politics and Drug Regulation, Center for the Study of Drug Development, University of Rochester Medical Center, Publication Series PS-7701, Rochester, N.Y., 1977.
6. Hutt, P.B.: Balanced Government Regulation of Consumer Products, Ibid., Publication Series PS-7601, 1976.
7. Swisher, S.N.: The introduction of adenine fortified blood preservatives: Introduction and an interpretation of its history. Transfusion 17:309, 1977.
8. Report of Panel on Review of Blood and Blood Derivatives, Bureau of Biologics, Food and Drug Administration. Federal Register. (In Press.)
9. An Evaluation of the Utilization of Human Blood Resources in the United States, Panel Report, Swisher, S.N., Chairman, National Academy of Sciences, National Research Council, Washington, D.C., 1970.
10. Titmuss, R.M.: The Gift Relationship: From Human Blood to Social Policy. Pantheon Books, New York, 1971.
11. Surgenor, D., Mac, N., Wallace, E.L., Cumming, P.D., Mierzwa, B.D., and Smith, F.A.: Blood services: Prices and public policy. Science 180:384, 1973.
12. Cherubin, C.E. and Prince, A.M.: Serum hepatitis specific antigen (Sh) in commercial and volunteer sources of blood. Transfusion 11:25, 1971.
13. Surgenor, D. and Mac, N.: Progress toward a national blood system. N. Engl. J. Med. 291:17, 1974.
14. Swisher, S.N.: A national blood program for the United States; A case study. Arch. Intern. Med. 135:1344, 1975.
15. George, R.O. and Wagner, H.N.: Ten years of brain tumor scanning at Johns Hopkins: 1962-1972. In: Noninvasive Brain Imaging:

Completed Tomography and Radionuclides, DeBlanc, H.J. and Sorenson, J.A., eds., Society of Nuclear Medicine, New York, 1975, p. 3.

16. Gift, D.A. and Schonbein, W.R.: An Introduction to "Entropy-Minimax" Pattern Detection and Its Use in the Determination of Diagnostic Test Efficacy. Dept. of Radiol., Michigan State University, Technical Report #1, East Lansing, MI, 1979.

17. Rosenshein, M.S., Farewell, V.T., Price, T.H., Larson, E.B., and Dale, D.C.: The cost effectiveness of therapeutic and prophylactic leukocyte transfusions. N. Engl. J. Med. 302:1058, 1980.

18. Editorial: Can We Afford To Treat Acute Leukemia? Ibid., p. 1084.

19. Annual Report of the Blood Transfusion Service, Perrault, R.A., M.D., Ph.D., National Director, Toronto, Ontario, Canada, 1979.

20. Surgenor, D. and Mac, N.: Comments on the Titmuss-Anderson debate over the gift relationship. Human blood and the renewal of altruism; Titmuss in retrospect. Int. J. Health Sciences 2:443, 1972.

III. Transfusion in Specific Clinical Settings

21

Hemorrhage, Shock, and Burns: Pathophysiology and Treatment

John A. Collins, M.D.

Our understanding of the course, effects, diagnosis, and treatment of hemorrhagic shock has developed at an uneven pace throughout this century. The great wars provided strong stimuli while they were in progress, but it has been the general advance of the scientific basis of medicine plus careful observations in man that have been most responsible for our present state of knowledge.

The nature of the vascular collapse that follows hemorrhage and especially that which follows serious injury was largely obscure. Theories centering on dysfunction of the central nervous vasomotor centers enjoyed some popularity about the time of World War I. Various toxins were thought to be responsible for the vascular collapse so common in seriously injured patients who did not appear to have lost large amounts of blood. Around 1930, classical experiments by Phemister and by Blalock firmly established that loss of fluid from the circulation was the primary cause of shock in most injured patients. These studies established the concept and demonstrated the importance of "third space" losses—that is, fluid lost from the circulation but still contained within the body proper. By the time of World War II, plasma was a favored solution for resuscitation from hemorrhage and serious injury, but direct battlefield and field hospital experience demonstrated the superiority of whole blood.

Certain civilian "experts" were difficult to convince, however, and the United States nearly embarked on the invasion of Europe during World War II without provisions for a supply of blood in the combat area!

From almost the beginning of this century, various experiments and some clinical experience demonstrated the efficacy of simple salt solutions for limited hypovolemia; except in pediatrics, the practice of treating hypovolemia with simple salt solutions was not common. After the Second World War, great advances were made in defining the hormonal and metabolic changes that occurred after hemorrhage and serious injury. Many of these responses cause a significant retention of salt and of water. This hormonal setting was considered to be a strong indication to limit the administration of salt and water to patients following significant injuries including operation. This was the prevailing opinion at the time of the Korean War. In the early 1960s, a series of experiments indicated that there might be a large shift of extracellular fluid into the intracellular space after serious hemorrhage, and that proper resuscitation from such hemorrhage required the administration of large amounts of saline in addition to replacing the shed blood. Studies in hemorrhaged animals showed improved survival when saline was given in addition to reinfusion of the blood. These studies led to a rather remarkable reversal of practice; instead of restricting the use of salt and water, salt solutions were then used in very large volumes. Ironically, both lines of investigation were flawed. Subsequent studies showed that the apparently large shifts of fluid out of the extracellular space after major hemorrhage were at best rather small. What was observed was a delay in the equilibration of certain markers which had been misinterpreted as a decrease in the volume of distribution of the marker. The improved survival after hemorrhage when supplemental salt and water were used was observed in dogs, an animal which sequesters large volumes of fluid in the enteric circulation in response to hemorrhage. Similar results in other species were not as apparent.

At about this time, the American involvement in the war in Vietnam escalated. Many casualties were treated with very large amounts of salt and water, and many developed pulmonary edema. Since then, there has been continued improvement in the monitoring of circulatory changes in seriously ill patients, and a better understanding of the advantages and limitations of the use of supplemental salt and water. Some significant controversies remain, and these will be discussed later.

This chapter is organized as follows: the changes that occur in response to hemorrhage or hypovolemia are discussed first, then the complications of hemorrhage in various organs and systems, then the means of establishing the diagnosis of hypovolemia, and finally treatment. Use of blood itself is treated in Chapter 22. Burns, which are a special circumstance, are discussed separately at the end of this chapter.

THE RESPONSE TO HEMORRHAGE IN MAN

A great deal of experimental work has been done on the circulatory, metabolic, and endocrine responses to hemorrhage, but much of the work in animals is of limited value because of species differences and the use of anesthesia. However, there have been several studies directed at man, both injured patients and normal volunteers.[1,2,3] The following brief and oversimplified version of the sequence of events that follows blood loss is based whenever possible on such studies (Table 21-1).

The initial response to blood loss is contraction of the great veins, the "capacitance" system. This is both intrinsic and under neural control and results in a smaller vascular space on the venous side of the circulation. The decreased blood volume can thus still serve adequately, with little change needed elsewhere in the system. It is therefore a very efficient response, similar to an internal transfusion. However, it can buffer the loss of only about 10 to 15 percent of the normal blood volume. At the same time some shift of extracellular fluid into the vascular space begins. Cardiac output and oxygen consumption do not change, and the endocrine and metabolic changes are minimal.

At loss of about 15 to 30 percent of blood volume, more extensive adjustments occur. The compensatory ability of the venous capacitance system has been exceeded. The ability of the extracellular space to replenish plasma volume is still intact, assuming a normally nourished and hydrated individual, but this takes hours to be completed. Triggered by atrial and arterial wall receptors, sympathetic stimulation of the heart increases both rate and force of contraction so that output is maintained despite a decreasing filling pressure. This involves more work by the heart muscle, requiring coronary arterial dilation and an increased fraction of the cardiac output diverted to the heart itself. Blood flow to skin and muscle may be reduced by sympathetically mediated arteriolar constriction. Endocrine responses become more evident with increased excretion of aldosterone and antidiuretic hormone, resulting in retention of salt and water and a lower urinary output. Blood sugar and free fatty acid levels in-

Table 21-1. General Pattern of Response to Hemorrhage

Blood Loss*	Vascular Response	Endocrine Response	Metabolic Response	Signs and Symptoms
Mild (10–15% of blood volume, 500–700 ml).	Contraction of great veins; recruitment of ECF	Slight	Slight	Usually transient
Moderate (30% of blood volume, 1500–2000 ml).	All of above, plus: Arteriolar constriction with reduced flow to skin and muscle; decreased cardiac output; narrow pulse pressure; tachycardia (occas. bradycardia).	Increase in aldosterone, ADH, growth hormone. Variable increase in cortisol, catecholamines. No increase in insulin.	Increased glycolysis and mild hyperglycemia. Increased lipolysis and free fatty acid levels. Small increase in lactate levels. Hyperventilation with alkalemia. Oxygen consumption may be increased. Decreased urinary sodium and volume.	Thirst, orthostatic hypotension, apprehension, weakness, pallor, cool skin.
Severe (greater than 30% of blood volume; greater than 2000 ml).	All of above. Cardiac output less than 50% normal. Hypotension. Most of remaining cardiac output to heart and brain.	All of above. Marked increase in catecholamines.	Severe lactic acidosis. Severe oliguria. Mixed venous PO_2 approaching 20 mm Hg or less.	Air hunger. Deteriorating state of consciousness.

* Volumes given refer to average adults.

crease, oxygen consumption increases, and lactate levels may rise slightly as anaerobic metabolic pathways begin to be utilized. Hyperventilation begins with a resulting alkalemia. It is in this range of blood loss that cardiac output begins to decrease, and systolic blood pressure and central venous pressure fall. The patient may experience thirst, weakness, and some apprehension. He will begin to look pale, and his skin will get cool. If moved or sat up, he may exhibit orthostatic hypotension and become lightheaded, nauseated, or even lose consciousness. This is also the range of blood loss (15 to 20 percent) with the greatest individual variability of response, varying from partial decompensation and a clinical picture of severe shock in some patients to a deceptively normal appearance in others. This latter situation is treacherous because decompensation may occur suddenly with relatively small further losses and will almost certainly occur if the patient is given general anesthesia without some form of ef-

fective volume replacement. Studies in young adult men indicate that bradycardia or at least a slowing pulse rate is a fairly common response to acute blood loss of this magnitude. "Paradoxical" bradycardia was noted in a number of combat casualties in Korea.

At a loss of 30 percent of blood volume, practically all patients will exhibit some if not most of the signs and symptoms of shock: thirst, pallor, cool skin, severe orthostatic hypotension, tachycardia, oliguria, and a systolic blood pressure below 100, even when supine. Cardiac output is now significantly reduced despite the institution of perfusion priorities by selective regional arteriolar constriction. Blood flow to the viscera is maintained at the expense of the carcass, and even the distribution of visceral flow is altered to protect the heart and brain. Renal blood flow decreases as renal vascular resistance increases. The endocrine responses become more marked, catecholamines and 17-hydroxysteroids are secreted, and lactic acid levels are significantly elevated.

If blood loss continues, all of the compensatory responses are exceeded, and blood flow to the heart and brain decreases. Air hunger is marked, and the patient will lose consciousness. Metabolic acidosis becomes profound as blood flow to the liver falls below a critical level. A blood volume 50 percent of normal cannot be tolerated for long. Even with a loss of 50 percent which has been stopped, expansion of plasma volume from endogenous sources alone may not occur in time. When central aortic pressure falls below the level at which adequate coronary perfusion can be maintained, cardiac output falls with further fall in central aortic pressure (the adrenergic neural and humoral responses already at maximum levels cannot increase further to maintain pressure), which in turn causes a further fall in coronary perfusion. Once this vicious circle is entered, death rapidly ensues.

Of the various responses to hemorrhage, one of the more commonly misunderstood are the changes in acid-base response. The response to hemorrhage is not a simple, more-or-less linear worsening of acidosis as hemorrhage progresses. In fact, the earliest response to even severe hemorrhage is almost always a significant hyperventilation with resulting alkalemia if the patient is not severely obtunded or anesthetized. The degree of metabolic acidosis in combat casualties in Vietnam did roughly correlate with the degree of circulatory impairment (Table 21-2).[4] Even profound hypotension was not always associated with a strong metabolic acidosis or

lactic acidemia, however. More detailed analysis showed that there was probably a strong temporal component in the acid-base response to injury (Table 21-3).[5] The early hyperventilatory response was apparent, but an unexpected feebleness of the respiratory compensation for lactic acidosis was found. This relative impairment seemed worse in those casualties with the longest interval between injury and study. This suggested a pattern of response to a metabolic acid load in hypoperfused patients that is the opposite of that seen in metabolic acidosis in well perfused patients. In the latter, the respiratory response is usually initially incomplete with better respiratory compensation occurring later.

The "classical" pathophysiologic interpretation of hemorrhagic shock as a circulatory phenomenon is incomplete. A prolonged, severe reduction of peripheral and visceral blood flow will also lead to a number of serious impairments or breakdowns in various organs and systems, distinct from the circulatory decompensation.

COMPLICATIONS OF HEMORRHAGE

There is a pertinent quotation attributed to Cannon: "Shock not only stops the machine, it wrecks the machinery." This implies persisting damage after the hypovolemia has been corrected. This, in fact, is one of the worst effects of hemorrhage and is a major cause of failure of treatment. In a recent autopsy study of trauma victims, almost 50

Table 21-2. Acid-base Status on Admission of Combat Casualties in Vietnam Classified by Blood Pressure; Mean Data

Blood pressure	Number of Patients	pH	PaCO$_2$ (mm Hg)	Base Deficit (mEq/L)	Blood Lactate (mgm/dl)	Time from injury (hours)	Pulse (beats/ min)
Unobtainable	28	7.25	34.1	−9.6	64.2	2.4	135
∠ 90 mm Hg	101	7.34	34.1	−5.4	33.9	1.9	114
> 90 mm Hg	322	7.41	35.0	−2.1	16.3	1.9	91

(Collins JA et al: Acid-base status of seriously wounded combat casualties. I. Before treatment. Ann. Surg. *171*:595–608, 1970.)

Table 21-3. Acid-base Status on Admission of Combat Casualties in Vietnam, Classified by Ventilatory Response; Mean Data

	Hyperventilation N = 75	Normal Ventilation N = 123	Relative Hypoventilation (pH < 7.36)	
			PaCO$_2$ > 30 N = 45	PaCO$_2$ < 30 N = 7
pH	7.51	7.40	7.30	7.31
PaCO$_2$(mmHg)	25.6	36.2	38.4	23.6
Base Deficit (mEq/L)	−1.3	−2.3	−6.3	−12.1
Blood Lactate (mgm/dl)	19	18	32	70
Blood Pressure (mmHg)	129	120	95	61
% of patients hypotensive	15	11	40	86
Time from injury (hours)	1.2	1.6	3.2	2.5

(Hyperventilation means pH > 7.42, PaCO$_2$ < 36 mmHg; normal ventilation means pH 7.36–7.42)
(Collins, JA: The ventilatory response to metabolic acidosis in hemorrhagic shock, in Shock in Low- and High-Flow States, Proc. Symp. Brook Lodge, Augusta, Michigan, 1971, Excerpta Medica, Amsterdam, pp. 212–216.)

percent of deaths were due to brain injury, but 35 percent were due to the effects of hemorrhage.[6] Of the latter group, most died of either single- or multiple-organ failure. In fact, multiple-organ failure following resuscitation and treatment of traumatic shock now seems to be the major barrier to salvaging these patients. In spite of publications emphasizing the statistical importance of a particular organ or system, most of these patients die of multisystem failure. In some patients, a single event or organ failure has clearly led to the others, but this type of analysis is usually missing in statistics which are focused primarily on one or another organ system.

Lungs

For the past 15 years, there has been persistent interest in the impairment of pulmonary function that follows serious injury or major hemorrhage. The war in Vietnam focused much of this attention, but persistence of posttraumatic pulmonary insufficiency in civilian practice throughout the 1970s clearly established this as more than a peculiarity of combat injury. A great deal of experimental work was performed which, along with careful clinical observation, helped to better define the problem and resulted in a changed attitude toward this lesion. Not all questions have been answered, however.[7]

In the mid-1960s, the term "shock lung" gained considerable popularity, reflecting a general belief that posttraumatic pulmonary functional impairment was the result of hemorrhage. Many experiments in animals, however, failed to produce a similar lesion after hemorrhage alone. Scattered hemorrhagic lesions were produced by some but not all investigators in dogs but with minimal functional impairment. Little change of any kind was produced in other species. Studies in primates in particular have yielded little evidence of posthemorrhagic pulmonary impairment.

During hemorrhage, compliance and shunt usually improve while dead space increases. Pulmonary blood volume and extravascular lung water decrease. Following treatment there have been varying, usually unimpressive, decreases in compliance and little if any impairment in oxygenation. Most studies did not closely parallel clinical practice, however. The effects of treatment, in fact, may be more important than the effects of hemorrhage itself.[8,9] Pertinent studies on the effects of treatment are discussed in the several sections of this chapter.

The most attractive hypothesis linking hemorrhage with pulmonary insufficiency is that of damage to the lungs by hypoperfusion. The lungs are rather unique, however, in that they are able to tolerate total ischemia for several hours with surprisingly little detrimental effect, provided alveolar ventilation is maintained. An atelectatic lung tolerates ischemia poorly. Even static inflation with nitrogen is at least partly protective.

Increased permeability of the pulmonary capillary membrane is now considered the central derangement in posttraumatic pulmonary insufficiency in man. Most studies in several other species have shown no increase in permeability to protein after treated or untreated hemorrhagic shock, although such can be produced by increased pulmonary capillary pressure.[8]

Clinical evidence relating hemorrhage to pulmonary insufficiency is, in fact, difficult to find. Pulmonary insufficiency is not a common sequel of hemorrhage alone or of the hypovolemic shock of cholera. Most clinical studies indicate that the element most strongly associated with posttraumatic pulmonary insufficiency is sepsis, especially septic peritonitis. One detailed clinical study contrasted pulmonary functional changes in patients sustaining severe hemorrhage with those in patients with major infections.[10] The differences were striking, favoring sepsis as a cause of pulmonary insufficiency. The only hemorrhaged patients who developed pulmonary insufficiency were those who also became infected. The causal link between infection and pulmonary insufficiency is probably the inflammatory mediators released locally at the site of infection or within the lungs by the action of septic products. Abundant experimental evidence in animals supports such a relationship and has demonstrated the ease with which gram-negative bacteria or endotoxin can produce increased pulmonary capillary permeability,[11] in sharp contrast to the studies on hemorrhaged animals.

There are some aspects of severe hemorrhage in man that indirectly alter pulmonary function but that are not widely discussed. Many patients with repeated hematemesis aspirate significant amounts of blood, especially if they are obtunded, supine, or have tubes traversing the esophagus. Blood is a very irritative agent when aspirated into the lower airway and produces severe reaction and consolidation. Hemorrhagic shock in the elderly is more likely to damage the left ventricle because of the higher incidence of coronary arteriosclerosis in this age group. Patients with ruptured abdominal aortic aneurysms, for example, show a high incidence of left ventricular dysfunction after operation.[12] These patients may develop pulmonary edema with normal central venous pressures, similar to patients with classical myocardial infarctions. Measurement of pulmonary arterial wedge pressures has identified this mechanism in this group of patients formerly thought to have pulmonary impairment as a direct effect of hemorrhage.

Experimentally, there are provocative reports that some of the metabolic patterns of pulmonary tissue are altered after severe hemorrhage.[13,14] More such studies are needed because the metabolic activities of the lungs are also of great importance. It may be that hemorrhage does damage the lungs, but not in the simple and readily evident manner that was assumed only a relatively few years ago.

As with stress ulceration, the incidence and severity of posttraumatic pulmonary insufficiency seems to be decreasing in recent years. There are various guesses but no proof of the reasons for this decline. Earlier use of mechanical ventilatory support may be helpful, but it is likely that greater care and sophistication in the use of resuscitative fluids is the main reason.

Kidneys

If the war in Vietnam focused attention on the lungs as the site of complications after serious injury, the Korean War focused attention on the kidneys even more. Posttraumatic renal failure was relatively common among casualties during the Korean War; hemodialysis and peritoneal dialysis were newly developed techniques, and considerable experimental work on acute renal failure was already underway, having been stimulated by experiences in World War II. During the Korean War, the natural history of posttraumatic renal failure became well documented; the ability to control some of the metabolic complications by dialysis was well demonstrated, and the persistent high mortality despite frequent and seemingly adequate dialysis was noted. Not much has changed in the intervening 25 years. Despite all the advances since then, the mortality from posttraumatic renal failure remains practically the same.[15]

Various reported series differ in the types of patients studied, but some patterns are apparent. Renal failure in man can clearly occur after hemorrhage alone, with gastrointestinal hemorrhage dominating in many civilian series. Crushing injuries without dramatic hypotension can also result in renal failure, presumably by rhabdomyolysis. As with pulmonary insufficiency, infection is a major and seemingly increasingly important associated condition. Disseminated intravascular coagulation and hemolytic transfusion reactions are often followed by acute renal failure. The role of various drugs, especially antibiotics, is not clear, but many antibiotics unquestionably increase the incidence and worsen the degree of renal impairment. Radiologic contrast materials given intravascularly are another iatrogenic threat to renal function after serious hemorrhage or injury. Acute renal failure after injury, however, is most often correlated with significant sustained hypotension; most of the time, it represents failure to restore blood volume rapidly enough.

The classical form of posttraumatic renal failure is severe oliguria—beginning within hours of injury, persisting for 3 to 4 weeks, and resolving (if the patient recovers) through a diuretic phase. More common, in fact, is the nonoliguric form of renal failure which can go undetected until rather advanced if the volume of urine is used to monitor renal function.[16]

Mortality in acute renal failure is rarely due to the uremia itself, which is well con-trolled by dialysis. The commonest cause of death is sepsis, followed by multiple-organ failure. Certain concurrent conditions or antecedent events are associated with even higher mortality: jaundice, infection, pulmonary insufficiency, gastrointestinal stress ulceration, diabetes, heart failure, ruptured abdominal aortic aneurysm, and extensive burns. The mortality rate even without these conditions is probably at least 60 percent, with the nonoliguric form only slightly better than the oliguric form. This is at least double the mortality rate of acute renal failure that does not follow hemorrhage or injury. The greater catabolism in injured patients is usually cited as the reason for this striking difference in outcome, but this is a totally inadequate explanation. The added metabolic load of catabolism is easily handled by dialysis. It is more likely that the initial injury either allowed significant bacterial contamination, which is poorly controlled by the patient in renal failure, or significantly impaired other organs and defense systems, or both. It is also not at all clear why renal failure so impairs antibacterial defenses, but this may be the effect that most often causes the death of the patient.

There is still no general agreement on the mechanisms by which acute renal failure becomes established.[17] A variety of models have been established in animals, falling largely into the categories of metabolic poisons (e.g., heavy metals), intraluminal tubular toxins (e.g., myoglobin), and severe hypoperfusion (e.g., temporary renal arterial occlusion). Four main mechanisms of pathophysiology have been studied: vasomotor alterations, renal tubular obstruction, backflow of glomerular filtrate through damaged tubular epithelium, and decreased glomerular permeability. Others have been proposed, but even among these four extensively studied factors there has been little agreement as to which are most or least important. It is likely that the different models represent different diseases, and that clinical posttraumatic renal failure may also result from a variety of mechanisms.

In many experimental models, prior salt loading or the establishment of a saline diuresis at the time of the insult protects the animal against the occurrence of renal failure. Drugs that inhibit the formation of prostaglandin increase the incidence of renal failure in experimental settings. Acute renal failure in humans is accompanied by high circulating levels of renin, which can be inhibited by saline loading or diuresis. Prostaglandins are thought to counteract the effects of renin on the renal vasculature; together with renin, they form a balanced local humoral control mechanism regulating the amount and distribution of renal blood flow.

Because the expected mortality from acute renal failure after hemorrhage or injury is so high, prevention is extremely important. Persistent oliguria in the recently hemorrhaged or injured patient is therefore a true emergency requiring vigorous and correct diagnosis and immediate treatment. If the oliguria is in response to hypovolemia, as is often the case, rapid administration of the proper fluids is corrective. Administration of a tubular diuretic is a serious error in this setting because this will worsen the hypovolemia and possibly damage the renal tubular epithelium directly. If the oliguria represents established renal failure, however, administration of large amounts of fluid is a serious mistake, because the fluid can be removed only by dialysis. The differential is obviously of great importance. The adequacy of restoration of the blood volume can be estimated as already described, but these methods are not absolute. In the patient with multiple severe injuries, assessing the adequacy of volume replacement can be particularly difficult. The urine itself will offer some clues as to whether the oliguria is nephrogenic or hypovolemic in origin. The usual differentiating values are shown in Table 21-4. Usually, the values are clearly in one category or the other and are consistent with the clinical estimation of the adequacy of volume replacement. Prior administration of a tubular diuretic can lessen the differential value of these tests by

Table 21-4. Differentiating Features in Oliguria

	Hypovolemic	Nephrogenic
Urine Na	< 20 meq/l	> 30 meq/l
Urine/Plasma Creatinine	> 30	< 15
Urine/Plasma Urea	> 10	< 5
Urine/Plasma Osmolality	> 1.5	< 1.2
Urine Osmolality	> 500	< 400

moving the values for hypovolemic patients closer to those seen in acute renal failure.

As noted, there is strong experimental evidence that saline loading protects against posthemorrhagic and posttraumatic acute renal failure. There is indirect but consistent clinical evidence that the same is true in man. The incidence of acute renal failure in combat injuries in Vietnam was strikingly less than in Korea. There were several significant differences in the care given the casualties in the two wars, but the much more aggressive use of saline loading in Vietnam was one of the more significant. The greater incidence of pulmonary insufficiency in Vietnam may have been related to the same factor.

Heart

There have been a fairly large number of experimental studies on the function of the heart during and after hemorrhage. The results at first seem contradictory, but in fact a fairly consistent pattern has emerged. Most of the reported myocardial dysfunction during hypovolemia and soon after reinfusion of shed blood can be explained on the basis of decreased coronary perfusion. If this is controlled, myocardial dysfunction becomes evident only after severe, prolonged hypovolemia, and is relatively mild.[18,19] There was considerable interest in the early 1970s in a specific myocardial depressant factor released from ischemic tissue, but subsequent studies have failed to confirm the presence of such a substance.[20,21] Most of the cardiac dysfunction that occurs during and after severe hemorrhage experimentally is therefore due to reduced coronary perfusion and its aftereffects. There is more involved, however, as indicated by characteristic structural changes that occur in the left ventricle after severe hemorrhage.[22] More recently, changes in left ventricular compliance following hemorrhage and resuscitation have been described.[23]

The particular stresses placed upon the heart during hemorrhage deserve some emphasis. The heart is obviously the central organ of the circulation. As blood volume decreases with hemorrhage, the heart is driven harder in order to maintain blood flow. This hormonal and neurogenic effect helps maintain cardiac output despite decreasing filling pressures, but at the cost of increased work by the heart. The heart thus has a relative increase in its oxygen requirements in response to hemorrhage. Blood flow and oxygen delivery occur mainly during diastole. With progressively worsening hemorrhage, heart rate increases and diastolic time decreases. Diastolic pressure also falls. The physical forces determining oxygen supply to the heart are thus adversely affected at a time when oxygen requirements are increased. Most other organs in the body can work at lower mixed venous oxygen tensions, thereby extracting more oxygen from the available perfusing blood. The human heart, however, works all the time near its lowest mixed venous oxygen tension so that this compensatory mechanism is not available. The ability of the coronary arteries to dilate thus becomes critical. Major hemorrhage in patients with coronary arteriosclerosis or preexisting heart disease is tolerated very poorly.

Treatment must be rapid and precise, and hemorrhage must be stopped quickly. This sometimes creates the paradoxical situation in which an operation may be indicated sooner in patients with an increased operative risk than in those in better general health. This occurs most often in patients with gastrointestinal bleeding and known coronary artery disease. A recent study demonstrated

severe left ventricular dysfunction in patients who survived rupture of abdominal aortic aneurysms.[12] Such patients usually have significant arteriosclerosis involving the coronary arteries, and rupture of the aneurysm is usually a major hemorrhage.

Gastrointestinal Tract

The primary gastrointestinal complication of hemorrhage is stress ulceration of the stomach. Other sequelae include paralytic ileus, various ulcerative lesions of the colon, scattered ischemic lesions of the small and/or large intestine, vascular thrombosis with mesenteric infarction, noncalculous gangrenous cholecystitis, and others, but most of these are unusual. Stress ulceration is relatively common after serious injury or major hemorrhage.[24] It can be seen within a few hours of the inciting event. It is usually seen after persistent hypovolemia and therefore is more properly considered a complication of failure to achieve adequate resuscitation promptly. The lesions are characteristic: multiple superficial erosions primarily in the fundus of the stomach. Experimentally, the disease can be produced reliably in several species by prolonged hemorrhagic shock, but in man it is often also found in association with jaundice, acute renal failure, persistent intraabdominal infection, acute ventilatory insufficiency, and other acute, life-threatening disorders.

The relative importance of mucosal ischemia and of an alteration in the protective properties of the gastric mucus are debated; but it is clear, both in animals and in man, that raising the intraluminal pH of the gastric contents to a level that prevents activation of pepsin minimizes the bleeding associated with stress ulceration and probably minimizes the formation of the ulcers themselves. Both H_2-receptor blockade (cimetidine) and titration of gastric contents with antacids have been reported as effective, with contradictory data on the relative efficacy of each.[25,26] If either approach is to be used prophylactically, however, it will be more effective if started as soon as possible, and both approaches require monitoring the pH of the gastric contents hourly for maximum effect. The pH should be kept above 3.5 if necessary by increasing dosage, increasing frequency of administration, or combining the methods of treatment. Prevention is important, because bleeding severe enough to require operative control is associated with a high mortality rate.

Although there are no truly "hard" data, it is apparent that the incidence of severe bleeding from this serious complication of hemorrhagic shock is much less than it was ten or more years ago. This is probably due to better understanding, monitoring, and treatment of hypovolemia and its other complications. Because the overall incidence of peptic ulcer disease in the United States is declining significantly for unknown reasons, even this explanation is not certain.

Liver

The liver is one of the organs critical to the patient's ability to recover successfully from a major hemorrhage because of its enormous biochemical and metabolic activity, its central role in regulating coagulation and fibrinolytic factors, and its position guarding the systemic curculation against septic products released from the intestinal tract. Much investigative work on changes in the liver after hemorrhage has been done in dogs, a particularly poor model because of the odd sphincteric mechanism in the hepatic veins. Other species also show marked changes in hepatic structure and function after hemorrhage, however, and it is likely that the damage rendered to the livers of seriously hemorrhaged patients has been greatly underestimated clinically. For example, the prolonged but "mild" jaundice that follows extensive transfusion for hemorrhage is often attributed to extravascular hemolysis of the nonviable fraction of the transfused red cells. An intact liver should easily handle the load of pigment so produced, however, and at best any increase in bilirubin should be quite transient. This one common observation strongly indicates an impairment of hepatic function following hemorrhage that is often ignored clinically.

The structural changes in the liver after severe hemorrhage resemble those seen after any severe hypoxemic insult: centrolobular necrosis without central venous congestion. Earlier, there is probably a relatively nonspecific fatty infiltration of the hepatocytes.

Antibacterial Defenses

It has become increasingly clear that there is a serious impairment of antimicrobial defenses in patients following serious hemorrhage or injury. This impairment is manifested by an increased incidence of invasive infection, and in recent times by multiple system failure. As series of patients with multiple system failure following hemorrhage or injury are analyzed, it becomes apparent that infection is a common feature in the majority of instances. Abundant experimental and clinical evidence links infection to impairment of these organs individually. These observations imply a causal relationship collectively or sequentially. Lung, kidneys, liver, GI tract, central nervous system, body cell mass and body fuels, coagulation, and antimicrobial defenses themselves all seem part of this unfortunate constellation. Experimental investigation of this phenomenon is increasing, and much more work is needed.

There is a significant derangement of function of the granulocytes after injury; this is best studied in burned patients. This seems to correlate with the extent of the burn and with the presence of known infection. The defects improve as the wound heals. Incubation of these malfunctioning granulocytes from burned patients with fresh normal plasma restored at least some of their functional capacity.[27] This observation led to a trial of fresh frozen plasma in burned patients.[28] The functional chemotactic index was twice as great in five burned patients given 2 to 12 units of fresh frozen plasma during the first week following injury as was that of four comparably burned patients who received no fresh frozen plasma. In a separate group of burned patients whose granulocytes manifested a low functional chemotactic index, similar improvement was induced by the administration of three units of fresh frozen plasma per day. The groups were too small, however, to demonstrate a clinical effect.

The ability of the lungs to clear and kill inhaled bacteria is adversely effected by serious injury and hemorrhage.[29,30] The pulmonary defense mechanisms are rather complex and, although it is not clear how hemorrhage produces this effect, the effect is reproducible. Considerable older experimental work focused on the reticuloendothelial system (RES). We have recently found in rats that the impairment of antibacterial defenses after hemorrhage persists long after RES function returns to normal (unpublished observations). Moreover, the type of fluid used for resuscitation influenced the extent and duration of impairment of antibacterial defenses.

DIAGNOSIS OF HYPOVOLEMIA

Most physicians consider themselves very familiar with the signs and symptoms of hypovolemia. The sequence of changes implied in Table 21-1 can, in fact, serve as a useful guideline for most patients. In specific situations, however, there can be great variation in responses and manifestations, and other conditions may be active which can mislead in either direction. The diagnosis of hypovolemia can be more difficult and subtle than many clinicians are aware of. In some situations, blood pressure does not fall until renal function has already been seriously impaired;

in others, hypotension occurs without hypovolemia. Pulse rate and urinary output can be seriously misleading. Even central venous pressure is not a "gas gauge" for the circulation. Mental status can be influenced by drugs or injury. In short, there is no foolproof method of diagnosing hypovolemia, and there is certainly no *single* criterion which should be relied upon. It is the weight of available evidence, carefully collected and interpreted with mature clinical judgment, which determines when the patient is hypovolemic and, just as important, when hypovolemia has been corrected. The data are sometimes contradictory.

Two recently applied monitoring devices can be of great help in very difficult situations. One is the balloon-tipped catheter, which can be used in the wedged position to measure pulmonary "capillary" pressure, which in turn reflects left atrial pressure. This is a much more informative measurement than is central venous pressure, but even this can be artefactually high if the patient is being ventilated with continuous positive pressure. Balloon-tipped catheterization carries its own risks and is usually not necessary in managing the hypovolemic patient. With persistent uncertainty of the diagnosis despite one's best efforts, with failure to respond to treatment, or with known or anticipated serious cardiac or pulmonary complications, its use becomes more firmly indicated and it can be extremely helpful under these circumstances.

Another useful procedure is the measurement of central or mixed venous oxygen tension. These values reflect the adequacy of oxygen delivery to the peripheral tissues. The absolute values for normal vary with the position of the catheter and the activity of the patient (40 mm Hg for true mixed venous blood at rest), but it is the direction of change that is important. A rising mixed or central venous PO_2 generally means that the circulatory status of the patient is improving. The opposite applies equally. Measurements of oxygen tension are available rapidly in most hospitals; in difficult situations, some kind of central venous catheter will probably be in use anyway.

The indications of adequacy of blood volume are thus indirect; what we really look for is adequacy of the circulation. Also helpful are all of the following: arterial blood pressure, pulse rate, respiratory rate, mental status, color of mucous membranes, color and temperature of skin, urinary output, changes in urinary composition, and, if measured, central venous pressure, pulmonary artery wedge pressure, and central or mixed venous oxygen tensions. Hematocrit or hemoglobin are relatively poor monitoring devices in this context. They are measures of concentration; thus, any observed changes reflect rate of refilling the plasma volume, not direct changes in blood volume.

Differential Diagnosis

The differential diagnosis of hypovolemia is also not always simple. The causes of hypotension or of vascular collapse are very numerous. Only a few will be discussed here that are sometimes involved in situations in which they might be confused with hypovolemia. *Pulmonary embolism* and *acute myocardial infarction* can both result in inadequate cardiac output and thus mimic hypovolemia. In both, however, the filling pressures in the heart should be high, not low. Forcing fluids to establish the differential from hypovolemia could be a serious error.

There is a situation in which hypovolemia can mimic pulmonary embolism. *Acute ileofemoral venous thrombosis* is often followed by sequestration of large volumes of fluid in the leg and thigh. The unilateral swelling indicates the diagnosis of venous thrombosis. The hypotension, tachycardia, hyperpnea, and oliguria that may accompany are often interpreted as evidence of a large pulmonary embolus when in fact they reflect acute hypovolemia. It must be remembered that a

swollen leg and thigh represents the loss of liters of fluid.

Myocardial infarction can be interrelated *with hemorrhage* in the same patient. Serious hypovolemia in a patient with preexisting coronary arterial disease is likely to cause an acute myocardial infarction, which can then confuse further diagnosis and management. Conversely, an acute myocardial infarction may have led to the accident for which an injured patient is admitted. In any case, the patient with a recent myocardial infarction who becomes hypovolemic must be treated quickly and with precision. Both blood volume and oxygen carrying capacity need to be maintained much more carefully than in patients with normal hearts because the margin for error in overtransfusion is much narrower. An increasingly common finding in blunt trauma victims, particularly motor vehicle accident victims, is *myocardial contusion*.[31] This is associated with steering wheel or dashboard injuries to the sternum. It is impossible in some situations to differentiate between myocardial infarction and myocardial contusion. Arrhythmias are common following this injury and are the predominant cause of early death.

Among acutely injured patients, there are several conditions that occasionally must be distinguished from hypovolemia. Some of these can be rapidly lethal unless correctly diagnosed and treated.

Pericardial tamponade is most important, since it can be so rapidly lethal yet can be treated so quickly. The usual signs of distant heart sounds, paradoxical pulse, narrow pulse pressure, distended neck veins, and large globular heart shadow on x-ray are of very limited value in the acutely injured patient. Concomitant blood loss may mask some of the circulatory signs. Heart sounds can be hard to evaluate in many circumstances. The heart shadow may change very little acutely even with significantly increased pressure in the pericardial sac. Thus, absence of any or all of the above signs does not rule out tamponade. It must be considered in the differential diagnosis in all hypotensive patients who are known to have sustained a penetrating or significant blunt injury to the chest. The key to detection in most patients is accurate determination and monitoring of the central venous pressure. The concurrence of an elevated or even high normal central venous pressure with systemic hypotension in a patient with chest trauma dictates that pericardial tamponade be seriously considered.

Tension pneumothorax may also be a cause of severe hypotension. In this condition, the hemithorax becomes overdistended with air causing collapse of the lung and a shift of the mediastinum to the opposite hemithorax. This shift in the mediastinum causes compression and distortion of the great veins and impedes venous return to the heart. Compression of the lungs and their low pressure vascular system also adds significantly to this damming up of blood in the central circulation. If it develops quickly enough, occurs in the face of concomitant volume loss, or occurs in children whose mediastinum is less firm, tension pneumothorax can quickly produce death by the above mechanism. Signs that aid in differentiating this condition from similar causes of shock include shift of the trachea to the contralateral side, percussion tympany and decreased breath sounds on the ipsilateral side. If there is even a strong index of suspicion of this diagnosis, it is better to insert a chest tube or needle than to wait for more obvious signs or x-ray confirmation. This is a complication that occurs in patients on ventilatory support with continuous positive pressure, as well as in injured patients.

An *acute spinal cord injury* can cause hypotension by the same mechanism as spinal anesthesia—i.e., the sudden removal of the neural control of vasomotor tone in much of the vascular system. This is usually well tolerated unless central aortic pressure drops markedly or unless there has been significant associated blood loss. It is surprising how easy it is to temporarily overlook a spinal cord injury when other, more attention-getting injuries are present. Needless to say, intact motion and sensation can be quickly and easily determined, even in injured legs. Although spinal injuries can cause hypotension, it is a good policy never to consider a head injury as the cause of hypotension or shock. While it is true that the head, scalp, and face have a rich blood supply and that blood loss from injuries to these structures can be severe, this should be clinically evident. Intracranial bleeding and brain injury do not cause hypotension, except terminally when there is decompensation or compression of the medullary centers. The usual response to increased intracranial pressure is peripheral vasoconstriction and a rising blood pressure. Hemorrhage may, of course, mask this response. Nevertheless, the occurrence of hypotension in a patient with serious head injury necessitates a careful search for other causes. If the central venous pressure is low and other evidence indicates hypovolemia, blood loss must be assumed and its source found. In this regard, the abdomen is difficult to evaluate in patients with head injury. Thus, if no other site of blood loss is found, objective evidence must be sought to diagnose or rule out intraabdominal bleeding—e.g., paracentesis with peritoneal lavage.

TREATMENT

Control of Hemorrhage

The most important aspect of the treatment of hemorrhage is sometimes never mentioned in discussions of treatment, and occasionally does not receive the priority it deserves in actual clinical management. When there is ongoing hemorrhage, every effort to control it must be taken. External bleeding can be controlled in most instances by the application of direct pressure. Rarely, a tourniquet will be necessary for extremity wounds, usually when a traumatic amputation has occurred. Pelvic and abdominal bleeding in an injured patient may be temporarily controlled using the "MAST" or G-suit which is now undergoing trial in various centers.[32] This three-compartment pressure suit is inflated to 80 mm Hg, but the safety of this device and the allowable duration of inflation have not been completely determined. Removal of the suit may prove hazardous, particularly if the suit has been applied in the "field" and the patient arrives without having received intravenous fluids. Therefore, two large-caliber intravenous catheters should be inserted prior to deflation and then each of the compartments should be deflated separately with concomitant restoration of volume. The opportunity for definitive operative intervention must be available at the time the G-suit is deflated.

In any bleeding patient, immediate operative intervention may become an essential part of resuscitation. The operation should be undertaken sooner rather than later in a number of other circumstances—including cases where the rate of bleeding is more rapid than can be replaced, or where associated conditions make continued hemorrhage especially dangerous, or where available blood supplies are being depleted, or hemorrhage is unlikely to stop without operation. In some conditions—e.g., rupture of an abdominal aortic aneurysm—reexpanding the blood volume without being able to immediately stop the hemorrhage may in fact be a serious error. It is sometimes necessary to begin the operation in a seriously hypovolemic patient, achieve control of the hemorrhage, then replace the lost blood and complete the resuscitation. In some extraordinary circumstances, it is necessary to perform an emergency thoracotomy and clamp the descending thoracic aorta (if the hemorrhage is occurring distal to this) in order to resuscitate the nearly empty heart and to preserve or restore perfusion of the heart and brain while more specific measures of control are applied. It is not clear what is the true salvage rate in patients who require

such heroic measures, but an occasional patient seems to be saved from otherwise certain death.

Starting Intravenous Fluids

The more serious the situation is or might be, the greater the need for multiple large intravenous lines. It is well, if possible, to avoid inserting central venous catheters initially, as the contracted great veins make insertion more difficult and complications such as pneumothorax more likely. There is often discussion about avoiding inserting intravenous lines in the upper or lower parts of the body if the corresponding vena cava or immediate branches are likely to be injured. However, such suggestions are probably not well founded. The flow through the cavae is such that the addition of resuscitative fluid at the achievable rates of administration is not likely to make much difference. If either cava is freely venting into a body cavity, as is sometimes assumed in these discussions, the position of the lines will have little effect because such a patient will soon be dead unless the holes are closed. If there are reasonable routes available for intravenous lines, they should be used unless there is an obvious obstruction to venous return.

The most important blood drawn on the bleeding patient is that for type and cross-match. If the patient is hypovolemic from loss of other than blood, the hematocrit can help estimate the magnitude of contraction of the plasma component. If disorders of the hemostatic mechanism are suspected, appropriate samples should be drawn before blood or blood products are administered, if possible. If the patient is in shock, simple salt solutions should be given as rapidly as possible. With plastic bags, compression devices, and multiple ports, it is possible to give a liter in a few minutes. If the patient does not respond even after 3 to 4 liters, the diagnoisis must be questioned, immediate operation must be considered, uncrossmatched blood should be used—or, as is most likely, all three things should occur.

Restoration of Perfusion

The second most important principle in the treatment of hemorrhage is that restoration of perfusion is initially more important than restoration of oxygen-carrying capacity. This is based on extensive clinical and experimental observation, on the significant functional reserve of the oxygen delivering system, and on the demonstrated ability of most tissues to withstand hypoxemia much better if some form of perfusion is maintained. This is the justification for the immediate use of a nonblood fluid which expands plasma volume. The choice of fluids for use after the immediate fluid loading is somewhat controversial and will be considered a bit later in this chapter.

Estimation of Blood Loss

It would be helpful to have a reasonably accurate estimate of the extent of loss of blood or fluid when beginning treatment. The uncertainties are often greatest in the patient with multiple injuries, but unfortunately even approximate estimates of loss can be seriously wrong. Many guidelines and rules of thumb have been devised for estimating the blood loss with "typical" injuries, but the variations are too great in individual patients to make them reliably useful.[1,3,33] An awareness of the potential magnitude of hidden blood loss can be gained from simple geometry. If a thigh of average dimensions is consdiered to be a cylinder for computational purposes, an increase of only one cm in the radius of that thigh represents a net gain of two liters in volume. In the acutely injured patient, immediate changes in dimensions are largely due to bleeding into injured tissues. Even the rela-

tively small upper arm can contain a significant amount of extravasated blood. When a limb such as the thigh has a fracture of its main support bone (femur), the extremity loses its cylindrical shape and assumes a more spherical shape. The volume of a sphere is much more than that of a cylinder.

With the abdomen, the situation may be particularly misleading because the length of the abdominal cavity can and does change in an inapparent manner by raising of the diaphragms. In fact, this may be the dominant dimensional change early after abdominal injury. With concurrent and equal changes in both the radius and length of our typical abdominal "cylinder," a gain of 1 cm represents a change in volume of 2.9 liters. Changes of this magnitude are not usually evident externally. Abdominal swelling in an injured patient may also be due to the accumulation of air in the gastrointestinal tract and the sequestration of a predominantly extracellular type of fluid in the enteric lumen and/or peritoneal space. Nevertheless, a briskly bleeding intraabdominal vessel can quickly fill that cylinder before these other contents can add to the dimensional changes. Thus, a patient can exsanguinate into the peritoneal cavity without any dramatic change in abdominal dimensions or appearance. Therefore, it can be a tragic blunder to assume that, because the abdomen is not distended, hypotension is not due to intraabdominal bleeding.

The cranial vault, because of its fixed volume, is not considered an important site for sequestration of hidden blood. Each hemithorax, on the other hand, may contain 2 to 3 liters of blood, a fact that emphasizes the importance of physical examination and x-ray of the chest, even in the most critically injured patient. The pelvis is also notorious as a source of hidden blood loss, particularly if the bleeding is retroperitoneal. Six to eight units of whole blood can easily be sequestered in the pelvis without externally visible signs. Any sizeable area can, of course, "hide" lost blood, including retroperitoneal areas, the buttocks, and the shoulder girdle.

Type of Fluid Lost

In addition to the volume of fluid lost, the types of fluid lost can be variable and partly unknown. Specific types of injury may result in losses of fluid other than blood. Burns are the best example in which extracellular type fluid and plasma are lost in very large amounts, producing profound shock in the extensively burned individual. Burns will be considered further in the last section of this chapter. Crushing types of injury can produce losses of all three types of fluid. In a situation that has fortunately become rare, tight tourniquets left on limbs for too long a time can result in rapid sequestration of plasma and extracellular fluid in the ischemic limb after release. It is rare to see venous return so extensively interrupted at the time of injury that it produces massive fluid sequestration, but this can be a life-threatening complication of acute iliofemoral venous thrombosis. Whatever the mechanism of injury, the presence of extravasated blood in body cavities or in soft tissue evokes an inflammatory response which is accompanied by the sequestration of extracellular-type fluid in varying amounts. With time, then, blood which is "shed internally" and the responses of the tissues to the injuring force can cause the loss of additional volumes in the form of extracellular fluid which may well exceed the volume of the blood originally lost.

Adequacy of Replacement

The adequacy of replacement is judged largely on clinical grounds, as outlined under *Diagnosis of Hypovolemia.* Some interesting observations about what constitutes adequate reexpansion of blood volume exist that challenge some old concepts.[2] The "traditional wisdom" in treating hemorrhage has been

that a greater than normal blood volume is required for adequate resuscitation from severe hypotension. Measurements of blood volume in apparently well-resuscitated, stable patients following severe hemorrhage, however, have almost always shown less than the predicted normal blood volumes for at least the first day, with (often) greater than normal blood volumes by the third day. This pattern has been very consistent in studies on severely injured combat casualties, even when central venous pressure was included as a guide for fluid replacement. Data in reports on postoperative civilian patients have often been obscured by the inclusion of septic patients, who usually require and develop blood volumes greater than normal. When data on hemorrhage alone can be extracted, however, a pattern similar to that reported in combat casualties is apparent, again even when central venous pressure is included as a criterion for adequate replacement of blood loss.

This pattern suggests that there may be a fixed contraction of the capacitance system (great veins) following severe blood loss. The classic study on the relationship of blood volume to central venous pressure showed no evidence of such a phenomenon but was performed on normal volunteers in the supine position who were bled less than 15 percent of expected blood volume.[34] In a study on combat casualties, looking especially at this possibility, the degree of "undertransfusion" despite clinical stability and normal central venous pressure was directly related to the amount of blood lost at injury.[35] Of great interest is the fact that four of these casualties developed pulmonary edema when measured blood volumes were at predicted normal or less. It appears that the pulmonary artery may also participate in the loss of vascular compliance that occurs in the response to stress. Earlier studies showing that blood volumes after resuscitation were less than normal were taken as evidence of clinical error in managing the patient. It may be that persistent contraction of the capacitance and pulmonary arterial systems, plus some impairment of left ventricular function, make the severely hemorrhaged patient much more susceptible to overtransfusion.

Crystalloid Solutions

Of the various nonblood fluids that are used to treat hemorrhage, by far the most widely used in the United States are the "crystalloid" solutions. These are simple electrolyte solutions that mimic interstitial fluid. They are basically isotonic sodium chloride with variations, which are generally of little importance except when very large volumes are infused rapidly or when renal function is poor. The United States Navy Surgical Research Team compared acid-base and electrolyte changes in combat casualties resuscitated with large amounts of saline solution and with lactated Ringer's solution.[36] There was little difference in the average blood electrolyte and acid-base values for the two groups. However, when patients with cholera were resuscitated with saline solution, the metabolic acidosis persisted.[37] These patients are unusual in that they have a severe subtraction metabolic acidosis (loss of alkaline gastrointestinal secretions), a situation very different from the usual injured or hemorrhaging patient whose acidosis is due to an accumulation of organic acids that are rapidly "burned off" when circulation is restored.

The crystalloid solutions have a number of important advantages as resuscitative fluids. They are cheap, plentiful, easily stored, and readily available. They can be administered instantly; they do not transmit communicable diseases; they are nonimmunogenic; and they are essentially nontoxic except for total fluid load. They do not impede replenishment of albumin levels after resuscitation, although there is some contrary evidence. A broad clinical experience indicates that simple saline solutions are effective plasma volume expanders in many clinical situations. Careful studies on blood volume changes in volunteers with moderate hemorrhages indicate a somewhat preferential retention of infused saline solution in the plasma space, approaching 35 to 40 percent of the initially infused fluid.[38,39] The longer-term effects on plasma volume are less clear and may be strongly influenced by individual renal function, prehemorrhage protein stores, and associated abnormalities. The effectiveness of crystalloid replacement for very large hemorrhages is much less certain. Judicious use of saline solutions has reduced the amount of blood used in resuscitation and in the operating room, with little apparent loss of effectiveness.[40] The United States Navy Surgical Research Team favored a blood-plus-saline regimen over a blood-plus-colloid approach after a direct clinical comparison of the two in the war in Vietnam. Less objectively analyzed experience throughout this combat zone agreed with this practice.

The disadvantages of simple saline solutions are those of all nonoxygen-carrying plasma expanders, plus the important feature of lack of plasma-specific osmotic activity. These fluids expand the extracellular fluid space, with plasma volume expansion resulting as it is a compartment of this extracellular space. To the extent that the plasma volume is expanded, its specific osmotic activity relative to the interstitial space is reduced. The specific disadvantages of these fluids are flooding of the extracellular space and reduction in plasma-specific osmotic activity. Both of these promote the development of interstitial edema, which can be damaging in the lungs.

Several factors increase the chance of inadvertent flooding unless great care is taken in the use of these fluids. First, the greater the blood loss, the greater is the relative requirement of crystalloid solution needed to restore the circulation. This is at least due partly to the loss of plasma-specific osmotic activity. The relationship is not a constant one, nor does it run in a straight line. Rather, it is a sharply rising curve, with ever-increasing amounts of saline solution required to replace succeeding increments of blood loss. In a situation of continuing hemorrhage in which saline solution is being given to maintain blood pressure, gross flooding can easily occur unless one keeps track of the amount of blood lost and the amount of crystalloid solution given. Second, the central venous pressure may not indicate gross overloading with crystalloid infusions. The central venous pressure measures a result of the interaction of blood volume, venous tone, and the efficiency of the right heart as a pump. Crystalloid solutions expand the extracellular volume primarily, and relatively small fractions remain in the plasma space if blood loss has been extensive or if plasma-specific osmotic activity is low. The central venous pressure does not measure changes in the interstitial fluid space, which is where flooding occurs with the use of saline solution. After pulmonary edema occurs, the central venous pressure may rise as a result of increased pulmonary vascular resistance and myocardial hypoxia. Third, seriously injured patients will retain infused salt and water to an abnormal degree, perhaps even greater than is evident from input and output data.[41] The kidneys cannot be relied on to make up for therapeutic excesses.

Maintenance of Colloid Osmotic Pressure

As the primary "toxicity" of the crystalloid fluids is pulmonary edema, there has been considerable investigation of the relationship between infusion of such fluids and changes in pulmonary function. One of the significant current controversies in this field is the extent to which supplementation with albumin or artificial colloids is necessary to minimize pulmonary edema. This will be considered in some detail, because it also bears importantly on the question of the proper use of albumin.

Several recent publications review the mechanisms for maintaining an appropriate content and distribution of fluids in the lungs, the effects of alterations in plasma-oncotic pressure and in capillary hydrostatic pressure, and the impact of alterations in pulmonary capillary permeability.[42-44] These articles can provide the physiological principles needed to understand what may be happening in some of the very complex interrelationships discussed in this chapter.

Although there is some disagreement on details, it is clear that overloading the circulation produces pulmonary edema by elevating capillary hydrostatic pressure. This form of edema is associated with a prominent leak of protein along with fluid. Dilution of plasma-specific osmotic pressure allows edema to form at lower hydrostatic pressures. Such edema usually begins in the pulmonary interstitial space but can extend to alveolar flooding with increased capillary permeability. The earliest practical way of detecting interstitial edema is probably through changes in compliance. Interstitial pulmonary edema clearly need not cause hypoxemia, but, if alveolar flooding occurs, shunting is inevitable. Even before alveolar flooding develops, the effects of interstitial edema on the closing of terminal airways could conceivably lead to atelectasis and shunting.

The fact that excessive retention of salt and water results in pulmonary edema is neither new nor surprising. Fatal pulmonary edema can be produced by extensive infusions of salt water in animals with normal central venous pressures; clinical examples of the same phenomenon have been too common. An important component of the clinical situation may be the ability of the patient to excrete the excess quantities of salt and water after resuscitation.[41,45,46]

Proper Use of Albumin

The role of the concentration of albumin in plasma in the genesis of pulmonary edema and respiratory failure after resuscitation is one of the most controversial areas in the entire field of resuscitation from hemorrhage. There are at least two main opposing arguments: (1) plasma-specific osmotic pressure (colloid osmotic pressure, or COP) should be kept near normal during resuscitation to minimize the risk of pulmonary edema, and (2) abundant use of simple salt solutions without supplemental albumin ("crystalloid") poses no threat to pulmonary function. Recently, another provocative concept has been offered—namely, that use of supplemental albumin may in fact increase the risk of postresuscitative pulmonary insufficiency.

The conservative position, favoring preservation of near-normal COP, has firm theoretical and some experimental and clinical support. Ironically, the isolated, perfused lung has proved to be one of the easiest organs in which to demonstrate Starling's principles of fluid exchange across capillary membranes. Reducing the COP of the perfusate allows pulmonary edema to occur at lower perfusion pressures. Adding albumin to the resuscitative regimen of primates treated for hemorrhagic shock minimized the amount of fluid that accumulated in the lungs,[47] but there is disagreement on this point. A similar study in dogs did not measure lung water content. Another, which dealt with hemodilution with saline, concluded that accumulation of fluid in the lungs could be partly reversed by giving albumin.[48]

Evidence from clinical studies is confirmatory. Elective hemodilution preoperatively with salt solutions produced greater impairment of oxygenation than when colloid was used, but the studies were not simultaneous.[49] Giordano et al.[50] and Skillman et al.[51] reported improved oxygenation in patients on ventilatory support who were given albumin and diuretics. Patients on mechanical ventilators may retain fluids excessively, however. An earlier study showed significant improvement in pulmonary function in some injured patients from the use of diuretics alone.[52] I know of no such study in which patients were given albumin alone. Skillman et al. later reported a prospective, controlled study in which patients undergoing operations on the abdominal aorta were given salt water either alone or with supplemental albumin.[53] Those given the supplemental albumin had less impairment of oxygenation postoperatively. The patients were treated by a predetermined protocol, however, and not on the basis of clinical signs and measured pressures. In addition, the method for measuring oxygenation was one that is influenced by changes in mixed venous oxygen tension, which was not measured.

Rackow et al.[54] and Weil et al.[55] have reported findings that are very similar: COP correlates inversely with survival in patients in ventilatory failure and is very low in patients with noncardiogenic pulmonary edema. Chest radiographs were rated independently, and a correlation was found between low COP and radiologic evidence of pulmonary edema. Interestingly, measured intrapulmonary "shunt" did not correlate with COP or with the radiologic changes. All patients on ventilators with a COP of less than half normal died, while those with a COP of 75 percent of normal or above survived. Other studies have indicated similar patterns. The trouble with many of these studies is that, although they document concurrence, they don't necessarily indicate cause. It is likely that dying patients have a low COP from a variety of causes, including sequestration in infected areas, failure of synthesis, and occasionally widespread loss of capillary integrity. What is needed is a controlled study showing that death can be prevented or ventilatory failure reversed by the administration of albumin. A "clean" study of this type has not yet been reported.

The argument that abundant salt solution can be administered without causing pulmonary edema has considerable experimental and clinical support. A large number of experimental studies document the efficacy of salt solutions in replacing up to half the expected blood volume in patients with acute hemorrhages.[2,56] With greater hemorrhages, the need for red blood cells overrides the issue of the need to restore COP. If normal animals are deliberately overloaded with salt solutions, very large excesses are needed to produce pulmonary edema. A number of investigators are finding that it is very difficult to produce pulmonary edema in intact animals solely by lowering COP. Most of these studies have not yet been published. Even when COP is lowered and large amounts of salt water are infused, a surprisingly large amount of fluid can be sequestered in nonpulmonary sites, especially the skin, fat, and muscle, thus protecting the lungs.[57]

The clinical evidence largely supports this position. It is difficult to produce severely lower COP in previously healthy subjects. The study by the U.S. Navy Surgical Research Team in Vietnam demonstrated this point very well: there was little difference in total protein levels 24 hours after resuscitation in groups treated with or without supplemental albumin.[58] Recently, a number of prospective studies have compared albumin-rich and albumin-poor treatment regimens and have studied pulmonary function in detail. Lowe et al. found no differences between the two groups.[59] It is noteworthy, however, that the difference in total protein concentration between the two groups was rather small, as in the Navy study, and that the total protein (and presumably COP) in the nonalbumin group was not greatly depressed. It is also interesting that there was very little postresuscitative pulmonary insufficiency in either group in this study of 141 seriously injured patients. A similar prospective study by Virgilio et al. duplicated many of the conditions of the Skillman study but also calculated "shunt," which eliminated the effect of varying mixed venous oxygen tensions, and treated all patients according to vital signs and measured pressures.[60] Pulmonary capillary wedge pressure was monitored very closely. There were no differences between the two groups. COP was reduced below the level in the Lowe study but was still above half normal. In this study, even when pulmonary capillary wedge pressure exceeded COP, pulmonary edema was not evidenced as long

as the wedge pressure was not elevated. Weil's group has claimed this difference is critically important in avoiding pulmonary edema.

There are a number of similar studies now in press, but, to the author's knowledge, all match this pattern except those noted below. These studies, if they can be summarized, showed little difference between patients treated with and those treated without supplemental albumin, but either COP was not drastically lowered or pulmonary capillary wedge pressures were very carefully monitored and kept well within normal ranges.

Possible harmful effects of albumin. Finally, there is the interesting question of whether supplemental albumin might make a pulmonary lesion worse. Theoretically, if the capillary membrane becomes permeable to albumin, no effect on fluid exchange would be expected from administering albumin. In fact, the higher concentrations produced in the interstitial or intraalveolar fluid might delay recovery, but this concept is unproven. Furthermore, the pulmonary interstitial fluid is normally relatively rich in albumin, so that there is a lower intravascular-extravascular gradient than in most organs studied. The pulmonary lymphatics seem to play an important role in protecting the lungs from becoming overloaded with fluid. Early flooding of the interstitial space with protein-poor filtrate might lower the concentration of albumin in the interstitial fluid by a washout effect and thus be partly protective. Gump et al.[61] and Smith et al.[62] have documented that the lungs of surgical patients dying with ventilatory insufficiency have several times the normal amount of albumin, but clearly this represents advanced disease. Teplitz has suggested, on the basis of ultrastructural studies of patients dying with posttraumatic pulmonary insufficiency, that the capillary lesions are skip lesions, in which there are normal-appearing areas interspersed with areas of obvious damage.[63] If these normal areas are keeping the patient alive, they should be protected from pulmonary edema if possible. Furthermore, the real questions about the use of albumin arise early in the process of resuscitation, when there is little evidence of pulmonary vascular injury.

The possibility that a paradoxically harmful effect may occur from administering albumin during resuscitation is based almost entirely on experimental observations. We found increased fluid in the lungs of rats treated for hemorrhage with plasma compared to those treated with simple electrolyte solutions.[9] These rats were treated by protocol, not by measured pressures, although rather small volumes of fluid were used by modern criteria. Plasma was used as the protein solution, and there is provocative older evidence that plasma components become denatured during storage and may be detrimental. Schloerb et al. found more fluid in the lungs of rats when they were overloaded with albumin (human) than with salt solutions in equal volume, but this is what one would expect from the plasma volume-expanding properties of these fluids.[64] Holcroft et al.,[65] and Moss et al.[66] found increased fluid early after resuscitation in the lungs of baboons treated for hemorrhage with protein solution, compared to those treated with lactated Ringer's solution. Both studies unfortunately used human protein. Holcroft et al.[65] used human plasma protein fraction, in which about 20 percent of the protein is alpha and beta globulin. These preparations contain variable and sometimes considerable levels of bradykinin. Recently, these protein fractions have been associated in man with cardiovascular collapse, which may be due to very high levels of prekallikrein activator.[67] This might trigger extensive activation of the kinin system in a "primed" recipient; hemorrhage might be such a prime. As they now stand, the results are not clearly interpretable.

Most published and to-be-published clinical studies comparing albumin-supplemented regimens with albumin-free regimens do not show increased pulmonary complications from the use of albumin. One exception is a study by Lucas et al., reporting that injured patients treated with albumin had much greater dependency on mechanical ventilatory support than those treated with saline.[68] This study has several features that must be noted, however. Plasma volumes were nearly 10 percent greater in the albumin-treated group, and both central venous pressures (15.4 vs. 8.4) and pulmonary capillary wedge pressures (11.2 vs. 5.5) were also significantly higher. The plasma albumin concentration in the "albumin-poor" group was 3 g per 100 ml. Thus, no group was notably hypoalbuminemic, and the treated group had remarkably high concentrations for seriously injured patients. All patients in fact received considerable amounts of albumin in blood and fresh frozen plasma; in addition, the "albumin" group apparently received 900 grams over the first six days! If anything, what this study shows is that it is possible to give too much albumin to an injured patient. There are states of congenital hypoalbuminemia, and even analbuminemia, with reasonable duration of survival. To this author's knowledge, there are no documented instances of spontaneous, sustained hyperalbuminemia. As with many substances, albumin should be considered as potentially dangerous in excess. One of the interesting facets of the Lucas study, in fact, was the finding of impaired renal excretion of salt and water in these overloaded patients. There is growing experimental evidence indicating that the concentration of albumin in the plasma has an important effect on renal function. One of the built-in protections against fluid overload, in fact, may be a greater ease of renal excretion of excessive amounts of salt and water in the presence of acute dilutional hypoalbuminemia.

Summary. It is difficult to summarize such a controversial area. The evidence seems clear that a lower COP allows pulmonary edema to occur more easily but that, without elevation of perfusion pressure, pulmonary edema is difficult to produce simply by lowering COP. A reasonable position seems to be that, if one is going to lower COP during resuscitation, pulmonary perfusion pressure should be monitored and elevation of left atrial pressure should be avoided. There is currently no clinical evidence that adding albumin is harmful, except for one study in which excessive amounts of albumin and salt solutions apparently were used. In practical terms, there may well be a threshold COP above which little is gained by administering albumin, but below which there is increasing risk of pulmonary edema.[69] Some investigators estimate this threshold at a COP somewhat above half normal, or concentrations of albumin somewhere around 25 grams per liter. Even in patients with leaking pulmonary capillaries, the proper use of albumin remains obscure because of the possibility that the leaking may not be uniform throughout the pulmonary vascular bed. The available experimental evidence indicates that use of salt solutions alone increased edema in areas of pulmonary contusion, but there are not many studies on this point. The ability of the patient to excrete salt and water in the urine if needed can be an important variable.

Plasma

Plasma, once the favored resuscitative solution, is hardly used at all now for the treatment of hypovolemia. Plasma as the sole resuscitative fluid yields results that are clearly inferior to those obtained with a number of other resuscitative fluids in most experimental studies.[9,70] On the other hand, the plasma-expanding and flow properties of the native proteins are superior to those of the artificial substitutes. The risk of hepatitis is so real and the evidence of benefit so poor, that in the context of hemorrhage it is mainly albumin that is used and discussed currently. For correction of coagulation deficiencies, of course, fresh frozen plasma can be useful, but

it is not an acceptable fluid for the treatment of hypovolemia.

Artificial Colloids

Artificial colloids are substances that can substitute for the osmotic activity of plasma proteins.[71] They have the advantage of being either wholly manufactured or nonhuman biological products. They are therefore less expensive, more easily supplied, and do not transmit communicable diseases. Their disadvantages are those of all nonoxygen-carrying plasma expanders, with certain additions. There are functions of plasma proteins for which these materials cannot substitute: clotting, carrier (especially of albumin), immunologic, and probably others. These functions are absent to some degree in all "natural" plasma protein products, but some are always present. The artificial colloids do not last as long in the plasma space as do natural plasma proteins, although homologous proteins may sometimes be removed at rapid rates, and albumin may be cannibalized for calories. Artificial colloids appear to delay the endogenous replenishment of lost albumin.

The artificial colloids have toxicities that are significant. The dextrans and hydroxyethyl starch (HES) are mildly immunogenic, and allergic reactions occur in a low but significant percentage of recipients. Serious reactions to low molecular weight dextran continue to be reported but are rarely fatal. The dextrans and HES share the characteristic of interfering with the normal formation and maturation of a fibrin clot.[72] This characteristic is detectable in the clinical dosage range and is a dosage-dependent response. Potentially serious bleeding disorders after extensive use of dextran were observed during the Korean War, and recommendations for limiting the total dose to 1 to 1.5 liters in 24 hours seemed reasonable.[73] This is clearly a major disadvantage to the use of dextran and HES in the acutely injured or bleeding patient. There is variable interference with subsequent typing and crossmatching, which seems to be minimal with HES and low-molecular-weight dextran (LMD). Nevertheless, if these substances are to be used, a specimen of blood should be drawn for crossmatching before administration.

One of the reasons advanced for using LMD (and one heavily emphasized in the promotions of the supplier) is its specific rheologic properties—that is, it has the ability to disaggregate blood cells and improve flow by lowering the resistance to flow which is intrinsic in the blood of injured patients. The studies advanced in support of this concept are largely poorly controlled. The dextrans, particularly LMD, are hyperoncotic relative to plasma. They produce a plasma volume expansion that is greater than the infused volume. They concurrently lower the hematocrit, a major determinant of whole blood viscosity as currently measured. Most studies showing hemodynamic benefit have not adequately considered or controlled blood volume changes or have not used truly comparable groups of patients; some studies on viscosity do not even mention hematocrit changes; some use concentrations of dextran that should not be achieved clinically. It is noteworthy that many of the studies that do control the important variables fail to demonstrate a specific rheologic advantage of LMD in the clinically usable dosage range.[74] In addition, there have been serious questions raised about the renal toxicity of LMD in states of low renal blood flow.[2] It is not likely that use of these materials for the treatment of hemorrhage will increase significantly in the United States in the foreseeable future. They remain relatively popular in parts of Europe, and Gruber has reviewed the dextrans in considerable detail.[71]

An extensive evaluation of various gelatins as plasma substitutes is underway in Europe.[75] These substances are less well characterized than the dextrans or HES.[71] Viscosity and/or cell-aggregating effects may be detrimental, but effects on blood clotting may be less marked.

BURNS

In several respects, burns represent a special kind of injury, especially as regards fluid dynamics and resuscitation. For this reason burns are dealt with separately. The recent excellent review by Pruitt is recommended for more detail on all aspects of the care of the burned patient.[28] Only the nature and treatment of the hypovolemia associated with burn injury will be discussed here.

Pathophysiology of Hypovolemia

There is extensive loss of interstitial fluid and protein into the burned area. This loss persists for at least the first day after injury, usually stabilizes in the second day, and may begin to be reabsorbed by the third or fourth day. A marked increase in vascular permeability seems to account for most of these changes initially. Various drugs have been tried in attempts to control these changes in permeability, but none have proven to be of benefit and many involve significant risks. A seemingly unique feature of major burn injury is that capillary permeability increases in remote (unburned) areas as well.[76] This phenomenon creates special problems in treatment. Hypovolemia is profound soon after major burn injury, and particularly large volumes of fluid are required to reverse it because of the diffusely leaking vascular system.

The hemodynamic changes early after major burns have been well documented.[77] Cardiac output is initially severely depressed. Blood volume is lower than normal and continues to decrease unless vigorously supported with parenteral fluids. Even with continuous administration of fluids at rapid rates, blood volume remains significantly below expected normal (about 80 percent) throughout the first day, recovers to about 90 percent by the second day and to normal and often above normal thereafter. Cardiac output begins recovering with the first administration of fluids, even when an increase in blood volume cannot be detected. Cardiac output is back to normal by the end of the first day in the successfully resuscitated patient and remains well above normal thereafter until the wounds are healed. The discrepancy between the changes in blood volume and the changes in cardiac output, especially the profound early depression of the latter, is not completely explained. A marked increase in vascular resistance contributes significantly. Evidence of toxic factors that depress myocardial function has been sought, but without convincing evidence of their existence. Pulmonary vascular resistance remains significantly elevated after systemic vascular resistance returns to normal. Most of the regimens for administration of fluids described subsequently produce similar changes in plasma volume.

Use of Crystalloid

Salt water was accepted as the key element in resuscitation from major burns quite early, and was widely used as such well before it became accepted as treatment for blood loss. Various analytical and empiric clinical data have led to the formation of a number of "formulas" for the treatment of seriously burned patients. These are intended as no more than guidelines, with clinical signs and urinary output determining the details of treatment. Three of the most widely used "formulas" are shown in Table 21-5 along with two newly proposed approaches. The recommended procedure is to administer half the total requirement for the first 24 hours in the first 8 hours and the other half in the remaining 16 hours, always subject to the carefully monitored condition of the patient. Total requirements by any of the standard "formulas" are surprisingly large. An 80-kg patient with a 50 percent burn would require 16 liters of fluid during the first 24 hours according to the most aggressive of the formulas (Parkland). Requirements during the second 24 hours are much less.

Use of Colloid

The first point of controversy in the resuscitation of the burned patient is what kind and how much protein-containing fluid to use. The earlier formulas were based on analyses of the kinds of fluids lost into and from the burn wound. This fluid is unquestionably a protein-rich fluid, but the concept that straightforward replacement is the best treatment may not be as logical as it appears. If protein is lost into the wound because of loss of capillary integrity, it may be futile to pour more into a circulation in which the classical Starling forces no longer apply because large molecular substances move freely across a major part of the vascular bed. Evidence in favor of such an interpretation has come from the two major burn units in Texas, Parkland and Brooke Army Medical Center. In similar studies, administration of colloid (albumin or plasma) during the first 24 hours after a major

Table 21-5. Various "Formulas" for Use as Guides for Resuscitation of the Burned Adult Patient, First 24 Hours Only

	Electrolyte	Colloid	"Free" Water
Evans	1 ml/Kg/% burn	1 ml/Kg/% burn	2000 ml as 5% dextrose
Brooke I	1.5 ml/Kg/% burn	0.5 ml/Kg/% burn	2000 ml as 5% dextrose
Parkland	4 ml/Kg/% burn as lactated Ringer's	none	none
Hypertonic (Monafo)	Sodium 250 meq/l, sufficient to maintain urinary output 30 ml/hr	none	none
Brooke II (Pruitt)	2 ml/Kg/% burn as lactated Ringer's	none	none

burn had no detectable effect on the plasma volume of the recipient provided the administration of salt and water remained constant. In the second 24 hours, an increase in plasma volume was detected which was greater than that seen with salt and water alone, confirming the return of at least sufficient capillary integrity to allow the intravascular retention of large molecular substances. If colloid adds nothing to the expansion of plasma volume during the early resuscitation from a major burn, why should it be used? No reliable answer is apparent, but established practice dies hard. Considerations of cost alone should dictate less use of colloid. A very large experience has been gained in several excellent burn centers whose published results are admirable in which only simple electrolyte solutions are used for the early resuscitation from burns. Most agree with the use of colloid after the first 24 hours, and in fact the subsequent need for albumin can be quite large because of great losses through the wound, poor intake of food, and the metabolic diversion of energy and protein to other priorities.

The controversy over the need for colloid early after burns has recently been rekindled by a published report of significantly better results in patients given colloid during early resuscitation.[78] The number of patients was very small, however, and the trial needs to be expanded and repeated. A detailed study of cardiac function early after burn injury also found some evidence of higher cardiac output, but the differences may have been due to effects of the colloid toward the end of the first burn day. To repeat, the great weight of current clinical and experimental evidence does not establish the need to administer colloid solutions during the first 24 hours after a major burn injury. Clinical studies in this area are continuing.

Replacement Volume Requirements

The second controversy regarding the treatment of hypovolemia due to burns involves the amounts of salt and of water needed for adequate and safe resuscitation. The burned patient is not an infinite sponge into which salt and water can be poured without limit. Pulmonary edema is rare in the first two days after burn unless the lungs have been injured directly. Pulmonary complications are very common later. It is hard to distinguish the effects of the administration of fluids from the effects of remote sepsis, hematogenous or airborne direct infection, and the general impairment of antibacterial defenses, but retrospective studies have indicated that patients over 50 years of age are much less tolerant of fluid loading. For these reasons, Pruitt has revised the recommended guidelines for fluids during the first 24 hours (labeled Brooke-II in Table 21-5) and has advocated the use of colloid and salt-free water thereafter to maintain blood volume and urinary output. This is an attempt to limit the total load of sodium administered during resuscitation. Mobilization and excretion of these large loads of sodium are not complete until several weeks after injury and are delayed by septic complications.

Hypertonic Saline

Another approach to this problem has been to limit the total amount of fluid given by using hypertonic sodium solutions during the first 24 hours.[79] The current recommended concentration is 250 meq/l. Such an approach produces hypernatremia and hyperosmolality of the plasma. Plasma volume is maintained at the cost of cellular dehydration and at the risk of renal impairment. The advantage is a lack of the gross edema characteristic of the burned patient resuscitated by the usual methods and perhaps less need for escharotomy. However, because the total amount of sodium administered is not substantially different, it is hard to appreciate the longer-term value of this approach. Accelerated loss of water through the burn wound is characteristic of the period following early resuscitation,[80] and hypernatremia is a frequent complication even in patients resuscitated with large volumes of mildly hypoosmolar fluid (lactated Ringer's solution contains 135 meq Na/l). Children, on the other hand, show a tendency to develop hyponatremia in the early days after injury and resuscitation. Hypertonic saline is not widely used at present as the primary means of treating hypovolemia due to burns.

Changes in Red Cell Mass

The changes in red cell mass after major burns are interesting.[81,82] With the early contraction of plasma volume there is little need for transfusion of red cells even in most patients with extensive burns unless hemorrhage has occurred for other reasons. Patients with exceptionally deep burns involving a lot of muscle (this is common in electrical injuries) may require transfusion of red cells soon after injury. There is a significant continuing loss of red cell mass, however, which is proportional to the extent of full-thickness burns. In addition to the immediate loss, there is a continued daily loss of up to 10 percent or more per day for at least four days. Subsequent operative procedures, especially operative debridement of burns, involve significant blood loss and transfusion of red cells is usually required. In addition, the relative unresponsiveness of the bone marrow to erythropoietin which is seen in a variety of acute and chronic illnesses, is also found in patients who have unhealed burn wounds.[83] Aggressive programs of early operative debridement of burn wounds can create the need for very large amounts of red cells by transfusion.

REFERENCES

1. Beecher, H.K., Burnett, C.H., Shapiro, S.L., Simeone, F.G., Smith, I.D., Sullivan, E.R., and Mallory, T.B.: The physiologic effects of wounds. Med. Dept. U.S. Army: Surgery in WW II. Office of the Surgeon General, Dept. Army, Washington, D.C., 1952.

2. Collins, J.A. and Ballinger, W.F.: The treatment of shock. In: The Management of Trauma, 2nd ed., Ballinger, W.F., Rutherford, R.B., and Zuidema, G.D., eds. W.B. Saunders, Philadelphia, 1973, pp. 70-95.

3. Grant, R.T. and Reeve, E.B.: Observations on the general effect of injury in man. Spec. Report Series, Medical Res. Council (London), No. 277, 1951.

4. Collins, J.A., Simmons, R.L., James, P.M., Bredenberg, G.E., Anderson, R.W., and Heisterkamp, G.A.: Acid-base status of seriously wounded combat casualties. I. Before treatment. Ann. Surg. 171:595, 1970.

5. Collins, J.A.: The ventilatory response to metabolic acidosis in hemorrhagic shock. In: Shock in Low- and High-Flow States, Proc. Symp. Brook Lodge, Augusta, Michigan, Excerpta Medica, Amsterdam, 1971, pp. 212-216.

6. Trunkey, D.D. and Lim, R.C.: Analysis of 425 consecutive victims of trauma: an autopsy study. J. Am. Coll. Emerg. Phys. 3:368, 1974.

7. Collins, J.A.: The acute respiratory distress syndrome. Adv. Surg. 11:171, 1977.

8. Anderson, R.W. and DeVries, W.C.: Transvascular fluid and protein dynamics in the lung following hemorrhagic shock. J. Surg. Res. 20:281, 1976.

9. Collins, J.A., Braitberg, A., and Butcher, H.R.: Changes in lung and body weight and lung water content in rats treated for hemorrhage with various fluids. Surgery 73:401, 1973.

10. Clowes, G.H., Hirsch, E., Williams, L., Kwasnik, E., O'Donnell, T.F., Cuevas, P., Sani, V.K., Moradi, I., Farizan, M., Sarovis, C., Stone, M., and Kuffler, J.: Septic lung and shock lung in man. Ann. Surg. 181:681, 1975.

11. Clowes, G.H.: Pulmonary abnormalities in sepsis. Surg. Clin. N. Am. 54:993, 1974.

12. Weisel, R.D., Dennis, R.C., Manny, J., Mannick, J.A., Valeri, C.R., and Hechtman, H.B.: Adverse effects of transfusion therapy during abdominal aortic aneurysmectomy. Surgery 83:682, 1978.

13. Henry, J.N., McArdle, A.H., Buonous, G., Hampson, L.G., Scott, H.J., and Gurd, F.N.: The effect of experimental hemorrhagic shock on pulmonary alveolar surfactant. J. Trauma 7:691, 1967.

14. Rohatgi, P., Tauber, I., and Massaro, D.: Hemorrhagic hypotension and the lung: in vitro respiration. Am. Rev. Respir. Dis. 113:763, 1976.

15. Etheredge, E.E. and Hruska, K.A.: Acute renal failure in the surgical patient. In: The Management of Trauma, 3rd ed., Zuidema, G.D., Rutherford, R.B., and Ballinger, W.F., eds. W.B. Saunders, Phila., 1979, pp. 148-180.

16. Baxter, C.R., Zedlitz, W.H., and Shires, G.T.: High output acute renal failure complicating traumatic injury. J. Trauma 4:567, 1964.

17. Thurau, K. and Boylan, J.W.: Acute renal success: The unexpected logic of oliguria in acute renal failure. Am. J. Med. 61:308, 1976.

18. MacDonald, J.A.E., Milligan, G.E., Mellon, A., and Ledingham, I.M.: Ventricular function in experimental hemorrhagic shock. Surg., Gynecol., Obstet. 140:572, 1975.

19. Wilson, J.M., Gay, W.A., and Ebert, P.A.: The effects of oligemic hypotension on myocardial function. Surgery 73:657, 1973.

20. Lefer, A.M., Glenn, T.M., Wangensteen, S.L., Ramey, W.G., Ferguson, W.W., and Starling, J.R.: Editorial comments: controversy over myocardial depressant factor in shock. J. Trauma 13:746, 1973.

21. Wangensteen, S.L., Ramey, W.G., Ferguson, W., and Starling, J.R.: Plasma myocardial depressant activity (shock factor) identified as salt in the cat capillary muscle bioassay system. J. Trauma 13:181, 1973.

22. Martin, A.M., Hackel, D.B., and Kurtz, S.M.: The ultrastructure of zonal lesions of the myocardium in hemorrhagic shock. Am. J. Pathol. 44:127, 1964.

23. Alyono, D., Ring, W.S., and Anderson, R.W.: The effects of hemorrhagic shock on the diastolic properties of the left ventricle in the conscious dog. Surgery 83:691, 1979.

24. Lucas, C.E., Sugawa, C., Riddle, J., Rector, F., Rosenberg, B., and Watt, A.J.: Natural history and surgical dilemma of "stress" gastric bleeding. Arch. Surg. 102:266, 1971.

25. Menguy, R.: The prophylaxis of stress ulceration. N. Engl. J. Med. 302:461, 1980.

26. Priebe, H.J., Skillman, J.J., Bushnell, L.S., Long, P.C., and Silen, W.: Antacid versus cimetidine in preventing acute gastrointestinal bleeding: a randomized trial in 75 critically ill patients. N. Engl. J. Med. 302:426, 1980.

27. Warden, G.D., Mason, A.D., and Pruitt, B.A.: Evaluation of leukocyte chemotaxis in vitro in thermally injured patients. J. Clin. Invest. 54:1001, 1974.

28. Pruitt, B.A.: The burn patient: I. Initial Care. Vol. 16, No. 4, p. 1, 1979. II. Later care and complications of thermal injury. Vol. 16, No. 5, p. 10, 1979.

29. Esrig, B.C. and Fulton, F.L.: Sepsis, resuscitated hemorrhagic shock and "shock lung": an experimental correlation. Ann. Surg. 182:218, 1975.

30. Roth, R.R., Mullane, J.F., Huber, G.L., Phelps, T.D., and Wilfong, R.G.: Blood loss and factors affecting pulmonary antibacterial defenses. J. Surg. Res. 17:36, 1974.

31. Jones, J.W., Hewitt, R.L., and Drapanas, T.: Cardiac contusion: a capricious syndrome. Ann. Surg. 181:567, 1975.

32. Batalden, D.J., Wichstrom, P., Ruez, E., and Gustilo, R.: Value of the G suit in patients with severe pelvic fracture: controlling hemorrhagic shock. Arch. Surg. 109:326, 1974.

33. Clarke, R., Topley, E., and Flear, C.T.G.: Assessment of blood loss in civilian trauma. Lancet i:629, 1955.

34. Gauer, D.H., Henry, J.P., and Sieker, H.O.: Changes in central venous pressure after moderate hemorrhage and transfusion in man. Circ. Res. 4:79, 1956.

35. Simmons, R.L., Heisterkamp, C.A., and Doty, D.B.: Postresuscitative blood volumes in combat casualties. Surg., Gynecol., Obstet. 128:1193, 1969.

36. Carey, L.C., Cloutier, C.T., and Lowery, B.D.: The use of balanced electrolyte solution for resuscitation. In: Body Fluid Replacement in the Surgical Patient. Fox, C.L., Jr. and Nahas, G.G., eds. Grune and Stratton, New York, 1970, pp. 200-207.

37. Carpenter, C.C.J., Biern, R.O., Mitra, P.P., Sack, R.B., Dons, P.E., Wells, S.A., and Khaura, S.S.: Electrocardiogram in Asiatic cholera; separate studies of effects of hypovolemia, acidosis, and potassium loss. Br. Heart J. 29:103, 1967.

38. Moore, F.D., Dagher, F.J., Boyden, C.M., Lee, C.J., and Lyons, J.H.: Hemorrhage in normal man: I. Distribution and dispersal of saline infusions following acute blood loss—clinical kinetics of blood volume support. Ann. Surg. 163:485, 1966.

39. Pruitt, B.A., Moncrief, J.A., and Mason, A.D.: Efficacy of buffered saline as the sole replacement fluid following acute measured hemorrhage in man. J. Trauma 7:767, 1967.

40. Rush, B.F. and Stewart, R.A.: More liberal use

of a plasma expander: impact on a hospital blood bank. New Engl. J. Med. 280:1202, 1969.

41. Gump, F.E., Kinney, J.M., Iles, M., and Long, C.C.: Duration and significance of large fluid loads administered for circulatory support. J. Trauma 10:431, 1970.

42. Fishman, A.P.: Pulmonary edema: the water-exchanging function of the lung. Circulation 46:390, 1972.

43. Robin, E.D., Cross, C.E., and Zelis, R.: Pulmonary edema. N. Engl. J. Med. 288:239, 292, 1973.

44. Staub, N.C.: Pulmonary edema. Physiol. Rev. 54:678, 1974.

45. Abrams, J.S., Deane, R.S., and Davis, J.H.: Adverse effects of salt and water retention on pulmonary function in patients with multiple trauma. J. Trauma 13:788, 1973.

46. Lucas, C.E., Ledgerwood, A.M., Shier, M.R., and Bradley, V.E.: The renal factor in the post-traumatic "fluid overload" syndrome. J. Trauma 17:667, 1977.

47. Gaisford, W.D., Pandey, N., and Jensen, C.G.: Pulmonary changes in treated hemorrhagic shock. II. Ringers lactate solution versus colloid infusion. Am. J. Surg. 124:738, 1972.

48. Cooper, J.D., Marder, M., and Lowenstein, E.: Lung water accumulation with acute hemodilution in dogs. J. Thorac. Cardiovasc. Surg. 69:957, 1975.

49. Laks, H., O'Connor, N.E., Anderson, W., and Pilon, R.N.: Crystalloid versus colloid hemodilution in man. Surg., Gynecol., Obstet. 142:506, 1976.

50. Giordano, J.M., Joseph, W.L., Klingmaier, C.H., and Adkins, P.C.: The management of interstitial pulmonary edema. Significance of hypoproteinemia. J. Thorac. Cardiovasc. Surg. 64:739, 1972.

51. Skillman, J.J., Parikh, B.M., and Tanenbaum, B.J.: Pulmonary arteriovenous admixture: improvement with albumin and diuresis. Am. J. Surg. 119:440, 1970.

52. Fleming, W.H. and Bowen, J.C.: The use of diuretics in the treatment of early wet lung syndrome. Ann. Surg. 175:505, 1972.

53. Skillman, J.J., Restall, D.S., and Salzman, E.W.: Randomized trial of albumin vs. electrolyte solutions during abdominal aortic operations. Surgery 78:291, 1975.

54. Rackow, E., Fair, A., and Leppo, J.: Colloid osmotic pressure as a prognostic indicator in critically ill patients. Chest 70:429, 1976.

55. Weil, M.H., Henning, R.J., Morisetta, M., and Michaels, S.: Relationship between colloid osmotic pressure and pulmonary artery wedge pressure in patients with cardiorespiratory failure. Am. J. Med. 64:643, 1978.

56. Lowe, R.J. and Moss, G.S.: Pulmonary failure after trauma. In: Surgery Annual, Vol. 8. Nyhus, L.M., ed., 1976, pp. 63-90.

57. Pappova, E., Bachmeier, W., Crevoisier, J.L., Kollar, J., Kollar, M., Tobler, P., Zahler, H.W., Zaugg, D., and Lundsgaard-Hansen, P.: Acute hypoproteinemic fluid overload: its determinants, distribution, and treatment with concentrated albumin and diuretics. Vox Sang. 33:307, 1977.

58. Cloutier, C.O., Lowery, B.D., and Carey, G.C.: The effect of hemodilutional resuscitation on serum protein levels in hemorrhagic shock. J. Trauma 9:514, 1969.

59. Lowe, R.J., Moss, G.S., Jilek, J., and Levine, H.D.: Crystalloid vs. colloid in the etiology of pulmonary failure after trauma: a randomized trial in man. Surgery 81:376, 1977.

60. Virgilio, R., Smith, D.E., Rice, C.L., Hobelmann, C.L., Zarins, C.K., James, D.R., and Peters, R.M.: Effect of colloid osmotic pressure and pulmonary capillary wedge pressure on intrapulmonary shunt. Surg. Forum 27:168, 1976.

61. Gump, F.E., Mashima, Y., Ferenczy, A., and Kinney, J.M.: Pre- and postmortem studies of lung fluids and electrolytes. J. Trauma 11:474, 1971.

62. Smith, P.C., Frank, H.A., Kasdon, E.J., Dearborn, E.C., and Skillman, J.J.: Albumin uptake by skin, skeletal muscle and lung in living and dying patients. Ann. Surg. 187:31, 1978.

63. Teplitz, C.: The core pathobiology and integrated medical science of adult respiratory insufficiency. Surg. Clin. N. Am. 56:909, 1976.

64. Schloerb, P.R., Hunt, P.T., Plummer, J.A., and Cage, G.K.: Pulmonary edema after replacement of blood loss by electrolyte solution. Surg., Gynecol., Obstet. 135:893, 1972.

65. Holcroft, J.W., Trunkey, D.D., and Lim, R.C.: Further analysis of lung water in baboons resuscitated from hemorrhagic shock. J. Surg. Res. 20:291, 1976.

66. Moss, G.S., Siegel, D.C., Cochin, A., and Fresquez, V.: Effects of saline and colloid solutions on pulmonary function in hemorrhagic shock. Surg., Gynecol., Obstet. 183:53, 1971.

67. Alving, B.M., Hojima, Y., Pisano, J.J., Mason, B.L., Buckingham, R.E., Mozen, M.M., and Finlayson, J.S.: Hypotension and Hageman-factor fragments in plasma protein fraction. N. Engl. J. Med. 299:66, 1978.

68. Lucas, G.E., Weaver, D., Higgins, R.E., Ledgerwood, A.M., Johnson, S.D., and Bowman, D.G.: Effects of albumin versus non-albumin resuscitation on plasma volume and renal excretory function. J. Trauma 18:564, 1978.

69. Schüpbach, P., Pappova, E., Schilt, W., Kollar, J., Kollar, M., Sipos, P., and Vucic, D.: Perfusate oncotic pressure during cardiopulmonary bypass. Vox Sang. 35:332, 1978.

70. McCarthy, M.D.: A comparison of plasma expanders with blood and plasma as a supplement to electrolyte solutions in the treatment of rats undergoing third-degree burns of fifty percent of the body surface. Ann. Surg. 136:546, 1952.

71. Gruber, U.F.: Blood Replacement. Springer-Verlag, Berlin, 1969.

72. Alexander, B.: Recent studies on plasma colloid substitutes: their effects on coagulation and hemostasis. In: Body Fluid Replacement in the Surgical Patient. Fox, C.L., Jr. and Nahas, G.G., eds. Grune and Stratton, Inc., New York, 1970, pp. 157-169.

73. Langdell, R.D., Adelson, E., Furth, F.W., and Crosby, W.H.: Dextran and prolonged bleeding time: results of a sixty-gram, one-liter infusion given to one hundred sixty-three normal human subjects. J.A.M.A. 166:346, 1958.

74. Chien, S., Usami, S., and Gregersen, M.I.: Effects of plasma expanders on blood viscosity. In: Body Fluid Replacement in the Surgi-cal Patient. Fox, C.L., Jr., and Nahas, G.G., eds. Grune and Stratton, New York, 1970, pp. 138-148.

75. Lundsgaard-Hansen, P., Hässig, A., and Nitschmann, H.: Modified gelatins as plasma substitutes, Bibl. Haematol. No. 33, 1969.

76. Arturson, G.: Capillary permeability in burned and nonburned areas in dogs. Acta. Chir. Scand. (suppl. 274):55, 1961.

77. Asch, M.J., Feldman, R.J., Walker, H.L., Foley, F.D., Popp, R.L., Mason, A.D., and Pruitt, B.A.: Systemic and pulmonary hemo-dynamic changes accompanying thermal injury. Ann. Surg. 178:218, 1973.

78. Jelenko, C., Williams, J.B., Wheeler, M.I., Calloway, B.D., Fackler, V.K., Albers, G.A., and Barger, A.A.: Studies in shock and resuscitation. I. Use of a hypertonic, albumin-containing, fluid demand regimen (HALFD) in resuscitation. Crit. Care Med. 7:157, 1969.

79. Monafo, W.W., Chuntrasakul, C., and Ayva-zian, V.H.: Hypertonic sodium solutions in the treatment of burn shock. Am. J. Surg. 126:778, 1973.

80. Harrison, H.N., Moncrief, J.A., Duckett, J.W., and Mason, A.D.: The relationship between energy metabolism and water loss from vaporization in severely burned patients. Surgery 56:203, 1964.

81. Loebl, E.C., Baxter, C.R., and Curreri, P.: The mechanism of erythrocyte destruction in the early postburn period. Ann. Surg. 178:681, 1973.

82. Topley, E., Jackson, D.M., Cason, J.S., and Davies, J.W.L.: Assessment of red cell loss in the first two days after severe burns. Ann. Surg. 155:581, 1962.

83. Andes, W.A., Rogers, P.W., Beason, J.W., and Pruitt, B.A.: The erythropoietin response to the anemia of thermal injury. J. Lab. Clin. Med. 88:584, 1976.

22

Surgical Problems of Transfusion Therapy, Including Cardiopulmonary Bypass

John A. Collins, M.D.

Were I to list the main problems facing the surgeon relative to transfusion therapy, I believe that three would easily stand out. By far the most serious problem is not having blood available when and in the amount needed. Other problems are relatively small compared to this one. The second might be argued among surgeons, but I suspect that the accidental misadministration of blood deserves that (dis)honor. There are few things that even surgeons do that are as potentially hazardous for their patients as giving them blood intended for someone else. It is imperative that all members of the team caring for surgical patients, and in particular the surgeons themselves, be aware of this fact. The third leading problem is probably the transmission of hepatitis, even though many surgeons seem blissfully unaware that such things still happen. This is dealt with in Chapter 36. It is hoped that significant further protection for patients will be possible in the foreseeable future.

Beyond these three are the usual array of "standard" transfusion reactions, discussed in Chapter 37, which tend not to be serious problems in surgical patients because transfusion is usually an acute rather than a chronic and repetitive event. There are several subsets of surgical patients, however, who become involved in special situations.

Exsanguinating hemorrhage, whatever that means, usually rapidly becomes a surgical problem. The requirement for rapid administration of large amounts of stored blood brings with it a host of potential, putative, mistaken, or as yet barely thought of problems which will be considered briefly. Cardiopulmonary bypass is one of the more recent advances in surgery. It is very closely linked to transfusion therapy and has a set of special problems that will also be considered.

MASSIVE TRANSFUSION

There is an often-told story of a surgeon of the old school who looked up from a bloody operative field and saw some clear liquid running rapidly through the intravenous tubing. "What's that?" he growled.

The anesthesiologist answered, "Lactated Ringer's."

"Look down here, sonny—is this patient bleeding Lactated Ringer's? The patient is losing blood, so blood is what you should be giving him."

"Well, that seems logical enough, but I sure hope this patient doesn't develop diarrhea."

Things are often not as simple as they seem. Stored blood is not the equivalent of the patient's own blood. It differs antigenically, metabolically, functionally, and in a number of other ways. Most of these differences are ordinarily well tolerated; however, when exsanguinating hemorrhage occurs and is treated by massive transfusion, these differences from normal become imposed on the recipient rapidly and in large amounts, and many then represent potential causes of trouble. Clear evidence of when and to what extent these differences become important has been very difficult to obtain, however.[1]

Mathematics

The mathematics of exchange transfusion have been worked out for several types of situations.[2,3] The simplest expression for incremental exchange in which equal volumes are withdrawn and infused in that sequence is

$$X_n = X_o(1 - \frac{b}{v})^n$$

when X_n = the amount or concentration of the substance in question remaining in the recipient's circulation, X_o = the starting amount or concentration, b = the volume of a unit of blood, v = the recipient's blood volume, and n = the number of units transfused.

For continuous exchange with equal rates of withdrawal and infusin at constant blood volume, the following formula applies:

$$X_n = X_o \, e^{-\frac{bn}{v}}$$

Any endogenous replacement during transfusion or the presence of the substance in question in the blood transfused would result in higher levels in the recipient at the end of transfusion. Even assuming no replacement and complete absence in the transfused blood and using the circumstances that must apply to ensure the patient's survival (e.g., blood volume must not drop to half normal), one can make a reasonable estimation of the amount of original blood elements still remaining in the recipient after the transfusion of various volumes (Table 22-1). Both for-

Table 22-1. Percent Replacement of the Recipient's Blood Volume with Transfused Blood under Three Assumptions of Massive Transfusion; Blood Volume Transfused Refers to Volumes Equivalent to the Patient's Normal Blood Volume

Assumption	1 Blood Volume	2 Blood Volumes	3 Blood Volumes
Perfect exchange	63%	86%	95%
Usual (?) situation	70 to 75%	90%	97%
Fatal delay	82%	97%	99%

mulas give very similar results under clinical conditions. Even after two blood volumes in transfusion, most recipients will have at least 10 percent of their original blood elements remaining; or conversely, no more than 90 percent of the circulating blood volume will be donor blood. At a transfusion volume equal to the recipient's blood volume, no more than 70 percent of the circulating blood will be donor blood. The difficulty in obtaining complete exchange under clinical circumstances is widely underestimated; stated another way, the extent of replacement of the recipient's blood with donor blood is usually grossly overestimated. These considerations are important for evaluating the potential impact of stored blood on the recipient. They are particularly important in trying to evaluate the coagulation disorders associated with transfusion and any abnormalities resulting from defects in transfused red cells.

Hemostatic Disorders

The breakdown in hemostasis that occurs in some patients during extensive transfusion is a particularly distressing event because it contributes to the bleeding for which the transfusions are being given. To the extent that the transfusions themselves are contributing to the hemostatic defect, a vicious circle exists. Many clinicians are convinced (wrongly) that this in fact is what occurs in these patients, and that the blood used to treat the hemorrhage also contributes to causing the hemorrhage. The implications are clinically very important: less blood is better if the transfused blood interferes with hemostasis.

The hemostatic deficiencies in stored blood are significant. Platelets are probably essentially absent unless the blood is very fresh. Factors V and VIII deteriorate during storage at rates that are variously described. By the third week of storage in citrate, both Factors are probably at no more than 10 to 15 percent normal activity, perhaps less. Thus, extensive transfusion with whole blood (even more with red cell concentrates plus salt water or albumin) involves significant dilution of these hemostatic factors. A moderate number of studies on the changes in coagulation during extensive transfusion have been reported.[1] When platelets or Factors V or VIII have been measured, however, the degree of depletion in abnormally bleeding patients has usually been far greater than can be accounted for by exchange transfusion alone. For example, an adult patient transfused 10 units of blood should not have a platelet count below $50,000/\mu L$ on the basis of dilution unless that patient began with a platelet count below $150,000/\mu L$, yet many pathologically bleeding patients have levels lower than this. Even more inconsistent with a mechanism of exchange transfusion are the observations of very low fibrinogen levels in many such patients. Fibrinogen levels are normal in stored blood; even with red cell concentrates, at least one-third the normal concentrations of fibrinogen should be found in extensively transfused recipients. Fibrin degradation products and/or fibrin-fibrinogen complexes are often found in such patients. Finally, in Vietnam we studied a number of patients who had significant coagulopathies when transfusion was begun. The coagulation abnormalities improved during transfusion with 3-week-old blood, then worsened when the transfusion was stopped. All of these observations point toward some kind of consumption of coagulation components and of platelets in many of these patients, most likely disseminated intravascular coagulation (DIC).

An important confirmation of this hypothesis has recently been published.[4] Injured, heavily transfused patients were studied for hemostatic disorders. There was no relationship between the observed disorders and the amount of blood transfused. For heavily transfused patients, however, there was a strong correlation between the recorded duration of hypotension and the degree of coagulation abnormality. This further indicates that it is something in the patient rather than in the blood which causes the coagulation abnormalities. DIC is well known to result from or be worsened by hypoperfusion.

The implications of this hypothesis are quite different from those of the transfusion-dilution sequence. If DIC is the causative factor, then a contributing factor is too little blood and too late—not too much blood. Stored blood, however, may not be completely innocent. A hemolytic transfusion reaction is a well-documented cause of DIC. It is possible that partial activation of some coagulation components occurs during storage, and that a heavily transfused patient is more susceptible to the development of DIC, but this is purely speculative at present.

Several investigators have postulated or reported impaired function of platelets in heavily transfused patients. It is not clear that the functional studies were properly controlled for differences in the concentration of platelets. Even so, there is increasing evidence that DIC is associated with a platelet functional defect.

The disorders of hemostasis that occur in the massively transfused patient are difficult to categorize and are probably far from simple. They are almost certainly not due to simple exchange transfusion-dilution. They likely involve DIC, in at least some of these patients, and if so may result from combinations of tissue damage and poor perfusion.

Impaired Function of Hemoglobin

The main reason to transfuse red cells in treating the exsanguinating patient is to restore oxygen delivering capacity to the circulation. During storage in citrate in the liquid form, however, the function of hemoglobin as an oxygen-delivering agent becomes progressively more impaired because of a progressive decrease in the concentration of 2,3-diphosphoglyceric acid (2,3-DPG) in the stored red cells. Given the time to respond, the concentrations of 2,3-DPG in erythrocytes almost always increases in response to stress on the oxygen delivering system. The changes induced by storage are thus opposite in direction from the usual compensatory response. Restoration of 2,3-DPG back to and even above normal does occur after transfusion into the recipient, but this requires hours and sometimes a day or longer. Even given the mathematics of exchange transfusion, it is quite possible to drive the recipient's oxygen delivering capacity in the direction of the impaired level of the stored cells with rapid, extensive transfusion. There has understandably been concern about this aspect of transfusion therapy, as the impairment occurs when survival is threatened by circulatory insufficiency.

Attempts to demonstrate a clearly harmful effect from impaired function of hemoglobin have been surprisingly difficult. Numerous studies have shown the expected changes in such things as cardiac output, mixed venous oxygen tension, tissue oxygen tension, etc., but a harmful effect on the individual has not been apparent. Probably the closest was a study of two patients with abnormal red cell glycolysis and hemolytic anemias.[5] One had high levels of 2,3-DPG and the other had very low levels. When stressed by exercise, the patient with the high levels had greater aerobic work capacity, and could work at lower cardiac outputs and higher mixed venous oxygen tensions. Two separate reports referred to higher mortality in stressed animals treated with red cells depleted of 2,3-DPG compared to those treated with normally functioning cells; but details of these experiments were never published.[6,7]

There is surprisingly abundant evidence against a critical role for the depletion of 2,3-DPG, in spite of the persuasive theoretical evidence. There are a variety of congenitally aberrant hemoglobins characterized by increased affinity for oxygen, in some instances exactly equal to the affinity of normal hemoglobin in red cells completely depleted of 2,3-DPG.[8] These patients are characterized by normal longevity, asymptomatic activity, and normal fertility, but all have moderately increased hematocrits (mid-50s). One report describes casualties in Vietnam who were massively transfused with blood stored 2 to 3 weeks in ACD and therefore completely depleted of 2,3-DPG. These casualties showed no clinical evidence of impaired delivery of oxygen, and metabolic studies showed rapid clearance of preexisting lactic acidosis and of infused loads of lactate, implying efficient aerobic metabolism.[9]

More direct studies have been reported in which rats and humans were exchange-transfused with red cells depleted of 2,3-DPG.[10,11] There was only minimal impairment of maximum aerobic work performance. Exercise may not be a challenge equivalent to hemorrhage, however; marked gradients between lung and working muscle in pH and temperature would act to increase the efficiency of the delivery of oxygen by hemoglobin, thus offsetting the effects of depletion of 2,3-DPG. Studies using hemorrhage as a challenge and also varying the hematocrit reported a significantly increased mortality in rats treated with red cells depleted of 2,3-DPG and also anemic.[12,13] There was some disagreement about whether depletion of 2,3-DPG in the absence of anemia was associated with increased mortality; the studies showing higher mortality allowed little time for the animals to recover from the prior exchange transfusion.

These observations, although reassuring regarding the effects of storage-induced depletions of 2,3-DPG, dealt largely with otherwise normal individuals. Coronary arterial insufficiency would be a very worrisome abnormality for a patient treated for hemorrhage with depleted cells. The human heart works near its lowest tolerable mixed venous oxygen tension and thus cannot strip much more oxygen off available hemoglobin. Blood (and oxygen) supply occurs largely during diastole; both diastolic pressure and the time spent in diastole tend to decrease during serious hemorrhage. The oxygen requirements of the heart may be increased in response to hemorrhage because of the effects of adrenergic stimulation. These circumstances indicate that the ability of the coronary vessels to dilate is critical for the ability to withstand hemorrhage.

Clinical experience confirms this connection. Experiments on isolated heart preparations showed that banding the coronary arteries made the function of the left ventricles very sensitive to the concentration of hemoglobin in the blood perfusing the hearts.[14] Attempts to prove the same thing for changes in 2,3-DPG were not properly controlled. Comparisons between patients receiving normal red cells and those receiving red cells augmented in 2,3-DPG during and after coronary arterial bypass operations showed such marked differences between the two groups (due to poor results in the controls) that the entire study is very difficult to interpret.[15] A separate study found better cardiac function after resection of abdominal aortic aneurysms in patients given relatively normal red cells as opposed to those given red cells depleted of 2,3-DPG.[16] The former patients were operated upon electively, however, while the latter patients had sustained rupture of their aneurysms with attendant greater hypotension and loss of blood. Conclusions are therefore impossible regarding the effects of the transfused blood. In spite of the lack of proof, however, it remains quite likely that patients with impairment of coronary arterial flow are especially sensitive to the functional properties of the red cells transfused in treatment of hemorrhage.

Impaired flow in organs other than the heart, especially the brain, may also be important. With the use of CPD-stored blood in the United States, the problem of the functional properties of the red cells was not really tested because about half of the blood transfused was still in the period of storage when levels of 2,3-DPG were relatively normal. With extensive transfusion, fresher stocks are usually required as the supply of the appropriate ABO and Rh type is consumed. If adenine-supplemented storage becomes popular, depletion of 2,3-DPG will have to be considered more seriously in these special situations as concentrations of 2,3-DPG decline earlier. Various methods have been described for augmenting levels of 2,3-DPG in cells depleted during storage. Most involve some kind of additive, but if the need is demonstrated the extra efforts may be worthwhile. The need, however, is likely to be demonstrable only in certain special circumstances. Under most conditions, depletion of 2,3-DPG seems not to be of great importance if the hematocrit is preserved near normal.

Acid-Base Imbalance

Blood becomes progressively more acidic during storage in citrate in the liquid state. By 3 weeks of storage, blood contains a metabolic acid load of 25 to 30 meq/l. Patients dying of exsanguination are often severely acidotic. Transfusing one into the other might be expected to result in a worsened acidosis and possibly harmful effects. Some studies in dogs indicate that such reactions might occur and that administration of alkalinizing agents during extensive transfusion would prevent this "transfusion acidosis." Alkalinizing agents have a number of potential harmful effects, however, and in general acidosis seems better tolerated than alkalosis.

Studies on massively transfused casualties in Vietnam did not confirm the occurrence of transfusion-caused acidosis;[9] quite the opposite was found. Even patients initially profoundly hypotensive and severely acidotic transfused with large volumes of 3-week-old blood not only handled the infused acid load but improved their acid-base status to nearly normal during transfusion. The only patients to show worsening acidosis were those in whom hemostasis was not obtained. These patients were bleeding to death, and the acidosis was likely because of that, not because of transfusion. It is also doubtful that such acidosis was a major factor in causing their deaths. Administration of alkalinizing agents to this group was largely futile and could not even control the acidosis itself.

Retrospective analysis showed that routine use of alkalinizing agents in accordance with guidelines proposed at the time would have resulted in the administation of enormous amounts to casualties who did perfectly well without them. Several casualties in that study would have received well over 1000 meq sodium bicarbonate on the day of injury. Ironically, soon after resuscitation most casualties were alkalotic even without supplementation. This is a well-recognized response to injury and involves both renal and respiratory mechanisms. ACD-stored blood (used in Vietnam) contains about 15 meq of sodium citrate per unit of blood, so that massive transfusion represents a significant infusion of alkalinizing material, even without supplementation. CPD contains slightly less.

It is disturbing to think what would have happened to those casualties if what seemed like logical and sound advice had been followed. Severe alkalosis and a great excess load of sodium would certainly have caused serious problems. Several conclusions seem obvious. Empirical treatment should be well-founded by documentation of need and effectiveness; it should not be resorted to when measurement of the variable in question is possible and practical, as is now the case with acid-base balance. The metabolic effects of massive transfusion may not be easily predictable. The patient-recipient is not a simple system involving addition or subtraction. In the case of acid-base balance, the acidosis of the exsanguinating casualty and of the blood used for treatment is due in both instances to organic acids that are normal intermediary metabolites and that are rapidly "burned off" when perfusion is restored.

Once again, a complication attributed to the blood used for treatment is more properly attributed to lack of that blood.

Citrate Toxicity

Citrate is an excellent anticoagulant for storing blood. It binds ionized calcium and so prevents clotting. It is not consumed during storage. It is a normal intermediary metabolite and is rapidly metabolized by the recipient after transfusion. The anticoagulant effect is reversed almost instantly on infusion by the recipient's level of ionized calcium. The problem with citrate is that the binding equilibrium with calcium is such that a significant molar excess of citrate is required to keep ionized calcium levels low enough to prevent coagulation during storage. The infusion of citrated blood thus represents infusion of "free" citrate into the recipient. It was shown long ago that rapid exchange transfusion with blood that is free of calcium will not produce much change in animals, but that rapid exchange with citrated blood can be lethal. The lethal effect is due to binding of ionized calcium in the recipient. This lethal effect of citrated blood is dependent on the rate of infusion, as citrate is metabolized relatively rapidly in every nucleated cell in the body. Its rate of removal is largely limited by its rate of diffusion into the intracellular space. Citrate is also excreted in the urine when blood levels are elevated, but this route of removal will depend on urinary output. In addition to its removal, infusion of citrate causes the mobilization of calcium from skeletal stores, presumably via the action of parathyroid hormone. Parathyroid hormone is released very soon after beginning infusion of a solution containing citrate.[17] Its effects depend on skeletal perfusion which is reduced in response to hemorrhage. It is not known if the ability of the parathyroid glands to rapidly synthesize new hormone can be overcome by prolonged rapid transfusion. There are conflicting reports on the effect of hypovolemia on the ability to metabolically remove infused citrate.

In spite of these uncertainties, it is clear that rapid transfusion of citrated blood causes a significant depression of the level of ionized calcium in the recipient's plasma.[1] Recovery tends to occur fairly quickly when the transfusion is stopped. It is not clear if these changes interfere with cardiac function and represent an abnormality that should be treated. At least one study in heavily transfused patients found little evidence of impaired cardiac function despite ionized calcium concentrations as low as one-third normal.[18] Several recent studies in animals indicate that cardiac output may be well maintained despite low levels of ionized calcium, but that more sophisticated studies such as measurement of dP/dt show changes much earlier. At least one group strongly advocates the use of supplemental calcium during rapid transfusion, but their own data show only small differences in cardiac output, deal only with the period of actual transfusion, and are derived from patients undergoing cardiopulmonary bypass.[19] The problems with supplemented calcium are that "routine" use has probably been lethal in the past,[20] and that even with documentation of decreased ionized calcium levels administration of calcium has not always been helpful.[21] Low ionized calcium has been reported in acutely, severely ill patients who have not been transfused; administration of calcium has had only a transient effect.[22,23]

Objective guidelines for the use of supplemental calcium would be very helpful, since it is a potentially dangerous method of treatment. It was hoped that the well-known effect of hypocalcemia on the electrocardiogram might provide such on-line information. Unfortunately, studies in infants and adults have shown that, while a relationship exists between the concentration of ionized calcium and the duration of the Q-T interval, it is not consistent enough to be predictive.[24,25] For the moment, it is probably best to reserve use of supplemental calcium for situations in which the patient seems not to be responding to adequate treatment (keeping in mind that the most common cause for such a situation is hypovolemia) or when there is objective evidence of acute heart failure. Calcium should be tried cautiously by giving small doses in the ionized form by a route different from that in which the blood is being administered. Laboratory measurement of ionized calcium is usually too slow to be useful in what is a rapidly changing situation. Measurement of total calcium is not only too slow, it is inappropriate. Total calcium usually increases in the plasma during infusion of citrate, and can be above normal when the patient or animal dies of a decreased concentration of ionized calcium.

Hyperkalemia

The concentration of potassium in the plasma of stored blood increases steadily throughout storage, reaching up to 25 to 30 meq/l by the end of the third week. Because hemorrhaging, hypoperfused patients often exhibit hyperkalemia, concern over the effects of transfusion seems warranted. Once again, however, direct measurements in transfused patients yielded paradoxical results. Most such patients seem to be hypokalemic after extensive transfusion.[26-28] The main reason is probably the alkalosis already referred to. In addition, the load of potassium administered by transfusion is much less than it appears to be. The concentrations refer to the plasma phase, so that 10 units of blood contain a plasma total in excess of normal of only about 75 meq. Moreover, most of that represents potassium which has left viable stored red cells and which returns to those red cells after transfusion.[29] The actual load of additional potassium is very small.

In spite of these reassuring observations, there are two points of concern regarding potassium during massive transfusion. The first is that hyperkalemia may occur transiently during very rapid transfusion, especially if the patient is acidotic and hypoperfused. Hyperkalemia worsens the cardiovascular effects of hypocalcemia, both electrical and mechanical.[30, 31] Both complications are unusual, but probably occur in the same setting: very rapid transfusion of large volumes into poorly perfused patients. The potential for harmfully synergistic effects is real. The second problem is that prolonging the period of storage in the liquid state will presumably cause higher concentrations of potassium in the plasma phase.

It should be emphasized that potassium is usually not a problem during massive transfusion, but that a potential for harmful effects certainly exists.

Hypothermia

The specific heat of blood is such that it requires about 150 K cal to warm the usual adult blood volume from 4 °C to 37 °C.[1] This is the amount of heat equivalent to that produced by a half hour of moderately heavy muscular work and requires about 30 liters of oxygen plus the fuel substrates for production. Many studies have shown that patients heavily transfused with refrigerated blood become hypothermic, especially if paralyzed in air-conditioned operating rooms with open body cavities. Core temperatures commonly go into the low 30s C.

Theoretically, hypothermia can be a very serious complication because all of the problems discussed so far are made worse by hypothermia. Hypothermia impairs coagulation in ways not completely clear. Lower temperatures cause a further increase in the affinity of hemoglobin for oxygen. Metabolism of both lactate and citrate are impaired at lower temperatures. Potassium tends to shift from the intracellular to the extracellular space as temperatures decline. Viscious circles are possible because the acidosis of hypothermia will make hyperkalemia worse, which could worsen the effects of hypocalcemia, resulting

in poorer perfusion with worsened acidosis and hyperkalemia.

Clinical studies have strongly suggested better results if hypothermia is avoided or lessened during transfusion, but these studies were not tightly controlled.[32] Controlled studies in animals[31] and in newborn infants[33] failed to show any advantage of avoiding hypothermia. The excellent results obtained in Vietnam may have been in part due to the avoidance of hypothermia because of the hot environment and relative lack of air conditioning.

The question is important enough to receive more definitive study; the theoretical potential for harm is great. Mechanical methods for heating blood during transfusion are available, although all have some drawbacks. The clinical situation dictates rapid warming from 4 °C to 37 °C, but the temperature of contact should not exceed 40 to 42 °C because of the danger of hemolysis. This requires good control of temperature and rapid transfer of heat. Microwave devices have so far proven dangerous. The currently used devices accept a large, dead space to achieve adequate heating of the blood without overheating the contacting surface. Once the dead space is filled, the rate of transfusion can remain rapid. On the basis of currently available evidence, safe heating of blood used for transfusion seems strongly indicated, but more studies are needed.

Pulmonary Insufficiency

Many massively transfused patients develop acute pulmonary insufficiency within a few days following transfusion. The sequence has led many to speculate on a cause-effect relationship. It is possible to construct a list of potential mechanisms by which transfusion might cause pulmonary insufficiency. The most extensively studied is microembolization. Stored blood develops particulate debris of a wide range of sizes. Much of this is small enough to pass through the standard filters used for transfusion (170 micron pores) and presumably lodges in the pulmonary circulation. It is unlikely that this is helpful, but it is not clear to what extent it is harmful.

A fair amount of experimental work in dogs is supportive of microembolization as a mechanism of injury due to extensive transfusion, but studies in primates have been unconvincing at best. One of the early clinical studies seemed to show a lesser degree of impairment of pulmonary function in patients transfused through special fine filters.[34] The two groups in the controlled part of the series, however, were not strictly comparable; all the patients without injury to the chest or abdomen fell into the fine filter group. Another series found differences in patients transfused with only a few units of blood, but the differences were based on differences among groups in the preoperative measurements of pulmonary function; the postoperative values were the same among the different groups.[35] More detailed studies of pulmonary function in transfused patients were interpreted as showing an increased dead space in transfused patients, presumably reflecting pulmonary embolization, but the data reveal that the changes could have been due to differences in cardiac output.[36] Several recent clinical trials have shown no benefit from the use of fine filters, including one well-controlled study involving elderly patients receiving significant volumes of transfused blood.[37-39]

There are other mechanisms whereby transfusion might cause pulmonary edema even during the transfusion of a single unit of blood via changes in pulmonary capillary permeability.[40] A hemolytic transfusion reaction can cause DIC, which is itself a potential cause of pulmonary insufficiency. Certain fractions of stored plasma can be lethal in certain experimental models, and harshly handled blood can be worse than no treatment at all in some models of hemorrhagic shock in dogs. These indicate that some components of plasma may be altered during handling and storage in ways that produce harmful effects on the recipient. Many activated inflammatory mediators cause increased capillary permeability and thereby could cause pulmonary insufficiency. Certain experiments implicate the plasticizer diethylhexylphthalate as a cause of increased pulmonary capillary permeability in transfused rats,[41] but other studies do not support such an interpretation.

Possibly the most common link between transfusion and pulmonary insufficiency is simple hypervolemia with resulting pulmonary edema. It is easy to overshoot in replacing blood volume when the losses are hidden or variable. Some severely hemorrhaging patients develop very significant impairment of left ventricular function, probably as a result of ischemic damage to the left ventricle from reduced supply of oxygen because of coronary arterial insufficiency during periods of increased demand.[16] Finally, patients vomiting large volumes of blood tend to aspirate and to develop a rather severe pneumonitis. In such patients pulmonary insufficiency would follow transfusion, but the two events are only indirectly related.

Whatever the potential mechanisms, the existence of posttransfusion pulmonary insufficiency has been controversial. Several studies from Vietnam found no evidence of such a lesion in heavily transfused combat casualties.[42-44] Other studies found strong evidence of such a connection, usually in the postoperative period, and with a clear dose-response relationship in one study.[45,46] Because of the importance of the question and the obscurity of the answer, we reviewed the records of the first three Army Surgical Research Teams in Vietnam and found a complex pattern.[47] There was no evidence of transfusion-related hypoxemia in the preoperative period. In casualties with injuries limited to the extremities, there was no evidence of transfusion-related hypoxemia in the postoperative period, even in a significantly large group given several blood volumes in transfusion. In casualties with injuries involving the lungs, however, there was a strong dose-response relationship between transfusion and the development and extent of hypoxemia during the first few postoperative days. We interpreted this pattern as indicating that it was the magnitude and site of the injury that were responsible for the apparent relationship. Extensive damage to the lungs caused progressively worsening hypoxemia for several days and also created the need for extensive transfusion. When the chest or abdomen was not injured directly, no relationship was seen despite the use of very large amounts of blood.

As all the transfusions involved in the study[47] were done with 3-week-old blood with only gross filters and involved large numbers of patients receiving very large amounts of blood, the results are very reassuring regarding any of the potential mechanisms whereby transfusion might cause pulmonary insufficiency. The patients studied, however, were the healthiest possible, aside from the recent injuries: 18 to 22 years old, medically screened, and athletically conditioned. A study in a much older civilian population also found very little evidence of pulmonary insufficiency in those heavily transfused with or without fine filters,[39] but a recent study found moderate degrees of pulmonary insufficiency in patients transfused with or without fine filters.[37] There thus may be some relationship, but it is almost certain that, if any lesion at all is produced by transfusion, it is not a severe one.

Other Problems

Many other problems are possible as a result of massive transfusion. In fact, every way in which stored blood differs from normal blood is potentially a source of difficulty. Concentrations of phosphate and of ammonia are moderately high in stored blood; but, in terms of the total body stores, these levels are not very significant. Plasticizer leaches from the plastic bag into the stored blood at about .25 mgm per 100 ml of blood per day of storage. This is not desirable. Various studies have indicated that these plasticizers can be biologically harmful; however, there has been very little evidence of toxicity in the amounts and forms encountered as a result of transfusion. Exposure to the same plasticizers occurs significantly in the course of living in the United States. One alternative, returning to glass containers, has such great disadvantages that it is not seriously considered. The other alternative, developing of plastic containers without leachable plasticizers, is being explored.

Potential problems from altered protein components have already been referred to in the discussion of pulmonary insufficiency. Both kinins and Hageman-factor fragments have been identified in plasma protein fractions and may have been responsible for serious adverse reactions in human recipients.[48] There is some experimental evidence that transfusion may impair reticuloendothelial function.[49] The phagocytic cells in stored blood do not function after several days of storage.[50] The problem of impaired antibacterial defenses after major injury or massive transfusion is unquestionably of great clinical significance. Recently, there has been a resurgence of interest in the effects of various plasma components on antibacterial defenses. The effects of using red cell concentrates instead of whole blood have been investigated with reports of impaired opsonic activity in animals[51] but little or no evidence of such effect in man.[52] Reports of depletion of opsonic factors in serious illness which can be replaced by administering cryoprecipitate are being evaluated. The entire field of the effects of treatment with blood and blood components on antibacterial defenses is an extremely important one that deserves considerable attention. It may be second in importance only to control of transfusion-associated hepatitis.

Infants

Massive transfusion is rarely a surgical problem in infants. Most of the above discussions refer to adults. Extensive transfusion is occasionally used to treat various nonsurgical conditions in infants, especially as exchange transfusion. Some of the problems that are relatively well managed by adults may be much less well tolerated or compensated for by the immature systems of the newborn (see Ch. 33).

CARDIOPULMONARY BYPASS

Cardiopulmonary bypass by means of extracorporeal circulation represents a unique situation in surgery. The entire circulating blood volume is continuously and simultaneously being withdrawn and reinfused. This requires extensive dilution and extensive contact of the blood with foreign surfaces and with a gas interface. There is no comparable clinical situation. It is not surprising that there are special problems associated with this procedure.

In the early experience with extracorporeal circulation, whole blood was used to "prime" the device so that the circulation was maintained largely undiluted but with extensive mixing with donor blood, often equal or exceeding the patient's normal blood volume. There was extensive contact with metallic surfaces as well as plastic, gas, and topical silicone. Mechanical damage to circulating red cells tended to be greater than at present; perfusion of the patient was usually poorer; the procedures were longer; and higher pressure suction was commonly used to return shed blood to the system. Compared to current results, patients then were more acidotic and poorly perfused, had more embolization by tissue particles, fat and silicone particles, had a higher incidence of postoperative pulmonary and renal failure, and had a peculiar series of febrile disorders variously labeled "pump syndrome," "homologous blood syndrome," and "postcardiotomy syndrome." Some of these cases were due to infection by cytomegalovirus, but many were not.

There were probably many reasons for these poorer results. Results seemed to improve markedly, however, when an unconventional approach was used: dilution with nonblood fluids by "priming" the device with simple electrolyte solutions with or without albumin. Other improvements were occurring simultaneously, but there was certainly a strong impression that dilutional bypass produced much less damage. The reasons are largely speculative, but a number of experiments demonstrated in animals that circulating citrated whole blood through an extracorporeal circulatory device made it capable of producing harmful effects in recipient animals. Among the factors proposed as likely mechanisms were hemolysis, denaturation of proteins, activation of various coagulation factors, aggregation of platelets, disruption of leukocytes, and activation of inflammatory mediators. A variety of effects may in fact have been involved. Hemodilution presumably lessened many of these effects. While results are now better, they are still far from perfect, and prolonged bypass is still poorly tolerated. Attention is now being directed toward extracorporeal devices that have less potential for altering circulating blood, such as membrane oxygenators and refined pumping systems, for situations requiring prolonged cardiopulmonary bypass.

Perhaps the most common persisting aberration after bypass is the disruption of normal hemostasis. This, too, seems less severe now than in the early days of the technique, but it is clearly a persisting problem. There have been many studies reported of hemostatic function in patients after bypass, and the results are not always consistent. There have been many proposed mechanisms for the hemostatic abnormality, but no single convincing pattern is evident. One of the problems inherent in comparing these studies is the large number of potential variables among the different studies. Often, no basis exists for judging comparability because some of the pertinent factors are not described in the reports. Some of the pertinent variables include: the preoperative status of the patient; the type of pump used; the type of oxygenator used; the type of priming solution; the extent of total dilution and the nature of the diluting solutions; the operative procedure; the experience of the operative team; the duration of bypass; the details of the use of heparin and of protamine; the temperatures of the patients; the time after bypass when the studies were done; the extent of postoperative blood loss; the incidence of reoperation for hemorrhage; the use of blood or components postoperatively; and the use of drugs that interfere with platelet function. Almost no reported study gives details on all of these points. It is not surprising, then, that interpretation of results has been difficult.

One of the first large series evaluated specifically for bypass hemorrhage found the following correlations[53]:

1. Total blood loss after extracorporeal circulation was greater in patients having ventriculotomy than in those having atriotomy or arteriotomy.

2. Longer duration of bypass was associated with greater postoperative blood loss, with about 1 ml additional blood loss per minute of bypass above 60 minutes. (However, duration of bypass is also a function of the complexity of the procedure.)

3. Cyanotic congenital heart disease was associated with three times greater blood loss than acyanotic congenital heart disease, perhaps reflecting the well-known effect of erythrocythemia, but again there were proba-

bly differences in types of procedure and duration of bypass.

Surprisingly, repeat cardiotomies were associated with only slightly greater blood loss than the same procedures done for the first time. The incidence of reoperation for bleeding was three percent. Experiences reported from different centers are not identical, but the above is reasonably representative.

Detailed studies of the coagulation system and of platelet function after cardiopulmonary bypass have yielded generally similar patterns.[54-58] There is a significant decrease in the concentration of all coagulation factors and in the number of platelets immediately after cessation of bypass, with significant recovery back toward normal by 3 to 4 hours postoperatively. In addition, various aspects of platelet function are impaired. There does not appear to be a single, dominant cause of excessive bleeding following cardiopulmonary bypass. At least three different patterns have been reported: mechanical causes, platelet dysfunction, and coagulation defects. The last group includes patients who have lingering effects of heparin, or in whom the protamine has been metabolized more rapidly than the heparin so that initially adequate reversal of the effects of heparin disappears a few hours postoperatively.

The postulated causes for the platelet dysfunction include aggregation on the foreign surfaces during bypass, dilution with nonfunctioning platelets from recently drawn citrated blood, aggregation by ADP from hemolyzed red cells during bypass (aggregation by ADP is often the most markedly abnormal function), and others.[56,57] Coagulation defects have been assumed to be due to: dilution (which can account for part but not all of a defect); lingering heparin; heparin-protamine complexes; circulating inhibitors; fibrinolysis; DIC; and other factors. Apart from the dynamics of heparin, DIC has received the most attention as a potential cause for hemostatic failure following bypass. In fact, there is surprisingly little solid evidence to support the occurrence of DIC in more than a very occasional patient who is doing badly and may be in DIC from hypoperfusion rather than bypass. One study demonstrated high levels of fibrin degradation products in the chest tube drainage of patients after cardiotomy and also patients following thoracotomy without cardiopulmonary bypass.[58] The simultaneous blood levels of fibrin degradation products were very low.

One large retrospective study reported on the value of various studies of hemostasis done soon after operation in predicting which patients would bleed excessively.[59] Prolonged prothrombin times, partial thromboplastin times, and low fibrinogen concentrations correlated roughly with the extent of postoperative bleeding. Platelet counts and the levels of fibrin(ogen) degradation and split products had no predictive value. The overall rate of reoperation for bleeding in this large series was a remarkably low 0.5 percent, a result the authors attributed to prompt use of appropriate supplemental blood components in the 20 percent of patients found to have more than the usual degree of coagulation abnormality. This, however, was not a controlled trial.

Several other large series found that measured coagulation abnormalities correlated poorly with clinical bleeding. The most useful role for coagulation studies in the patient bleeding excessively after cardiopulmonary bypass is in detecting the patient who needs immediate reoperation. The patient with rapid bleeding and only mild coagulation abnormalities almost certainly needs to be reexplored to establish better mechanical hemostasis. Most authors seem to agree that marked coagulation abnormalities should be corrected promptly despite the poor correlation with clinical bleeding, and that the bleeding patient with a markedly prolonged bleeding time should be given platelets. Following bypass is one situation in which heparin assays and/or titration tests with pro-

tamine can be helpful; however, the adequacy of reversal by protamine may be temporary because its metabolic removal is more rapid than that of heparin.

A comment is called for on the use of blood in cardiopulmonary bypass. Most of the centers with the largest experience and most admirable results use nonblood primes. It is difficult to justify the use of whole blood for priming bypass equipment in the face of these reported results. This is becoming less common in the United States but still persists in some areas. On the basis of the published record, it seems to represent waste of blood, needless exposure of the patient to hepatitis and immunization, and, ironically, perhaps a higher risk of a variety of complications.

REFERENCES

1. Collins, J.A.: Massive blood transfusion. Clin. Haematol. 5:201, 1976.
2. Massaglia, G. and Thomas, E.D.: Mathematical consideration of cross-circulation and exchange transfusion. Transfusion 11:216, 1971.
3. Wiener, A.S. and Wexler, I.B.: The use of heparin when performing exchange blood transfusions in newborn infants. J. Lab. Clin. Med. 31:1016, 1946.
4. Harke, H. and Rahman, S.: Haemostatic disorders in massive transfusion. Bibl. Haematol. 46:179, 1980.
5. Oski, F.A., Marshall, B.E., Cohen, P.J., Sugerman, H.J., and Miller, L.J.: Exercise with anemia: the role of the left-shifted or right-shifted oxygen-hemoglobin equilibrium curve. Ann. Intern. Med. 74:44, 1971.
6. Huggins, C.E., Suzuki, H., and Grove-Rasmussen, M.: Life support by liquid and frozen blood. Abstr. 24th Ann. Meeting, Am. Assn. Blood Banks, 1971, p. 94.
7. Oski, F.A., Gottlieb, A.J., and Miller, L.D.: The influences of heredity and environment on the red cell's function of oxygen transport. Med. Clin. N. Am. 54:731, 1970.
8. Bellingham, A.J.: Haemoglobins with altered oxygen affinity. Br. Med. Bull. 32:234, 1976.
9. Collins, J.A., Simmons, R.L., James, P.M.,

Bredenberg, C.E., Anderson, R.W., and Heisterkamp, C.A.: The acid-base status of seriously wounded combat casualties. II. Resuscitation with stored blood. Ann. Surg. 173:6, 1971.

10. Woodson, R.D., Wranne, B., and Delter, J.C.: Effect of increased blood oxygen affinity on work performance of rats. J. Clin. Invest. 52:2717, 1973.

11. Wranne, B., Nordgren, L., and Woodson, R.D.: Increased blood oxygen affinity and physical work capacity in man. Scand. J. Clin. Lab. Invest. 33:347, 1974.

12. Collins, J.A. and Stechenberg, L.: The effects of the concentration and function of hemoglobin on the survival of rats after hemorrhage. Surgery 85:412, 1979.

13. Malmberg, P., Hlastala, M.O., and Woodson, R.D.: The effect of increased blood oxygen affinity on oxygen transport in hemorrhagic shock. J. Appl. Physiol. 47:889, 1979.

14. Case, R.B., Berglund, E., and Sarnoff, S.J.: Ventricular function. VII. Changes in acute coronary resistance and ventricular function resulting from acutely induced anemia and the effect thereon of coronary stenosis. Am. J. Med. 18:397, 1955.

15. Dennis, R.C., Vito, L., Weisel, R.D., Valeri, C.R., Berger, R.L., and Hechtman, H.B.: Improved myocardial performance following high 2,3-DPG red cell transfusion. Surgery 77:741, 1975.

16. Weisel, R.D., Dennis, R.C., Manny, J., Mannick, J.A., Valeri, R., and Hechtman, H.B.: Adverse effects of transfusion therapy during abdominal aortic aneurysmectomy. Surgery 83:682, 1978.

17. Miller, R.N., Engelhardt, R., Collins, J.A., Slatopolsky, E., and Ladenson, J.H.: Observations on the biochemical effects of transfusion of citrate-phosphate-dextrose stored blood in man. Laryngoscope 86:1272, 1976.

18. Howland, W.S., Schweizer, O., Carlon, G.C., and Goldiner, P.L.: The cardiovascular effects of low ionized calcium during massive transfusion. Surg., Gynecol., Obstet. 145:581, 1977.

19. Olinger, G.N., Hottenrot, C., Mulder, D.G. et al.: Acute clinical hypocalcemic myocardial depression during rapid blood transfusion and postoperative hemodialysis. J. Thorac. Cardiovasc. Surg. 72:503, 1976.

20. Wolf, P.L., McCarthy, L.J., and Hafleigh, B.: Extreme hypercalcemia following blood transfusions combined with intravenous calcium. Vox Sang. 19:544, 1970.

21. Carlon, G.C., Howland, W.S., Goldiner, P.L., Kahn, R.C., Bertoni, G., and Turnbull, A.D.: Adverse effects of calcium administration. Arch. Surg. 113:882, 1978.

22. Drop, L.J. and Lower, M.B.: Low plasma ionized calcium and response to calcium therapy in critically ill man. Anesthesiol. 43:300, 1975.

23. Taylor, B., Sibbald, W.J., Ydmonds, M.W. et al.: Ionized hypocalcemia in critically ill patients with sepsis. Canad. J. Surg. 21:429, 1978.

24. Giacoia, G.P. and Wagner, H.R.: Q-oTc interval and blood calcium levels in newborn infants. Pediatrics 61:877, 1978.

25. Ladenson, J.H., Miller, W.V., and Sherman, L.A.: Relationship of physical symptoms, ECG, free calcium, and other blood chemistries in reinfusion with citrated blood. Transfusion 18:670, 1978.

26. Bunker, J.P., Stetson, J.B., Coe, R.C. et al.: Citric acid intoxication. J.A.M.A. 157:1361, 1955.

27. Schweizer, O. and Howland, W.S.: Potassium levels, acid base balance and massive blood replacement. Anesthesiology 23:735, 1962.

28. Wilson, R.F., Mammon, E., and Walt, A.J.: Eight years of experience with massive blood transfusion. J. Trauma 11:275, 1971.

29. Valeri, C.R. and Hirsch, N.M.: Restoration in vivo of erythrocyte adenosine triphosphate, 2,3-diphosphoglycerate, potassium ion, and sodium ion concentrations following the transfusion of acid-citrate-dextrose-stored human red blood cells. J. Lab. Clin. Med. 73:722, 1969.

30. Lee, Y.C.P., Richman, H.G., and Visscher, M.B.: $[Ca^{++}]$ and $[K^{+}]$ interrelations influencing mechanical and electrical events in cardiac activity. Am. J. Physiol. 210:499, 1966.

31. Taylor, W.C., Gillis, C.N., Nash, C.W., and Kallman, G.L.: Experimental observations on cardiac arrhythmia during exchange transfusion in rabbits. J. Pediatr. 58:470, 1961.

32. Boyan, C.P.: Cold or warmed blood for massive transfusions. Am. Surg. 160:282, 1964.

33. Milner, R.D.G., Fekete, M., Hodge, J.S., and Assau, R.: Influence of donor blood tempera-

ture on metabolic and hormonal changes during exchange transfusion. Arch. Dis. Child. 47:933, 1972.

34. Reul, G.J., Greenburg, S.D., Lefrak, E.A., McCollum, W.B., Beall, A.C., and Jordan, G.L.: Prevention of post-traumatic pulmonary insufficiency: fine screen filtration of blood. Arch. Surg. 106:386, 1973.

35. Barrett, J., Tahir, A.H., and Litwin, M.S.: Increased pulmonary arteriovenous shunting in humans following blood transfusion. Arch. Surg. 113:947, 1978.

36. Takaori, M., Nakajo, N., and Ishii, T.: Changes of pulmonary function following transfusion of stored blood. Transfusion 17:615, 1977.

37. Durtschi, M.B., Haisch, C.E., Reynolds, L., Pavlin, E., Kohler, T.R., Heimbach, D.M., and Carrico, C.J.: Effects of micropore filtration on pulmonary function after massive transfusion. Am. J. Surg. 138:8, 1979.

38. Snyder, E.L., Underwood, P.S., Spivack, M., DeAngeles, L., and Haberman, E.T.: An in vivo evaluation of microaggregate blood filtration during total hip replacement. Ann. Surg. 190:75, 1979.

39. Virgilio, R.W.: A prospective controlled study on the effect of fine filters on postoperative pulmonary function in heavily transfused patients. In: Proc. Symp. on Microaggregates, U.S. Army R+D Command. Geelhoed, G., ed. (in press).

40. Wolf, C.L. and Canale, V.C.: Fatal pulmonary hypersensitivity reaction to HL-A incompatible blood transfusion: report of a case and review of the literature. Transfusion 16:135, 1976.

41. Berman, I.R., Iliescu, H., and Stachura, I.: Pulmonary effects of blood container materials. Surg. Forum 28:182, 1977.

42. Carey, L.C., Lowery, B.D., and Cloutier, C.T.: Hemorrhagic shock. Curr. Probl. Surg. 8:23, 1971.

43. Collins, J.A., Gordon, W.C., Hudson, T.L., Irvin, R.W., Kelly, T., and Hardaway, R.M.: Inapparent hypoxemia in casualties with wounded limbs: pulmonary fat embolism? Ann. Surg. 167:511, 1968.

44. Martin, A.M., Simmons, R.L., and Heisterkamp, C.A.: Respiratory insufficiency in combat casualties. I. Pathologic changes in the lungs of patients dying of wounds. Ann. Surg. 170:30, 1969.

45. McNamara, J.J., Molot, M.D., and Stremple, J.F.: Screen filtration pressure in combat casualties. Ann. Surg. 172:334, 1976.

46. Simmons, R.L., Heisterkamp, C.A., Collins, J.A., Gensler, S., and Martin, A.M.: Respiratory insufficiency in combat casualties. IV. Hypoxemia during convalescence. Ann. Surg. 170:53, 1969.

47. Collins, J.A., James, P.M., Bredenberg, C.E., Anderson, R.W., Heisterkamp, C.A., and Simmons, R.L.: The relationship between transfusion and hypoxemia in combat casualties. Ann. Surg. 188:513, 1978.

48. Alving, B.M., Hojima, Y., Pisano, J.J., Mason, B.L., Buckingham, R.E., Mozen, M.M., and Finlayson, J.S.: Hypotension associated with prekallikrein activator (Hageman-factor fragments) in plasma protein fraction. N. Engl. J. Med. 299:66, 1978.

49. Wilson, J.D., Taswell, H.F., and Didisheim, P.: Effects of washed cell and whole-blood transfusion on reticuloendothelial function in dogs. Transfusion 9:289, 1969.

50. McCullough, J., Benson, S.J., Yunis, E.J., and Quie, P.G.: Effect of blood-bank storage on leukocyte function. Lancet 2:1333, 1969.

51. Alexander, J.W.: Hemotherapy and antibacterial defense mechanisms. Bibl. Haematol. 46:26, 1980.

52. Pappova, E., Lundsgaard-Hansen, P., Senn, A., and Tschirren, B.: Serum levels of IgG and C_3, postoperative infections, and blood component therapy. Bibl. Haematol. 46:37, 1980.

53. Gomes, M.M.R. and McGoon, D.C.: Bleeding patterns after open-heart surgery. J. Thorac. Cardiovasc. Surg. 60:87, 1970.

54. Bachman, F., McKenna, R., Cole, E.R., and Najafi, H.: The hemostatic mechanism after open-heart surgery. I. Studies on plasma coagulation factors and fibrinolysis in 512 patients after extracorporeal circulation. J. Thorac. Cardiovasc. Surg. 70:76, 1975.

55. Kalter, R.D., Saul, C.M., Wetstein, L., Soriano, C., and Reiss, R.F.: Cardiopulmonary bypass: associated hemostatic abnormalities. J. Thorac. Cardiovasc. Surg. 77:427, 1979.

56. McKenna, R., Bachman, F., Whittacker, B., Gilson, J.R., and Weinberg, M.: The hemo-

static mechanism after open-heart surgery. II. Frequency of abnormal platelet functions during and after extracorporeal circulation. J. Thorac. Cardiovasc. Surg. 70:298, 1975.

57. Salzman, E.: Blood platelets and extracorporeal circulation. Transfusion 3:274, 1963.

58. Umlas, J.: Fibrinolysis and disseminated intravascular coagulation in open heart surgery. Transfusion 16:460, 1976.

59. Marengo-Rower, A.J., Lambert, C.J., Leveson, J.E., Thiele, J.P., Geisler, G.F., Adam, M., and Mitchell, B.F.: The evaluation of hemorrhage in cardiac patients who have undergone extracorporeal circulation. Transfusion 19:426, 1979.

23

Anesthesiologic Perspectives of Blood Transfusion

William S. Howland, M.D.

The anesthesiologist requires blood bank products to correct significant preoperative anemia, sustain intravascular volume, replace operative blood loss, and reverse blood coagulation deficits.

PREOPERATIVE ANEMIA

The correction of significant preoperative anemia is usually accomplished before the anesthesiologist makes his preoperative visit. The origin of the traditional recommended requirement of 10 grams of hemoglobin in order to receive anesthesia is shrouded in obscurity, unsubstantiated by clinical investigation, and yet a standard in anesthetic practice. In these days of fear of unjustified malpractice claims, anesthetizing a patient with a hemoglobin level below 10 grams for an elective operation is seldom done. More significant to the anesthesiologist than the level of hemoglobin is the cause of the anemia. Adequate tissue oxygenation can be accomplished with a hemoglobin level less than 10 grams if it is appreciated that oxygen delivery is a function of the paO_2 which is elevated during anesthesia, hemoglobin saturation, hemoglobin level, hemoglobin oxygen affinity, cardiac output, peripheral vascular resistance, and blood volume. Therefore, the as-sessment of hemoglobin in the preoperative period should also correlate the cause and duration of the anemia, the patient's cardiac status, the status of lung function, and the type and probable duration of the surgery.

VOLUME OF BLOOD ADMINISTERED

The administration of banked blood with its "storage lesion" should be considered in relation to the size of the patient and the rate of transfusion. If the patient's weight is considered, two common misapprehensions can be negated. The first is to avoid the "single" blood transfusion. Common sense will allow that the administration of one unit of blood to a 10-kg child with a blood volume of 800 ml is not malfeasance. Similarly, 10 units of blood administered to a 100-kg patient will have different effects than the same volume administered to a 50-kg individual. Also, it is apparent that the term "massive" transfusion really means "rapid" transfusion as far as deleterious effects on the patient are concerned. Ten units given in 10 hours will have different effects than 10 units administered in one hour. Thus, the therapeutic effectiveness of blood replacement depends upon the ability of the recipient to reverse the "storage" lesion of bank blood relative to the speed of transfusion. The principal conditions which must be reversed to restore the normal physiologic status of red cells and plasma after transfusion into the recipient include: (1) the outward shift of potassium from the red cells and the depletion of intraerythrocytic 2,3-DPG and ATP levels; (2) the elevated pCO_2 and acid content of the blood unit; (3) the absence of ionized calcium from banked blood; (4) the temperature of the administered blood (4° C ± 2); (5) the partial depletion of plasma coagulation factors, particularly V and VIII; and (6) the decrease in viable and functional thrombocytes.

As will be discussed later, (1) the hyperkalemia of transfused blood does not require specific treatment in adults; (2) 2,3-DPG levels rise with return of the cells to in vivo conditions; (3) the elevated $paCO_2$ is eliminated by the lungs; (4) the decreased bicarbonate may require buffering; (5) the hypocalcemia will correct itself; (6) the temperature can be corrected with blood warmers; (7) the decrease of coagulation factors can be corrected with fresh frozen plasma or specific concentrates; and (8) defective platelet "functional" activity and/or decreased numbers can be treated with platelet concentrates. Infrequently, replacement of coagulant factors and platelets is necessary in routine practice.

The management of the patient who receives rapid and massive blood transfusion will be presented and the rationale for it discussed later.

BLOOD COMPONENTS

Modern blood banking techniques have resulted in the anesthesiologist being supplied with blood components instead of whole blood for replacement therapy in the operating and recovery rooms. Although the anesthesiologist will use many of the blood components often, some infrequently, and a few only in special instances, he should be familiar with the components available and their indications for use.

Red Cell Preparations

Whole Blood. 450 ml donor blood plus 63 ml anticoagulant, hematocrit 42 ± 2.0 percent. This is the material of choice for use whenever possible for blood volume loss replacement.

Concentrated Red Cells. 300 ± 20 ml with hematocrit of 70 to 90 percent, depending upon preparation by sedimentation or centrifugation. Concentrated red cells may have to be reconstituted with compatible single unit plasma or albumin if administration of a large volume is necessary and whole blood is not available.

Leukocyte-poor Red Cells. These are usually administered to patients to prevent white cell reactions in the previously sensitized patient.

Modified Whole Blood. This material has had the platelets and, in some instances, the cryoprecipitate removed from the plasma. Its use is much the same as concentrated red cells.

Frozen Red Cells. These are principally used to preserve rare blood types for long periods.

Washed Red Cells. These are used for patients who have anaphylactoid reactions to IgA, or to remove white cells to prevent febrile reaction.

Platelet Preparations

Platelet Concentrates. These are prepared by pooling platelets from six to eight random donors. One unit contains about 50 ml, and 5×10^{10} to 10×10^{10} platelets. Pooled concentrated platelets may ultimately alloimmunize patients and decrease the efficiency of further platelet transfusions.

HLA-Typed Single Donor Platelets. These platelets collected by mechanical means are used to minimize antigenic differences between donor and alloimmunized recipients. (See Chs. 26 and 27.)

Coagulation Factor Products

Cryoprecipitate. This product contains Factor VIII and Fibrinogen; the Factor VIII content is 80 to 120 units, and the Fibrinogen content is 300 to 400 mgm in 10 to 15 ml of plasma.

Fresh Frozen Plasma. This material contains all plasma coagulation factors.

Whole Blood. Only factors V and VIII decrease to any extent with storage in CPD solution. Although whole blood is usually regarded as primarily a red cell replacement material, it also replaces some coagulation factors quite efficiently.

Concentrated Factor VIII. This material is of use primarily in hemophilia A patients undergoing surgery.

Prothrombin Complex Concentrates. These contain factors II, VII, IX and X. They are of use primarily in hemophilia B patients.

White Blood Cell Products

These are principally granulocytes, for use in granulocytopenic recipients with severe infections.

Plasma Volume Expanders

Natural Albumin

1. Single donor plasma
2. Fresh frozen plasma

Manufactured Albumin

1. 5% plasma protein fraction (250 ml)
2. 5% human albumin (250 ml)
3. 25% human albumin (50 ml). This material is almost always administered with electrolyte solutions.

Artificial Volume Expanders. These are largely obsolete in practice in the U.S. (See Ch. 35.)

The starting product for most component therapy is whole blood drawn into a multi-compartment container containing an anticoagulant. At present, the principal anticoagulant in use is CPD or CPD-A1, a mixture of sodium citrate, citric acid, a phosphate buffer, and dextrose with or without supplemental adenine. The blood bank routinely provides primarily packed red blood cells for the anesthesiologist and surgeon to use in the operating room or emergency room and to the internist to use on the wards of the hospital if a total program of component therapy is to be successful. In specific circumstances, the following products are available: granulocytes, platelets, fresh frozen plasma, salt poor albumin, cryoprecipitates, or frozen red blood cells.

RED CELL CONCENTRATES

Concentrated red blood cells can be prepared by centrifugation or sedimentation. Centrifugation now can be performed at any time after collection without producing cell injury. The hematocrit of this component should not be more than 70 percent to maintain sufficient available plasma glucose, to preserve red blood cell viability, and provide adequate fluidity during transfusion. Many anesthesiologists feel that this procedure does not, in fact, provide adequate flow properties for use in the operating room, when they are required to administer cold, high-hematocrit, slowly flowing blood to patients requiring large volumes in a hurry. One solution to this problem is to reconstitute the packed red blood cells with either a plasma volume expander or crystalloid. This presupposes that the anesthesiologist has available sufficient ventilating and monitoring equipment to obviate need for his constant attention to the patient. Better yet, ancillary assistance should be available to reconstitute the packed red blood cells. Sedimented red cells can be diluted easily with normal saline solution to decrease viscosity.

To the anesthesiologist, the ambiguous term "packed red blood cells" usually means a unit of whole blood from which the plasma has been removed. To the blood banker, the designation of a whole blood component as "packed red blood cells" is generally assumed to mean red blood cells from which most of the plasma has been removed by sedimentation or centrifugation. However, the term can also include centrifuged red cells from which the buffy coat (leukocytes and platelets) have been largely removed, and also washed red cells in which plasma and buffy coat have been removed by at least three washings. Thus, four products are available to the clinician, all with somewhat different characteristics: gravity-sedimented red cells, centrifuged red cells with or without the buffy coat removed, and washed red cells.

Sedimented red blood cells are the most readily available because no mechanical equipment is needed to prepare them. They also contain practically all of the leukocytes and platelets,[1] and have almost the same (less than 1 meq/l difference) plasma potassium[2] as whole blood. The reduction in plasma volume (hematocrit 65 to 70 percent) is insufficient to prevent IgA allergic reactions or hepatitis.[3] Centrifuged red blood cells permit harvesting of more plasma (hematocrit 80 percent), but this increases problems associated with elevated viscosity.

Centrifuged red blood cells with the buffy coat partially but not competely removed should contain a maximum of about 30 percent of the leukocytes present in the original donor unit. The percentage can be reduced further with scrupulous attention to procedures. This product provides no protection against the development of hepatitis.[4] Also, sufficient leukocytes and platelets are present to cause alloimmunization in the previously unsensitized patient. However, this degree of leukocyte removal is adequate to prevent febrile reactions in most patients.

For many patients, washed red blood cells have little to offer over "buffy coat poor" red blood cells. Washed red blood cells are more expensive to prepare and increase the risk of bacterial contamination. Machine-washed red cells are preferable to batch-washed cells because machine washing is more efficient and effective. Patients who develop anaphylactoid reactions to IgA must receive red blood cells almost completely free of plasma. Even the small amount of plasma, less than 1 percent, that remains in well-washed red blood cells can cause transfusion reactions in some of these patients.

It has been stated that fewer febrile transfusion reactions occur with "concentrated red blood cells," but it should be emphasized that this refers to "buffy coat poor" red blood cells or previously frozen, washed, and concentrated red cells. These products are usually not easily available to the clinician and are quite different from the concentrated red blood cells available in most blood banks. In one report, 59 percent of transfusion reactions were caused by the usual concentrated red blood cells.[5]

Recent work in dogs has suggested that whole blood may be preferable to packed red cells for resuscitation of acute hemorrhagic shock when the effect on resistance to infection is considered.[6] Dogs subjected to a high level of controlled blood loss experienced depressions in serum protein, C3, IgG, and total opsonic activity when resuscitated with packed red cells in saline. This did not occur where whole blood was used. The significance of these observations in the case of man is unclear. Such findings could be of significance in blood replacement practices in patients who might have preexistent diminished opsonic activity and defense against infection as a result of other causes.

The problems associated with use of concentrated red blood cells are two-fold. The first is the need to use reasonably a source which is produced as a product of the preparation of other valuable blood components. This product may be more expensive than whole blood if plasma substitutes are also necessary to replace surgically induced blood volume loss. About 60 percent of blood is used intraoperatively in the U.S. The second is that, while concentrated red blood cells are completely adequate to treat the deficiency in oxygen-carrying capacity associated with anemia not related to acute blood loss, they are difficult to administer rapidly and often must be reconstituted or diluted if sudden, rapid blood loss occurs.

INDICATIONS FOR RED CELLS

It is now generally accepted that the primary indication for red blood cell concentrate transfusion is to replace a deficient red blood cell oxygen-carrying capacity. Many transfusion therapists have advocated that one-third to one-half of all transfusions in the operating room be given as packed red blood cells.[7] This can be accomplished by giving the first several units as packed red cells. This may require that they be diluted with saline solution or plasma protein products if whole blood is not available, and to provide adequate rheological properties. The claim that the incidence of hepatitis with use of concentrated red blood cells is less than that with whole blood appears to be incorrect.

Cryopreserved red cells have a number of specific uses. Although the available methods of cryopreservation vary, they have one common major requirement—the necessity of adding the cryoprotective agent, glycerol, prior to freezing. Since the intravenous administration of substantial amounts of glycerol is undesirable, glycerol-protected blood must be washed prior to transfusion. The cost of washing in both dollars and time has restricted severely the routine use of previously frozen red cells in clinical practice. Furthermore, red cell freezing and washing require multiple entries into the blood pack, thereby restricting the post-thaw shelf life to 24 hours.

For many transfusion situations, contamination of the red cell preparation with leukocytes is undesirable and sometimes dangerous. Compared with liquid-stored blood, frozen washed red cells have few leukocytes and virtually no platelets. Frozen washed red cell preparations are also essentially free of detectable plasma proteins. Thus, febrile and IgA-induced allergic transfusion reactions are largely eliminated by using frozen blood.

PLASMA PRODUCTS: COAGULATION FACTORS

The plasma that is separated from the red blood cells is a source material for a number of products such as albumin, plasma protein fraction (PPF), Factor VIII concentrate, and Factor IX complex. Fresh-frozen plasma is the blood component most useful for hemostasis in the operating room which is usually easily available to the anesthesiologist. Fresh-frozen plasma preserves the maximal levels of the labile coagulant proteins, Factors V and VIII. Fresh-frozen plasma can be prepared routinely in the blood bank and is generally more practical to use than either fresh plasma or frozen lyophilized plasma. Anti-A and Anti-B antibodies normally are present in the plasma of individuals lacking the corresponding antigen. Thus, although plasma transfusion may be given without a crossmatch, it must be compatible with the recipient's ABO group. In order to preserve the clotting factors, the plasma should be transfused within 6 hours after it is thawed. Additionally, the anesthesiologist must be alert to the fact that some single donor frozen plasma has had Factor VIII removed. Thus, it is a practice in some hospitals to order single donor fresh-frozen plasma with clotting factors and single donor plasma without clotting factors. It is also the practice at Memorial Hospital to administer one unit of fresh frozen plasma with clotting factors present for each five units of packed red blood cells or whole blood administered. It is our experience, after studying many thousands of these cases, that coagulation deficiencies of Factors

V and VIII or other plasma clotting factors do not occur if this routine is followed. The need for this has been questioned, however. (See Ch. 24.)

Fresh-frozen plasma is also useful when a patient on Coumadin therapy must be operated on as an emergency. Fresh frozen plasma will achieve the desired hemostatic levels of vitamin K-dependent coagulation factors before parenterally administered vitamin K_1 will be effective.

Although hemophilia is seldom encountered by the anesthesiologist, he must be prepared to treat such patients. At the present time, therapy of hemophilia A is accomplished with Factor VIII concentrate or with cryoprecipitate which is prepared by thawing of a unit of fresh frozen plasma under controlled conditions and recovering the cold precipitated factors. Each bag of cryoprecipitate[8] has about 30 to 50 percent of the Factor VIII activity of the original unit of plasma and less than 3 to 5 percent of the original volume as well as substantial amounts of fibrinogen. Cryoprecipitate is useful in the treatment of patients with classic hemophilia, Von Willebrand's disease, Factor XIII deficiency, and decreased fibrinogen levels. An additional component available to the anesthesiologist is Factor IX complex, which contains Factors II, VII, IX, and X. Factor IX complex is indicated in any congenital deficiency of Factors II, VII, IX, or X, and it is of particular benefit to those patients with Christmas disease or Factor IX deficiency (Hemophilia B). Although Factor IX complex would be of value in treating acquired coagulation deficiencies such as in severe liver disease, the risk of hepatitis and of induced thrombosis is so great that its use should be reserved for only the most exceptional circumstances. (See Ch. 25.)

USE OF ALBUMIN PRODUCTS

Albumin is one of the most important of the plasma components. The functions of albumin, in addition to providing volume expansion, are those of specific oncotic activity and as an agent to transport various substances in a bound state. It has been our belief and that of others[9] that the incidence and severity of pulmonary insufficiency in the postoperative period is decreased if combinations of colloid and crystalloid are used for volume replacement rather than large volumes of crystalloid alone. This is especially true in patients with interstitial lung disease who may have received chemotherapy or radiation therapy in the preoperative period. Infusion of fresh frozen plasma appears to have a greater oncotic activity when compared with 25 percent albumin appropriately diluted or 5 percent albumin. In a study comparing fresh frozen plasma, 5 percent albumin, and normal saline in patients with interstitial lung disease, it was found that fresh frozen plasma resulted in more oxygen availability as defined by arteriovenous O_2 content difference and had a greater and more prolonged oncotic effect than albumin solutions. Normal saline alone appeared to decrease both oxygen availability and oncotic pressure.[10] It is obvious from the literature that the crystalloid vs. colloid controversy has not been completely resolved. In the practice at Memorial Hospital in which surgery often produces large third-space volume deficits, we have found that some colloid administration is necessary to correct intravascular volume deficits, oliguria, hypotension, and tachycardia in patients who have experienced rapid or large losses of blood volume. (See Ch. 21 for further discussion.)

PLASMA SUBSTITUTES

Attempts to minimize the need for fresh human plasma products for volume replacement have resulted in the production of gelatins, dextrans, hydroxyethyl starch, and manufactured human albumin products that are effective but do not require refrigeration. However, all plasma expanders except albumin compromise hemostasis.[11] The explanation for these hemostatic defects remains obscure, since conventional clotting parameters are not sufficiently affected. Dextran, hydroxethyl starch, and other macromolecules precipitate fibrinogen, Factor VIII, and Von Willebrand factor from plasma. Dextran reduces platelet adhesiveness, spreading, and reactivity to ADP, resembling that found in Von Willebrand's disease. The abnormal bleeding of this disorder, as well as that consequent to administration of dextran, can be corrected by the administration of cryoprecipitate. Alexander[12] concludes that dextran and other synthetic plasma expanders adversely affect hemostasis by depletion of Von Willebrand factor(s).

AVAILABLE ALBUMIN PRODUCTS

The significant coagulation defects and allergic reactions produced by synthetic plasma expanders have forced physicians to rely on human albumin for volume expansion. Synthetic expanders are now rarely used in the U.S. There are two forms of fractionated albumin available. Of course albumin is also provided by single donor plasma, frozen or unfrozen. Manufactured albumin has been subjected to an extensive manufacturing process and results in highly purified albumin (Cohn fraction V) or plasma protein fraction (Cohn fraction IV and V or PPF).[13]

The protein composition of PPF is determined by methods that have been approved for each manufacturer. The protein content is set at 5.00 ± 0.30 percent. In addition to the alpha and beta globulins present in the PPF which usually are in the range of about 12 percent, the albumin exists both as monomer and as some dimers and other oligomers. The effect of albumin dimers and oligomers on the oncotic characteristics and drug-binding properties of the albumin has not been determined. PPF must be composed of at least 83 percent (usually about 88 percent) albumin, no more than 1 percent gamma globulin, 130 to 160 meq/l of sodium, less than 2 meq/l of potassium, with a pH of 7.0 ± 0.3.

This solution is stabilized with 0.004 molar sodium acetyltryptophanate and 0.004 molar sodium caprylate. After being introduced into the final container, the PPF solution is heated at an attained temperature of $60^\circ C \pm 0.5^\circ C$ for 10 hours for sterilization. The shelf dating period is 5 years when stored at $5^\circ C$ or 3 years when stored at $30^\circ C$ or less.

Production of plasma protein fraction (PPF) and albumin require manufacturing methods that include low temperatures (-3 to $+5^\circ C$), various concentrations of ethyl alcohol (8 to 30 percent), varying hydrogen ion concentrations (pH 4.6 to 7.2) and several centrifugal separations of precipitates. Virtually every step in the manufacturing process has the potential for causing protein denaturation—i.e., an alteration in the protein's molecular structure which may effect its stability or in vivo function.

PPF AND HYPOTENSION

Other usually labile proteins may proceed through the fractionation process in variable ways into the final product. For example, several lots of PPF that produced hypotension when administered rapidly were found to have high levels of prekallikrein activator (PKA).[14] PKA is perhaps better known as Hageman Factor Fragment (Table 23-1). Activated Hageman Factor can act to trigger blood coagulation and fibrinolysis, and also can activate prekallikrein to kallikrein, which in turn acts upon higher molecular weight kininogen to produce bradykinin (Fig. 23-1).

Bradykinin is a nonapeptide with a molecular weight of about 1,000 which has vasodilator activity and causes smooth muscle contraction. In the normal circulation, bradykinin is rapidly inactivated largely by kinases, proteolytic enzymes that degrade kinins to inactive forms. The half-life of bradykinin in blood is about 20 seconds; it is almost totally destroyed in one passage through the pulmonary circulation.

In the original work of Bland[15] and associates on this problem, it was postulated that

Table 23-1. Components of the Kallikrein-Kinin System

1. Hageman Factor	—Factor XII—MW about 80,000
2. Prekallikrein Activator(s) or Hageman Factor Fragment(s)	—"PKA"—MW about 28,000 Generated from Factor XIII; Catalyze(s) Prekalikrein—Kallikrein
3. Plasma Prekallikrein	—"PK"—MW about 100,000
4. Plasma Kallikrein	—MW about 100,000 Catalyzes release of BK from HMWK
5. High-Molecular Weight Kininogen(s)	—"HMWK"—MW about 200,000 Preferred substrate from plasma kallikrein
6. Bradykinin	—"BK"—A nonapeptide, MW about 1,000. Has vasodilatory activity; causes smooth muscle contraction.
7. Kininases	—Proteolytic enzymes that degrade kinins to inactive forms

bradykinin caused the hypotension occasionally produced by PPF. Recent studies at the Bureau of Biologics with samples of PPF retained from Bland's original studies were found to be high in PKA activity.[16] It has been shown that there is a direct correlation between levels of PKA and the amount of hypotension produced in animal models.[17]

PKA activity has been found in only a few lots of albumin. Indeed, this is reasonably to be expected because a further fractionating process is necessary to produce albumin isolated in Cohn Fraction V. Most of the PKA is removed by these additional fractionation steps. Precise control of manufacturing and testing of lots of albumin products for PKA before release have largely eliminated this as a clinical problem. PKA is present in all plasma and tends to concentrate in Cohn Fraction IV, but it also may be found in albu-

min, the Cohen Fraction V precipitate. After heating to 60° C for pasteurization, bradykinin may still be present, kallikrein is not found, kininogen is still present but at very low levels, and prekallikrein activator is present in various amounts and maintains its activities. PKA exerts its effect by activation of the patient's own kinin system.

It is well known that the administration of PPF fractions does not cause adverse responses in all patients. Individuals differ in their ability to destroy bradykinin, and they may have differing levels of PKA already circulating as the result of the trauma of surgery which activates Hageman Factor. Potentially, chemical reactions producing PKA can occur at almost any stage in plasma derivative manufacture, in the source plasma, during the fractionation, in the partially fractionated products, in the paste or dried pow-

Figure 23.1 The relationship of proteins of the Kinin-generating pathway to Hageman Factor.

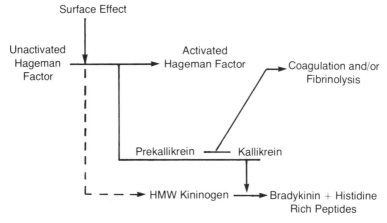

der stages, in the bulk, and finally, perhaps, even in bottles on the shelf.

MASSIVE BLOOD REPLACEMENT

The principal complications of massive blood replacement are pulmonary insufficiency, citrate toxicity, hyperkalemia, red cell 2,3-DPG depletion, acidosis, and hypocoagulability. Since many of these factors are discussed elsewhere, only those factors which are of major interest to the anesthesiologist and which he can control will be considered here.

PULMONARY INSUFFICIENCY

Pulmonary insufficiency during and after massive transfusion has been considered to be due to administration of microemboli or plasticizers found in stored blood, disseminated intravascular coagulation, and circulatory overload. Although there is little or no clinical evidence of the value of 40μ or finer filters for the removal of microemboli, they are in widespread use and, in our opinion, are of value in conjunction with fluid restriction and adequate colloid administration. The opinion of other authorities differ (see Chs. 22 and 24). The plasticizer diethylhexylphthalate (DEHP) has been shown to accumulate in blood stored in plastic containers and to cause increased capillary permeability in rats, but there is no evidence that this occurs in humans.[18]

Pulmonary insufficiency after massive transfusion is uncommonly encountered at Memorial Hospital. It rarely occurs in patients in whom the central venous pressure and urinary output are measured regularly, concomitantly with blood and fluid administration, and an accurate record of weighed and volumetric blood loss is maintained. If pulmonary insufficiency occurs as evidenced by early decreases in PaO_2, the patient usually responds to diuresis with furosemide

and, if necessary, positive end-expiratory pressure (PEEP) ventilation.

HYPOCALCEMIA

We have repeatedly shown that "citrate intoxication"[19] or, as should be more accurately termed, citrate-induced decrease in ionized calcium, does not occur at a level that will produce depression of myocardial function or interfere with hemostasis after massive transfusion. Many years ago, it was demonstrated that the administration of large volumes of ACD solution alone at a rate equivalent to 20 units of whole blood per hour did not produce myocardial depression as measured by the methods then available. These results have since been corroborated by studies employing intraoperative cardiac output measurements and wedge pressure measurements, even though prolongation of electrocardiographic Q-T intervals was observed.[20] It was previously shown that there is a decrease in Ca++ associated with speed of transfusion and the recipient's plasma citrate level but that neither rate or volume of transfused blood bore significant relation to final citrate levels.[21] Rate of citrate metabolism appears to be the major determinant of citrate concentration in plasma. Since the institution of blood warming and the withholding of calcium administration, no cases of ventricular fibrillation during massive and rapid blood administration have been encountered at Memorial Hospital.

HYPERKALEMIA

Hyperkalemia during massive transfusion has been postulated to be the result of administration of whole blood, the plasma of which contains an excess of K. In the patient, hyperkalemia of this source is counteracted by the alkalosis that results from the metabolism of citrate to bicarbonate, the return of the potassium to the red cell when banked blood is circulating, and renal elimination if an adequate urinary output is maintained during massive transfusion. This paradox is clarified if one considers the potassium load of the infused blood products. Numerous measurements of the potassium content of one-week-old CPD bank blood have shown plasma potassium levels in the range of 13 to 15 meq/l. Fresh frozen plasma, removed from red cells which have not developed ATP deficiency due to storage, averaged only 3.0 ± 0.20 meq/l of potassium. Since there are about 300 ml of plasma in a unit of bank blood, the infused potassium "load" of each unit is approximately 5 meq/unit. Similarly, for fresh frozen plasma 0.6 meq of K is administered for each 200-ml unit. The plasma from one-week-old concentrated red cells contains 1 to 2 meq/unit of K.

If a level of 3.5 to 5.0 meq/l of serum potassium is assumed in the bleeding patient or 1.0 to 1.5 meq/450 ml of blood lost, the net gain of potassium on an exchange basis is only 2.5 to 4.0 meq/unit replaced. Assuming no urinary excretion, the transfusion of 20 units of whole blood would result in the administration of 50 to 80 mEq of potassium; this will occur over a period of time. The concomitant use of warmed blood will aid RBC membrane ATPase to become active as it approaches 37 ° C. Additionally, the more alkaline pH which develops as citrate is metabolized will also lower potassium.

Finally, it has been shown that, with adequate renal function, the majority of net potassium gain (bank blood plasma K level minus patient's plasma K level) will be excreted as the transfusion proceeds. Indeed, potassium must be administered in many operations in which the patient's potassium level falls during the operative procedure.[21] Hyperkalemia of massive transfusion in adults is neither a real nor a theoretical occurrence. Repeated studies have shown that the end results of massive transfusion in adults is usually hypokalemia.

RED CELL 2,3-DPG LEVELS

The significance of a fall in 2,3-DPG in banked blood arises from the fact that this red blood cell glycointermediate is one of the factors which influences the position of the oxyhemoglobin dissociation curve and the value of P_{50}, the partial pressure of oxygen at which 50 percent of the hemoglobin is oxygenated. In ACD-preserved blood, 2,3-DPG decreases up to 95 percent after 10 days of storage. In CPD-preserved blood, the level of 2,3-DPG is maintained at a relatively high level but primarily only during the first 7 days of storage.[22] While, theoretically, transfused blood with higher levels of 2,3-DPG should be beneficial, this has not been shown unequivocally to occur in man in vivo. In 1973, Schweizer was unable to demonstrate a correlation between serum lactate levels and red cell 2,3-DPG levels in 10 patients who received an average of 33 units of ACD blood (range 20 to 62 units).[23] Neither was there an observable correlation with the clinical condition of the patient. Collins was unable to demonstrate any deficiency in oxygen delivery to the tissues in young battle casualties who received two to three blood volume exchanges of low 2,3-DPG red cells.[24] Weisel found no evidence of impairment of oxygen transport in the first 24-hour period postoperatively in high-risk elderly patients (average age 70 years), despite the stress of major surgery.[25] There may be circumstances in which anemia and/or impaired function of hemoglobin become important, such as in coronary artery disease. At the present time, the administration of 2,3-DPG-depleted bank blood is probably not deleterious if anemia is corrected at the same time.

ACIDOSIS

Acidosis during massive transfusion is probably deleterious. For many years we have recommended that the acid load of bank blood (8 to 12 meq/l) be routinely reversed with the administration of 50 mEq of NaHCO$_3$ for every five units of blood, but this may not be necessary. Acidemia still may occur during massive transfusion, but the ready availability of blood gas determinations should guide NaHCO$_3$ administration to those patients with demonstrated acidemia.

HEMOSTATIC AND COAGULATION DEFECTS

The hypocoagulability occurring as a result of massive transfusion can be an exceedingly complex phenomenon. The most noticeable hemostatic defect found in bank blood is progressive loss of platelets in the unit of whole blood. Yet, after administration of 20 units of blood, the platelet level may be found to be in the range of 40 to 60 thousand/cu ml, and the patient often has no abnormal bleeding. Indeed, routine administration of platelet concentrates during massive transfusion is not practiced in Memorial Hospital and in our experience is seldom needed. There is evidence of decay of platelet viability in stored cold blood (see Chs. 24 and 26). Some of the remaining platelets survive in recipients after storage of blood for up to 72 hours but are of unproven functional capability.[26] Postoperative bleeding due to dilutional platelet deficiency is uncommon unless more than one and a half blood volumes are exchanged. Where thrombocytopenic bleeding occurs intraoperatively for whatever cause, platelet concentrates should be administered. (See Ch. 24.)

Plasma coagulation Factors V and VIII are the only factors significantly lost during blood storage at 4° C. After an initial rapid drop, they decay slowly, are above the level required for hemostasis for 24 hours, and may continue to be adequate for 21 days.[27] The average age of banked blood administered is usually seven days. The practice at Memorial Hospital is to administer two units of fresh frozen plasma for every 10 units of blood. The rationale for this procedure is to prevent or correct plasma coagulation defects, which may or may not be associated with abnormal bleeding. Other authors do not recommend this use of fresh frozen plasma. (See Ch. 24.)

Reference to Figure 23-1 demonstrates that coagulation can be initiated by activation of the early steps of the process, induce disseminated intravascular coagulation (DIC) and then fibrinolysis. This in turn results in the formation of fibrinogen/fibrin (FDP/fdp) degradation products. By utilizing the Thrombo-Welco Test for fibrin degradation products, it has been possible to demonstrate in our laboratory measurable levels of FDP/fdp in 26 of 50 units of CPD blood (range 10 to 80 mg/ml). The same proportion of positive units was found in concentrated red cells. Only two positive results were found among 30 units of fresh frozen plasma. This suggests that some activation of the fibrinolytic system occurs in the process of blood collection and storage, and possibly after separation of the plasma.

The diagnosis of DIC is usually made when a patient has thrombocytopenia, hypofibrinogenemia, prolongation of thrombin, prothrombin, and partial thromboplastin times; in addition, the presence of FDP/fdp and soluble fibrin monomer has been demonstrated in the patient's plasma. In the perioperative period, decreased plasma coagulation factors secondary to massive transfusion may prolong the prothrombin and partial thromboplastin times, and an elevation of FDP/fdp may be caused by that present in banked blood. The platelet count may fall solely on the basis of hemodilution. Thus, studies of coagulation changes which occur during massive transfusion should also include methods for determining the presence of soluble fibrin monomers, such as the ethanol gel test, the protamine serial dilution, or methods employing Reptilase, and the thrombin time.

MANAGEMENT OF THE PATIENT RECEIVING MASSIVE BLOOD REPLACEMENT

During the last 25 years, massive blood replacement has been a continuing challenge at Memorial Hospital. Even at the present time, when a number of radical cancer surgery operative procedures have been perfected, blood loss of 5000 ml or more is commonly incurred. In the last two years prior to preparation of this chapter, 210 patients received 10 or more units of CPD-preserved banked whole blood or packed red cells in the operating room. Of these, 15 received 30 or more units. Over the last 25 years, mortality has been reduced from 50 percent after replacement of 12 units to less than 10 percent by using the program described here. No immediate mortality is now anticipated, except in those instances in which severe and rapid hemorrhage cannot be controlled and blood replacement is inadequate. These results have been obtained in a population which on average is mainly over 40 years of age and has a high incidence of cardiovascular and pulmonary disease. Nevertheless, these figures compare favorably with those from the Vietnam War experience in healthy young men who were battle casualties. No similar published civilian experience is available with which to compare these results. Granted that most of blood loss occurs during operative procedures in these cases and that for the most part hypovolemic shock can be avoided, the techniques that have been evolved should apply to all cases of rapid and massive blood replacement.

MASSIVE TRANSFUSION MANAGEMENT PROTOCOL

When massive transfusion is required, several monitoring devices should be in place in all cases. These monitors should include:

1. An accurate method for determining blood loss. A method of weighing used sponges with subtraction of the weight of wet or dry sponges should be routinely used. The circulating nurse cannot be permitted to be too busy to perform this function. The suction bottles for volumetric determination of blood loss should be visible to the anesthesiologist. A record must be kept of the amounts of irrigation fluid used so that overestimation of blood loss, excessive replacement, and subsequent circulatory overload do not occur.

2. Massive transfusion patients require insertion of a catheter for continuous central venous pressure monitoring and the insertion of a urinary catheter as well, the drainage of which should be visible to the anesthesiologist. This is essential for continuous evaluation of the patient's intravascular volume.

3. Estimated blood loss, fluid and blood replacement, central venous pressure, and urinary output should be recorded regularly, at least on the anesthesia record.

4. Administration of large volumes of blood, over 3 units in Memorial Hospital, requires the use of a blood-warming device. The advantages of this are two-fold: the complications of hypothermia are avoided, especially cardiovascular depression; and peripheral vasoconstriction is also avoided. (Peripheral vasoconstriction would result in the measurement of a falsely low blood pressure and might lead to resultant overtransfusion.)

5. The acid load of bank blood does not usually require buffering, except in the presence of shock and in some elderly patients. With the easy availability of acid-base determinations, buffer is not administered until metabolic acidosis develops. However, at times when little laboratory support is available, a former routine of administering 50 meq of sodium bicarbonate for every 5 units of bank blood is employed.

6. Two units of fresh frozen plasma with coagulation factors are administered for every 10 units of banked blood. This is suffi-

cient to correct the depressed levels of Factors V and VIII, which occur in bank blood but which may be inadequate in the face of DIC.

7. Supplemental calcium salts are not given.

8. Platelet concentrates are not routinely administered for the dilutional thrombocytopenia that usually occurs unless significant abnormal capillary bleeding occurs.

9. Careful monitoring of the patient's electrolyte levels is necessary because hypokalemia may occur during prolonged operations. Also, since the sodium level of bank blood is of the order of 160 to 165 meq/l, care must be taken that sodium overloading and/or hypernatremia do not occur.

10. If rapid and massive transfusion is commonly encountered in any hospital, laboratory facilities should be available for sophisticated analysis of hemostatic abnormalities. Unfortunately, a reliable method of determining bleeding times in the operating room has not yet been devised, despite substantial efforts in this direction.

REFERENCES

1. Chaplin, H.: Packed red blood cells. N. Engl. J. Med. 281:364, 1969.
2. Simon, G.E. and Bove, J.R.: The potassium load from blood transfusion. Postgrad. Med. 49:61, 1971.
3. Leikola, J., Kostinen, K., and Lehtien, M., et al.: IgA induced anaphylactic transfusion reactions: A report of four cases. Blood 42:111, 1973.
4. Kliman, A.: No hepatitis after packed red blood cells. N. Engl. J. Med. 297:1290, 1968.
5. Grindon, A.J.: The use of packed red blood cells. J.A.M.A. 235:389, 1976.
6. Beiting, C.V., Kozak, K.J., and Dreffer, R.L., et al.: Whole blood vs packed red cells for resuscitation of hemorrhagic shock: an examination of host defense parameters in dogs. Surgery 84:194, 1978.
7. Kliman, A.: Letter to the Editor. J.A.M.A. 235:2586, 1976.
8. Bidwell, E., Dike, G.W.R., and Sharpe, T.J.: Therapeutic materials. In: Human Blood Coagulation, Haemostasis and Thrombosis, 2nd Edition. Biggs, R., ed., Blackwell Scientific, Oxford, 1976, p. 249.
9. Skillman, J.J., Restall, S., and Salzman, E.W.: Randomized trial of albumin vs electrolyte solutions during abdominal aortic operation. Surgery 78:291, 1975.
10. Carlon, G.C., Kahn, R.C., Bertoni, G., Campfield, P.B., Howland, W.S., and Goldiner, V.L.: Rapid volume expansion in patients with interstitial lung diseases. Anesth. Analg. 58:13, 1979.
11. Thompson, W.L.: Hydroxyethyl starch. In: Blood Substitutes and Plasma Expanders, Jamieson, G.A. and Greenwalt, T.J., eds. Alan R. Liss, Inc., New York, 1978, p. 283.
12. Alexander, B.: Effects of plasma expanders on coagulation and hemostasis: Dextran hydroxyethyl starch, and other macromolecules revisited. In: Blood Substitutes and Plasma Expanders, Jamieson, G.A. and Greenwalt, T.J., eds. Alan R. Liss, Inc., New York, 1978, p. 293.
13. Cohn, E.J., Strong, L.E., Hughes, W.L., Mulford, Ashworth, J.N., Melin, M., and Taylor, H.L.: Preparation and Properties of Serum and Plasma Proteins. IV. A System for the Separation into Fractions of the Protein and Lipoprotein Components of Biological Tissues and Fluids. J. Am. Chem. Soc. 68:459, 1946.
14. Alving, B.M., Hojima, Y., Pisano, J.J., Mason, B.L., Buckingham, R.E., Mozen, M.M., and Finlayson, J.S.: Hypotension associated with prekallikrein activator (Hageman-factor fragments) in plasma protein fraction. N. Engl. J. Med. 299:66, 1978.
15. Bland, J.H.L., Laver, M.B., and Lowenstein, E.: Vasodilator effect of commercial 5 percent plasma protein fraction solutions. J.A.M.A. 224:1721, 1973.
16. Proceedings of the Workshop on Measurement of Potentially Hypotensive Agents. Bureau of Biologics, Food and Drug Administration, Bethesda, MD, September 15-16, 1977, pp. 23 and 172.
17. Proceedings of the Workshop on Measurement of Potentially Hypotensive Agents. Bureau of Biologics, Food and Drug Adminis-

tration, Bethesda, MD, September 15–16, 1977, p. 61.

18. Collins, J.A.: Massive Transfusion: What is current and important? In: Massive Transfusion. Nusbacher, J., ed. American Association of Blood Banks, Washington, D.C., 1978, pp. 1–16.

19. Howland, W.S., Schweizer, O., Carlon, G.C., and Goldiner, P.L.: The cardiovascular effects of low levels of ionized calcium during massive transfusion. Surg. Gynecol. Obstet. 145:581, 1977.

20. Howland, W.S., Bellville, J.W., Zucker, M.B., Boyan, P., and Cliffton, E.E.: Massive blood transfusion. V. Failure to demonstrate citrate intoxication. Surg. Gynecol. Obstet. 105:529, 1957.

21. Howland, W.S., Schweizer, O., Carlon, G.C., and Goldiner, P.L.: The cardiovascular effects of low levels of ionized calcium during massive transfusion. Surg. Gynecol. Obstet. 145:581, 1977.

22. Schweizer, O. and Howland, W.S.: 2,3-Diphosphoglycerate levels in CPD-preserved bank blood. Anesth. Analg. 53:516, 1973.

23. Schweizer, O. and Howland, W.S.: Factors influencing the level of 2,3-DPG during anesthesia and operation. Anesth. Analg. 52:542, 1973.

24. Collins, J.A.: Massive blood transfusion. Clinics in Haematology 5:201, 1976.

25. Weisel, R.D., Dennis, R., and Manny, J., et al.: Adverse effects of transfusion therapy during abdominal aortic aneurysectomy. Surgery 83:682, 1978.

26. Perkins, H.A., Osborn, J.J., and Gerbode, F.: The role of exchange transfusion in the production of abnormal bleeding following extracorporeal bypass. Proc. 7th Congr. Int. Soc. Blood Trans., 1958, p. 25.

27. Perkins, H.A.: The use of "fresh" blood. In: Massive Transfusion. Nusbacher, J., ed. Amer. Assoc. of Blood Banks, Washington, D.C., 1978, pp. 71-79.

24

Strategies for Massive Transfusion

Herbert A. Perkins, M.D.

Massive transfusion is defined here as administration of a volume of blood or components equal to or greater than the blood volume of the recipient. Massive transfusion and its associated problems are seen most commonly in the trauma service, in vascular surgery including heart-lung bypass, and with exchange transfusions. The problems encountered in patients who are massively transfused may relate to the condition for which the blood is administered, complications associated with that condition, underlying patient defects and/or abnormalities in the transfused blood.

Blood for transfusion differs significantly from the blood in the donor's circulation in several ways: (1) It has been mixed with an anticoagulant-preservative solution, and (2) further changes occur during storage. At the usual rate of blood transfusion, the biochemical changes in stored blood are corrected by the recipient as the blood is transfused or shortly thereafter. Massive amounts of banked blood can, however, introduce amounts of abnormal constituents faster than the recipient's compensatory mechanisms are able to operate. Both the volume of transfused blood and the rate of transfusion determine the outcome. For most defects in stored blood, both a high volume and rapid rate of transfusion are required before physiologically significant abnormalities occur in the patient. Volume alone may lower the recipient's platelet count simply by dilution. Platelet reserves are limited and, once exhausted, may take four to five days for replacement through synthesis by megakaryocytes.

ANTICOAGULANT-PRESERVATIVE SOLUTIONS AND THEIR SIGNIFICANCE IN MASSIVE TRANSFUSION

The anticoagulant-preservative solutions in general use are listed in Table 24-1.[1] A standard blood collection consists of 450 ml donor blood mixed with 63 ml of CPD or CPDA-1. The anticoagulant-preservative solution dilutes the donor blood constituents to 88 percent of their original concentration. The solution adds 18 meq of sodium and 3 meq of phosphorus to each unit. The pH of freshly collected CPD anticoagulated blood is 7.0 to 7.2 when measured at 37° C.

The citrate concentration is sufficient to bind the ionized calcium of the unit with excess citrate remaining available to complex with calcium in the recipient. Early experiences with massive transfusion led to the belief that "citrate toxicity" could result in cardiac standstill, and attempts were made to compensate for this with intermittent injec-

Table 24-1. Anticoagulant-Preservative Solutions in General Use

	CPD	CPDA-1
Na₃ citrate	26.3 gm	26.3 gm
Citric acid	3.27 gm	3.27 gm
Dextrose	25.2 gm	31.9 gm
NaH₂PO₄•H₂O	2.22 gm	2.22 gm
Adenine	—	0.275 gm
Water to make	1000 ml	1000 ml
Volume per 100 ml	14 ml	14 ml
Red cell storage limit	21 days	35 days

Citrate-Phosphate-Dextrose Solution (CPD)
Citrate-Phosphate-Dextrose-Adenine Solution (CPDA-1)

(Codes of Federal Regulations. #21 Food and Drugs, 640:4, 1979.)

tions of calcium. Recently available techniques for measuring ionized calcium, the fraction which has physiologic activity, demonstrated lowering of ionized calcium levels by massive infusion of citrated blood. Moreover, current experience with plateletpheresis and leukapheresis of alert healthy donors revealed symptoms attributable to low levels of ionized calcium when red cells and citrated plasma were rapidly reinfused. Rates of reinfusion of 70 to 80 ml per minute are routine in this procedure; in small donors particularly, symptoms of tingling about the lips and even carpopedal spasm have been noted. Nonetheless, these symptoms are usually easily and quickly controlled by slowing the rate of infusion. More serious adverse effects attributable to citrate infusion have not been noted with cytapheresis.

In massive transfusion of bleeding patients, it is most unusual to infuse blood at the rate used in cytapheresis (70 to 80 ml/min) and certainly unlikely that such a rate would be required for a period of several hours. Additional protection of the ionized calcium level of the transfused recipient occurs when red cell concentrates are transfused supplemented by at least some fluids which lack citrate. These facts all suggested that "citrate toxicity" was not the explanation for episodes of cardiac standstill occurring during rapid transfusion. Instead, hypothermia resulting from rapid transfusion of refrigerated blood was the likely cause. Hypothermia can be

avoided by warming the transfused blood either immediately before or during infusion.

The practice of injecting calcium salts intermittently to counter the citrate effects—while seemingly plausible therapy—has been discouraged by studies in massively transfused patients. Measurement of ionized calcium levels during massive transfusion confirmed the expected fall, but intermittent injection of calcium resulted in a sharp increase of both total and ionized calcium with rapid return of the ionized calcium concentration to levels close to those before the injection.[2] The transitory hypercalcemia induced by intermittent injections may well be more dangerous than hypocalcemia. In fact, Howland has shown that the mortality rate was higher in those patients who received calcium than in those who did not.[3]

CHANGES IN BLOOD ON STORAGE: RED BLOOD CELLS

Further changes which occur in bank blood on storage at 4° C are outlined in Table 24-2. Red cell viability decreases on storage. Transfused cells which were irreparably damaged are removed from the circulation within hours. The remainder are restored to biochemical normalcy and live out the remainder of their normal lifespan in the circulation of the recipient. The proportion of transfused cells remaining in the circulation of the recipient 24 hours after transfusion is considered as the percent viability. Regulations of the Food and Drug Administration require that at least 70 percent of the red cells remain viable in the anticoagulant-preservative solution at the end of the permitted storage period. For CPD blood, the viability of red cells after 21 days of storage averages 80 to 85 percent, but there is considerable variability based largely on the characteristics of the cells of the individual donors. Thus, an older unit may under some circumstances contain more viable red cells than a fresher unit.[4]

Table 24-2. Changes in Bank Blood on Storage at 4°C

I. Decrease of essential components
   A. Red cell viability
   B. Red cell 2,3 diphosphoglycerate (DPG)
   C. Platelet viability
   D. Granulocyte viability
   E. Coagulation factors
     1. Factor V
     2. Factor VIII

II. Increase in toxic materials
   A. Plasma lactate
   B. Plasma potassium
   C. Plasma ammonia
   D. Plasticizers

III. Formation of microaggregates

The primary function of the red blood cell is to deliver oxygen to the tissues. With storage, red cell oxygen release to the tissues becomes impaired as 2,3-diphosphoglycerate (DPG) falls. The 2,3-DPG remains at normal levels in CPD or CPDA-1 blood for at least a week. If oxygen-releasing capacity of the blood does decrease as a result of DPG depletion, the recipient may compensate by increasing the rate of blood flow to the tissues and will biochemically restore DPG to normal levels within hours. Therefore, in most cases requiring massive transfusion, the level of DPG in the transfused blood is of no significance. There is potential danger for the patient only in the following circumstances: 1) when the volume transfused results in an almost complete exchange within a few hours; 2) when all or almost all of the transfused blood has been stored more than one to two weeks; and 3) when the recipient has no reserve to increase his cardiac output. This subject is discussed in greater detail in Chapters 22 and 23.

CHANGES IN BLOOD ON STORAGE: HEMOSTATIC FACTORS

The changes which occur in hemostatic factors on storage have long been established. Most of the plasma coagulation factors are completely stable on storage, and even plasma from outdated blood has levels of activities within the range required for normal hemostasis. Of particular note is the fact that fibrinogen retains its clottability virtually intact. This has diagnostic implications in that a low fibrinogen level in a massively transfused patient is usually secondary to factors other than dilution—for example, disseminated intravascular coagulation.

The labile factors are Factor VIII and Factor V, and the lability of even these factors has been overemphasized by extrapolation from conditions where a rise in pH accelerated their rate of decay—conditions not present in units of blood collected for transfusion in the usual way. Rapaport[5] showed that Factor V in acid-citrate-dextrose (ACD) blood after storage for 21 days ranged from 20 to 60 units/dl. Only 10 to 15 units/dl are required for normal hemostasis.[6] Factor VIII levels at the same point ranged from 20 to 50 units/dl. The hemostatic level for Factor VIII is 25 to 30 units/dl,[6] and patients under stress are stimulated to raise their own Factor VIII concentration.

All of the above data have been widely corroborated. The recent report by Counts et al.[7] is in agreement with one notable exception: Counts demonstrated a much more accelerated loss of Factor VIII. It should be noted, however, that Counts used modified whole blood in which most of the Factor VIII had already been removed to prepare cryoprecipitate. Moreover, Counts reported that even the small amount of Factor VIII in his transfused blood did not result in significant deficiency of Factor VIII in the circulation of his patients.

The data just presented lead to the inevitable conclusion that massive transfusion with stored blood or plasma will not by itself reduce the activity of any plasma coagulation factors to a level at which hemostasis is compromised. This conclusion has important implications regarding demands for fresh whole blood or fresh-frozen plasma for these patients.

Normal hemostasis, however, also requires

viable and functional platelets, and the data on platelets lead to different conclusions. Platelet viability seems best preserved at 20 to 24° C; under the best conditions yet devised, platelets have been satisfactorily preserved for only 72 hours. At the 1 to 6° C required for storage of red cells, the microtubules of platelets are disrupted, and the lifespan of transfused platelets becomes abbreviated. However, the common assumption that there are no viable platelets at any time in refrigerated whole blood is not correct. Kissmeyer-Nielsen[8] showed many years ago that the recovery of platelets in recipients transfused with ACD whole blood was 45 percent after storage for 24 hours, compared with 54 percent using fresh blood. Even after 72 hours, recovery was 20 percent. The ability of platelets to be aggregated by adenosine diphosphate becomes impaired in only a few hours, even after storage at 20 to 24° C. However, this is irrelevant for hemostasis because, as Slichter and Harker have shown,[9] platelets stored for 72 hours are still effective in correcting the bleeding time of thrombocytopenic recipients. These conclusions are further corroborated by the demonstrable efficacy of stored platelet concentrates in widespread routine use.

Although it must be accepted that platelets can be stored in a functional state for a limited period, all would agree that blood stored more than a day or two lacks viable platelets and should be regarded as platelet-free. Replacement of recipient blood with platelet-free blood results in dilution of the recipient's platelet count as soon as his limited reserves have been exhausted. Once platelet reserves are exhausted, four to five days are required before synthesis of new platelets can restore the platelet count. From these facts, it is obvious that significant thrombocytopenia will result from transfusions per se if the volume of platelet-free materials is sufficiently large. In an uncomplicated situation, an adult will maintain an adequate platelet count until 15 to 20 units of blood have been administered.[10] Lomanto and Howland[11] reported that no

patient transfused with less than about 1.3 blood volumes had a platelet count below 100,000/μl. The persistence of severe thrombocytopenia increased with larger amounts of blood, but even when 1.3 to 4.0 blood volumes were replaced, only 50 percent of the patients had platelet counts below 100,000/μl. Similar data are available from the study of Counts[7] (Fig. 24-1).

CHANGES IN BLOOD ON STORAGE: TOXIC MATERIALS

The closed container in which blood is stored prevents elimination of waste products of metabolism. Red blood cell viability is dependent on glycolysis, the end product being lactate. The pH of blood is already relatively acidic from addition of the anticoagulant-preservative solution. Lactate further depresses the pH to approximately 6.8 at the end of 21 days of storage. Although transfused blood initially presents the patient with excess acid, subsequent metabolism of citrate results in a net excess of base.

Plasma potassium concentration increases at a rate of approximately 1 meq/l per day during 21 days' storage of whole blood. In Chapter 23, Howland presents convincing evidence that the increased plasma potassium is of no significance in massive transfusion of adult patients. In fact, the recipient is most likely to have a plasma potassium below normal. Transfusions in neonates will be discussed in Chapter 33. Ammonia accumulates rapidly in stored blood,[12] but this is of significance, if at all, only for patients in severe liver failure. Plasticizers are known to leach from the polyvinyl chloride generally used for blood containers,[13] but no evidence that they are harmful to the recipient has yet been presented.

The only significant difference between CPD and CPDA-1 for the massively transfused patient is the better red cell viability in CPDA-1. During the additional two weeks of

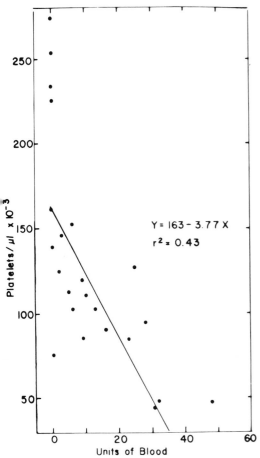

Fig. 24-1. Plot of platelet counts against the number of units of blood transfused to the patient prior to the time the sample was obtained for the platelet counts. No platelet transfusions had been given to any of the patients represented on the graph. (Counts, R.B., Haisch, C., and Simon, T.L., et al.: Hemostasis in massively transfused trauma patients. Ann. Surg. 190:91, 1979.)

storage of CPDA-1 blood, there are further but minimal rises in plasma potassium and hydrogen ion. The adenine in CPDA-1 is believed to be safe even in massive transfusion. The concentration of adenine in CPDA-1 is half that employed in an earlier trial where a rare patient had crystals of an adenine metabolite in his kidney.[14] Adenine at the higher concentration has been routinely employed in Sweden since 1964.[15]

When plasma is removed from red cells at the beginning of storage, the concentration of potassium and other potentially toxic materials rises faster in the remaining plasma because of its smaller volume; however, the total amount of these materials in the plasma is no greater. The pH does not fall significantly faster in red cell concentrates than in whole blood, since the red cells provide most of the buffering capacity.

Microaggregates composed of platelets, granulocytes, and fibrin increase progressively in stored blood and are larger if red cells with the buffy coat have been prepared by centrifugation. Microaggregate filters are available and often recommended if more than five to ten units of blood must be transfused in rapid succession. However, there is little evidence that microaggregate filters have a significant role to play in preventing "shock lung" in humans, and several recent clinical studies have shown no benefit from the use of fine filters. (See Ch. 22.)

Most microaggregate filters remove particles above 10 to 20 microns in diameter, primarily by adsorption to densely packed fibers. Such filters remove platelets and granulocytes as well and should never be used when these cells are required. A major problem with these filters is their tendency to become obstructed and require replacement following passage of several units of blood. Another type of microaggregate filter has 40-micron pore screens. This filter permits platelets to pass and does not easily become obstructed, but it does permit passage of microaggregates in the 10 to 40 micron range. Whether these smaller aggregates are harmful to the recipient remains to be established.

COMPLICATIONS ASSOCIATED WITH MASSIVE TRANSFUSION

We have summarized the well-documented alterations that occur in blood during collection and storage and the extent of their expected effects on the recipient of massive amounts of blood. Clinical studies of patients receiving massive transfusions, however, have often presented conflicting and confusing conclusions about the effects of massive transfusion because of inability to distinguish between the effects of the blood itself and the effects of the condition requiring transfusion and its complications. Disagreements abound, particularly in relation to the kinds of hemostatic defects which occur in massively transfused patients, their cause, and the best way to treat them. The information presented earlier in this chapter results in the conclusion that massive transfusion per se should not result in significant deficiency of plasma coagulation factors, but may very well result in a deficiency of platelets. However, massive transfusions are required in situations where additional therapy or complications may further compromise hemostasis.

Plasma substitutes in very large amounts may aggravate a bleeding tendency. More than one liter of dextran can prolong the bleeding time of an adult, presumably because dextran coats the platelets and impairs their function. Hydroxyethyl starch appears to have somewhat lesser effect; and hemostasis is not impaired by albumin, plasma protein fraction or electrolytes—except for the effect of dilution.

The major complication impairing hemostasis during massive transfusion is disseminated intravascular coagulation (DIC). DIC is almost inevitable when extensive tissue damage is accompanied by prolonged shock and resulting poor perfusion. DIC leads to further loss of platelets as well as consumption of plasma coagulation Factors V and VIII, prothrombin, and fibrinogen. Secondary fibrinolysis adds to the problem by dissolving fibrin clots and by releasing fibrin breakdown products which inhibit coagulation and platelet plug formation.

Attempts to control DIC by heparin in situations where there is massive tissue injury, large open wounds, or incisions in high-pressure blood vessels may serve only to aggravate blood loss. The basic rule of treatment of DIC is to remove the cause, if possible. Correction of shock and improvement of the circulation by restoring blood volume to normal is the safest and most effective therapy in this situation. With improved circulation, activated clotting factors can be removed by the reticuloendothelial system or neutralized by normal circulatory inhibitors. As the patient's blood volume is being restored, it may also be necessary to replace platelets and coagulation factors. Although plasma of any storage age will maintain adequate levels of plasma coagulation factors in an uncomplicated situation where there is no increased rate of consumption, the levels of fibrinogen and Factor VIII may be so low following DIC that they can be effectively raised only by concentrates.

COMPONENT THERAPY IN SURGERY

Blood banks separate the vast majority of blood donations into a variety of components, each having markedly different optimal storage conditions. Specific deficiencies are best met by supplying the required materials in the most concentrated form practical. This permits correction of the deficiencies by intravenous therapy without overexpansion of blood volume. The advantages of red cell concentrate over whole blood for the patient who needs increase of his oxygen-carrying capacity but has a normal or expanded blood volume are obvious. Before concentrates were available, patients with very low levels of platelets and hemophiliacs with very low levels of Factor VIII had no possibility to correct their defects to a safe level. The required amount of missing factor must be concentrated to permit an adequate dose in a volume that the recipient's circulation can tolerate. Once the effectiveness of platelet and Factor VIII concentrates was established, the demands for them increased so that they can now be met only by dividing most units of collected blood into components. Inevitably, whole blood becomes less and less available. It has never been possible to recruit blood donors in numbers that permit wasteful usage of blood, and in recent years the needs of patients have been met only by benefiting multiple patients from each donation of blood. Thus, it is possible with a single donation to provide red cells for one patient, platelet concentrate for a second, Factor VIII and/or fibrinogen (cryoprecipitate) for a third, and then to fractionate the remaining plasma into albumin and gammaglobulin.

For the patient going to surgery, with a normal blood volume but with a hemoglobin level which must be raised before he can tolerate the stress of surgery, transfusion of red cell concentrate is the only sensible option. Once surgery begins, however, and transfusions are required to replace blood lost, the surgeon commonly argues that his patient lost whole blood, and that the loss should therefore be replaced with whole blood. This argument is an oversimplification. The patient may be losing whole blood, but he will very often have a greater deficit of red cells than of plasma, either because his hemoglobin level was not normal in the first place, because he has received a significant volume of parenteral fluids, or because there has been transudation of extravascular fluids into the circulation. Whole blood is diluted somewhat by the anticoagulant-preservative solution. An equal volume of red cells has the same volume-expanding capabilities as whole blood but will result in a higher hematocrit in the recipient (Table 24-3). One report suggests that a higher hematocrit slows blood loss from surgical wounds, presumably because of the increase in blood viscosity.[16] This appears logical but requires confirmation.

Packed red cells may be appropriate therapy during surgery even if there is not a relatively greater deficit of red blood cells. Since whole blood will have much more limited availability, red cell concentrates should be used whenever possible. In the usual surgical case, where the number of units of blood transfused may be two to four, patient recovery is unaffected by transfusion of red cells instead of whole blood. The red cells may require supplementation with parenteral fluids, but electrolyte solutions are usually adequate, and routine supplementation with albumin or plasma protein fraction is never justifiable. It is now common practice at many hospitals to require that the first three or four units crossmatched for surgery be in the form of red cell concentrates.

The limited supplies of whole blood should be reserved for the situations where they will be most useful. The massively bleeding patient will require replacement of his red cells and of plasma volume. With massive transfusions, some authorities believe that replacement with electrolytes may be insufficient and that colloid will be required. Simultaneous transfusion of red cells and colloid is accomplished most conveniently by transfusing whole blood. Although it would appear to be a waste of time and money to take blood apart into components and then have to put them back together for transfusion, it would be even more wasteful to make whole blood of all types available at all sites in quantities to meet any unexpected emergencies. Most of it would never be transfused before it became outdated. In any case, blood supplies are not sufficient to permit this.

There will, therefore, be frequent situations where sudden loss of blood must be treated with components. The first issue to recognize

Table 24-3. Red Blood Cell Components

	Whole Blood	Red Blood Cells	Modified Whole Blood
Volume of blood	450 ml		
Volume of CPD	63 ml		
Total volume	513 ml	271 ml	453 ml
Hematocrit	40 %	75 %	45 %
Volume of red cells	203 ml	203 ml	203 ml
Volume of plasma	310 ml	68 ml	250 ml

is that red cells, with their higher hematocrit, are more viscous than whole blood and cannot be forced through a needle as rapidly. Wide-bore intravenous lines or dilution of red cells may be required in such situations. The surgical team will be prepared for such a situation if red cells are transfused through a Y administration set with saline on the other arm. If rapid flow is suddenly required, 25 to 50 ml of saline can be quickly transferred through the Y set and mixed with the red cells. The red cells can then be rapidly transfused into the patient.

Where time permits, red cells can be diluted before they are hung for transfusion. In that case, dilution may be with saline, with compatible plasma (usually stored fresh-frozen) or with albumin. An alternative approach, which allows preparation of most required components but results in larger stockpiles of whole blood, is favored by some blood banks. Platelet concentrate and/or cryoprecipitate is prepared from a unit of whole blood, and then the remaining plasma is returned to the red cells. This can be accomplished without breaking the sterile seal and without limiting the subsequent period of storage. The resulting product is referred to as "modified" whole blood. A comparison of the contents of whole blood, red cells, and modified whole blood is shown in Table 24-3. Note that all three components contain the same volume of red cells but differ in the volume of plasma and resulting hematocrit. Modified whole blood is not widely available, since it requires an additional step in component preparation and limits the amount of plasma available for fractionation into albumin. More important, separated red cells and plasma provide optimal flexibility for patient care, permitting the two components to be used separately or together as required.

EVALUATION FOR HEMOSTATIC DEFECTS

When time permits, surgical procedures should always be preceded by a careful evalu-

ation of the patient's history to detect a bleeding tendency. Prior surgery with no hemostatic problems is the best evidence of normal capabilities. If there is any question as to whether hemostasis is normal, a battery of simple tests should be performed (Table 24-4).[17]

Initial evaluation of the actively bleeding patient must include an assessment of the type of bleeding that is occurring. If a patient has large amounts of blood emerging from an operative site without any evidence of defective hemostasis in other areas of the body, a local surgical lesion is most likely responsible. In contrast, indications of a more diffuse derangement of hemostasis consist of generalized, uncontrolled oozing at multiple sites.

In the course of massive transfusion, there are predictable effects on the patient even in the absence of complications. As indicated above, significant thrombocytopenia may occur when the volume of blood transfused approaches 1.5 to 2 times the blood volume of the recipient. The need for platelet concentrates can be established by monitoring the platelet count at intervals once the volume of blood transfused has reached the dangerous range.

The bleeding time test has always been considered too imprecise and too difficult to perform in the operating room to recommend its use here. Recently, however, investigators in Seattle[7,18] have shown that the template bleeding time (which does provide acceptably reproducible results) can be performed on the leg with results identical to those obtained using the more traditional arm. Counts[7] did not find that the bleeding time discriminated well between bleeding and nonbleeding trauma cases. Although all eight patients with abnormal bleeding had a bleeding time of 13

Table 24-4. Recommended Screening Tests for Hemostasis prior to Surgery

1. Template bleeding time
2. Platelet count
3. Prothrombin time
4. Partial thromboplastin time
5. Thrombin time
6. Inspection of clot for stability

minutes or more (seven were 17 minutes or more), 63 percent of his 19 nonbleeding patients had a bleeding time ⩾10 minutes and 47 percent had a bleeding time ⩾15 minutes at some time in their course. However, as will be discussed below, the bleeding time proved to be more useful in cases involving cardiopulmonary bypass.

The prothrombin and partial thromboplastin times have proven to be less helpful than platelet counts in the massive transfusion situation. Although one would expect them to be prolonged by the consumption coagulopathy of DIC, they are often modestly prolonged in the absence of significant bleeding, and a number of clinical studies have failed to show a correlation between the prothrombin time (PT) or partial thromboplastin time (PTT) and the occurrence of abnormal bleeding. McNamara et al.[19] compared two groups of battle casualties: One group had major trauma requiring massive transfusion (mean number of units = 8.5) and one group had minor injuries requiring minimal transfusion (mean number 1.1 units). Both groups developed prolongations of PT and PTT with mild reduction of platelet levels, and normal to elevated fibrinogens, and did not significantly differ from each other in test results. Twenty percent of the major trauma group manifested diffuse bleeding, even though the mean values of the laboratory tests in this subgroup were not different from either of the two major groups. In a recent study of civilian trauma victims, Counts et al.[7] found the PT and PTT to be fair predictors of bleeding only when they were markedly prolonged. Of six samples where the PT and PTT were >1.5 times control, four were from patients with abnormal bleeding and two from patients without abnormal bleeding. On the other hand, of the 12 samples where the PT was <1.3 times control, only one had generalized bleeding; of the 18 patients whose PTT was <1.3 times control, only three had generalized bleeding. Thus, it may be concluded that the PT and PTT tests, although not always helpful, can serve a useful function. If markedly prolonged, they provide evidence of plasma coagulation factor deficiencies.

The most useful test to document consumption coagulopathy from DIC is estimation of the fibrinogen level. In these emergencies, fibrinogen is best measured by the less specific but rapid and inexpensive techniques based on precipitation or on the thrombin time. Since fibrinogen levels will be raised by severe stress, serial estimations may be more useful as an index of consumption than a single test.

Specific coagulation factor assays, other than for fibrinogen, play no useful role during massive transfusion. The only exception to this statement is the patient with a congenital coagulation factor deficiency. In hemophilia, frequent assays of the specific factor will be required to monitor replacement therapy in major trauma or surgery until the wound is well healed.

Counts et al.[7] showed that the levels of Factors V and VIII correlated poorly with the number of units of modified whole blood transfused. Counts' study involved 27 patients who received 893 units of blood (mean number was 33 units per patient). Only nine of the units (1 percent) were administered within 24 hours of the time that they were collected. The level of Factor VIII was rarely below 50 percent. The data indicated a large physiologic reserve of Factor VIII with higher than normal levels in patients after trauma or operations. The level of plasma coagulation factors in individuals could not be predicted from the volume of blood transfused. The concordance between levels of Factor VIII, Factor V, and fibrinogen suggest that consumption of these proteins is the major cause of the occasional deficiencies noted.

STRATEGIES FOR MASSIVE TRANSFUSION: GENERAL COMMENTS

With massive loss of blood, the first priority in therapy is the restoration of blood volume.

If the blood volume can be restored quickly, DIC may be prevented or aborted and, with adequate blood pressure, oxygen and nutrients can be delivered to the essential organs. The blood volume can be raised with blood, components, plasma substitutes, or electrolytes. Usually, electrolytes are most readily available and the first to be started. Normal saline is the preferred electrolyte solution, but a balanced salt solution may be used—provided that solutions containing calcium, such as Ringer's lactate, are not infused through the same tubing as citrated blood. Neutralization of citrate by its calcium may result in clotting of the blood in the tubing or, more likely, activation of clotting factors which are then swept into the circulation of the recipient where they may aggravate the tendency to DIC. Low-ionic-strength solutions (e.g., 5 percent dextrose in water or 1/4 strength saline in dextrose) may cause red cell aggregation or, on prolonged contact, hemolysis, and are also not recommended for routine use. Electrolytes leave the circulation of the recipient rapidly, and must be infused in volumes approximately three times the volume of blood lost if they are to maintain the circulation unassisted. Many surgeons faced with a patient who is obviously losing more than 10 to 15 percent of his blood volume would infuse colloids as soon as possible. There is, of course, considerable difference of opinion as to whether the risk of pulmonary edema is greater with colloids or with electrolytes. If colloids are used, dextran or hydroxyethyl starch may be used within limits; but albumin or the crude albumin preparation known as plasma protein fraction is usually preferred. The albumin preparations have no effect on hemostasis (beyond dilution), but the plasma protein fraction has been implicated in the etiology of unexpected drops in blood pressure because of its content of vasoactive peptide stimulators.[20] Electrolyte solutions are far cheaper than colloids, and there is increasing evidence that they may be as safe, or safer than, colloid solutions when the patient is properly monitored.[21]

None of these emergency volume replacement solutions will restore the oxygen-carrying capacity of the recipient's blood; nonetheless, restoration of the hemoglobin level is of secondary importance. As long as the circulation is effective, oxygen can usually be released in adequate quantities to the tissues, compensating for the lower level of hemoglobin by increasing rates of flow. The next priority is restoration of a reasonably normal level of hemoglobin in order to ensure that oxygen-carrying capacity does not drop below the level at which compensation is possible and in order to remove the strain from the heart caused by the increased demand for cardiac output.

Whole blood, red cells, or modified whole blood will provide volume-expanding effects as well as oxygen-carrying capacity, and replacement with blood should begin as early as possible. At the time the first needle is inserted into the patient's vein to begin fluid infusion, a properly labeled blood sample should be taken for typing and crossmatching. In general, the preferred component for transfusion is of the ABO and Rh types of the patient; it takes only several minutes to establish this. If time permits, a complete crossmatch should be done before transfusion begins, but the surgeon should never hesitate to accept uncrossmatched blood if waiting for the completion of the tests will increase the risk to the patient. Type O, Rh-negative blood is often held in emergency rooms for immediate transfusion into patients whose ABO and Rh type are not known. It is usually safer to wait a few minutes for blood of the recipient's ABO type. If type O blood is to be used for patients of unknown type, it should be in the form of red cell concentrate. The larger plasma volume of whole blood may contain dangerous amounts of anti-A or anti-B, which can destroy red cells of the recipient and delay subsequent administration of type-specific blood.

In the emergency situation created by the rapidly bleeding patient, blood components should be chosen first on the basis of compatibility of blood type. If whole blood of the appropriate blood type is immediately available, that could be the first choice for transfusion, since it would provide not only red cells but also plasma. If whole blood is not available, red blood cell concentrates will have to be used. These must be supplemented, especially if large numbers of units are transfused, with additional intravenous fluids. These fluids may be electrolyte solutions, plasma substitutes, or plasma itself. The plasma used for volume replacement can be of any storage age, but it is often most convenient to store plasma for emergency situations in the frozen state. Such plasma has its normal complement of coagulation factors, although, as already indicated, they are usually not required.

With severe tissue damage, prolonged shock, and generalized bleeding, DIC should be suspected. Although primary control of DIC should be directed to restoration of normal blood volume, replacement of hemostatic factors may accelerate recovery. If the fibrinogen level is low, cryoprecipitate should be transfused. Each bag of cryoprecipitate contains approximately 250 mg of fibrinogen,[22] and the transfusion of 4 grams (16 bags) should raise the fibrinogen level of the average adult by more than 100 mg/dl. The cryoprecipitates will, in addition, provide large amounts of Factor VIII. Cryoprecipitates also contain the α_2 glycoprotein fibronectin, which provides essential opsonins. Recent work suggests that transfusion of cryoprecipitate into the injured patient with sepsis reverses the opsonin deficiency and this is paralleled by a decline in the septic state as well as marked improvement in cardiopulmonary function.[23]

Many blood banks provide cryoprecipitate with 10 to 20 ml of plasma into which it can be dissolved on thawing. Thus, the fibrinogen and Factor VIII concentrate is in fresh-frozen plasma. Sixteen bags of cryoprecipitate containing an average of 15 ml fresh-frozen plasma each provide 250 ml of plasma, the equivalent of a unit of fresh-frozen plasma. Therefore, cryoprecipitates as well as fresh-frozen plasma may be used to supplement red cell concentrates to provide volume as well as plasma coagulation factors.

Platelet transfusions may be required to prevent or correct the dilutional thrombocytopenia of uncomplicated massive blood transfusion or to correct the thrombocytopenia caused by DIC. Prophylaxis may be accomplished by using fresh whole blood which still contains viable platelets. There are a significant number of viable platelets in whole blood stored not more than 24 hours and, when available, such blood could be administered once the patient has received an equivalent of 1.5 to 2 times his blood volume in replacement therapy. Of course, fresh blood should never be wasted by transfusing it before it is needed. The suggestin that fresh, unrefrigerated blood has unique hemostatic capabilities[24] has no scientific support. The argument for fresh, warm blood was based on the fact that platelets lose their ability to be aggregated by ADP within hours of blood collection. It was assumed, therefore, that fresh, warm blood would provide effective platelets, whereas platelet concentrates stored for up to 72 hours might not. No studies were ever done to compare the hemostatic effect of fresh, warm, whole blood vs. routine platelet concentrates; it is of course now well established by published data[9] and general experience that platelet concentrates are hemostatically effective when stored for periods up to 72 hours. In summary, then, there is no justification for demanding fresh unrefrigerated blood for massive transfusion, and requests for whole blood stored less than 24 hours can be met only to the extent that such units happen to be available. The simplest and most direct method of providing the patient with effective platelets is to transfuse platelet concentrates. These can be routinely stockpiled and made available with a minimum of delay. Of course, if the platelet count of the recipient is already low enough to cause bleeding problems, it will not be possible to raise it adequately with whole blood. Platelets must then be transfused as concentrates.

Seattle have confirmed these observations,[7] demonstrating correction of the defect with transfusion of platelet concentrates.

STRATEGIES FOR MASSIVE TRANSFUSION: THE TRAUMA PATIENT

The trauma patient can present the most severe problems. He is likely to be admitted with no history as to previous transfusion or hemostasis problems, and often with inadequate history of the nature of his injury. He may have spent far too long with reduced blood volume and arrive in severe shock. Massive tissue damage will aggravate the tendency to DIC. Control of large bleeding vessels is the first concern. Such patients are obviously best handled in a trauma service with adequate experienced personnel and supplies to handle such problems.

Obtaining a blood sample for typing and crossmatching and starting intravenous infusions is the first priority. The choice of electrolytes vs. colloids, whole blood vs. packed red cells, etc., will depend on the previous experiences of the surgeons and the relative availability of the different products.

Bleeding from the site of trauma does not, of course, imply a generalized hemostatic defect; but, if generalized oozing occurs at all cut surfaces and all needle puncture sites, a hemostatic defect can be assumed to be present. Studies both in the combat casualties of Viet Nam[25] and in civilian casualties in this country[7] have made it clear that the most likely cause when generalized bleeding occurs is a deficiency of platelets. In the Viet Nam experience, abnormal bleeding did not correlate with results of the prothrombin time or partial thromboplastin time tests, and bleeding was not controlled by infusion of fresh-frozen plasma. In contrast, bleeding was associated with low platelet counts and was controlled by transfusion of fresh whole blood. Recent studies on trauma patients in

STRATEGIES FOR MASSIVE TRANSFUSION: CARDIOPULMONARY BYPASS

Cardiopulmonary bypass adds the further complications of exposure of blood to large foreign surfaces, including a gas interface, and the use of heparin. All of the problems previously described for massive transfusion situations may also be encountered. However, in recent years there has been a marked decrease in the volumes of blood transfused during open heart surgery and, in any case, the volume employed to prime the extracorporeal circuit is not large enough to have by itself a significant effect on the patient. Recognition of this fact has resulted in extensive use of hemodilution, where electrolytes provide a large proportion or all of the priming solution, with the expectation that most or all of the red cells in the extracorporeal circuit will be returned to the patient at the end of the operation. The volume of blood used for priming and to replace blood lost by hemorrhage is often as low as two to three units and is rarely more than ten. Therefore, it makes little sense for the heart surgeon to insist on fresh whole blood for the procedure. Packed red cells of any storage age may be used and, in fact, many patients have been operated on successfully using frozen-thawed red cells. These cells are suspended in saline with no platelets and no coagulation factors.

Defects in hemostasis are more common after cardiopulmonary bypass, however, than in other types of major surgery. Innumerable publications have proposed a welter of explanations and corrective therapy. In all likelihood, the causes of abnormal bleeding in this situation can be attributed to inadequate heparin neutralization, DIC, and platelet problems. Heparin neutralization is usually well controlled with experience. DIC is a rare complication, but there are situations in which poor flow coupled with inadequate levels of heparin can induce defibrination during bypass. Moreover, inadequate cardiac output following bypass can potentiate DIC, especially if the heparin is neutralized too quickly. Such situations are so rare that the routine use of fresh-frozen plasma cannot be justified in this situation.

Platelets present a special problem in cardiopulmonary bypass. As soon as bypass begins, the platelet count of the recipient will drop approximately 50 percent. This occurs even if the circuit was primed with fresh whole blood which, therefore, offers no advantages. At the end of bypass, the platelet count is almost always below normal but usually greater than $90,000/\mu l$. Even counts as low as 60,000 are not usually associated with more bleeding than are higher counts. Only in the rare cases where DIC has occurred or very large amounts of stored blood were administered will there be sufficient thrombocytopenia to require platelet transfusion. Prophylactic use of platelets in this situation does not decrease blood loss,[26] is a waste of a valuable commodity, and exposes the patient to additional sources of hepatitis.

Very recently, Harker et al.[18] presented the best evidence that a significant qualitative platelet defect may occur during cardiopulmonary bypass. Harker showed that the template bleeding time became progressively prolonged during bypass and was always over 30 minutes if the bypass lasted long enough. The prolonged bleeding time was associated with a loss of alpha granules from the platelets, presumably because they were activated by exposure to the foreign surfaces. In almost all cases, the prolonged bleeding time was quickly corrected when bypass was discontinued. The rare patient with a generalized bleeding tendency after bypass had a persistently prolonged bleeding time. In all of those cases, transfusions of platelet concentrates normalized the bleeding time and controlled

Table 24-5. Most Useful Screening Tests for Hemostasis When Abnormal Bleeding Follows Cardiopulmonary Bypass

1. Platelet count
2. Fibrinogen
3. Template bleeding time

hemostasis. It is important to note that many of these patients who benefitted from platelet transfusions had a platelet count in excess of $100,000/\mu l$.

From Harker's studies, the conclusion is that the most useful tests of hemostasis during and following heart surgery are those listed in Table 24-5. As already indicated, it is possible to do a bleeding time on a patient during surgery by performing it on a leg.

Finally, if we compare the studies of Counts on trauma patients[7] with those of Harker on cardiopulmonary bypass,[18] it appears that the qualitative platelet defect noted by Harker in open heart surgery was not recognized to be a problem in the trauma series. Both of these studies were carried out by personnel from the same institution. Counts did not find the bleeding time to be helpful in managing the patients in the trauma series. Both authors concluded, however, that there was no need for fresh whole blood and no need for fresh-frozen plasma in massive transfusion situations. Both demonstrated the usefulness of platelet concentrates for dilutional thrombocytopenia in trauma as well as for the qualitative platelet defect in cardiopulmonary bypass.

FINAL COMMENTS

During surgery or trauma, rapid blood loss from the site of injury alone should not be assumed to indicate a generalized defect of hemostasis unless there is profuse oozing from all of the exposed surfaces.

When hemostatic breakdown seems likely, therapy is best guided by appropriate laboratory tests, with primary emphasis on the platelet count and fibrinogen level. Supplementation of these tests with a bleeding time, prothrombin time (PT) or partial thromboplastin time (PTT) is probably wise, provided that they are used as indications for transfusion of specific components only when markedly abnormal. The usefulness of the bleeding time to document a qualitative platelet defect after cardiopulmonary bypass has been documented, but even in the trauma situation a bleeding time greater than 15 to 25 minutes would logically call for platelet concentrates. A decreased fibrinogen level may indicate consumption coagulopathy and levels below 60 to 100 mg/dl should be treated with cryoprecipitates. The PT and PTT may provide further evidence of DIC, especially in situations where the fibrinogen concentration was originally very high and consumption reduced it to levels still within normal limits. If the PT and PTT are prolonged more than 1.5 to 2 times control values, cryoprecipitate should be supplemented with fresh-frozen plasma to ensure adequate levels of Factor V. All of the above recommendations for specific hemostatic therapy assume that the patient is bleeding in a manner which suggests defective hemostasis.

The laboratory tests should not be used as an arbitrary indication for therapy. Abnormal test results are frequently found in patients who are not bleeding abnormally. Moreover, no specific test results can be offered as a goal of therapy. The patient with a large open wound requires approximately 100,000 platelets per μl; far lower levels are required before abnormal bleeding will occur spontaneously. Similar considerations involve plasma coagulation factors. Bleeding will occur at the operative site or in other potential bleeding sites (e.g., stress ulcers) with levels of clotting factors otherwise adequate for control of spontaneous bleeding.

When laboratory tests are not feasible, or not available in time, transfusion therapy must be empirical. Platelet concentrates (8 to 10 units) should be given after transfusion of more than 15 units of blood. Routine administration of fresh-frozen plasma at intervals is often recommended; for example, Gill et al.[27] recommend two units of fresh-frozen plasma with every ten units of red cells. However, no evidence is available to support the necessity for this regime. When there is generalized oozing and other evidence of defective hemostasis, transfusion of platelet concentrates should be the first consideration. If these fail to correct the bleeding tendency, cryoprecipitates, supplemented if necessary with fresh-frozen plasma, should be administered.

Correction of the hemostatic defects is important, but equal effort must be addressed to maintenance of the blood volume and an adequate level of hemoglobin. Platelet concentrates, cryoprecipitates, and fresh-frozen plasma will provide part of the volume replacement, but red cells and possibly other fluids will also be necessary.

REFERENCES

1. Codes of Federal Regulations. #21 Food and Drugs, 640:4, 1979.
2. Perkins, H.A., Snyder, M., Thacher, C., and Rolfs, M.R.: Calcium ion activity during rapid exchange transfusion with citrated blood. Transfusion 11:204, 1971.
3. Howland, W.S., Jacobs, R.G., and Goulet, A.H.: An evaluation of calcium administration during rapid blood replacement. Anesth. Analg. 39:557, 1960.
4. Dern, R.J., Gwinn, R.P., and Wiorkowski, J.J.: Studies on the preservation of human blood. I. Variability in erythrocyte storage characteristics among healthy donors. J. Lab. Clin. Med. 67:955, 1966.
5. Rapaport, S.I., Ames, S.B., and Mikkelsen, S.: The levels of antihemophilic globulin and proaccelerin in fresh and bank blood. Am. J. Clin. Pathol. 31:297, 1959.
6. Rizza, C.R.: Management of patients with coagulation factor deficiencies. In Biggs, R. (ed.): Human Blood Coagulation, Haemostasis and Thrombosis. Blackwell, Oxford, 1976, p. 392.
7. Counts, R.B., Haisch, C., Simon, T.L., Max-

well, N.G., Heimbach, D.M., and Carrico, C.J.: Hemostasis in massively transfused trauma patients. Ann. Surg. 190:91, 1979.

8. Kissmeyer-Nielsen, F. and Madsen, C.B.: Platelets in blood stored in untreated and siliconed glass bottles and plastic bags. II. Survival studies. J. Clin. Pathol. 14:630, 1961.

9. Slichter, S.L. and Harker, L.A.: Preparation and storage of platelet concentrates. II. Storage variables influencing platelet viability and function. Br. J. Haematol. 34:403, 1976.

10. Krevans, J.R. and Jackson, D.P.: Hemorrhagic disorder following massive whole blood transfusions. J.A.M.A. 159:171, 1955.

11. Lomanto, D. and Howland, W.S.: A re-evaluation of massive blood replacement. Clin. Anesthesiol. 9:33, 1972.

12. Greenberg, J.R., Rosenman, L.D., and Lewis, A.E.: Ammonia content of stored blood. J.A.M.A. 165:348, 1957.

13. Jaeger, R.J. and Rubin, R.J.: Migration of a phthalate ester plasticizer from polyvinyl chloride blood bags into stored human blood and its localization in human tissues. N. Engl. J. Med. 287:1114, 1972.

14. Falk, J.S., Lindblad, G.T.O., and Westman, J.M.: Histopathologic studies on kidneys from patients treated with large amounts of blood preserved with ACD-adenine. Transfusion 12:376, 1972.

15. Åkerblom, O., De Verdier, C.-H., Finnson, M., Garby, L., Högman, C.F., and Johansson, S.G.O.: Further studies on the effect of adenine in blood preservation. Transfusion 7:1, 1967.

16. Hopkins, R.W., Fratianne, R.B., Rao, K.V., and Damewood, C.A.: Effects of hematocrit and viscosity on continuing hemorrhage. J. Trauma, 14:482, 1974.

17. Perkins, H.A.: Postoperative coagulation defects. Anesthesiology 27:456, 1966.

18. Harker, L.A., Branson, H.E., Malpass, T.W., Hessel, E.A., II, and Slichter, S.J.: Mechanism of abnormal bleeding in patients undergoing cardiopulmonary bypass: Acquired transient platelet dysfunction associated with α granule release. Blood (in press).

19. McNamara, J.J., Burran, E.L., Stremple, J.F., et al.: Coagulopathy after major injury. Ann. Surg. 176:243, 1977.

20. Alving, B.M., Hojima, Y., Pisano, J.J., Mason, B.L., Buckingham, R.E., Jr., Mozen, M.M., and Finlayson, J.S.: Hypotension associated with prekallikrein activator (Hageman-factor fragments) in plasma protein fraction. N. Engl. J. Med. 299:66, 1978.

21. Virgilio, R.W., Rice, C.L., Smith, D.E., James, D.R., Zarins, C.K., Hobelmann, C.F., and Peters, R.M.: Crystalloid vs. colloid resuscitation: Is one better? Surgery 85:129, 1979.

22. Ness, P.M. and Perkins, H.A.: Cryoprecipitate as a reliable source of fibrinogen replacement. J.A.M.A. 241:1690, 1979.

23. Saba, T.M. and Jaffe, E.: Plasma fibronectin (opsonic glycoprotein): Its synthesis by vascular endothelial cells and role in cardiopulmonary integrity after trauma as related to reticuloendothelial function. Am. J. Med. 68:577, 1980.

24. Lim, R.C., Jr., Olcott, C., Robinson, A.J., et al.: Platelet response and coagulation changes following massive blood replacement. J. Trauma 13:577, 1973.

25. Miller, R.D., Robbins, T.O., Tong, M.J., and Barton, S.L.: Coagulation defects associated with massive blood transfusions. Ann. Surg. 174:794, 1971.

26. Woods, J.E., Taswell, H.F., Kirklin, J.W., and Owen, C.A., Jr.: The transfusion of platelet concentrates in patients undergoing heart surgery. Mayo Clin. Proc. 42:318, 1967.

27. Gill, W., Champion, H.R., Long, W.B., et al.: Volume resuscitation in critical major trauma. J. Roy. Coll. Surg. (Edin.) 20:166, 1975.

25

Blood Component Therapy for Patients with Coagulation Disorders

John A. Penner, M.D.

The hemostatic potential of blood components has been recognized for well over a century; however, the therapeutic use of blood components had to await developments in the field of coagulation as well as in the technical sciences associated with protein separation. With the rapid advances in both areas over the past 30 years, it has become possible to produce concentrates of many of the blood clotting elements. As a result, replacement therapy now has become an accepted practice in the management of hemorrhagic disorders. The complexities of the coagulation mechanism, however, have presented problems, and the clinical use of these components often has suffered from the physician's failure to understand principles of hemostasis. The following brief review of some of the historical events in blood coagulation, with a discussion of the practical aspects of the clotting mechanism and the characteristics of the available products, will provide a basis for a better understanding of our present therapeutic use of concentrated blood products.

HISTORICAL DEVELOPMENTS

Initial observations on the process of hemostasis recognized that a gelatinous clot formed after blood was withdrawn from the circulation and that the clot consisted of cells held together by a fibrous structure—Fibrin. The presence of an enzyme in blood, responsible for the formation of this fibrous material, was postulated by Alexander Schmidt in 1861[1,2] as he developed his theory of blood coagulation based on the proteolytic enzyme thrombin's role in converting the soluble fibrinogen to the gel-like fibrin. Recognition of other plasma factors involved in the clotting of blood for the most part arose from the clinical descriptions of the familial bleeding disorders. Hemophilia, for example, was well recognized in writings of the Koran as early as the second century, A.D., as a transmitted hemorrhagic disorder which appeared in male offspring. The rite of circumcision was abrogated in families with this disorder if death occurred in the first two males of the family as a result of bleeding. The postulation that a deficiency of a specific clotting factor was responsible for failure of clot formation and bleeding in this disorder was not established until Dr. John Otto in 1803[3] described the clinical manifestations and noted that blood obtained from these patients would not clot. Hemophilia B, Factor IX deficiency, was not identified as a separate entity from classical hemophilia until well over 100 years later. Dr. Pavlovsky in Argentina identified a family with a sex-linked hemorrhagic disorder whose plasma would correct the clotting time of plasma from families considered to have a classical form of hemophilia.[4] Dr. Biggs and coworkers in England subsequently described a similar sex-linked disorder in a family with the surname Christmas.[5] With the aid of a newly developed two-stage clotting assay—the thromboplastin generation test (TGT), which required a mixture of plasma and serum to generate clotting activity—they demonstrated that the plasma of the patient with classical hemophilia was defective and could be corrected by adding plasma from members of the Christmas family. On the other hand, the Christmas family's serum was found to be defective in the TGT, and this defect could be corrected by adding normal serum or serum from patients with classical hemophilia.[6] The Christmas factor deficiency—Hemophilia B, therefore—was characterized, and another factor was added to the clotting mechanism. A number of years prior to the discovery of the Christmas factor, several investigators working independently in the late 1930s approached the clotting system by different paths and discovered the requirement for a labile globulin subsequently termed Factor V.

Dr. Walter Seegers, a pioneer in the field, participated in much of the early work on thrombin and antithrombin with the University of Iowa group. While pursuing his investigation of the properties of purified prothrombin at Wayne State University in Detroit, Seegers recognized that a labile plasma factor accelerated the conversion of prothrombin to thrombin. He separated this factor from plasma and characterized it as a globulin, which he termed Accelerator Globulin (AC-G).[7] Dr. Armand Quick in Milwaukee devised a new clotting test, the prothrombin time, which employed tissue thromboplastin and calcium to produce a clot in plasma. While using the prothrombin time test, Quick realized that plasma lost activity when stored, and that a labile plasma factor was necessary to promote rapid clot formation in his test.[8] At almost the same time in Oslo, Norway, Dr. Paul Owren encountered a patient with a serious bleeding disorder whose blood clotted slowly and could be corrected by the addition of fresh but not aged plasma.[9] Initially, he named the deficient substance Factor V and later Accelerin. These observations were reported during World War II. Owren, Seegers, and Quick were all unaware of the others' findings until several years after their discoveries.

Many of the clotting factors have had similar histories—recognition and description by several investigators and, as a result, multiple terminologies. Factor VII, for example, was known initially as serum prothrombin conversion accelerator (SPCA) by Dr. Alexander[10]; as proconvertin by Dr. Owren[8]; and as autoprothrombin I by Dr. Seegers.[11] A conference of many of the investigators in this field resolved the problem by compromising on a Roman numeral system. The currently accepted factors are listed in Table 25-1. Factors VII, X, and XI, like Factor V, were identified by investigating patients who demonstrated autosomal recessive transmission of a bleeding disorder in which the patient's plasma could be corrected by the addition of other defective plasmas. Systems using purified reagents have substantiated the requirement for these factors in the clotting mechanism. Note that two of the factors as-

Table 25-1. Plasma Clotting Factors

I	Fibrinogen	IX	PTC, Christmas, Auto II (IXa)*
II	Prothrombin (IIa)*	X	Stuart-Prower, Auto III (Xa, Auto C)*
III	Thromboplastin	XI	PTA (XIa)*
IV	Calcium	XII	Hageman (XIIa)*
V	Accelerator globulin (VI or Va)*	XIII	Fibrin stabilizer, Fibrinase (XIIIa)*
VII	SPCA, Auto I (VIIa)*	—	Fitzgerald, High molecular weight kininogen
VIII	Antihemophilic, AHF (VIIIa)*	—	Fletcher, Prekallikrein

* Active form

sociated with Factor XII[12]—the Fletcher[13] and Fitzgerald[14] Factors—comprise the contact activation system and have not as yet received a Roman numeral designation. The contact factors are unique in that the patients with these deficiencies do not have bleeding disorders; they were discovered as a result of abnormalities observed in coagulation screening procedures obtained prior to surgery. The characterization of these factors is proceeding, and additional members of this group continue to be identified.[15]

THERAPY

The beginnings of replacement therapy, the administration of blood or plasma—even for the well-known hemophilic disorders—had to await the development of blood typing and transfusion techniques. As soon as the mysteries of the blood groups were mastered, however, the approach to the management of hemorrhagic problems proceeded as expected with transfusion of whole blood containing all of the elements presumably required for hemostasis. With the recognition that certain of these factors, V and VIII, were labile—that is, their activity was not sustained on storage at 5°C for periods longer than 12 to 24 hours[16]—the demand for large quantities of fresh plasma and blood arose. Initially, the demand was met by preparing fresh plasma and freezing it for future use. The advent of fractionation techniques for separating some of these elements from plasma permitted long-term storage in lyophilized form and reduced the heavy burden on the blood bank for fresh blood.

Plasma fractionation evolved in 1946 with the application of a new technique to precipitate plasma proteins, Cohn and coworkers[17] found that ethanol precipitated proteins from plasma without denaturing them and that, as the concentration of ethanol increased, different groups of proteins precipitated. Thus, by adjusting the amount of ethanol added, it was possible to separate plasma proteins that could be concentrated and employed as therapeutic agents. Cohn's fraction I, consisting of fibrinogen, and Factor VIII, was one of the first products produced for therapeutic use. The Michigan Department of Health in 1951 prepared quantities of this fraction and made it available as a dry frozen concentrate for the treatment of hemophilic patients in the state. Subsequently, a commercial product, Fibro-AHF, was marketed by Merck-Sharpe and Dohme and employed for treatment of patients with hemophilia as well as those with fibrinogen deficiencies. The Ethanol precipitation process produced a seven-fold concentration. The final product, when reconstituted to a volume of 200 ml, contained approximately 2 grams of fibrinogen and 300 units of Factor VIII. Additional steps in the fractionating process were added later in the form of glycine[18] and, most recently, in the form of polyethylene glycol precipitation, which permitted further purification of the crude Cohn fractions without a significant decrease in yield. The demand for Factor VIII by the 100,000 or so patients with classical hemophilia throughout the world has made these products commercially profitable for a number of manufacturers. The initial Cohn fraction produced primarily for its fibrinogen content has been discontinued as a result of the high incidence of hepatitis associated with its use and the availability of other sources of fibrinogen and Factor VIII.

Factor VIII Concentrates

A unique contribution to the preparation of Factor VIII was the development of cryoprecipitation techniques. Fibrinogen was recognized for many years as cryoglobulin which appeared as a precipitate in thawed, frozen plasma. This precipitate dissolved as the plasma was brought to room temperature. It also was known that Factor VIII adhered to fibrinogen, and attempts to produce a Factor VIII free of fibrinogen had met with considerable difficulty. The brilliant discovery by Dr.

Judith Poole that Factor VIII also separated from plasma in the cold along with the fibrinogen[20] led to the development of a method for producing Factor VIII. This process and its modifications[21] suddenly made available a greatly expanded capacity for production of Factor VIII and stimulated blood banking facilities in this country to provide large quantities of Factor VIII from our blood resources. With cryoprecipitation techniques, it also was possible to separate Factor VIII for immediate use or for further concentration by other methods and to proceed with processing the remaining plasma for prothrombin complex (prothrombin and Factors VII, IX, and X), albumin, and gamma globulin. Albumin has been the most profitable plasma fraction and perhaps has provided the major incentive for manufacturers to consider preparing clotting factors, since the processing of additional fractions from the same plasma source reduced the cost of plasma for each product.

Prothrombin Complex

Previous investigational experience with preparation of prothrombin permitted the rapid development of methods using tricalcium phosphate and DEAE resins for concentrating all of the vitamin K-dependent clotting factors—prothrombin and Factors VII, IX, and X.[22] This prothrombin complex became available as a concentrate as soon as the hemophilia B patient's therapeutic need materialized.[23] Considerable interest also was shown in possible use of the complex for hemorrhagic disorders associated with liver disease and warfarin therapy, although the product's potential for causing hepatitis and thrombosis has virtually eliminated this application.

"Activated" Prothrombin Complex

The newest and perhaps most innovative development in the field of replacement therapy has been the preparation of a product specifically designed to combat the bleeding problems that occur in the hemophilic patient with a Factor VIII inhibitor. The potential use of products containing activated factors for bypassing the Factor VIII requirements of the coagulation process was well recognized from laboratory experience that defined the role of Factor Xa and its activators in the clotting cascade. The initial studies by Fecete and coworkers[24] and by Kurczynski and Penner[25] demonstrated the antiinhibitor properties of a prothrombin complex concentrate which contained a number of spontaneously generated active factors; this led to the preparation of the first plasma fraction tailored for use in a specific disorder. The new approach, "bypassing therapy," represents a significant change from our concept of using blood components in their native state as "replacement" for deficient factors.

Many other products containing concentrates of plasma factors remain to be developed or are in the process of development. Concentrates of Factor V, for example, are difficult to prepare and useful only for a small number of patients with congenital deficiencies, while the plasma protease inhibitors, antithrombin III, and the fibrinolytic agent, plasminogen, could be in great demand provided they prove to be efficacious in thrombotic disorders.

HEMOSTASIS

The hemostatic mechanism, from a practical aspect, must be examined in relation to the various components involved in maintaining the integrity of the vascular bed. Bleeding develops with injury to the vessel wall resulting in extravasation of blood into extraendothelial and extravascular tissues. The role of the vessel in this process is recognized but not completely understood. Contraction of large as well as small vessels, some without surrounding muscle cells, occurs almost immediately with injury decreasing blood flow and producing stasis. The platelet's role in this process also must be acknowledged. Much of the vasoconstriction observed may represent a response to substances released from platelets activated by contact with a damaged vessel wall. Plasma factors become involved relatively late in the hemostatic process eventually providing the fibrin structure which serves as mesh work for the clot enclosing incorporated erythrocytes and leukocytes. The reparative phase is ushered in by the fibrinolytic system, which also interacts with complement and other elements of inflammation.

Table 25-2 lists these major phases of hemostasis. Note that vascular response occurs in the first few seconds, as do platelet adhesion and release of vasoactive substances. Fibrin formation begins shortly after the platelets accumulate at the site of injury and slowly progresses over a period of minutes. Fibrinolysis and reendothelization develop much more slowly, requiring days for completion.

Platelet function has been described in another section; however, for purposes of continuity here, the platelets' contributions to hemostasis must be recognized—particularly their unique ability to seal the damaged vascular bed by adhering to subendothelial collagen and elastin to form a plug. The Von-Willebrand's factor, along with its associated Factor VIII,[26] is required for this function and is attached to the platelet membrane. A deficiency of the VonWillebrand's factor or its binding site on the platelet membrane

(Bernard-Soulier Syndrome) impairs platelet adhesion, producing a bleeding disorder comparable to that of severe thrombocytopenia.[27]

The platelet's ability to *aggregate* and *release* in response to physiologic and non-physiologic agents—thrombin, ADP, epinephrine, collagen, endotoxin, and the Von-Willebrand's cofactor, Ristocetin—also contributes to hemostasis. When these agents bind to or stimulate the platelet membrane, metabolic processes are activated which initiate prostaglandin synthesis through the action of a specific phospholipase which breaks down dietary fatty acids in the membrane (Fig. 25-1).[28] When thromboxane, the major end product of prostaglandin synthesis in the platelet, is released, it produces a powerful vasoconstriction and induces additional platelet aggregation, while prostacyclin, the major product of the endothelial cell, inhibits this response. Release of serotonin, another vasoconstricting agent, also occurs during platelet aggregation. In addition, the membrane phospholipid, platelet factor 3, becomes exposed while a similar substance in the platelet granule is released, providing a binding surface for calcium on which prothrombin, Factor X, and other procoagulants interact to form thrombin. Defects in aggregation, prostaglandin synthesis, or release result in ineffective hemostasis demonstrated by a variety of hereditary disorders such as thrombasthenia and storage pool disorders, and by acquired drug-induced dysfunctions.[29]

Table 25-2. Phases of Hemostatis

Vascular: (2–5 sec)	1. Contraction
	2. Loss of endothelial integrity and capacity to release prostacycline, fibrinolysin activator, and antithrombin
	3. Attachment and activation of contact factors XII, prekallikrein.
Platelet: (3–10 sec)	1. Adhesion to damaged area and release of thromboxane A_2
	2. Aggregation and release of ca++, factor 3, factor 4, thromboxane A_2, Serotonin, ATP, ADP.
Plasma: (30–120 sec)	1. Activation intrinsic path XII_a-X_a-Thrombin
	2. Fibrin clot formation
Repair: (6–48 hr) (10–60 days)	1. Fibrinolysis
	2. Endothelialization

PROSTAGLANDIN GENERATION

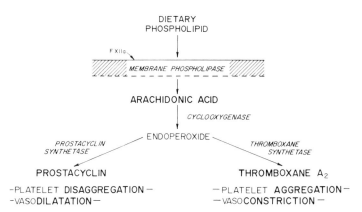

Fig. 25-1. Prostaglandin Generation: Formation of thromboxane A$_2$, the major product of platelet and prostacyclin, the major product of endothelial cells.

Plasma Clotting Factors

The plasma clotting factors[30] involved in hemostasis are listed in Table 25-1. The list has been expanded recently to include substances which interact with the surface proteases and in turn affect the fibrinolysin and complement systems. The complex interaction of these clotting factors can best be explained by examining several of the major reactions involved: (1) activation of Factor X; (2) thrombin formation; and (3) fibrin formation.

Contact activation initiates the cascade of the intrinsic system (Fig. 25-2). Factor XII becomes bound to negatively charged surfaces and undergoes a conformational change with the help of small amounts of kallikrein (active Fletcher factor) formed in the circulation. The resulting protease, Factor XIIa, activates both Factor XI and prekallikrein, which in turn catalyze the formation of more Factor XII. Factor XIa in the presence of platelet phospholipid (platelet factor 3) participates along with other members of the intrinsic clotting system, Factors VIII and IX (Fig. 25-3A) in the formation of Factor Xa, the amplifier for the clotting mechanism. Small amounts of Factor X also can be activated directly by Factor XII, while much larger quantities are generated when Factor VIII interacts with tissue thromboplastin and

Factor V. This latter reaction has been termed the extrinsic pathway (Fig. 25-2), recognizing the extrinsic nature of tissue products as opposed to the intrinsic system (Fig. 25-2) in which all of the factors required in coagulation are available within the blood stream. Once the very potent Factor Xa is formed in the presence of Factor V and platelet factor 3, a rapid conversion of prothrombin to thrombin occurs (Fig. 25-4).

Thrombin then acts on fibrinogen by cleaving fibrinopeptides A and B from the alpha and beta chain of the three-chained dimer to form monomers which precipitate as a gel. The presence of the transamidase, XIIIa, activated by thrombin from its precursor state, transforms the monomer gel into a cross-linked, structured clot (Fig. 25-5).

Despite the potency of activating agents, inhibitors for this process also are present and are able to control the reactions. Antithrombin III (ATIII), the naturally occurring inhibitor for serine proteases, inactivates thrombin, Xa, XIa, XII, but not VIIa. It is a progressive inhibitor, binding proteases slowly over a period of minutes. However, in the presence of heparin, ATIII becomes an immediate inhibitor, inactivating thrombin and other proteases within seconds.[31]

Fibrinolysin (plasmin) is a serine protease similar to thrombin and can cleave fibrinogen as well as fibrin into multiple fragments in a

COAGULATION CASCADE

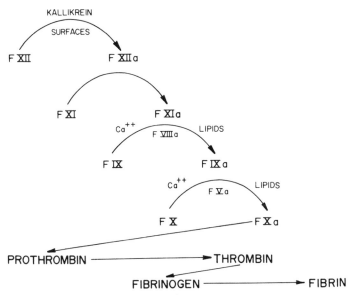

Fig. 25-2. Coagulation Cascade: Activation of the contact factors when they become attached to surfaces that develop a negative charge, leads to activation of the other serine proteases from their precursors and terminates with the formation of thrombin and conversion of fibrinogen into a fibrin clot. Many of these proteases interact with each other as well as other systems to provide a much more complex set of reactions as depicted in the illustration.

slowly progressive manner to form fragments designated X and Y (initial larger forms) and D and E (smaller later forms) (Fig. 25-6). Plasminogen can be activated by the active Fletcher factor (kallikrein) or by Factor XII in addition to tissue and bacterial kinases (Urokinase, Streptokinase). Antiplasmin, an alpha-2 glycoprotein, like ATIII inhibits plasmin but, unlike ATIII, does not interact with heparin.

INVESTIGATION OF BLEEDING DISORDERS

Laboratory Procedures

The investigation of hemorrhagic disorders is dependent on the use of several general co-agulation screening procedures,[32] although more specific assays may be required to establish a diagnosis. The various procedures available for laboratory investigation of coagulation problems are listed in Table 25-3.

Platelets can be enumerated by phase microscope count or by electronic counting devices, while platelet function can be assessed by the bleeding time. In major centers, more sophisticated procedures are available to define platelet dysfunctional states and provide measurements of adhesion, aggregation, and release as well as clot retraction.[33]

Plasma clotting factors can be evaluated by two simple assays that are routinely available in most hospitals. The prothrombin time (PT) is a measure of coagulation via the extrinsic system (Fig. 25-3) and requires the addition of the tissue extract-thromboplastin and Ca++ to the patient's citrated plasma. Defi-

A. *Extrinsic*

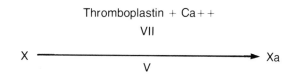

B. *Intrinsic*

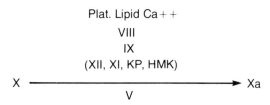

Fig. 25-3. Coagulation Reactions: a) the extrinsic system requires tissue substances (thromboplastin) to convert factor X to Xa and is assayed by the prothrombin time procedure. b) the intrinsic system require elements contained within the blood stream, platelet phosphatides providing the surface for plasma factor interaction and is assayed by the partial thromboplastin time. Activation of the contact factors is provided by surfaces—in the laboratory assay elliagic acid, Kaolin or celite usually are added.

ciencies of fibrinogen, prothrombin, or Factors VII, V, or X can prolong the prothrombin time clotting test, as can anticoagulants such as heparin and specific factor inhibitors arising in various clinical disorders. The partial thromboplastin (APTT) is essentially a lipid activated clotting time and provides a measure of intrinsic coagulation (Fig. 25-2). the addition of a platelet phospholipid (platelet factor 3 substitute), calcium, and an activating surface for Factor XII (Celite, Kaolin, or ellagic acid) to the patient's plasma, activates Factor XII and the cascade with generation of thrombin. The clotting time is prolonged by the deficiency of fibrinogen or any of the in-

trinsic factors or by the presence of heparin or inhibitors (i.e., antibodies to Factor VIII in patients with Lupus Erythematosus). Thrombin evolves more slowly in this procedure; therefore, it is more sensitive to the action of heparin but less sensitive to fibrinogen deficiency than the prothrombin time.

Specific factor assays can be undertaken with either procedure by employing a commercially available factor-deficient plasma as a substrate for the test. For example, the patient's plasma in different dilutions can be added to Factor VIII-deficient plasma. The APTT values obtained with these additions can be compared with those obtained with

Final Pathway

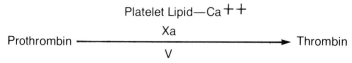

Fig. 25-4. Final Pathway: Factor Xa once formed in the intrinsic or extrinsic system acts as an amplifier for thrombin formation molecule of Xa in the presence of lipid and factor V can produce 50 to 100 molecules of thrombin from its precursor prothrombin.

Fibrin Formation

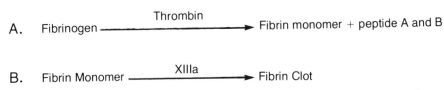

Fig. 25-5. Fibrin formation: (*A*) Fibrin monomer precipitate or gel forms after thrombin clips peptide A and B from the Fibrinogen Dimer. (*B*) A structured fibrin clot occurs when factor XII is converted to XIIIa, fibrinase, by thrombin. XIIa is able to interact with the fibrin monomer.

similar mixtures containing normal plasma to provide a measure of Factor VIII in the patient's plasma. Fibrinogen can be assayed directly by determining rate of clot formation following addition of thrombin, while the presence of heparin can be assessed also by adding thrombin and determining the clotting time (thrombin clotting time-TCT).[34] Correction of a prolonged TCT by the addition of protamine sulfate increases the specificity of the assay for heparin. Fibrinolysin activity can be evaluated by determining the lysis time of the patient's plasma euglobulin precipitate after reconstitution and clotting with thrombin (euglobulin lysis time). A number of new procedures which use chemical chromogenic substrates as a substitute for fibrinogen are proving useful for specific assays of various factors. The end point is determined by a spectrophotometer rather than by a clot timing device.[35]

Diagnostic Approach

Although the approach to the bleeding patient is dependent upon the laboratory and its ability to provide the procedures described above, the patient's clinical history is of considerable importance in the selection of the appropriate laboratory procedures and in assessing the severity and form of the hemorrhagic problem. A history of a congenital or familial disorder in a male will focus attention on a single plasma factor deficiency, Factor VIII or IX, recognizing that the hemophilias are the most frequently encountered inherited disorder in a male. A similar bleeding disorder in a female suggests Von Willebrand's disease or, if the patient is Jewish, Factor XI deficiency (both conditions also can be seen in males). Older patients without a history of bleeding problems most likely have an acquired hemorrhagic problem as-

Fibrinolysin

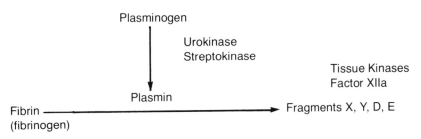

Fig. 25-6. Fibrinolysin: Plasminogen (prekallikrein) can be activated by a number of substances to form the protease plasmin which attacks fibrin splitting off fragments identified by their size and ability to precipitate or interfere with thrombin activity.

Table 25-3. Clinical Laboratory Procedures

PLATELET COUNT
    Bleeding Time
    Clot Retraction
    Prothrombin Consumption
    Platelet Aggregation
    Platelet Adhesion
PROTHROMBIN TIME
    Factor Assay (V, VII, X)
PARTIAL THROMBOPLASTIN TIME (Activated)
    Factor Assay (V, VII, IX, X, XI, XII, Fitzgerald, Fletcher, etc.)
THROMBIN CLOTTING TIME
    (Heparin, Fibrinogen)
FIBRINOGEN ASSAY
FIBRIN SPLIT PRODUCTS
EUGLOBULIN LYSIS TIME (Fibrinolysin)
    Plasminogen Chromogenic Assay (Plasminogen, plasmin activator
    and Inhibitors)

sociated with liver disease or perhaps a collagen-vascular disorder.

The laboratory procedures of most value for screening are (1) the platelet count and the bleeding time, for identifying platelet deficiency or dysfunction and (2) the prothrombin time and activated partial thromboplastin time, for determining the adequacy of the plasma factors. These procedures will provide information required to establish the need for treatment and to select appropriate blood component. Assays for specific factors and platelet functions will further define the disorder, but such information is seldom necessary to initiate therapy.

HEMOSTATIC BLOOD COMPONENTS

Blood products currently available for use in hemorrhagic disorders are listed in Table 25-4. The effectiveness of these hemostatic agents is dependent upon the accuracy of the diagnosis and the selection and administration of the appropriate product. With respect to administration, rapid infusion by vein is recommended in order to ensure a maximum circulating level of the product sufficient to correct an existing deficiency. Specific orders to this effect often are necessary to discourage

infusion at a slow rate which may fail to provide an effective level.

Factor activity is defined on the basis of a plasma equivalent unit. One unit represents the activity of a given factor in 1 ml of pooled fresh normal plasma. For example: 800 units of Factor VIII are equivalent to the Factor VIII present in 800 ml of plasma.

PLATELET CONCENTRATES

Preparation

Platelets currently are obtained from plasma prepared by plasmapheresis technique or from whole blood.[36] "Double or triple pak" plastic bags are employed to maintain a closed system which allows separation of platelet-rich plasma from the erythrocytes by centrifugation. An additional centrifugation of the platelet-rich plasma concentrates the platelets and either permits the displacement of the supernatant plasma into a separate satellite bag for further processing or returns the plasma to the original bag to reconstitute the red cells. Platelet concentrates must contain at least 5.5×10^{10} platelets (50 percent of the platelets available from a unit of whole blood) in a plasma volume of approximately 50 ml. A slightly acidic antico-

Table 25-4. Coagulation Components of Blood

Product	Content (approximate)	Clinical Use	Comments
Platelet Concentrate	0.5×10^{10} platelets/50-ml bag	Thrombocytopenia 1 bag/10 kg	Loss of function on storage. Outdated after 72 hours. Low incidence of hepatitis.
Plasma	240 ml	All deficiency disorders 5–10 ml/kg	Low incidence of hepatitis. Store frozen.
Factor VIII Concentrate	300 μ/10 ml 1000 μ/30 ml	Hemophilia A 10–20 μ/kg	High frequency of non-A, non-B hepatitis. Store at room temp. or 5°C.
Cryoprecipitate	Factor VIII-100 μ/20 ml VonWillebrand's factor-150 μ Fibrinogen-200 mg	Hemophilia A or Von-Willebrand's Disease 1 bag/10 kg	Low incidence of hepatitis. Store frozen.
Prothrombin Complex	Factor IX-500 μ/30 ml Factor X-300 μ, II Prothrombin-200 μ Factor VII-300 μ	Hemophilia B 10–20 μ/kg	High incidence non-A, non-B hepatitis. Thrombogenicity may be a problem. Store at 5°C.
Anti-inhibitor Complex	Factor IX-400 μ/30 ml Factor X-200 μ Prothrombin-150 μ Factor VII-800 μ Factor Xa 4–6 μ	Factor VIII and Factor IX Inhibitor Disorders 50–100 μ/kg	High incidence non-A, non-B hepatitis. Expect thrombogenicity as a potential problem. Store at 5°C.
Antithrombin III	500 μ/10 ml	Thrombotic Disorders 20 μ/kg	Low incidence, if any, of hepatitis. Experimental product.
Plasminogen	Unknown	Thrombotic Disorders	Low incidence of hepatitis. Experimental product.

agulant (CPD) generally is used in order to reduce the tendency for platelet clumping. Concentrates are maintained at room temperature in most blood banks and are discarded after 72 hours of storage.

Administration and Dosage

Each concentrate is administered rapidly within 15 minutes through a filter to prevent clumped platelets from entering the circulation. Although dosage requirements will depend on the clinical situation and the existing platelet count, one concentrate per 10 kg of body weight usually will increase the circulating platelet count 30,000 to 50,000/mm³. If platelet antibodies are present in high concentration, these levels may not be achieved.

Bleeding may be controlled despite the lack of significant elevation in platelet count, according to some but not all observers (see Ch. 26).

Indications

Platelet concentrate therapy is recommended for thrombocytopenic disorders. Spontaneous bleeding may occur with platelet counts of less than 10,000/mm³. Providing platelet function is normal, values ranging from 10,000 to 50,000/mm³ usually are not associated with spontaneous bleeding and are not an indication for platelet concentrate administration unless active bleeding is present, presumably from a localized source (i.e., bleeding ulcer). Platelets with normal function and in excess of 50,000/mm³ provide effective hemostasis for minor surgery; values of 100,000/mm³ or more are preferred for major procedures, particularly when large areas of granulation tissue may be exposed or when extensive dissection is required.

The relationship of platelets to bleeding in patients suffering from thrombocytopenia of various etiologies is illustrated in Figure 25-7. Bleeding severity is indicated on a scale of 1 to 4, with 1 representing minimal activity (usually localized petechia), and 4 representing extensive bleeding from mucosal surfaces and skin not controlled by local measures. The platelet count has been plotted in relation to the bleeding scale and demonstrates the adequacy of platelet levels above 10,000/mm³ as well as the fact that many patients with values below 10,000/mm³ do not develop serious bleeding.

The function of the circulating platelets is of even greater significance than the platelet count. Clinical signs, appearance of new petechiae or mucosal bleeding, hematuria, etc. indicate a lack of functionally effective platelets. The bleeding time provides a very simple and direct test of platelet function and can be employed to determine needs for platelet concentrates. Figure 25-8 examines the same thrombocytopenic patients seen in Fig. 25-7. In Figure 25-8, clinical signs of bleeding are correlated with the bleeding time by the IVY method using a long, disposable lancet. Note that serious bleeding is associated with bleeding times of 15 minutes or greater. Most of these patients had platelet counts of less than 10,000/mm³. Patients with platelet dysfunction and bleeding times in excess of 15 minutes, therefore, would have a bleeding risk comparable to that of severe thrombocytopenia and may require platelet concentrate therapy, despite platelet counts that are in a nonbleeding range (see Ch. 26).

Hazards

Platelet concentrates may carry the hepatitis viruses. The risk is comparable to the administration of single units of blood. Platelets may clump when damaged; if infused, they can act as microemboli-occluding vessels or can generate and release sufficient thromboxane A_2 to induce vasospasm with resulting ischemia. Release of platelet factor 4 from damaged platelets also can neutralize heparin present in the circulation. Immunization frequently occurs following repeated administration of platelet concentrates. This problem is discussed in Chapters 26 and 27.

Clinical Disorders Which May Require Platelet Concentrates

Thrombocytopenic Disorders. These disorders can be categorized as familial or acquired. Familial conditions include May-

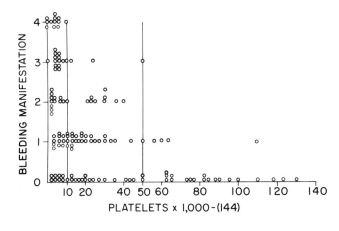

Fig. 25-7. Bleeding in thrombocytopenic patients: Bleeding manifestations rated on a scale of 1 to 4 (see text) are plotted in relation to platelet count in patients with thrombocytopenia.

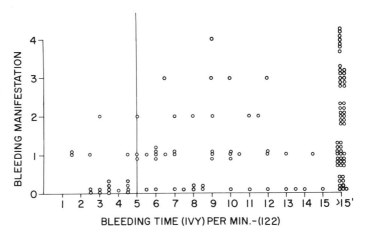

Fig. 25-8. Bleeding in thrombocytopenic patients: Bleeding manifestations rated on a scale of 1 to 4 (see text) are plotted in relation to the IVY Bleeding Time obtained on patients with thrombocytopenia.

Hegglin anomaly, TAR syndrome (thrombocytopenia with absent radius), and a group with a moderate thrombocytopenia and dysfunctional platelets—Wiskott-Aldrich Syndrome, Glanzmann's thrombasthenia, and Bernard-Soulier Disorder (Giant Platelet Syndrome). Acquired forms can be further classified on the basis of their etiology. Production disorders (megakaryocytopenic) may be secondary to chemical or drug toxicity or associated with bone marrow displacement by leukemia or lymphoma. Immune platelet destruction occurs in the form of idiopathic or autoimmune thrombocytopenia (ITP), post-transfusion purpura (PTP), and drug-induced thrombocytopenia. Increased utilization develops as a result of disseminated intravascular coagulation, particularly in the presence of endotoxins and in conditions in which endothelial damage predominates—e.g., thrombotic thrombocytopenia purpura (TTP) and homocystinuria. Dilutional thrombocytopenia also should be considered in the diagnosis of acquired thrombocytopenia; it is a finding in patients who receive large amounts of blood following a massive hemorrhage. Fresh blood is seldom available in large quantities, and bank blood is relatively platelet-poor after the first few days of storage.

Platelet Dysfunction Disorders. These disorders also can be classified as familial and acquired as well as by the function affected.

Most of the familial disorders listed above are characterized by a mild-to-moderate thrombocytopenia.

Qualitative disorders are primarily drug-induced, resulting from the use of aspirin, antiinflammatory drugs, and a large miscellaneous drug group which includes diuretics, tranquilizers, antihistamines, antibiotics, and barbiturates. Platelet aggregation and release are affected because most of these agents interfere with prostaglandin formation by inactivating cyclo-oxgenase, the enzyme that converts arachidonic acid and other fatty acids to endoperoxides prior to transformation into thromboxane (Fig. 25-1).

Recommendations

Platelet concentrates should be administered to patients with thrombocytopenia or thrombocytopathic disorders if active bleeding is present and can be demonstrated clinically, or if surgery is contemplated and platelet number or function are not adequate for hemostasis. Administration of one concentrate per 10 kg body weight ordinarily will be effective, although larger amounts at frequent intervals may be necessary when platelets are being destroyed or utilized rapidly.

Major procedures, such as open heart surgery where large vascular areas of the chest are exposed, may be associated with increased platelet utilization and impaired function. Platelet concentrates may prove necessary to control bleeding on occasion, even when counts are in excess of 100,000/mm^3. Apparently, defects induced by the oxygenator as well as by the anesthetic agents impair platelet function to the extent that additional platelets are required (see Ch. 24).

PLASMA FACTOR CONCENTRATES

Plasma can be fractionated by a number of techniques to provide semipurified concentrates of a variety of coagulation factors. The major products, Factor VIII and the prothrombin complex (Factors II, VII, IX, and X) are available from a number of manufacturers of biologicals. Preparation of additional therapeutic agents from plasma is possible; several potential products have been included in Table 25-4. All of these fractions will be discussed, in addition to a new product processed to contain active coagulants for use in the inhibitor disorders.

Factor VIII Concentrates

Historical aspects of hemophilia therapy have been discussed. Products currently available from at least six manufacturers in this country provide adequate amounts of Factor VIII for management of hemophilia A patients. Cryoprecipitate produced by blood banks throughout the country provides an additional source of Factor VIII, as well as fibrinogen and VonWillebrand's factor for patients suffering from deficiencies of these factors. The cost of such products as a result of competition has decreased over the past few years, while coverage for these costs by major insurance companies and state funds have expanded. At present, most of the hemophilic patients in this country, estimated at 25,000, have access to these therapeutic agents.

Preparation

Cryoprecipitate prepared by regional or community blood banks contains Factor VIII, fibrinogen, and VonWillebrand's factor in a 20 to 30-ml volume. The latter two factors, being stable, are found in good concentration. Approximately 200 mg of fibrinogen is present in each bag. This product can be employed for treatment of patients with fibrinogen deficiencies of a congenital type, afibrinogenemia, and dysfibrinogenemia, as well as for patients with acquired forms resulting from increased utilization (DIC) or destruction (fibrinolysis). Most of the VonWillebrand's factor also is retained in the precipitate—approximately 100 to 200 plasma-equivalent units. The amount of Factor VIII, however, is variable, depending upon the concentration in the original plasma and the care with which the product is thawed and separated. Some bags have been found to contain as little as 10 units, although, with reasonable care, the contents range from 100 to 150 units. Cryoprecipitate also serves as a source of fibronectin or cold-insoluble globulin, a factor important for cell adhesion and a source of opsonin.[37]

The technique of preparation of cryoprecipitate is relatively simple. Red cell-free plasma, separated by centrifugation from units of whole blood or obtained by plasmapheresis, is fast-frozen in ethanol and dry ice or placed in a −40°C freezer. It is then allowed to thaw, usually overnight in a refrigerator at 5°C. The bag is then placed in a press, and the supernatant plasma is restored to the packed cells or squeezed into a satellite bag for further processing. The precipitate which remains in the original bag is frozen and maintained at −40°C for no longer than 6 months.

Commercial Factor VIII concentrates generally are prepared from a starting cryoprecipitate, although some manufacturers continue to use ethanol fractionation as a first step. Glycine or polyethylene glycol separation is followed by a washing procedure, reconstitution, and lyophilization (a number of different methods have been described[19]). Several package sizes are available—a 200 to 300-unit bottle which can be reconstituted with 10 ml of distilled water and a 30-ml size containing 800 to 1000 units. The VonWillebrand's factor and fibrinogen content vary with the technique of preparation. However, both factors generally are present in a much lower concentration than is found in cryoprecipitate. Factor VIII activity identified on the bottle label is verified by the Bureau of Biologics. Some discrepancies have been noted in the past, depending on the type of Factor VIII assay employed—a two-stage procedure (thromboplastin generation test) or a one-stage procedure (activated partial thromboplastin time). The one-stage procedure is more physiologic, but it is less specific and tends to provide higher values.

At least six different manufacturers produce Factor VIII. Most products have similar half-lives in the circulation—approximately 10.5 hours—and appear to be equally effective. A comparison of three products administered to three different hemophilic patients is shown in Figure 25-9. A much higher level of Factor VIII activity was achieved with one product because its Factor VIII content was well above the label claim, which was used as the basis for dosage. The rate of disappearance, however, was similar to the others. Experiments carried out in bleeding and non-bleeding hemophilic patients have failed to demonstrate a difference in Factor VIII survival. Thus, there is no evidence to indicate an increased Factor VIII utilization during bleeding episodes.[38]

Administration and Dosage

All products should be administered rapidly to achieve effective levels of Factor VIII. Cryoprecipitate should be infused within a few hours after it is thawed, while commercial lyophilized concentrates (see individual

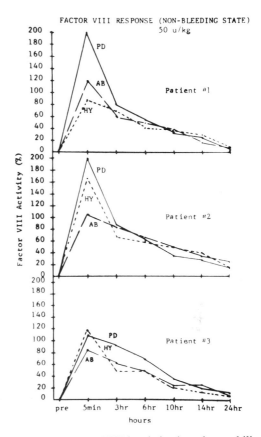

Fig. 25-9. Factor VIII levels in three hemophilic patients receiving three factor VIII concentrates. The products were administered on the basis of label claim. One product was found to contain a much higher value than identified on the label and therefore peak activity was much greater than achieved with the other concentrates. Circulating half-lives were approximately the same for all products.

product information inserts), usually are stable for several days after reconstitution and can be infused as a pulse dose or as a constant drip.

Acute bleeding episodes will require 10 to 20 u/kg of Factor VIII for control, depending upon the extent and site of the bleeding and the duration of the symptoms. Minor bleeds, if treated early as the first symptoms appear, usually will respond to a single dose of 10 u/kg. More extensive bleeding into hip joints or the retroperitoneal area may require multiple doses of 20 u/kg. Much larger quantities are recommended for major surgery; for example, a pulse dose of 30 u/kg immediately before surgery, followed by a continuous infusion of 3 u/kg/hr for 3 to 5 days, then a single daily dose of 30 u/kg for another 5 to 7 days provides a high constant circulatory level of Factor VIII over a total course of 10 to 12 days of therapy. This program can be altered depending on the extent of the surgical procedure and complications that may arise. An antifibrinolytic agent, epsilon amino caproic acid (Amicar-Lederle) has been employed to reduce fibrinolytic activity following surgery. Note that a large number, perhaps 20 percent, of the hemophilic patients in the United States participate in home care programs and maintain a supply of Factor VIII at home for use as needed. The hemophilia centers are responsible for training the patients and for following their care. The HEW Hemophilia Comprehensive Evaluation Program provides funding for some 17 centers throughout the U.S. The National Hemophilia Foundation also lists additional centers.

Indications

These products are recommended for the treatment of Hemophilia A (Factor VIII deficiency). Their use in hemophilic patients has been restricted primarily to treatment of acute bleeding episodes, although in some cases prophylactic administration has been employed on a daily or every other day basis to prevent bleeding. A unique use—induction of immune tolerance in patients with Factor VIII antibodies (inhibitors)—has been described.[39] Cryoprecipitate also has been effective in management of VonWillebrand's disease and fibrinogen deficiencies.

Hazards

Hepatitis remains a major problem. A relatively high incidence of infection has been noted with use of commercial products which generally are prepared from large (600-liter) batches of plasma. Most infections are now non-B types, as a result of the use of hepatitis screening procedures for products and donors. Cryoprecipitates, however, carry a lower risk of infectivity because they are obtained from single, usually volunteer donors.

Hemolysis also is of concern when large amounts of Factor VIII are required for managing surgical cases. The presence of erythrocyte isoagglutinin can produce sufficient hemolysis to lower hemoglobin and hematocrit values, making it difficult to determine if blood loss has occurred.[40] A Coombs test and measurement of serum bilirubin and haptoglobin will help to differentiate hemolysis from blood loss in a patient whose hematocrit is dropping rapidly. Hemolysis resulting from hyperfibrinogenemia also has been reported.[41] Although hyperfibrinogenemia is primarily related to the use of a Cohn fraction preparation no longer on the market, it may occur with the use of large quantities of cryoprecipitate. Red cell membranes as well as isoagglutinins often are found in cryoprecipitate. Preferably, such products should be ABO type-specific for the patient receiving them.

Circulatory overload with pulmonary edema, which occurred frequently when plasma was the only therapeutic agent available, is no longer a problem now that concentrates are in common use.

Protein reactions consisting of uticaria, headache, fever, and backache usually are mild and are encountered in perhaps 5 percent of hemophilic patients immediately after infusion of the product. Most patients will respond promptly to administration of Diphenhydramine 25 mg or Hydrocortisone 50 mg. Often the symptoms will simply disappear without treatment in 30 to 60 minutes. Severe reactions, hypotension, respiratory distress, and shock have been observed rarely, sometimes appearing several hours after infusion. Immediate administration of diphenhydramine, hydrocortisone, and/or epinephrine may be required to control this complication. Possible substances in the product which may be responsible for these reactions include prekallikrein (kinin release), endotoxin from bacterial contamination (induction of DIC and shock), and aggregated protein (activation of complement and basophil release of histamine). Allergens such as penicillin or shellfish metabolites present in donor blood also can produce reactions if the hemophilic recipient is allergic to these substances. Patients should be carefully observed after administration of the product, and appropriate medications should be available if needed.

Patients who regularly react to products should receive prophylactic medication with oral or I.V. Dephenhydramine prior to product administration.

Clinical Examples of Disorders Requiring Factor VIII Concentrates

Hemophilia. This is a familial sex-linked hemorrhagic disorder that occurs as a result of a defect in the Factor VIII molecule which renders it nonfunctional in the coagulation mechanism. A small-molecular-weight component appears to contain the clotting activity and is attached to a much larger protein presumed to be VonWillebrand's factor. Antibodies developed against Factor VIII and currently used to assay Factor VIII antigen combine with the larger VonWillebrand portion of the molecule. Thus, patients with Hemophilia A will demonstrate very little Factor VIII clotting activity but normal amounts of the Factor VIII antigen. The VonWillebrand patient, on the other hand, usually lacks the larger carrier protein for Factor VIII and will have decreased amounts of both clotting activity and antigen.[42]

The hemophilic's lack of Factor VIII clotting activity results in a bleeding diathesis. Patients with severe deficiencies, less than 1 percent of Factor VIII, frequently hemorrhage into large joints spontaneously or after only minor trauma. Hematuria and soft tissue bleeding also are common problems. Patients

with milder disease with Factor VIII levels of 2 percent or more have much less difficulty and bleed only as a result of trauma, and seldom into joints.

The following cases serve to illustrate the present use of Factor VIII in the treatment of bleeding in hemophilia.

Case #1. One of our "home care" patients, a 12-year-old male with a family history of a sex-linked bleeding disorder (the mother's brother was a bleeder) and a Factor VIII clotting activity of less than 1 percent (Factor VIII antigen 100 percent) twisted his ankle on the way home from school. He immediately reconstituted a 350-unit bottle of Factor VIII, withdrew it into a syringe, and administered it intravenously while his mother observed. His mother reported the treatment to our home care center. He resumed normal activities the next day.

Case #2. A 38-year-old male with a well-documented severe form of Hemophilia A and knee joint deformities from recurrent hemarthrosis was admitted for joint replacement. Laboratory studies prior to surgery did not reveal Factor VIII inhibitor activity. He received a 30 u/kg dose of Factor VIII (2100 u) preoperatively and 3 u/kg/hr (210 u) during surgery. Surgery was uneventful. For the first 5 days postoperative, Factor VIII was administered as a constant infusion (concentrate prepared and administered from bottles over 3 to 6 hours). After 5 days, the constant infusion was changed to an intermittent dose of 30 u/kg daily. The patient was discharged on the 12th day after surgery to continue to receive a dose of 10 u/kg/day for the next week while pursuing a program of physical therapy at home. During his hospitalization, a partial thromboplastin time (APTT) was obtained daily to provide assurance that therapy was effective (the APTT should remain in the normal range during constant Factor VIII infusion) and that an inhibitor had not developed.

VonWillebrand's (VW) Disease. This disorder was characterized by VonWillebrand in 1926[43] but was described also by Minot and Lee in Boston in 1920.[44] It is an autosomal disorder which usually is transmitted in a mild heterozygous form and occasionally appears in the homozygous state with severe manifestations. The VW factor as previously described is required for platelet adhesion to collagen and serves as a carrier protein for Factor VIII. The classical pattern is characterized by a prolonged bleeding time, and decreased levels of Factor VIII clotting activity (VIIIc), Factor VIII antigen (VIIIa), and ristocetin cofactor activity (VWr). VWr is measured by a platelet clumping assay using formalin-fixed platelets to measure the patient's plasma VW activity when ristocetin is added.[45] Severe disorders exhibit a bleeding time in excess of 15 minutes and have little if any Factor VIIIc, Factor VIIIa, or VWr activity. Milder forms may have a variable prolongation of bleeding time and only a modest decrease in VIIIc and VIIIa. (A significant lengthening of the bleeding time may be produced by repeating the test 2 hours after ingestion of two tablets of aspirin.[46] Platelet aggregation in response to ristocetin also may be normal. A number of variants of VonWillebrand have been described with normal Factor VIIIc and normal or decreased Factor VIIIa and/or VWr activity. In some patients, platelet function actually is *enhanced,* and two dimensional electrophoresis techniques are required to identify the immunological variant of the Factor VIIIa.[47]

The milder forms of VW generally exhibit mucosal bleeding with recurrent epistaxis in addition to increased ease of bruising. Bleeding after dental extraction or with certain forms of surgery—tonsillectomy for example—may be severe, while little if any bleeding may occur following surgery where the wound site can be sutured and vessels can be tied off easily.

Cryoprecipitate is the therapeutic agent of choice and usually produces prompt improvement in bleeding time and in ristocetin cofactor activity. Factor VIII gradually increases after infusion of the concentrate and appears to have a very prolonged half-life although the hemostatic effect is not prolonged

and disappears within 4 to 8 hours. An average therapeutic dose is 1 concentrate per 10 kg body weight and can be repeated at 8-hour intervals. Some of the severe cases do not respond to cryoprecipitate but may improve when platelets with their attached VW factor are administered as concentrates (1 unit per 10 kg body weight). The use of cryoprecipitate in VW disease is illustrated by the following case:

A 23-year-old woman with VW disease was in her last trimester of pregnancy. The diagnosis made prior to pregnancy had been based on a bleeding time of 7 minutes (12 minutes after 10 grains of aspirin), a Factor VIIIc of 38 percent, Factor VIIIa of 39 percent, and VWr activity of 28 percent. Ristocetin-induced aggregation of the patient's platelets was normal, a likely occurrence when VW factor activity exceeds 3 to 5 percent. One parent had a decreased Factor VIIIa and VWr activity. At time of delivery, she received 6 concentrates of cryoprecipitate. A similar dose was repeated after delivery and daily for the next 3 days. The patient did not experience any excessive bleeding.

Following delivery, the episiotomy site may bleed, while uterine bleeding is less common as a result of contraction stimulated by ergotamine or similar agents and the abundance of tissue thromboplastin in this site. Occasionally, a fibrinolysin blocking agent, epsilon amino caproic acid (Amicar) has been employed to prevent rapid resolution of formed clots. This medication has been found to be particularly efficacious for dental extractions in patients with either VW disease or hemophilia.

Hypofibrinogenemia. This abnormality is found in a variety of inherited and acquired disorders. Dysfunctional syndromes (*dysfibrinogenemia*) with dominant autosomal transmission have been described and are being encountered with increasing frequency. Most of these patients are asymptomatic; the abnormality is identified only on laboratory screening procedures usually obtained for reasons unrelated to hemostasis. The fibrinogen, when measured by a thrombin clotting type of an assay, is found to be low, ranging from 40 to 80 mg%, while the immune assay and clotting assays which permit gradual formation of fibrin after addition of an excess of thrombin often provide a normal value. The prothrombin time usually is prolonged, while the partial thromboplastin time with its slower clot formation may be normal. Hemostasis is adequate for these patients, and fibrinogen concentrate administration is unnecessary unless major surgery is contemplated or the patient has been exposed to serious trauma. In contrast, *afibrinogenemia,* an autosomal recessive disorder, may be associated with serious bleeding similar to Von-Willebrand's disease. The total lack of fibrinogen observed in these cases is responsible for a prolonged bleeding time and a markedly prolonged prothrombin time, partial thromboplastin time, and thrombin clotting time. Fibrinogen levels usually are less than 30 mg% by both clotting and immune assays. Administration of plasma or cryoprecipitate containing fibrinogen corrects the abnormal coagulation studies and effectively controls bleeding. The half-life of fibrinogen is approximately 3 days, and a single administration of 2 to 4 concentrates provides a prolonged effect.

Acquired hypofibrinogenemia results most frequently from consumption associated with disseminated intravascular coagulation (DIC). The loss of platelets in this disorder usually is more critical than the fibrinogen depletion. In instances where fibrinogen levels decrease to 50 mg% or less, cryoprecipitate Factor VIII concentrates may be required to improve hemostasis.

Hypofibrinogenemia also occurs with increased fibrinolysin activity and can be seen in the presence of certain malignancies (prostate or pancreas) in association with some forms of DIC or following open heart surgery, major trauma, and use of fibrinolytic agents. Cryofactor VIII can be expected to improve hemostasis in these conditions as well after administration of 10 to 12 concentrates. The beneficial effect may be transient if fibrinolysin activity is marked. Epsilon amino caproic acid (EACA) also may be employed and usually is effective, as it reduces fibrinogen destruction by blocking the activation of plasminogen. It is essential, however, that primary fibrinolytic disorders be identified and distinguished from DIC. In the case of DIC, EACA is contraindicated and could lead to additional severe thrombotic complications.

Recommendations and Comments

Factor VIII concentrates—both commercial lyophilized products and cryoprecipitate—have revolutionized the treatment of hemophilia. Home care programs are now commonplace throughout the United States, and patients who treat themselves promptly prevent the crippling arthropathies that often developed in the past. Patients are able to maintain normal activities with minimal time spent in recuperation.[48] The hazards of major surgery also have been eliminated. Hepatitis remains a problem. Cryoprecipitates, with their reliable content of VonWillebrand's factor, fibrinogen, and fibronectin, have a broader use than commercial concentrates in the treatment of VonWillebrand's disease and some of the hypofibrinogenemias. The lowered risk of hepatitis also makes this product appealing for the mild hemophilic patient who requires infrequent treatment and has not yet contracted hepatitis. The usefulness of fibronectin has not been identified or defined sufficiently to consider it of value as a therapeutic agent, although as a source of opsonin it may be effective in the treatment of sepsis and associated shock.

PROTHROMBIN COMPLEX CONCENTRATES

Concentrates of the vitamin K-dependent factors synthesized in the liver—prothrombin and Factors VII, IX, and X—have proven effective in the management of hemophilia B, Factor IX deficiency. They also have received considerable attention as a result of their thrombogenic properties,[49] their use in non-hemophilic patients with bleeding disorders, and in patients who have developed inhibitor or antibodies to Factor VIII or Factor IX.[50] Thrombogenic activity in the two major commercially available concentrates has been reduced recently,[51] while a new product prepared to contain active forms of Factors X and VII has been developed and licensed for treatment of patients with inhibitor disorders (see anti-inhibitor coagulant complex).[52]

Preparation

Ordinarily, the cryoprecipitate containing Factor VIII is removed from plasma before further processing. In one method of preparation, cryo-poor plasma is mixed with polyethylene glycol, the supernatant absorbed with DEAE resin, eluted, and lyophilized. Some products also are prepared using tricalcium phosphate as an adsorbing agent.[22,23] Each 30-ml bottle contains approximately 500 units of Factor IX and somewhat lesser quantities of Factors II, VII, and X. Heparin and/or antithrombin III have been added to several products to prevent procoagulant activation and formation of thrombin. Each lot is tested for thrombogenicity in a recalcified clotting assay, and factor activity is verified by the Bureau of Biologics before release. The commercial products available in the U.S. are Konyne (Cutter Lab, Los Angeles) and Proplex (Hyland Lab, Costa Mesa, Calif.).

The half-life of Factor IX in the circulation is approximately 14 hours.

Administration and Dosage

Products are reconstituted in 30 ml distilled water and infused promptly to prevent formation of thrombin in the solution. A relatively rapid administration, 3 to 5 minutes per bottle, is recommended to achieve hemostatic levels. Constant infusion is never employed, and the use of inhibitor to fibrinolysin activation such as epsilon amino caproic acid (EACA) is contraindicated.

Acute bleeding episodes in Factor IX-deficient patients will respond to doses of 10 to 20 u/kg, depending on the extent and severity of the bleed. Doses can be repeated at 8- to 12-hour intervals, although there is some risk that other factors in the product will accumulate in the circulation and accelerate coagulation, increasing the risk of thrombosis.

Indications

Prothrombin concentrate is approved only for use in patients with hemophilia B, Factor IX deficiency, although it is considered acceptable for treatment of the few rare cases of congenital Factor X and Factor VII deficiency. Despite its potential effectiveness in the treatment of bleeding associated with liver disease and overdose of the oral anticoagulant, warfarin, prothrombin concentrate has not been approved for use in these conditions.

Hazards

Fatal hepatitis has been reported in hemophilic as well as nonhemophilic patients who have received prothrombin concentrate.[53] Often, the milder nature of hemophilia B results in less frequent treatment during childhood, with reduced exposure to hepatitis. Infection, when it occurs in the older hemophilic patient, may be more serious and is associated with a much higher mortality. A tragic example of this problem recently occurred when a 9-year-old hemophilia B patient in our clinic died as a result of hepatitis contracted from his first exposure to commercial Factor IX concentrates.

Thrombogenic complications following administration of the product have been reported predominantly in patients with liver disease who can be presumed to have a deficiency of antithrombin III. In a few instances, however, hemophilia B patients also have developed thrombosis, pulmonary emboli, or DIC as a result of treatment with these concentates.[54] Many physicians, therefore, have preferred to use plasma instead of the concentrate to treat their patients. As noted previously, thrombogenicity for both commercial products now available in this country has been reduced, although some clinicians continue to advocate addition of heparin 50 u/bottle prior to administration.

Clinical Examples of Disorders Requiring Prothrombin Complex Concentrates

Hemophilia B. This disorder is much less common than hemophilia A and makes up approximately 15 percent of the estimated 25,000 hemophilic patients in the U.S. The sex-linked transmission of a bleeding disorder, prolonged activated partial thromboplastin time, and a normal prothrombin time suggest the diagnosis of hemophilia which can be defined further by determining Factor IX activity. Clinical manifestations often are less severe than for hemophilia A. Some cases will have very few hemarthroses but develop soft tissue bleeding only, usually as a result of trauma. Others, however, are not clinically distinguishable from hemophilia A and have required synovectomy and joint replacements for recurrent hemarthrosis. Use of the prothrombin complex concentrate to manage bleeding in hemophilia B is illustrated by the following case report:

A 17-year-old male, one of two brothers with a history of bleeding at circumcision, had no other family history of a bleeding disorder. His laboratory values included a partial thromboblastin time of 60 seconds (control <30 sec) and Factor IX activity of 3 percent. He was injured when a baseball hit his right forearm. He was unable to receive immediate treatment and 6 hours later was given prothrombin complex concentrate in a dose of 20 u/kg of Factor IX (1400 u). A large, painful hematoma was present over the upper wrist and forearm. Loss of sensation and weakness of the hand developed. Surgery was required to alleviate pressure over a nerve. He received a dose of 20 u/kg of Factor IX prior to surgery and again 8 hours later. Two doses of 20 u/kg were administered during the next 24 hours and one dose daily thereafter for one week. He recovered completely without loss of function. An APTT assay was obtained daily immediately before a dose to insure that some residual Factor IX activity was present at a level sufficient to shorten the clotting time.

Nonhemophilic Bleeding Disorders. Nonhemophilic patients with life-threatening bleeding as a result of severe liver disease or warfarin therapy overdose have benefited from treatment with these products, although they are aproved only for use in hemophilia B. Some of these patients have succumbed later to hepatitis. Therefore, the risk of such complication must be discussed with the patient, the patient's family, and an appropriate human investigation committee before initiating such an approach.

Factor VIII Inhibitor Disorders. These also have responded to prothrombin complex concentrate in the past and may continue to do so. However, recent changes in these preparations, designed to reduce thrombogenicity, appear also to have reduced their effectiveness in the management of these disorders.[51] At present, their antiinhibitor activity can be considered weak and far inferior to the activated products described below.

Recommendations

The prothrombin complex concentrate is effective for the treatment of paients with hemophilia B and may be useful for patients with Factor VIII inhibitors. The risk of hepatitis and thrombogenicity, although now reduced, limits its use to patients with frequent need of treatment. The product is not approved for nonhemophilic bleeding disorders, although it may be beneficial in circumstances where life-threatening hemorrhage has not responded to other measures.

ANTI-INHIBITOR COAGULANT COMPLEX

During the past few years a new approach has been conceived to provide an alternative to "replacement" therapy in patients who have developed inhibitors or antibodies to clotting factors. The concept, "bypassing" therapy, recognizes the potential of the activated procoagulants in the clotting cascade and their ability to bypass requirements for Factor VIII in hemophilic and nonhemophilic patients who have developed Factor VIII inhibitors. Initially, prothrombin complex concentrates considered to have developed thrombogenic activity during preparation were employed successfully in patients with both Factor VIII and Factor IX inhibitors.[50,55] These active products were found to contain Factor Xa and probably Factors VIIa and IXa as well. Their ability to bypass the Factor VIII requirements for coagulation was demonstrated in vitro as well as in vivo in a large number of cases.[25] Attempts to produce a consistent product with such bypassing activity has been accomplished only recently; as a result, a new licensed protease complex— Autoplex (Hyland Laboratories, Costa Mesa, Calif.)—is now available for managing this disorder. The product no longer consists of the *natural* procoagulants as they are found in plasma, but rather a mixture of procoagulants and coagulants.[52]

Preparation

The product is prepared in a manner similar to the standard prothrombin complex concentrate but allowed to activate and develop specific quantities of Factors VIIa, IXa, and Xa. This coagulant mixture is tested for a "bypassing activity" by addition to Factor VIII-deficient plasma. Factor VIII correction is employed to identify potency, one unit representing that amount which will correct the partial thromboplastin time of hemophilic plasma using an elaigic acid activator (equivalent to 50 percent level of Factor VIII).[52]

Administration and Dosage

Bottles containing approximately 400 Factor VIII correction units are reconstituted with 30 ml of distilled water and infused rapidly within 5 to 20 minutes; thrombin may develop on standing. A dose of 50 to 100 u/kg is recommended for the treatment of acute bleeding episodes in patients with inhibitors. The dose can be repeated at 8-hour intervals until subjective or objective improvement is achieved. Monitoring this therapy is difficult. The partial thromboplastin time can be expected to improve, although generally not to control values, and the prothrombin time will become shorter than normal; preferably, it should not be allowed to decrease to less than 50 percent of control value.

Indications

The product is designed for use in patients who have developed inhibitors to Factor VIII. The level of inhibitor should be in excess of 2 Bethesda Units (4 Oxford Units). Both hemophilic and nonhemophilic patients with inhibitors to Factor VIII have been shown to respond to the complex. At least one case of hemophilia B, Factor IX inhibitor and another with Factor XI inhibitor have benefited from therapy with the original spontaneously activated Factor IX product.[55,56] Presumably, such patients will respond to the controlled activated product now available.

Hazards

The risk of viral hepatitis is similar to that of other products. Thrombogenicity, although not observed during the initial clinical studies, must remain a major concern. Studies in animals have consistently demonstrated this characteristic in the form of disseminated intravascular coagulation. The use of the fibrinolysin activator inhibitor, epsilon amino caproic acid (Amicar) should be prohibited while patients are receiving this therapy.

Clinical Examples of Disorders Requiring Anti-inhibitor Coagulant Complex

Factor VIII inhibitors are antibodies which develop in approximately 15 percent of the hemophilic patients who require frequent treatment with concentrates.[57] Most likely, a similar number of Factor IX inhibitors occur in hemophilia B. Nonhemophilic patients also have acquired inhibitors to Factor VIII in association with lupus erythematosus, drug reactions (especially Penicillin), following pregnancy, or spontaneously in the absence of known disease. These inhibitors may disappear within several months or may persist for years.

Several therapeutic approaches have been considered for the inhibitor disorders, including massive Factor VIII therapy, immunosuppression, and exchange transfusion. These measures, although successful in part, generally have been unreliable.[58,59] Concentrates of the prothrombin complex, however, have proven effective in controlling bleeding in many of these patients. The response is not as consistent as that obtained when Factor VIII concentrates are administered to hemophilic patients without inhibitors. The following case will serve to illustrate the use of this new product:

An 18-month-old male with classical Hemophilia A lacerated his tongue and developed active bleeding that failed to respond to replacement therapy with Factor VIII concentrate. A partial thromboplastin time following infusion of Factor VIII 50 u/kg dose remained prolonged. Addition of normal plasma to the patient's plasma also failed to correct the prolonged APTT. An inhibitor assay provided a value of 48 Bethesda Units. Anti-inhibitor complex, 75 Factor VIII correction units/kg, was administered, and the bleeding gradually stopped over a period of one hour. Additional protease complex was administered, 50 u/kg at 8-hour intervals for the next 2 days and daily for the next 3 days. No further bleeding occurred, and the patient was discharged. Following the first dose, the prothrombin time decreased to 9 seconds (control 11 sec), and the APTT decreased to 46 seconds (previously 90 sec). The platelet count and fibrinogen level remained unchanged. Fibrin degradation products were not present as measured by the protamine sulfate floculation method.

Recommendations

Activated prothrombin concentrates have been developed for a specific problem: the management of patients with Factor VIII inhibitors. The factor or factors responsible for the clinical effect—"bypassing activity"—have not been identified, although active species of Factors VII and X appear to be involved. The Factor VIII correction unit correlates with clinical effectiveness, and a dosage of 50 to 100 units/kg can be administered and repeated as necessary at 8-hour intervals for acute bleeding episodes. Surgery has been accomplished using this product to control hemostasis, although responses have not been as consistent as those of hemophilic patients without inhibitors who receive Factor VIII. Thrombogenicity remains a problem and should be considered before initiating therapy. At present, no useful procedures for monitoring therapy are available, although the effects of the product can be demonstrated by following the prothrombin time and activated partial thromboplastin time.

OTHER PLASMA PRODUCTS

A number of additional hemostatic products could be extracted from plasma, providing the demand is sufficient to make production reasonable. Unfortunately, many of the known clotting factors are of value only for a few rare congenitally deficient patients; therefore, commercial preparation is not feasible. Protease inhibitors such as antithrombin III, however, could be in great demand if they prove to be effective as prophylactic and therapeutic agents in the management of thrombotic disorders. Several clinical studies are under way to determine the efficacy of antithrombin III in the prevention of postoperative thrombosis.[60,61] In addition, antithrombin III prepared by the American Red Cross has been employed in the management of disseminated intravascular coagulation and in congenital deficiencies. The potential use of this product as an antithrombotic agent is unlimited; presumably, commercial preparations eventually will be available. Other protease inhibitors, α_1 antitrypsin and α_2 macroglobulin, are less promising but also may be of value.

Plasminogen represents another highly regarded plasma protein that could prove useful in the management of thrombosis. This protease precursor may be more effective when altered to increase selective binding to fibrin—in which case it could have marked advantages over our present plasminogen-activating agents, Urokinase and Streptokinase, which induce fibrinogen as well as fibrin degradation.

SUMMARY

It is evident from this discussion that the use of blood component therapy has become well established and that platelet concentrates as well as plasma factor concentrates have become essential to the management of the various hemorrhagic disorders. This development has had a major impact on our hemophilic population, transforming the care and the complications of the disorder to the extent that most patients are able to lead a near-normal life, completing their education and maintaining a work schedule with little if any need for time off to recover from bleeding episodes.

In addition, component therapy itself has undergone dramatic changes over the past few years, not only with respect to improvement in product purity and yield but also in relation to the development of more creative uses. "Bypassing" therapy has been developed as a result of production of products containing active factors, manufactured in a controlled manner for the specific purpose of managing inhibitor disorders. In the future, it may be possible to create other protease mixtures that can be employed for specific as well as nonspecific hemostatic problems. The protease inhibitors have yet to be fully evaluated and may become the most valuable of our blood by-products if they can be shown to be useful in treating thrombotic disorders.

REFERENCES

1. Schmidt, A.: Ueber den Faserstoff und die Ursachen: Selner Gerinnung. Arch. F. Anat. u Physiol., 1861, p. 545.
2. Morowitz, P.: The Chemistry of Blood Coagulation. Bethel, F.H., Ed. Charles C. Thomas, Springfield, 1958. Reprinted Ergebnisse der Physiologie 4:307, 1905.
3. Otto, J.C.: An account of an hemorrhagic disposition existing in certain families. Med. Reposit. 6:1, 1803.
4. Pavlovsky, A.: Contributions to the pathogenesis of hemophilia. Blood 2:185, 1947.
5. Biggs, R. and Douglas, A.S. et al.: Christmas disease: A condition previously mistaken for haemophilia. Br. Med. J. 2:1378, 1952.
6. Biggs, R. and Douglas, A.S.: The thromboplastin generation test. J. Clin. Pathol. 6:23, 1953.
7. Ware, A.G., Guest, M., and Seegers, W.H.: Plasma accelerator factor and purified prothrombin activation. Science 106:41, 1947.
8. Quick, A.J.: On the constitution of prothrombin. Am. J. Physiol. 140:212, 1943.
9. Owren, P.A.: Parahemophilia: Hemorrhagic diathesis due to absence of a previously unknown clotting factor. Lancet 1:446, 1947.
10. Alexander, B. and Goldstein, R., et al.: Congenital SPCA deficiency. J. Clin. Invest. 30:596, 1951.
11. Seegers, W.H., Johnson, S.A., and Penner, J.A.: Quantitative concepts related to prothrombin and autoprothrombin I activity. Can. J. Biochem. & Physiol. 34:887, 1956.
12. Ratnoff, O.D. and Colopy, J.E.: A familial

hemorrhagic trait associated with a deficiency of a clot promoting fraction of plasma. J. Clin. Invest. 34:602, 1955.

13. Hathaway, W.E. and Alsever, J.: The relation of Fletcher factor to Factor XI and XII. Br. J. Haematol. 18:161, 1970.

14. Donaldson, V.H., et al.: Kininogen deficiency in Fitzgerald trait. J. Lab. Clin. Med. 87:327, 1976.

15. Coleman, R.W., et al.: Williams trait: Human kininogen deficiency with diminished levels of plasminogen proactivator and prekallikrein. J. Clin. Invest. 56:1650, 1975.

16. Fahey, J.L., Ware, A.G., and Seegers, W.H.: Stability of prothrombin and Ac Globulin in stored plasma. Am. J. Physiol. 154:122, 1948.

17. Cohn, E.J., et al.: Preparation and properties of serum and plasma proteins. J. Am. Chem. Sci. 68:549, 1946.

18. Wagner, R.H., Smith, M., and McLester, W.D.: Precipitation of Factor VIII with aliphatic amino acids: The Hemophilias. KM Brinkhous ed. Chapel Hill, U. of N. Carolina Press, 1964, p. 81.

19. Johnson, A.J., Newman, J., and Karpatkin, M.H.: Preparation of a high purity AHF with polyethylene glycol. Brinkhous, K.M., ed. Hemophilia and New Hemorrhagic States. U. of N. Carolina Press, Chapel Hill, N.C., 1970.

20. Poole, J.G. and Shannon, A.E.: Production of high potency concentrates of antihemophilic globulin in closed bag system. N. Engl. J. Med. 273:1443, 1965.

21. Simson, L.R., Oberman, H.A., and Penner, J.A.: A method for preparing plasma factor VIII concentrate. Am. J. Clin. Path. 45:373, 1966.

22. Bidwell, E. and Booth, J.M., et al.: The preparation for therapeutic use of a concentrate of factor IX containing also factors II, VII and X. Br. J. Haematol. 13:568, 1967.

23. Hoag, M.S., et al.: Treatment of Hemophilia B with a new clotting factor concentrate. N. Engl. J. Med. 280:581, 1969.

24. Fecete, L.F., Holst, S.L., Peetom, F., and Deveber, L.: Auto factor IX concentrate: A new therapeutic approach to the treatment of Hemophilia A patients with inhibitors. XIV Int. Cong. Hemat. Abst. #295, 1972.

25. Kurczynski, S.M. and Penner, J.A.: Activated prothrombin concentrate for patients with factor VIII inhibitors. N. Engl. J. Med. 291:164, 1974.

26. Tschopp, T.B., Weiss, H.J., and Baumgarther, H.R.: Decreased adhesion of platelets to subendothelium in VonWillebrand's disease. J. Lab. Clin. Med. 83:296, 1974.

27. Bithell, T.C., Parekh, S.J., and Strong, R.R.: Platelet function studies in Bernard-Soulier Syndrome. Ann. N.Y. Acad. Sci. 201:145, 1972.

28. Moncada, S. and Vane, J.R.: Arachidonic acid metabolites and the interactions between platelets and blood vessel walls. N. Engl. J. Med. 300:1142, 1979.

29. Burch, J.W., Stanford, N., and Majerus, P.W.: Inhibition of platelet prostaglandin synthesis by oral aspirin. J. Clin. Invest. 61:314, 1978.

30. Davie, E.W. and Fujikawa, K.: Basic mechanisms in blood coagulation. Ann. Rev. Biochem. 44:799, 1975.

31. Penner, J.A. and Hunter, M.: Antithrombin III: Isolation and clinical characteristics. In: Progress in Clinical and Biological Research. Vol. 5, p. 277, 1976. Jamieson, G. and Greenwalt, T., eds. A. Liss, Inc., N.Y.

32. Owen, C.A. and Bowie, E.J.: The diagnosis of bleeding disorders. Little Brown, Boston, 1975.

33. Triplet, D.A., et al.: Platelet function and laboratory evaluation and clinical applications. Educational Products Division, American Society of Clinical Pathology, 1978.

34. Penner, J.: Experience with a thrombin clotting time assay for measuring heparin activity. Am. J. Clin. Pathol. 61:654, 1974.

35. Bang, N.U. and Mattler, L.E.: Sensitivity and specificity of plasma serine protease chromogenic substrates. Haemostasis 7:158, 1978.

36. Mourad, N.: A simple method for obtaining platelet concentrates free of aggregates. Transfusion 8:48, 1968.

37. Chen, A.B., Amrani, D.L., and Mosesson, M.W.: Heterogeneity of the cold insoluble globulin of plasma; a circulating cell surface protein. Biochim. Biophys. Acta. 493:310, 1977.

38. Penner, J.A.: Unpublished data.

39. Brachmann, H. and Gormsen, J.: Massive factor VIII infusion in hemophiliacs with factor VIII inhibitor, high responder. Lancet 2:933, 1977.

40. Rosati, L.A., Barnes, B., Oberman, H., and Penner, J.: Hemolytic anemia due to anti-A in concentrated antihemophilic factor preparations. Transfusion 10:139, 1970.

41. Kekwick, R.A. and Wolf, P.: A concentrate of human antihemophilic factor: Its use in six cases of hemophilia. Lancet 1:647, 1957.

42. Zimmerman, T.S., Ratnoff, O.D., and Powell, A.E.: Immunologic differentiation of classic hemophilia and VonWillebrand's disease. J. Clin. Invest. 50:244, 1971.

43. VonWillebrand, E.A.: Hereditarpseudo-namofili finsk lakarsallsk. Handl. 68:87-112, 1926.

44. Minot, G.R. and Lee, R.I.: Miscellaneous hemorrhagic conditions. In: Nelson's New Loose Leaf of Medicine. New York: Nelson, Vol. 8, Chapt. 6, 1920, p. 155.

45. Weiss, H.J., et al.: Quantitative assay of a plasma factor deficient in VonWillebrand's disease. J. Clin. Invest. 52:2708, 1973.

46. Quick, A.J.: Salicylates and bleeding: The aspirin tolerance test. Am. J. Med. Sci. 252:265, 1966.

47. Zimmerman, T.S., Abildgaard, C.F., and Meyer, D.: The factor VIII abnormality in severe VonWillebrand's disease. N. Engl. J. Med. 301:1307, 1979.

48. Rabiner, S.F. and Telfer, M.C.: Home transfusion for patients with Hemophilia A. N. Engl. J. Med. 283:1011, 1970.

49. Cedarbaum, A.I., Blatt, P.M., and Roberts, H.: Intravascular coagulation with the use of human prothrombin complex concentrates. Ann. Intern. Med. 84:683, 1976.

50. Abildgaard, C.F., Britton, M., and Harrison, J.: Prothrombin complex concentrate in the treatment of hemophilic patients with inhibitors. J. Pediat. 88:200, 1976.

51. Penner, J.A. and Abildgaard, C.F.: Ineffectiveness of certain commercial prothrombin concentrates in the treatment of patients with inhibitors of factor VIII and IX. N. Engl. J. Med. 300:565, 1979.

52. Abildgaard, C. and Penner, J.: Anti-inhibitor coagulant complex (Autoplex) for treatment of factor VIII inhibitors in hemophilia. Blood (in press).

53. Hoofnagel, J.H., Gerety, R.J., Thiel, J., and Barker, L.: The prevalence of hepatitis B surface antigen in commercially prepared plasma products. J. Lab. Clin. Med. 88:102, 1976.

54. Kasper, C.K.: Postoperative thrombosis in Hemophilia B. N. Engl. J. Med. 289:160, 1973.

55. Penner, J. and Kelly, P.E.: Management of patients with factor VIII or IX inhibitors. Sem. in Thromb. and Hemost. 1:386, 1975.

56. Bick, R.L., Thompson, A., and Radack, K.: Surgical Hemostasis with Factor XI Containing Concentrate. J.A.M.A. 229:163, 1974.

57. Kasper, C.K.: Incidence and course of inhibitors among patients with classic hemophilia. Thromb. Diath. Haemorr. 30:263, 1973.

58. Green, D.: Factor VIII antibodies: Immunosuppressive therapy. Ann. N.Y. Acad. Sci. 240:389, 1975.

59. Hultin, M.D. and Shapiro, S.S., et al.: Immunosuppressive therapy of factor VIII inhibitors. Blood 48:95, 1976.

60. Kakkar, V.V.: The clinical use of Antithrombin III. VIIth Int. Cong. Thromb. and Haemost. London Abst. #0629, 1979.

61. Coon, W. and Penner, J.: Evaluation of Antithrombin III in total hip surgery (in progress).

26

Platelet Transfusions for Nonmalignant Diseases

Peter A. Tomasulo, M.D.

INTRODUCTION

In the early 1960s, platelet transfusions were only available at large hospitals supporting special programs in cancer therapy. Even in these hospitals, platelets were often "rationed" in small quantities among the many patients in need of them. At the present time, almost all hospitals have the capacity to provide platelet transfusion therapy, either with platelet concentrates prepared in their own blood banks or with concentrates provided by full-service regional blood centers.

There has been a marked increase in platelet transfusion therapy. One hospital reports an increase in transfusions from fewer than 800 units in 1968 to more than 20,000 units during 1977.[1] The National Red Cross Blood Program distributed 196,000 units of platelets in 1972 and 965,000 units in 1978.[2] In the past, bleeding was the leading cause of death in patients with hematologic malignancies. The appropriate use of platelet transfusion therapy has helped to control bleeding complications, and now infection is the most frequent cause of death in these patients.[3,4] In spite of the benefits of platelet transfusion therapy, the dramatic increase in platelet administration indicates the possibility that some platelet concentrates may be adminis-

tered to patients who do not benefit from them.

Objective clinical and laboratory criteria for platelet administration are not generally agreed upon in detail. There is no systematic approach which is consistently applied to transfusion. Platelet transfusion strategies have usually been developed locally and are often based more on "what appears to have worked" than on comprehensive, controlled studies of platelet transfusion. Learning to use platelets in this fashion has pitfalls. If the aggressive use of platelet concentrates during experimental chemotherapy or during a new surgical procedure is found to be associated with a minimal need for red blood cell (RBC) replacement, physicians might assume that the platelet transfusions prevented excess hemorrhage.

However, the conclusion that platelet transfusions are necessary cannot be justified unless a control group of patients treated without platelets is available for comparison. Much of current platelet transfusion practice has grown based on experiences such as this hypothetical one. If there were more widespread use of platelet transfusion protocols in situations other than therapy for acute leukemia, it would be possible to compare one strategy with another, and we might increase our understanding more quickly. Of course, research protocols of this type are difficult to design and implement.

COMPARING RED CELL TRANSFUSION TO PLATELET TRANSFUSION

Indications for whole blood and red cell transfusion are well accepted, but it is not possible to extrapolate from red cell transfusions directly to platelet transfusions. There are many significant differences. Red cells are given to improve the oxygen-carrying capacity of the blood and are administered until the patient improves clinically and his hemoglobin is elevated. Platelets are administered not only to stop active thrombocytopenic bleeding but also to prevent hemorrhage during stress (e.g., surgery) in patients who are not presently bleeding. Platelets can be administered to patients with normal platelet survival or to patients with extremely short platelet survival. (Short survival occurs more commonly with platelets than with red cells.) Some patients in need of platelet transfusion have normal platelet counts but abnormal platelet function. Because such different clinical situations exist, physicians must have different transfusion strategies to match each clinical situation as well as specific plans for the evaluation of each platelet transfusion.

Although it is acknowledged that each red blood cell transfusion has the potential to influence future red cell transfusion results by inducing the formation of antibodies to non-ABH antigens, this is not generally a significant worry in routine transfusions. Antigens other than A, B, and $Rh_o(D)$ on the red cell surface are not very immunogenic.[5,6] The simplicity and sensitivity of compatibility testing for red cells, coupled with extensive knowledge of RBC antigens, tends to diminish the significance of red cell alloantibodies since it is generally possible to obtain compatible blood even in the minority of patients who become immunized.[6-8]

This is not the case with platelet transfu-

sions. More than 70 percent of patients become refractory after repeated platelet transfusions.[9,10] Platelets are highly immunogenic, and we cannot prevent the formation of potent, platelet-destroying alloantibodies. Further, our knowledge of platelet antigen systems is primitive compared to the extensive body of knowledge available concerning red cell antigens. There are no accepted crossmatch procedures with which to select compatible donors or to detect preformed platelet antibodies,[11] although this is presently an area of intense research interest. Thus, the adverse effect of each transfusion on subsequent platelet transfusions is very different from the effect in red cell transfusion therapy. Physicians must be aware of this and should administer platelets only when appropriate indication is present and when there is genuine hope for success.

Almost all red blood cell transfusions are effective—that is, hemolytic transfusion reactions occur rarely and subsequent reactions can almost always be prevented by appropriate selection of donor red cells. This is not the case with platelet transfusions. Many factors influence the survival and recovery of transfused platelets, and a significant proportion of all platelet transfusions administered do not raise the platelet count and therefore have *no* beneficial effect. Unless the success or failure of each platelet transfusion is evaluated, there will be no basis for rational decisions during future situations in which platelet transfusion may be required. If there is no chance for benefit from random-donor platelet transfusion therapy, specially matched donors should be sought. Patients should not be subjected to the risks of febrile transfusion reactions, fluid overload, hepatitis, allergic reactions, etc. if previous experience indicates no chance of beneficial effect.

INDICATIONS FOR PLATELET TRANSFUSIONS

In general terms, the decision to transfuse platelets must be made after a review of the patient's clinical condition. In a bleeding patient, one should ask, "How low is the platelet count, and how much is the thrombocytopenia contributing to the blood loss?" For example, a patient with a lacerated radial artery and a platelet count of 60,000/μl would not benefit from platelet transfusion; the appropriate therapy is the repair of the vessel. Similarly, not all moderately thrombocytopenic patients need prophylactic platelet transfusion for surgery, and not all severely thrombocytopenic patients should be placed on prophylactic therapy for their routine daily activities.

Generally, spontaneous bleeding does not occur until very low platelet counts are reached (i.e. less than 20,000/μl), and transfusions are thus usually reserved for those thrombocytopenic patients who are bleeding, or for prophylaxis against bleeding. Some patients, however, may not demonstrate evidence of hemorrhage despite prolonged thrombocytopenia with levels as low as 5,000 to 10,000, while some other patients may show evidence of active hemorrhage with platelet counts of 40,000 to 50,000/μl. Also, there is some evidence to suggest that rapidly falling platelet counts are more likely to be associated with spontaneous bleeding.[12] Thus, the indications for platelet transfusion cannot be rigid and need to be individualized. A clinical examination, a platelet count, and occasionally a bleeding time will give enough information to make a correct decision about the potential benefit of platelet transfusions in most clinical situations.

CLINICAL ASSESSMENT

The clinical assessment of a bleeding patient in regard to the appropriateness of platelet transfusion therapy should take into account the volume and nature of the bleeding. Blood loss exceeding 5 ml/kg of body weight per hour is unlikely to be caused exclusively by thrombocytopenia or thrombocytopathy. Particularly in the postsurgical setting, inadequate surgical hemostasis and mechanically

correctable problems should be considered as additional factors.[12] Clinical evidence of a platelet deficit includes diffuse oozing from surgical incisions and venepuncture sites, scattered petechiae, and ecchymoses in areas not associated with trauma or a surgical incision.

PLATELET COUNT

The platelet count is the most commonly utilized and most practical laboratory test both for determining the need for platelet transfusions and for assessing their efficacy.[13,14]

Severe Thrombocytopenia

Patients with platelet counts in the range of 5,000 to 20,000/μl require different platelet transfusion strategies than those with higher platelet counts. Patients with counts in this low range may need regularly scheduled prophylactic platelet transfusions to prevent mucous membrane hemorrhage and severe bruising while pursuing daily activities at home or even while at bed rest in a hospital. Patients with acute leukemia and severe aplastic anemia often fall into this group. It must be remembered, however, that some patients with leukemia and many patients with milder forms of aplastic anemia do not bleed and therefore do not require any platelet transfusions, even with counts as low as 5,000 to 10,000/μl (see also Chapter 27). At times of anticipated stress, such as during elective surgery or after injury leading to clinically significant hemorrhage, patients with platelet counts lower than 20,000/μl should be treated with platelets.

Moderate Thrombocytopenia

Patients who are clinically stable and who have platelet counts in the range of 20,000 to 60,000/μl do not require prophylactic platelet transfusions when they are at bed rest or during routine daily activity. Nevertheless, if a patient in this range requires surgery or is severely injured, platelet transfusions may be beneficial after the major sites of blood loss are repaired. Elective surgery in patients with platelet counts in the lower part of this range usually should not be attempted without platelet transfusion support (see Surgery in Thrombocytopenic Patients, p. 537).

Mild Thrombocytopenia

Patients with normal platelet function and platelet counts between 60,000 and 100,-000/μl rarely bleed excessively from injuries but might occasionally respond favorably to platelet transfusion. These patients should *not* be treated routinely with platelets at the time of injury or surgery; rather, there should first be a careful clinical assessment. Only rarely is surgery or injury complicated by excessive generalized hemorrhage which might be related to thrombocytopenia in this range. Platelet transfusions are indicated in such patients when there is excessive bleeding and when the template bleeding time is outside of the hemostatic range (see below). If these criteria are not met, an alternative explanation for the bleeding should be sought rather than wasting time and valuable resources by futile platelet transfusions.

Patients with 100,000/μl or more normally functioning platelets do not require platelet transfusion therapy.

TEMPLATE BLEEDING TIME (TBT)

A significant limitation of the platelet count is its failure to detect acquired or congenital defects of platelet function, which may cause serious hemorrhage in association with platelet counts which would be hemostatic if platelet function were normal. While the platelet count provides valuable data, the template bleeding time is the test which most accurately indicates the in vivo significance of qualitative platelet disorders. The normal

range for the template bleeding time in most laboratories is from 2 to 8 minutes. However, *normal values* are not synonymous with *hemostatic values,* and many studies indicate adequate platelet-related hemostasis so long as the template bleeding time does not exceed twice the upper limit of normal, with excessive bleeding encountered only when the template bleeding time is longer than 12 to 15 minutes.[12]

The template bleeding time ordinarily correlates reasonably well with the platelet count[15] (see Fig. 26-1). In general, the bleeding time is normal if the patient has more than 100,000 normally functioning platelets per microliter. When the bleeding time is in the normal range, the patient does not have abnormal risk of hemorrhage in the absence of other coagulation defects, and no platelet therapy is indicated even at times of severe stress or injury. As the platelet count decreases below 100,000/μl, the bleeding time increases until it becomes nearly infinite below 10,000/μl.

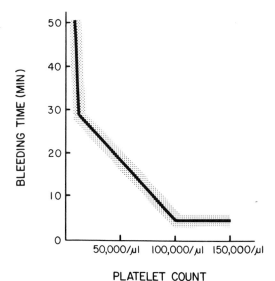

Fig. 26-1. The relation of platelet count to bleeding time (assuming normal platelet function). Not all observers feel the relationship is linear between 100,000 platelets/μl and 10,000/μl. (Adapted from Harker, L. A., and Slichter, S.J.: The bleeding time as a screening test for evaluation of platelet function. N. Engl. J. Med. 287:155, 1972.)

Rarely, patients with histories of serious bleeding will show normal template bleeding times until given a dose of aspirin, after which their bleeding times may show excessive prolongation. A consistently normal template bleeding time, before and after aspirin challenge, may rule out a clinically significant disorder of platelet function.

Bleeding times are superfluous and should not be performed on patients who are severely thrombocytopenic. In contrast, the template bleeding time may be helpful in patients with moderate thrombocytopenia in that platelet transfusions will not correct or prevent a bleeding diathesis in any patient whose template bleeding time does not exceed twice the upper limit of normal.

The bleeding time is helpful in the detection of congenital and acquired causes of abnormal platelet function in which cases there is little correlation between the platelet count and the risk of hemorrhage (see Platelet Dysfunction).

Despite the sensitivity and predictive value of the template bleeding time, certain limitations restrict its usefulness in clinical settings. Foremost among these is the problem of attempting to perform the test on patients in the operating suite or recovery room, where multiple IV's and arterial lines may preclude use of the forearm area and requirements for sterile protocol limit physical access to the patient by persons trained to perform the test. The effect of elevated central venous pressure, anesthetics, fluid load, and hypothermia further complicate interpretation during the postoperative period. The template bleeding test may be difficult to perform on uncooperative patients, particularly infants and children, while patients with edema, scars, and skin lesions may have erratic and nonreproducible results.

PLATELET TRANSFUSION IN SPECIFIC CLINICAL SETTINGS

Although the clinical examination, platelet count, and bleeding time are very helpful in deciding whether to administer platelets, one must also carefully consider other aspects of the clinical situation. The cause of the thrombocytopenia influences the potential for successful platelet support.

LOW PLATELET COUNT WITH DECREASED RATE OF PLATELET PRODUCTION

The most common diseases in this category (see Table 26-1) are: acute leukemia; aplastic anemia; marrow-infiltrative diseases; and bone marrow aplasia induced by intensive chemotherapy for malignancies. In these situations, the survival of endogenous platelets is normal or nearly normal in the absence of other complications. Normal platelet survival is generally associated with successful platelet transfusion therapy; but, unfortunately, patients with these clinical conditions are at risk for frequent and/or prolonged periods of bone marrow aplasia, serious infections, drug toxicity, and other factors which make planning for platelet support very difficult. Platelets should be administered to these patients only when necessary as part of a carefully planned transfusion strategy to help support them through thrombocytopenic periods. (This topic is discussed in more detail in Ch. 27.)

LOW PLATELET COUNT WITH NORMAL OR INCREASED RATE OF PLATELET PRODUCTION

In most clinical situations in this category (see Table 26-2), the effective survival of en-

Table 26-1. Situations Involving Low Platelet Count with Decreased Platelet Production

1. Leukemia
2. Chemotherapy
3. Aplastic Anemia
4. B_{12} or Folic Acid Deficiency*
5. Marrow Infiltrative Diseases

* Thrombocytopenia from these is rarely severe enough to require platelet transfusion.

Table 26-2. Situations Involving Low Platelet Count with Normal or Increased Platelet Production

1. Massive Transfusion
2. Splenomegaly
3. Infection,* DIC, and Other Nonimmunologic Processes
4. Thrombotic Thrombocytopenic Purpura and other Angiopathic processes
5. Idiopathic Thrombocytopenic Purpura
6. Drug-Induced Immune Thrombocytopenia
7. Other Syndromes with short platelet survival

* Infection also suppresses platelet production.

dogenous platelets is shortened, and this makes platelet transfusion therapy difficult. Nevertheless, platelet transfusions can be useful in many patients with thrombocytopenia and normal marrow function. Occasionally, diagnostic information may be a by-product of platelet transfusion as well (see ITP).

Massive Transfusion

Patients receiving massive red cell transfusions (more than 15 to 18 units in a few hours) may suffer a moderate degree of thrombocytopenia.[16,17] The platelet count rarely drops below 50,000/μl and, therefore, massive bleeding on the basis of thrombocytopenia is infrequent.[18,19] The cause of the thrombocytopenia is loss of endogenous platelets from the body through bleeding and replacement with banked blood which either contains nonviable platelets or no platelets at all (whole blood modified). The bone marrow of a bleeding patient who requires very rapid replacement transfusion cannot make platelets fast enough to compensate for this loss. Patients receiving massive red cell transfusion should be examined periodically for signs of thrombocytopenic hemorrhage (generalized oozing, petechiae, ecchymoses). If these signs are present or if thrombocytopenia is likely (e.g., platelet count was borderline at the onset of surgery), a platelet count should be performed. If widespread thrombocytopenic hemorrhage occurs in these patients, platelet transfusion is the proper therapy. The ques-

tion of when to use platelet transfusions is complicated by the lack of controlled studies and the difficulty of interpreting the template bleeding time in patients who are often in shock with fluctuating abnormalities in central and peripheral venous pressure, acid-base status, and fluid and electrolyte balance. Patients with counts below 50,000 to 60,-000/μl with a template bleeding time outside the hemostatic range should receive platelet transfusions if clinical evidence of platelet-related bleeding is present.

The timing of the platelet replacement is important because attempting to raise the platelet count while the massive hemorrhage and red blood cell replacement continue is usually unsuccessful. As long as the bleeding is uncontrolled, maximum transfusion effort should be directed at maintenance of the intravascular volume and the oxygen-carrying capacity. The use of platelet concentrates during this period will generally be wasteful but, of course, in life-threatening situations it should be tried (see Fig. 26-2). After the vascular damage is repaired and the major bleeding controlled, the necessity for red cell replacement will be reduced. One platelet transfusion (1 unit/10 kg; see below for complete discussion of platelet transfusion dose) at this time is usually sufficient to terminate the bleeding due to thrombocytopenia until the patient's own bone marrow can supply sufficient platelets to prevent future hemorrhage (approximately 2 to 3 days).[20] During the recovery period, the patient should be examined frequently for signs of thrombocytopenic hemorrhage. If necessary, the clinical examination can be supported by platelet counts. If the thrombocytopenia recurs or does not respond to platelet transfusions after the red cell replacement has been terminated, another mechanism for the thrombocytopenia should be sought.

Thrombocytopenic hemorrhage does not occur in every patient receiving large quantities of blood.[16,19,20] Indeed, Counts et al.[21] have pointed out that clinically significant thrombocytopenia may be anticipated only

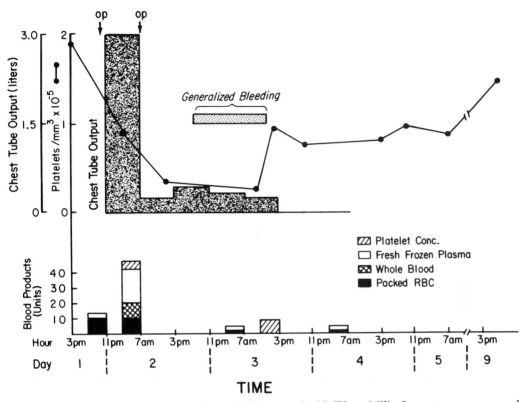

Fig. 26-2. This middle-aged female, who was being treated with IV penicillin for acute pneumococcal aortic endocarditis, ruptured her aortic valve and was taken to surgery (OP) on an emergency basis. During surgery, she lost 4,700 cc of blood and received 10 units of packed cells. A prosthetic valve was placed; however, in the Intensive Care Unit, she lost more than 3,000 cc of blood from her chest tubes over the next 8 hours. During this entire period, 10 more units of packed cells and 10 units of whole blood were administered. The patient's platelet count was 97,000 and the PT and PTT were normal. In spite of these values, many units of fresh-frozen plasma and platelet concentrates were administered. This therapy failed to stop the bleeding from the chest tubes. At 7 a.m., the patient was taken back to the operating room (second OP) where major hemorrhage was detected from the aortic incision. The chest tube drainage decreased dramatically after corrective surgery; however, during the next 8 hours, *generalized* hemorrhage (multiple petechiae and blood in the urine and tracheal secretions as well as a slight increase in the chest tube output) was noted. At this time, the platelet count was 10,000 and thrombocytopenic hemorrhage was correctly diagnosed. Platelet concentrates were administered. The generalized hemorrhage and the drainage from the chest tubes stopped. The platelet count returned to normal. The platelet concentrate and fresh frozen plasma administered after the first operation during the massive hemorrhage did not decrease the blood loss because the patient was bleeding from a surgical site. After the surgical defect was corrected (second operation), *generalized* bleeding, caused by severe dilutional thrombocytopenia, occurred. This was treated successfully with one platelet transfusion. (Levin, J. and Tomasulo, P.A.: Unpublished observations, Baltimore, 1975.)

after an adult has received 15 to 20 units of blood (about 1.5 to 2.0 times his blood volume). Only 2 of 27 massively transfused patients had a platelet count of less than 100,000/µl after having received up to 18 units of blood, and one of these patients had a platelet count of 76,000/µl before any blood was transfused. It is therefore not appropriate to routinely transfuse platelets to patients on the basis of the number of units of red cells transfused. Patients receiving many units of blood should be examined for the signs of thrombocytopenic hemorrhage; platelet counts should be performed; and, if necessary, after these evaluations, platelet transfusions should be administered.

Fresh Blood as a Source of Platelets

Some clinicians have attempted to use "ultrafresh," unrefrigerated blood to maintain the viability of donor platelets and keep the recipient's platelet count high.[22] However, there is no convincing evidence to date to show that patients benefit preferentially from using ultra-fresh, unrefrigerated blood rather than banked blood plus platelet concentrates. (Also see Ch. 24.) In addition, the experience with this technique is limited, and the logistic complications of attempting to use ultra-fresh blood in modern, active hospitals or in regional blood systems make such programs impractical. Further, there is an increased likelihood of technical error when extreme demands are made on the blood collectors and processors attempting to provide ultra-fresh blood for a transfusion emergency.

While the request for ultra-fresh warm blood is rare, some physicians caring for patients requiring massive transfusion request "the freshest blood available" in order to maintain the platelet count and clotting factors. However, platelets rapidly lose their viability during storage at $4°C$. Kissmeyer-Nielsen and Madsen[23] showed that recovery of platelets in recipients transfused with acid-citrate-dextrose whole blood was 45 percent after storage for 24 hours, compared with 54 percent using fresh blood; after 72 hours, recovery was 20 percent.

Moreover, it is unreasonable to place unnecessary demands on blood donors and blood banks, since the patient's platelet needs can be reliably satisfied by the use of banked blood supplemented as necessary with plate-

let concentrates. Although the use of "fresh blood" has been interpreted in anecdotal reports as being beneficial in the prevention of bleeding due to thrombocytopenia during massive transfusion, this is likely due to the fact that thrombocytopenic bleeding is very unusual in this setting. (For a discussion of protein clotting factors during massive transfusion, see Ch. 24.)

Splenomegaly

In normal individuals, about one-third of the total body platelet mass is sequestered in the spleen.[24] As the spleen increases in size, the percentage of the body's platelets which is sequestered increases.[25] Patients with massively enlarged spleens (and often decreased bone marrow function, as in myeloproliferative disease) may have moderate to severe thrombocytopenia at least partially on the basis of increased sequestration of platelets. Some patients with myeloproliferative diseases have poor platelet function as well.[26,27]

Therapy is complicated by splenomegaly because an increased proportion of transfused platelets is sequestered. Transfused platelets have a normal or nearly normal survival time in the presence of splenomegaly, but the immediate posttransfusion recovery is moderately reduced.[25] Because of this expected poor posttransfusion recovery, large doses of platelets (1.5 units/10 kg) should be administered to these patients when platelet transfusion support is necessary. Subsequently, the appropriate dose can best be determined by observing the result of each transfusion and basing future decisions on these results. Unfortunately, some patients with enlarged spleens are transfused frequently enough with both red blood cells and platelets to become sensitized to platelet antigens (alloimmunized) and refractory to random-donor platelet transfusions. After many transfusions, it is difficult to decide which factor (alloimmunization or splenomegaly) is more important in reducing transfusion responses, and often an empiric trial of HLA-matched platelets is necessary (see Ch. 27).

Infection and Disseminated Intravascular Coagulation (DIC)

In severely infected patients (especially with gram-negative organisms) even without DIC, thrombocytopenia is a frequent complication.[28,29] The degree of thrombocytopenia does not regularly lead to excessive bleeding and, therefore, platelet transfusion may not be necessary in these patients.[30] Successful therapy for the infection corrects the platelet deficit. Although there is agreement that platelet survival in thrombocytopenic septic patients is shortened, the mechanism of the thrombocytopenia is controversial. Some investigators feel that platelet-bound antibody or immune complexes produce the thrombocytopenia, but other explanations are possible.[31,32] If the platelet count falls to very low levels and serious thrombocytopenic blood loss occurs, platelets should be administered in large doses (1.5 units/10 kg). Transfusion results should be monitored to determine the appropriate dosage for future transfusions.

In some patients with DIC, the platelet count may occasionally reach very low levels. In this syndrome, bleeding can be life-threatening. Appropriate therapy for patients with DIC is treatment of the underlying cause of the syndrome. If the cause of the DIC cannot be corrected, hemostatic replacement therapy is not often helpful.[33] Life-threatening hemorrhage in patients with DIC is not always caused by severe thrombocytopenia but, when it is, platelet transfusion therapy may be beneficial if the cause of the DIC is reversible. Frequent large doses of platelets (1.5 units/10 kg) may maintain the platelet count in the hemostatic range.[34] Because platelets act early in the clotting sequence, it may be possible to reduce blood loss during the time that the basic process is being treated. Platelet

transfusion should be monitored with frequent platelet counts to assure that the desired therapy has been obtained and to plan future transfusions (see Practical Aspects of Platelet Transfusion Therapy).

Platelet transfusion is not definitive therapy for any patient with DIC but rather is part of supportive care for the most severely affected patients *with thrombocytopenic hemorrhage*. Platelet transfusion should be administered rarely and then only for serious clinical situations characterized by severe thrombocytopenic blood loss and other signs of clinical instability.

Thrombotic Thrombocytopenic Purpura (TTP)

The very low platelet counts in TTP are probably produced by consumption of platelets in multiple thrombotic lesions.[35] Microthrombi consisting of hyaline material are found in the microvasculature. Special staining has demonstrated that these thrombi are made primarily of platelet materials.[36] One report of three patients suggested that platelet transfusion does not increase the platelet count and is not appropriate therapy for patients with this syndrome.[37] Plasma exchange or whole blood exchange, certain drug protocols including antiplatelet agents, as well as splenectomy and prednisone have apparently improved survival in patients with TTP.[38,39] Because platelets appear to be part of the vascular lesions, blood products containing platelets probably should not be administered to patients with acute TTP, unless necessary for therapy of life-threatening, platelet-related bleeding.

Idiopathic Thrombocytopenic Purpura (ITP)

Thrombocytopenia in ITP is caused by an agent, probably an antibody, which leads to a profound decrease in the survival of endogenously produced platelets. The specificity of the agent is broad, and it reacts in in vitro systems with the platelets of most normal individuals.[40–42] Many studies of platelet transfusion in patients with ITP have demonstrated that survival of transfused platelets is also profoundly shortened.[25] Platelet transfusion, therefore, is usually not of great therapeutic benefit to ITP patients, but there is a role for carefully planned platelet transfusions in certain patients with ITP.[43]

Therapeutic Use of Platelets in Patients with ITP. Platelet transfusions should be administered only to those patients with ITP who have life-threatening hemorrhage. These transfusions will probably not be beneficial, but there is little else that can be done for an ITP patient with an intracranial hemorrhage or a hemorrhage which may cause airway obstruction.

Minor surgery can usually be accomplished in ITP patients without platelet transfusions. It is usually not necessary to administer platelets to a patient with uncomplicated ITP at the time of splenectomy.[44,45] Prior to the time when platelet concentrates were easily available, many patients with ITP underwent splenectomy without the need for red blood cell transfusions or prolonged hospitalization.[46–48] Indeed, splenectomy has been performed uneventfully without transfusions in patients with counts as low as 2,000/μl.[12] However, it is preferable to control the underlying disease prior to surgery with corticosteroids or immunosuppressive drugs, if possible.

A few patients with more chronic forms of ITP may occasionally respond to platelet transfusion therapy. Certainly, if the platelet count is profoundly depressed and *major* elective surgery is planned on a patient with chronic ITP, the effects of platelet transfusions can be assessed prior to the operation (see Surgery in Thrombocytopenic Patients). Some patients can be supported for a short period after the procedure.

Diagnostic Information after Therapeutic Platelet Transfusion in Patients with ITP. Many patients with this disease have no significant health problems other than thrombocytopenia. At present, there is no definitive diagnostic test which can confirm or rule out the diagnosis of ITP.[49] If a patient thought to have ITP is bleeding seriously enough to consider platelet transfusion before the benefits of steroid therapy or splenectomy can be available, much diagnostic information can be obtained by observation of the patient during and shortly after the transfusion of a large concentrate of platelets (1.5 units/10 kg). Platelet transfusions should never be administered for purely diagnostic purposes; however, if catastrophic hemorrhage requires platelet transfusion therapy, and if platelet counts done immediately prior to and at various intervals after transfusion indicate very low recovery and short (a few hours or less) survival, this strengthens the diagnostic impression of ITP (see Assessing the Effects of Platelet Transfusion). A normal half-life of transfused platelets appears incompatible with a diagnosis of ITP.[50]

Drug-Induced Immune Thrombocytopenia

Certain frequently prescribed drugs are associated with the production of antibodies which shorten platelet survival and lead to thrombocytopenia. At times, the thrombocytopenia is profound, although, generally, it is more moderate. Appropriate therapy for drug-induced immune thrombocytopenia consists of supportive care and withdrawal of the offending drug. After the drug has been stopped, the platelet count generally returns to normal within 4 to 14 days.[51,52] Because in most circumstances drug-induced thrombocytopenia is associated with short platelet survival, and because patients recover rapidly, platelet transfusion has little or no role in the therapy of patients with this syndrome. Occasionally, severe thrombocytopenia and generalized, life-threatening hemorrhage occur in these patients, and then platelet transfusions might be administered. Platelet transfusions should not be admininstered to these patients for minor bleeding or bruising.

Surgery in Thrombocytopenic Patients

Patients with platelet counts between 60,-000 and 100,000/μl usually tolerate surgical procedures without excessive blood loss. These patients do not require routine prophylactic platelet transfusions. Sometimes, patients with counts between 40,000 and 60,-000/μl bleed excessively during major surgery. If there is excessive, thrombocytopenic blood loss, platelets should be administered therapeutically.

Thrombocytopenic patients with decreased platelet production and platelet counts below 40,000/μl who are scheduled for surgery may occasionally require prophylactic platelet transfusions, but insufficient experience is available to suggest routine transfusion.[53] If on the basis of the patient's history it is considered necessary, administration of platelets to these patients on the evening prior to surgery allows the determination of the post-transfusion increment and survival. Knowledge of the response to platelet transfusion prior to the operation allows the surgical team to plan for normal hemostasis during the surgery and the 3- to 4-day postoperative period during which the patient will be at risk for thrombocytopenic hemorrhage. If the patient does not respond to the presurgery transfusion, the causes of this poor response should be investigated and alternative plans should be made before the surgery is begun.

Although correction and maintenance of the template bleeding time into the normal range allows hemostatically safe operations, it is not always necessary to achieve complete correction. Many studies indicate adequate platelet-related hemostasis so long as the template bleeding time does not exceed twice the upper limit of normal, with excessive bleeding encountered only when the TBT was longer than 12 to 15 minutes.[54-60]

While these guidelines apply to most thoracic, abdominal, and orthopedic procedures, an important exception may occur in patients undergoing central nervous system surgery. In this setting, the major concern is not the hazard of massive blood loss but rather the risk of damage to vital structures which may occur from even minute extravasations. It may be advisable to attempt correction of the TBT into the normal range with maintenance of the platelet count at higher levels than those needed simply to avoid excessive bleeding in other types of surgery. Similar considerations may apply to retinal surgery and to surgery on structures such as the ureter, where small organizing clots or hematomas may cause serious damage or obstruction.[12] Although this approach is logical, at present there are no data documenting the benefits of this "extra attention" during certain surgical procedures.

Cardiopulmonary Bypass

Excessive bleeding in patients during and shortly after cardiopulmonary bypass (CPB) is rare but can be a serious management and puzzling diagnostic problem. The cause for the bleeding is usually a surgical one, but in some instances it is associated with abnormalities in hemostasis.[60] Mild thrombocytopenia is regularly observed during CPB but is not often clinically significant. Studies of the relationship between low platelet counts and blood loss during CPB have shown that these two factors are not significantly correlated. A mild platelet functional abnormality seems to be regularly induced by CPB, but this defect does not consistently contribute to excessive blood loss.[61,62]

The routine administration of platelets to

patients undergoing cardiopulmonary bypass is an unnecessary practice which exposes the patient to the risk of transfusion without significant hope of beneficial effect. Indeed, it has been demonstated that platelet transfusions are only rarely necessary during cardiac surgery.[63] In many well-controlled series, patients given platelet transfusions or fresh blood show no significant difference in postbypass blood loss when compared to patients receiving only bank blood or frozen red cells.[56,64-72] There is at best a very poor correlation—and usually no correlation at all—between excessive bleeding and the platelet count, or the severity of the abnormality observed in platelet function tests.[12]

Furthermore, the overwhelming majority of bypass patients do not experience abnormal blood loss despite consistent changes in the platelet count and in vitro tests, and most bypass patients have hemostatically adequate, although not always normal, template bleeding times.[12]

Nevertheless, rarely, patients do have significant blood loss as a result of thrombocytopenic and/or thrombocytopathy-related to CPB. It has been suggested that patients with excessive blood loss in the immediate postoperative period should be carefully examined, both clinically and with the help of the coagulation laboratory.[62] The coagulation laboratory can usually provide diagnostic information useful in monitoring and treating postoperative patients with serious blood loss. The same indications should be applied to the use of platelet transfusions in bypass patients as in any other surgical situation. Thus, platelet transfusions are indicated when excessive bleeding consistent with a platelet deficiency is accompanied by a platelet count of less than 40,000 to 60,000/μl and a template bleeding time outside the hemostatic range. When severe platelet functional abnormalities and/or thrombocytopenia appear to be related to excessive blood loss, a platelet transfusion (1 unit/10 kg) may be administered. It is best to administer the platelet transfusion *after* surgery.[62] If the transfusion

is administered *during* surgery, the beneficial effect will be less than if the transfusion is administered after major surgical bleeding is controlled and the patient's blood is no longer exposed to the bypass pump. The clinical and laboratory result of these postoperative platelet transfusions should be observed and recorded in the progress notes (see Assessing the Effects of Platelet Transfusion).

Disorders Associated with Platelet Dysfunction

Acquired Defects of Platelet Function. Most forms of acquired platelet functional abnormalities do not, in themselves, produce serious hemorrhage (see Table 26-3). Therapy for patients with reversible defects of platelet function is different from therapy for patients with permanent defects.

Reversible Acquired Defects of Platelet Function. *Drugs.* Many drugs induce changes in platelet metabolism and platelet function which prolong the bleeding time and increase the risk of hemorrhage at times of stress. Aspirin is the most common drug involved in the production of these abnormalities. Normal individuals during normal activity do not ordinarily suffer any negative effects when taking aspirin, but aspirin-treated individuals may bleed excessively at the time of *severe* injury or *major* surgery. For this reason, patients who may require blood transfusions during elective major surgery should be questioned about medications and be instructed to stop taking drugs which affect platelet function one week or more prior to surgery.[73,74] An alternative drug without platelet effect—e.g., acetaminophen—should be substituted if necessary during the time the patient is at risk. If surgery must be performed on a patient whose platelet function is inhibited by a drug, a template bleeding time and close clinical examination during surgery will allow an appropriate decision concerning platelet transfusion. Only rarely will platelets be necessary but, if they are, 0.5 to 1 unit of

Table 26-3. Acquired Defects of Platelet Function

Irreversible Defects	Reversible Defects
1. Idiopathic Thrombocythemia	1. Drug-Induced Platelet Functional Abnormality
2. Polycythemia Rubra Vera	2. Uremia
3. Myelofibrosis	3. Disseminated Intravascular Coagulation
4. Chronic Myelogenous Leukemia	4. Scurvy
5. Acute Leukemia	

platelets/10 kg is appropriate, assuming the response to platelet transfusions is normal. In aspirin-treated patients with normal platelet counts, normal function in 20 percent of the platelets will provide adequate hemostasis and, therefore, large doses of platelets may not be necessary.[75]

Uremia. Uremia is accompanied by a variable degree of platelet dysfunction,[76,77] and serious bleeding may occur in the face of a normal platelet count.[78] The template bleeding time is often markedly prolonged and provides the best index of the patient's platelet status.[15,79] Peritoneal dialysis and hemodialysis are the only effective means of correcting the hemorrhagic diathesis, and there is preliminary evidence to suggest that peritoneal dialysis corrects platelet dysfunction better than hemodialysis.[80] Platelet transfusions are only temporarily effective in uremic patients.

Patients being prepared for nephrectomy, transplant, renal biopsy, or other surgical procedure should undergo preoperative dialysis until the template bleeding time is returned to the hemostatic range.[78]

Many patients with uremia and platelet functional defects are candidates for renal transplantation, and therefore attempts have been made to prevent the sensitization of the recipient to issue (HLA) antigens. Experience has shown, however, that prior transfusion actually improves the survival of compatible kidney grafts. Therefore, early requests for HLA-matched platelets to prevent sensitization of renal transplant candidates are not justified.

Whether individuals awaiting renal transplantation should be intentionally transfused before transplantation is controversial.[81–84]

This topic is discussed more fully in Chapter 29.

Irreversible Acquired Defects of Platelet Function. *Myeloproliferative disorders.* Patients with myeloproliferative disease may have platelet defects of variable severity.[26,27] Spontaneous and surgical bleeding associated with normal or elevated platelet counts but prolonged TBT's have been described in polycythemia vera, acute myelogenous leukemia, acute monocytic leukemia, and chronic myelogenous leukemia. In most instances, effective treatment of the underlying disease corrects the bleeding diathesis, although platelet transfusions may be required in acute surgical situations for bleeding associated with a prolonged TBT.[12] Since the consequences of sensitization to platelet antigens and refractoriness to platelet transfusions are severe, platelet transfusions should be used conservatively. Minor bleeding events—for example, nose bleeds—should be treated with local measures when possible.

Congenital Defects of Platelet Function. Some patients with congenital defects of platelet function (see Table 26-4) bleed excessively from birth after even minor trauma, and others are not diagnosed until they bleed excessively at the time of major surgery. Although other therapeutic modalities have been tried, platelet transfusion is appropriate therapy for most of these patients.[85] The administration of an appropriate dose of normally functioning platelets provides adequate hemostasis. However, the transfusion of blood and/or platelets induces the formation of antiplatelet antibodies and refractoriness to random-donor platelets. Refractory patients with poorly functioning platelets are candidates for specially matched platelet

Table 26-4. Congenital Disorders Which May Be Associated with a Prolonged Template Bleeding Time and a Bleeding Diathesis

1. vonWillebrand's Disease*
2. Glanzmann's Thrombasthenia
3. Bernard-Soulier Syndrome
4. Marfan's Syndrome
5. Ehlers-Danlos Syndrome
6. Wiscott-Aldrich Syndrome
7. Albinism
8. Storage-pool Disease
9. Defects of platelet release reactions

* There is no intrinsic platelet function abnormality in Von Willebrand's Disease, and platelet transfusion is *not* appropriate therapy.

transfusions but are very difficult management problems. Platelets should be administered to patients with congenital defects of platelet function only at times of extreme need. When hemorrhage is minor, local therapy should be used.

The probability of alloimmunization appears to be greater in association with Glanzmann's thrombasthenia and Bernard-Soulier syndrome than with other platelet functional defects.[86,87] The platelets of Glanzmann's and Bernard-Soulier patients lack specific membrane glycoproteins.[88-91] These patients are known to make antibodies to the missing glycoproteins. The specificity of such antibodies is broad. In the case of one Glanzmann's patient, the antibody reacted with all normal platelets tested, precluding the possibility of obtaining compatible platelet concentrates.[92]

When a patient with a *severe* inherited platelet functional disorder is scheduled for major surgery, the blood bank, coagulation laboratory, and clinical team must work closely together to provide adequate hemostasis (see Table 26-5). There is no well-documented experience upon which to base a rational plan of therapy for these patients. Patients with mild disorders probably should

Table 26-5. Considerations in Planning for the Patient with Qualitative Platelet Defect

1. Bleeding Time
2. In Vitro Platelet Function Test
3. Increment and T½ of Transfused Platelets
4. T½ of Correction of Qualitative Defect

only receive platelet transfusions if they bleed excessively at surgery. A plan can be suggested for patients with severe platelet defects and a past history of serious bleeding episodes.

The platelet defects can usually be monitored by the in vitro platelet function studies which characterize the patient's platelet defect, and by template bleeding times. Because these patients may have normal, or nearly normal, platelet counts, the in vitro studies and/or the bleeding times must be followed as well as the degree of hemorrhage and the platelet count (Table 26-6). If the patient has been tansfused or pregnant in the past, it is difficult to predict accurately the response to transfusion of random-donor platelets, and therefore difficult to choose the appropriate dose of platelets to correct the hemostatic defect prior to surgery. The dose should be calculated on the basis of the transfusion history and the previous response to platelet transfusions. The platelets should be administered on the evening or the afternoon prior to surgery and should be accompanied by platelet counts, in vitro studies, and bleeding times immediately before and at varying intervals after the transfusion. The interpretation of these laboratory tests permits the correlation of the platelet count and the dose of platelets with the appropriate correction of the platelet functional defect. The survival of the platelets and the duration of the correction of the platelet defect give an indication of the necessary frequency of platelet transfusion in the immediate postoperative period.

If the presurgical transfusion leads to an increment in platelet count insufficient to correct the bleeding abnormality, surgery should be delayed until matched or compatible platelet donors can be found. HLA typing and/or platelet crossmatch tests,[93-97] if available, should be used to select compatible donors either within nonaffected members of the patient's family or within a pool of unrelated volunteers.

If the trial transfusion is successful, a plan for platelet transfusion before and after sur-

Table 26-6. Suggestions for Monitoring Transfusion of Patients with Abnormal Platelet Function

	Bleeding Time	Aggregation (Epinephrine, ADP)		The Outcome of Platelet Transfusion Should be Monitored by Platelet Counts and:
		1st Wave	2nd Wave	
Aspirin Ingestion	Prolonged	Normal	Decreased	Bleeding Time[b] Aggregation
Uremia	Prolonged	Sometimes Abnormal	Sometimes Abnormal	Bleeding Time[b]
Myeloproliferative Disease	Prolonged	Sometimes Abnormal	Sometimes Abnormal	Bleeding Time[b, c]
Glanzmann's Thrombasthenia	Prolonged	Absent	Absent	Bleeding Time Aggregation
Bernard Soulier	Prolonged	Normal[a]	Normal[a]	Bleeding Time
Storage Pool Disease	Prolonged	Normal	Decreased	Bleeding Time[b] Aggregation
von Willebrand's Disease	Prolonged	The prolonged bleeding time in von Willebrand's disease is not caused by a platelet function abnormality, and platelet transfusion is not appropriate therapy.		

[a] Aggregation with ristocetin is abnormal.
[b] Platelet transfusion is rarely necessary.
[c] Some bleeding patients have elevated platelet counts, and platelet transfusion may not be appropriate.

gery can be made. The in vitro test which detects the abnormality in platelet function should be performed on a daily or a twice daily basis. In combination with the platelet count, template bleeding time, and an assessment of blood loss, it can be used to monitor the patient after surgery. It is unlikely that platelets will be needed after the third or fourth postoperative day.

Presurgical study of patients with inherited platelet functional abnormalities can prevent unnecessary morbidity associated with surgery. In some situations, there will be no potential for improving the platelet performance (even with specially matched donors); in these circumstances, the risks and the potential benefits must be weighed before a decision to operate is reached.

PRACTICAL ASPECTS OF PLATELET TRANSFUSION

ABO AND Rh COMPATIBILITY

Platelet membranes express the antigens of the ABO system, but at present it is not clear whether these antigens are absorbed from the plasma in which they circulate or are synthesized on the platelet.[98,99] The expression of the A, B, and H antigens is much weaker on the platelet surface than on the red cell surface. The antigens can be demonstrated best by absorption and elution studies but, rarely, very potent anti-A or anti-B antibody agglutinates platelets. There are conflicting observations concerning the effect of ABO incompatibility between donor and recipient on the result of platelet transfusions.[14,100,101] There is also conflicting evidence concerning the relationship of the titer of antibody and the magnitude of the effect of ABO incompatibility on the survival of transfused platelets.[102,103] Nevertheless, years of clinical practice have demonstrated that ABO-incompatible platelets provide adequate hemostasis. In carefully done studies analyzing the result of platelet transfusions to a highly selected group of patients, ABO-compatible transfusions appear to give better results than ABO-incompatible ones. The differences are minor and, therefore, it is appropriate medical practice to transfuse ABO-incompatible platelets when ABO-compatible ones are not available.[104]

The antigens of the Rh system are probably not on platelet surfaces.[105-107] However, red cell alloimmunization due to contamination of the platelet transfusion by red cells, and hemolytic reactions caused by antibodies in the donor plasma have been reported.[108] Since units of platelets contain significant amounts of red cells (approximately 0.4 ml per unit), Rh immunization by contaminating red cells is a potential problem. The risk of forming anti-Rh_o(D) has been shown to be approximately 8 percent after transfusion with 80 to 110 units of platelets. If platelets from an Rh-positive donor have to be given to an Rh-negative woman of childbearing age, it is recommended that Rh immunoglobulin be administered shortly after the platelet transfusion. The use of Rh immunoglobulin for other Rh-negative recipients should be considered on an individual basis.

SINGLE-DONOR PLATELET TRANSFUSION

Many investigators have demonstrated that HLA-matched platelets often provide good platelet increments and effective hemostasis in highly alloimmunized patients who are unresponsive (refractory) to pooled platelet concentrates from random donors, and to single-donor concentrates from non-HLA-matched donors.[103,104] Because of this success with HLA-matched donor recipient pairs, some clinicians have begun using HLA-matched platelets or concentrates of platelets obtained from one donor by plateletpheresis for patients who have not been previously sensitized and are still responsive to random-donor platelet concentrates. The use of random single donors or HLA-matched single donors is intended to prevent or delay sensitization and the development of refractoriness to platelet transfusion.[109]

However, there is no evidence to suggest that the use of single-donor platelets before alloimmunization is beneficial.[110] Patients being supported by HLA-matched platelets from nonrelated donors and from HLA-matched siblings may eventually become sensitized by these donors and stop responding, no matter how closely the donor and recipient are matched at the HLA loci.[97,111,112] Indeed, in a canine model it has been shown that the incidence of alloimmunization is similar in dogs supported by a single random donor as compared to a pool of multiple random donors. Of note, however, was that alloimmunization actually developed earlier in the dogs receiving single-donor platelets.[113]

Refractoriness to HLA-matched, nonrelated donors may be produced by closely linked antigens for which we have no assays at present. Single-donor platelets are more expensive than pools of routinely collected platelet concentrates, and the demands on the donors are extraordinary.[114] Until well-controlled studies are completed, patients requiring long-term platelet support should receive pools of random-donor platelets until they become refractory to this form of transfusion therapy. Thereafter, special efforts should be made to select specific donors either on the basis of platelet-specific antigens or on the basis of the HLA type (see Ch. 27, Management of the Alloimmunized Patient).

ADMINISTRATION OF PLATELETS

Platelet concentrates are stored either at 4°C in approximately 30 ml of plasma or, with agitation, at 22°C in 50 ml or more of plasma. A seven-unit pool of random-donor concentrates stored at 22°C will approximate 400 ml (or more). Many patients with cardiovascular disease may not tolerate large infusions of plasma. Volume overload can be prevented by an additional concentration step in the blood bank. The platelet pool may be subjected to a second "hard" centrifugation and then resuspended in 50 ml to 100 ml of plasma rather than 400 ml. This allows the infusion of large doses of platelets to patients with precariously balanced cardiovascular systems. These "superconcentrates" should be infused at once because platelets stored at 22° C in small volumes of plasma deteriorate rapidly.

Platelet pools should be administered immediately after preparation from single-donor concentrates. They should be infused as rapidly as is appropriate for the cardiovascular system of the patient. Platelets should be administered through routine blood filters or platelet/component filters (170μ).[115,116] Platelets must not be administered through some "microaggregate" filters because these filters have been shown to remove platelets from blood and thereby reduce the therapeutic effectiveness of platelet transfusions.[117-119]

DOSE OF PLATELETS

The number of platelets in a "unit" (the number of platelets prepared from 450 ml of routinely donated whole blood) may be highly variable, depending on such things as method of separation and donor count. Some investigators use a figure of 5.5×10^{10} platelets as a unit since minimum standards of quality control require that periodic counts on randomly selected platelet preparations reveal at least 5.5×10^{10} platelets per unit in 75 percent of units counted.[120] However, the standards require that platelet counts be performed on only 4 units per month, regardless of the number of units produced at a given facility. Since the number of platelets per unit is variable, precise calculation of expected increments is impossible unless platelet counts are performed on each concentrate. Even without this information, clinically important estimates of response can be described.

If the platelet count of a bleeding thrombocytopenic patient can be increased by 50,000 to 70,000 platelets per μl, this is generally sufficient to provide hemostasis. An increment of this magnitude one hour after trans-fusion can be provided to an uncomplicated, nonrefractory patient by administering one unit of platelets for each 10 kg of body mass. A 70-kg man usually responds satisfactorily to a pool of 7 platelet concentrates. The half-life of the transfused platelets is 36 to 48 hours in an uncomplicated patient. There are few studies which have specifically addressed the question of dosage, and some clinical experience suggests that fewer units (4 to 5 per transfusion) may be given without increasing transfusion frequency or hemorrhagic complications. If the clinician carefully observes and records response to platelet transfusions, he can select the minimum number of units that can provide hemostasis. This approach has seemingly saved platelet units and has decreased the number of donors to which the patient is exposed.[121]

Many factors influence the recovery of transfused platelets and their intravascular survival time. Physicians ordering platelets should assess the patient's previous response to platelet transfusions and should be cognizant of those factors which affect platelet recovery and survival when they choose a dose of platelets for a bleeding thrombocytopenic patient. Patients with a history of multiple pregnancies or multiple transfusions (red cell, white cell, or platelet transfusions) may be sensitized to platelet antigens and, on this basis, have a decreased response to platelet transfusion.[9,10,100] Patients with markedly enlarged spleens sequester an increased proportion of transfused platelets in this organ and have a decreased response to platelet transfusions.[24] Increased turnover, as might be seen with fever and infection, and even fever alone will result in poor response to transfused platelets.[14] Patients with DIC and other syndromes leading to rapid platelet destruction also respond poorly.[33] Physicians ordering platelets for these patients should increase platelet orders to approximately 1.5 or 2 platelet units/10 kg for the first transfusion in a bleeding episode. Close observation of this first transfusion plus a review of previous responses can then be used to determine the dose of platelets necessary for future platelet transfusions. The review of previous platelet transfusion responses is the most important factor leading to the selection of the appropriate dose of platelets.

ASSESSING THE EFFECTS OF PLATELET TRANSFUSION

Transfusions administered to prevent hemorrhage cannot be evaluated in the same fashion as those administered to reduce active hemorrhage. Complete evaluation of both situations requires clinical and laboratory examination. A bleeding patient must be examined to detect changes in the rate of blood loss, and the patient to whom platelets are administered prophylactically must be examined to assure that no thrombocytopenic hemorrhage has begun. Neither examination is complete without platelet count determinations.

Although some physicians feel that a thrombocytopenic patient may benefit from platelet transfusions even if there is no increment in the platelet count, the majority of the evidence and clinical experience is to the contrary.[13,14,44,122] If bleeding slows or stops after a platelet transfusion which does not increase the platelet count, one should not assume that the platelet transfusion was causally associated with the cessation of hemorrhage. In fact, even though the bleeding stopped, one should consider the platelet transfusion a "failure" and analyze the possible explanations as well as seek new methods of donor selection to improve future platelet transfusion results if necessary. Every platelet transfusion should be followed by a clinical evaluation and platelet counts.

The recipient of platelet transfusions should routinely have three platelet counts: one immediately prior to platelet transfusion; one approximately 1 hour after the administration of the platelet concentrate; and a third the next morning (8 to 24 hours later). This combination of platelet counts allows the de-

termination of the peak expected recovery after transfusion and the survival of transfused platelets. The knowledge of the 1-hour posttransfusion increment is helpful when choosing a dose of platelets and may be an important method for determining refractoriness due to alloimmunization (also see Ch. 27). Also, the knowledge of the survival allows the clinician to determine the period of protection from hemorrhage associated with each platelet transfusion. The cost of the platelet counts is minimal in comparison with the cost of unnecessary platelet transfusions. This two-part assessment is desirable, whether platelets are administered therapeutically to stop acute thrombocytopenic hemorrhage or for prophylactic purposes. The platelet count is the only convenient objective measure of the success or failure of a prophylactic platelet transfusion.

Platelet transfusions are all too often administered without adequate documentation in the progress notes of the indications for transfusion or the results of transfusion. Because many patients require platelet transfusion over many months, the progress notes can be of great help in making therapeutic decisions. If platelet transfusion is unsuccessful, possible explanations (infection, fever, DIC, ITP, splenomegaly, etc.) should be considered, and plans for future transfusions should be indicated. If the transfusion is successful, this also should be noted, as a dose of platelets given will be helpful for planning future transfusions. Careful attention to this detail can reduce excessive exposure to platelets and can lead to a timely switch to HLA-matched products when random-donor platelets are no longer effective as a result of alloimmunization.

The topic of Adverse Effects of Platelet Transfusion is discussed in the next chapter.

SUMMARY

Platelet transfusion therapy has been shown to be highly beneficial for patients with malignant and nonmalignant thrombocytopenic diseases. There has been a dramatic improvement in survival of patients at risk for thrombocytopenic hemorrhage. Therapy is complicated by the fact that platelets are highly alloimmunogenic and induce the formation of platelet antibodies. A significant proportion of all platelet transfusions administered is ineffective, and there are many factors which reduce the response to platelet transfusion. Careful attention to the needs of patients receiving platelet transfusion and careful assessment of the results of platelet transfusion will prolong the period of response to random-donor and matched platelets as well as reduce the risks of ineffective platelet transfusions. An organized approach to the problems of patients with thrombocytopenic hemorrhage will increase our knowledge of the effects of platelet transfusion and allow the further development of this already very beneficial therapeutic modality.

REFERENCES

1. McCullough, J., Undis, J., and Allen, Jr., J.W.: Platelet production and inventory management. In: Platelet Physiology and Transfusion. Schiffer, C.A., ed., American Association of Blood Banks, Washington, D.C., 1978.
2. Blood Services Operations Report. American National Red Cross, July 1, 1977-June 30, 1978.
3. Hersh, E.M., Bodey, G.P., Nies, B.A., and Freireich, E.J.: Causes of death in acute leukemia. A ten-year study of 414 patients from 1954-1963. J.A.M.A. 193:105, 1965.
4. Chang, H.Y., Rodriguez, V., Narboni, G., Bodey, G.P., Luna, M.A., and Freireich, E.J.: Causes of death in adults with acute leukemia. Medicine 55:259, 1976.
5. Giblett, E.R.: Blood group alloantibodies: An asessment of some laboratory practices. Transfusion 17:299, 1977.
6. Aster, R.H.: Matching of blood platelets for transfusion. Am. J. Hematol. 5:373, 1978.
7. Pineda, A.A., Brzica, Jr., S.M., and Taswell, H.F.: Hemolytic transfusion reaction. Recent experience in a large blood bank. Mayo Clin. Proc. 53:378, 1978.
8. Mollison, P.L.: Blood Transfusion in Clinical Medicine. 6th edn. Blackwell Scientific Publications, London, 1979.
9. Shulman, N.R.: Immunological considerations attending platelet transfusion. Transfusion 6:39, 1966.
10. Howard, J.E. and Perkins, H.A.: The Natural history of alloimmunization to platelets. Transfusion 18:496, 1978.
11. Filip, D.J., Duquesnoy, R.J., and Aster, R.H.: Predictive value of cross-matching for transfusion of platelet concentrates to alloimmunized recipients. Am. J. Hematol. 1:471, 1976.
12. Simpson, M.B.: Platelet Function and Transfusion Therapy in the Surgical Patient. In: Platelet Physiology and Transfusion. Am. Assoc. Blood Banks, Washington, D.C., 1978, pp. 51-67.
13. Gaydos, L.A., Freireich, E.J., and Mantel, N.: The quantitative relation between platelet count and hemorrhage in patients with acute leukemia. N. Engl. J. Med. 266:905, 1962.
14. Freireich, E.J., Kliman, A., Gaydos, L.A., Mantel, N., and Frei, E. III: Response to repeated platelet transfusions from the same donor. Ann. Intern. Med. 59:277, 1963.
15. Harker, L.A. and Slichter, S.J.: The bleeding time as a screening test for evaluation of platelet function. N. Engl. J. Med. 287:155, 1972.
16. Krevans, J.R. and Jackson, D.P.: Hemorrhagic disorder following massive whole blood transfusions. J.A.M.A. 159:171, 1955.
17. Lim, Jr., R.C., Olcott, IV, C., Robinson, A.J., and Blaisdell, F.W.: Platelet response and coagulation changes following massive blood replacement. J. Trauma. 13:577, 1973.
18. Simmons, R.L., Collins, J.A., Heisterkamp, C.A., Mills, D.E., Andren, R., and Phillips, l.L.: Coagulation disorders in combat casualties: I. Acute changes after wounding. II. Effects of massive transfusion. III. Post-Resuscitative changes. Ann. Surg. 169: 455, 1969.
19. Collins, J.A.: Problems associated with the massive transfusion of stored blood. Surgery 75:274, 1974.

20. Gardner, F.H. and Cohen, P.: The use of platelet transfusions. Med. Clin. North. Am. 50:1559, 1966.

21. Counts, R.B., Haisch, C., Simon, T.L., Maxwell, N.G., Heimbach, D.M., and Carrico, C.J.: Hemostasis in massively transfused trauma patients. Ann. Surg. 190:91, 1979.

22. Davis, R.W. and Patkin, M.: Ultrafresh blood for massive transfusion. Med. J. Aust. 1:172, 1979.

23. Kissmeyer-Nielsen, F. and Madsen, C.B.: Platelets in blood stored in untreated and siliconed glass bottles and plastic bags. II. Survival studies. J. Clin. Pathol. 14:630, 1961.

24. Aster, R.H.: Pooling of platelets in the spleen: Role in the pathogenesis of "hypersplenic" thrombocytopenia. J. Clin. Invest. 45:645, 1966.

25. Aster, R.H. and Jandl, J.H.: Platelet sequestration in man. II. Immunological and clinical studies. J. Clin. Invest. 43:856, 1964.

26. Inceman, S. and Tangun, Y.: Platelet defects in the myeloproliferative disorders. Ann. N.Y. Acad. Sci. 201:251, 1972.

27. Adams, T., Schutz, L., and Goldberg, L.: Platelet function abnormalities in the myeloproliferative disorders. Scand. J. Haematol. 13:215, 1974.

28. Cohen, P. and Gardner, F.H.: Thrombocytopenia as a laboratory sign and complication of gram-negative bacteremic infection. Arch. Intern. Med. 117:113, 1966.

29. Levin, J., Poore, T.E., Young, N.S., Margolis, S., Zauber, N.P., Townes, A.S., and Bell, W.R.: Gram-negative sepsis: Detection of endotoxemia with the limulus test. Ann. Intern. Med. 76:1, 1972.

30. Emerson, W.A., Zieve, P.D., and Krevans, J.R.: Hematologic changes in septicemia. Johns Hopkins Med. J. 126:69, 1970.

31. Oppenheimer, L., Hryniuk, W.M., and Bishop, A.J.: Thrombocytopenia in severe bacterial infections. J. Surg. Res. 20:211, 1976.

32. Kelton, J.G., Neame, P.B., Gauldie, J., and Hirsch, J.: Elevated platelet-associated IgG in the thrombocytopenia of septicemia. N. Engl. J. Med. 300:760, 1979.

33. Sharp, A.A.: Diagnosis and management of disseminated intravascular coagulation. Br. Med. Bull. 33:265, 1977.

34. Hattersley, P.G. and Kunkel, M.: Cryoprecipitates as a source of fibrinogen in treatment of disseminated intravascular coagulation (DIC). Transfusion 16:641, 1976.

35. Lerner, R.G., Rapaport, S.I., and Meltzer, J.: Thrombotic thrombocytopenic purpura. Serial clotting studies, relation to the generalized Shwartzman reaction, and remission after adrenal steroid and dextran therapy. Intern. Med. 66:1180, 1967.

36. Berkowitz, L.R., Dalldorf, F.G., and Blatt, P.M.: Thrombotic thrombocytopenic purpura. A pathology review. J.A.M.A. 241:1709, 1979.

37. Berberich, F.R., Cuene, S.A., Chard, R.L., and Hartmann, J.R.: Thrombotic thrombocytopenic purpura. Three cases with platelet and fibrinogen survival studies. J. Pediatr. 84:503, 1974.

38. Byrnes, J.J. and Lian, E.C.Y.: Recent therapeutic advances in thrombotic thrombocytopenic purpura. Semin. Thromb. Hemostas. 5:199, 1979.

39. Myers, T.J., Waken, C.J., and Ball, E.D., et al.: Thrombotic Thrombocytopenic Purpura: Combined Treatment with Plasmapheresis and Antiplatelet Agents. Ann. Intern. Med. 92:149, 1980.

40. Shulman, N.R., Marder, V.J., and Weinrach, R.S.: Comparison of immunologic and idiopathic thrombocytopenia. Trans. Assoc. Am. Physicians. 77:65, 1964.

41. Shulman, N.R., Marder, V.J., and Weinrach, R.S.: Similarities between known antiplatelet antibodies and the factor responsible for thrombocytopenia in idiopathic purpura. Physiologic, serologic, and isotopic studies. Ann. N.Y. Acad. Sci. 124:499, 1965.

42. Donnell, R.L., McMillan, R., Yelenosky, R.J., Longmire, R.L., and Lightsey, A.L.: Different antiplatelet antibody specificities in immune thrombocytopenic purpura. Br. J. Haematol. 34:147, 1976.

43. Aisner, J.: Platelet transfusion therapy. Med. Clin. North. Am. 61:1133, 1977.

44. Jackson, D.P.: Treatment of disorders of blood platelets. In: Treatment of Hemorrhagic Disorders. Ratnoff, O.D., ed., Harper & Row, New York, Evanston and London, 1968.

45. Hoak, J.C. and Koepke, J.A.: Platelet transfusions. Clin. Haematol. 5:69, 1976.

46. Christensen, B.E., Hansen, L.K., Krisiensen, J.K., and Videbak, A.A.: Splenectomy in haematology. Indications, results, and com-

plications in 41 cases. Scand. J. Haematol. 7:247, 1970.

47. Scharfman, W.B., Tartaglia, A.P., and Propp, S.: Splenectomy preceding surgical intervention in idiopathic thrombocytopenic purpura. Arch. Intern. Med. 116:406, 1965.

48. Schwartz, S.I., Bernard, R.P., Adams, J.T., and Bauman, A.W.: Splenectomy for hematologic disorders. Arch. Surg. 101:333, 1970.

49. Mueller-Eckhardt, C.: Idiopathic thrombocytopenic purpura (ITP): Clinical and immunologic considerations. Semin. Thromb. Hemostas. 3:125, 1977.

50. Ries, C.A. and Price, D.C.: ^{51}Cr-Platelet kinetics in thrombocytopenia: Correlation between splenic sequestration of platelets and response to splenectomy. Ann. Intern. Med. 80:702, 1974.

51. Gynn, T.N., Messmore, H.L., and Friedman, I.A.: Drug-induced thrombocytopenia. Med. Clin. North. Am. 56:65, 1972.

52. Miescher, P.A.: Drug-induced thrombocytopenia. Semin. Hematol. 10:311, 1973.

53. Becker, G.A. and Aster, R.H.: Platelet transfusion therapy. Med. Clin. North. Am. 56:81, 1972.

54. Kahan, B.D., Green, D., and Ruder, et al.: Single donor, HL-A matched platelet transfusions for thrombocytopenic patients undergoing surgery. Surgery 77:241, 1975.

55. Laros, R.K., Jr., and Sweet, R.L.: Management of idiopathic thrombocytopenic purpura during pregnancy. Am. J. Obstet. Gynecol. 122:182, 1975.

56. Umlas, J.: In vivo platelet function following cardiopulmonary bypass. Transfusion 15:596, 1975.

57. Brown, C.H. III, Weisberg, R.J., and Natelson, E.A., et al.: Glanzman's thrombasthenia: assessment of the response to platelet transfusions. Transfusion 15:124, 1975.

58. McKenna, R., Bachman, F., and Whittaker, B., et al.: The hemostatic mechanism after open heart surgery. J. Thorac. Cardiovasc. Surg. 70:298, 1975.

59. Dieter, R.A., Jr., Neville, W.E., and Pifarre, R., et al.: Preoperative coagulation profiles and posthemodilution cardiopulmonary bypass hemorrhage. Am. J. Surg. 121:689, 1971.

60. Bachmann, F., McKenna, R., Cole, E.R., and Najafi, H.: The hemostatic mechanism after open-heart surgery. I. Studies on plasma coagulation factors and fibrinolysis

in 512 patients after extracorporeal circulation. J. Thorac. Cardiovasc. Surg. 70:76, 1975.

61. Pike, O.M., Marquiss, J.E., Weiner, R.S., and Breckenridge, R.T.: A study of platelet counts during cardiopulmonary bypass. Transfusion 12:119, 1972.

62. Bick, R.L.: Alterations of hemostasis associated with cardiopulmonary bypass: Pathophysiology, prevention, diagnosis, and management. Semin. Thromb. Hemostas. 3:59, 1976.

63. Thurer, R.L., Lytle, B.W., Cosgrove, D.M., and Loop, F.D.: Autotransfusion following cardiac operations: a randomized prospective study. Ann. Thorac. Surg. 27:500, 1979.

64. Harding, S.A., Shakoor, M.A., and Grindon, A.J.: Platelet support for cardiopulmonary bypass surgery. J. Thorac. Cardiovasc. Surg. 70:350, 1975.

65. Hardesty, R.L., Bayer, W.L., and Bahnson, H.T.: A technique for the use of autologous fresh blood during open-heart surgery. J. Thorac. Cardiovasc. Surg. 56:683, 1968.

66. Schmidt, P.J., Peden, J.C., Jr., and Brecher, G., et al.: Thrombocytopenia and bleeding tendency after extracorporeal circulation. N. Engl. J. Med. 265:1181, 1961.

67. Umlas, J. and Sakhuja, R.: The effect on blood coagulation of the exclusive use of transfusions of frozen red cells during and after cardiopulmonary bypass. J. Thorac. Cardiovasc. Surg. 70:519, 1975.

68. Woods, J.E., Tasell, H.F., and Kirklin, J.W., et al.: The transfusion of platelet concentrates in patients undergoing heart surgery. Mayo Clin. Proc. 42:318, 1967.

69. Grindon, A.J. and Schmidt, P.J.: Platelet-poor blood in open heart surgery. N. Engl. J. Med. 280:1337, 1969.

70. Hallowell, P., Bland, J.H.L., and Buckley, M.J., et al.: Transfusion of fresh autologous blood in open heart surgery. J. Thorac. Cardiovasc. Surg. 64:941, 1972.

71. Litwak, R.S., Jurado, R.A., and Lukban, S.B., et al.: Perfusion without donor blood. J. Thorac. Cardiovasc. Surg. 64:714, 1972.

72. O'Brien, T.G., Haynes, L.L., and Hering, A.C., et al.: The use of glycerolized frozen blood in vascular surgery and extracorporeal circulation. Surg. 49:109, 1961.

73. Torosian, M., Michelson, E.L., Morganroth, J., and MacVaugh III, H.: Aspirin- and

Coumadin-related bleeding after coronary-artery bypass graft surgery. Ann. Intern. Med. 89:325, 1978.

74. Rubin, R.N.: Aspirin and postsurgery bleeding. Ann. Intern. Med. 89:1006, 1978.

75. Stuart, M.J., Murphy, S., Oski, F.A., Evans, A.E., Donaldson, M.H., and Gardner, F.H.: Platelet function in recipients of platelet from donors ingesting aspirin. N. Engl. J. Med. 287:1105, 1972.

76. Eknoyan, G., Wacksman, S.J., Glueck, H.I., and Will, J.J.: Platelet function in renal failure. N. Engl. J. Med. 280:677, 1969.

77. Weiss, H.J.: Platelet physiology and abnormalities of platelet function. N. Engl. J. Med. 293:531, 580, 1975.

78. Rabiner, S.F.: Uremic bleeding. Progress in Thrombosis and Hemostasis. 1:233, 1972.

79. Stewart, J.H. and Castaldi, P.A.: Uraemic bleeding: a reversible platelet defect corrected by dialysis. Quart. J. Med. 36:409, 1967.

80. Nenci, G.G., Berrettini, M., Agnelli, G., Parise, P., Buoncristiani, U., and Ballatori, E.: Effect of peritoneal dialysis, haemodialysis and kidney transplantation on blood platelet function. I. Platelet aggregation by ADP and epinephrine. Nephron 23:287, 1979.

81. Russell, P.S.: Steps toward immediate progress in clinical transplantation. Transplant. Proc. 9:1327, 1977.

82. Vincenti, F., Duca, R.M., Amend, W., Perkins, H.A., Cochrum, K.C., Feduska, N.J., and Salvatierra, Jr., O.: Immunologic factors determining survival of cadaver-kidney transplants. The effect of HLA serotyping, cytotoxic antibodies and blood transfusions on graft survival. N. Engl. J. Med. 299:793, 1978.

83. Opelz, G. and Terasaki, P.I.: Improvement of kidney-graft survival with increased numbers of blood transfusions. N. Engl. J. Med. 299:799, 1978.

84. Feduska, N.J., Vincenti, F., Amend, Jr., W.J., Duca, R., Cochrum, K., and Salvatierra, Jr., O.: Do blood transfusions enhance the possibility of a compatible transplant? Transplantation 27:35, 1979.

85. Gerritsen, S.W., Akkerman, J.W.N., and Sixman, J.J.: Correction of the bleeding time in patients with storage pool deficiency by infusion of cryoprecipitate. Br. J. Haematol. 40:153, 1978.

86. Bucher, U., de Weck, A., Spengler, H., Tschopp, L., and Kummer, H.: Platelet transfusions: Shortened survival of HL-A-identical platelet and failure of *in vitro* detection of anti-platelet antibodies after multiple transfusions. Vox Sang. 25:187, 1973.

87. Tobelem, G., Levy-Toledano, S., Nurden, A.T., Degos, L., and Caen, J.P.: Further studies on a specific platelet antibody found in Bernard-Soulier syndrome and its effects on normal platelet function. Br. J. Haematol. 41:427, 1979.

88. Nurden, A.T. and Caen, J.P.: An abnormal platelet glycoprotein pattern in three cases of Glanzmann's thrombasthenia. Br. J. Haematol. 28:253, 1974.

89. Degos, L., Dautigny, A., Brouet, J.C., Colombani, M., Ardaillou, N., Caen, J.P., and Colombani, J.: A molecular defect in thrombasthenic platelets. J. Clin. Invest. 56:236, 1975.

90. Kunicki, T.J. and Aster, R.H.: Deletion of the platelet-specific alloantigen Pl^{A1} from platelets in Glanzmann's thrombocytopenia. J. Clin. Invest. 61:1225, 1978.

91. Kunicki, T.J., Johnson, M.M., and Aster, R.H.: Absence of the platelet receptor for drug-dependent antibodies in the Bernard-Soulier syndrome. J. Clin. Invest. 62:716, 1978.

92. White, G.C., Tomasulo, P.A., Kunicki, T.J., and Aster, R.H.: Unpublished Observation, 1979.

93. Wu, K.K., Hoak, J.C., and Thompson, J.S., et al.: Use of platelet aggregometry in selection of compatible platelet donors. N. Engl. J. Med. 292:130, 1975.

94. Gockerman, J.P., Bowman, R.P., and Conrad, M.E.: Detection of platelet isoantibodies by (^{3}H) serotonin platelet release and its clinical application to the problem of platelet matching. J. Clin. Invest. 55:75, 1975.

95. Sugiura, K., Steiner, M., and Baldini, M.: Platelet antibody in idiopathic thrombocytopenic purpura and other thrombocytopenias. J. Lab. & Clin. Med. 96:640, 1980.

96. Tosato, G., Appelbaum, F. R., and Deisseroth, A. B.: HLA-matched platelet transfusion therapy of severe aplastic anemia. Blood 52:846, 1978.

97. Brand, A., van Leeuwen, A., Eernisse, J.G.,

and van Rood, J.J.: Platelet transfusion therapy. Optimal donor selection with a combination of lymphocytotoxicity and platelet fluorescence tests. Blood 51:781, 1978.

98. Gurevitch, J. and Nelken, D.: ABO groups in blood platelets. J. Lab. Clin. Med. 44:562, 1954.

99. Lewis, J.H., Draude, J., and Kuhns, W.J.: Coating of "O" platelets with A and B group substances. Vox Sang. 5:434, 1960.

100. Baldini, M., Costea, N., and Ebbe, S.: Studies on the antigenic structure of blood platelets. Proc. Eighth Cong. Europe Soc. Haematol., S. Karger, Basel, 1962, p. 378.

101. Bosch, L.J.: Studies on Platelet Transfusion in Man, J.B. Wolters, Groningen, 1965.

102. Aster, R.H.: Effect of anticoagulant and ABO incompatibility on recovery of transfused human platelets. Blood 26:732, 1965.

103. Lohrmann, H.P., Bull, M.I., Decter, J.A., Yankee, R.A., and Graw, Jr., R.G.: Platelet transfusions from HL-A compatible unrelated donors to alloimmunized patients. Ann. Intern. Med. 80:9, 1974.

104. Duquesnoy, R.J., Anderson, A.J., Tomasulo, P.A., and Aster, R.H.: ABO compatibility and single-donor platelet transfusion therapy of alloimmunized thrombocytopenic patients. Blood 54:595, 1979.

105. Gurevitch, J. and Nelken, D.: Studies on platelet antigens. III. Rh-Hr antigens in platelets. Vox Sang. 2:342, 1957.

106. Dausset, J., Colombani, J., and Evelin, J.: Presence de l'antigène Rh (D) dans les leucocytes et les plaquettes humaines. Vox Sang. 3:266, 1958.

107. Lawler, S.D. and Shatwell, H.S.: Are Rh antigens restricted to red cells? Vox Sang. 7:488, 1962.

108. Zoes, C., Dube, V.E., and Miller, H.J., et al.: Anti-A_1 in plasma of platelet concentrates causing a hemolytic reaction. Transfusion 17:29, 1977.

109. Reiss, R.F. and Katz, A.J.: Statewide support of thrombocytopenic patients with ABO matched single donor platelets. Transfusion 16:312, 1976.

110. Slichter, S.J. and Harker, L.A.: Thrombocytopenia: Mechanisms and Management of Defects in Platelet Production. Clin. Haematol. 7:523, 1978.

111. Duquesnoy, R.J., Filip, D.J., Rodey, G.E., Rimm, A.A., and Aster, R.H.: Successful transfusion of platelets "mismatched" for HLA antigens to alloimmunized thrombocytopenic patients. Am. J. Hematol. 2:219, 1977.

112. Herzig, R.H., Terasaki, P.I., Trapani, R.J., Herzig, G.P., and Graw, Jr., R.G.: The relationship between donor-recipient lymphocytotoxicity and the transfusion response using HLA-matched platelet concentrates. Transfusion 17:657, 1977.

113. O'Donnell, M.R. and Slichter, S.J.: Platelet (PLT) Alloimmunization—Correlation with Donor Source. Clin. Res. 27:390A, 1979.

114. Wieckowicz, M.: Single donor platelet transfusions: Scientific, legal, and ethical considerations. Transfusion 16:193, 1976.

115. Morrison, F.S.: The effect of filters on the efficiency of platelet transfusion. Transfusion 6:493, 1966.

116. Arora, S.N. and Morse, E.E.: Platelet filters—An evaluation. Transfusion 12:208, 1972.

117. Cullen, D.J. and Ferrara, L.: Comparative evaluation of blood filters: A study in vitro. Anesthesiology 41:568, 1974.

118. Mason, K.G., Hall, L.E., Lamoy, R.E., and Wright, C.B.: Evaluation of blood filters: Dynamics of platelets and platelet aggregates. Surgery 77:235, 1975.

119. Marshall, B.E., Wurzel, H.A., Neufeld, G.R., and Klineberg, P.L.: Effects of Intersept micropore filtration of blood on microaggregates and other constituents. Anesthesiology 44:525, 1976.

120. Code of Fed. Regulations. 21:Food and Drugs 640.24 p. 119, April 1, 1979.

121. Aisner, J.: Clinical Use of Platelet Transfusions for Patients with Cancer. In: Platelet Physiology and Transfusion. Am. Assoc. Blood Banks, Wash., D.C., 1978, p. 39.

122. Higby, D.J., Cohen, E., Holland, J.F., and Sinks, L.: The prophylactic treatment of thrombocytopenic leukemic patients with platelets: A double blind study. Transfusion 14:440, 1974.

27

Platelet and Granulocyte Transfusion Therapy for Patients with Cancer

Charles A. Schiffer, M.D., and Joseph Aisner, M.D.

Advances in the design of aggressive combination chemotherapy regimens for patients with cancer and in the technology available for the blood transfusion support of such patients have occurred in parallel in the last decade. Whereas previously granulocyte transfusion and more specialized aspects of platelet transfusion were confined to cancer centers, there has been a significant shift in recent years to the regional and general hospital blood bank as the major suppliers of this type of transfusion support. As has been discussed elsewhere in this volume, the facilities for platelet and granulocyte transfusion are expensive to develop and maintain. They involve the training of large numbers of skilled personnel and require particularly careful attention to quality control, both with regard to the final cell product and to the collection technique in order to eliminate any chance of significant donor side effects.

Prior to undertaking the development of such "pheresis centers," consideration should be given to the potential patient population being supplied. Thus, despite combination chemotherapy and multimodality therapy administered to patients with the most common forms of cancer (i.e., gastrointestinal, lung, and breast carcinomas), such patients infrequently require platelet transfusion and very rarely require granulocyte transfusion

because the marrow aplasia is of relatively short duration following therapy. Conversely, primary bone marrow disorders such as adult acute leukemia and aplastic anemia are characterized by prolonged pancytopenia measured in weeks to months, therefore requiring the availability of specialized transfusion capabilities. It does not appear necessary or appropriate for sophisticated technology to be set up at smaller blood centers to supply occasional patients who may require specialized support. Rather, it makes economic sense that such patients should be supplied by regional blood centers. This in turn suggests that careful organization and rapid lines of communication be present in these centers such that their large geographic catchment areas can be supplied efficiently.

In terms of the clinical use of platelet and granulocyte transfusion, almost all of the published experience deals with patients with leukemia or aplastic anemia. The same principles apply, however, to the larger group of patients with cancer receiving intensive therapy.

PLATELET TRANSFUSION

Some aspects of platelet transfusion such as donor/recipient compatibility, dose, and method of administration are similar in patients with malignant or nonmalignant disorders and have been discussed in the previous chapter. This chapter will emphasize those topics of particular importance in patients with cancer.

Indications for Transfusion

As shown in Table 27-1, abnormalities in platelet number and function as well as the presence of potential bleeding sites which are unique for each patient can contribute to the development of hemorrhage in patients with cancer. Although occasional patients with myeloproliferative syndromes and normal numbers of abnormal platelets may bleed and benefit from platelet transfusion, most other causes of abnormal platelet function initially require correction of the underlying disorder (e.g., dialysis for uremia) with platelet transfusion being reserved only for patients who are concurrently severely thrombocytopenic.

The major cause of thrombocytopenia in patients with cancer is impaired platelet production due to the effects of systemic chemotherapy in combination with bone marrow involvement by the tumor (Table 27-1). In some patients with inadequate dietary intake, folate deficiency can also be a factor resulting in decreased production. Accelerated platelet destruction, most commonly caused by disseminated intravascular coagulation (DIC) and occasionally by immune mechanisms can also contribute to the development of severe thrombocytopenia. This is particularly true in patients with concurrent impairment of platelet production. Thrombocytopenia can also be exacerbated by the rapid administration of large volumes of platelet-poor red blood cells to patients with brisk hemorrhage.

There is a direct relationship between the platelet count and the bleeding time, the only currently available method of assessing in vivo platelet function.[1] Although bleeding times begin to increase at platelet counts less than 100,000/μl, a number of studies have

Table 27-1. Causes of Hemorrhage in Cancer Patients

I. THROMBOCYTOPENIA
  A. Decreased platelet production
    1. Bone marrow involvement by tumor
    2. Chemotherapy
    3. Nutritional (e.g. folate deficiency)
  B. Accelerated platelet destruction
    1. Disseminated intravascular coagulation
    2. Immune destruction (occasional patients with lymphoid neoplasm; rarely drug mediated)
    3 Splenomegaly
  C. Hypertransfusion of platelet poor stored blood (rare)

II. THROMBOCYTOPATHY (Impaired platelet function)
  A. Multiple myeloma; paraproteinemias
  B. Myeloproliferative disorders
  C. Renal, hepatic dysfunction
  D. Medications (e.g., salicylates)

III. POTENTIAL BLEEDING SITES
  A. Tumor sites
  B. Mucosal ulcerations due to therapy
  C. Diagnostic procedures.

demonstrated that a large "buffer" zone exists and that significant spontaneous hemorrhage tends to occur predominantly at profoundly thrombocytopenic levels less than 10-20,-000/μl.[2-4] Because life-threatening hemorrhage can develop rapidly in the absence of prior signs of minor hemorrhage such as bruising, petechiae, microscopic hematuria, etc., it has become the practice at most cancer centers to administer platelets prophylactically at counts of 10-20,000/μl to prevent serious hemorrhage, particularly while antineoplastic therapy is being given. The validity of this approach has been established in patients with leukemia in two prospectively randomized studies, those of Higby et al.[5] and Murphy et al.[6] Because many clinical factors influence the development of hemorrhage at a given platelet count (Table 27-2), it is often appropriate to administer platelets at higher platelet counts to seriously ill patients. This increased risk of bleeding is particularly true in the presence of severe infections or rapid tumor lysis, probably because of the development of overt or subclinical DIC, and it is advisable to maintain higher platelet counts

Table 27-2. Factors Increasing the Risks of Hemorrhage

1. Coagulation abnormalities (e.g., DIC)
2. Serious infection
3. Sites of tumor involvement (e.g., intracranial and ulcerative GI tumors)
4. Rapid tumor lysis
5. Uremia
6. Rapid falls in platelet count
7. Protracted vomiting
8. Mucosal injury following chemotherapy

in the range of 30 to 50,000/μl during these acute episodes by increasing the dose or frequency of transfusions as necessary.

Conversely, some patients who are clinically stable remain free of hemorrhage despite persistent counts less than 10,000/μl. This is often the case in patients with aplastic anemia or in patients who are not concurrently granulocytopenic and hence not at increased risk of acquiring infections. In this regard, Slichter and Harker[7] studied the concentration of platelets necessary to prevent spontaneous bleeding in aplastic thrombocytopenic patients by measuring fecal blood loss. The patients' red cells were labeled with ^{51}Cr and stools were collected for 1 to 2 weeks. In patients receiving no medications except anabolic steroids who had platelet counts greater than 10,000/μl, stool blood loss was no different from values found in normal subjects—i.e., less than 5 ml/day. At levels between 5,000 and 10,000/μl, blood loss was only slightly increased above normal (9 ml ± 7/day) but in 4 patients with platelet counts of less than 5,000/μl, daily stool blood loss was 50 ml ± 20/day. Semisynthetic penicillins and prednisone were found to have a marked effect on enhancing gastrointestinal blood loss. Overall, therefore, this study confirms clinical impressions that not all patients require platelet transfusions at rigidly predetermined count levels. This observation is of importance because a strict prophylactic approach generally results in increased platelet usage with an increased potential for the oc-

currence of the many side effects to be described below.

Of interest, however, is the finding that in patients with leukemia the development of alloimmunization (perhaps the most serious consequence of platelet transfusion) may not be related to the number of transfusions given.[8] Furthermore, because of the administration of chemotherapeutic agents which affect mucosal integrity and the presence of sites of tumor which can serve as foci for bleeding, most patients with leukemia and other types of cancer are not comparable to patients with stable aplastic anemia. In addition, more rapid fluctuations in platelet and granulocyte count, with a resultant increased risk of infection, are also noted more commonly in patients with leukemia. In an effort to individualize the decision about the proper timing of platelet transfusion, Solomon et al.[9] performed a prospective randomized study in which patients with leukemia either were given prophylactic platelets or were transfused only for specific indications—i.e., clinically significant bleeding or a rapidly falling platelet count (a decline of 50 percent or more in a 24-hour period). Although the "specific indications" group required fewer platelets than the prophylactic group, the overall results of therapy in terms of mortality and complete remission rate were similar. The authors concluded that giving platelets for specific indications may protect patients with acute leukemia during induction therapy as effectively as does giving platelets at predetermined platelet levels.

Based on our experience and interpretation of the available data, it is our present policy to utilize prophylactic transfusion for most cancer patients undergoing treatment at platelet counts of 10 to 20,000/μl, with particular attention focused on those patients who have an increased risk of bleeding due to the factors listed in Table 27-2.[10] Prophylactic platelet transfusions are withheld in certain patients who are stable and usually not concurrently severely granulocytopenic. This latter policy requires, however, that platelets are readily available and that the patients are followed closely by physicians and hospital staff experienced in the management of thrombocytopenia.

For the average clinically stable adult patient, approximately 2 to 3 transfusions of between 4 and 8 units of platelets are required per week, with increased transfusion requirements during periods of accelerated platelet destruction. In children, approximately 1 unit/10 kg of body weight is a reasonable "starting dose." In all patients, platelet counts should be monitored daily during active portions of a patient's treatment course. It is not necessary to ABO match for platelet transfusion, although some platelet concentrate preparations may have high red blood cell contamination—in which case it is advisable to centrifuge the pooled concentrates (180 g × 3 min) to eliminate incompatible erythrocytes. In ABO-incompatible transfusions prepared by certain of the pheresis machines, this step is mandatory because of the larger number of red blood cells in these preparations.

Side Effects of Platelet Transfusion

The aggressive use of platelet transfusion has markedly decreased the incidence of serious hemorrhage in patients with leukemia undergoing initial induction treatment, thereby allowing the delivery of effective doses of chemotherapy and contributing significantly to the increased remission rates now achievable in adult acute leukemia. A number of side effects related to the platelet transfusions themselves can occur, some of which can be ameliorated or prevented by close cooperation between the blood bank and the clinicians (Table 27-3).

1. *Transfusion reactions* following platelet transfusion can be due to sensitization to either histocompatibility antigens, RBC antigens, or plasma proteins. Sensitization to plasma proteins probably occurs most com-

Table 27-3. Hazards of Platelet Transfusion

1. Transfusion reactions
2. Circulatory congestion
3. Transmission of blood-borne infectious diseases
4. Graft versus host disease
5. Transfusion of red cell alloantibodies
6. Sensitization to RBC antigens
7. Granulocytopenia with (?) marrow suppression (alloimmunized patients)
8. Alloimmunization

monly in IgA-deficient recipients.[11-13] Transfusion reactions most commonly occur during or shortly after the infusion and are usually mild, consisting of a sensation of chilliness and rarely shaking chills, or occasionally by rises in temperature with or without urticaria. Premedication with antihistamines and acetaminophen can ameliorate these reactions but need not be administered pretransfusion to the majority of patients who do not have reactions. Rarely, the reactions are very severe and may even be associated with pulmonary symptomatology. When these reactions are observed in IgA-deficient patients, the administration of washed platelet concentrates may prove successful, although washing will only remove the plasma proteins.[14] Alloimmunization to HLA or leucocyte antigens is the most common cause of reactions; in some patients, reactions can be prevented by centrifugation of the pooled platelet concentrates at 180 × g for 3 minutes, which removes the majority of contaminating leucocytes.[15] Although this procedure usually prevents the febrile reaction it generally does not result in improved post-transfusion platelet increments or survival in our experience.

2. *Circulatory congestion*, particularly in children or elderly recipients, can occur because a pool of 4 to 6 units of platelet concentrate represents a volume load of 200 to 300 ml of plasma. If necessary, the volume of plasma can be reduced prior to infusion by centrifugation of the pooled concentrates with resuspension of the platelet button in a smaller volume. These concentrated transfusions should be administered shortly after

preparation because of the decreased platelet viability after storage at higher platelet concentrations. In addition, the platelets will no longer be in a totally closed system after these manipulations.

3. *Transmission of infectious diseases* is a well-known complication of blood transfusion and can be a particular problem in immunosuppressed patients. Although type B hepatitis has decreased in incidence, non-A, non-B hepatitis remains a problem in recipients exposed to large numbers of units of blood.[16,17] Toxoplasmosis, cytomegalovirus and rarely malaria[18] and salmonella[19] infections have been described in recipients of platelets. Another unusual problem is the transfusion of bacteria which have proliferated in platelet concentrates stored at room temperature.[20] The clinical clue to this complication is the occurrence of a severe febrile reaction shortly after the infusion is begun. Such a reaction mandates cessation of the infusion, blood, and platelet bag cultures and strong considseration for institution of antibiotic therapy in granulocytopenic recipients. Fortunately, experience with room temperature storage has shown that the transmission of bacterial infection is exceedingly uncommon.[21-24] Careful attention to skin cleansing at the time of blood collection and inventory rotation designed to provide the freshest available platelets should help to further decrease the incidence of this unusual complication.

4. *Graft versus host disease* (GVHD) can occur in heavily immunosuppressed patients because of the presence of sufficient numbers of viable lymphocytes in standard platelet concentrates. Furthermore, single-donor platelets prepared by a variety of methods and in particular by the Haemonetics Model 30 contain as much as a 10-fold greater number of lymphocytes (often 3 to 4×10^9/transfusion), thereby potentially increasing the risk of GVHD. Presently GVHD has been described in marrow transplant recipients, patients with congenital immune deficiencies, and only rarely in patients with leukemia or other types of cancer. Although it is mandatory to irradiate all blood products for the two former groups of patients, it is premature to recommend this for all platelet recipients. Nonetheless, as single-donor transfusions are used more frequently and more immunosuppressive therapy is utilized, GVHD may become more common, and clinicians should be alert for the many unusual clinical manifestations of this disease. (See Ch. 37, Adverse Effects of Transfusion.)

5. *Hemolysis of Recipient Red Cells:* The transfusion of large volumes of plasma increases the probability of producing a positive direct Coombs test in the recipient if ABO incompatible platelets must be administered. Since pools consist of the plasma from many different donors, only a few of whom can be expected to have high-titer antibodies, the risk of significant recipient hemolysis is very low, even when group O platelets must be administered to a group A patient. However, hemolytic transfusion reactions have been reported.[25]

6. *Sensitization to Rh_o (D) and other RBC antigens* can occur in recipients of multiple transfusions because of the small number of RBCs present in essentially all platelet preparations. Fortunately, this infrequently results in clinically important future difficulties in obtaining compatible RBCs for transfusion. The antigens of the Rh system are not detectable on the platelet surface; but, if platelets from an Rh-positive donor are given to an Rh-negative patient, it is possible that the recipient will become sensitized to Rh_o (D) and will produce an antibody in response to the red cells. If platelets from Rh-positive donors must be administered to a young Rh-negative recipient or an Rh-negative female recipient in the child-bearing age, the formation of anti-Rh_o (D) can be prevented by the administration of Rh immune globulin.[26] Care must be taken when administering intramuscular injections to thrombocytopenic patients however. If anti-Rh_o (D) is present in the recipient's serum prior to transfusion of Rh-positive platelets, one would not expect a

shortened survival of the transfused platelets or a transfusion reaction in association with the transfusion.

7. *Granulocytopenia,* lasting for a few days and therefore suggesting possible bone marrow suppression, has been described following the transfusion of mismatched platelets to alloimmunized patients with otherwise stable aplastic anemia.[27] The suggested mechanism is "innocent bystander" destruction of host granulocytes in association with immune lysis of transfused platelets. This represents an important potential complication of platelet transfusion because of the possibility of an acquired infection increasing the likelihood of hemorrhage.

However, this complication is probably exceedingly rare as indicated by the data of Tomasulo et al.,[28] who monitored leukocyte and granulocyte counts after 109 single-donor platelet transfusions to 10 alloimmunized patients with aplastic anemia who were refractory to random-donor platelet transfusions. The posttransfusion granulocyte counts 24 to 72 hours following unsuccessful platelet transfusions (platelet recoveries <20 percent of predicted) were not significantly different from the posttransfusion granulocyte counts following successful platelet transfusions (platelet recoveries $\geq$ 20 percent of predicted).

8. *Alloimmunization* to histocompatibility antigens occurs in the majority of recipients of multiple random donor platelet transfusions and represents the most important long-term complication of platelet transfusion.[28a] Estimates of the frequency of alloimmunization following random-donor platelet transfusion vary from approximately 50 to 100 percent, depending in part on the patient population being studied and the intensity of cytotoxic and immunosuppressive therapy being administered.[29-32] The management of alloimmunized patients is one of the most difficult and frustrating problems in platelet transfusion and will be discussed in detail.

Management of Alloimmunization

Diagnosis. Following the transfusion of fresh or properly stored platelets to a clinically stable adult of average size, one should achieve a platelet increment one hour post-transfusion of approximately 6000 to 8000/μl per unit of platelets transfused. In thrombocytopenic recipients, posttransfusion counts provide excellent assessments of platelet recovery and in some patients platelet survival, so that isotopic labeling is not required to measure posttransfusion kinetics. Because recipients differ in size and the number of platelets/unit vary, it is helpful to express increments in a standardized fashion such as the "corrected count increment" (CCI) where:

$$CCI = \frac{\text{Absolute increment} \times \text{Body surface area (m}^2)}{\text{Number of platelets transfused } (\times 10^{11})}$$

Using this formula one would expect a CCI of approximately 20,000/μl one hour after transfusion of fresh, random pooled platelet concentrates. If platelet counts are not available on the final bag, a value of 0.7×10^{11} platelets/unit may be used. For example, if a patient with a body surface area of 1.7 m^2 has a platelet count increment of 45,000/μl after a transfusion of 6 units of platelets, the calculations are as follows:

$$CCI = \frac{45,000 \times 1.7}{6 \times 0.7} = 18,210/\mu l$$

The hallmark of the clinical diagnosis of alloimmunization is a failure to achieve adequate platelet count increments following transfusion. Frequently, but not invariably, transfusion reactions accompany the onset of platelet refractoriness. The diagnosis of alloimmunization can be difficult in the presence of other clinical factors such as severe infection, brisk hemorrhage, DIC, fever, and hepatomegaly or splenomegaly which accelerate platelet utilization and decrease posttransfusion recovery. The presence of anti-HLA (lymphocytotoxic) or antiplatelet antibodies can help confirm the diagnosis, but these tests are usually not available in general hospitals or on an emergency basis. As a rapid, rough clinical guide, the measurement of platelet increments 1 hour posttransfusion can often help in the differential diagnosis because, with the exception of massive organomegaly or septic shock, immunologic destruction is the only cause of such rapid platelet destruction which can eliminate increments immediately posttransfusion.[33] In an analysis of 79 platelet transfusions given to 73 thrombocytopenic patients with leukemia, Daly et al.[33] noted that a CCI 1 hour posttransfusion of 10,000/μl or greater was generally associated with absence of lymphocytotoxic antibody, whereas CCI of less than 10,000/μl were invariably associated with high levels of strongly cytotoxic antibody except in patients with organomegaly or shock. HLA-matched transfusions produced no improvement in increments when the previous 1-hour CCI had been 10,000/μl or greater, whereas in the other groups significantly better increments were obtained. In these patients, a platelet count at 18 to 24 hours after transfusion was useless in distinguishing alloimmunization from other clinical conditions that result in accelerated platelet destruction.

The use of this approach is shown in Figure 27-1, which outlines the course of a patient with acute progranulocytic leukemia and DIC with accompanying infection and high fevers. Although the platelet counts had returned to pretransfusion values the day after the first few transfusions, it can be seen that good increments were obtained at 1 hour therefore suggesting rapid destruction due to causes other than alloimmunization. Subsequently, transfusion reactions, high levels of lymphocytotoxic antibodies, and poor 1-hour increments were noted, indicating the development of alloimmunization and the need for histocompatible platelets. Thus, measurement of count increments immediately post-

transfusion is indicated in patients in whom day-to-day increments have been unsatisfactory. Although occasionally the clinical course of patients is so complex as to make the interpretation of poor 1-hour increments difficult, the converse (i.e., normal increments in the face of high levels of anti-HLA antibody) is an unusual finding. It should also be emphasized that fresh platelets should be used in these evaluations because storage conditions in many blood banks are not optimal and such inadequately stored platelets can have decreased viability and function post-transfusion.

Donor Selection

Platelets have HLA antigens which are shared with all other tissues and tested for most easily on lymphocytes, as well as platelet specific antigens expressed on their surface. Most of the platelet-specific antigens characterized to date are present in the vast majority of the population and are therefore an uncommon cause of platelet refractoriness. Nonetheless, antibodies to these and presumably other, as-yet-undiscovered platelet antigens can develop.[34] In such patients, selection of donors by a variety of antiplatelet antibody tests is necessary.[35-39] Unfortunately, most of these tests are either cumbersome or inaccurate, and it often is difficult to obtain suitable donors for these patients.[40] This is presently an area of intense research interest, and practical and reliable crossmatch techniques may become available in the future.

In the vast majority of cases, however, successful transfusions of platelets can be accomplished using platelets matched at the HLA-A and B loci using both family members as well as nonrelated donors.[41,42] In general, it is ideal to choose donors who are either HLA identical with the recipient or who do not possess any HLA-mismatched antigens; this is because the recipient's antibody is

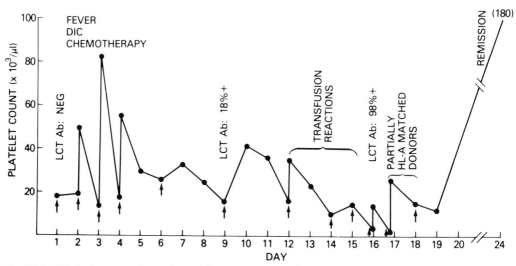

Fig. 27-1. Clinical course of a patient with acute progranulocytic leukemia who developed lymphocytotoxic (LCT) antibodies and became refractory to random donor platelets. The arrows indicate platelet transfusions and the vertical lines on the day of transfusion indicate one hour count increments. (Schiffer, C.A., Aisner, J., and Wiernik, P.H.: Platelet transfusion for patients with leukemia. In: The Blood Platelet in Transfusion Therapy. Greenwalt, T.J. and Jamieson, G.A., eds. Alan R. Liss, Inc., New York, 1978. Reprinted with permission.)

usually multispecific (i.e., directed against most of the HLA antigens). Logistically, this can represent a considerable problem because of the large number of antigens expressed at these loci (genetic "polymorphism"). Depending on the genetic frequency of the recipient's particular antigens, it may thus be impossible to obtain large numbers of suitable donors without developing large files of potential "on call" donors. Such files have been recruited at many blood centers in the United States and presently a national HLA donor file with provision for shipping HLA-matched platelets country-wide is available.[43]

The number of available donors can also be increased by a strategy of "selectively mismatching" for antigens which are serologically cross-reactive with one of the patient's antigens and hence may not be recognized as "foreign."[44] Similarly, one can often mismatch for HLA-B12, a common antigen which in many individuals is expressed strongly on lymphocytes but not on platelets.[45] Table 27-4 illustrates the expansion of the number of donors produced by this approach. Of note is that a pool of 5000 donors would provide an average of only 1.5 A-matched nonfamily donors for each of 48 patients, and that for many recipients there are no perfect A-matched donors. Thus, even with a very large pool of HLA-typed donors, it is difficult to find donors who will be an A-match with a given patient, thereby emphasizing the importance of the "selective mismatch" approach for some patients. Unfortunately, this strategy is usually less successful in heavily transfused, severely alloimmunized patients.[46]

If appropriate matched donors cannot be located for refractory patients, it is inadvisable to continue to administer random donor platelets prophylactically because the risks and discomforts of transfusion outweigh the benefits. Significant bleeding in such patients can sometimes be managed by infusions of massive amounts of unmatched platelets,[47] although heavily sensitized patients usually do not develop count increments and continue to bleed. The possible mechanisms operative in the patients who do respond to this

Table 27-4. Results of Histocompatibility Donor Availability Analysis in HLA Typed Donor Pools of Different Sizes

	A Matches Only	A Matches & B Matches with "Blanks" Only	A Matches & B Matches with "Blanks" and/or Crossreactive Antigens
500	0.20[a] (0–3)[b]	2.4 (0–14)	27 (0–102)
750	0.25 (0–3)	3.75 (0–20)	43 (0–152)
1000	0.30 (0–4)	5.2 (0–26)	59 (0–213)
1500	0.40 (0–5)	8.8 (0–44)	89 (1–334)
2000	0.54 (0–7)	12 (0–53)	120 (1–443)
3000	0.88 (0–10)	18 (0–72)	183 (4–667)
4000	1.1 (0–14)	24 (0–98)	243 (4–907)
5000	1.5 (0–21)	31 (0–132)	306 (7–1129)

a. Mean value calculated from data on 48 patients
b. Range

Donor availability for 48 patients
A = 4 antigen match
B = 3 antigen match where fourth donor antigen is either unknown ("blank") or crossreactive
(Duquesnoy, R.J., Vieira, J., Aster, R.H.: Donor Availability for Platelet Transfusion Support of Alloimmunized Thrombocytopenic Patients. Transplant Proc. 9:519, 1977. By permission.)

maneuver may be the fortuitous presence of a small number of matched platelets in the random donor pool or a temporary reduction in antibody titer by the large amounts of infused antigen allowing platelets transfused subsequently to survive.

Platelet Cryopreservation

The availability of technology allowing long-term platelet storage is of considerable potential assistance in the management of alloimmunized patients. Both autologous and HLA-typed platelets have been frozen for subsequent use in alloimmunized patients, thereby decreasing the crisis atmosphere which frequently occurs when an HLA-matched donor is required on short notice.[48] In the autologous setting, platelets are obtained from patients between courses of chemotherapy during remission of their leu-kemia, frozen and stored, and transfused during subsequent periods of thrombocytopenia.[49] Cryopreservation techniques using both dimethylsulfoxide (DMSO) and glycerol[50] have been described, but to date only the DMSO methodology has been reproducible enough for general usage. Using 5 percent DMSO, polyolefin freezing bags, and a variety of freezing rates and conditions, recoveries varying between 60 and 70 percent of fresh platelets with satisfactory hemostatic results have been noted in a number of laboratories.[10,30,51,52] Because the DMSO is largely removed following thawing, there are no side effects following these transfusions, and the technology is simple enough for use outside of research laboratories. Successful transfusion of platelets which have been frozen at liquid nitrogen temperatures ($-120°$ C) for 3 or more years has been described (Figure 27-2) and should therefore permit long-term storage of HLA matched

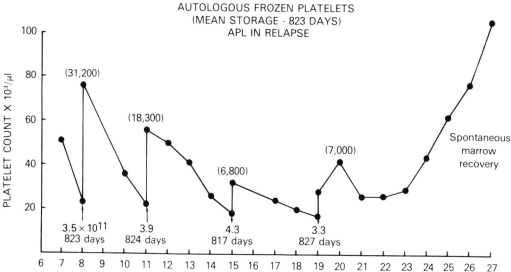

Fig. 27-2. Platelet count increments (CCI in parentheses) following transfusion of autologous frozen platelets stored an average of 823 days administered to a patient with acute progranulocytic leukemia (APL) in relapse. The patient was febrile and infected during the last two transfusions, possibly accounting for the decreased increments.

platelets as well as random-donor platelets for emergency use.[53]

Single-Donor Platelet Transfusion

Single-donor platelets have been used predominantly in the setting of recipient alloimmunization that developed following transfusion of more readily available random-donor platelets. With the development of efficient plateletpheresis procedures, there has been an increased interest in the use of single-donor platelets from the initiation of transfusion with the goals of decreasing hepatitis acquisition and possibly modifying the pattern of recipient alloimmunization. Although long-term support of leukemic children is possible using family members,[54] there is little contemporary data available concerning the rate of alloimmunization in patients receiving platelets with higher degrees of leucocyte contamination prepared using pheresis machines. There are also certain theoretic considerations in addition to increased cost and donor risk which may make the provision of single-donor platelets equivalent to or actually worse than random-donor platelets. If an attempt is made to provide closely HLA-matched platelets from nonrelated donors, one may select for the development of antibodies against non-HLA platelet antigens which are not easily detectable and which could make further donor selection difficult if not impossible. Similarly, providing partially matched platelets in order to produce a "narrow range" of sensitization only against the mismatched antigens may not be successful because of the considerable serologic cross-reactivity in the HLA system. Thus, antibody formed by exposure to a single HLA antigen may have activity against a broad range of HLA antigens, resulting in a situation analogous to that which occurs following random donor transfusion. Indeed, in a canine model, it has been shown that the incidence of alloimmunization is similar in dogs supported by a single random donor as compared to a pool of multiple random donors. Of note, however, was that alloimmunization actually developed earlier in the dogs receiving single-donor platelets.[55] Certainly, further careful research is necessary before single-donor platelet transfusion is utilized as "standard" supportive care, with the exception of the requirements of the alloimmunized patient.

GRANULOCYTE TRANSFUSION

Patients with cancer are at increased risk of acquiring serious infections because of a number of interrelated factors listed in Table 27-5. Infection acquisition in cancer patients can be decreased by instituting certain simple measures, such as scrupulous attention to oral and cutaneous hygiene, along with more investigative approaches such as gastrointenstinal tract sterilization with oral antibiotics or sequestration in laminar flow "germ free" rooms. Nonetheless, because of advances in platelet transfusion support, infection is the leading cause of death in cancer patients receiving aggressive chemotherapy.[56] This is particularly true in patients with leukemia and other causes of prolonged marrow aplasia, and it is in this group of patients that granulocyte transfusions are most often utilized. Although there was considerable debate about the efficacy of granulocyte transfusion in the earlier years of their investigative use, a number of recent studies, including four prospectively randomized controlled studies, have clearly demonstrated their effectiveness, resulting in increased and more widespread use of granulocyte transfusion.[57-62] This chapter will not review this

Table 27-5. Predisposing Factors for Infection in Cancer Patients

1. Granulocytopenia
2. Chemotherapy: Erosive mucosal and gastrointestinal tract lesions
3. Obstructive tumors (e.g. pulmonary → pneumonia; retroperitoneal → urinary tract infections)
4. Altered state of consciousness (CNS metastases; metabolic abnormalities)
5. Immunosuppressive effects of therapy and of the malignancy
6. Indwelling venous or urinary catheters

evidence further but rather will suggest guidelines for the proper use of granulocyte transfusion.

Indications for Granulocyte Transfusion

There is a direct relationship between the absolute granulocyte count and the risk of developing bacterial or mycotic infections in leukemia patients.[63] As with the platelet count, however, there is a considerable "buffer" zone such that the infection rate does not increase appreciably until the granylocyte count is < 500/ml. Furthermore, when reasonable infection prevention measures are taken, serious bacteremic infections are unusual except in the presence of severe (< 100 to 150/μl) granulocytopenia. In addition, despite even profound granulocytopenia, the majority of infections will respond to the administration of appropriate broad spectrum parenteral antibiotics at the first sign or symptom of infection.[64] Thus, only a minority of leukemia patients and an even smaller percentage of other patients with cancer will become candidates for granulocyte transfusion.

As has been emphasized in Chapter 9, the technology of granulocyte procurement, although formidable and improving steadily, is not comparable to the relative "ease" with which it is possible to obtain physiologic doses of normally functional platelets. With the available differential centrifugation devices, even with corticosteroid premedication and rouleaux producing agents, one can collect doses of granulocytes from single donors which are marginal at best for the treatment of seriously infected adults. Procurement techniques currently available allow for the collection of 0.8 to 3.5 × 10^{10} granulocytes from a normal donor in 2 to 4 hours. This contrasts with the normal rate of granulocyte production in an adult, which is 10^{11} cells per day and which can rise several-fold in the face of stress. Without donor premedication the yield is even less, and it is unclear whether such low doses can be effective. There is inferential evidence that, in an adult, at least 10^{10} functional granulocytes must be administered to be assured of a therapeutic effort.[65]

Although the dose of granulocytes obtained by filtration leukopheresis tends to be higher, there are significant functional and morphologic abnormalities present in these preparations such that the "effective dose" of granulocytes administered may be considerably lower than crude computations of cell yield would lead one to believe.[65a]

Because of the limitations imposed by the granulocyte dose and the problems with histocompatibility to be discussed below, it would appear logical to initiate granulocyte transfusion as promptly as possible in the group of patients who are unlikely to respond to antibiotics alone in an attempt to eradicate or halt the progression of the infection before it has become overwhelming. Analysis of granulocyte transfusion and empiric antibiotic trials have helped to identify clinical characteristics of this small group of patients (Table 27-6). Of particular importance is the expected duration of granulocytopenia because it has been shown that almost all patients who develop marrow recovery and a rise in granulocyte of as little as 100 to 200/μl within a week of onset of the infection[64] will recover from the infection and will not require or benefit from granulocyte transfusions.[61,62] The criteria listed are not intended to be all-inclusive, and it should be empha-

Table 27-6. Indications for Consideration of Early Administration of Granulocyte Transfusion

1. Expectation of prolonged, profound granulocytopenia
2. Any suggestion of infection unresponsive to antibiotics
3. Gram-negative bacteremia
4. Infection in life threatening or parenchymal sites
5. Other complicating medical factors
6. Antibiotic resistant organisms
7. Fungal infections (?)
8. Expectation of responsiveness of underlying malignancy to therapy

sized that all such patients do not necessarily require granulocyte transfusions. It is prudent, however, to tentatively identify donors for these "high-risk" patients so that granulocyte transfusion can be initiated if there is any suspicion of failure to respond to antibiotic therapy alone. It is generally possible for experienced clinicians to predict the clinical course in these patients within 24 hours of beginning antibiotics, or even sooner in some seriously ill patients. Thus, in the noncritical candidate, a 1- or 2-day trial of broad spectrum antibiotics should precede institution of granulocytes to determine whether this alone might be sufficient for infection control.[65] Such an approach requires close coordination between the clinicians and the blood center. In this regard, it is also helpful to anticipate problems and tissue type and medically screen potential family member donors for each patient with leukemia at the time of the patient's admission.

An example of this decision-making process is illustrated in Fig. 27-3. This patient was an elderly female who had completed induction chemotherapy for acute nonlymphocytic leukemia approximately 3 weeks before and developed high spiking fevers (days 2 and 3) due to an extensive cellulitis in the vulval area. Blood cultures were positive for Pseudomonas aeruginosa. Because of the poor prognostic factors (elderly patient, severe granulocytopenia, gram negative bacteremia), a donor was contacted and placed "on call" for the next day. Because myeloid recovery was possible at this stage of the patient's induction therapy, a bone marrow aspirate was done on day 4 which revealed a regenerative marrow with myeloid maturation to the myelocyte-metamyelocyte stage. Although the patient remained febrile, her condition and the local lesion were stable and because of the likelihood of early marrow recovery granulocyte transfusions were not given. As can be noted, the circulating white blood cell count increased on day 6 and the patient recovered uneventfully. Thus, it was possible to make a rational clinical decision

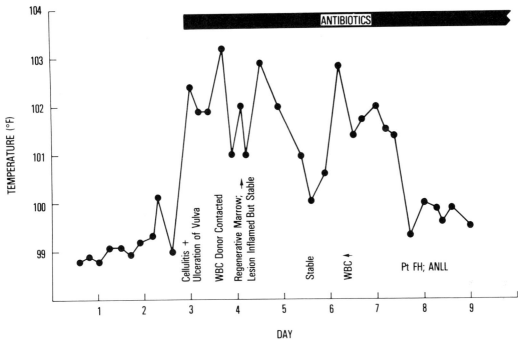

Fig. 27-3. Clinical course of an elderly patient with acute nonlymphocytic leukemia (ANLL) and a vulval infection with associated bacteremia (see text).

about the need for granulocyte transfusion within 24 hours of the onset of infection.

Frequently, the clinical situation is less clear-cut than in this patient and in some cases may result in some transfusions to patients who may well have recovered with antibiotics alone. Nonetheless, it is hoped that, given the limitations of current technology, larger numbers of patients can be benefited by employing all effective therapies at a time prior to life-threatening spread of infection. Conversely, granulocyte transfusion has been demonstrated to be ineffective in certain circumstances. Patients with cancer frequently become febrile from noninfectious causes, and a number of studies have indicated that administering granulocytes to patients without documented infection (so-called "fever of unknown origin") is of no therapeutic benefit.[60,66] Similarly, there is no proven benefit from granulocyte transfusions given to moderately granulocytopenic (500 to 1,000/µl) patients. Transfusion should therefore be re-

served for profoundly aplastic patients, with the possible exception of patients who become severely infected with rapidly falling granulocyte counts in the <500/µl range.

In contrast to the convincing human and animal evidence documenting their effectiveness in bacterial infections, there is relatively little data available concerning the utility of granulocyte transfusion in fungal infections (hence the "question mark" concerning fungal infections in Table 27-6). Furthermore, the nonphagocytic mechanisms by which granulocytes kill filamentous fungi such as *Aspergillus* species are poorly understood, although there is a clearcut relationship between the acquisition of most fungal infections and prolonged granulocytopenia in the leukemic population. A single animal study indicates that granulocyte transfusions can decrease the severity of experimentally induced Candida albicans infections in dogs;[67] there exist some suggestive, but inadequately documented, observations suggesting a similar salutary effect in Candidal infections in humans.[57] Although clearly more data are needed in this area, one would predict success with adequate doses of granulocyte transfusion in combination with appropriate antifungal antibiotic therapy, in view of the clinical observations that fungal infections usually respond promptly when bone marrow recovery with endogenous granulocyte production occurs.

Granulocyte Donors

Prior to the development of devices suitable for the separation of granulocytes from normal donors, donors with chronic myelogenous leukemia (CML) were utilized because it was possible to obtain large numbers of leukocytes from these patients by simple centrifugation of units of whole blood. Although histocompatibility considerations and unpredictable availability of such donors have resulted in a shift to the use of normal donors, it should be recalled that striking clinical responses were noted using CML cells.[68] Furthermore, CML donors with high white blood cell counts represent the only source from whom one can predictably obtain near-physiologic doses (routinely $>10^{11}$ leukocytes) for transfusion. Because myeloid precursors capable of further division are transfused, short-term "engraftment" occurs in occasional nonalloimmunized recipients such that a single transfusion can result in adequate numbers of circulating granulocytes in the recipient for a number of days. Although GVHD has been a rare accompaniment of this therapeutic "bonus,"[69] most institutions would not routinely irradiate CML preparations except when they are administered to severely immunosuppressed marrow transplant recipients.

As reviewed elsewhere, normal donors should satisfy standard blood bank donor criteria in addition to having no specific contraindications to the various premedications utilized. It is desirable that donors be ABO-compatible with the recipient because there is significant red blood cell contamination of most granulocyte preparations, and this contamination is difficult to eliminate without significantly compromising granulocyte yields. In addition, ABO antigens are expressed on granulocytes, and there are data suggesting that posttransfusion granulocyte count increments are decreased following ABO-incompatible transfusions.[57,70] Thus, both normal and CML donors and recipients should be ABO-compatible whenever possible.

Duration of Granulocyte Transfusion Support

The decision to initiate granulocyte transfusion should be made with great care because, in addition to the expense and possibility of recipient side effects, one must also consider the inconvenience to the donor as well as the possibility of more significant donor morbidity. Because of dosage considerations, it is ideal to administer granulocyte transfusions as frequently as possible with a minimal goal of one transfusion per day. If available, particularly in patients with severe infections, it may be desirable to give transfusions from multiple donors per day so as to maximize the dose and approach the physiologic response to infection.[71] In general, one should plan on at least 3 to 4 days of granulocyte transfusion support with a less clearly definable upper limit to the duration of transfusions. Although there is controversy about this latter point with relatively little relevant data available, the following situations represent reasonable general guidelines for the cessation of granulocyte transfusion:

1. any spontaneous and sustained rise in recipient granulocyte count to $>200/\mu l$ or evidence of marrow myeloid regeneration.

2. eradication of the clinical signs of infection being treated.

3. severe transfusion reactions suggesting alloimmunization (unless histocompatible donors can be located as described below).

4. obvious progression of infection despite granulocyte transfusion.

5. progressive refractoriness of the patient's underlying tumor.

When the clinical situation is unclear, it is sometimes appropriate to withhold transfusion for 1 to 2 days in order to observe the patient's course and to reinstitute transfusion should clinical deterioration occur.

Assessment of the Results of Granulocyte Transfusions

A number of factors have made it difficult to accurately measure the effects of granulocyte transfusion, thereby complicating the evaluation of individual transfusions as well as making it difficult to perform discriminating research in this area. As is easily appreciated, the clinical course of seriously infected, granulocytopenic patients is highly variable. The ultimate outcome depends in part on the primary diagnosis and likelihood of marrow recovery, patient age, presence of other medical illnesses, infecting organism and site of infection, appropriateness of antibiotics used, concurrent hemorrhage, and quality of platelet support. Because each of these factors can individually determine the outcome of an infection, it is often impossible to separate out the possible beneficial (or deleterious) effects of granulocyte transfusions. In addition, because the number of granulocytes administered is generally a small fraction of the response of normals to a pyogenic infection, it is unusual to observe unquestionable profound clinical changes following granulocyte transfusion.

Nonetheless, it is important to monitor the results of transfusion as best as possible in order to decide about the necessity of continuing transfusions, the advisability of utilizing different donors, etc. As shown in Table 27-7,

Table 27-7. Methods of Assessing the Results of Granulocyte Transfusion

1. Posttransfusion count increments
2. Transfusion reactions
3. Migration to infected sites or skin chambers
4. Clinical response
5. Isotopic labeling

there are a number of parameters to be monitored posttransfusion:

1. *Posttransfusion count increments.* Measurement of blood counts posttransfusion is the standard test of the viability of blood products and has been a simple tool for the study of the effectiveness of platelet transfusion. Following granulocyte transfusion, however, recoveries are usually less than 10 percent of predicted with absolute increments usually less than 200 to 300/μl, thereby limiting the value of count increments as a clinical tool. Furthermore, obvious clinical responses can be seen in the absence of count increments. This is particularly true when filtration leukopheresis granulocytes were utilized,[58,59] possibly because activation of the complement system occurs during the collection procedure, which may modify the migratory pattern of these granulocytes posttransfusion.[72] The explanation for the reduced granulocyte recovery is unclear, although animal experiments suggest that transfused granulocytes may be preferentially attracted to inflammatory sites at the expense of the circulating pool.[73] Recent experiments using radio-labeled granulocytes have confirmed this observation in humans.[78]

2. *Transfusion reactions* following granulocyte transfusion can occur during or shortly following the infusion and can be of life-threatening severity characterized by fever, chills, tachycardia, hypertension, or hypotension, and occasionally by immunologically mediated pulmonary infiltrates. The reactions can usually be ameliorated by premedication or treatment with acetaminophen, antihistamines, and corticosteroids or by slowing the infusion rate. As a rough

guide, it is advisable to administer centrifugation-collected granulocytes over at least 1 to 2 hours with filtration leukopheresis granulocytes infused over 3 to 4 hours. The slower rate is recommended for the filtration granulocytes because of the well-documented increased incidence of transfusion reactions using these cells, which is presumably caused by damage to the cells during the collection procedure.[59,74,75] Transfusion reactions should not be regarded as a "routine" occurrence but should rather be regarded as a "clue" that something is awry with the granulocyte preparation. Thus, if severe transfusion reactions consistently occur with filtration leukopheresis preparations, it is incumbent upon the transfusion laboratory to review and modify their collection procedures so as to improve the quality of the product. With centrifugation-collected granulocytes, transfusion reactions strongly suggest the presence of recipient alloimmunization and donor-recipient incompatibility which may require a switch to other donors. Close, day-to-day liaison between the clinicians and transfusion service is necessary to monitor the incidence of transfusion reactions so as to implement the necessary changes in patient management or collection technique.

3. *Migration of granulocytes to infected sites* (or in the research setting to skin chambers) should be monitored in patients with accessible infected areas (usually cutaneous lesions). The presence of granulocytes in areas which were previously acellular strongly suggests that the transfused cells were viable and survived in the circulation.

4. *Clinical response*, as assessed by physical examination, radiographic clearing, lysis of fever, etc., is usually difficult to quantitate because of the many factors described above which also modify the course of the infection. Obviously, however, the patient and the blood counts must be monitored at least daily in order to make decisions about the need for further transfusions.

5. An ideal *isotopic label* would permit simultaneous measurement of granulocyte kinetics and migration to infection sites. Both ^{51}Chromium and diisopropylfluorophosphate (DF^{32}P) have not been suitable research tools for this purpose because DF^{32}P is a beta emitter which does not permit surface scanning to be performed while ^{51}Cr is not tightly bound to the granulocyte. Recently, ^{111}Indium oxine has been successfully utilized as a granulocyte label. It also has the advantage of being a gamma emitter, thereby allowing semiquantitative analysis by scans of migration of transfused granulocytes to sites of infection or destruction.[76] Preliminary studies indicate that transfused granulocytes are transiently sequestered in the pulmonary vasculature for up to a few hours posttransfusion,[77] although other recent observations also demonstrate that some labeled granulocytes can be detected in infected sites as early as 30 minutes after transfusion.[78]

HISTOCOMPATIBILITY TESTING

Granulocytes have antigens on their surface which are shared with other tissues such as HLA A and B loci antigens and ABH, as well as antigens specific for granulocytes themselves.[79] A variety of techniques of varying complexity and sensitivity, including agglutination, cytotoxicity, fluorescent labeling,[80] complement fixation, and granulocyte opsonization are available to detect these antigens. Most of the assays require purification of the granulocyte preparations prior to testing and 4 to 24 hours to perform and are therefore not ideally suitable for immediate crossmatching purposes. In addition, it has been difficult to correlate these in vivo tests with clinical outcome, in part because of the difficulties involved in measuring the results of transfusion and possibly in part because of the unreliability of some of the assay systems.[81,82] Certain points are clear, however. It is known that granulocytes are highly antigenic and that the majority of recipients of multiple granulocyte transfusions will develop antigranulocyte antibodies[83] which will be manifested clinically by the development of transfusion reactions.[94] In earlier studies in humans, the incidence of severe transfusion reactions was much increased in patients with leucoagglutinins, and granulocyte recovery and migration to infected sites were decreased in such patients.[84,85] In animals it has been demonstrated that transfusion of non-matched granulocytes to sensitized granulocytopenic dogs results in no migration to skin chambers, markedly decreased granulocyte recovery, and accompanying falls in recipient platelet count.[86] In another dog model, survival following experimental septicemia was markedly inferior in alloimmunized granulocytopenic dogs compared to nonimmunized controls given random-donor granulocytes.[87]

Thus, while there is no available evidence that "nonmatched" granulocytes administered to alloimmunized recipients are of benefit, there is ample evidence that such transfusions are associated with significant recipient side effects. As with platelet transfusion recipients, a significant percentage of potential granulocyte recipients are alloimmunized, the clinical diagnosis of which has been discussed previously. At the time of first considering granulocyte transfusions, one must therefore determine—by clinical evaluation, and by measurement of lymphocytotoxic antibody if possible—the likelihood of recipient alloimmunization. If the recipient is not alloimmunized, one can utilize ABO-compatible donors without regard for other histocompatibility considerations. If alloimmunization is suspected, then "matched" donors, the definition of which is problematic, should be searched for. Although there is controversy about this issue, all studies to date[81,88-90] have demonstrated a correlation between donor-recipient HLA compatibility and posttransfusion count increments (an admittedly imperfect measurement). HLA typing does not take into consideration granulocyte-specific antigens, a well-known cause of febrile transfusion reactions, probably best (although inconsistently) detected by leucoagglutination. Because reliable granulo-cyte-specific antigen testing is not generally available, it may be preferable to utilize HLA-matched family members as donors on the assumption that non-HLA granulocyte antigens are more likely to be identical in the family setting. If there are no family donors, closely HLA-matched nonrelated donors are the next choice, accompanied by careful monitoring for transfusion reactions and clinical response. Granulocytes prepared by centrifugation techniques frequently contain large numbers of accompanying platelets, and measurement of posttransfusion platelet increments can provide a rough estimate of compatibility. However, transfusion reactions, presumably due to granulocyte-specific antigens, can still occur in the setting of good platelet increments. If even partially matched donors cannot be located, then it is often advisable to withhold granulocyte transfusions because the high probability of an ineffective transfusion may not justify the expense and potential donor risk. Lastly, it should be appreciated that the reliance on histocompatible donors frequently severely limits the number of donors available per alloimmunized patient. Although the feasibility of consecutive daily donation is well documented,[91] this approach mandates close donor monitoring and also increases donor inconvenience and possible side effects.

Prophylactic Granulocyte Transfusion

In view of the association between the level of granulocyte count and the risk of infections, it would appear logical, analogous to the platelet transfusion situation, to administer granulocyte transfusion prophylactically to prevent infection. However, prophylactic granulocyte transfusion represents a greater undertaking than does prophylactic platelet transfusion; this is because of the shorter half-life of granulocytes and the resultant need to administer transfusions more frequently. Two prospectively randomized studies have been completed to date which suggest that daily administration of granulocyte transfusion over a 2 to 3 week period of time can decrease infection acquisition following bone marrow transplantation or intensive induction therapy of adult acute leukemia.[92,93] No improvement of overall survival was noted, however, suggesting that most of the infections acquired by the control group could be effectively treated with antibiotics and/or therapeutic granulocyte transfusion. In addition, a high rate of recipient alloimmunization which complicated subsequent patient management has been noted in studies in which nonrelated, non-HLA-matched donors were used.[93,94] In view of these findings as well as the expense, the potential donor morbidity, and the possibility of GVHD which has been described in a leukemic recipient of prophylactic granulocyte transfusion,[95] the use of prophylactic granulocytes should be considered a strictly investigational procedure which should not be utilized outside of research settings.

CONCLUSIONS

Proper utilization of specialized platelets and granulocyte transfusion support depends on an understanding of the great variety of clinical problems encountered by patients with cancer as well as the complexities of cell procurement and storage and donor selection. In order to provide such a service for their patients, there must be close, day-to-day cooperation and consultation between the clinicians and the transfusion service with the flexibility to rapidly modify the blood product as the patient's condition varies. In addition to the consideration for the patient's problems, careful consideration must be given to the stresses and risks faced by the donor, particularly common in the situation where the alloimmunized patient is dependent on the availability of a small number of donors. Lastly, it should be emphasized that there are few aspects of platelet and granulo-

cyte transfusion which are strictly "routine." Rather, there are large gaps in our knowledge of the proper use of platelet and granulocyte transfusion which require continued laboratory and clinical investigation.

REFERENCES

1. Harker, L.A. and Slichter, S.J.: The bleeding time as a screening test for evaluation of platelet function. N. Engl. J. Med. 287:155, 1972.
2. Gaydos, L.A., Freireich, E.J., and Mantel,N.: The quantitative relation between platelet count and hemorrhage in patients with acute leukemia. N. Engl. J. Med. 266:905, 1962.
3. Roy, A.J., Jaffe, N., and Djerassi, I.: Prophylactic platelet transfusions in children with acute leukemia: A dose response study. Transfusion 13:283, 1973.
4. Belt, R.J., Leite, C., Haas, C.D., and Stephens, R.L.: Incidence of hemorrhagic complications in patients with cancer. J.A.M.A. 239:2571, 1978.
5. Higby, D.J., Cohen, E., Holland, J.F., and Sinks, L.: The prophylactic treatment of thrombocytopenic leukemic patients with platelets: A double blind study. Transfusion 14:440, 1974.
6. Murphy, Koch, and Evans: Randomized trial of prophylactic vs. therapeutic platelet transfusion in childhood acute leukemia. Clin. Res. 24:379a, 1976.
7. Slichter, S.J. and Harker, L.A.: Thrombocytopenia: mechanisms and management of defects in platelet production. Clin. Haematol. 7:423, 1978.
8. Dutcher, J.P., Schiffer, C.A., Aisner, J., and Wiernik, P.H.: Alloimmunization following platelet transfusion: The absence of a dose response relationship. Blood, 1981 (in press).
9. Solomon, J., Bofenkamp, T., and Fahey, J.L., et al.: Platelet prophylaxis in acute non-lymphoblastic leukemia. Lancet i:267, 1978.
10. Schiffer, C.A., Aisner, J., and Wiernik, P.H.: Platelet transfusion therapy for patients with leukemia. In: The Blood Platelet in Transfusion Therapy. Greenwalt, T.J. and Jamieson, G.A., eds. Alan R. Liss, Inc., New York, 1978, pp. 267-279.
11. Kevy, S.V., Schmidt, P.J., McGinniss, M.H.,

and Workman, W.G.: Febrile, nonhemolytic transfusion reactions and the limited role of leukoagglutinins in their etiology. Transfusion 2:7, 1962.

12. Thulstrup, H.: The influence of leukocyte and thrombocyte incompatibility on non-haemolytic transfusion reactions. I. A retrospective study. Vox Sang. 21:233, 1971.

13. Pineda, A.A. and Taswell, H.F.: Transfusion reactions associated with anti-IgA antibodies: Report of four cases and review of the literature. Transfusion 15:10, 1975.

14. Silvergleid, A.J., Hafleigh, E.B., Harabin, M.A., Wolf, R.M., and Grumet, F.C.: Clinical value of washed-platelet concentrates in patients with non-hemolytic transfusion reactions. Transfusion 17:33, 1977.

15. Herzig, R.H., Herzig, G.P., Bull, M.I., Decter, J.A., Lohrmann, R.-P., Stout, F.G., Yankee, R.A., and Graw, R.G., Jr.: Correction of poor platelet transfusion responses with leukocyte-poor HLA-matched platelet concentrates. Blood 46:743, 1975.

16. Alter, H.J., Holland, P.V., Purcell, R.H., Lander, J.J., Feinstone, S.M., Morrow, A.G., and Schmidt, P.J.: Posttransfusion hepatitis after exclusion of commercial and hepatitis-B antigen-positive donors. Ann. Intern. Med. 77:691, 1972.

17. Meyers, J.D., Huff, J.C., Holmes, K.K., Thomas, E.D., and Bryan, J.A.: Parenterally transmitted hepatitis A associated with platelet transfusions. Epidemiologic study of an outbreak in a marrow transplantation center. Ann. Intern. Med. 81:145, 1974.

18. Garfield, M.D., Ershler, W.B., and Maki, D.G.: Malaria transmission by platelet concentrate transfusion. J.A.M.A. 240:2285, 1978.

19. Rhame, F.S., Root, R.K., MacLowry, J.D., Dadisman, T.A., and Bennett, J.V.: Salmonella septicemia from platelet transfusions. Study of an outbreak traced to a hematogenous carrier of salmonella cholerae-suis. Ann. Intern. Med. 78:633, 1973.

20. Buchholz, D.H., Young, V.M., Friedman, N.R., Reilly, J.A., and Mardiney, M.R., Jr.: Bacterial proliferation in platelet products stored at room temperature. N. Engl. J. Med. 285:429, 1971.

21. Silver, H., Sonnenwirth, A.C., and Beisser, L.D.: Bacteriologic study of platelet concentrates prepared and stored without refrigeration. Transfusion 10:315, 1970.

22. Katz, A.J. and Tilton, R.C.: Sterility of platelet concentrates stored at 25° C. Transfusion 10:329, 1970.

23. Mallin, W.S., Reuss, D.T., Bracke, J.W., Roberts, S.C., and Moore, G.L.: Bacteriological study of platelet concentrates stored at 22° C and 4° C. Transfusion 13:439, 1973.

24. Wrenn, H.E. and Speicher, C.E.: Platelet concentrates: Sterility of 400 single units stored at room temperature. Transfusion 14:171, 1974.

25. Zoes, C., Dube, V.E., Miller, H.J., and Vye, M.V.: Anti-A_1 in the plasma of platelet concentrates causing a hemolytic reaction. Transfusion 17:29, 1977.

26. Goldfinger, D. and McGinniss, M.H.: Rh-incompatible platelet transfusions—risks and consequences of sensitizing immunosuppressed patients. N. Engl. J. Med. 284:942, 1971.

27. Herzig, R.H., Poplack, D.G., and Yankee, R.A.: Prolonged granulocytopenia from incompatible platelet transfusions. N. Engl. J. Med. 290:1220, 1974.

28. Tomasulo, G., Duquesnoy, R.J., and Zandt, D., et al.: Do mismatched platelet transfusions induce granulocytopenia in refractory alloimmunized patients? Blood 53(Suppl): 304, 1978 (Abstract).

28a. Tomasulo, P.A.: Management of the alloimmunized patient with HLA-matched platelets. In: Platelet Physiology and Transfusion. Schiffer, C.A., ed. Am. Assoc. Blood Banks, Washington, D.C., 1978, pp. 69–82.

29. Tejada, F., Bias, W.B., Santos, G.W., and Zieve, P.D.: Immunologic response of patients with acute leukemia to platelet transfusions. Blood 42:405, 1973.

30. Schiffer, C.A., Lichtenfeld, J.L., Wiernik, P.H., Mardiney, M.R., Jr., and Joseph, J.M.: Antibody response in patients with acute nonlymphocytic leukemia. Cancer 37:2177, 1976.

31. Green, D., Tiro, A., Basiliere, J., and Mittal, K.K.: Cytotoxic antibody complicating platelet support in acute leukemia. J.A.M.A. 236:1044, 1976.

32. Howard, J.E. and Perkins, H.A.: The natural history of alloimmunization to platelets. Transfusion 18:496, 1978.

33. Daly, P.A., Schiffer, C.A., Aisner, J., and Wiernik, P.H.: The value of 1-hour post transfusion counts in predicting the need for HLA matched platelet transfusions. J.A.M.A. 243:435, 1980.

34. Wu, K.K., Thompson, J.S., Koepke, J.A., Hoak, J.C., and Flink, R.: Heterogeneity of antibody response to human platelet transfusion. J. Clin. Invest. 58:432, 1976.

35. Wu, K.K., Hoak, J.C., Thompson, J.S., and Koepke, J.A.: Use of platelet aggregometry in selection of compatible platelet donors. N. Engl. J. Med. 292:130, 1975.

36. Brand, A., van Leeuwen, A., and Eernisse, J.G., et al.: Platelet transfusion therapy. Optimal donor selection with a combination of lymphocytotoxicity and platelet fluorescence tests. Blood 51:781, 1978.

37. Gockerman, J.P., Bowman, R.P., and Conrad, M.E.: Detection of platelet isoantibodies by (^{3}H) serotonin platelet release and its clinical application to the problem of platelet matching. J. Clin. Invest. 55:75, 1975.

38. Slichter, S.J.: Selection of compatible platelet donors. In: Platelet Physiology and Transfusion. Schiffer, C.A., ed. Am. Assoc. Blood Banks, Washington, D.C., 1978, p. 83–92.

39. Sugiura, K., Steiner, M., and Baldini, M.: Platelet antibody in idiopathic thrombocytopenic purpura and other thrombocytopenias. J. Lab. & Clin. Med. 96:640, 1980.

40. Filip, D.J., Duquesnoy, R.J., and Aster, R.H.: Predictive value of crossmatching for transfusion of platelet concentrates to alloimmunized recipients. Am. J. Hematol. 1:471, 1976.

41. Yankee, R.A., Grumet, F.C., and Rogentine, G.N.: Platelet transfusion therapy: The selection of compatible platelet donors for refractory patients by lymphocyte HL-A typing. N. Engl. J. Med. 281:1208, 1969.

42. Lohrmann, H., Bull, M.I., Decter, J.A., Yankee, R.A., and Graw, R.G., Jr.: Platelet transfusions from HL-A compatible unrelated donors to alloimmunized patients. Ann. Intern. Med. 80:9, 1974.

43. Graw, R.G., Jr., Herzig, R.H., Langston, M.G., Perdue, S.T., and Terasaki, P.I.: National donor registry and computer transfusion programs for platelet transfusions. Transplant. Proc. 9:225, 1977.

44. Duquesnoy, R.J., Filip, D.J., Rodey, G.E., Rimm, A.A., and Aster, R.H.: Successful transfusion of platelets "mismatched" for HLA antigens to alloimmunized thrombocytopenic patients. Am. J. Hematol. 2:219, 1977.

45. Aster, R.H., Szatkowski, N., Liebert, M., and Duquesnoy, R.J.: Expression of HLA-B12, HLA-B8, w4, and w6 on platelets. Transplant. Proc. 9:1695, 1977.

46. Tosato, G., Appelbaum, F.R., and Deisseroth, A.B.: HLA-matched platelet transfusion therapy of severe aplastic anemia. Blood 52:846, 1978.

47. Nagasawa, T., Kim, B.K., and Baldini, M.G.: Temporary suppression of circulating antiplatelet alloantibodies by the massive infusion of fresh, stored, or lyophilized platelets. Transfusion 18:429, 1978.

48. Schiffer, C.A., Aisner, J., and Wiernik, P.H.: Clinical experience with transfusion of cryopreserved platelets. Br. J. Haematol. 34:377, 1976.

49. Schiffer, C.A., Aisner, J., and Wiernik, P.H.: Frozen autologous platelet transfusion for patients with leukemia. N. Engl. J. Med. 299:7, 1978.

50. Dayian, G. and Rowe, A.W.: Cryopreservation of human platelets for transfusion: A glycerol-glucose, moderate rate cooling procedure. Cryobiology 13:1, 1976.

51. Kim, B.K. and Baldini, M.G.: Biochemistry, function, and hemostatic effectiveness of frozen human platelets. Proc. Soc. Exper. Biol. and Med. 145:830, 1974.

52. Valeri, C.R., Feingold, H., and Marchionni, L.L.: A simple method for freezing human platelets using 6% dimethylsulfoxide and storage at −80° C. Blood 43:131, 1974.

53. Daly, P.A., Schiffer, C.A., Aisner, J., and Wiernik, P.H.: Successful transfusion of platelets cryopreserved for more than 3 years. Blood 54:1023, 1979.

54. Freireich, E.J., Kliman, A., Gaydos, L.A., Mantel, N., and Frei, E., III: Response to repeated platelet transfusion from the same donor. Ann. Intern. Med. 59:277, 1963.

55. O'Donnell, M.R. and Slichter, S.J.: Platelet (PLT) alloimmunization-correlation with donor source. Clin. Res. 27:390A, 1979.

56. Levine, A.S., Schimpff, S.C., Graw, R.G., Jr., and Young, R.C.: Hematologic malignancies and other marrow failure states: progress in the management of complicating infections. Sem. in Hematol. 11:141, 1974.

57. McCredie, K.B., Hester, J.P., Freireich, E.J., Brittin, G.M., and Vallejos, C.: Platelet and leukocyte transfusions in acute leukemia. Hum. Pathol. 5:699, 1974.

58. Higby, D.J., Yates, J.W., Henderson, E.S., and Holland, J.F.: Filtration leukapheresis for granulocyte transfusion therapy. N. Engl. J. Med. 292:761, 1975.

59. Schiffer, C.A., Buchholz, D.H., Aisner, J., Betts, S.W., and Wiernik, P.H.: Clinical experience with transfusion of granulocytes obtained by continuous flow filtration leukopheresis. Am. J. Med. 58:373, 1975.

60. Alavi, J.B., Root, R.K., Djerassi, I., Evans, A.E., Gluckman, S.J., MacGregor, R.R., Guerry, D., Schreiber, A.D., Shaw, J.M., and Koch, P.: A randomized clinical trial of granulocyte transfusions for infection in acute leukemia. N. Engl. J. Med. 196:706, 1977.

61. Herzig, R.H., Herzig, G.P., Graw, R.G., Jr., Bull, M.I., and Ray, K.K.: Successful granulocyte transfusion therapy for gram-negative septicemia: A prospectively randomized controlled study. N. Engl. J. Med. 296:701, 1977.

62. Vogler, W.R. and Winton, E.F.: A controlled study of the efficacy of granulocyte transfusions in patients with neutropenia. Am. J. Med. 63:548, 1977.

63. Bodey, G.P., Buckley, M., Sathe, Y.S., Freireich, E.J.: Quantitative relationships between circulating leucocytes and infection in patients with acute leukemia. Ann. Intern. Med. 64:328, 1966.

64. EORTC International Antimicrobial Therapy Project Group: Three antibiotic regimens in the treatment of infection in febrile granulocytopenic patients with cancer. J. Infect. Dis. 137:14, 1978.

65. Higby, D.J. and Burnett, D.: Granulocyte transfusions: current status. Blood 55:2, 1980.

65a. Schiffer, C.A.: Filtration leukapheresis: Summary and perspectives. Exper. Hematol. 7:42, 1979.

66. Fortuny, I.E., Bloomfield, C.D., Hadlock, D.C., Goldman, A., Kennedy, B.J., and McCullough, J.J.: Granulocyte transfusion: A controlled study in patients with acute non-lymphocytic leukemia. Transfusion 15:548, 1975.

67. Ruthe, R.C., Andersen, B.R., Cunningham, B.L., and Epstein, R.B.: Efficacy of granulocyte transfusions in the control of systemic candidiasis in the leukopenic host. Blood 52:493, 1978.

68. Freireich, E.J., Levin, R.H., Whang, J., Carbone, P.P., Bronson, W., and Morse, E.E.: The function and fate of transfused leukocytes from donors with chronic myelocytic leukemia in leukopenic recipients. Ann. N.Y. Acad. Sci. 113:1081, 1964.

69. Schwarzenberg, L., Mathe, G., Amiel, J.L., Cattan, A., Schneider, M., and Schlumberger, J.R.: Study of factors determining the usefulness and complications of leukocyte transfusion. Am. J. Med. 43:206, 1967.

70. Graw, R.G., Jr., Herzig, G., Perry, S., and Henderson, E.S.: Normal granulocyte transfusion therapy: Treatment of septicemia due to gram-negative bacteria. N. Engl. J. Med. 287:367, 1972.

71. Higby, D.J., Freeman, A., Henderson, E.S., Sinks, L., and Cohen, E.: Granulocyte transfusions in children using filter-collected cells. Cancer 38:1407, 1976.

72. Nusbacher, J., Rosenfeld, S.I., MacPherson, J.L., Thiem, P.A., and Leddy, J.P.: Nylon fiber leukapheresis: Associated complement component changes and granulocytopenia. Blood 51:359, 1978.

73. Rosenshein, M., Price, T., and Dale, D.: Neutropenia, inflammation, and the kinetics of transfused neutrophils. Clin. Res. 26:507A, 1978.

74. Aisner, J., Schiffer, C.A., and Wiernik, P.H.: Granulocyte transfusion: evaluation of factors influencing results and a comparison of filtration and intermittent centrifugation leukapheresis. Br. J. Haematol. 38:121, 1978.

75. Herzig, G.P.: Leukocyte donor and recipient reactions with filtration leukapheresis: The character, frequency, and management. Exper. Hematol. 7:31, 1979.

76. Thakur, M.L., Lavender, J.P., Arnot, R.N., Silvester, D.J., and Segal, A.W.: Indium-111-labeled autologous leukocytes in man. J. Nuclear Med. 18:1012, 1977.

77. Weiblen, B.J., Forstrom, L., and McCullough, J.: Studies of the kinetics of indium-111 labeled granulocytes. J. Lab. Clin. Med. 94:246, 1979.

78. Dutcher, J.P., Schiffer, C.A., and Johnson, G.: Rapid migration of Indium-111 labeled granulocytes to infected sites (submitted for publication).

79. Lalezari, P.: Neutrophil antigens: Immunology and clinical implications. In: The Granulocyte: Function and Clinical Utilization. Greenwalt, T.J. and Jamieson, G.A., eds. Alan R. Liss, Inc., New York, 1977, pp. 209-225.

80. Verheught, F.W.A., Borne, A.E.G.Kr. von dem, van Noord-Bokhorst, J.C., and Engelfriet, C.P.: Autoimmune granulocytopenia: The detection of granulocyte autoantibodies with the immunofluorescent test. Br. J. Haematol. 39:399, 1978.

81. Hester, J.P. and Rossen, R.O.: Multiple granulocyte transfusions (TX): Role of HLA compatibility and leukoagglutinins. Proc. Am. Assoc. Cancer Res. 15:53, 1974.

82. Ungerleider, R.S., Appelbaum, F.R., Trapani, R.J., and Deisseroth, A.B.: Lack of predictive value of antileukocyte antibody screening in granulocyte transfusion therapy. Transfusion 19:90, 1978.

83. Thompson, J.S., Burns, C.P., and Herbick: Stimulation of granulocyte antibodies by granulocyte transfusion. Blood 50(Suppl):303, 1977.

84. Goldstein, I.M., Eyre, H.J., Terasaki, P.I., Henderson, E.S., and Graw, R.G., Jr.: Leukocyte transfusions: Role of leukocyte alloantibodies in determining transfusion response. Transfusion 11:19, 1971.

85. Eyre, H.J., Goldstein, I.M., Perry, S., and Graw, R.G., Jr.: Leukocyte transfusions: Function of transfused granulocytes from donors with chronic myelocytic leukemia. Blood 36:432, 1970.

86. Appelbaum, F.R., Trapani, R.J., and Graw, R.G., Jr.: Consequences of prior alloimmunization during granulocyte transfusion. Transfusion 17:460, 1977.

87. Westrick, M.A., Debelak-Fehir, K.M., and Epstein, R.B.: The effect of prior whole blood transfusion on subsequent granulocyte support in leukopenic dogs. Transfusion 17:611, 1976.

88. Graw, R.G., Jr., Goldstein, I.M., Eyre, H.J., and Terasaki, P.I.: Histocompatibility testing for leucocyte transfusion. Lancet 2:77, 1970.

89. Higby, D.J., Mishler, J.M., Cohen, E., Rhomberg, W., Nicora, R.W., and Holland, J.F.: Increased elevation of peripheral leukocyte counts by infusion of histocompatible granulocytes. Vox Sang. 27:186, 1974.

90. McCullough, J., Wood, N., Weiblen, B.J., Fortuny, I.E., and Yunis, E.J.: The role of histocompatibility testing in granulocyte transfusion. In: The Granulocyte: Function and Clinical Utilization. Greenwalt, T.J. and Jamieson, G.A., eds. Alan R. Liss, Inc., New York, 1977, pp. 321-328.

91. Buchholz, D.H., Schiffer, C.A., Wiernik, P.H., Betts, S.W., and Reilly, J.A.: Granulocyte harvest for transfusion: Donor response to repeated leukapheresis. Transfusion 15:96, 1975.

92. Clift, R.A., Sanders, J.E., Thomas, E.D., Williams, B., and Buckner, C.D.: Granulocyte transfusions for the prevention of infection in patients receiving bone-marrow transplants. N. Engl. J. Med. 298:1052, 1978.

93. Mannoni, P., Rodet, M., Radeau, E., Beaujean, F., and Brun, B.: Granulocyte transfusion: Efficiency of prophylactic granulocyte transfusions in care of patients with acute leukemia. In: Blood Leucocytes: Function and Use in Therapy. Hogman, C.S., Lindahl-Kiessling, K., and Wigzell, H., eds. Almquist and Wiksell International, Stockholm, 1977.

94. Schiffer, C.A., Aisner, J., Daly, P.A., Schimpff, S.C., and Wiernik, P.H.: Alloimmunization following prophylactic granulocyte transfusion. Blood 54:766, 1979.

95. Ford, J.M., Lucey, J.J., Cullen, M.H., Tobias, J.S., and Lister, T.A.: Fatal graft-versus-host disease following transfusion of granulocytes from normal donors. Lancet 2:1167, 1976.

28

Transfusion in Transplantation with Emphasis on Bone Marrow Transplantation

Rainer Storb, M.D., and Paul L. Weiden, M.D.

Marrow transplantation, once considered a desperate therapeutic maneuver in terminally ill patients, has now become a therapeutic option to some patients with aplastic anemia, acute leukemia, or other hematologic malignancies.[1-3] Accordingly, the number of transplantations has steadily increased. For example, in Seattle alone, 145 transplants were carried out in 1978 and 175 in 1979 and in 1980. It is now feasible to extend marrow transplantation to the treatment of patients with genetic disorders of hematopoiesis. Cure of paroxysmal nocturnal hemoglobinuria by allogeneic and syngeneic marrow transplantation showed that this disease is an acquired stem cell defect.[4,5] The longest survivor with congenital Fanconi's anemia cured by a marrow transplant is, as of this writing, more than 6 years after grafting.[5] Cure of genetic disorders associated with hemolytic anemia and neutropenia has been reported in animal models. The obvious target disorders in man are thalassemia major and sickle cell disease.

Until recently, marrow donors have been almost exclusively siblings identical with the recipient for the antigens of the major human histocompatibility complex (HLA). More recently, however, the feasibility of marrow grafts from HLA-nonidentical family members has been explored with some success.[6,7] Since donor and recipient are not genetically identical, patients must have some form of immunosuppressive preparation so that they will not reject the graft. The type of preparation is influenced by the nature of the underlying diseases. Most patients with aplastic anemia have been prepared with a regimen of cyclophosphamide administered at doses of 50 mg/kg on each of 4 days. In patients with hematologic malignancies, the conditioning regimen not only must be immunosuppressive but must also serve to eradicate leukemic cells. Leukemic patients, therefore, have been treated not only with cyclophosphamide but also with total body irradiation (TBI) given in doses of 800 to 1,000 rad midline tissue at 4 to 26 rads per minute. Following the preparative regimen and the intravenous infusion of 2 to 6 $\times$ 10^8 donor marrow cells per kg, most marrow grafts are initially successful. Increasing marrow cellularity and rising peripheral blood counts of donor origin are evident in 2 to 4 weeks. Subsequent graft rejection has been a considerable problem in patients with aplastic anemia, and this complication has been linked to pretransplant transfusions.[8]

Before transplantation, almost all marrow transplant recipients go through periods of no marrow function owing to their disease or its treatment with chemotherapeutic agents. After grafting, there is a period of 14 to 30 days before the graft begins to function. Effective supportive measures during these periods of marrow aplasia are absolutely essential to success in a marrow transplantation program. The principles guiding the transfusion support before transplantation are to some extent different from those used after transplantation. The two periods will, therefore, receive separate consideration.

TRANSFUSION SUPPORT BEFORE MARROW TRANSPLANTATION IN PATIENTS WITH APLASTIC ANEMIA

Sensitization to Non-HLA Antigens by Blood Transfusion

The principles of transfusion support for patients with aplastic anemia are primarily derived from experience in the management of iatrogenic marrow failure induced in the course of chemotherapy of patients with malignant hematologic diseases, especially acute leukemia. There are some obvious and important differences between such patients with malignant diseases and patients with aplastic anemia. Patients with iatrogenic marrow failure are usually immunosuppressed during periods of chemotherapy and blood cell support; thus, they are less likely to be sensitized to minor and major histocompatibility antigens. On the other hand, patients with aplastic anemia are more likely to have protracted pancytopenia with little expectation of prompt recovery.

Recent developments in the field of experimental and clinical marrow transplantation have emphasized a new factor which must be considered when designing support by transfusions. This is the possibility of sensitizing the transfusion recipient with tissue antigens that are not recognized by current histocompatibility typing techniques. Sensitization to these antigens may jeopardize attempts at marrow transplantation even when

the marrow donor is a sibling matched with the recipient for the known antigens of the major histocompatibility complex. In the following section we will present evidence that multiple transfusions, particularly from members of the family, may have a negative influence on the outcome of a subsequent marrow graft. We will also develop specific recommendations for transfusion support of the patient with aplastic anemia who is a potential candidate for marrow transplantation.

Blood Transfusions and Rejection of Subsequent Marrow Grafts in Experimental Animals

In mice, allogeneic marrow engraftment was prevented when the recipients were given several whole blood transfusions from the prospective marrow donor before conditioning of the recipient by TBI and transplantation.[9] Immunization against subsequent marrow transplants and failure of the infused marrow to take was also observed in rhesus monkeys and dogs after transfusions with blood from the intended donor and after multiple transfusions from third party donors.[10-12] Transfusions were harmful regardless of whether they were given 3 months or 24 hours before TBI. The data so far reported refer to randomly selected donor-recipient pairs or pairs that were mismatched for the major histocompatibility antigens.

Loutit and Micklem[13] showed that prior immunization by allogeneic H-2 compatible donor spleen cell injections caused increased mortality in X-irradiated recipient mice following marrow grafting, thus indicating that minor antigenic differences may also be important. In view of the importance of HLA-identical human siblings for platelet transfusions and for marrow grafting, we evaluated the effect of preceding blood transfusions in dog leukocyte antigen (DLA)-identical canine sibling pairs.[14,15] All 58 untransfused recipients in that study successfully engrafted. In contrast, dogs given one or more transfusions of whole blood from the marrow donor before transplantation, as a rule, rejected. This must be explained by sensitization of the recipient to currently undetected non-DLA antigens contained in the transfused blood. TBI, approximately two and one-half times the lethal dose, was not sufficient to suppress sensitization to the grafted marrow. The finding of a 100 percent incidence of marrow graft rejection (19 of 19 instances) after only three transfusions of whole blood from the marrow donor suggested that at least two polymorphic histocompatibility systems outside of DLA were involved in sensitization. The probability of encountering 19 of 19 rejections if only one polymorphic locus were involved is smaller than 0.008 (binomial significance test). Therefore, attempts at unraveling the genetics of these antigen systems by in vitro tests of immunity will be difficult to interpret.

The conclusion that polymorphic "minor" antigen systems are involved is consistent with the additional observation that transfusions from unrelated donors can immunize a recipient against a subsequent marrow graft from a DLA-identical littermate. In that situation, rejection of the marrow might be expected only when one or more of the blood transfusion donors and the marrow donor share "minor" antigens not present in the recipient. Exposure to very large numbers of unrelated transfusion donors before grafting would, therefore, increase the danger of graft rejection even in DLA-identical sibling pairs.

It has been suggested that frozen, thawed, leukocyte-depleted red blood cells (RBCs) diminish the incidence of immunization of recipients to transplantation antigens. In a recent controlled clinical trial it was demonstrated that patients receiving only leukocyte-poor blood were significantly less likely to produce lymphocytotoxic antibodies than patients who received ordinary packed RBCs.[16] Earlier marrow graft studies using DLA-nonidentical unrelated recipients had failed to show a clear-cut reduction in the rejection rate among animals receiving leuko-

cyte-poor RBC transfusions. More recent studies, however, in DLA-identical littermate pairs have been encouraging with most dogs showing sustained marrow engraftment after transfusion of leukocyte-poor red blood cells.[15] Similarly, most dogs given leukocyte-poor platelet transfusions showed sustained engraftment. These data could mean (1) that platelets and RBC exhibit only some but not all of the non-DLA antigens involved in sensitization and rejection, or (2) that platelets and RBCs express none of the antigens, and sensitization and rejection were due to mononuclear cell contamination on the order of 1.5×10^5 cells per dog.

The latter explanation was supported by preliminary observations in this same canine model showing that rejection can be seen in some dogs after injections of 1.5×10^5 mononuclear peripheral blood cells from the marrow donor. Other preliminary studies have shown that none of six dogs studied so far have rejected their marrow grafts after preceding transfusion of marrow donor granulocytes that were depleted of mononuclear cells. These findings in DLA-identical canine marrow graft recipients are of potential practical importance for the platelet, RBC, and granulocyte support of human marrow graft candidates. The incidence of rejection after marrow transplantation for aplastic anemia could perhaps be reduced if techniques could be developed for producing platelets, RBCs, and granulocytes poor in mononuclear cells for use during the phase of conventional management before transplantation. The nature of the mononuclear cells involved in sensitization and rejection is currently under investigation. The antigens are apparently also expressed on skin epithelial cells, since dogs presensitized with cultured skin epithelial cells all rejected subsequent marrow grafts from their DLA-identical littermates.[15] Furthermore, in vitro marrow-lymphocyte coculture studies have shown that erythroid progenitor cells share the antigens involved in sensitization. In fact, the coculture test proved to be very accurate in predicting the fate of subsequent marrow grafts in transfused dogs.[17]

Transfusions and Graft Rejection in Clinical Marrow Grafting

The current experience in human marrow grafting has justified the concern with respect to the harmful effects of preceding transfusions. Rejection rates ranging from 25 to 60 percent have been reported in multiply transfused patients with aplastic anemia given marrow grafts from HLA-identical siblings.[5, 17a, 18-23] Rejection has been the most prominent cause of failure in marrow transplantation. As a result, in most series only 45 to 50 percent of all transplanted patients have become long-term survivors with functioning grafts.

Based on the data in experimental animals and on the cumulative human transplant experience, it was hypothesized that marrow graft rejection could be dramatically decreased and survival accordingly increased if patients with aplastic anemia were treated by marrow grafts before sensitization to non-HLA antigens by transfusion of blood products. We have recently reported the results of 30 patients with severe aplastic anemia who had received no transfusions of blood products until just before marrow transplantation from HLA-identical family members.[8] As of November 1980, 25 of the 30 are alive between 24 to 100 (median 35) months. The actual projection of survival for 2 to 8 years is 83 percent. Twenty of the 25 surviving patients have no problems. Five have chronic graft-versus-host disease, resolving in two and active in three. Five patients died with infection or hemorrhage, four of whom had graft-versus-host disease. These data indicate that early transplantation should be carried out before transfusions are given for any patient with severe aplastic anemia who has an HLA-identical family member available to serve as a donor.

However, most patients with aplastic anemia will have had transfusion support before the option of bone marrow transplantation is considered. It seemed important to develop tests to determine which patient was sensitized against the intended marrow donor and which one was not. Sensitized patients would need to be subjected to more intensive immunosuppressive conditioning regimens such as a procarbazine/antithymocyte serum/TBI regimen found to be effective in dogs[11] or a cyclophosphamide/TBI regimen used in patients with leukemia.[2, 3, 24] Such regimens are potentially more toxic and also prolong the pregrafting period during which the patient is at risk. One report suggested that the presence of lymphocytotoxic antibodies against random individuals was predictive of marrow graft rejection.[25] However, others were unable to confirm this report in larger series of patients.[26, 27] Work with two in vitro tests of cell-mediated immunity—the relative response index in mixed leukocyte reaction (MLR)[1] and the ^{51}Cr release assays[22, 27a]—has been encouraging. Results of both tests showed a strong correlation with rejection or acceptance of the bone marrow transplant. The results support the concept that an important factor involved in marrow graft rejection is immunization of the patient against minor histocompatibility antigens of the donor, presumably through preceding blood transfusion. However, with many other additional factors possibly predictive of marrow graft rejection—e.g., age of recipient, donor-recipient ABO groups, etc.—it was clear that a multifactorial analysis was needed to isolate those factors that really predicted graft rejection.

A binary logistic regression analysis of the first 73 consecutive patients transplanted at our center in Seattle showed that, of 24 possible predictive factors, only two correlated strongly with graft rejection:[22] (1) a positive relative response index in MLR indicating sensitization of patient against donor; and (2) a low number of marrow cells used for transplantation. Sensitization to the minor antigens involved in rejection appeared to be independent of refractoriness to random donor platelets.

The Seattle Marrow Transplant Team met with success in its initial attempts to avoid rejection in multiply transfused patients with positive in vitro tests by more powerful immunosuppressive conditioning with TBI combined with cyclophosphamide or procarbazine and antithymocyte globulin; however, overall survival was poor because of complicating graft-versus-host disease and interstitial pneumonia.[1] This led to the Team's discontinuation of the use of TBI for patients with nonmalignant diseases. Other groups are still using TBI regimens, either at reduced doses or with lung shielding to avoid lung damage. One center has used cyclophosphamide and total lymphoid irradiation with reduction in the rejection rate. More time is needed to evaluate the effect of these maneuvers on survival.

Having demonstated that graft rejection was less likely with a larger number of marrow cells, we turned to the donor's peripheral blood as an added source of cells. These cells are of interest because they might contribute (1) additional hemopoietic stem cells,[28,29] and (2) additional lymphoid cells shown experimentally to facilitate engraftment in vivo or increase erythropoiesis in vitro.[1] For these reasons we decided to give additional donor buffy coat cells for patients who were shown by in vitro tests to be sensitized and, thus, at great risk of graft rejection. Thirteen of 16 such sensitized recipients given marrow only rejected the graft, while 3 of 23 of those given marrow plus buffy coat rejected.[1] Survival in the two groups was 25 and 71 percent, respectively. The addition of buffy coat did not appear to increase the incidence of graft-versus-host disease. Consequently, the survival among patients transplanted in Seattle over the past three years has risen to over 70 percent. However, rejection is still observed in a considerable proportion of transfused patients. Clearly, emphasis must be placed on measures to prevent sensitization by blood transfusions.

Recommendations for Pretransplant Transfusion Support in Patients with Aplastic Anemia

One important step to improve the overall clinical results of marrow grafting is for the physician to be aware of the possibility of transplantation when a patient with aplastic anemia is first seen. HLA typing of patient and family should be done immediately. If no HLA-identical family member is available, marrow transplantation should not be attempted at present and more conventional treatment can be instituted. If, on the other hand, an HLA-identical family member is available, early transplantation should receive prime consideration. Transfusions of blood products should not be given unless indicated by urgent medical necessity. All transfusions from family members should be avoided, and a transplant center should be contacted immediately to secure admission of the patient. If transfusions are necessary, an attempt to prevent alloimmunization should be made by using only leukocyte-poor RBCs prepared by machine-washing RBCs using large volumes of saline, or, if available, RBCs passed through nylon fiber columns or tightly packed cotton fiber filters. Similarly, leukocyte-poor platelets should be used when necessary.

With regard to the level at which platelet support should be instituted, some guidance can be obtained from studies of stool blood loss in patients with thrombocytopenia on no medication except androgenic steroids which revealed the following:[30] Patients with platelet counts greater than 10,000/μl showed stool blood loss not different from normal— i.e., less than 5 ml per day. At platelet levels between 5,000 and 10,000/μl, blood loss was only slightly increased above normal (9 $\pm$ 7 ml per day). However, platelet counts of less than 5,000/μl were associated with markedly elevated blood loss in the stool (50 ± 20 ml per day). Semisynthetic penicillins and prednisone were found to markedly enhance blood loss in some patients.[30] It was concluded from these studies that platelet transfusions should not be given prophylactically to thrombocytopenic patients unless counts are below 5,000/μl and that all drugs should be avoided except for essential medications. Indeed, another study suggested that prophylactic platelet transfusions may not be warranted and that platelet transfusions should only be given for specific indications such as clinically significant bleeding.[31] (Also see Ch. 27.)

Transfusion Support Before Marrow Transplantation in Patients with Acute Leukemia

The principles of blood support for patients with acute leukemia and other hematologic malignancies were discussed in Chapter 27. Blood support is usually necessary when the patients are undergoing chemotherapy-induced remission—i.e., at a time when they are usually severely immunosuppressed and thus less likely to become sensitized to blood products than are the patients with aplastic anemia. Studies in mice given preceding transfusions from their marrow donors in the presence of 6-mercaptopurine treatment had a significantly reduced marrow graft rejection rate when compared to mice not given 6-mercaptopurine.[32] Therefore, perhaps because transfusions are usually given during chemotherapy or because more powerful immunosuppressive conditioning regimens are used in pretransplant conditioning of leukemic patients, the rate of marrow graft rejection in leukemic patients has been low—on the order of 1 to 2 percent.[24] Thus, at the time of this writing, there is no indication to restrict the transfusion support for leukemic patients in the pretransplant period. If possible, however, transfusions from family members should be avoided, since they carry the highest risk of immunizing the recipient to non-HLA antigens present in the marrow donor.

TRANSFUSION SUPPORT AFTER MARROW TRANSPLANTATION

This portion of the chapter will not deal with the rare patient with aplastic anemia and a syngeneic marrow donor or with children who have severe combined immunodeficiency. These patients, in general, do not require the administration of immunosuppressive conditioning agents, and thus, present no unique problems of postgrafting transfusion support. We rather will consider here the most common marrow transplant situation involving patients with allogeneic or syngeneic marrow grafts for treatment of malignant diseases, such as leukemia, or allogeneic marrow grafts for nonmalignant hematologic disorders, such as severe aplastic anemia. These patients share the need for intensive cytoreductive and immunosuppressive conditioning regimens before infusion of the marrow graft. Hematopoietic suppression following these regimens is severe. However, its duration is limited to 4 to 6 weeks, the time needed for the infused marrow to function. Thus, intensive transfusion support is required for a finite period of time. No precise set of criteria for transfusion support would be universally accepted by all centers undertaking marrow transplantation; we shall, however, outline the current approaches of the Seattle Marrow Transplant Team.

Irradiation of Transfusions

Viable lymphocytes capable of causing graft-versus-host disease in severely immunosuppressed individuals are present in all cellular transfusion products, including stored RBCs. All blood products transfused into marrow graft recipients should therefore be irradiated in vitro with 1500 rad to prevent the unwanted proliferation of lymphoid cells.[24]

Red Blood Cell Transfusions

Patients are given standard units of ABO-compatible packed RBCs obtained from random, community donors to maintain their hematocrit at 25 to 30 percent. Patients generally require RBC support for 6 to 12 weeks posttransplantation until graft erythropoiesis is adequate to sustain the hematocrit. A relatively unusual source of RBC loss seen in 5 to 10 percent of marrow transplant recipients is hemorrhagic cystitis secondary to high-dose cyclophosphamide used in the conditioning regimen. However, recent data suggest that the incidence of this complication is markedly decreased by continuous bladder irrigation during the period of cyclophosphamide therapy and for 48 hours thereafter.[33]

Platelet Transfusions

Platelet transfusions are administered after transplantation whenever the platelet count is less than 20,000/μl. Platelets are transfused at this level because their transfusion requirement is anticipated to be of relatively short, finite duration in contrast to the longer, indefinite duration of platelet support, and thus increased risk of sensitization, in patients with aplastic anemia before marrow transplantation. Patients are transfused with room temperature-stored, pooled, random-donor platelets prepared by standard techniques[30, 33a] (see Ch. 9) until they become refractory to random platelet transfusions. Patients are considered refractory when a 1-hour posttransfusion platelet increment of less than 5 percent of the expected is obtained on two separate occasions following the transfusion of a pool of 6 units of random-donor platelets.

When patients become clinically refractory to random-donor platelets, platelets are obtained by plateletpheresis from family members. An HLA-identical donor, generally the marrow donor, is utilized for family member platelet support whenever possible—i.e., of sufficient size and age, without medical or social contraindications, and not serving as a granulocyte donor. Parents frequently serve as platelet donors for younger children. Since many factors can contribute to poor recovery and survival of random-donor platelets, family member platelet transfusions are continued only if such transfusions appear to provide more satisfactory platelet support—i.e., higher platelet counts with greater platelet increments and/or longer survival of transfused platelets—than random-donor platelets. If patients require massive platelet support because of septicemia, surgery, etc., both random donor and family member platelet support are provided. HLA-selected, unrelated donor platelets obtained by pheresis are utilized, if available, for the occasional patient with no suitable family donor.

As pointed out in the first portion of this chapter, transfusion support from family members should be avoided before transplantation. If necessary, however, family member transfusion support for the patient with aplastic anemia can be initiated 24 to 48 hours before the first dose of cyclophosphamide is administered, owing to the special immunosuppressive properties of the drug. In patients treated with total body irradiation, family member support should not begin until the day of marrow grafting.

The number and sources of platelet support required in 60 allogeneic marrow transplant recipients (20 with aplastic anemia, 20 with acute lymphoblastic leukemia, and 20 with acute myelogenous leukemia) are depicted in Figure 28-1. The number of platelet units transfused ranged from 16 to 531 (mean = 171) units per patient.[34] Two-thirds of the total number of units transfused were obtained from random donors—i.e., pooled platelets from single-unit whole blood dona-

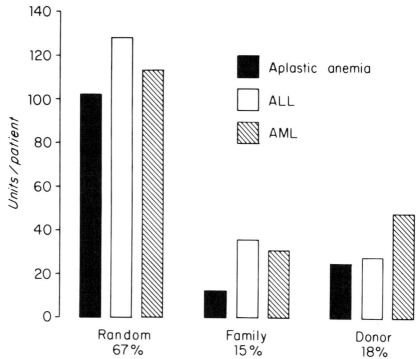

Fig. 28-1. The number of units per patient and the sources of platelet support required during the immediate pre- and posttransplantation periods for 20 patients with aplastic anemia, 20 patients with acute lymphoblastic leukemia (ALL) and 20 patients with acute myelogenous leukemia (AML). Random donor platelets were pooled from single unit whole blood donations; family and marrow donor platelets were obtained from multiple unit plateletpheresis. (Weiden, P.L., Slichter, S.J. and Banaji, M.: Marrow transplantation for aplastic anemia and leukemia—a review of results and blood product support required. In: The Blood Platelet in Transfusion Therapy. Vol. 28. Alan R. Liss, Inc., New York, 1978.)

tions, while one-third of the units were obtained from the marrow donor or other family members by plateletpheresis.

Although the clinical course of most marrow transplant recipients is complex and it may be difficult to categorize every patient, three general patterns of platelet support have been observed:

1. patients supportable entirely by random donor platelets.

2. patients refractory to random-donor platelets, but supportable by HLA-identical sibling platelets.

3. patients refractory to both random-donor platelets and HLA-identical sibling platelets.[30,34]

The platelet requirements of a representative patient supported by random donors is illustrated in Figure 28-2. Note that both the 1-hour platelet count increment and the survival varied, but that transfusion of approximately 4 units of platelets/m^2 every 2 to 4 days maintained the count above 20,000/μl. This can be expected in the absence of septicemia or other causes of platelet consumption. In this patient, platelet production by the marrow graft was adequate to maintain the count after day 25 postgrafting. Although the patient had received no transfusions before the marrow transplant, this pattern can also be observed in patients who have received extensive prior transfusions.

The platelet support of a patient refractory to random donors but supportable by HLA-identical sibling (marrow donor) platelets is illustrated in Figure 28-3. Transfusion of

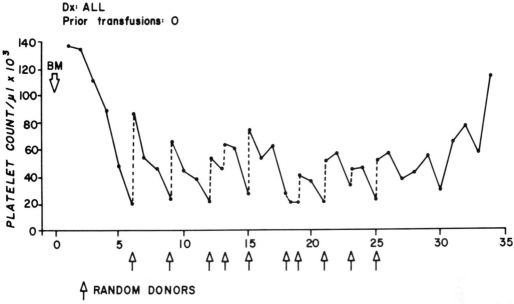

Fig. 28-2. Pattern of platelet support in a marrow transplant recipient supported adequately by pooled, random donor platelets. Each transfusion (*open arrows*) represents a pool of 6 to 8 platelet concentrates. Day of transplantation is day 0.

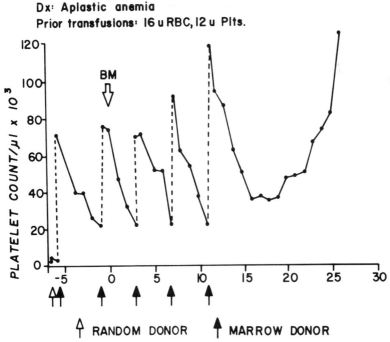

Fig. 28-3. Pattern of platelet support in a marrow transplant recipient refractory to random donor platelets (*lower left corner*), but adequately supported by platelets from the HLA-identical sibling marrow donor (*solid arrows*).

pooled random platelets before transplantation resulted in no rise in platelet count, but both the increment and the survival of HLA-identical sibling platelets were satisfactory. This pattern of support occurs most commonly in extensively transfused patients and is presumably the result of sensitization to HLA antigens.

The platelet support of a patient refractory to both random-donor and HLA-identical sibling platelets is illustrated in Figure 28-4. The patient had no prior transfusions, yet he responded poorly to his first random-donor transfusion given several days before transplantation. During the first week posttransplantation, refractoriness to both random-donor and marrow donor platelets was demonstrated on numerous occasions. Since the marrow donor provided no better support than random donors, random-donor platelets were used. Approximately coincident with the institution of prednisone therapy, platelet recovery and survival improved somewhat, and the patient could be maintained until marrow graft function was adequate.

The mean platelet support required per week before and after allogeneic marrow transplantation for patients with aplastic anemia and acute leukemia is depicted in Figure 28-5. As expected, the period of maximum support was in the second and third posttransplant weeks when the patients' own platelet production had been eliminated by the intensive conditioning regimen and marrow graft function was not yet adequate. Since the platelet counts of many patients with leukemia were normal or only minimally suppressed before transplantation, the platelet support requirement for patients with leukemia increased postgrafting. In contrast, patients with aplastic anemia showed no increase in their platelet transfusion requirement postgrafting since most had been severely thrombocytopenic pregrafting. By the third posttransplant week, patients with aplastic anemia required fewer units of platelets than they did before transplantation.

Fig. 28-4. Pattern of platelet support in a marrow transplant recipient refractory to both random donor and HLA-identical sibling platelets. Multiple transfusions from both random and sibling sources failed to achieve satisfactory platelet increments or survival. Administration of prednisone was associated with some increase in platelet recovery and survival from either random or sibling donors.

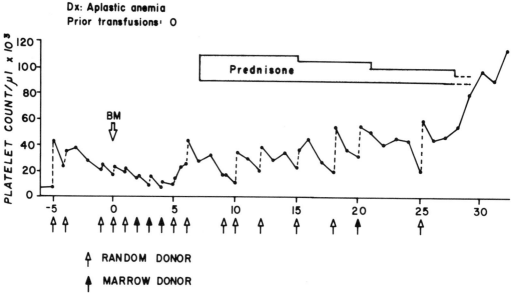

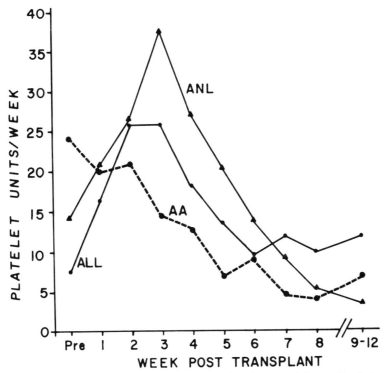

Fig. 28-5. Mean number of platelet units per patient transfused per week immediately before and after allogeneic marrow transplantation. Patient groups as in Fig. 28-1, except that ANL indicates acute myelogenous leukemia. (Weiden, P.L., Slichter, S.J., and Banaji, M.: The Blood Platelet in Transfusion Therapy. Vol. 28. Alan R. Liss, Inc., New York, 1978.)

Thus, although the magnitude of platelet support required by allogeneic marrow transplant recipients is great, it probably does not exceed and may even be less than that required in the treatment of severe aplastic anemia or advanced acute leukemia without marrow transplantation.

Granulocyte Transfusions

There is a high probability of bacterial or fungal infection with considerable morbidity and risk of mortality during the period of granulocytopenia postgrafting. Granulocyte transfusions can be utilized in two ways during this period to decrease the morbidity and mortality of infection: (1) therapeutically to treat established infections, and (2) prophy-

lactically to prevent the development of infection.

The marrow transplant setting provides a high likelihood of obtaining an optimal granulocyte donor. Transplant recipients have frequently had exposure to HLA antigens by transfusion prior to transplantation and therefore may not respond well to randomly selected, histoincompatible granulocyte transfusions. Furthermore, intensive granulocyte transfusions from one or a small number of histoincompatible granulocyte donors would be likely to lead to immunity with poor granulocyte recovery and associated "transfusion reactions," even in the absence of preexisting alloimmunity. Both of these potential problems can be minimized by selection of the single granulocyte donor most likely to be compatible with the recipient. Ideally, the HLA-identical sibling marrow donor can serve as the granulocyte donor. If the marrow donor or other HLA-identical siblings are unsuitable because of age, medical or social contraindication, etc., other relatives sharing at least one HLA haplotype (parent, sibling, child, etc.) can be utilized. The use of a single granulocyte donor also reduces the risk of patient exposure to cytomegalovirus, hepatitis, and other blood-borne infections (Ch. 36). This may be particularly important because both cytomegalovirus and hepatitis have been important causes of death among marrow transplant recipients.[24, 34a, 35-37]

Family member granulocyte donors are also well motivated to donate daily during the 2 to 3 week period of severe granulocytopenia (less than 200 granulocytes/μl). Straight Teflon-Silastic arteriovenous shunts are inserted into the donor's forearm under local anesthesia to permit such intensive granulocyte support from a single donor. Approximately 20 billion granulocytes daily are collected using either continuous flow centrifugation (or reversible leukoadhesion to nylon columns), irradiated, and transfused immediately into the marrow graft recipient.[6, 35]

The value of therapeutic granulocyte transfusion in treating established infections in severely granulocytopenic patients with leukemia treated by conventional chemotherapy has been clearly established in several controlled trials (see Ch. 27). The experience of the Seattle Marrow Transplant Team is consistent with a clinical benefit of granulocyte transfusions in the treatment of established infection in this specialized setting as well.[19, 24] At present, bacterial or fungal infection during the initial postgrafting period is a rare cause of patient mortality, although the precise contribution of therapeutic granulocyte transfusions to the low mortality cannot be objectively determined.

Documented bacterial or fungal infection which does not respond rapidly to appropriate antibiotic therapy in a marrow transplant recipient with fewer than 200 granulocytes/μl is now regarded as an indication for therapeutic granulocyte transfusions. Persistent high fever, unresponsive to antibacterial and antifungal therapy and without culture documentation of infection, is also an indication for therapeutic granulocyte transfusion, particularly if accompanied by clinical deterioration. Once initiated, therapeutic granulocyte transfusions are continued until the marrow graft is capable of sustaining the granulocyte count at greater than 200/μl—i.e., the granulocyte count of the patient rather than the apparent status of the infection determines the duration of granulocyte transfusion therapy.

The prophylactic transfusion of granulocytes during the period of agranulocytosis has been shown in a randomized study to be effective in the prevention of infection in marrow graft recipients.[19] Patients were assigned either to receive or not receive granulocyte transfusions when their circulating granulocyte levels fell to less than 200/μl. During the first 21 posttransplant days, there were 2 local infections and no septicemias in 29 transfused patients, compared to 7 local infections and 10 septicemias in 40 control patients. There was, however, no substantial effect of prophylactic granulocyte transfusions on patient survival. Thus, the use of prophylactic granulocyte transfusion in marrow transplantation should not be regarded as routine.

Protective Environment and Transfusion Requirement

Transfusion requirements for RBCs, platelets, and granulocytes are not entirely independent. The relationship between peripheral platelet count and gastrointestinal blood loss discussed earlier in this chapter indicates that effective platelet support is likely to decrease the amount of RBC support required. Infection can be a major cause of decreased platelet survival and hence of increased platelet transfusion requirement.[38] Furthermore, some antibiotics—e.g., semisynthetic penicillins—have been shown to increase gastrointestinal blood loss in thrombocytopenic patients.[30] Thus, effective prevention or treatment of infection by granulocyte transfusions is likely to decrease the platelet and RBC support required.

Prevention of infection by other modalities might also be expected to contribute to a decreased requirement for platelet and therapeutic granulocyte transfusions. One method to prevent infection in patients with agranulocytopenia is laminar air flow isolation with skin and intestinal decontamination. This approach was evaluated during the first 50 posttransplant days in a prospective randomized study involving 90 allogeneic marrow transplant recipients.[39] Prevention of infection was documented because patients transplanted in the protective environment had significantly fewer episodes of septicemia and major local infections than did control patients. Patients in the protective environment were given platelet transfusions on 28 percent of the "on-study" days, compared to 39 percent among those in the control group. Only 11 percent of the patients in the protective environment received therapeutic granulocyte transfusions, compared to 50 percent of the patients in the control group.

ABO-Incompatible Marrow Transplants

Marrow transplantation can be performed without difficulty between siblings who have "minor" ABO incompatibilities—i.e., recipients who are blood group A or B with donors who are blood group O. There is no apparent increase in graft-versus-host disease and no effect on patient survival.[40]

Marrow transplantation across major ABO incompatibilities—e.g., recipients who are group O with donors who are group A or B—presents a more formidable problem. First, if AB blood group antigens were present on marrow stem cells, an increased incidence of marrow graft rejection would be expected. Increased rejection, however, has as yet not been observed,[22, 40] suggesting that the A and B antigens are absent on the hematopoietic stem cell.

Marrow transplantation across major ABO incompatibilities still entails two potential risks: (1) acute hemolytic transfusion reaction at the time of marrow infusion, and (2) persistent hemolysis posttransplantation if the production of isohemagglutinins and other RBC antibodies cannot be suppressed. In order to prevent acute transfusion reactions, we have decreased antibody titers before marrow infusion by plasma and whole blood exchanges using a continuous flow centrifuge.[40] Pooled cryoprecipitate-poor plasma was utilized for most of the exchanges, with fresh frozen plasma occasionally used at the end of an exchange. Exchanges were completed by infusion of platelet-rich plasma and infusion or exchange of whole blood of donor type. Plasma and whole blood exchanges were generally performed daily for 3 days prior to marrow transplantation. Preexchange A or B antibody titers (up to 1:512 IgM and 1:2048 IgG) were eliminated in approximately one-third of the patients and reduced significantly (titers up to 1:16) in the remainder. Marrow was infused without incident or evidence of hemolysis in all patients.

Plasma and whole blood exchanges obviously impose heavy demands for both plasma and RBC support. Recently, other bone marrow transplant teams have tried to prevent acute transfusion reactions by a less costly alternative procedure involving differential centrifugation and multiple or continuous washes to eliminate or greatly reduce incompatible RBCs in the marrow graft.[41]

Posttransplantation, several patterns of antibody titer have been observed.[40] An occasional patient had no evidence of persisting antibody or antibody production after transplantation. More commonly, patients have had positive direct antiglobulin (Coombs') tests caused by IgG and/or complement sensitization without detectable circulating antibody. Most patients, however, had detectable circulating antibody and positive antiglobulin tests after transplantation, generally associated with increased RBC transfusion requirements. Hematocrits could be maintained with group O RBC without difficulty. In some patients, circulating antibody was present for 3 months after transplantation and the direct antiglobulin test was positive for even longer. In all patients, however, host type antibody production ultimately ceased as the patient's immune system and plasma cells were replaced by donor cells.

Plasma and Protein Transfusions

The conditioning regimens employed for allogeneic marrow transplantation frequently result in anorexia, nausea, vomiting, intestinal food intolerance, and severe mucositis. After transplantation, infection and graft-versus-host disease may contribute to persistence of these symptoms and in addition cause abdominal pain, profound diarrhea, and liver dysfunction. As a consequence, patients are frequently in negative caloric and nitrogen balance. Parenteral hyperalimentation, therefore, has become a standard component of the general supportive care administered to marrow transplant recipients. Since hypoalbuminemia is frequently observed in these patients, albumin infusions are commonly added empirically to the usual parenteral hyperalimentation regimen.

Allogeneic marrow recipients are profoundly immunodeficient, especially during the initial 3 to 4 months after transplantation.[42] Viral and other opportunistic infections are frequent causes of patient morbidity and mortality. Interstitial pneumonia secondary to cytomegalovirus is the single most frequent cause of death in allogeneic marrow recipients transplanted for leukemia.[36] Herpes zoster occurs in close to one-half of marrow transplant recipients within 1 year of transplantation but has rarely progressed to fatal

pneumonitis. Herpes simplex and measles virus have also resulted in fatal infections. Unfortunately, no modality for the prevention or treatment of these viral infections is of proven efficacy in marrow graft recipients. Among the approaches which have been utilized are the prophylactic or therapeutic administration of adenosine arabinoside, human leukocyte interferon,[43] and immune plasma or globulin. Immune plasma or globulin is of established value in the prevention of varicella in immunosuppressed patients, but the value of passive administration of antibody in the prevention of cytomegalovirus infection has not been established. Since the procurement of sufficient amounts of cytomegalovirus or other viral immune plasma or globulin represents a major commitment of resources, these agents should not be routinely administered until efficacy is established. Clearly, however, allogeneic marrow transplant recipients represent an ideal group in which well-designed clinical trials of the efficacy of immune plasma or globulin can be undertaken.[37]

Peripheral Blood Lymphocytes and Stem Cell Transfusions

The bone marrow alone provides an adequate source of allogeneic or syngeneic cells to result in complete repopulation of the recipient hematopoietic and lymphoid systems.[2,3,5,8,20,24,42] Even in successful transplants, however, complete reconstitution of the immune system requires many months,[20,42] and during this period the risk of opportunistic infection is great.[24,35-37] Furthermore, not all transplants result in successful engraftment, especially among patients with aplastic anemia. As discussed earlier in this chapter, donor peripheral blood cells have, therefore, recently been added to the marrow for patients with aplastic anemia. Donor buffy coat cells are obtained daily for the first 5 posttransplant days using pheresis techniques, either continuous flow centrifugation or discontinuous, differential centrifugation, and infused without irradiation.[1] The addition of buffy coat cells to the marrow has resulted in a decreased incidence of allogeneic graft rejection without any apparent increase in incidence or severity of graft-versus-host disease in patients with aplastic anemia.[1]

Transfusion of viable, nonirradiated peripheral blood lymphoid cells might accelerate the recovery of immune competence following marrow transplantation. Studies in canine marrow graft recipients have documented that normal donor lymphoid cells can be infused into stable marrow graft recipients without precipitating graft-versus-host disease.[44] Preliminary observations in man also suggest that this approach is feasible. Controlled trials will be necessary, however, to establish whether infusion of viable donor peripheral blood lymphocytes can contribute to a decrease in the morbidity or mortality of opportunistic infection in allogeneic marrow graft recipients.

CONCLUSION

In this chapter we have suggested guidelines for the transfusion support of potential marrow graft candidates before transplantation and for marrow graft recipients during the initial posttransplantation period. It is important to recognize that any transfusions given before initiation of the transplant conditioning regimen may jeopardize the cure of severe aplastic anemia by marrow transplantation. After transplantation, *all* patients will be profoundly pancytopenic for a limited period of time, and intensive transfusion support is vital to patient survival.

REFERENCES

1. Storb, R., for the Seattle Marrow Transplant Team: Decrease in the graft rejection rate and improvement in survival after marrow transplantation for severe aplastic anemia. Translant. Proc. 11:196, 1979.

2. Thomas, E.D., Sanders, J.E., Flournoy, N., Johnson, F.L., Buckner, C.D., Clift, R.A., Fefer, A., Goodell, B.W., Storb, R., and Weiden, P.L.: Marrow transplantation for patients with acute lymphoblastic leukemia in remission. Blood 54:468, 1979.

3. Thomas, E.D., Buckner, C.D., Clift, R.A., Fefer, A., Johnson, F.L., Neiman, P.E., Sale, G.E., Sanders, J.E., Singer, J.W., Shulman, H., Storb, R., and Weiden, P.L.: Marrow transplantation for patients with acute non-lymphoblastic leukemia in first remission. N. Engl. J. Med. 301:597, 1979.

4. Fefer, A., Freeman, H., Storb, R., Hill, J., Singer, J., Edwards, A., and Thomas, E.D.: Paroxysmal nocturnal hemoglobinuria and marrow failure treated by infusion of marrow from an identical twin. Ann. Intern. Med. 84:692, 1976.

5. Storb, R., Thomas, E.D., Buckner, C.D., Clift, R.A., Johnson, F.L., Fefer, A., Glucksberg, H., Giblett, E.R., Lerner, K.G., and Neiman, P.: Allogeneic marrow grafting for treatment of aplastic anemia. Blood 43:157, 1974.

6. Clift, R.A., Hansen, J.A., Thomas, E.D., Buckner, C.D., Sanders, J.E., Mickelson, E.M., Storb, R., Johnson, F.L., Singer, J.W., and Goodell, B.W.: Marrow transplantation from donors other than HLA identical siblings. Transplantation 28:235, 1979.

7. Dupont, B., O'Reilly, R.J., Pollack, M.S., and Good, R.A.: Use of HLA genotypically different donors in bone marrow transplantation. Translant. Proc. 11:219, 1979.

8. Storb, R., Thomas, E.D., Buckner, C.D., Clift, R.A., Deeg, H.J., Fefer, A., Goodell, B.W., Sale, G.E., Sanders, J.E., Singer, J., Stewart, P., and Weiden, P.L.: Marrow transplantation in thirty "untransfused" patients with severe aplastic anemia. Ann. Intern. Med., 92:30, 1980.

9. Barnes, D.W.H. and Loutit, J.F.: What is the recovery factor in spleen? Nucleonics. 12:68, 1954.

10. van Putten, L.M., van Bekkum, D.W., de Vries, M.J., and Balner, H.: The effect of preceding blood transfusions on the fate of homologous bone marrow grafts in lethally irradiated monkeys. Blood 30:749, 1967.

11. Storb, R., Floersheim, G.L., Weiden, P.L.,

Graham, T.C., Kolb, H.J., Lerner, K.G., Schroeder, M.L., and Thomas, E.D.: Effect of prior blood transfusions on marrow grafts: abrogation of sensitization by procarbazine and antithymocyte serum. J. Immunol. 112:1508, 1974.

12. Elfenbein, G.J., Anderson, P.N., Humphrey, R.L., Mullins, G.M., Sensenbrenner, L.L., Wands, J.R., and Santos, G.W.: Immune system reconstitution following allogeneic bone marrow transplantation in man: a multiparameter analysis. Transplant. Proc. 8:641, 1976.

13. Loutit, J.F. and Micklem, H.S.: Active and passive immunity to transplantation of foreign bone marrow in lethally irradiated mice. Brit. J. Exp. Path. 42:577, 1961.

14. Storb, R., Epstein, R.B., Rudolph, R.H., and Thomas, E.D.: The effect of prior transfusion on marrow grafts between histocompatible canine siblings. J. Immunol. 105:627, 1970.

15. Storb, R., Weiden, P.L., Deeg, H.J., Graham, T.C., Atkinson, K., Slichter, S.J., and Thomas, E.D.: Rejection of marrow from DLA identical canine littermates given transfusions before grafting: antigens involved are expressed on leukocytes and skin epithelial cells but not on platelets and red blood cells. Blood 54:477, 1979.

16. Miller, W.V., Schmidt, R., Luke, R.G., and Caywood, B.E.: Effect on cytotoxicity antibodies in potential transplant recipients of leucocyte-poor transfusions. Lancet i:893, 1975.

17. Torok-Storb, B.J., Storb, R., Deeg, H.J., Graham, T.C., Wise, C., Weiden, P.L., and Adamson, J.W.: Growth in vitro of donor marrow cultured with recipient lymphocytes predicts the fate of marrow grafts in transfused DLA-identical dogs. Blood 53:104, 1979.

17a. Camitta, B.M., Thomas, E.D., Nathan, D.G., Gale, R.P., Kopecky, K.J., Rappeport, J.M., Santos, G., Gordon-Smith, E.C., and Storb, R.: A prospective study of androgens and bone marrow transplantation for treatment of severe aplastic anemia. Blood 53:504, 1979.

18. Bone Marrow Transplant Registry: Bone marrow transplantation from histocompatible, allogeneic donors for aplastic anemia. J.A.M.A. 236:1131, 1976.

19. Clift, R.A., Sanders, J.E., Thomas, E.D., Williams, B., and Buckner, C.D.: Granulocyte transfusions for the prevention of infection in patients receiving bone-marrow transplants. N. Engl. J. Med. 298:1052, 1978.

20. Elfenbein, G.J., Anderson, P.N., Klein, D.L., Schacter, B.Z., and Santos, G.W.: Difficulties in predicting bone-marrow graft rejection in patients with aplastic anemia. Transplant. Proc. 10:441, 1978.

21. Gluckman, E., Devergie, A., Marty, M., Bussel, A., Rottembourg, J., Dausset, J., and Bernard, J.: Allogeneic bone marrow transplantation in aplastic anemia—report of 25 cases. Transplant. Proc. 10:141, 1978.

22. Storb, R., Prentice, R.L., and Thomas, E.D.: Marrow transplantation for treatment of aplastic anemia. An analysis of factors associated with graft rejection. N. Engl. J. Med. 296:61, 1977.

23. U.C.L.A. Bone Marrow Transplant Team: Bone-marrow transplantation in severe aplastic anaemia. Lancet ii:921, 1976.

24. Thomas, E.D., Storb, R., Clift, R.A., Fefer, A., Johnson, F.L., Neiman, P.E., Lerner, K.G., Glucksberg, H., and Buckner, C.D.: Bone-marrow transplantation. N. Engl. J. Med. 292:832 and 895, 1975.

25. Gale, R.P., Fitchen, J.H., Cahan, M., Opelz, G., and Cline, M.J.: Pretransplant lymphocytotoxins and bone-marrow graft rejection. Lancet i:170, 1978.

26. Gluckman, E.: Pretransplant lymphocytotoxins and bone-marrow graft rejection. Lancet i:443, 1978.

27. Storb, R., Hansen, J.A., Weiden, P.L., Clift, R.A., and Thomas, E.D.: Pretransplant lymphocytotoxins do not predict bone marrow graft rejection. Transplantation 26:423, 1978.

27a. Parkman, R., Rosen, F.S., Rappeport, J., Camitta, B., Levey, R.L., and Nathan, D.G.: Detection of genetically determined histocompatibility antigen differences between HL-A identical and MLC nonreactive siblings. Transplantation 21:110, 1976.

28. Storb, R., Epstein, R.B., Ragde, H., Bryant, J., and Thomas, E.D.: Marrow engraftment by allogeneic leukocytes in lethally irradiated dogs. Blood 30:805, 1967.

29. Storb, R., Graham, T.C., Epstein, R.B., Sale, G.E., and Thomas, E.D.: Demonstration of hemopoietic stem cells in the peripheral blood of baboons by cross circulation. Blood 50:537, 1977.

30. Slichter, S.J. and Harker, L.A.: Clinics in

Haematology. Thrombocytopenia: mechanisms and management of defects in platelet production. 7:523, 1978.

31. Solomon, J., Bofenkamp, T., Fahey, J.L., Chillar, R.K., and Beutler, E.: Platelet prophylaxis in acute non-lymphoblastic leukemia. Lancet i:267 and 278, 1978.

32. Mathé, G.: Réduction par l'azathioprine de l'inhibition de la greffe de moelle osseuse allogénique par des transfusions sanguines antérieures. Rev. Franc. Études Clin. et Biol. 11:1026, 1966.

33. Blume, K.G.: Unpublished observations.

33a. Slichter, S.J. and Harker, L.A.: Preparation and storage of platelet concentrates. I. Factors influencing the harvest of viable platelets from whole blood. Br. J. Haematol. 34:395, 1976.

34. Weiden, P.L., Slichter, S.J., and Banaji, M.: Marrow transplantation for aplastic anemia and leukemia—review of results and blood product support required. In: The Blood Platelet in Transfusion Therapy. Greenwalt, T.J., and Jamieson, G.A., eds. Alan R. Liss, Inc., New York, 1978, p. 295.

34a. Meyers, J.D., Huff, J.C., Holmes, K.K. Thomas, E.D., and Bryan, J.A.: Parenterally transmitted hepatitis A associated with platelet transfusions. Epidemiologic study of an outbreak in a marrow transplantation center. Ann. Intern. Med. 81:145, 1974.

35. Clift, R.A., Buckner, C.D., Fefer, A., Lerner, K.G., Neiman, P.E., Storb, R., Murphy, M., and Thomas, E.D.: Infectious complications of marrow transplantation. Transplant. Proc. 6:389, 1974.

36. Neiman, P.E., Reeves, W., Ray, G., Flournoy, N., Lerner, K.G., Sale, G.E., and Thomas, E.D.: A prospective analysis of interstitial pneumonia and opportunistic viral infection among recipients of allogeneic bone marrow grafts. J. Infect. Dis. 136:754, 1977.

37. Young, L.S. and Jordan, M.C.: Infection in marrow transplantation: problems and perspectives. Transplant. Proc. 10:259, 1978.

38. Harker, L.A. and Slichter, S.J.: Platelet and fibrinogen consumption in man. N. Engl. J. Med. 287:999, 1972.

39. Buckner, C.D., Clift, R.A., Sanders, J.E., Meyers, J.D., Counts, G.W., Farewell, V.T., Thomas, E.D., and the Seattle Marrow Transplant Team: Protective environment for marrow transplant recipients. A prospective study. Ann. Intern. Med. 89:893, 1978.

40. Buckner, C.D., Clift, R.A., Sanders, J.E., Williams, B., Gray, M., Storb, R., and Thomas, E.D.: ABO-incompatible marrow transplants. Transplantation 26:233, 1978.

41. Braine, H.G., Sensenbrenner, L.L., and The Bone Marrow Transplant Team: RBC incompatible bone marrow transplants. Exp. Hematol. 6(Suppl. 3):9 (Abstract), 1978.

42. Noel, D.R., Witherspoon, R.P., Storb, R., Atkinson, K., Doney, K., Mickelson, E.M., Ochs, H.D., Warren, R.P., Weiden, P.L., and Thomas, E.D.: Does graft-versus-host disease influence the tempo of immunologic recovery after allogeneic human marrow transplantation? An observation on 56 long-term survivors. Blood 51:1087, 1978.

43. O'Reilly, R.J., Everson, L.K., Emodi, G., Hansen, J., Smithwick, E.M., Grimes, E., Pahwa, S., Pahwa, R., Schwartz, S., Armstrong, D., Siegal, F.P., Gupta, S., Dupont, B., and Good, R.A.: Effects of exogenous interferon in cytomegalovirus infections complicating bone marrow transplantation. Clin. Immunol. Immunopathol. 6:51, 1976.

44. Weiden, P.L., Storb, R., Tsoi, M.S., Graham, T.C., Lerner, K.G., and Thomas, E.D.: Infusion of donor lymphocytes into stable canine radiation chimeras: implications for mechanism of transplantation tolerance. J. Immunol. 116:1212, 1976.

ACKNOWLEDGMENT

This work was supported by Grant Numbers CA 18221, CA 18029, CA 15704, and CA 18047 awarded by the National Cancer Institute, U.S. Department of Health, Education and Welfare.

29

Transfusion of Patients with End-Stage Renal Disease

Herbert A. Perkins, M.D.

Anemia is an inevitable and often severe complication of chronic renal failure. When uremia is severe, red cell production in the marrow is depressed, and the survival of cells in the peripheral blood is shortened. Each hemodialysis loses a small amount of blood, which inevitably is left in the extracorporeal circuit at the end of the treatment, and accidental leaks from the circuit can result in larger losses. Uremia causes defective platelet plug formation, which can result in spontaneous bleeding. Repeated loss of red blood cells can lead to iron deficiency. Hypersplenism is occasionally an additional recognized complication.

The degree of anemia is often severe enough to limit patient activity and occasionally great enough to be life-threatening. Treatment with iron can correct iron deficiency, and splenectomy will cure hypersplenism. Androgens may result in a small but significant increase in the hematocrit. In many cases, however, the only effective therapy is red cell transfusions, and these were formerly prescribed with little hesitation. Repeated red cell transfusions may have two types of undesired effects. Allosensitization may occur to the various foreign constituents of the donor blood, and chill-fever reactions caused by antibodies to donor leukocytes are especially common. Many of these patients are candidates for renal transplantation, and prior transfusions may have a marked effect on the possibility of a successful graft.

LEUKOCYTE ANTIBODIES

The importance of antibodies to leukocytes has been recognized since the studies of Dausset[1] in the 1950s. Payne[2] and others confirmed that these were alloantibodies induced by blood transfusion. Subsequently, similar antibodies were shown to result from pregnancy[3,4] and from skin grafting and organ transplantation. Since leukocytes had been shown to induce allograft sensitization in rabbits,[5] recognition that the human leukocyte antigens might be shared by other tissues and could be of critical importance in tissue grafting came early.[6] Patients with chronic uremia have evidence of impaired immune responses, but their ability to form antibodies to transfused leukocyte antigens is not obviously reduced.[7]

Many centers quickly recognized the correlation between antibodies to leukocytes and the occurrence of febrile nonhemolytic transfusion reactions in recipients of blood. The cause and effect relationship was demonstrated when red cells rendered leukocyte-poor were shown to minimize or eliminate the reactions.

HLA SYSTEM

Investigation of the specificity of the antibodies and inheritance of the leukocyte antigens led to definition of the HLA histocompatibility system (see Ch. 6). The HLA antigens were shown to be shared by most cells of the body, and HLA typing of organ transplant donors and recipients established the HLA system as the major histocompatibility system in man. In early studies, HLA typing was performed by an agglutination technique using mixed leukocytes (primarily granulocytes) from the peripheral blood as the target. More recently, a cytotoxic technique with lymphocytes as the target cells has become standard.

TRANSFUSION AND GRAFTING

In the previous chapter on bone marrow transplantation, it was pointed out that transfusion of blood components prior to marrow transplantation has a potential only to increase the possibility of graft rejection. The more transfusions given, the higher the probability of an unsuccessful result. Early studies in renal transplantation resulted in similar conclusions. More recently, however, it has been clearly established that transfusions prior to renal transplantation can have a second effect, completely opposite to the first: they may result in improved renal graft survival. This discussion will be limited to kidney transplantation, but it is probable that all of the comments to be made apply equally well to all solid organ grafts. In fact, one of the earliest bits of evidence that prior transfusions might enhance survival of solid organ grafts came from the recognition that patients who had had previous open heart surgery had a better prognosis for survival of a cardiac allograft.[8]

Lymphocytotoxic Crossmatch

Blood transfusions given to patients with end-stage renal disease stimulate production of lymphocytotoxic alloantibodies; the more transfusions given, the larger the number of patients with detectable antibodies and the larger the proportion of random cells with which the patients' sera react.[7] If the serum of a potential graft recipient contains cytotoxic antibodies reacting with the lymphocytes of the intended kidney donor, hyperacute rejection of the graft is an almost inevitable result.[9,10] In the small proportion of cases with positive crossmatches where graft failure did not occur, the lymphocytotoxic antibodies presumably reacted with antigens other than products of the HLA-A and B loci. They may have been antibodies reacting primarily in the cold, autoantibodies, or antibodies to only the B lymphocytes of the donor (see below).

In any case, the very frequent occurrence of early rejection when the patient's serum was cytotoxic to the donor's lymphocytes led to routine adoption of a lymphocytotoxic crossmatch test prior to transplantation. A positive crossmatch is now accepted as a contraindication to renal transplantation. Antibodies may become undetectable in a patient's serum in time if they are not restimulated, but it has been shown that rejection is likely if the crossmatch with an earlier serum is positive, even though the current serum has no demonstrable in vitro effect. This further increases the chance of contraindication to transplantation.

Many patients with end-stage renal disease have produced a large variety of antibodies to random lymphocytes. It may become very difficult, if not impossible, to find an unrelated kidney donor whose cells are crossmatch-compatible. Most patients waiting for a kidney transplant are dependent on unrelated cadaver donors, since they do not have a possible donor who is an immediate relative. Since transfusions may result in an incompatible crossmatch with unrelated kidney donor cells, and since the more transfusions given the more likely it is that a compatible kidney will never be found, nephrologists recognized that they should avoid or limit transfusions to patients waiting for a kidney transplant.

Antibodies to Random Cells but with Negative Crossmatch

Further argument for limiting blood component transfusions derived from reports from many centers[11,12] which showed a poorer rate of graft survival in patients who had formed lymphocytotoxic antibodies to the cells of random individuals even though the crossmatch with the cells of the intended kidney donor was nonreactive. These same studies showed even worse graft survival in those patients whose antibodies reacted with the cells of the majority of random individuals. In contrast to the situation with a positive crossmatch, the effect of antibodies to random cells is more controversial, and there is much disagreement about explanations for the phenomenon. A number of centers, including our own,[13–15] do not find graft survival impaired in patients with antibodies to random cells if the crossmatch is negative. In fact, we find somewhat superior graft survival in those patients whose antibodies react with a majority of random cells.

We have offered the following hypothetical explanation: Patients may vary in their ability to be sensitized by specific HLA antigens, presumably because of their different immune response (Ir) genes. If they receive multiple transfusions, they are exposed to most HLA antigens to which they easily respond. They will not be transplanted with kidneys containing those antigens because the crossmatch test will be positive. If a negative crossmatch is obtained, one could assume that the donor kidney contains antigens to which the patient does not readily respond and that the chance for graft survival will be better than average.

How can one account for the discrepant findings which show in some studies that antibodies to random cells impair graft prognosis and in other studies that they do not? Patients who form antibodies to random cells are more likely to have formed antibodies to donor cells, and the latter may be missed by an insensitive crossmatch technique. Evidence favoring this explanation comes from two sources. Fuller has published data[16] showing that antibodies to random cells impaired graft prognosis in earlier studies, but that they no longer did so when a more sensitive crossmatch technique was adopted. Terasaki, who has presented the most convincing evidence that antibodies to random cells impair graft prognosis,[11] assembled his data from multiple centers, with presumably variable efficiency in their crossmatch techniques. More recently, he reported that the detrimental effect of antibodies to random cells is less evident than it was in earlier years.[17]

At the time Terasaki published his original data on the effect of antibodies to random cells, he speculated that patients who make antibodies after transfusion are hyperresponders who may also be more likely to respond to the graft. Nothing stated above eliminates this as an additional possibility.

TRANSFUSION POLICY

Whether or not antibodies to random cells impair graft prognosis, the possibility of inducing antibodies to all potential kidney donor cells is sufficient grounds for the general policy which was adopted approximately 10 years ago: Patients waiting for a kidney transplant were not transfused unless absolutely necessary. In many centers, when transfusions were mandatory, the red cells were given as deglycerolized, previously frozen red cells. The assumption was that frozen-stored red cells were contaminated by few, if any, white cells and would be less likely to induce leukocyte antibodies. At the time this remained to be proven, but subsequent reports have confirmed that, the fewer the leukocytes in a red cell component, the less likely the formation of alloantibodies to white cells.

Leukocyte-Poor Blood

Red blood cells may be deprived of their leukocytes in a variety of ways, all of which remove platelets even more efficiently. The term "leukocyte-poor red cells" refers most commonly to products from which the white cells have been separated by centrifugation and removal of the buffy coat, but these may be prepared also by filtration of heparinized blood through nylon fiber columns. Alternatively, washed red cells may be used, provided that the buffy coat is removed at each wash. Frozen-stored red cells are rendered leukocyte-poor because the thawed cells must be washed free of the cryoprotective agent glycerol and many, if not all, of the white cells have been killed by freezing conditions which are not optimal for their survival. The Huggins technique for deglycerolizing red blood cells agglomerates the red cells at low ionic strength and settles them by gravity.[18] The Meryman technique uses a centrifuge and freezing solutions of normal ionic strength.[19] The Huggins product has more leukocytes, but none of these appears viable; white cells can be cultured from the red cells deglycerolized by the Meryman technique.

The number of white cells contaminating the final red cell concentrate can thus vary widely (Fig. 29-1) from nearly 5 billion to less than 10 million, and their immunogenicity may vary according to conditions of storage. Transfusion of leukocyte-poor red blood cells prepared by differential centrifugation results in fewer immunized recipients than transfu-

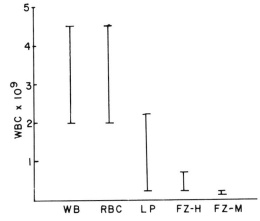

Fig. 29.1. Range of leukocyte numbers contained in various red blood cell components. Wb = whole blood; RBC = concentrated red cells; LP = leukocyte-poor red cells prepared by centrifugation and removal of the buffy coat. FZ = frozen red cells; H = Huggins cytoglomerator technique; M = Meryman centrifuge technique.

sion of whole blood or red cell concentrates which retain the buffy coat (Table 29-1).[20,21] Leukocyte-poor red cells also have less tendency to sensitize a recipient to reject the donor's skin graft.[22] Moreover, the antibodies resulting from leukocyte-poor red cells are more likely to be limited in the proportion of random cells with which they react. On the other hand, the more leukocyte-poor units transfused, the more antibodies stimulated, and recipients of leukocyte-poor red cells only may be eventually be immunized in a proportion indistinguishable from recipients of components with the buffy coat (Table 29-1).[23]

Frozen-stored red cells are even less likely to stimulate production of antibodies to leukocytes[24] (Table 29-1), whether deglycerolized by agglomeration or by centrifugation. The cytoglomerator product is less immunogenic than red cells prepared by differential centrifugation, even though the degree of leukocyte contamination is similar (Table 29-1). Leukocytes are killed under the unfavorable freezing conditions of the low-ionic-strength agglomeration technique and may

Table 29-1. Lymphocytotoxic Antibodies in Relation to Specific Red Cell Components Transfused (San Francisco Data)

Date of Analysis	Total No. of Cases	Any WB	WB Only	LP Only	FZ Only	No Transfusions
1975	246	10/46 (22%)		5/55 (9%)	3/39 (8%)	2/106 (2%)
1977	369	17/107(16%)		5/56 (9%)	2/41 (5%)	10/165 (6%)
1979	409	84/179(46%)	31/65(48%)	18/41(44%)	6/33(18%)	33/154(21%)

Analysis restricted to patients with no antibody on entrance to study.
WB = whole blood or red cells with buffy coat
LP = leukocyte-poor red cells prepared by differential centrifugation
FZ = frozen red cells prepared by cytoglomerator technique

Note progressive increase in patients who developed antibody as more of them remained on prolonged dialysis. Cytotoxic antibodies appeared even in the absence of transfusion.

then be less immunogenic. The data in Table 29-1 show that, in our experience, frozen-stored red cells did not result in a significant increase in detectable antibodies to leukocytes compared with patients who had not been transfused.

On the basis of the above evidence, it is reasonable to conclude that induction of lymphocytotoxic alloantibodies will be greatest in recipients of red cell components containing the buffy coat, less in recipients of leukocyte-poor red cells, and least in recipients of frozen red cells. These findings supported the practice of transfusing a leukocyte-poor red cell product into patients awaiting a renal transplant whenever it was impossible to avoid transfusion altogether.

Effects of Transfusion on Renal Graft Survival

The decision to avoid transfusing these patients whenever possible had unexpected consequences. Renal allograft survival became progressively worse from one year to the next,[17] and sharply lower one-year graft survival[25] became apparent in contrast to the usual improvement in clinical results as experience increases. This decrease in graft survival was not clearly obvious for years. There is no direct proof that it is the result of changing transfusion practices, but no alternative explanation can be offered.

Although there were several earlier reports suggesting that patients who had never been transfused had a worse prognosis for graft survival, it was not until the report of Opelz and Terasaki in *Lancet* in 1974[26] that widespread serious attention was paid to the possibility that blood transfusions prior to transplantation might in some way exert a protective effect on the graft, provided that they did not induce formation of cytotoxic antibodies reacting with the cells of the kidney donor.

In their *Lancet* report, Opelz and Terasaki noted a strikingly poor one-year cadaver graft survival of 32 percent in patients who had never been transfused. Patients who received frozen red cells had equally bad results. Opelz and Terasaki repeated their analyses a number of times on sequential series of transplants.[27-29] Each time, those patients who were never transfused had very poor graft survival. In later studies, frozen-stored red cells had an effect on graft survival intermediate between other red cell components and no transfusions. Leukocyte-poor red cells were not distinguished in these studies from standard packed cells or whole blood, but a previous paper indicates that over 90 percent of the red cells transfused by the centers in the study were in the form of leukocyte-poor red cells.[30]

The poor graft survival in patients who have never been transfused has been confirmed in so many laboratories that it would be impossible to cite them individually.[31] In most centers, blood transfusions have resulted in improved survival of subsequent renal allografts. The effect of transfusion is less obvious when a related kidney donor is used, probably because related grafts have superior survival.

Prior pregnancies probably have a similar, but less obvious, protective effect.[29,32,33] In a preliminary analysis of data at this center,[34] graft survival was improved in patients with a prior history of pregnancy. As more data have been collected, the protective effect of prior pregnancies has become less obvious. In most patients, the possible protective effect of prior pregnancies is obscured by blood transfusions.

The majority of reports indicate that graft survival progressively improves, the larger the number of prior transfusions[29] (Fig. 29-2). This quantitative effect is not apparent in all studies, however.[35-40] Persijn et al.[39] and our own results indicate that a single unit of blood provides as much protection as multiple units. In any case, it seems evident that a single prior transfusion results in a measurable increase in graft survival. The greater protective effect of larger numbers of transfusions is balanced by the tendency of the larger numbers to induce multiple cytotoxic antibodies which may prevent transplantation. Solheim[37] indicates that, if patients who die on dialysis while waiting for a transplant are included in the equation, no overall benefit can be attributed to prior transfusion.

The type of blood administered prior to transplantation is not usually taken into account in most reports. Many of them indicate that the vast majority of transfusions were with leukocyte-poor red cells. This may indicate that leukocyte-poor red cells are fully protective, but the good responses may result from occasional transfusion of red cells containing the buffy coat. At this center, those patients who have received all of their transfusions in the form of leukocyte-poor red cells have had graft survival in the same range as those who received only components containing the buffy coat or a mixture of the two.

The protective effect of leukocyte-poor red cells on the subsequent survival of human renal allografts is consistent with data obtained on the dog in which leukocyte-poor red cells resulted in marked prolongation of kidney allograft survival.[41]

Effect of Frozen-stored Red Cells

The effect of frozen-stored red cells is more controversial. As outlined above, Terasaki's studies have consistently shown that graft survival is less good when recipients have received frozen-stored red cells only, compared with those receiving leukocyte-poor or standard packed cells. The data of Briggs et al.[40] and in our center are in agreement with this finding. In contrast, Polesky[42] and Fuller[24] find graft survival in patients who have received only frozen-stored red cells to be equal or superior to that in recipients of components containing the buffy coat. Polesky's frozen-stored red cells were prepared by the Meryman technique. Fuller reports better graft survival when the frozen red cells were deglycerolized by the Huggins technique than by the Meryman technique. It may well be that red cell components have a parallel effect in their ability to induce formation of the unwanted cytotoxic antibodies and in their desired effect of inducing better graft survival.

Timing of Transfusions

Most studies have analyzed the protective effect of prior transfusions without consideration of when they were given within the lifetime of the patient. As will be discussed below, animal experiments suggest that the timing of transfusions could be of considerable importance. If given too shortly before transplantation, they may have no effect; if given too long before transplantation, their effect may wear off. Stiller et al.[43] reported

Fig. 29-2. Actuarial graft survival rates in recipients of first cadaver-kidney transplants separated by the number of pretransplant blood transfusions that the recipients had received. The number of blood units transfused is indicated at the end of each curve. All types of blood products (whole, packed, or frozen) were included. Numbers of patients in each subset are given in parentheses. Statistical significance was calculated by weighted regression analysis. (Opelz, G. and Terasaki, P.I.: Improvement of kidney-graft survival with increased numbers of blood transfusions. Reprinted by permission N. Engl. J. Med. 299:799, 1978.)

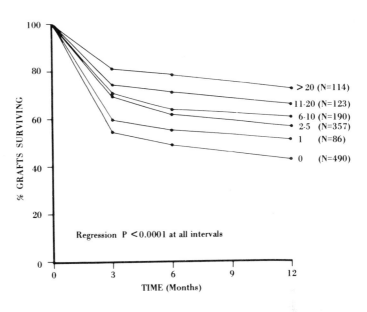

that transfusions given at the time of transplantation also have some protective effect, but this is not apparent in all studies.[29] Buy-Quang et al.[33] analyzed the timing of transfusions given prior to transplantation and found (as would be expected from the animal data) that transfusions are more protective of the graft when administered within 6 months prior to surgery. Opelz reported a similar analysis at the 1979 meeting of the American Association for Clinical Histocompatibility Testing but was unable to find a significant correlation with the time at which transfusions were given.

MECHANISM OF PROTECTIVE EFFECT OF TRANSFUSIONS

The mechanism by which prior transfusions protect the graft is not known, but numerous hypotheses have emerged from the human data and animal studies. Many of the studies have been done in rats, an animal in which hyperacute rejection of an organ graft does not occur. Animal studies have shown protection from whole blood, lymphocytes, and plasma or serum.

Enhancing Antibody

A favored explanation is that transfusion may induce, in addition to the dangerous cytotoxic antibodies, antibodies or resulting antigen-antibody complexes which can protect the graft. In animals, graft protection can be induced by passive transfusion of serum obtained from recipient strain animals sensitized by donor strain antigens. Moreover, active enhancement of the graft can be induced by active immunization of the recipient with donor strain antigens. In some instances, of course, these procedures accelerate rejection, depending on the type of antibody formed. The timing of active immunization for protection is critical. Active enhancement is difficult to demonstrate until 1 to 2 weeks after the initial antigen stimulus[44] and may wear off rapidly.[45]

The exact target of the enhancing antibodies is not established, but the two favorite theories are (1) that they are directed against antigens on B lymphocytes and (2) that they are autoantibodies directed against the antigen-combining sites of cell receptors or antibodies specific for the donor antigens (anti-idiotypes).

Cellular Immunity

There is clear evidence that serum antibodies can interfere with the in vitro expression of cellular immunity. They can block mixed lymphocyte reaction (MLR) responses.[46] Of course, lymphocytotoxic antibodies can do this by killing the stimulator or responder cells in the MLR, but antibodies to B lymphocytes block MLR by reacting only with stimulator cells. The role of antibodies to B lymphocytes in human renal transplantation is controversial, although it does seem clear that matching donor and recipient for the DRw B lymphocyte antigens of the HLA region results in superior graft survival.[47-50] Despite this, a positive lymphocytotoxic crossmatch to donor B cells may have no effect on graft survival.[51] Terasaki has shown that human antibodies to B cells fall into two classes: those which react best at body temperature and are directed primarily against DRw antigens, and those which react best in the cold and are usually autoantibodies. He finds that graft survival is impaired in those recipients who have antibodies reacting in the warm temperature region with a panel of B cells, whereas those with antibodies which react best in the cold with B cells have a better-than-average graft survival.[52] He proposes that the cold-reacting antibodies to B cells may be the graft-enhancing antibodies.

Anti-idiotype Antibodies

The possiblility that anti-idiotype antibodies might explain the improved graft survival has been suggested by Binz and Wigzell.[53] They have clearly shown that anti-idiotype antibodies can protect animals. Their anti-idiotype antibodies, however, were induced by a highly artificial system. No evidence has been presented that successful grafts in humans are associated with anti-idiotypic antibodies.

Tolerance

The phenomenon of tolerance, defined as deletion of the clones committed to react against graft antigens, does not appear to be a likely explanation for the improved graft survival of renal allografts after blood transfusion. Animals so protected still show pathological evidence of cellular infiltration, indicating that the host does recognize the graft as foreign. Moreover, the same animals will still reject a skin graft from the donor.[54]

Effects of Red Cells

The enhancing effects of frozen-stored red cells at some centers have led to speculation that red cells per se might be responsible for the effect. Van Es and Balner have used Rhesus monkeys to confirm the protective effect of prior blood transfusions in a highly standardized prospective study.[45] They then transfused red cells which had been totally deprived of leukocytes by passage through tightly packed cotton fiber filters.[31] These leukocyte-free transfusions were still protective. Theoretical support for a protective effect of red cells was offered by Keown and Descamps,[55] who showed that damaged red cells were engulfed by macrophages in the reticuloendothelial system, with resulting impairment of the immune response of bystander lymphocytes. Presumably, the lymphocytes were no longer able to obtain the cooperation of the neighboring macrophages. Further in vitro studies indicated that cellular responses could be impaired by free hemoglobin or even by ferric hydroxide.

Unfortunately for this theory, van Rood transplanted seven patients who had been transfused with cotton fiber-filtered blood only (in the same manner as Balner's monkeys), and six of the recipients lost their grafts by early rejection.[56] Van Rood concluded that the protective effect of transfusions required the equivalent of 50 ml of whole blood. This would be in the range of leukocytes supplied by a unit of leukocyte-poor red cells.

Suppressor T Lymphocytes

Still another hypothesis which would not require an antigen-specific effect of prior transfusions is that transfusions may nonspecifically stimulate production of suppressor T lymphocytes.[57] In a few isolated instances, patients have been shown to produce suppressor cells which inhibit mixed lymphocyte reaction responses.[58] However, there is no evidence that this suppressor effect correlates with graft enhancement by transfusion.

Specificity

It is still not at all clear whether the enhancing effect of transfusions is specific (i.e., directed against donor antigens) or nonspecific. The human data are based almost entirely on the transfusion of blood from donors unrelated to the kidney donor. Protective effect of a single or limited number of transfusions argues for nonspecificity, unless the response is to very common antigens not yet identified. On the other hand, the majority of animal experience with graft enhancement by transfusion has employed transfusions from the kidney donor strain. Little effort has been made in humans to see whether donor-specific blood would have a greater enhancing potential, largely because of the fear of inducing antibodies which will accelerate graft rejection.

Newton and Anderson[59] injected four potential kidney allograft recipients with lymphocytes from the kidney donor. None rejected the graft. This approach has been further followed at the University of California in San Francisco by Cochrum et al.,[60] coupled with careful testing of serial recipient samples for the appearance of antidonor antibodies against T cells and B cells at 4°C, room temperature, and 37°C. Eighteen recipients have thus far been transfused with 200 ml of donor blood on three occasions at 2-week intervals. All recipients had family donors who differed for one HLA haplotype, and all had a relatively high MLR response with donor lymphocytes indicating a relatively poor prognosis for graft survival.[61] Of the 18 recipients, four formed cytotoxic antibodies against donor T cells which contraindicated the transplant. Six of the others have been transplanted. Only two had recognized mild rejection crises which were easily reversible. All six grafts are functioning well at periods up to 1 year.

RECOMMENDATIONS

On the basis of the above findings, what recommendation can be made at this time in regard to the deliberate transfusion of patients who are waiting for a kidney transplant? It seems clear that patients who have never been transfused have a very bad prognosis for graft survival. Therefore, it does not seem in the patient's best interest to transplant if he has had no prior blood transfusions. At the very least, the strict program of withholding transfusions could be relaxed somewhat to obtain a more comfortable life for patients on chronic dialysis. On the other hand, the more transfusions given, the more likely the patient will form cytotoxic antibodies which will prevent transplantation. The ideal number of pretransplant transfusions cannot be stated at the present time, but it could be in the range of two or three. Minimal evidence suggests that these are best given more than 2 weeks but less than 6 months prior to transplantation. If more than 6 months has elapsed and the patient is still waiting for a transplant, some centers would give one further transfusion.

The type of red cell component to be transfused is more debatable. Fuller[24] and

Polesky[42] recommend frozen-stored red cells, arguing that they are fully protective but have less likelihood of inducing cytotoxic antibodies. Whether they are fully protective is controversial, and more centers use leukocyte-poor red cells, which do appear to be fully protective and do have a lesser tendency to induce cytotoxic antibody formation than components with the buffy coat. The latter should probably never be transfused into patients waiting for a renal transplant except in uncontrollable emergencies.

A reasonable compromise which is consistent with current information would be to transfuse 2 or 3 units of leukocyte-poor red cells into patients who have never received prior transfusions. For those patients who require a larger number of transfusions because of medical indications, the subsequent use of frozen-stored red cells would be appropriate. Transfusion of blood from the intended kidney donor should be considered strictly experimental at the present time.

These recommendations are made with the knowledge that many controversies remain in this field and that new information, which is accumulating at a rapid rate, may well require them to be changed.

REFERENCES

1. Dausset, J.: Leuco-agglutinins. IV. Leuco-agglutinins and blood transfusion. Vox Sang. 4:190, 1957.
2. Payne, R.: Leukocyte agglutinins in human sera. Arch. Intern. Med. 99:587, 1957.
3. Payne, R. and Rolfs, M.R.: Fetomaternal leukocyte incompatibility. J. Clin. Invest. 37:1756, 1958.
4. Van Rood, J.J., van Leeuwen, A., and Eernisse, J.G.: Leucocyte antibodies in sera of pregnant women. Vox Sang. 4:427, 1959.
5. Medawar, P.B.: Immunity to homologous grafted skin. II. The relationship between the antigens of blood and skin. Br. J. Exper. Pathol. 27:15, 1946.
6. Van Rood, J.J., van Leeuwen, A., Eernisse, J.G., Frederiks, E., and Bosch, L.J.: Relation-

ship of leukocyte groups to tissue transplantation compatibility. Ann. N.Y. Acad. Sci. 120:285, 1964.
7. Perkins, H.A., Howell, E., Gantan, Z., Mims, M.C., Dickerson, T., and Senecal, I.: Variation in cytotoxic antibody response to transfusion in prospective renal allograft recipients. Transplantation 17:216, 1974.
8. Dong, E., Jr., Griepp, R.B., Stinson, E.B., and Shumway, N.E.: Review of four years experience with clinical heart transplantation at Stanford University Medical Center. Transplant. Proc. 4:787, 1972.
9. Kissmeyer-Nielsen, F., Olsen, S., Petersen, V.P., and Fjeldborg, O.: Hyperacute rejection of kidney allografts, associated with pre-existing humoral antibodies against donor cells. Lancet 2:662, 1966.
10. Patel, R. and Terasaki, P.I.: Significance of the positive crossmatch test in kidney transplantation. N. Engl. J. Med. 280:735, 1969.
11. Terasaki, P.I., Kreisler, M., and Mickey, R.M.: Presensitization and kidney transplant failures. Postgrad. Med. J. 47:89, 1971.
12. Van Hooff, J.P., Schippers, H.M.A., van der Steen, G.J., and van Rood, J.J.: Efficacy of HL-A matching in Eurotransplant. Lancet 2:1385, 1972.
13. Belzer, F.O., Salvatierra, O., Jr., Cochrum, K.C., and Perkins, H.A.: Good kidney graft survival in hyperimmunized patients. Transplant. Proc. 7 (suppl. 1):71, 1975.
14. Salvatierra, O., Perkins, H.A., Amend, W., Jr., Feduska, N.J., Duca, R.M., Porter, D.E., and Cochrum, K.C.: The influence of pre-sensitization on graft survival rate. Surgery 81:146, 1977.
15. Ferguson, R.M., Simmons, R.L., Noreen, H., Yunis, E.J., and Najarian, J.S.: Host presensitization and renal allograft success at a single institution: First transplants. Surgery 81:139, 1977.
16. Fuller, T.C., Cosimi, A.B., and Russell, P.S.: Use of an antiglobulin-ATG reagent for detection of low levels of alloantibody: Improvement in renal allograft survival in presensitized recipients. Transplant. Proc. 10:463, 1978.
17. Terasaki, P.I., Opelz, G., and Mickey, M.R.: Analysis of yearly kidney transplant survival rates. Transplant. Proc. 8:139, 1976.
18. Huggins, C.E.: Frozen blood: Principles of

practical preservation. Monogr. Surg. Sci. 3:133, 1966.

19. Meryman, H.T. and Hornblower, M.: A method for freezing and washing red blood cells using a high glycerol concentration. Transfusion 12:145, 1972.

20. Caseley, J., Moses, V.K., Lichter, E.A., and Jonasson, O.: Isoimmunization of hemodialysis patients: Leukocyte-poor versus whole blood transfusions. Transplant. Proc. 3:365, 1971.

21. Miller, W.V., Schmidt, R., Luke, R.G., and Caywood, B.E.: Effect on cytotoxicity antibodies in potential transplant recipients of leukocyte-poor blood transfusions. Lancet 1:893, 1975.

22. Hattler, B.G., Jr., Miller, J., and Amos, D.B.: Antibody and allograft reactivity following administration of blood. Surg. Forum 23:284, 1972.

23. Suarez-Ch., R. and Jonasson, O.: Isoimmunization of potential kidney transplant recipients: General frequency and some associated factors. Transplant. Proc. 4:577, 1972.

24. Fuller, T.C., Delmonico, F.L., Cosimi, A.B., Huggins, C.E., King, M., and Russell, P.S.: Impact of blood transfusion on renal transplantation. Ann. Surg. 187:211, 1978.

25. Van Hooff, J.P., Kalff, M.W., Poelgeest, A.E., Persijn, G.G., and van Rood, J.J.: Blood transfusions and kidney transplantation. Transplantation 22:306, 1976.

26. Opelz, G. and Terasaki, P.I.: Poor kidney-transplant survival in recipients with frozen-blood transfusions or no transfusions. Lancet 2:696, 1974.

27. Opelz, G. and Terasaki, P.I.: Prolongation effect of blood transfusions on kidney graft survival. Transplantation 22:380, 1976.

28. Opelz, G. and Terasaki, P.I.: Enhancement of kidney graft survival by blood transfusions. Transplant. Proc. 9:121, 1977.

29. Opelz, G. and Terasaki, P.I.: Improvement of kidney-graft survival with increased numbers of blood transfusions. N. Engl. J. Med. 299:799, 1978.

30. Opelz, G., Mickey, M.R., and Terasaki, P.I.: Blood transfusions and unresponsiveness to HL-A. Transplantation 16:649, 1973.

31. van Es, A.A. and Balner, H.: Effect of pretransplant transfusions on kidney allograft survival. Transplant. Proc. 11:127, 1979.

32. Tiilikainen, A., Kock, B., Kuhlbäck, B., and Wallenius, M.: Transfusions and kidney graft survival in Finland. Scand. J. Urol. Nephrol. suppl. 42:70, 1977.

33. Buy-Quang, D., Soulillou, J.-P., Fontenaille, C.H., Guimbretière, J., and Guenel, J.: Rôle bénéfiques des transfusions sanguines et des grossesses dan la survie des allogreffes rénales. Nouv. Presse Méd. 6:3503, 1977.

34. Perkins, H.A. and Salvatierra, O.: Correlation of renal allograft survival with previous blood transfusions. Transplant. Proc. 9 (suppl. 1):209, 1977.

35. Murray, S., Dewar, P.I., Uldall, P.R., Wilkinson, R., Kerr, D.N.S., Taylor, R.M.R., and Swinney, J.: Some important factors in cadaver-donor kidney transplantation. Tissue Antigens 4:548, 1974.

36. Husberg, B., Lindergård, B., Lindholm, T., and Löw, B.: Blood transfusion and kidney transplantation. Scand. J. Urol. Nephrol. suppl. 42:73, 1977.

37. Solheim, B.G., Flatmark, A., Jervell, J., and Arnesen, E.: Influence of blood transfusions on kidney transplant and uremic patient survival. Scand. J. Urol. Nephrol. suppl. 42:65, 1977.

38. Walter, S., Poulsen, L.R., Friedberg, M., Afzelius, R., Federspiel, B.H., Larsen, H.W., and Petersen, K.: The effect of blood transfusions on renal allograft survival. Scand. J. Urol. Nephrol. suppl. 42:62, 1977.

39. Persijn, G.G., van Hooff, J.P., Kalff, M.W., Lansbergen, Q., and van Rood, J.J.: Effect of blood transfusions and HLA matching on renal transplantations in the Netherlands. Transplant. Proc. 9:503, 1977.

40. Briggs, J.D., Canavan, J.S.F., Dick, H.M., Hamilton, D.N.H., Kyle, K.F., Macpherson, S.G., Paton, A.M., and Titterington, D.M.: Influence of HLA matching and blood transfusion on renal allograft survival. Transplantation 25:80, 1978.

41. Currier, C.B., Jr. and Pierce, J.C.: Effects of blood transfusions on antibody formation and canine renal allograft survival. Surg. Gynecol. Obstet. 139:241, 1974.

42. Polesky, H.F., McCullough, J.J., Yunis, E., Helgeson, M.A., Andersen, R.C., Simmons, R.L., and Najarian, J.S.: The effects of transfusion of frozen-thawed deglycerolized red cells on renal graft survival. Transplantation 24:449, 1977.

43. Stiller, C.R., Lockwood, B.L., Sinclair, N.R., Ulan, R.A., Sheppard, R.R., Sharpe, J.A., and Hayman, P.: Beneficial effect of operation-day blood-transfusions on human renal-allograft survival. Lancet 1:169, 1978.

44. Zimmerman, C.E.: Enhancing potential of whole blood. Transplant. Proc. 9:1081, 1977.

45. van Es, A.A., Marquet, R.L., van Rood, J.J., Kalff, M.W., and Balner, H.: Blood transfusions induce prolonged kidney allograft survival in Rhesus monkeys. Lancet 1:506, 1977.

46. Sengar, D.P.S., Rashid, A., and Harris, J.E.: Relationship of blood transfusions to appearance of mixed lymphocyte culture blocking factor activity in plasma of uraemic patients and renal allograft recipients. Vox Sang. 27:1, 1974.

47. Ting, A. and Morris, P.J.: Matching for B-cell antigens of the HLA-DR series in cadaver renal transplantation. Lancet 1:575, 1978.

48. Albrechtson, D., Flatmark, A., Jervell, J., Solheim, B., and Thorsby, E.: HLA-DR antigen matching in cadaver renal transplantation. (Letter) Lancet 1:825, 1978.

49. Martins Da Silva, G., Vassalli, P., and Jeannet, M.: Matching renal grafts. (Letter) Lancet 1:1047, 1978.

50. Persijn, G.G., Gabb, B.W., van Leeuwen, A., Nagtegaal, A., Hoogeboom, J.J., and van Rood, J.J.: Matching for HLA antigens of A, B and DR loci in renal transplantation by Eurotransplant. Lancet 1:1278, 1978.

51. Ettenger, R.B., Terasaki, P.I., Opelz, G., Malekzaden, M., Pennisi, A.J., Vittenbogaart, C., and Fine, R.: Successful renal allografts across a positive crossmatch for donor B-lymphocyte alloantigens. Lancet 2:56, 1976.

52. Iwaki, Y., Terasaki, P.I., Park, M.S., and Billing, R.: Enhancement of human kidney allografts by cold B-lymphocyte cytotoxins. Lancet 1:1228, 1978.

53. Binz, H. and Wigzell, H.: Successful induction of specific tolerance to transplantation antigens using autoimmunization against the re-cipient's own natural antibodies. Nature 262:294, 1976.

54. Ockner, S.A., Guttman, R.D., and Lindquist, R.R.: Renal transplantation in the inbred rat. XIII. Modification of rejection by active immunization with bone marrow cells. Transplantation 9:30, 1970.

55. Keown, P.A. and Descamps, B.: Improved renal allograft survival after blood transfusion: A nonspecific, erythrocyte-mediated immunoregulatory process? Lancet 1:20, 1979.

56. van Rood, J.J., Persijn, G.G., van Leeuwen, A., Goulmy, E., and Gabb, B.W.: A new strategy to improve kidney graft survival: The induction of CML nonresponsiveness. Transplant. Proc. 11:736, 1979.

57. Thomas, J., Thomas, F., and Lee, H.M.: Why do HLA-nonidentical renal allografts survive 10 years or more? Transplant. Proc. 9:85, 1977.

58. Engleman, E.G., McMichael, A.J., Bates, M.E., and McDevitt, H.O.: A suppressor T cell of the mixed lymphocyte reaction in man specific for the stimulating alloantigen. Evidence that identity at HLA-D between suppressor and responder is required for suppression. J. Exper. Med. 147:137, 1978.

59. Newton, W.T. and Anderson, C.B.: Planned preimmunization of renal allograft recipients. Surgery 74:430, 1973.

60. Cochrum, K.C., Hanes, D., Potter, D., Vincenti, F., Amend, W., Feduska, N., Perkins, H., and Salvatierra, O.: Donor specific blood transfusions in HLA-D disparate 1-haplotype related allografts. Presented at the annual meeting of the American Association for Clinical Histocompatibility Testing, San Diego, May, 1979.

61. Cochrum, K.C., Hanes, D., van Speybroeck, J., Perkins, H., Ferrone, S., Indeveri, F., Amend, W., Vincenti, F., Feduska, N., and Salvatierra, O.: HLA-D antigen disparity and HLA-DRw antibodies in intrafamilial renal allograft survival. Transplant. Proc. 11:404, 1979.

30

Transfusion Therapy of Chronic Anemic States

Scott N. Swisher, M.D., and Lawrence D. Petz, M.D.

INTRODUCTION

Chronic anemia of variable severity is associated with a wide range of illnesses; it is thus a problem which frequently confronts the clinician. In many instances, the associated anemia is insignificant because of adequate compensatory physiological adjustments. In these situations, it is more important to understand the pathogenesis of the anemic state than it is to correct it per se; clarification of the cause of the anemia may disclose the presence of a serious and potentially treatable underlying disorder such as an occult tumor or chronic infection. Anemia is no longer an acceptable diagnosis. It is the *cause* of the anemia that is important for the rational management of the anemic patient.

Similarly, the appropriate treatment of chronically anemic patients varies widely; elimination or control of an underlying disease leads all strategies in importance and effectiveness. Where this is not possible, replacement of substances necessary for hematopoiesis such as vitamin B_{12}, folic acid, and iron, or of blood itself by transfusion are secondary strategies of therapy, again of variable effectiveness. Replacement of vitamin B_{12}, folic acid, or iron deficiencies is effective only if there is a significant lack of the specific substance and in the absence of other mechanisms which will suppress

normal hematopoiesis. Transfusion, particularly chronic transfusion, then becomes a strategy of final resort in the management of patients with chronic anemia.

Chronic transfusion may be a life-long commitment in many patients. It frequently leads to a number of hazardous complications, including some which are life-threatening. At times, these patients become effectively untransfusable. The decision to transfuse chronically is thus of great importance. It is usually much preferable to have the patient somewhat limited and symptomatic than exposed to the risks of chronic transfusion.

Many of the major causes of chronic anemia are dealt with in other parts of this book where an effort has been made to integrate transfusion into general strategies of patient management. Disorders such as malignant diseases, hemolytic states, and chronic renal insufficiency are examples of such problems where transfusion provides a major component of a complex pattern of treatment. This chapter deals with a broad group of disorders, listed in Table 30-1, which share a number of common problems related to transfusion therapy. It is equally important to integrate transfusion therapy in a thoughtful way into the program of management of patients with

Table 30-1. Chronic Anemic States Which May Require Chronic Transfusion Therapy*

I. Hypoproliferative Anemias.
   A. Hypoplastic or aplastic states of unknown cause.
      1. With pancytopenia.
      2. Pure red cell aplasia.
   B. Drug or chemical induced hypoplastic or aplastic disorders.
   C. Radiation induced marrow destruction.
   D. Marrow destruction secondary to myelofibrosis or myelophthisic processes.
   E. Aplastic or hypoplastic phase of paroxysmal nocturnal hemolytic anemia.

II. Chronic Dysplastic Disorders of the Bone Marrow.
   A. Preleukemic states including unresponsive megaloblastic anemia.
   B. Sideroblastic anemias not due to pyridoxine deficiency.
   C. Congenital dyserythropoietic anemias.
   D. Congenital hyporegenerative disorders of bone marrow.
      1. Fanconi syndrome.
      2. Diamond-Blackfan syndrome of congenital red cell aplasia.
   E. "Constitutional" anemia, (adult acquired Fanconi syndrome).

III. Anemias of Chronic Disease; Anemia Associated With:
   A. Renal insufficiency.
   B. Chronic inflammation.
   C. Hepatic failure.
   D. Malignant tumors.
   E. Endocrine failures.

IV. Anemia Due to Chronic Blood Loss Uncontrolled by Iron Therapy.
   A. Hereditary hemorrhagic telangiectasia.
   B. Chronic gastrointestinal blood loss, multiple causes.
   C. Chronic uterine blood loss, multiple causes.
   D. Iron deficiency with associated marrow hyporegeneration.

* Table does not include the major congenital and acquired hemolytic disorders or anemias associated with malignant diseases, which are dealt with elsewhere in this book.

these disorders, although the problems encountered in doing this may be somewhat less difficult. The discussion here will be based upon some general principles, pertinent to all of these disorders, followed by comments upon the transfusion problems encountered in the specific diseases listed in Tables 30-1 and 30-2.

ASSESSMENT OF THE ANEMIC PATIENT

Three kinds of information are usually available for assessment of the anemic patient: (1) laboratory measurements of levels of hemoglobin and/or hematocrit; (2) evaluation of the patient's symptoms; and (3) physiological assessments of the patient's functional capacities. The first of these is clearly the most objective, but may not be the most informative for making decisions about the need for transfusion. The latter two are less

objective, and are more likely to be influenced by factors such as: the rapidity of onset of anemia; the presence of other physiological abnormalities such as fever, cardiovascular, or pulmonary disease; and the nature of the patient's underlying illness. Nevertheless, these data are probably of greater value in determining the need for red cell transfusion than are the measurements of hemoglobin and hematocrit. Once an unacceptable level of physiological impairment due to anemia has been associated with a specific level of hemoglobin or hematocrit, these laboratory measurements become of more value as guidelines for management of future transfusion schedules. Evaluation of the need for transfusion in a given patient is thus a sophisticated, clinically based process of decision which requires skilled interviewing, refined physical examination, and, at times, physiological testing. It should rarely be based upon measurements of hemoglobin and hematocrit alone.

Table 30-2. Other Acute or Chronic Anemic States in which Transfusion Therapy is Required Only under Exceptional Circumstances

I. Anemias of Nutritional Deficiency
   A. Megaloblastic Anemias.
      1. Vitamin B_{12} deficiency.
      2. Folic acid deficiency.
   B. Chronic severe malnutrition.
II. Hemolytic anemias.*
   A. Microangiopathic hemolytic disorders.
   B. Hemolytic-Uremic syndrome.
   C. Traumatic cardiac hemolytic anemia.
   D. Hemolytic anemia due to chemical or physical agents.
   E. Hemolytic anemia secondary to infection.
   F. Associated with hypersplenism.
III. Anemia Associated with Pregnancy and Delivery.
   A. Megaloblastic anemia of pregnancy.
   B. Postpartum anemia.

* Table does not include major congenital and acquired hemolytic states, anemia associated with malignant disease, or acute blood loss dealt with elsewhere in this book.

Hemoglobin and Hematocrit Levels and Red Cell Mass

Hemoglobin and hematocrit levels nevertheless do provide a general indication of the probability of significant physiological impairment of a patient. A physician, conservative in the use of transfusion, might employ the guidelines shown in Table 30-3.

Although hemoglobin and hematocrit are the usually available laboratory measurements for the assessment of anemia, they are useful because they are relatively highly correlated with the patient's red cell mass.[1] It is red cell mass which is of greater physiological significance rather than the blood's concentration of hemoglobin. Situations in which the red cell mass is lower or higher than would be indicated by the hematocrit are usually recognizable clinically. These are situations in which the plasma volume is reduced, as in "stress" polycythemia, excessive diuresis or dehydration, in which case the hematocrit will be higher in relation to red cell mass than normal. Conversely, states of hydremia associated with intravascular fluid retention, as in the last trimester of pregnancy, will have a lower hematocrit even in the presence of a normal red cell mass.

Red cell mass or plasma volume can be measured by radioisotopic methods employing ^{51}Cr-labeled red cells or radioiodinated serum albumin. These measurements are rarely necessary in the clinical setting where transfusion is under consideration. Even in marked states of hydremia of pregnancy, the normal red cell mass is infrequently diluted to an hematocrit of less than 30 percent. In situations where a patient's red cell mass is in fact reduced, hydremia or loss of plasma volume will confuse the evaluation of the severity of anemia by the hematocrit. This may be a sig-

Table 30-3. Guidelines for Assessing Physiological Impairment of the Anemic Patient and Prescribing Transfusion Strategy

Average Hemoglobin Level (gm%)	Probability of Significant Impairment	Transfusion Strategy
10 or more	very low	Avoid
8 to 10	low	Avoid; transfuse only if demonstrably better after transfusion trial.
6 to 8	moderate	Try to avoid by decreased activity; if impossible, transfuse.
6 or less	high	Frequently requires transfusion.

nificant difficulty. A comprehensive evaluation of the patient will usually provide the information needed to estimate the true state of the red cell mass. In rare instances, direct measurements of red cell mass may be of value.[2,3]

In situations where blood is lost acutely, the hemoglobin concentration and hematocrit are recognized to be unreliable guides to the size of the red cell mass. The correlation between these measurements and red cell mass will not be reestablished until the blood volume has again stabilized and the red cell mass deficit has been replaced by additional plasma. This may require 24 to 48 hours or more to occur after an acute blood loss, depending upon the availability of fluid and other physiological factors. Virtually by definition, this problem does not occur in chronic anemic states where a relatively stable blood volume is usually present, and the hemoglobin concentration and hematocrit again reasonably and usefully reflect the size of the red cell mass.

The need for chronic transfusion and the level of hemoglobin which should be maintained are greatly influenced by the level of the patient's activity. Younger people who are strenuously active in daily living or employment may require higher levels of hemoglobin if they are unable or unwilling to reduce this level of activity; conversely, they usually have the greatest capacity for physiological compensation of anemia in the absence of significant cardiovascular or pulmonary disease. Sedentary people may require less transfusion, but with substantial individual variation from patient to patient. These factors strongly influence the decision to transfuse or not, and the level of hemoglobin that should be maintained in the patients who are given blood.

The first step in the decision process is to determine the minimum level of hemoglobin at which the patient can function satisfactorily. This decision should not be made by the physician alone. The several risks, costs, and inconveniences of transfusion and its avoidance should be explained. The patient's feelings should strongly influence the physician's ultimate recommendations for a program of management. Availability of transfusion facilities, blood, and costs involved are other important but secondary factors in the decision.

Evaluation of Patient's Symptoms of Anemia

The most important pieces of historical information from the anemic patient are those related to the level of activity that can be sustained and what happens when this level is exceeded. If other factors which limit functional capacity coexist, it may be difficult or impossible to untangle those symptoms due primarily to anemia. In general, the most informative data are those which reveal the level of cardiorespiratory compensation evoked by exertion in the anemic state.

It is important that these questions be asked in an open-ended, nonleading way. Initial questions, such as "Tell me about your physical activities at present?" "What happens if you climb two flights of stairs rapidly?" or "What happens when you exert yourself?" do not lead the patient into an expected answer or focus attention on a specific system. An initial question such as "Do you become short of breath and have to stop when you try to climb two flights of stairs rapidly?" suggests that this is the principal symptom of interest to the physician. The patient then might or might not reveal his observations about a pounding heart or chest pain caused by the exertion. More specific questions such as the last can be asked appropriately after the patient has had an opportunity to tell of his own observations as he sees and evaluates them.[4]

Specificity of Symptoms of Anemia

A number of other symptoms are traditionally associated with anemia by both physicians and the public alike. They are very much less specific for anemia, and in fact may not be statistically associated with anemia in large populations until levels of hemoglobin lower than 7 to 8 gm% have developed. At this point, significant cardiovascular changes may be evoked. Elwood et al.[5] studied the symptoms of irritability, palpitation, dizziness, breathlessness, fatigue, and headache in a population of iron-deficient women in England with hemoglobin levels between 8 and 12 gm% after effective iron therapy and placebo treatment. They found no evidence to support a significant relationship of these symptoms to iron deficiency or the associated anemia. Other studies have reached similar conclusions.[6,7]

These results corroborate the views of experienced clinicians who recognize the nonspecific nature of many of these symptoms based upon their daily contacts with patients. The frequency of a symptom such as fatigue alone, estimated to be present in over 90 percent of patients consulting a general internist for all causes in one study, documents its lack of specificity.[8] Psychological mechanisms may be responsible for many of these symptoms. Elwood and colleagues obtained some data to suggest that the six symptoms they evaluated were more clearly related to "neurotic" phenomena than to hemoglobin level.[5] These data and common experience indicate that it is no simple task to evaluate the symptoms presented by the anemic patient in terms of the need for transfusion. Nevertheless, these data are among the most important in making the required decisions.

Physiological Compensations for Anemia and Their Evaluation

The physiological adjustments caused by acute blood loss—i.e., acute anemia—are mainly due to an acutely decreased blood volume. In contrast, the blood volume of the chronically anemic patient is normal or only moderately and slowly decreased in most instances. These two circumstances evoke different physiological adjustments. There are three principal adjustments caused by chronic anemia: (1) shift of the hemoglobin oxygen dissociation curve; (2) cardiovascular compensations; and (3) respiratory compensations.

Shift of the Hemoglobin Oxygen Dissociation Curve. In order to transport an equivalent volume of oxygen, the cardiac index (cardiac output in liters per minute per meter squared of body surface area) would have to rise in inverse proportion to the level of blood hemoglobin if no other compensations occurred. There is, however, in most states of chronic anemia an increase in oxygen abstraction from the blood as it passes through the low-oxygen tension areas of the systemic microcirculation. That is, a larger proportion of the oxygen being transported bound to hemoglobin is released in these areas. This is accomplished by shifting the oxygen dissociation curve (O_2 tension plotted against hemoglobin saturation) to the right (Fig. 30-1).

This means that, at a given level of oxygen tension in the tissues which is lower than that in the lung capillaries and pulmonary arteries, more oxygen is removed from a gram of hemoglobin in chronically anemic blood

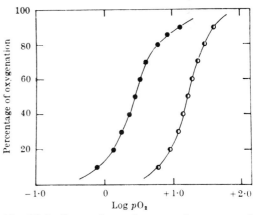

Fig. 30-1. Comparison of oxygenation curves of hemoglobin and whole blood; ● 0.3 percent "stripped" hemoglobin in 0.01 M NaCl at 30 °C, pH 7.0 (before deoxygenation) ○, whole blood at 30 °C plotted from the data of Astrup et al. 1965. (Harris, J.W. and Kellermayer, R.W.: The Red Cell. Revised ed., Harvard University Press, Cambridge, Mass., 1970.)

than would be the case with a gram of hemoglobin from normal blood. This remarkable effect is due to the role of intracellular erythrocyte, 2,3-diphosphoglyceric acid (2,3-DPG), an intermediate of red cell glucose metabolism, in controlling the position of the oxygen dissociation curve. Binding of oxygen to hemoglobin within the red cell involves formation of a complex of oxygen, hemoglobin, and 2,3-DPG, with the latter having the effect of decreasing the hemoglobin affinity for oxygen; the affinity of hemoglobin for oxygen is thus inversely related to the red cell concentration of 2,3-DPG. The exact mechanism by which the compensatory rise in 2,3-DPG occurs is not clear; it may be due to intracellular alkalosis.[9-14] The effect may be responsible for a substantial part of the overall adjustment in oxygen transport resulting in a major saving of cardiac work.[15,16] Metabolic disorders such as diabetic ketoacidosis reduce the red cell 2,3-DPG concentration and may unfavorably influence oxygen transport in the patient who is also chronically anemic. Other disorders characterized by hypoxemia, such as high-altitude adaptation and anoxia due to lung or heart disease, also result in a rise in red cell 2,3-DPG concentration. Blood pH also influences the position of the oxygen dissociation curve by the Bohr effect (Fig. 30-2). An acid pH decreases oxygen affinity, whereas a higher pH within the physiological range increases oxygen binding. These changes partially offset the increased oxygen affinity associated with 2,3-DPG depletion in the presence of ketoacidosis.[17]

In spite of an apparently important role in adapting certain patients to states of chronic anemia, the value of transfusing red cells with high 2,3-DPG (as compared with stored erythrocytes, in which this compound has been depleted) has not been convincingly demonstrated. Some 2,3-DPG is regenerated within hours of transfusing stored depleted red cells, and it is virtually normal in concentration after 24 hours. It is clear that the concentration of blood hemoglobin, and thus

oxygen-carrying capacity, is of greater physiological importance than is 2,3-DPG level in correcting the oxygen transport deficits of anemic patients. Thus, it is rarely justified to use fresh blood with high 2,3-DPG levels for transfusing anemic patients.

Cardiovascular Compensations. Increased cardiac output is the other major mechanism of compensation for severe anemia. Both stroke volume and cardiac rate increase, with the former predominating.[18,19] Significant cardiovascular compensations are not evoked until the hemoglobin level has decreased about one-half in otherwise normal persons. Exercise increases cardiovascular compensations which may be minimal in the resting state.

If symptoms and findings of congestive heart failure occur with levels of hemoglobin around 7 gm% or higher, it is almost always due to associated intrinsic heart disease—most frequently coronary artery disease or hypertensive heart disease.[20-24] The coronary circulation is increased in the normal heart as the left ventricular work load rises. In severe anemia, however, with hemoglobin levels less than 5 gm%, coronary blood flow may become relatively inadequate and ventricular function is decreased. This may lead to congestive heart failure with decreased renal blood flow and sodium retention.[25]

The clinical assessment of the adequacy of cardiovascular compensations for anemia rarely needs to go beyond standard clinical techniques. A careful evaluation of the patient's history regarding exercise tolerance, anginal pain or other chest discomfort, edema, dyspnea, and orthopnea are of great importance. The main observations of importance in the physical examination are heart rate, cardiac rhythm, precordial activity, heart size, venous pressure, presence or absence of hepatojugular reflux, pulmonary rales, and peripheral edema. Systolic flow murmurs are not uncommon in anemic patients; their importance lies in differentiating them from murmurs of valvular or other origin. Gallop rhythms of S_3 or S_4 type may be

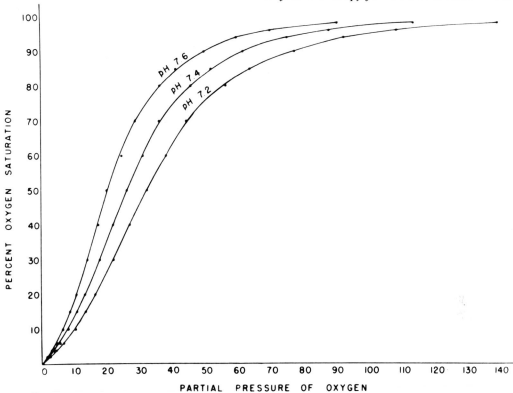

Fig. 30-2. Oxygen dissociation curves of human hemoglobin at various pH values. (Harris, J.W. and Kellermeyer, R.W.: The Red Cell, Revised ed., Harvard University Press, Cambridge, Mass., 1970.)

heard and raise the question of early onset of cardiac decompensation. The blood pressure may show a wide pulse pressure, and the pulse may be bounding; peripheral resistance is usually decreased in chronic anemia, in contrast to its increase in acute blood loss.[26]

At times, electrocardiography, including stress tests, may be useful in evaluating these patients. Chest radiographs may also be useful, and a wide range of the present-day noninvasive diagnostic technology will be useful on occasion. Usually these procedures are directed toward assessment of the nature and extent of underlying heart disease, rather than the effects of anemia itself upon the heart.

The importance of detecting early cardiac failure is two-fold: a transfusion may increase blood volume rapidly and precipitate acute pulmonary edema;[23] if the patient is severely anemic, heart failure may signal the need for increased amounts of transfusion to reduce the need for cardiac work and improve the patient's state of compensation. The anemic patient in congestive heart failure requires transfusion with sedimented red cells at very slow rates. At times it is useful to remove 250 to 500 ml of blood, following infusion of a unit of red cells with a hematocrit of about 70 percent. If the blood is anticoagulated and handled in a sterile fashion, the patient's own red cells can be concentrated by centrifugation and reinfused after removal of most of the plasma. This results in an increase in hematocrit with little or no change in blood volume. If necessary, the blood volume can be decreased, while increasing the hemoglobin concentation. Other appropriate measures for control of congestive failure should also be employed.

Respiratory Compensations. Changes in pulmonary function generally occur in parallel with those of the cardiovascular system. The respiratory rate and depth may be increased, with a rise in minute volume. The arterial oxygen tension may be reduced with increased oxygen gradient to alveolar air. There is usually decreased maximal oxygen uptake, but this does not reflect abnormal lung function. Anemic subjects incur a higher oxygen debt at a given work load when compared to nonanemic persons.[18,27-29] These observations indicate that all compensations available for anemia are unable to transport the oxygen required for work loads above a certain level, and that the compensations themselves impose a significant work load.[30]

Any limitation of respiratory function—particularly those disorders which decrease maximum ventilation or decrease gas diffusion between alveoli and lung capillaries—will limit the effectiveness of the integrated compensations for anemia. Again, clinical techniques of evaluation of respiratory function are usually adequate for assessment of the average anemic patient. Arterial blood gas measurements, along with spirometry, may be useful when there is some uncertainty about a patient's pulmonary function. When there are clear-cut abnormalities, a more complete pulmonary function study may be in order.

THE STRATEGY OF CHRONIC TRANSFUSION THERAPY

Accurate periodic assessments of chronically anemic patients are critical in making the decision to transfuse them and deciding how much blood to administer. One must differentiate between tolerable levels of physiological compensation, particularly those of the cardiovascular system, and excessive requirements for compensation which the patient is unable to maintain within reasonable physiological costs. Existence of intrinsic cardiovascular or pulmonary disease frequently limits these compensations. Such patients usually require institution of chronic trans-

fusion therapy at higher levels of hemoglobin than patients without these limitations for a given level of activity. Requirements for transfusion may be increased by life-styles which involve high levels of exertion, if the level of activity cannot be reduced. Coexistence of many other diseases may also limit the effectiveness of the compensatory mechanisms; these diseases must be factored into the decisions about transfusion. The aim of a transfusion program should be to reduce the requirement for compensation to a tolerable point, not to remove the need for all compensation. The least amount of blood required to accomplish this is the proper amount.

There is an unfortunate tendency to overtransfuse many chronically anemic patients who do require blood and to transfuse patients who are adequately adjusted to living with a low hematocrit. This is done many times with the laudable goal of "making the patient feel better" and with inadequate recognition of the hazards and inconvenience of long-term transfusion. It is important that transfusions meet the patient's real needs, not the physician's concepts of what those needs should be. It is usually better for the patient to live with even significant symptoms or limitations than to face the hazards of life-long transfusion.

TRANSFUSION SCHEDULES

If the decision has been made to institute chronic transfusion, the initial several months of this program should be regarded as a therapeutic trial. The patient should be evaluated carefully and frequently to determine if the desired effects are being obtained. The level of hemoglobin or hematocrit which adequately reduces the undesirable effects of chronic anemia can usually be determined within 3 months, and the amount of blood required to maintain this level can be approximated. The goal is to minimize variations in the hematocrit around a target level, while administering the least amount of blood needed to do this.

After these factors have been determined, it is nearly always better long-term strategy to schedule transfusion at regular intervals, rather than to follow the hematocrit with transfusion after it reaches a predetermined level. Scheduled transfusions usually result in a higher average hematocrit with less administered blood and avoid the oscillations frequently encountered when the hematocrit is being "chased." Regular, scheduled transfusions are generally better integrated into the patient's pattern of daily living, since they can be planned for in advance. They reduce the need for medical or laboratory visits. When the patient is transfused on indication of a low hematocrit, visits to the laboratory and then to the physician are required in order for the decision to give blood to be made. Frequently, a second visit to a transfusion facility must be made to receive the transfusion.

Transfusion of the patient on the basis of the recurrence of symptoms is usually quite unsuccessful. Wide swings of hematocrit usually occur. The hematocrit is usually well below the target level when unacceptable symptoms occur, and a number of transfusions may be required over several days to restore an adequate red cell mass. This strategy has little to be said for it, except possibly in those few patients whose need for transfusion is relatively unpredictable. Even in these patients, periodic surveillance of the hematocrit may be preferable, with transfusion at a predetermined low level.

Two variables can be manipulated to achieve the best results of chronic transfusion: the amount of blood administered and the interval between transfusions. Most patients are able to receive two units of sedimented red cells at one sitting. The circulatory volume increase is usually tolerable, and the time required for infusion is not excessive. As a reference point and general rule of thumb, it can be calculated that a requirement for 2 units of red cells every 2 weeks in an average adult reflects the situation encountered with essentially total failure of red cell production. More frequent weekly transfusions of 1 unit might result in reduction in the variations of the hematocrit, but at the cost of greater inconvenience for the patient. Thus, it is our policy to transfuse most patients 2 units at a time and to determine the interval between transfusion on the basis of total need for blood. In the absence of blood loss, alloimmunization, or other causes of inefficient transfusion, this usually results in an interval of 2 to 4 weeks between transfusions.

INEFFICIENT TRANSFUSIONS

Transfusion requirements above the level of about 2 units every 2 weeks in an adult suggest inefficiency of the transfusion for one or more reasons. The expected rise in hematocrit following a transfusion should be calculated; if it is not met, further evidence of inefficient transfusion is present. Does the patient have an occult alloimmunization to a red cell antigen with destruction of the transfused erythrocyte at an increased rate, but not so rapidly as to result in an overt hemolytic transfusion reaction? Investigation of this possibility may be very difficult (see Ch. 7). The responsible alloantibody may be present in only very small amounts in the patient's serum, since much of it may be bound to incompatible transfused red cells. It may be necessary to allow the patient to become quite anemic by destroying a large proportion of the transfused cells before the responsible alloantibody becomes detectable. It may be detectable by a direct antiglobulin test of the patient's red cells with observation of so-called "mixed field" of agglutination; in this case, it may be recoverable by elution from the red cells. Unfortunately, in some instances donor red cells are destroyed without serological evidences of donor-recipient incompatibility. Investigations of this type are in the domain of a sophisticated transfusion service and laboratory, but the clinician caring for the patient is responsible for determining that a problem may be present, and for obtaining the necessary consultative help.

Before beginning a program of chronic transfusion, one should consider typing the patient's red cells for the four additional major antigens of the Rh system, and for the major antigens of the Kell, S., Kidd, and Duffy systems. These data may be useful in the search for suspected alloimmunization, in that they limit to some extent the possibilities to be looked for and may suggest the most probable antigenic responses.[31] Extended typing is of little value after transfusion has begun, because donor and recipient cells are then admixed. Storage of a pretransfusion specimen of the donor's red cells in the frozen state should be considered where possible.

Although the practice of extended pretransfusion typing has a rationale, it is infrequently of major help in identification of alloimmunization. In most instances, standard serological methods will identify the responsible antibody and permit selection of a compatible donor. For this reason, most transfusion services transfuse patients chronically without preliminary extended red cell typing.

The presence of autoimmune acquired hemolytic anemia of the warm autoantibody type may also account for increased blood requirements and inefficient transfusion. This disorder may develop insidiously, particularly in patients with an underlying neoplastic disease of the lymphoreticular system or another autoimmune disorder. Usually, but not in all instances, the direct red cell antiglobulin test will be positive, for either γ globulin or complement components or both. Again, the assistance of a sophisticated transfusion service, transfusion reference laboratory, or general immunodiagnostic laboratory will frequently be needed to define this problem adequately before further transfusion therapy can proceed.

Administration of blood nearing its outdating is a second reason for relative inefficiency of transfusion. By definition, as blood reaches outdating, only about 70 percent of the infused red cells will be viable. This means that approximately 4 units of blood near expiration of dating will be equivalent to 3 units of blood within a few days of its drawing. Transfusion services should be encouraged to provide units that are no more than 5 days old for these patients whenever possible. There is no appreciable advantage in using blood that is in storage for shorter periods, and no major contraindication to administration of occasional units that are older. What should be avoided is a policy of employing short-dated bloods regularly for these recipients. Nathan et al. have recently shown that most recently produced donor red cells collected by a procedure of differential centrifugation have a longer in vivo life span in patients with thalassemia major.[32] This collection technique is of investigative interest and may have some value to be defined in the future in occasional patients with specific transfusion problems.

Occult or overt blood loss from the gastrointestinal tract or other sources may be another cause of apparent inefficient transfusion and may result in an increased requirement for blood. Appropriate investigation of these possibilities should be carried out, particularly if the requirement for blood increases suddenly. This is most likely to occur in patients who also have thrombocytopenia in association with generalized bone marrow failure.

Nonimmunological mechanisms of hemolysis secondary to splenic enlargement, so-called "hypersplenism," may be responsible for high transfusion requirements. This can usually be evaluated on clinical grounds alone. The existence of portal hypertension, or substantial splenomegaly of any cause, may be a diagnostic cue in this direction. Preferential localization of [51]Chromium-labeled red cells in the spleen may corroborate this diagnostic suspicion. Hypersplenic destruction of red cells rarely occurs in the absence of a significantly enlarged and easily palpable spleen.

Coincident blood loss or hemolysis should be suspected, particularly if the patient has some evidence of blood regeneration, even though this is inadequate to meet his needs for red cells. Some degree of persistent or increasing reticulocytosis, in the face of a requirement for transfusion compatible with total red cell aplasia, may suggest one or more of these possibilities.

RISKS AND BENEFITS OF CHRONIC TRANSFUSION THERAPY

Categorical statements of risks and benefits cannot be made for groups of patients in various diagnostic categories. These assessments must be made for each patient in whom chronic transfusion therapy is considered. The policies of individual physicians seem to vary widely in these respects. There is little doubt that many chronically anemic patients are transfused beyond their real requirements. Since the risks of transfusion are largely linearly related to the amount of blood given, these patients face an unnecessary risk for little or no added benefit. Other patients would receive higher benefits from the same amount of transfusion if a more effective scheduling strategy were employed. In our experience, only a small number of chronically anemic patients are significantly undertransfused; however, when this occurs it usually presents a significant clinical problem.

The patient's overall prognosis, based upon the nature of the underlying disease or process causing anemia, is a major determinant of a rational transfusion policy. If the patient has a relatively short life expectancy, a year or less, those longer-term problems of chronic transfusion—such as iron overloading, recurrent severe febrile transfusion reactions and multiple red cell alloimmunizations—are of less importance. A policy of transfusion based upon the shorter-term risks—such as transmission of hepatitis, acute hemolytic reactions, transfusion of infected bloods, and circulatory overload—can be employed. This usually results in somewhat more liberal administration of blood in an effort to maximize the lethally ill patient's functional capacities for the remainder of his life. However, this consideration still does not justify transfusion beyond the patient's real physiological needs.

When the patient's prognosis for longer survival is more favorable, the physician formulating the transfusion policy must consider the long-term hazards of transfusion *plus* the short-term risks now aggregated over a longer time span with increased probability of their occurrence. This should lead to efforts to administer the least amount of blood compatible with an acceptable, even though reduced, functional capacity. Where the prognosis is uncertain, a conservative position of planning for the longest possible period of survival would seem reasonable.

There will certainly remain reasonable differences of opinion and practice in these decisions among competent physicians. Similarly, patients will vary in their decisions if the issues of risks and benefits of transfusion are clearly and accurately presented to them. While we urge a generally conservative policy of transfusion for all patients, it can be said that this therapeutic decision, like all therapeutic decisions, should also be subjected to careful and informed scrutiny of both patient and physician. Consultation may be helpful in doubtful situations. Decisions based upon hemoglobin levels alone are too frequently wrong, as are fixed policies applied to groups of patients in various diagnostic categories. The decision to transfuse chronically should include a plan for blood administration and for evaluation of its efficacy and safety. Only in this way does the patient receive maximal benefit from use of a precious and limited human resource.

SOME CLINICAL ASPECTS OF TRANSFUSION IN CHRONIC ANEMIC STATES

Transfusion therapy is employed in a wide range of hemotological disorders characterized by anemia. It is beyond the scope of this chapter to discuss in detail the many complexities of management of these anemic disorders. The reader may refer to any of the several excellent modern textbooks of hematology for more detailed discussions of the overall management problems posed by these disorders. Nevertheless, some comments with regard to specific aspects of transfusion therapy in certain of these anemic states may be of value. They are listed in Tables 30-1, 30-2, and 30-3.

Hypoproliferative Anemias

There are two major determinants of the strategy of transfusion of this very large and heterogenous group of patients:

1. Does the patient have primarily a deficit of red cells of clinically significant magnitude, or is the patient pancytopenic to a degree where significant thrombocytopenia and/or leukopenia are also present?

2. Is the prognosis of the patient's disorder favorable or unfavorable in the long term?

If the patient's only significant cytopenia is reflected by chronic anemia of clinically significant severity, the problem is manageable in a relatively straightforward fashion; the patient can be given transfusions on previously discussed indications for whatever period they are required. In some instances, this involves a life-long commitment to transfusion. By contrast, the patient with a pancytopenic state in which clinically significant thrombocytopenia and/or leukopenia are also present may require a very different strategy of management. Here, control of bleeding and/or infection with platelet and leukocyte transfusions may be of the greatest importance. As a practical matter, transfusion support of patients with severe and persisting thrombocytopenia and leukopenia is only effective for a relatively short period of time, on the order of a few months. Thus, these patients can for practical purposes be supported only during a period of transient

aplasia or hypoplasia under circumstances where there is a reasonably high probability that they will recover marrow function to a degree sufficient to eliminate or markedly reduce the need for chronic replacement of red cells, platelets, and leukocytes. Patients who have recoverable forms of severe hyporegenerative and hypoplastic states of the bone marrow tend to be those in whom a reasonably well-defined toxic response to a drug or chemical has occurred, or where extensive radiation exposure has induced marrow suppression and where recovery of some degree of marrow function is still possible.

It is now quite clear that patients with severe aplastic anemia have a poor prognosis with virtually all forms of medical therapy and that early marrow transplantation, in spite of its still somewhat experimental nature, seems to offer the best outlook in this situation. Unfortunately, suitable donors may not be available in many cases. Here, standard medical therapy utilizing transfusion as necessary seems reasonable, although very frequently it becomes ineffective in the long term. Many patients with relatively severe hyporegeneration of blood cells by the bone marrow are, fortunately, able to establish a functional if precarious balance and remain reasonably well and functional as long as this balance is maintained. If an episode such as an infection, trauma, or adverse drug response adds an element of further transient suppression of marrow blood cell production, the patient may need a period of transfusion support until the acute episode has subsided and the marrow function returns to its previous level. Such patients should be kept under careful surveillance, and their blood values should be followed during any such episodes.

Hyporegeneration with Normal Marrow Cellularity

A number of patients who are clinically categorized as having hyporegenerative bone marrow disorders do, in fact, have normally cellular or somewhat hypercellular marrows. Although the clinical problem presented by such patients may look very much like that associated with hypoplastic bone marrows, the long-term outlook is in general quite different. Many of these patients may need a variable amount of support by transfusion from time to time, although many also can be stabilized in a satisfactory functional condition without transfusion. Frequently, these patients who also have some evidence of dysplastic hematopoiesis along with the hyporegeneration of cellular elements will undergo transformation to a neoplastic disorder of the reticuloendothelium, commonly an acute leukemia. The need for increasing amounts of transfusion may herald this when it occurs in a patient who otherwise has been stable for some length of time. A careful reexamination of the blood and possibly the bone marrow in the face of increasing transfusion may establish the diagnosis of a malignant blood dyscrasia at an earlier point than would occur otherwise.

Myelofibrosis

The problem of transfusion therapy in patients with myelofibrosis of the type now recognized as a myeloproliferative disorder may also reflect significant changes in the character and clinical course of the underlying disorder. Relatively few of these patients will require chronic transfusion therapy, although they may require transfusion from time to time when hematopoiesis is suppressed by infection or other similar causes. These patients also are subject to transformation to a fully neoplastic reticuloendothelial disorder, particularly acute myeloblastic leukemia, myelomonocytic leukemia, and on occasion a wide variety of other leukemic and malignant reticuloendothelial disorders. This may be heralded by an increasing transfusion requirement, increasingly severe thrombocytopenia, or a rising or falling white blood cell count.

More commonly, as the spleen enlarges in patients with myeloid metaplasia there may be increasing severity of anemia and a requirement for increasing amounts of transfusion. When the amount of transfusion required by such patients exceeds that which total red cell aplasia would require (i.e., more than about 2 units of sedimented red cells every 2 weeks in the average adult), it is appropriate to suspect that the massive splenomegaly has induced a hypersplenic type of hemolysis. These patients may require splenectomy, now recognized to be useful in a large proportion of the very chronic patients in this disease category who have progressive increase in splenic size.

Patients with myeloid metaplasia who have increasing transfusion requirements should also be investigated for the presence of alloimmunization, as discussed in the first section of this chapter, where inefficient transfusions are considered. These patients also develop esophageal varices which may bleed chronically rather than massively.[33] They should also be investigated carefully for gastrointestinal blood loss.

Chronic Dysplastic Disorders of Bone Marrow

In this group of patients, the marrow is usually of normal cellularity. Anemia, thrombocytopenia, and leukopenia occur as a result of ineffective cell proliferation and differentiation, at times with evidence that cells are being destroyed in the bone marrow prior to their release. As a group, they are usually very long-term disorders, at times manifesting themselves shortly after birth. Their management must be developed with full consideration of the probable time course of the disorder.

In most instances, these patients are best managed without transfusion if that is at all possible. If not, it may be possible to transfuse them for relatively brief periods of severe anemia or to control transient episodes of thrombocytopenic bleeding by platelet transfusion. Chronic red cell transfusion may be required in some patients. This is the only type of chronic transfusion support which is practical for these patients over a long period of time. Because these patients in the several related groups are uncommon, there is relatively little critically collected information available about their long-term transfusion management. It nevertheless seems reasonable to apply the same general principles to their management as are employed in other chronic anemic disorders. The red cells produced by these patients generally do not have an excessively short life span. Thus, there is no need to suppress completely the patient's own red cell production (a strategy which may be appropriate in the chronic hemolytic states). Nevertheless, iron overload does develop in patients who may require chronic transfusion over long periods of time. The incidence of cardiac and hepatic dysfunction secondary to iron overload does not seem to constitute the same kind of serious limitation on life span that it does in disorders such as thalassemia major and sickle cell anemia. In general, it seems appropriate to transfuse these patients with the least amount of blood which is compatible with reasonable functional activity and normal growth and development during childhood. Transfusion requirements may change in later life, as puberty occurs in females, or as activity levels increase or decrease. The previously outlined principles of managing chronic transfusion will apply to such patients as adulthood is reached.

Virtually all of the disorders in this heterogenous group are at risk for the development of a fully neoplastic malignant blood dyscrasia. Again, worsening anemia, increasing thrombocytopenia, or changes in the white blood cell count and differential leukocyte count may herald this change in clinical course prior to the appearance of overt leukemic manifestations. If severe chronic thrombocytopenia is part of the picture, blood loss will add to the patient's transfusion requirement. Every effort should be made to minimize blood loss, including suppression of menstrual function in postpubertal women if menstrual blood loss is excessively heavy.

Anemias of Chronic Disease

With the exception of the anemia associated with severe renal insufficiency, most patients in this large category rarely require transfusion. Occasionally, additional factors such as blood loss, an acute infection, or an adverse drug effect may result in increasing anemia, and a brief period of transfusion therapy may be useful. In general, most patients in these groups have a poor long-term prognosis or are significantly limited by their primary disease so that they do not require transfusion for the primary purpose of improving their functional state. Transfusion given under these circumstances should be carefully evaluated for their objective clinical effect. The risk involved should be balanced against the utility to the patient of whatever improvement may have been produced.

Renal Failure

Patients with advanced renal failure who are not satisfactory candidates for renal transplantation and who are supported by hemodialysis or chronic peritoneal dialysis may require supplementation of their own inadequate hematopoiesis to achieve a satisfactory functional level of activity. Early in the experience with chronic hemodialysis, transfusion was given to these patients rather more liberally than at present. Through experience, it has been found that many patients will stabilize at hemoglobin levels between 5 and 8 g/100 ml, with need for only infrequent transfusion. It has thus become the policy in most clinics caring for significant numbers of these patients to give them the least possible amount of transfusion and to permit them to be as anemic as 5 g/% of hemoglobin unless there are major physiological evidences of distress at these levels. The additional complications of long-term transfusion—including febrile reactions, alloimmunization, and inefficient transfusions—in many instances appear to outweigh the advantages of maintaining these patients at higher levels of hemoglobin by transfusion. Although some individualization of this policy is necessary, it seems to be the best general management principle for dealing with the anemia of severe chronic renal insufficiency and dialysis therapy. The general problems associated with blood transfusion given to patients who are candidates for renal transplantation is discussed in Chapter 29.

Anemia due to Chronic Blood Loss, Uncontrolled by Iron Therapy

In this group of disorders of various etiologies, the common feature is chronic blood loss of such magnitude that, even with iron therapy, the patient cannot maintain a normal hematocrit. Again, the same criteria apply as to the indications for transfusion— namely, that the patient be functionally limited or seriously symptomatic in order to justify the risks of chronic transfusion. In many of these patients, blood loss is quite variable from time to time, and there may be substantial variation in the degree of anemia. In contrast to the usually preferable strategy of scheduled transfusions, these patients may be better managed and the amount of transfusion may be minimized by periodically determining the hematocrit and hemoglobin levels as well as keeping the patient under close surveillance for symptomatic anemia. Transfusions can then be administered on these indications rather than on a scheduled basis.

It is, of course, important to attempt to control the source of the abnormal blood loss

by whatever means are appropriate for the particular clinical situation presented by the patient. Control of blood loss is always a preferable strategy, and even substantial surgical risks can be accepted when contrasted with the serious cumulative risks of chronic transfusion.

If there is any degree of suppression of bone marrow responsiveness in these patients with severe and continuing blood loss, iron lack may not be the principal limitation on the regeneration of red cells. Any of the chronic diseases which cause anemia may also be present in the patient with chronic blood loss. Thus, if iron therapy has resulted in the normalization of the patient's iron stores, serum iron level, and iron-binding capacity but the anemia has not been corrected, it is well to look for other causes of limited red cell production. Folate deficiency is one such cause which is easily remediable.[34] Although the presence of folate deficiency can be documented biochemically with great certainty, it may be just as informative to carry out a therapeutic test with the administration of 5 mg of folic acid parenterally, followed by 1 mg per day orally for approximately 2 weeks, during which time the patient is observed for an increase in reticulocytosis and in hematocrit. It is of interest that blood and serum folate concentration may not reflect folate deficiency, particularly in the presence of iron deficiency, and may thus be misleading.[35]

Patients in whom oral iron therapy does not permit absorption of sufficient iron to compensate for iron lost by bleeding may justifiably be treated with parenteral iron. The risks of parenteral iron therapy, although not prohibitive, are nevertheless significant; most hematologists are conservative in the use of this modality of iron administration.[36,37] Uncompensated iron deficiency anemia secondary to uncontrollable chronic blood loss does constitute one of the legitimate indications for this treatment. It is only after all of these approaches to increasing the patient's own compensatory hematopoiesis that a program of transfusion therapy would appear to be justified.

OTHER DISORDERS WHICH MAY REQUIRE TRANSFUSION

In a number of other disorders characterized by acute or chronic anemia, transfusion is required only under exceptional circumstances. Some of these disorders are listed in Table 30-2.

Anemias of Nutritional Deficiency

Transfusion is rarely required in this group of disorders. An occasional patient with severe megaloblastic anemia (usually due to vitamin B_{12} deficiency) may be encountered in whom advanced heart failure is immediately life-threatening. In these patients, a program of partial exchange transfusion in which the plasma volume is reduced and partially replaced with donor red cells may be of immediate therapeutic value. The patient should of course be treated promptly with vitamin B_{12} or folate as indicated by the etiological mechanism responsible for anemia. All of the other necessary measures designed to control cardiac failure should be administered as well. It is of interest that transfusion does not correct the delirium associated with advanced vitamin B_{12} deficiency, even though the patient may be quite severely anemic. This manifestation of B_{12} depletion appears to depend upon some direct metabolic role of vitamin B_{12} in the central nervous system.[38] It should be noted that correction of the anemia does not correct the metabolic defects associated with folate depletion and in some instances these manifestations rather than anemia dominate the clinical picture.

Severe chronic malnutrition is a relatively uncommon disorder in the United States at present. Most patients so affected usually have a variety of other associated illnesses. Some have severe generalized malabsorption syndromes. Even in severely malnourished humans, rarely is anemia so severe as to require transfusion. It may be useful to administer serum albumin judiciously to assist in the mobilization of edema, but the primary problem in these patients is to reestablish a level of normal nutrition which will replete all of the associated nutritional deficiencies which they manifest.

Hemolytic Anemias

Chronic transfusion therapy is rarely necessary in this diverse group of patients. Severe traumatic hemolytic anemia secondary to cardiac abnormalities or artificial heart valves may be an infrequent exception to this generalization. These patients may require a program of minimal transfusion because of already impaired cardiac function which may limit the normal cardiovascular compensations for the anemia that occurs in most patients. They require most careful evaluation from this point of view. Hemolytic anemia patients should not be transfused unless (1) they are demonstrably improved following a trial administration of blood, and (2) it has been found that the rate of blood destruction is not increased to an unacceptable degree by the higher hematocrit.

Hemolysis secondary to chemical or physical agents or to a severe infection, particularly with a clostridial organism, may require acute short-term support by red cell transfusion as a life-saving measure. It should be recognized that the administration of normal red cells to these patients may increase the rate of hemolysis by providing an increased number of susceptible erythrocytes. Thus, the best strategy of transfusion may be to administer repeatedly small amounts of blood, sufficient to support the patient's oxygen transport while efforts are undertaken to control the cause of the acute hemolytic state. If the hemolysis associated with these disorders is severe enough to result in hemoglobinemia, the outlook for the patient is usually grave. Successful management will more likely depend upon interventions which limit the rate of hemolysis rather than the strategy of transfusion.

Transfusion is rarely justified by the phenomenon of hypersplenism alone. In most instances of hypersplenism due to congestive splenomegaly, hemolysis of such severity that the patient becomes seriously anemic does not occur in the absence of other disorders which limit the response of the bone marrow. Patients in whom hypersplenism is secondary to chronic liver disease and portal hypertension may also have chronic or recurrent gastrointestinal blood loss to account in part for their anemia. They should be carefully investigated for this and managed appropriately. Occasionally, the combination of splenic hyperfunction and hemolysis with recurrent blood loss and relatively marginal capability of the marrow to respond to anemia does produce a degree of anemia sufficient to justify transfusion, even chronically.

Anemias Associated with Pregnancy and Delivery

Complications of pregnancy associated with operative procedures or with excessive postpartum blood loss, while fortunately uncommon, can be dealt with in the same way that patients with other similar causes of blood loss are managed. Beyond these indications, transfusion is rarely justified or necessary in the course of even a complicated pregnancy. The megaloblastic anemia of pregnancy, a rare disorder, constitutes a bona fide emergency and requires prompt treatment with folic acid. If the patient's anemia has become so severe as to result in cardiac failure, she can be managed as suggested above in connection with the severe anemias of nutritional deficiency. This is rarely necessary.

In the past, transfusions unfortunately have been used all too frequently to correct mild-to-moderate degrees of postpartum anemia. The theory justifying this practice was that the new mother, going home with a newborn, would not tolerate anemia. At the very least, she would not "feel well" and would be less able to cope with her responsibilities as a mother. The practice of transfusing such patients unfortunately ignores an assessment of the real risks of transfusion. If there is no reason to believe that the patient will not adequately recover her red cell mass in a period of 6 weeks there is no reason to consider transfusing the postpartum patient. If, for example, the patient's anemia is so severe that she is symptomatic and truly limited from the physiological point of view, the probability is very high that there are other etiological factors involved which require investigation in depth. It can now be said with confidence that transfusing the postpartum patient without greater indication than a moderate level of tolerable symptoms does not justify the risk of transfusion.

Also, in the past, before the recognition of the phenomena of hydremia of pregnancy with hemodilution and a physiological fall in hematocrit during the last trimester, some patients were transfused in anticipation of delivery. Such patients, of course, are not truly anemic in that their total body red cell mass is usually within normal limits. The practice of transfusing such patients, or even treating them for "anemia" with a variety of hematinics, is presently unacceptable. The pregnant patient usually requires some iron supplementation in the diet, but for reasons other than anemia. She must transfer iron to the developing fetus and prepare for some iron loss during the period of lactation as well as a small amount of blood loss at the time of delivery. Fortunately, both of these practices of transfusing the pregnant woman either pre- or postpartum are now declining rapidly in the United States.

REFERENCES

1. Mollison, P.L.: Blood Transfusion in Clinical Medicine, 4th Ed. Blackwell, London, p. 134.
2. Berlin, N.I.: Laboratory evaluation of erythrokinetics. In: Hematology, 2nd ed. Williams, W., Beutler, E., Erslev, A., and Rundles,

W., eds. McGraw-Hill, New York, 1977, p. 237.

3. Erslev, A.: Erythrokinetics, ibid., 1977, p. 1621.

4. Enelow, A. J. and Adler, L. McK.: Basic Interviewing. In: Enelow, A.J., Swisher, S.N.: Interviewing and Patient Care, 2nd ed. Oxford University Press, New York, Oxford, 1979, p. 35.

5. Elwood, P.C., Waters, W.E., Greene, W.J.W., Sweetnam, P., and Wood, M.M.: Symptoms and circulating haemoglobin level. J. Chron. Dis. 21:615, 1969.

6. Wood, M.M. and Elwood, P.C.: Symptoms of iron deficiency: A community survey. Br. J. Prev. Soc. Med. 20:117, 1966.

7. Elwood, P.C. and Wood, M.M.: Effect of oral iron therapy on the symptoms of anemia. Br. J. Prev. Soc. Med. 20:172, 1966.

8. Kohn, L.A.: Unpublished observations communicated to authors.

9. Rodman, T., Clare, H.P., and Purcell, M.K.: Oxyhemoglobin dissociation curve in anemia. Ann. Intern. Med. 52:295, 1960.

10. Edwards, M.J., Novy, M.J., Walters, C.L., and Metcalfe, J.: Improved oxygen release: An adaptation of mature red cells to hypoxia. J. Clin. Invest. 47:1851, 1969.

11. Torrance, J., Jacobs, P., Lenfant, C., and Finch, C.A.: Intraerythrocytic adaptation to anemia. Blood 34:843, 1969.

12. Bellinghaus, A.J. and Grimes, A.J.: Red cell 2,3-diphosphoglycerate. Br. J. Haematol. 25:555, 1973.

13. Oski, F.A., Gottlieb, A.J., Miller, W.W., and Delivoria-Papadopoulas, M.: The effects of deoxygenation of adult and fetal hemoglobin on the synthesis of red cell 2,3-diphosphoglycerates and its *in vivo* consequences. J. Clin. Invest. 49:400, 1970.

14. Finch, C.A. and Lenfant, C.: Oxygen transport in man. N. Engl. J. Med. 286:407, 1972.

15. Oski, F.A., Gottlieb, A.J., Delivoria-Papadapoulas, M., and Miller, W.W.: Red Cell 2,3-diphosphoglycerate Levels in Subjects with Chronic Hypoxemia. N. Engl. J. Med. 280:1165, 1969.

16. Oski, F.A., Marshall, B.E., Cohen, P.J., Sugerman, H.H., and Miller, L.D.: Exercise with anemia: The role of the left-shifted on right-shifted oxygen-hemoglobin equilibrium curve. Ann. Intern. Med. 74:44, 1971.

17. Riggs, A.: Functional properties of hemoglobins. Physiol. Rev. 45:619, 1965.

18. Roy, S.B., Bhatia, M.L., Mathur, V.S., and Virmani, S.: Hemodynamic effects of chronic severe anemia. Circulation 28:346, 1963.

19. Roy, S.B., Bhatia, M.L., and Joseph, G.: Determinants and distribution of high cardiac output in chronic severe anemia. Indian Heart J. 18:325, 1966.

20. Bartels, E.C.: Anemia as the cause of severe congestive heart failure. Ann. Intern. Med. 11:400, 1937.

21. Whitaker, W.: Some Effects of Severe Chronic Anemia on the Circulatory System. Quart. J. Med. 25:175, 1956.

22. Zoll, P.M., Wessler, S., and Blumgart, H.L.: Angina pectoris: Clinical and pathological correlation. Am. J. Med. 11:331, 1951.

23. Graettinger, J.S., Parsons, R.L., and Campbell, J.A.: A correlation of clinical and hemodynamic studies in patients with mild and severe anemia with and without congestive heart failure. Ann. Intern. Med. 58:617, 1963.

24. Varat, M.A., Adolph, R.J., and Fowler, N.O.: Cardiovascular effects of anemia. Am. Heart J. 83:415, 1972.

25. Bradley, S.E. and Bradley, G.P.: Renal function during chronic anemia in man. Blood 2:192, 1947.

26. Fowler, N.O., Franch, R.H., and Bloom, W.L.: Hemodynamic effects of anemia with and without plasma volume expansion. Circulat. Res. 4:319, 1956.

27. Ryan, J.M. and Hickam, J.B.: The alveolar-arterial oxygen pressure gradient in anemia. J. Clin. Invest. 31:188, 1952.

28. Sproule, B.J., Mitchell, J.H., and Miller, W.F.: Cardiopulmonary physiological responses to heavy exercise in patients with anemia. J. Clin. Invest. 39:378, 1960.

29. Blumgart, H.L. and Altschule, M.D.: Clinical sigificance of cardiac and respiratory adjustments in chronic anemia. Blood 3:329, 1948.

30. Andersen, H.T. and Barkve, H.: Iron deficiency and muscular work performance. An evaluation of the cardio-respiratory function of iron deficient subjects with and without anaemia. Scand. J. Clin. Lab. Invest. 25:Suppl. 114, 1970.

31. Arlina, A.R., Unger, R.J., and Rosky, M.: Post-transfusion alloimmunization in patients

with sickle cell disease. Am. J. Hematol. 5:101, 1978.

32. Propper, R.D., Button, L.N., and Nathan, D.G.: New approaches to the transfusion management of thalassemia. Blood 55:55, 1980.

33. Rosenbaum, D.L., Murphy, G.W., and Swisher, S.N.: Hemodynamic studies of the portal circulation in myeloid metaplasia. Am. J. Med. 41:360, 1966.

34. Beck, W.S.: Folic acid deficiency. In: Hematology, 2nd ed., Williams, W., Beutler, E., Eslev, A., and Rundles, W., eds., McGraw Hill, New York, 1977, p. 334.

35. Das, K., Herbert, V., Colman, N., and Longo, D.L.: Unmasking covert folate deficiency in iron-deficient subjects with neutrophil hypersegmentation: IU suppression tests on lymphocytes and bone marrow. Br. J. Haematol. 39:357, 1978.

36. Becker, C.E., MacGregor, R.R., and Walker, K.S.: Fatal anaphylaxis after intramuscular iron dextran. Ann. Intern. Med. 65:745, 1966.

37. Jacobs, J.: Death due to iron parenterally. So. Med. J. 62:216, 1969.

38. Samson, D.C., Swisher, S.N., Christian, R.M., and Engel, G.L.: Cerebral metabolic disturbance and delerium in pernicious anemia: Clinical and electroencephalographic studies. Arch. Int. Med. 90:4, 1952.

31

Blood Transfusion in Acquired Hemolytic Anemias

Lawrence D. Petz, M.D., and Scott N. Swisher, M.D.

AUTOIMMUNE HEMOLYTIC ANEMIAS

Patients with autoimmune hemolytic anemia (AIHA) frequently present with anemia of sufficient severity as to suggest the possible need for blood transfusion. Indeed, when anemia of such severity is discovered, physicians frequently refer a sample of blood to the blood transfusion laboratory while simultaneously initiating diagnostic studies to determine the cause of the anemia. A diagnosis of AIHA is often first made by the blood transfusion service when autoantibodies are detected during performance of the compatibility ("crossmatch") test.

Nowhere in the management of patients with immune hemolytic anemias is the communication between clinician and laboratory personnel more important than in regard to blood transfusion. As with all clinical decisions concerning therapy, the possible benefits must be weighed in relationship to potential risks. The advisability of blood transfusion is related to the severity of the anemia, whether the anemia is rapidly progressive, and especially to the associated clinical findings. However, a clinical decision based on such facts must be tempered by the knowledge that blood transfusion has a greater than usual risk in patients with AIHA.

In this chapter, in regard to AIHA, we first discuss the indications (and lack of indications) for blood transfusion in specific clinical settings, and apply such principles to patients with AIHA. We then describe, from the point of view of practicing clinicians, the nature and clinical significance of the unique risks encountered when transfusion is necessary in a patient with AIHA. In essence, the risks relate to two factors. The autoantibody often complicates the compatibility test and may make it difficult to detect coexisting alloantibodies or to exclude their presence with confidence, thereby increasing the risk of an alloantibody-induced hemolytic transfusion reaction; secondly, the autoantibody itself may cause marked shortening of the survival of donor red cells. In spite of these added risks, we emphasize that blood should never be denied to a patient with a justifiable need (e.g., a progressively severe, life-threatening anemia), even though the compatibility test may be strongly incompatible. On the other hand, in discussing the difficulties faced by laboratory personnel, and adverse reactions to blood transfusion that are unique to patients with acquired hemolytic anemia, we hope to justify the view that frequently the course of lesser risk is to withhold blood transfusions in some settings where the initial clinical judgment would suggest their need.

We next review the principles and give technical details of the methods which should be utilized for the optimal selection of blood for patients with AIHA of various types. Finally, we discuss the optimal volume of blood to be transfused which may be of critical importance in safely treating patients with severe hemolytic anemia, consider the use of warm blood for patients with cold antibody AIHA, and discuss the use of washed red cells, autologous transfusions, and blood substitutes.

GENERAL PRINCIPLES CONCERNING INDICATIONS FOR TRANSFUSION IN ANEMIAS OF DIFFERENT CAUSES

It is useful to compare and contrast the indications for blood transfusion in AIHA with those of several more common causes of anemia which vary in abruptness of onset, alterations in blood volume, and in the need for transfusions. Acute blood loss, severe megaloblastic anemia, and chronic refractory anemias are three examples. In these instances, the requirements for blood transfusion are analogous to that in AIHA in that the most critical aspects of the clinical evaluation are the symptoms and signs resulting from the anemia or hypovolemia. Evidences of probable progression of manifestations of anemia are of crucial importance. The hemoglobin and hematocrit values are of significance but are too often overemphasized as criteria for transfusion in contrast to clinical criteria. The following familiar clinical settings illustrate fundamental principles.

Anemia with Hypovolemia

A patient with hematemesis, melena, a hemoglobin of 9 gm/dl, a blood pressure of 100/60 mm Hg, and a pulse of 128/minute should, of course, be transfused. Such anemia is producing life-threatening signs because of

hypovolemia; the manifestations of hypovolemia (hypotension and tachycardia) indicate that the anemia is acute in onset because compensatory increases in plasma volume will occur in slowly developing anemias, thus keeping total blood volume near normal.[1a] Further, the hematemesis and melena indicate that the anemia and hypovolemia are likely to become progressively and acutely more severe.

The severity of reduction in blood volume must be estimated and managed according to its effect on the cardiovascular system. The evaluation takes place at the bedside, with the assessments of volume loss, transfusion requirements, and response to therapy being made from the signs and symptoms of volume depletion.[2] Normally, the blood volume in an adult male is 69 ml per kg (30 ml RBC per kg and 39 ml plasma per kg); in an adult female, it is 65 ml per kg (25 ml RBC per kg and 40 ml plasma per kg).[3] Most patients can withstand an acute loss of up to 10 to 15 percent of their blood volume (about 750 ml in an adult of average size) without signs of vascular insufficiency. When the loss exceeds 1000 ml, rising to the range of 20 to 30 percent of blood volume, important signs of cardiovascular distress appear. At first, these are limited to tachycardia at rest and postural hypotension.[2] The pulse rate is an unreliable guide to hypovolemia, but a persistent rate of 100 or more per minute without other evident explanation (e.g., fever) may be caused by hypovolemia and suggests that the blood volume is less than 80 percent of normal.[4] A 70-kg patient may compensate for an acute loss of blood volume of up to about 1,500 ml by vasoconstriction and may appear normal if lying flat.[5] However, such a patient is in latent shock and may faint when placed in the upright position. If the systolic blood pressure is below 100 mm Hg as a result of acute blood loss, the blood volume is probably less than 70 percent of normal.[6] Loss of 40 percent of intravascular volume produces overt shock in most patients. Other clinical manifestations of hypovolemia include pallor, sweating, thirst, light-headedness, air-hunger, and restlessness.

TREATABLE ANEMIA OF SLOW ONSET

In contrast to the above example of a patient with acute blood loss, a patient with megaloblastic anemia with a hemoglobin of 8 gm/dl who has normal vital signs, no signs of hypovolemia, and whose symptoms are weakness, lethargy, and palpitations should not be transfused.[1b] The symptomatology and signs do not warrant blood transfusion, and effective and safer therapy is available. The stable vital signs with this level of hemoglobin indicate that the anemia cannot have been acute in onset. Unless there is concomitant evidence of blood loss, there are no indications that the anemia will rapidly become more severe.

REFRACTORY CHRONIC ANEMIA

A third familiar clinical example is that of a patient with a chronic anemia that may be quite severe but is stable and is not correctable by specific therapy (e.g., anemia associated with renal insufficiency, liver disease, carcinoma, chronic rheumatoid arthritis, and "refractory" anemias such as hypoplastic anemia and sideroblastic anemia). Such a patient should not be transfused unless required to correct associated symptoms of marked severity. Transfusions will temporarily improve the anemia and the patient's symptoms; but, if the underlying disease is not improved, anemia of similar severity will recur within weeks. For example, a 70-kg male has a red cell volume of about 2,100 ml (30 ml/kg). If, for convenience, we use a figure of 100 days as the normal red cell life span, he must produce 21 ml of red cells per day. To maintain a hemoglobin of 10 g/dl (about two-thirds of normal) requires 14 ml/day. Freshly obtained donor red cells are of all ages and therefore will have an average life expectancy of 100/2 or 50 days. Thus, the daily requirement of *transfused* red cells to maintain a hemoglobin level of 10 g/dl in a 70-kg male who is making no red cells is 14 × 2 or 28 ml/day or 196 ml/week. A unit of red cells contains about 200 ml, so that an average of one unit per week will need to be transfused. Thus, after transfusion of 3 units of red cells, the hemoglobin will return to the pretransfusion value in 3 weeks. Since transfusion does suppress erythropoiesis,[1b] such estimates often turn out to be clinical realities. The return of the patient's hemoglobin level to pretransfusion levels within weeks is often misinterpreted as an indication of poor survival of transfused red cells and as an indication that the hemoglobin will continue to decline. However, the marrow may be able to maintain a stable hemoglobin at a relatively low level, and optimal management may be the education of the patient to tolerate this degree of anemia rather than to repeatedly transfuse. Chronic transfusion therapy exposes the patient to all of the acute dangers of transfusion and may also result in iron overload and immunologic reactions which make subsequent transfusions more difficult. In some patients, multiple red cell alloantibodies may develop, thus making transfusion therapy much more difficult at a later time of urgent need.

PLACEBO EFFECT OF TRANSFUSION

Physicians should also consider that improvement in symptoms may be related to the strong placebo effect of blood transfusion, and its benefit may be exaggerated by the patient or by the physician himself. Patients with chronic anemia have compensatory increases in plasma volume, cardiovascular compensatory mechanisms, and increased red cell 2,3-diphosphoglycerate (2,3-DPG) which results in improved oxygen delivery to tissues, so that they usually manage quite well. For example, the results of controlled studies have indicated that patients with iron deficiency anemia with hemoglobin levels of 8 g per dl had no change in symptoms as a result of iron therapy and improvement in hemoglobin.[7-10] Indeed, large studies have failed to demonstrate any evidence of an association between hemoglobin levels above 8 g per dl and the severity of symptoms.[8,11]

THE DECISION TO TRANSFUSE

Nevertheless, it is certainly true that some patients with chronic severe anemia must be transfused to sustain a reasonable level of activity. Although it is impossible to give strict criteria for transfusion of such patients, some guidelines should be considered.

If the hemoglobin is above 10 g/dl, transfusion therapy for a chronic stable anemia is almost never indicated. If the patient's hemoglobin is stable at a level of 8 to 10 g/dl, transfusion is rarely necessary or desirable. Such patients may have mild symptoms, such as some decrease in exercise tolerance, but will do better ultimately if a program of chronic transfusions is not undertaken. For anemias of greater severity (hemoglobin of 5 to 8 g/dl), symptoms of anemia such as fatigue, a more marked decrease in exercise tolerance, and palpitations will usually be present and may prove intolerable to some patients. It is in this group of patients that clinical judgment is most critical. Many, but by no means all, such patients can make an adequate adjustment to their decreased exercise tolerance and thus avoid the problems associated with a program of chronic transfusion. At a level of hemoglobin below 5 g/dl, most patients will require repeated transfusions; but, even here, such a program must be embarked upon reluctantly and is not always necessary. Indeed, patients with chronic renal failure undergoing dialysis regularly sustain normal organ function in the presence of hemoglobin levels of 3 or 4 g/dl.[12] (See Ch. 30.)

These rather fundamental examples are cited as a basis for the following discussion which emphasizes that, although physicians may be somewhat ill at ease in the rather unfamiliar setting of AIHA, similar principles should be utilized in formulating a clinical decision concerning the advisability of blood transfusion. Thus, the clinician should assess the patient's symptoms and signs caused by the anemia, the acuteness of the hemolysis, the rapidity of progression of the anemia, and the probable effectiveness of therapy other than transfusion.

The clinical decision should be tempered by an assessment of the increased risk of transfusion, which varies depending on the type and severity of the hemolytic anemia, the difficulties imposed on the laboratory by the patient's autoantibodies, and the patient's history of prior transfusions and pregnancies.

ASSESSING THE NEED FOR TRANSFUSION IN AIHA

ASSESSING THE ACUTENESS OF ONSET AND RAPIDITY OF PROGRESSION OF AIHA

When a patient presents with AIHA and a moderately severe anemia, it is not possible to predict with certainty whether or not the anemia will rapidly become more severe. Thus, serial determinations of the hemoglobin and hematocrit should be performed at intervals determined by the results of the evaluation of the severity of the illness. In particular, the physician should note whether the patient appears acutely ill with symptoms attributable to acute hemolysis such as fever, malaise, and pain in the back, abdomen, and legs.[13] The presence or absence of hemoglobinuria and hemoglobinemia should be noted. These findings are usually manifestations of severe hemolysis.

If a patient is acutely ill, has a history of an abrupt onset of the illness, or has grossly evident hemoglobinuria, the hematocrit should be tested every 2 to 4 hours initially, whereas in less acutely ill patients, initial testing may be at 12 to 24-hour intervals. The frequency of testing may soon be decreased if the severity of the anemia proves to be essentially constant. In some cases of fulminant hemolysis, a significant fall in the hematocrit may occur within hours, whereas in a majority of patients with AIHA the anemia is essentially stable or only slowly progressive over a period of days.

THE APPROPRIATE USE OF BLOOD IN VARIOUS CLINICAL SETTINGS IN PATIENTS WITH AIHA

Severe but Stable Anemia During Initial Evaluation

Patients with an anemia that is essentially stable during the initial period of evaluation generally should not be transfused at this point even though they may have such symptoms as a marked decrease in exercise tolerance and palpitations with exertion. Even severe anemia found in AIHA is generally well tolerated, even in the elderly, if bed rest is employed.[14] Furthermore, response to therapy or spontaneous improvement may be rapid. For example, 50 percent of patients with warm antibody autoimmune hemolytic anemia will respond to adequate doses of corticosteroids during the first week of therapy,[14] and acute paroxysmal cold hemoglobinuria seldom lasts longer than 7 to 10 days.[15]

Progressively Severe Anemia

Some patients do, however, have an anemia that is steadily progressive in severity, thus leading to the development of symptoms of hypoxemia. Indeed, as emphasized by Pirofsky,[15a] progression of the severity of anemia frequently occurs in patients with warm antibody AIHA. Among 213 patients, the lowest hematocrit ranged from 7.5 percent to 41.5 percent, but with a median value of only 19 percent. A hematocrit of 15 percent or less

was observed in 49 of the patients! Even in severely anemic patients, there usually is no evidence of vascular collapse because blood volume remains near normal, but progressively more severe angina and cardiac decompensation may occur. Extremely anemic patients (hematocrit of 12 percent or hemoglobin of 4 g/dl) may develop neurological signs beginning as marked lethargy and weakness, and progressing to somnolence, mental confusion, obtundation, and death. In patients with anemia of such severity (or in those patients whose rate of progression of anemia indicates that this point will likely be reached), red cells are urgently needed and nothing can substitute for their use, although oxygen should also be administered. In the management of these acutely ill patients who have not yet had time to respond to therapy, the use of packed red cells sufficient to maintain a modest increase in hematocrit until therapy of the AIHA becomes effective is probably optimal (see below, *Optimal Volume of Blood to Be Transfused to Patients with AIHA*).

In some patients, in spite of adequate therapy, hemolysis proceeds chronically at a rate greater than that of their red cell production, resulting in a relentlessly progressive anemia. In this situation, chronic transfusion is necessary to sustain life, and the attendant risks, cost, and inconvenience must be accepted.

Chronic Stable Anemia

Many patients (especially those with cold agglutinin disease) are able to partially compensate for their shortened red cell survival and maintain a relatively stable (albeit occasionally quite severe) degree of anemia. In such patients, where transfusion may be considered as a means of relieving symptoms, the advantages and disadvantages of such management are similar to those with other "refractory anemias" and must be very carefully weighed. (Also see Ch. 30.)

As in any patient with chronic anemia,

transfusions should be given as packed red cells, although a leukocyte-poor red cell preparation may ultimately be required to prevent repeated febrile reactions.

Transfusions will at least partially suppress erythropoiesis, and the frequency of transfusions will need to be determined arbitrarily and will depend on the rate of hemolysis. It is usually convenient to give two or three units of packed red cells at a time when necessary. It is not advisable to completely correct the anemia; transfusion to a level of hemoglobin of 8 to 11 g/dl is perhaps optimal.

Fulminant Hemolytic Anemia

Least common among the indications for transfusion in immune hemolytic anemia is rapidly progressive anemia caused by acute massive hemolysis. Nevertheless, such fulminant hemolysis does occur, and such patients may even be hypotensive. Signs of shock should be sought in patients with acute hemolytic anemia in a manner similar to that described above regarding acute blood loss.

Patients who have AIHA of such severity can be expected to have gross evidences of hemolysis, particularly hemoglobinuria and hemoglobinemia. Diagnoses such as Clostridium perfringens (welchii) septicemia, and drug-induced immune hemolytic anemia caused by drug-antibody immune complexes (see below) should also be quickly investigated. The onset may be so acute that a reticulocytosis may not be present, since the bone marrow may not have had time to compensate. Indeed, a maximal increase in the reticulocyte count in response to a sudden decrease in red cell mass requires 7 to 10 days.[2]

Although such patients are uncommon, transfusion is urgent. If manifestations of shock are present, the immediate aim of transfusion is improvement in vital signs, which may be temporarily restored by the use of electrolyte or colloid solutions. Simultaneously, the physician should communicate a sense of urgency to the blood transfusion

laboratory (a maneuver rarely omitted) to find optimal red cells for transfusion. Rarely will these red cells be "compatible" in the crossmatch; nevertheless, their use is mandatory in this acutely life-threatening setting.

THE RISKS OF TRANSFUSION IN PATIENTS WITH AIHA

In AIHA, the risks of blood transfusion beyond the usual risks relate to the presence of the patient's red cell autoantibody. Autoantibodies usually will react with all normal red cells so that transfused cells usually have a shorter than normal life span. This cannot be avoided, assuming that optimal therapeutic measures are being utilized to treat the AIHA. The red cell autoantibody may react strongly in vitro (e.g., 2+ to 4+ by indirect antiglobulin test) with all available donor red cells to be transfused, thus making it impossible to obtain compatible blood for transfusion. Nevertheless, acute symptomatic transfusion reactions occur only infrequently. Subsequent survival is about as good as the patient's own red cells, and the net result is that transfusion generally causes temporary benefit. Thus, the reactivity in vivo of the autoantibody causes shortened survival of transfused red cells but usually does not contribute greatly to the acute risk of transfusion.

Although this is generally true, if the patient has very severe hemolysis, the autoantibody may cause striking destruction of transfused RBC, resulting in no benefit[16] or in dangerous degrees of hemolysis with hemoglobinemia, hemoglobinuria, renal failure,[17] and clinical deterioration.[18] This is probably particularly true if relatively large volumes of blood are given (see below: Optimal Volume of Blood to be Transfused).

In some patients, the autoantibody demonstrates clinically significant "relative specificity" in that it reacts stronger with red cells bearing certain common Rh antigens than with red cells lacking these antigens. Tests for determining autoantibody "relative specificity" should be performed, since red cells lacking the more strongly reactive antigen may survive significantly better than cells containing the more reactive antigen.

Further, when the patient's serum reacts with all red cells in routine crossmatch and antibody identification tests, the blood transfusion laboratory must utilize additional techniques in an attempt to demonstrate red cell antibodies other than the autoantibody. This is a critical aspect of selection of donor blood because, if the patient has previously been transfused or has been pregnant, and has developed red cell alloantibodies (e.g., anti-Rh, anti-Kell, anti-Kidd), donor red cells lacking such antigens must be selected for transfusion or a severe alloantibody-induced hemolytic transfusion reaction may ensue.

THE DIFFERENTIAL DIAGNOSIS OF IMMUNE HEMOLYTIC ANEMIAS

The problems relating to blood transfusion in patients with immune hemolytic anemias vary significantly, depending on the specific diagnosis. Table 31-1 lists a classification of acquired immune hemolytic anemias. Some characteristic features of autoimmune and drug-induced immune hemolytic anemias are indicated in Table 31-2. A detailed description of the laboratory tests necessary for definitive diagnosis of these disorders has recently been published[18a] and is briefly summarized in Table 31-3.

THE SELECTION OF DONOR BLOOD FOR TRANSFUSION IN SPECIFIC KINDS OF AIHA

WARM ANTIBODY AUTOIMMUNE HEMOLYTIC ANEMIA

The selection of blood for transfusion to patients with warm antibody AIHA is one of the most difficult tasks faced by a blood transfu-

sion laboratory. Also, laboratories vary in their resources, so that methods that are readily available in reference laboratories may not be feasible in many hospital blood banks. Thus, absorption of aliquots of a patient's serum with red cells of various types (e.g., Jk^a-negative, Fy^a-negative, and Kell-negative) may present no problem for reference laboratories, but it may be very impractical for hospital blood banks to obtain adequate supplies of the appropriate cells.

In addition, the problems presented by individual patients with warm antibody AIHA vary greatly. For example, if a patient has not been recently transfused, determination of the patient's Rh phenotype and the use of autoabsorption techniques are practical and are of significant value. However, some patients may be transferred to referral centers after first being transfused, in which case determining the Rh phenotype of the patient and the use of autoabsorption techniques may be unreliable.

The approach to selection of donor blood that is described below considers each of these factors. First, the various serologic techniques that are useful for red cell typing and alloantibody detection are described. Secondly, we indicate practical methods for determination of autoantibody specificity within the Rh system, and discuss the significance of the specificity in relation to blood transfusion. Finally, all of this information is used as the basis of making specific recommendations for the most appropriate and practical approaches to the selection of donor blood in various clinical settings.

ABO and Rh Grouping

ABO. There is usually no problem in determining the ABO and Rh type of patients with autoimmune hemolytic anemia if certain rules are followed; however, if these rules are not followed, serious errors can occur.

Because cold autoagglutinins reactive at room temperature are present in approximately 30 percent of the patients having

Table 31-1. Classification of Immune Hemolytic Anemias

I. Autoimmune Hemolytic Anemias (AIHA)
    A. Warm Antibody AIHA
        1. Idiopathic
        2. Secondary (chronic lymphocytic leukemia, lymphomas, systemic lupus erythematosus, etc.)
    B. Cold Agglutinin Syndrome
        1. Idiopathic
        2. Secondary
            a. Mycoplasma pneumoniae infection, infectious mononucleosis, virus infections
            b. Lymphoreticular malignancies
    C. Paroxysmal Cold Hemoglobinuria
        1. Idiopathic
        2. Secondary
            a. Viral syndromes
            b. Syphilis
    D. Atypical AIHA
        1. Antiglobulin test negative AIHA
        2. Miscellaneous and unclassifiable
II. Drug-Induced Immune Hemolytic Anemia
    A Immune Complex Mechanism
    B. Drug Adsorption Mechanism
    C. Drug-Induced AIHA

warm antibody autoimmune hemolytic anemia, the blood samples should preferably have been separated initially at 37° C and washed with warm saline before attempting grouping.

The cells are tested in the usual fashion with anti-A, anti-B, and anti-A,B, but a negative control of 5 to 10 percent albumin should also be used. This control should be compared with the tests; if positive, it indicates either nondispersed autoagglutination or spontaneous agglutination of heavily sensitized cells in albumin. Rarely, it may be necessary to wash the patient's cells using 45° C saline or to allow a short period of elution at 45° C before reliable typing can be attained.

Table 31-2. Some Characteristic Features of Autoimmune and Drug-Induced Immune Hemolytic Anemias

  I. Warm Antibody ATHA
    A. Clinical manifestations: Variable, usually symptoms of anemia, occasionally acute hemolytic syndrome
    B. Prognosis: Fair, with significant mortality
    C. Therapy: Steroids; splenectomy; immunosuppressive drugs
 II. Cold Agglutinin Syndrome
    A. Clinical manifestations: Moderate chronic hemolytic anemia in middle-aged or elderly person, often with signs and symptoms exacerbated by cold
    B. Prognosis: Good, usually a chronic and quite stable anemia
    C. Therapy: Avoid cold exposure; chlorambucil
III. Paroxysmal Cold Hemoglobinuria
    A. Clinical manifestations: Acute hemolytic anemia, often with hemoglobinuria, particularly in a child with history of recent viral or viral-like illness
    B. Prognosis: Excellent after initial stormy course
    C. Therapy: Not well defined; steroids empirically and transfusions if required
IV. Drug-Induced Immune Hemolytic Anemia
    A. Clinical manifestations: Variable, most commonly subacute in onset, but occasionally acute hemolytic syndrome
    B. Prognosis: Excellent
    C. Therapy: Stop drug; occasionally, a short course of steroids empirically

(Petz, L.D. and Garratty, G.: Acquired Immune Hemolytic Anemias. Churchill Livingstone, New York, 1980.)

Table 31-3. Classification and Differential Diagnosis of the Autoimmune Hemolytic Anemias

	Cells			Serum	
	Direct Antiglobulin Test	Eluate	Immunoglobulin Type	Serologic Characteristics	Specificity
Warm AIHA; about 80% of patients.	IgG (no complement) 20% IgG and complement 67% Complement (no IgG) 13%	IgG antibody	IgG (sometimes IgA or IgM present in addition, rarely alone)	Reacting by indirect antiglobulin test: 57% Agglutinating enzyme treated cells (37°C): 90% Hemolyzing enzyme treated cells (37°C): 13% Agglutinating untreated cells (20°C): 35% Agglutinating or hemolyzing untreated cells (37°C): (5%)	Usually within Rh system but often combined with a "non-specific" element. Other specificities include LW, U, Wr[b], En[a], I[T], K.
Cold agglutinin syndrome; about 18% of patients	Complement alone	No activity	IgM	High titer cold antibody (usually >1024 at 4°C). Reacts up to 30°C. Monoclonal protein (κ light chain) in the chronic disease.	Usually anti-I but can be anti-i or anti-Pr (very rare)
Paroxysmal cold hemoglobinuria; about 2% of patients	Complement alone (IgG cold antibody elutes off RBC at 37°C, e.g., in vivo, or even when RBC are washed at room temperature)	No activity	IgG	Potent hemolysin but will also agglutinate normal cells. Said to be biphasic (i.e., sensitizes cells in cold and then hemolyzes them when moved to 37°C). Usually only sensitizes cells up to 15°C.	Anti-P (i.e., only negative with p or P[k] cells)

(Petz, L.D. and Garratty, G: Acquired Immune Hemolytic Anemias. Churchill Livingstone, New York, 1980.)

Also, the patient's serum is tested against A, B, O, and his own cells as usual, although it may be necessary to perform these serum typings at 37° C if cold autoagglutination is simultaneously present. Problems in ABO typing patients with warm type autoimmune hemolytic anemia are not common.

Rh. If the cells have been separated and washed at 37° C, the main problem is that the cells may agglutinate spontaneously with the addition of albumin alone. This is particularly common if the patient's red cells are heavily sensitized with antibody as indicated by a strongly positive direct antiglobulin test. Therefore, antisera for "saline tube test" should always be used. Unfortunately, many commercial companies add a small amount of albumin (normally 5 to 10 percent) and/or other potentiating media to such sera, and therefore the patient's cells should always be added to albumin (e.g., 6 percent) as a negative control. An ideal negative control is the actual diluent that the manufacturer has used to dilute the antisera, but this diluent is not readily available for "saline tube test" reagents. If antisera fortified with albumin must be used (i.e., "slide and rapid tube" reagents), it is important that the diluent supplied by the same manufacturer of the antiserum be used as a negative control.

Alternatively, chemically reduced typing reagents may be used. These reagents allow for accurate typing by direct agglutination tests, even in patients who have a positive direct antiglobulin test.

If red cells are sensitized with complement but no IgG, the cells will not spontaneously agglutinate in the presence of albumin. Thus, the cheaper and more available slide and rapid tube reagents can usually be used safely.

Typing Red Cells for Antigens When Only Antiglobulin Test Reactive Antisera Are Available

Sometimes, only antiglobulin test reactive antisera are available for typing red cells for certain antigens (e.g., Duffy and Kidd). When patients have a strongly positive direct antiglobulin test, two approaches to typing can be used: (1) heating the patient's red cells to dissociate red cell-bound antibody, and (2) differential absorption procedures.

Heating Patient's Red Cells to Dissociate Red Cell-Bound Antibody

Heating red cells for 5 to 30 minutes at 45° C, or for 3 to 10 minutes at 50° C, sometimes will dissociate enough bound antibody to allow the red cells to be typed by strongly reactive antisera. Occasionally, one must heat the cells for about 3 to 5 minutes at 51 to 56° C. The main disadvantages of this method are that hemolysis often occurs, and red cell antigens may become weakened when they are heated above 37° C. This is particularly true at temperatures above 45° C. The degree of weakening depends on the antigens involved, the temperature, and the length of incubation. It is best to heat the cells for the shortest time at the lowest temperature that is effective. Unfortunately, heating at 45° C is not usually successful if the direct antiglobulin test is strongly positive; temperatures of at least 50° C must be used.

The direct antiglobulin test need not be made strictly negative, but, if possible, one should reduce it to 1+ to 1½+ at the strongest. This will allow for accurate typing providing that the typing sera react 3 to 4+ with positive controls. It is imperative that heterozygote (i.e., weakly positive) controls are heated under exactly the same conditions as the test red cells. It is best to try 45° C first; then, if the direct antiglobulin test is not reduced sufficiently, to try 50° C; and, finally, 51 to 56° C.

Unfortunately, many commercial antisera react rather weakly (2+) using the indirect antiglobulin technique, especially against red cells heterozygous for the antigen. This makes typing virtually impossible using the heat elution methodology unless the elution results in a negative or a very weakly positive direct antiglobulin test. When dealing with red cells that give a very strongly positive direct antiglobulin test, it is rare to be able to reduce the reactivity enough to perform reliable antigen typing with such weakly reactive typing reagents.

Differential Absorption Procedures. Equal aliquots of antisera and washed packed red cells—both positive (heterozygote and homozygote, preferably) and negative for the appropriate antigen—are incubated at 37° C, and the activity of the supernatant absorbed sera is compared with the absorbed sera from a similar mixture of the patient's red cells and the antisera. It is wise to titrate the absorbed serum against an appropriately positive red cell. If the patient's red cells contain the antigen—e.g., Jk^a—then the red cells will absorb antibody from the anti-Jk^a typing serum, leaving a lower titer. Heterozygote cells—Jk(a+b+)—will absorb some (or all) of the antibody, and homozygote cells—Jk(a+b−)—will be expected to absorb the antibody even more readily. Red cells lacking the appropriate antigen—i.e., Jk(a−)—will not absorb any anti-Jk^a; thus, the activity of the antibody will not be significantly changed after absorption. Titration scores of the absorbed sera from the control cells can be compared with those obtained using the patient's red cells for the absorption (see Table 31-4). Although this method is tedious and time-consuming, it will yield reliable results if carefully performed.

These methods can, of course, be used for Rh phenotyping if "saline tube test" antisera are not available and spontaneous agglutination is occurring using the "slide and rapid tube test" reagents.

Detection of Alloantibodies

If the patient's autoantibody reacts with all normal red cells, several techniques may be performed in order to detect alloantibodies which may also be present.

Comparison of Direct and Indirect Antiglobulin Tests. A comparison of the strength of reactivity of the direct and indirect antiglobulin tests sometimes affords extremely valuable information.

In patients with warm antibody AIHA, the indirect antiglobulin test caused by autoantibody is generally weaker than the direct antiglobulin test. Apparently, most of the antibody is absorbed to the patient's red cells in vivo. A coexisting alloantibody will not, of course, be absorbed by the patient's red cells, and may result in a strongly positive indirect antiglobulin test. Thus, if the indirect antiglobulin test is significantly stronger than the direct antiglobulin test, the presence of an alloantibody is highly suspect.

If the direct antiglobulin test is 4+, or if it is equal to or stronger than the indirect antiglobulin test, no conclusion can be reached concerning the presence or absence of alloantibodies.

Table 31-4. Jk^a Typing of Patient with Positive Direct Antiglobulin Test Using Differential Absorption

Red Cells Used to Absorb Anti-Jk^a Typing Serum	Dilutions of Absorbed Anti-Jk^a Tested Against Jk (a+b+) Red Cells*						Score
	1	2	4	8	16	32	
Jk(a+b+)	2+	1+	1+	½+	0	0	16
Jk(a+b−)	1+	1+	0	0	0	0	8
Jk(a−b+)	3+	3+	2+	2+	1+	0	32
Patient's	2+	1+	0	0	0	0	10

* These results indicate that the patient is probably Jk(a+).

(Petz, L.D. and Garratty, G.: Acquired Immune Hemolytic Anemias. Churchill Livingstone, New York, 1980.)

Testing of Patient's Serum Against a Red Cell Panel. If the screening tests for serum antibody reveal an antibody reactive at 37° C, the serum should be tested against a panel of phenotyped cells, as is routine in any blood bank determining specificities of alloantibodies. If a weakly reactive autoantibody and a strongly reactive alloantibody are present, the differences in the strength of the reaction of various cells of the panel will make this evident. For example, Table 31-5 shows a strong anti-Jk^a together with a weak autoantibody.

However, one has no assurance that a patient's alloantibody will react more strongly than the autoantibody; thus, additional tests to detect alloantibody are necessary.

Warm Autoabsorption Technique. The best technique currently available for determining if alloantibodies are present in addition to autoantibodies is to absorb the autoantibody from the patient's serum at 37° C using the patient's own RBC after first eluting some of the autoantibody. A simple elution-autoabsorption method was described in 1963 by Allen.[18b] This procedure was also suggested by Dorner, Parker, and Chaplin[19] and seemed to us to be a logical approach.[20] The technique may be modified by enzyme treatment of the patient's red cells after the elution procedure.[21] After absorption of the autoantibodies, the serum can then be tested for alloantibodies, since alloantibodies will, of course, not be absorbed onto the patient's own RBC. Details of the technique are listed in Table 31-6 and in Fig. 31-1.

Most autoantibodies have indirect antiglobulin test titers less than 16, and two autoabsorptions will remove all autoantibody, leaving any alloantibody present in the serum. If the autoantibody titer is higher than 16 by the indirect antiglobulin test, more autoabsorptions may be necessary to remove all autoantibody. If the autoantibody titer is not high, enzyme treatment of the eluted red cells is not necessary. Indeed, since the ratio of cells and serum is different in the in vitro absorption procedure than it is in vivo, autoabsorption without prior elution of the autoantibody (with or without enzyme treatment of the red cells) may suffice, particularly if the direct antiglobulin test is not strongly positive.

Following the autoabsorptions, the absorbed serum is retested. If a negative reaction is obtained, it is assumed that all the serum reactions were due to autoantibody. If a positive reaction still occurs, the absorbed serum should be tested against a panel of red cells to determine whether alloantibody is present or whether autoantibody is still present, thus requiring further warm autoabsorptions.

At the 1976 American Association of Blood Banks meeting, Morel and coworkers[21] presented data on 20 patients who had 3 + or 4+ direct antiglobulin tests, and indirect antiglobulin tests of 1+ to 4+. Twelve patients had autoantibodies that could be completely removed by two autoabsorptions. Eight other patients were shown to have alloantibodies present in addition to autoantibodies. The specificities involved were anti-E (three patients), anti-V^w (one patient), anti-c + E (two patients), anti-C^w (one patient), and anti-E + K (one patient).

Since the warm autoabsorption technique is so useful, we recommend storing some of the patient's red cells obtained at the time of the first transfusion episode so that they may be used in future autoabsorptions should continued transfusions be required. The red cells are best stored in ACD, CPD, or in the frozen state if facilities are available.

The Matuhasi-Ogata phenomenon may theoretically limit the usefulness of the warm autoabsorption technique (or the differential absorption technique described later). Matuhasi and Ogata suggested that antibodies of one specificity may adhere to antigen-antibody complexes of a different specificity.[22-25] Thus, one could envision the absorption of alloantibody onto red cells that are used to absorb autoantibody from the patient's serum. Experience indicates, however, that alloantibodies are indeed detectable after ab-

Table 31-5. Serum Containing Allo Anti-Jk^a and an Undefined Autoantibody When Reacted with a Panel of Red Cells

Donor No.	Rh Phenotype	Rh								Kell						Duffy		Kidd		Lewis		MNS				P	Lutheran		Sex Linked	Results		
		C	D	E	c	e	f	C^w	V	K	k	Kp^a	Kp^b	Js^a	Js^b	Fy^a	Fy^b	Jk^a	Jk^b	Le^a	Le^b	M	N	S	s	P1	Lu^a	Lu^b	Xg^a	IS	37°C	IAT
1	rr	0	0	0	+	+	+	0	0	0	0	0	0	0	+	+	0	+	+	+	0	+	0	+	0	0	0	+	+	0	0	3+
2	rr	0	0	0	+	+	+	0	0	0	+	0	+	0	+	0	+	+	+	0	+	0	+	0	0	+	0	+	+	0	0	3+
3	rr	0	0	0	+	+	+	0	0	+	0	0	+	0	+	+	+	+	0	+	0	0	+	+	+	+	+	+	+	0	0	3+
4	rr	+	0	0	+	+	+	0	0	+	0	0	+	0	+	0	+	+	+	0	+	+	0	0	+	+	0	+	+	0	0	3+
5	rr	0	0	0	+	+W	+	0	0	0	0	0	+	0	+	+	+	0	+	0	+	+	+	+	+	+	0	+	+	0	0	1+
6	R$_1^w$R$_1$	+	+	0	0	+	0	+	0	+	+	0	+	+	+	0	+	0	+	0	+	+	0	0	+	0	0	+	+	0	0	1+
7	R$_1$R$_1$	+	+	0	0	+	0	0	0	+	+	0	+	0	+	0	0	+	0	0	0	+	+	0	+	+	0	+	0	0	0	3+
8	R$_0$	0	+	0	+	+	+	0	+	+	+	0	+	0	+	+	0	+	+	0	0	+	0	+	+	+	0	+	0	0	0	3+
9	R$_2$R$_2$	0	+	+	+	0	0	0	0	0	+	0	+	0	+	+	0	+	+	0	0	0	+	+	+	+	0	+	0	0	0	3+
10	R$_2$R$_2$	0	+	+	+	0	0	0	0	0	+	0	+	0	+	0	+	0	+	+	0	0	+	0	0	+	0	+	0	0	0	1+

IS = "immediate Spin"; 37°C = Agglutination at 37°C; IAT = Indirect Antiglobulin Test.
Note that 3+ reactions are obtained with Jk^a positive red cells; all other cells yield 1+ reactions.
(Modified after Petz, L.D. and Garratty, G.: Acquired Immune Hemolytic Anemias. Churchill Livingstone, New York. 1980).

Table 31-6. Warm Autoabsorption Technique

a. Wash patient's red cells 4 times.

b. To packed washed cells add saline or 6% albumin (e.g., equal volume).

c. Incubate at 56 °C for 3 to 5 minutes.

d. Remove supernatant (eluate) after centrifugation.

e. Wash red cells 3 times.

f. Enzyme-treat red cells. (We routinely use papain, but ficin works well).

g. Add patient's serum to an equal volume of enzyme-treated cells.

h. Incubate at 37 °C for approximately 30 minutes.

i. Centrifuge. Remove serum.

j. Usually steps g–i must be repeated at least once more.†

k. Test autoabsorbed serum for activity. If negative: antibody was autoantibody. If still positive: antibody may be alloantibody or serum needs further autoabsorptions.

† Most autoantibodies do not have titers higher than 8; in these cases 2 autoabsorptions are usually sufficient. If the titer is higher than 16, 3 or more autoabsorptions may be necessary.

sorption of autoantibodies so that the extent of absorption of the alloantibody, if any, is not sufficient to nullify the usefulness of absorption techniques. Further, methods other than absorption techniques for detecting alloantibodies in the presence of autoantibodies are generally unreliable.

Use of the Warm Autoabsorption Technique in the Recently Transfused Patient. If a patient has been transfused in recent weeks, the warm autoabsorption test may not be absolutely reliable because it would seem possible that donor red cells that are still circulating could absorb alloantibody as well as autoantibody from the patient's serum in vitro. However, even if a patient has been recently transfused, we recommend performing the warm autoabsorption technique (although the differential absorption test is an adequate alternative when feasible—see below) because alloantibody may nevertheless be detected. Indeed, if alloantibody is not absorbed onto the circulating donor red cells in vivo, it may be true that it will not be absorbed in vitro either. However, in vitro conditions may not exactly mimic in vivo conditions—e.g., the ratio of cells and serum are different, and enzyme-treated red cells are usually recommended for in vitro autoabsorption. Therefore, failure to detect alloantibodies by the warm autoabsorption technique in a recently

transfused patient cannot be taken as definitive evidence of their absence.

In the recently transfused patient, it seems logical to omit the enzyme treatment of the red cells used for the warm autoabsorption to more closely mimic in vivo conditions. However, the significance of this recommendation has not been evaluated.

Dilution Technique. Dilutions of the patient's serum are tested against a pool of two screening cells containing most common red cell antigens. A dilution is selected that reacts approximately 1+, and that dilution is then tested against a panel of red cells. This technique is efficient when the alloantibody is of higher titer than the autoantibody, but cannot be used to confidently exclude the presence of alloantibody. Table 31-7 illustrates the results obtained in a case where the alloantibody of anti-E specificity has a titer of 64 and the autoantibody only a titer of 16. When the undiluted serum was tested, all cells reacted 3+, but a 1:64 dilution of the patient's serum only reacted with E-positive red cells.

Differential Absorption Technique. An approach that may be used instead of the warm autoabsorption method is the differential absorption technique—that is, the absorption of the autoantibodies from the patient's serum using red cells of varying

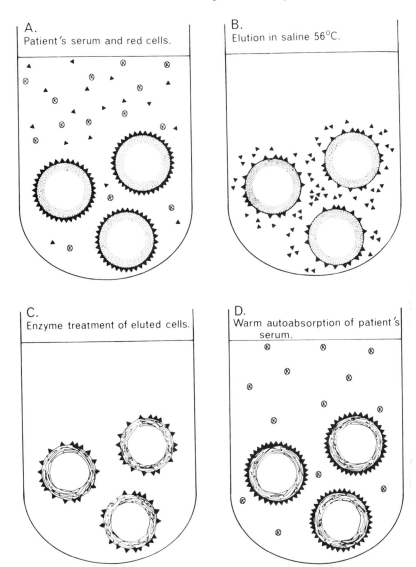

Fig. 31-1. The warm autoabsorption technique. Warm autoantibody molecules are illustrated by solid triangles, and anti-Kell alloantibody molecules are indicated by the symbol K. Fig. 31-1*A* indicates a Kell negative patient with warm antibody autoimmune hemolytic anemia who has formed anti-Kell as a result of previous transfusions. Autoantibody is present on the patient's red cells, and the serum contains both autoantibody and anti-Kell alloantibody. Fig. 31-1*B* indicates the first step of the warm autoabsorption technique. An aliquot of the patient's red cells is washed and incubated in saline at 56 °C for 5 minutes to elute some autoantibody. Fig. 31-1*C* illustrates alteration of the red cell membrane by proteolytic enzymes such as papain or ficin. This augments the ability of the red cells to absorb antibody. These red cells are then used to absorb the patient's serum at 37 ° C. As indicated in Fig. 31-1*D*, the autoantibody is removed from the serum, leaving only the alloantibody, which can then be identified by routine specificity testing against a panel of red cells. (Petz, L.D. and Garratty, G.: Acquired Immune Hemolytic Anemias. Churchill Livingstone, New York, 1980.)

Table 31-7. Results of Dilution Technique to Determine Presence of Alloantibody

	Dilutions of Patient's Serum									
	2	4	8	16	32	64	128	256	512	1024
IAT on screening cells (pooled)	3	3	3	2	2	1	0	0	0	0

	Panel of Group O Cells							
	rr	rr	r'r	R_1R_1	R_1R_2	R_1R_2	R_2R_2	r''r''
Undiluted serum	3	3	3	3	3	3	3	3
Serum diluted 1:64	0	0	0	0	1	1	1½	1½

Agglutination results are graded as 1+ to 4+.

phenotypes. For example, performing an absorption using a Jk^a-negative cell, of a serum containing a warm autoantibody and an anti-Jk^a alloantibody, will remove the autoantibody but not the anti-Jk^a. As with the warm autoabsorption technique, enzyme treatment of the red cells used for absorption will facilitate removal of the autoantibody but is not absolutely nececssary. The only practical limitation to the utilization of the differential absorption technique is obtaining an adequate supply of red cells of appropriate types for the absorption. Ideally, several ml of packed red cells of each type are needed. However, commercially available antibody detection cells and antibody identification panel cells may provide sufficient cell volumes to perform an abbreviated differential absorption using smaller volumes of the appropriate cell type with a concomitantly reduced volume of serum to be absorbed. The major disadvantage of using a reduced amount of serum for the differential absorption technique is that only a small volume of absorbed serum will be available for the subsequent testing for possible alloantibody specificity. For example, it may only be possible to test against three cells for anti-Jk^a specificity—two Jk(a+) and one Jk(a−). Although it is not possible to state definitively that anti-Jk^a is present if the two Jk(a+) cells are reactive and the Jk(a−) cell is not, Jk^a-negative blood should be used for transfusion. Further, anti-Jk^a may be excluded if all three cells give negative reactions with the absorbed serum.

Although this technique may seem hopelessly complicated since hundreds of red cell alloantibodies have been identified, alloantibodies of only a few specificities are responsible for a large majority of hemolytic transfusion reactions. That is, a large percentage of hemolytic transfusion reactions are caused by ABO, Rh, Kell, Kidd, and Fy^a antibodies.[26, 26a]

ABO alloantibodies will present no problem, providing proper cell typing is performed. Further, if the Rh phenotype of the patient is known, hemolytic transfusion reactions caused by Rh alloantibodies can be avoided by using blood of the same Rh phenotype as the patient. Thus, one may detect a large majority of potentially hemolytic alloantibodies by absorbing with several red cells—that is, Kell-negative, Jk^a-negative, Jk^b-negative, and Fy^a-negative. As a modification of this approach one could, for example, omit the absorption with Kell-negative red cells and, instead, select Kell-negative donor red cells for transfusion to assure lack of a Kell-related transfusion reaction. Although this principle could theoretically be extended to the other blood groups as well, it is obviously unrealistic to attempt to secure donor blood that is, for example, Kell-negative, Jk^a-negative, Fy^a-negative, and of the appropriate ABO and Rh type. If the cells used for absorbing are enzyme-treated and the autoantibody titer is less than 16 by indirect antiglobulin test, two absorptions will most likely remove all autoantibody.

In summary, then, in order to detect the most common clinically significant non-Rh alloantibodies, one needs only to absorb the autoantibody from the patient's serum with (enzyme treated) Jk^a-negative, Jk^b-negative, and Fy^a-negative red cells to exclude the presence of these alloantibodies. If no alloantibodies are detected in the absorbed aliquots of the patient's serum, one may then transfuse with donor red cells that are Kell-negative and of the same Rh phenotype as the patient. Although the possible presence of alloantibodies of numerous specificities is ignored, the probability of an alloantibody-induced hemolytic transfusion reaction is minimal.

If the patient's Rh phenotype is not known and cannot be determined accurately because of recent blood transfusion, hemolytic transfusions caused by Rh-related antibodies obviously cannot be avoided by selecting donor red cells of the same phenotype as the patient. In this case, one should also employ differential absorptions using R_1R_1 (CDe/CDe), R_2R_2 (cDE/cDE), and rr (cde/cde) red cells to detect Rh alloantibodies. One can reduce the total number of red cells used for these absorptions and maximize the information gained by selecting R_1R_1, R_2R_2, and rr red cells—all of which are Kell-negative and one of which is Jk^a-negative, one Jk^b-negative, and the other Fy^a-negative.[26b]

Absorption with the rr cells removes anti-c and anti-e; specificities remaining in the absorbed serum are anti-C, anti-D, and anti-E. The R_1R_1 cells absorb anti-C, anti-D, and anti-e; specificities left behind are anti-E and anti-c. The R_2R_2 cells absorb anti-D, anti-E, and anti-c; remaining are anti-C and anti-e. Depending on which other antigens were absent from the red cells used for the autoabsorptions, other important alloantibodies may also be detected in the absorbed serum. For example, the aliquot of serum absorbed with Jk^a-negative red cells may contain anti-Jk^a. Secondary eluates may also be helpful in defining specificities. The choice of red cells to be used may also be influenced by knowledge of the antigenic makeup of the patient's red cells, if known. For example, one may absorb with cells of the same Rh phenotype as the patient. Further, if, on the basis of the cell typing techniques described earlier, one is confident that the patient is Jk(a+), one need not absorb with Jk^a-negative red cells, since

the production of an alloantibody of anti-Jk^a specificity is, of course, impossible.

Although this method is cumbersome, it is the most reliable method to detect alloantibodies in the presence of autoantibodies in those most trying of times when a patient with warm antibody autoimmune hemolytic anemia has been recently transfused and has not had Rh phenotyping performed, and there are no pretransfusion red cells available for use in the warm autoabsorption technique.

Finally, as a note of reassurance, it should be emphasized that the probability of an alloantibody-induced hemolytic transfusion reaction is quite low in most instances. This is true because the incidence of alloantibodies capable of causing a hemolytic transfusion reaction in patients receiving blood of the same ABO and Rh types is a little over 1 percent.[26] The incidence of alloantibodies is lowest in patients who have never been pregnant or transfused, and increases with the number of exposures to blood.

Significance of Autoantibody Specificity

The only recommended method for determining clinically significant Rh specificity of an autoantibody is to titer the patient's serum or eluate against R_1R_1 (CDe/CDe), R_2R_2 (cDE/cDE) and rr (cde/cde) red cells.

Autoantibodies with Rh Specificity or "Relative Specificity." Serologists are frequently vague regarding the criteria used when reporting an autoantibody as having Rh specificity. Most warm autoantibodies react with all red cells of common Rh genotypes but may fail to react with gene deletion cells such as Rh_{null} cells. Other autoantibodies will react with all red cells tested but react to a higher titer or score against red cells bearing a particular Rh antigen. In either case, the autoantibody is usually said to have Rh specificity without distinguishing such reactions from each other or from the clear-cut specificity of Rh alloantibodies wherein cells

Table 31-8. Eluate Showing Anti-e "Relative Specificity"

	Dilutions of Eluate							
	2	4	8	16	32	64	128	256
rr (cde/cde)	4+	3+	3+	2+	2+	1+	0	0
R_1R_1 (CDe/CDe)	4+	3+	3+	2+	2+	1+	0	0
R_2R_2 (cDE/cDE)	3+	2+	1+	0	0	0	0	0

Agglutination reactions are graded as 1+ to 4+.
(Petz, L.D. and Garratty, G.: Acquired Immune Hemolytic Anemias. Churchill Livingstone, New York, 1980.)

lacking the appropriate antigen give strictly negative reactions. We will refer to antibodies that react with all normal red cells bearing common Rh antigens but that consistently react to a higher titer or score against red cells containing one or another Rh antigen as having "relative specificity."

Table 31-8 shows results of an eluate that would be interpreted as showing "relative specificity" against the e antigen. Such reactions should be confirmed by testing against several examples of red cells with and without the appropriate antigen before clinical decisions based on the "relative specificity" of the autoantibody are made.

Several investigators have studied the in vivo survival of red cells of varying Rh phenotypes in patients who have warm autoantibodies that were said to have Rh specificity. In most instances, detailed serologic data are not given and the autoantibodies are likely to have demonstrated "relative specificity."

Mollison has described a case in which survival of the patient's own e-positive red cells was markedly shortened, whereas transfused e-negative red cells survived almost normally. The patient's serum contained an autoantibody with anti-e specificity.[27]

Salmon[28] described two patients who had anti-e and anti-nl autoantibodies. In the first case, the T½ of ^{51}Cr-labeled red cells was 23 days for −D−/−D− red cells (e−,nl−), 24 days for cDE/cDE red cells (e−,nl+), and 12.5 days for cde/cde red cells (e+,nl+). In the second case, the T½ was 14 days for cDE/cDE red cells but only 4 days for CDe/cde red cells (Table 31-9).

Von dem Borne et al.[29] reported a patient who had autoanti-e and anti-nl antibodies. The [51]Cr T½ of CDe/CDe red cells was 1.9 days and that of cDE/cDE red cells was 4.0 days.

In Holländer's patient,[30] the autoantibodies had anti-D specificity; while cde/cde blood survived for at least 31 days, CDe/cde blood survived for only 3 days. In Crowley and Bouroncle's patient,[31] two autoantibodies, anti-D and anti-E, were present, and cde/cde cells survived normally. In the pa-

Table 31-9. Significance of Autoantibodies with Rh "Relative Specificity"

CASE 1
HALF-LIFE OF ^{51}Cr-LABELED RED BLOOD CELLS IN A cde/cde PATIENT WITH ANTI-e + nl AUTOANTIBODIES

—D—/—D—red blood cells: (e—nl—) = 23 days
cDE/cDE red blood cells: (e—nl+) = 24 days
cde/cde red blood cells: (e+nl+) = 12.5 days
The anti-e appears to be responsible for half-life diminution

CASE 2
HALF-LIFE OF ^{51}Cr-LABELED RED BLOOD CELLS IN A CDe/cde PATIENT WITH ANTI-e + nl AUTOANTIBODIES

cDE/cDE red blood cells: (e—nl+) = 14 days
CDe/cde red blood cells: (e+nl+) = 4 days
The anti-nl is less hemolytic in vivo than is anti-e

tient of Wiener, Gordon, and Russow,[32] the autoantibody reacted to highest titers with cells containing the rh′ (C) factor; when transfused with blood lacking this factor, the patient made a complete and lasting recovery. Previously, she had been treated with randomly selected Rh-positive donors and had failed to improve. Ley, Mayer, and Harris's patient[33] was group O cde/cde; cDE/cDE erythrocytes were demonstrated to survive normally (^{51}Cr T½ = 25 days), but cde/cde cells survived even less well than the patient's own cells (^{51}Cr T½ = 5 days and 13 to 14 days, respectively).

Högman, Killander, and Sjölin's case[34] was a 13-year-old child of genotype CDe/CDe, who had formed autoanti-e as well as an apparent "nonspecific" component. The latter component did not appear to be of much importance, as cDE/cDE red cells survived normally.

Bell et al.[17] mention one patient with anti-e who tolerated two e-negative units with the expected rise and maintenance of hemoglobin levels. No further details are given.

Habibi et al.[16] transfused cDE/cDE red cells to six patients with autoantibodies of e, ce, or Ce specificities. The blood "proved normally efficient in vivo," but two of six homozygous ee patients developed anti-E alloantibodies.

Clinical Approach Based on Autoantibody Specificity

Although the preceding data are scanty, we feel that if an autoantibody demonstrates "relative specificity" (e.g., the titer against red cells containing the e antigen is consistently two tubes higher than when tested against cells lacking the e antigen), it is preferable to avoid transfusion of blood containing the antigen in question at least during the first few days of hospitalization. An exception to this course is generally made if it would be necessary to give Rh-positive blood to an Rh-negative individual, especially in women who

have not passed child-bearing age, or if repeated transfusions are necessary. Another important although unusual exception concerns the patient who, in addition to the autoantibody, also has an alloantibody that would make it impossible to transfuse red cells simultaneously lacking antigens that the alloantibody and autoantibody are directed against. For example, if the patient has an alloanti-E and an autoanti-e, blood lacking the E antigen should be transfused.

The recommendation to select donor blood on the basis of autoantibody "relative specificity" is based in part on the fact that most patients with warm antibody AIHA respond to therapy quickly. That is, median duration of corticosteroid therapy before discernible response was only seven days in one large series.[14] Thus, patients can benefit from the more prolonged survival of transfused red cells lacking the antigen with which the autoantibody reacts preferentially during this time when dangers of alloimmunization are as yet minimal.

If transfusions are required over a more prolonged period of time, the development of alloantibodies becomes more likely. In this case, since a careful search for development of all clinically important red cell alloantibodies must be made at regular intervals (i.e., every 48 hours as is required for all patients requiring frequent transfusion[35]), it is probably more practical, if the patient's Rh phenotype is known, to change to the transfusion of red cells of the same Rh phenotype as the patient. This is true unless a supply of the patient's red cells obtained prior to the initial transfusion has been saved for use in the warm autoabsorption test. Without the availability of the patient's pretransfusion red cells for warm autoabsorption, the most reliable method for detecting alloantibodies requires absorption using red cells of varying antigenic types, and it may not be feasible to obtain an adequate supply of the appropriate cells. If the patient's Rh phenotype is not known and no alloantibody can be detected by the techniques described above, one may as well continue to transfuse with red cells lacking the more reactive antigen, providing one does not transfuse Rh-positive blood to an Rh-negative recipient.

In contrast to the above approach, some immunohematologists recommend ignoring the specificity of the autoantibody. This attitude is based on two considerations.

First, the evidence indicating good survival related to autoantibody "relative specificity" is not extensive and, in some reports, the benefit was minimal.[29] In other instances, good survival of donor blood lacking the more reactive antigen was not shown to be due to the autoantibody specificity, since survival of transfused cells containing the more reactive antigen was not studied.[16, 17, 31, 34]

Secondly, if one transfuses red cells that lack an antigen with which an autoantibody reacts, one may need to use red cells containing an antigen not found on the patient's own cells, thus causing the potential for alloimmunization. This does not seem to be a critical argument, since typing for Rh antigens other than Rh_o (D) is not part of routine blood transfusion practice, and we know of no data which convincingly demonstrate that patients with AIHA have an increased incidence of development of red cell alloantibodies after transfusion. However, it is true that there is some advantage to be gained by ignoring Rh "relative specificity" if one instead selects blood for transfusion that is the same Rh phenotype as the patient. This will avoid Rh alloantibody-induced hemolytic transfusion reactions and is particularly significant if a patient needs multiple transfusions over a period of days or weeks.

Autoantibodies without Demonstrated Specificity. If autoantibody specificity is not demonstrable, a seemingly logical approach is to do compatibility tests using as large a number of donor units as practical (e.g., 5 to 10 units) and then select for transfusion those units that are "least incompatible" in vitro. However, when such in vitro differences in reactivity are caused by variable

reactivity of the red cell autoantibody not related to a specific Rh antigen and not caused by the presence of alloantibody, there are no data indicating whether such comparatively weakly reactive units have better survival than more strongly reactive units. Pirofsky[14] states that the search for relatively weak incompatible units is of no value, whereas Rosenfield and Jagathambal[36] accept that it may be of some value.

AIHA without Serum Autoantibody. In contrast to the above problems frequently encountered in AIHA, it should also be pointed out that, in some patients with overt hemolysis, the autoantibody does not interfere with compatibility testing. This is true because the autoantibody may be undetectable in the patient's serum (apparently because it is entirely absorbed onto the patient's red cells) or detectable only by techniques more sensitive than those used in routine saline and albumin crossmatch tests. Even though the donor blood is apparently compatible, the transfused red cells cannot be expected to survive normally because the autoantibody, although detectable only with very sensitive techniques in vitro, will react with donor cells in vivo as it has with the patient's own cells.[18] Thus, precautions concerning transfusion in patients with warm antibody AIHA apply equally, even though the routine compatibility test would tend to falsely assure normal donor red cell survival.

When autoantibody is not detectable in the patient's serum by routine crossmatch tests, the use of more sensitive serologic techniques may be utilized (i.e., the use of enzyme-treated red cells). In addition, autoantibody is often readily detected in an eluate prepared from the patient's red cells and, in this case, tests for specificity against common Rh antigens may be performed by titrations against R_1R_1, R_2R_2, and rr cells as described above.

Patients who present with a positive direct antiglobulin test but who have no signs of an active hemolytic process need not receive any special consideration in the selection of donor blood unless there is detectable serum antibody or the patient has been recently transfused (see Ch. 7).

Selection of Donor Blood in Various Clinical Settings

On the basis of the preceding information, we feel that the following recommendations are appropriate. The extent of serologic testing that is required depends on (1) whether or not the patient has recently been transfused, and, if so, (2) whether pretransfusion red cells are available for performing the warm autoabsorption technique and (3) whether the patient's Rh phenotype has been determined.

Patient Not Recently Transfused. The procedures listed in Table 31-10 should be performed on all candidates for transfusion. These procedures are quite practical, are not excessively time-consuming, and should be omitted only when extreme urgency precludes adequate pretransfusion evaluation.

Determining the Rh phenotype of the patient is very important and should be performed in every patient. In addition, it is advisable to type the patient for K, Jk^a, Jk^b, and Fy^a antigens if feasible using the methods described previously.

If it is possible to obtain a generous aliquot of the patient's red cells, these may be used for subsequent warm autoabsorption tests if repeated transfusions are needed. As with any frequently transfused patient, a search for alloantibodies should be performed every 48 hours.[35]

Patient Recently Transfused; Pretransfusion Red Cells Not Available for Autoabsorption; Rh Phenotype of Patient Known. Table 31-11 indicates procedures recommended when the patient has been recently transfused, when pretransfusion red cells are not available for autoabsorption, and when the Rh phenotype of the patient is known. If a patient has been transfused recently, more extensive serologic testing is necessary to exclude the presence of alloantibodies. Further, even if all recommended procedures are performed, only Rh, Jk^a, Jk^b, Kell and Fy^a alloantibodies will be detected. Nevertheless, alloantibodies of other specificities that cause serious hemolytic transfusion reactions are very unusual, and more extensive testing is generally not practical.

The differential absorption test is the most reliable method for alloantibody detection because its effectiveness is not negated by prior transfusion. However, it is not often feasible for hospital blood banks to perform these absorptions and, in that case, the dilution technique and the warm autoabsorption test are the best techniques that are practical.

In regard to autoantibody specificity, it is generally preferable to ignore Rh "relative specificity" and transfuse blood of the same Rh phenotype as that of the patient. This approach would appear safer than selecting

---

Table 31-10. Warm Antibody AIHA Selection of Donor Blood

Patient Not Recently Transfused

A. Preliminary Steps
  1. Determine Rh phenotype of patient
  2. Compare strength of direct and indirect antiglobulin tests
  3. Save a generous aliquot of patient's red cells for subsequent warm autoabsorptions

B. Alloantibody Detection
  1. Test patient's serum against a red cell panel
  2. Warm autoabsorption technique

C. Autoantibody Specificity
  1. If Rh specificity or "relative specificity" present, give blood lacking the more reactive antigen, unless doing so would require giving D positive blood to a D negative patient or unless the patient has a specific alloantibody which necessitates antigen negative donor blood (e.g., one would not transfuse cDE/cDE red cells into a patient having autoanti-e and alloanti-E).

Table 31-11. Warm Antibody AIHA Selection of Donor Blood

Patient Recently Transfused and Pretransfusion Red Cells not Available for Autoabsorption; Rh Phenotype of Patient Known.

A. Preliminary Steps
   1. Compare strength of direct and indirect antiglobulin tests.
B. Alloantibody Detection
   1. Test patient's serum against a red cell panel.
   2. Dilution technique if autoantibody gives 3+ or 4+ reactions.
   3. Warm autoabsorption technique.
   4. Differential absorption technique if feasible, using Jk^a-negative, Jk^b-negative, Fy^a-negative, and Kell-negative red cells.
C. Autoantibody Specificity
   1. Rh "relative specificity" should be ignored and red cells of same Rh phenotype as patient should be transfused.

blood on the basis of Rh "relative specificity" of the autoantibody because the dangers of undetected Rh alloimmunization outweigh the possible advantage of better cell survival related to the autoantibody "relative specificity."

If, however, the patient's autoantibody demonstrates distinct Rh specificity or "relative specificity," one may wish to use donor blood lacking the more reactive antigen. In this case, the presence of Rh alloantibodies must be excluded with a high degree of confidence by performance of the differential absorption test using R_1R_1, R_2R_2, and rr red cells or by absorbing with cells of the same Rh phenotype as the patient.

If other information is available concerning the antigenic make-up of the patient's red cells, blood may be selected on this basis as well. If the patient is $Jk(a-b+)$, one may

transfuse with Jk^a-negative blood, in which case pretransfusion absorption with Jk^a-negative red cells would not be necessary. Also, since Kell-negative blood is common, it is easier to select donor units that are Kell-negative than it is to absorb the serum with Kell-negative cells.

If the patient's red cells cannot be typed for Jk^a, Jk^b, Kell, and Fy^a antigens, and if the differential absorption technique is not feasible, selection of Jk^a-negative and Kell-negative donor units that are of the same Rh phenotype as the patient is logical and may be practical. This is particularly important in patients who have received multiple transfusions in the past. It is probably more important to select Jk^a-negative red cells than Fy^a-negative cells, even though anti-Fy^a is somewhat more common because anti-Jk^a more often causes serious hemolysis. It is obviously

Table 31-12. Warm Antibody AIHA Selection of Donor Blood

Patient Recently Transfused and Pretransfusion Red Cells not Available for Autoabsorption; Rh Phenotype of Patient Not Known.

A. Preliminary Steps
   1. Compare strength of direct and indirect antiglobulin tests.
B. Alloantibody Detection
   1. Test patient's serum against a red cell panel.
   2. Dilution technique if autoantibody gives 3+ or 4+ reactions.
   3. Warm autoabsorption technique.
   4. Differential absorption technique if feasible using R_1R_1, R_2R_2, rr and Jk^a-negative, Jk^b-negative, Fy^a-negative, and Kell-negative red cells.
C. Autoantibody Specificity
   1. Since Rh phenotype of patient is not known, blood of any Rh phenotype may be given, except that D positive blood should not be given to a D negative recipient. Therefore, if the autoantibody demonstrates Rh specificity or "relative specificity," it is preferable to transfuse with red cells lacking the more reactive antigen.

not possible to extend this principle of using donor red cells lacking important antigens to other blood group systems ad infinitum.

Patient Recently Transfused; Pretransfusion Red Cells Not Available for Autoabsorption; Rh Phenotype of Patient Not Known. Recommendations are outlined in Table 31-12. They are similar to those indicated in Table 31-11 except that, in this case, if one performs the differential absorption technique one will need to use R_1R_1, R_2R_2, and rr cells for detection of Rh alloantibodies and red cells negative for Jk^a, Jk^b, Fy^a, and Kell antigens. As described previously, these may be the same carefully selected red cells. Since the patient's Rh phenotype is unknown, it is impossible to avoid Rh alloantibody-induced transfusion reactions by the simple expedient of transfusing cells of the same Rh phenotype of the patient. Thus, in regard to Rh autoantibody "relative specificity," one may as well transfuse red cells lacking the more reactive antigen to take advantage of the possibility of more prolonged survival.

COLD AGGLUTININ SYNDROME

Compatibility Testing at 37° C in Saline

There are several approaches to compatibility testing in patients with cold agglutinin syndrome. One method is to perform the compatibility test strictly at 37° C and to use only normal saline media (i.e., without using albumin or low-ionic-strength solutions). Cold agglutinins from only 7 percent of patients with cold agglutinin syndrome react at 37° C in saline, although positive reactions will be obtained about 30 percent of the time in albumin media.[37] If positive reactions occur at 37° C in saline, one must first suspect faulty technique. If cells and serum are not prewarmed before mixing, if the initial washes of the cells after incubation do not utilize saline at 37° C, or if centrifugation is performed at a temperature less than 37° C,

reactions may occur within seconds. Even if direct agglutination is not evident, complement may be bound by the antibody reactivity and result in a positive indirect antiglobulin test (one molecule of IgM antibody may bind several hundred molecules of complement). When cold agglutinins of very high thermal amplitude are present, it may be advantageous to use a monospecific anti-IgG antiglobulin serum in the antiglobulin phase of the compatibility test.

The advantages of this method are that time consuming autoabsorptions of the patient's serum are not necessary, and that the method can be utilized even if the patient has been recently transfused. The reliability of autoabsorption in the latter case is uncertain.

Several disadvantages are also apparent. First, it is obvious that red cell alloantibodies reacting at temperatures less than 37° C will not be detected. This is of little consequence since antibodies that do not react in vitro at temperatures less than 37° C are rarely, if ever, clinically significant. Giblett is emphatic about this point, stating that alloantibodies that do not react at 37° C are of no concern since she has observed no in vivo hemolysis associated with a cold-reacting alloantibody (such as anti-A_1, $-P_1$, $-M$, $-N$, $-Lu^a$, etc.) during a 20 year period, when over a million units of blood were transfused.[26] Mollison is somewhat more cautious in his conclusions but does state that, in view of the small amount of destruction caused by cold agglutinins which are weakly reactive at 37° C, it seems clear that those cold agglutinins that are active only at some lower temperature than 37° C can safely be ignored.[38] Indeed, the ninth edition of the American Association of Blood Banks Standards for Blood Banks and Transfusion Services[35] does not require a room temperature incubation phase of the crossmatch but, instead, states that, "Methods for testing for unexpected antibodies shall be those that will demonstrate significant coating, hemolyzing and agglutinating antibodies *active at 37° C,* and shall include an antiglobulin test" (emphasis added).

It is also true that antibodies reactive only in albumin media will be missed, but here, again, the risk is minimal because such antibodies are quite unusual.[39] Since compatibility testing at 37°C is quicker than other methods, can be utilized even if the patient has recently been transfused, and results in a very low risk of missing clinically significant alloantibodies, we feel it the method of choice. However, certain technical details are crucial in order to be certain that one is truly working *strictly* at 37°C.

A heated centrifuge or a centrifuge in a 37°C warm room may be used, a centrifuge may be placed in an incubator, or the tubes may be placed in centrifuge cups containing warm water. Samples transferred from a 37°C water bath and centrifuged immediately in a Serofuge at room temperature (20 to 25°C) drop approximately 7 to 8°C after only one minute of centrifugation. It is necessary to keep a Serofuge in an incubator at about 40°C, in which case the samples spin at about 37°C. Similarly, saline at 40°C may be used, since it drops a few degrees when it enters a test tube and when centrifuging is in progress. A few simple experiments with each laboratory's equipment is all that is required to determine the conditions required to be able to carry out all procedures strictly at 37°C.

Facilities not equipped with incubators in which centrifuges can be placed, may use 45°C prewarmed centrifuge cups and 45°C saline for washings as this will maintain the temperature during centrifugation at about 37°C. However, there is more chance that the temperature will dip below the required 37°C using this technique, and 45°C saline can sometimes elute significant IgG antibody off the red cells.

Cold Autoabsorption

An alternative approach is to absorb the cold autoantibody from the patient's serum before performing the crossmatch test. This method works well for low titer cold agglutinins. However, it is very time consuming when high titer antibodies causing cold agglutinin syndrome are present, requiring multiple absorptions even when using enzyme-treated red cells. This approach is therefore not optimal if blood is needed urgently. Further, as indicated previously, the reliability of autoabsorption tests in recently transfused patients is uncertain. However, the technique may be necessary in the small percentage of patients whose antibody is reactive at 37°C even in saline. When positive reactions are obtained at 37°C, one or two autoabsorptions, followed by compatibility testing at 37°C, is useful. Table 31-13 shows the results of autoabsorbing a serum with a cold agglutinin titre of 2048 (saline) and 8096 (albumin). After three absorptions for ½ hour each at 4°C using the patient's papainized red cells, the serum still reacted strongly (4+ with undiluted serum) at room temperature (25°C), but no longer reacted at 37°C.

Other Methods

Still another approach to compatibility testing in cold agglutinin syndrome is to inactivate the IgM cold agglutinin with 2-mercaptoethanol[40,41] or dithiothreitol (DTT).[42]

Pirofsky and Rosner[42] described the use of dithiothreitol at a concentration of 0.01M in a rapid fifteen minute, 37°C incubation test system. Dialysis was not required. They reported that this procedure caused at least a fourfold or greater decrease in IgM antibody titers, without affecting the activity of IgG antibodies.

Olson et al.[42a] used dithiothreital in a concentration of 0.01M, added equal volumes to test sera, and incubated for 30 minutes at 37°C. Thirty sera that contained red cell antibodies reactive by the indirect antiglobulin test showed virtually no alternation in activity after dithiothreital treatment, while 20 sera containing cold-reactive red cell antibodies showed almost total elimination of activity. However, none of the cold-reactive antibodies tested were pathologic high titer cold

**Table 31-13. Absorption of Cold Agglutinin
by Patient's Own Cells at 4 °C**

| | Titer Against Adult OI Cells | | | | | |
| | 4 ° C | | 25 ° C | | 37 ° C | |
	Saline	Albumin	Saline	Albumin	Saline	Albumin
Unabsorbed	2048	8096	1024	8096	0	32
Absorbed x 1	1024	2048	256	1024	0	16
Absorbed x 2	256	256	128	256	0	8
Absorbed x 3	128	128	16	64	0	0

(Petz, L. D. and Garratty, G.: Acquired Immune Hemolytic Anemias. Churchill Livingstone, New York, 1980.)

agglutinins from patients with cold agglutinin syndrome.

Freedman et al.[43] reviewed the optimal conditions for use of sulphydryl compounds in dissociating red cell antibodies. They noted that incubation at 37 ° C with 0.2M 2-mercaptoethanol provided the best conditions for inactivating IgM antibodies. However, it still failed to inactivate completely the extremely potent auto-anti-I (titer of 1,024,000) that was used. False positive reactions in the indirect antiglobulin test using anti-IgG or anti-complement antiglobulin serum were consistently obtained when sera which had been treated with 2-mercaptoethanol were not subsequently dialyzed. Although in many cases dialysis for as short as 30 minutes was sufficient, in others dialysis overnight was found to be necessary. Incubation of serum with DTT produced a slower effect than did 2-mercaptoethanol, and incubation for 2½ hours was necessary to reduce the anti-I titer from 1,024,000 to 1,024.

Using either reagent, IgM alloantibodies will, of course, be inactivated in addition to the cold agglutinins, and blood bank technologists are usually less confident with the use of such reagents than the use of 37 ° C apparatus or autoabsorptions.

Some investigators have suggested that adult i red cells be used for transfusion of patients with cold agglutinin syndrome who have anti-I autoantibodies. Van Loghem et al.[44] studied the survival of I and i red cells labeled with ^{51}Cr in one patient with chronic cold agglutinin syndrome. They demonstrated normal survival for the i donor cells with greatly shortened survival of both the patient's I cells and donor I cells. Woll et al.[45] reported one patient with transient cold agglutinin syndrome who responded to transfusion of warmed, freeze-thawed adult i red blood cells. However, they did not test the survival of adult I red cells. Bell et al.[17] reported unfavorable experiences transfusing two patients with cold agglutinin syndrome with adult i red cells. Two adult i units given a patient with strong anti-I survived for approximately the same period of time (i.e., 3 to 4 days) as several adult I units given subsequently. In a second patient with anti-I, no elevation of hematocrit was noted after transfusion of 2 units of adult i blood. These authors suggested that the minimal I antigen present on adult i erythrocytes seemed sufficient to render them biologically incompatible.

Experience indicates that transfusion of adult I red cells to patients with chronic cold agglutinin syndrome usually results in an appropriate rise in hemoglobin. Unusual patients may fail to respond to transfusion of adult I red cells, but a majority of available data indicate that the use of adult i cells is not a solution to the problem. In patients with chronic cold agglutinin syndrome, the repeated use of i cells is certainly not feasible because of their extreme rarity.

PAROXYSMAL COLD HEMOGLOBINURIA

Transfusion of compatible blood may be possible if the rare p or p^k cells are available through a rare donor file. Although the routine crossmatch test will appear to be compatible with other red cells since the antibody reacts only in the cold (usually <15 ° C), there is evidence indicating that p or p^k red cells will survive better.[15] Patients may require transfusion before such cells are available, and transfusion of RBC of common P types should not be withheld if transfusion is urgently needed. Although there are some reports of Donath-Landsteiner antibodies having other specificities, these are extraordinarily rare.

IN VIVO COMPATIBILITY TESTING

In vivo compatibility testing has been considered of value in AIHA by some investigators and is based on testing the in vivo survival of an aliquot of red cells. Red cell survival may be measured crudely by means of changes in serum bilirubin[46] or plasma hemoglobin,[19] or more precisely by utilizing [51]CR-tagged cells.[1c, 47-49] The methods have been described in detail elsewhere.[49,50]

There is some disagreement concerning the significance of in vivo survival studies in AIHA. In general, we feel that in most clinical settings an in vivo survival study does not provide information that would alter the decision concerning management of a patient with AIHA that is made on the basis of careful serologic technique and good clinical judgement. Further, an in vivo compatibility test must not be considered a substitute for meticulous in vitro compatibility testing as described previously. It is pertinent to consider the potential significance of in vivo compatibility tests in various clinical settings.

Critically Ill Patients

Patients with AIHA who have progressively severe and immediately life-threatening anemia must be transfused and results of in vitro and in vivo compatibility tests must not be used to dissuade one from this decision. For example, if a patient with overt he-

molysis has a hematocrit of 20 percent on a given morning, a hematocrit of 16 percent in the early afternoon and 12 percent by late afternoon, transfusion must be given. If a careful serologic study has been done using techniques and principles already described to select the best possible donor unit of blood, and an in vivo test nevertheless demonstrates a very short cell survival, there is no logical way to select a different unit of blood for transfusion. For the patient who is critically ill and is not yet responding to appropriate therapy such as high dose corticosteroids, such incompatible blood must still be given in the hope of obtaining temporary benefit.

Seriously Ill Patients

Many patients with AIHA are seriously ill but with hemolysis not as immediately or as definitely life-threatening as the patient described above. For example, if a 60 year old patient has a hematocrit that is stable at 15 percent during the first several days of hospitalization, EKG evidence of an old myocardial infarct, and a persistent tachycardia, transfusion to a somewhat higher hematocrit is probably desirable. Proponents of in vivo compatibility testing feel that an acceptable in vivo 1-hour survival of ^{51}Cr-labeled cells provides an important measure of reassurance in that an acute symptomatic transfusion reaction is unlikely to occur and that the transfusion will produce at least temporary benefit.[1d,47-50,50a] The available data support such a suggestion, the most extensive being that of Silvergleid et al.[48] who found that if the 1-hour survival was 85 percent or greater, none of 33 patients subsequently transfused with incompatible blood had an acute symptomatic transfusion reaction. However, there are two additional factors of importance which must be kept in mind.

First, even shorter in vivo survival studies do not preclude a beneficial effect of transfusion. Mollison[50] states that when survival of a test sample of radiolabeled red cells at 60 minutes is subnormal, it by no means follows that there will be clinically significant red cell destruction if a unit or more of blood is transfused. It is presumed that a small concentration of antibody which is able to cause the destruction of a small volume of incompatible red cells may not be capable of causing destruction of a larger volume of transfused cells. Indeed, Mayer[52] has reported that 11 patients with AIHA who had an in vivo survival of ^{51}Cr-labeled donor red cells of less than 70 percent at 24 hours nevertheless required transfusion. Only one of these patients had a complication directly attributable to the transfusion. Thus, one should not interpret short survival of an aliquot of ^{51}Cr-labeled red cells to mean that transfusion is contraindicated. Data are not available to determine the rate of destruction of a test dose of red cells that would be predictive of an acute symptomatic hemolytic reaction.

Secondly, even though "adequate" survival of an aliquot of ^{51}Cr-labeled cells (variously reported as greater than 70 or 85 percent at one hour[48,49] or greater than 70 percent at 24 hours[52]) apparently precludes an acute symptomatic transfusion reaction, nevertheless subsequent survival is unpredictable. Indeed, dangerous degrees of hemolysis may occur in subsequent hours unless 1-hour survival is strictly normal (normal survival is defined by Mollison[50] as 99 ± 5% at 1 hour). For example, Silvergleid et al.[48] reported one patient with warm antibody autoimmune hemolytic anemia who had a 1-hour red cell survival of 87 percent, a pretransfusion hematocrit of 10.5 percent, a posttransfusion hematocrit of 20.6 percent, but a hematocrit of only 10 percent just 16 hours posttransfusion. Another patient, with paroxysmal cold hemoglobinuria had a 1-hour survival of Tj(a+) red cells of 87 percent and was transfused with 0.5 units of blood; 53 percent of the radiolabeled cells survived to 48 hours. Still another patient with an alloantibody (anti-Jk[b]) had 94 percent survival of tagged cells at 1 hour but only 10 percent survival at 24 hours. That a 1-hour red cell survival study does not accurately predict

survival in subsequent hours is further indicated by an additional case report of a patient with anti-Lu[b]; survival of radiolabeled Lu[b] plus red cells was 84.4 per cent at 1 hour but only 48 percent at 5 hours and 8.5 percent at 24 hours.[51]

Thus, short survival does not contraindicate transfusion, and "adequate" but subnormal survival does not assure safety in spite of a high probability of temporary benefit without an immediate symptomatic hemolytic reaction. When survival of a small test volume of red cells is subnormal it is presently impossible to predict the survival of a therapeutic volume of transfused cells.

Clinically Insignificant Autoantibodies

Although not relevant to a discussion of autoimmune hemolytic anemia, chromium survival studies of red cell life span have provided useful information regarding a relatively common cause of in vitro incompatibility that cannot be resolved—i.e., the presence of autoantibodies in patients without hemolytic anemia. Silvergleid et al.[48] studied fourteen patients who had positive direct antiglobulin tests and "nonspecific warm autoantibodies" in their sera. In none of these patients was there clinical evidence of hemolytic anemia. In 13 of the cases ^{51}Cr-labeled red cell recovery at 1 hour was 99% ± 5%; in the other patient, it was 92 percent. Nine of these patients were subsequently transfused and there were no clinical signs of shortened red cell survival. Three of the patients who were transfused had been taking methyldopa. On the basis of these data, it appears that autoantibodies that are not causing hemolytic anemia will not cause shortened survival of transfused red cells.

Summary

In summary, if a patient is critically ill and transfusion must be given to sustain life, an in vivo compatibility test is inappropriate because even abnormal results should not preclude transfusion.

In patients who are seriously ill as a result of hemolytic anemia, 1-hour survival of labeled red cells is unlikely to be normal (99 ± 5%) and results of transfusion of a therapeutic volume of red cells are unpredictable when the survival of an aliquot of red cells is subnormal.

The available data indicate that patients who have weak autoantibodies but who do not have hemolytic anemia will not destroy transfused red cells at an accelerated rate in spite of in vitro incompatibility.

Decisions concerning transfusion of patients with AIHA that are reached on the basis of clinical judgment and careful in vitro serologic studies are generally not aided by an in vivo compatibility study.

In vivo compatibility tests in regard to alloantibodies are discussed in Chapter 7.

OPTIMAL VOLUME OF BLOOD TO BE TRANSFUSED TO PATIENTS WITH AIHA

The optimal volume of blood to be transfused to patients with AIHA varies with the clinical setting. In patients who have severe hemolysis but may only require transfusion temporarily until therapy becomes effective, the transfusion of only modest volumes of red cells just sufficient to maintain a tolerable hematocrit appears advisable. Indeed, Rosenfield and Jagathambal point out that the salutary effect of just 100 ml of packed red cells may be quite remarkable when given to a patient with cardiopulmonary embarrassment from anemia.[36] They suggest that 100 ml may be given as needed (perhaps twice daily, depending on the severity of hemolysis) and that there is no need to increase the hemoglobin even to a level of 8 g/dl. The aim of such transfusions is to supply just enough red cells to prevent hypoxemia while avoiding dangerous reactions resulting from overtransfusion.

The dangers of overtransfusion in patients

with AIHA are several. If the anemia is very severe (hematocrit 10 to 15 percent; hemoglobin 3.5 to 5.0 g/dl), and especially if the patient is elderly and/or if cardiac reserve may be reduced, transfusion may easily overload the circulation and precipitate cardiac failure. In such patients red cells should be administered slowly, not exceeding one ml/kg/hr.[1e] One must look for evidence of congestive heart failure during and following the transfusion, particularly elevated venous pressure and the presence of rales on auscultation of the chest. Cardiac failure after the administration of as little as 200 ml of red cells may develop up to 6 to 12 hours later and may be fatal.[1e] Although diuretics are of value and probably should be given to patients with diminished cardiac reserve, responses will vary, and their administration must not replace close clinical observation of the patient.

Some physicians recommend partial exchange transfusion which can be conveniently carried out by starting a venesection in one arm and infusing red cells in the other, and by keeping the rates of blood administration and removal nearly equal. Since the hematocrit in the blood removed is much lower than that in the blood administered, one may rapidly increase the patient's hematocrit without changing blood volume. This can also be accomplished with cell separation by exchanging plasma for red cells. However, such measures to acutely increase the patient's red cell mass are probably contraindicated in this clinical setting for the following reason.

An additional danger in patients with AIHA relates to the fact that the kinetics of red cell destruction always describe an exponential curve of decay indicating that the number of cells removed in a unit of time is a percentage of the number of cells present at the start of this time interval.[36] Thus, the more cells that are present at zero time, the more cells in absolute number will be destroyed in the unit time span. Indeed, Chaplin indicates that the most common cause of post-transfusion hemoglobinuria in AIHA may not be alloantibody induced hemolysis but instead may be the quantitative effect of transfusion in increasing the red cell mass subjected to on-going autoantibody mediated destruction.[50a] Such marked post-transfusion hemoglobinemia and hemoglobinuria has the potential for a significant degree of associated morbidity and possibly mortality. Patients undergoing severe post-transfusion intravascular hemolysis may develop disseminated intravascular coagulation, possibly as a result of procoagulant substances present in red cell lysates.[1f] Further, there is evidence that complement activation may also trigger coagulation. Such coagulation abnormalities may be fatal, again emphasizing the need for restraint in transfusion of patients with AIHA.[1f]

The following two case summaries were supplied by Chaplin[53]:

R.S., a 34-year-old white gravida-1, para-1, with relapsing primary autoimmune hemolytic anemia for 4 months, was hospitalized with a hemoglobin of 5.0 g/dl; reticulocytes of 16 percent; direct antiglobulin test strongly positive for C3d, moderately positive for IgM, negative for IgG; and all crossmatches "incompatible." Despite high-dose corticosteroids, she required 1 to 2 units of packed red cells daily to maintain her hemoglobin at 4.5 to 6.0 g/dl. She experienced increasingly severe hemoglobinemia and hemoglobinuria associated with transfusions, clearing within a few hours. No alloantibodies were demonstrable. On the 10th hospital day a splenectomy was performed without benefit. On the 12th hospital day, several hours following a transfusion, she developed acute respiratory distress, followed by cardiopulmonary arrest which did not respond to resuscitative measures. Autopsy revealed a single large para-aortic lymph node diagnosed as "plasmacytoid malignant lymphoma"; death was attributed to multiple fresh small pulmonary emboli.

L.F., a 56-year-old white woman, never previously pregnant or transfused, was semi-stuporous at time of admission to the hospital. She had a hemoglobin of 1.6 g/dl; hematocrit 6.2 percent; reticulocytes 19 percent; direct antiglobulin test strongly positive for C3d, moderately positive for IgG, weakly positive for IgM; and all crossmatches "incompatible." She was given corticosteroids and 3 units of packed group O, Rh-negative red cells. She developed fever and striking hemoglobinemia and hemoglobinuria which improved over the ensuing 3 hours. Her state of consciousness improved, and the hemoglobin rose transiently to 5.7 g/dl but was rapidly declining when she developed severe respiratory distress, followed by cardiopulmonary arrest which did not respond to resuscitation. At autopsy, no underlying cause for the autoimmune hemolytic anemia was found; death was attributed to multiple fresh small pulmonary emboli.

Patients who have a chronic hemolytic anemia that is unresponsive to therapy will, for practical purposes, require the transfusion of volumes of blood larger than 100 ml of RBC per transfusion. Patients with anemia causing signs and symptoms severe enough to require transfusion chronically may have only moderate degrees of hemolysis associated with a relatively poor marrow response—e.g., hemoglobin of 5 g/dl with less than 10 percent reticulocytes. Such patients can usually be managed as outlined above for patients with chronic anemia—i.e., with several units of red cells per transfusion as required.

Patients with chronic AIHA whose rate of hemolysis is significantly more severe and who require chronic transfusions are in greater danger of posttransfusion hemoglobinuria for reasons indicated above. Transfusion therapy will need to be individualized with an attempt being made to compromise between the impracticality of repeated use of small volumes of red cells, and the dangers inherent in transfusion of large volumes. Patients with marked shortening of red cell life span who require repeated frequent transfusions have a precarious outlook, at least in part because of the acute and chronic dangers of blood transfusions. Vigorous therapeutic measures for the AIHA are indicated, and every attempt should be made to wean the patient off transfusion if a stable, albeit low, hematocrit can be maintained.

THE USE OF WARM BLOOD FOR PATIENTS WITH COLD AGGLUTININ SYNDROME AND PAROXYSMAL COLD HEMOGLOBINURIA

Eminent authorities offer sharply differing opinions concerning the need for warm blood when transfusing patients with cold agglutinin syndrome. Dacie states that properly crossmatched blood can probably be transfused with safety if run in at a slow drip rate, in which case there is probably no need to attempt to warm it above room temperature.[54] In contrast, Rosenfield states that patients with cold agglutinin disease must receive warmed blood.[36] Mollison, in his comprehensive text,[1h] states that blood should be warmed before transfusion only in a few special circumstances, but does not list cold antibody autoimmune hemolytic anemia among these indications. He does recommend that the patient be kept warm.[1h] Wallace comments that hemolytic reactions are unlikely provided that the donor blood is warmed to body temperature and the recipient is kept warm.[55] Apparently the problem has not been studied in much depth, and no red cell survival studies are available comparing survival of blood transfused at various temperatures.

In regard to paroxysmal cold hemoglobinuria, Rawsen does report that even compatible Tj(a−) blood needs to be warmed to 37° C before transfusion.[15] Wallace, however, states that even transfusion of red cells of the common P groups (either P_1 positive or negative) is unlikely to precipitate an acute hemolytic transfusion reaction in PCH provided the donations are warmed to 37° C and the patient is maintained at a warm temperature.[55] Johnsen et al.[56] reported the results of transfusion of 150 ml of prewarmed packed red cells (P positive) to an 18-month-old boy with paroxysmal cold hemoglobinuria. The transfusion was followed by a temperature rise and passage of red-colored urine. How-

ever, the hemoglobin improved from 4.7 g/dl to 12.4 g/dl and remained at that level.

In the absence of extensive data, logic must prevail. Our experience in cold agglutinin syndrome has been consistent with Dacie's view, although in some instances we have empirically used an in-line blood warmer for seriously ill patients. The use of an "in-line" blood warmer would appear indicated if the patient has either severe paroxysmal cold hemoglobinuria or florid cold agglutinin disease. It is also logical to keep the patient warm even if the efficacy of such a maneuver has not been proven.

If blood is to be warmed, it must be done properly. Unmonitored or uncontrolled heating of blood is extremely dangerous and should not be attempted. Red cells heated too much are rapidly destroyed in vivo and can be lethal to the patient.[36] In the past, blood units were prewarmed by microwave units or by immersion in warm water. Neither practice is acceptable today. Nothing should be used but very efficient "in-line" blood warmers which are simple, efficient, and safe to use.[36]

USE OF WASHED RED BLOOD CELLS

Evans et al.[57, 57a] reported their experience using packed red cells or washed red cells in transfusing one patient with cold agglutinin syndrome. The cold antibody of one patient agglutinated red cells to a titer of 500,000 at 4° C and caused lysis of normal red cells both at room temperature and at 37° C (maximal at room temperature). A transfusion of two units of packed red cells was given without subjective reaction, although hemoglobinuria occurred following completion of the transfusion. A subsequent transfusion of three units of washed red cells was given without rise in plasma hemoglobin. The patient's serum complement was "always low." Although the data are far from conclusive, the authors speculated that the small amount of lasma present in the first transfusion of red ells provided the necessary complement for e hemolysis that followed. Further studies y Evans et al.[57a] indicated that transfusion of rge volumes of red cells to patients with old agglutinin syndrome caused a lowering f serum complement. ^{51}Cr-labeled normal d cells survived longer after red cell trans- sions than before, and the authors sug- ested that the reduction in serum comple- ent levels may have been responsible for the nproved survival. In our view, the phenome- on reported by Evans remains unexplained nd must be very uncommon. Serum com- lement is usually not strikingly reduced in atients with warm or cold antibody IHA,[18a] and we would not recommend the se of washed red cells for this rationale on he basis of the limited information available.

Some investigators recommend using ashed red cells for patients with AIHA to void febrile reactions caused by factors ther than red cell antibodies. This is reason- ble because the interpretation of a febrile re- ction in a seriously ill patient with AIHA is ifficult and could lead to unnecessary cessa- ion or delay of transfusion. These reactions nay largely be prevented by the use of leu- ocyte poor red cells, and it is true that one nethod of preparation of these cells is by nechanical washing. The justification for heir use in AIHA beyond that applicable to ther acutely ill patients is that the compati- ility test procedures may be much more time onsuming in AIHA. Thus, unnecessary ces- ation of the transfusion is more costly be- ause of the additional technical procedures, nd there may be a longer delay in selecting n alternative unit.

AUTOLOGOUS BLOOD TRANSFUSION IN AIHA

Three brief reports have suggested the use f autologous red cells for transfusion of pa- ients with AIHA. Goldfinger et al.[58] demon- trated that autologous frozen-stored red cells may be practical in some patients with AIHA. In one patient with IgM-mediated AIHA, normal in vivo recovery was demonstrated al- though in vitro red cell loss was 40 percent. In patients who had positive direct antiglobulin tests but not hemolytic anemia, in vitro red cell loss was only 2 to 14 percent and in vivo recovery and survival were normal. Storing red cells in the frozen state may be considered for patients who go into remission while on therapy for AIHA. In case of later relapse, the cells may be transfused without fear of al- loantibody induced hemolysis. However, be- cause of autoantibody in the patient's serum, red cell survival is not likely to be better than that of a homologous unit and conceivably could be worse if an antibody with a high degree of specificity for autoantigens is pres- ent. Until the efficacy of this approach can be demonstrated in more patients, it cannot be recommended other than for investigational programs.

Parr and Ballard[59] reported a patient with methyldopa-induced positive direct and in- direct antiglobulin tests who required sur- gery. The patient had equivocal evidence of hemolysis consisting of an elevated LDH with a normal hemoglobin and hematocrit. The patient's serum antibody reacted with all normal red cells tested. Rather than wait for a fall in the autoantibody titer, 3 units of au- tologous blood were stored in the liquid state and utilized during surgery. A similar ap- proach was used by Snyder and Spivack in two patients.[60] Although evidence indicates that methyldopa-induced autoantibody will not cause shortened survival of homologous blood if the patient's own red cell survival is normal, the use of autologous blood assures that an alloantibody induced transfusion re- action will not occur. In instances in which it is inconvenient or impossible to delay surgery until an adequate number of autologous units are collected, the warm autoabsorption tech- nique or other serologic methods as described above for patients with warm antibody AIHA may be used to exclude the presence of al- loantibody.

Table 31-14 Correlation between Mechanism of Red Cell Sensitization and Clinical and Laboratory Features in Drug-Induced Immunohematologic Abnormalities

Mechanism	Prototype Drugs	Clinical Findings	Serologic Evaluation	
			Direct Antiglobulin Test	Antibody Identification
I. Immune complex formation (drug and anti-drug antibody)	Quinidine, phenacetin	Small doses of drug, acute intravascular hemolysis usual; renal failure common; thrombocytopenia occasionally	Usually only complement components detected but IgG can be present	Drug + patient's serum + RBC (especially enzyme-treated) → hemolysis, agglutination or sensitization; antibody frequently IgM and capable of fixing complement; RBC eluate often non-reactive
II. Drug adsorbed onto red cell membrane; reacts with high titer serum drug antibody	Penicillins, cephalosporins	Large doses of penicillin (10 million units or more daily); other manifestations of allergy not necessarily present; usually subacute extravascular hemolysis; penicillin one of most common causes of drug induced immune hemolysis; rare cases of immune hemolytic anemia caused by cephalosporins	Strongly positive (IgG) when hemolytic anemia present; complement sensitization also in a minority of patients	Drug-coated RBC + serum → agglutination or sensitization (rarely hemolysis); high titer antibody associated with hemolytic anemia i always IgG; RBC eluate reacts only with antibiotic-coated RBC
III. Membrane modification (nonimmunologic absorption of proteins)	Cephalosporins	No cases of cephalosporin-induced hemolytic anemia caused by nonimmunologic mechanisms	Positive with antiserums to a variety of serum proteins	Drug-coated RBC + serum → sensitization to antiglobulin serums in low titer (nonimmunologic protein absorption); RBC eluate nonreactive
IV. Unknown	Methyldopa	Hemolysis in 0.8 percent of patients taking drug for at least 3 months; gradual onset of hemolytic anemia; most common cause of drug-induced immune hemolysis	Strongly positive (IgG) when hemolytic anemia present; rarely cells are sensitized with complement as well	Antibody sensitizes normal RBC without drug; antibody in serum and eluate identical to that found in warm antibody AIHA; no *in vitro* relationship to drug demonstrable

(Petz, L. D. and Garratty, G.: Acquired Immune Hemolytic Anemias. Churchill Livingstone, New York 1980.)

BLOOD SUBSTITUTES

A reasonable indication for the use of blood substitutes is the presence of severe autoimmune hemolytic anemia. This topic is discussed in Chapter 35.

COMPATIBILITY TESTING IN PATIENTS WITH DRUG-INDUCED IMMUNE HEMOLYTIC ANEMIA

Drugs result in the development of immune hemolytic anemia by several different mechanisms[18a,61-63] as outlined in Table 31-14. Drug induced hemolysis resulting from the immune complex mechanism or the drug absorption mechanism differs from AIHA in that the offending antibody is directed against the drug and not against intrinsic red cell antigens. Drugs that have been reported to cause immune hemolytic anemia and/or a positive direct antiglobulin test are listed in Table 31-15.

Immune Complex Mechanism

The immune complex mechanism is illustrated in Figure 31-2 and most drugs that cause immune hemolytic anemia do so by this mechanism. The immune complexes often activate complement on the red cell surface, with resultant intravascular hemolysis. The hemolysis usually subsides within 24 to 48 hours, as the plasma drug level falls.[50a] If transfusion is necessary, the major compatibility test will be compatible, unless coincidental red cell alloantibodies are present. This is true since the drug is necessary in the in vitro test system in order to demonstrate the drug-related antibody (Table 31-14). However, the transfused cells may not survive normally if drug administration is continued, or if the serum level of drug or drug-related immune complexes remains high.

Table 31-15. Drugs That Have Been Reported to Cause a Positive Direct Antiglobulin Test and Hemolytic Anemia.*

DRUG
Fuadin (stibophen)
Quinidine
P-aminosalicylic acid (PAS)
Quinine
Phenacetin
Penicillins
Chlorinated hydrocarbon insecticides (Dieldrin, Heptachlor, Toxaphene)
Antihistamines (Antazoline, Antistin)
Sulfonamides
Isoniazid (INH, Rifamate, Nydrazid)
Chlorpromazine (Thorazine)
Pyramidon (Aminopyrin)
Dipyrone
Methyldopa (Aldomet, Aldoril, Aldoclor)
Melphalan (Alkeran)
Cephalosporins
Mefenamic acid (Ponstel)
Carbromal (Carbrital, Carbropent)**
Sulfonylurea derivatives (Diabenese, Tolbutamide)
Insulin
Levodopa (L-dopa, Sinemet)
Rifampin (Rifadin, Rifamate, Rimactane)
Methadone**
Tetracycline
Methysergide (Sansert)
Acetaminophen
Hydrochlorothiazide
Streptomycin
Procainamide (Pronestyl, Sub-Quin)
Ibuprofen (Motrin)
Hydralazine (Apresoline, Hydralazide, Unipres, Serpasil)
Probenecid (Benamid)
Fenfluramine (Pondimin)
Triamterene (Dyrenium, Daiteren)
Trimellitic anhydride
Nomifensine

* Some brand names are listed, but it is impractical to list the name of all products containing each drug. For example the American Drug Index (J. B. Lippincott Co., Philadelphia, 1979) lists 235 products containing acetaminophen.

** Carbromal and methadone have been reported to cause positive direct antiglobulin tests but not hemolytic anaemia.

(Petz, L. D.: Drug-Induced Immune Haemolytic Anaemia. Clinics in Haematology, 9:455, 1980.)

Drug Adsorption Mechanism

The drug absorption mechanism of drug-induced hemolytic anemia is illustrated in Figure 31-3. Drugs causing immune hemolysis by this mechanism are primarily penicil-

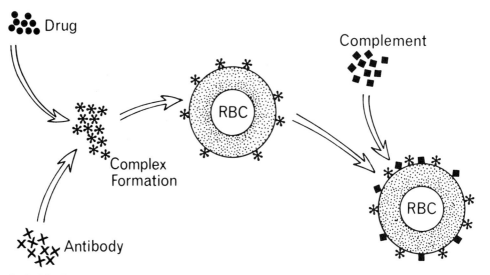

Fig. 31-2. The immune complex mechanism. Anti-drug antibody reacts with the drug to form an immune complex. The antibody-drug complex is then adsorbed onto red cells; the cell-bound complex may activate complement and result in intravascular hemolysis. Red cells have been considered "innocent bystanders" in this reaction. Quinidine and phenacetin are prototype drugs. (Petz, L.D. and Garratty, G.: Acquired Immune Hemolytic Anemias. Churchill Livingstone, New York, 1980.)

lins and cephalosporins. The fundamental difference in mechanism is that penicillins normally bind to the red cell membrane in the absence of antibody. This is readily demonstrable in vitro and also occurs in vivo when high doses of the drug are administered intravenously.[18a,64] As with the immune complex mechanism, the major crossmatch will be compatible. However, transfused red cells will become coated with drug in vivo and cannot be expected to survive any longer than the patient's red cells.

A therapeutic dilemma may occur when penicillin induced immune hemolytic occurs in that the clinical setting is usually one in which prolonged administration of high doses of penicillin are indicated—e.g., bacterial endocarditis. Often, penicillin induced hemolysis is mild and does not become progressively severe even with continued administration of the drug.

If hemolysis is mild and continuation of the drug is critical, one possible course is to continue the drug and to give occasional transfusions as necessary. However, severe and even fatal hemolysis caused by penicillin have been reported,[65,66] so very close observation is mandatory.

Penicillin and cepholosporin antibodies cross-react to a variable degree[67-70] and some investigators have studied the in vivo significance of this cross-reactivity in relationship to immune hemolytic anemia. Two reports suggest that shortened red cell survival may occur with both penicillins or cephalosporins.[71,72] However, recent experience indicates that hemolysis may resolve in a patient with penicillin induced hemolysis when cephalosporin is substituted even though the antibody demonstrates a high degree of in vitro cross-reactivity.[73]

Drug-Induced Autoimmune Hemolytic Anemia

Compatibility testing in patients with AIHA caused by methyldopa is similar to that described for warm antibody AIHA. Although no data are available, it is probable

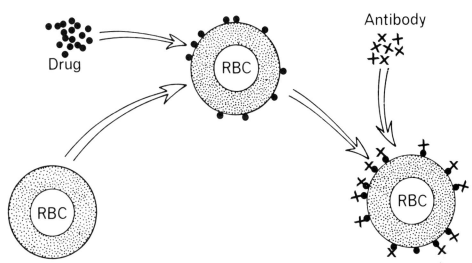

Fig. 31-3. The drug adsorption mechanism. Penicillin is the prototype drug. The essential feature is that the drug is nonspecifically bound to red cells and remains firmly adherent to the cells regardless of whether the patient develops an antibody to the drug. If a patient develops a potent anti-drug antibody, it will react with the cell-bound drug. Such red cells will yield a positive result in the direct antiglobulin test, and hemolytic anemia may ensue. Complement is usually not activated by anti-penicillin antibodies. (Petz, L.D. and Garratty, G.: Acquired Immune Hemolytic Anemias. Churchill Livingstone, New York, 1980.)

that donor red cells will survive as well as the patient's own red cells.

Other patients receiving methyldopa may have a positive direct antiglobulin test but no evidence of hemolysis. In many of these patients, the indirect antiglobulin test is negative so that the major compatibility test is compatible and donor blood can be expected to survive normally.

Still other patients receiving methyldopa have both positive direct and indirect antiglobulin tests caused by autoantibody, but have no evidence of hemolytic anemia or of compensated hemolysis.[18a] In performing the compatibility test, one must search for alloantibodies that may be present as described previously. However, even if alloantibodies do not appear to be present, all compatibility tests will be incompatible. The question then arises as to whether the autoantibody will cause shortened survival of donor red cells even though not causing shortened survival

of the patient's own red cells. Silvergleid et al.[48] studied the survival of radiolabeled donor cells in two such patients and demonstrated acceptable survival after one hour in each patient. Subsequent experience of our own and in association with Drs. J. Howard and F. C. Grumet at Stanford University indicates that, in such circumstances, donor units appear to survive normally, and clinical evidence of transfusion reactions does not result. In 21 transfusion episodes in 19 patients who were receiving methyldopa and who had positive direct and indirect antiglobulin tests caused by autoantibody but who did not have hemolytic anemia, there were no clinical manifestations of transfusion reactions, and adequate post-transfusion increments in the hemoglobin and hematocrit resulted in each case. Snyder and Spivack[60] have reported one additional similar case. Although this point merits further study, it presently appears that methyldopa induced red cell autoantibody does not cause hemolytic transfusion reactions if the patient's own red cell survival is normal.

Although no data are available concerning compatibility testing and blood transfusion in patients with drug-induced positive antiglobulin tests and autoimmune hemolytic anemia caused by drugs other than methyldopa— e.g., L-dopa and mefenamic acid—one might assume that similar principles would apply.

NONIMMUNOLOGICAL DRUG-INDUCED HEMOLYTIC ANEMIA

In addition to immunological mechanisms responsible for drug-induced hemolytic anemia, hemolysis may result from nonimmunological causes as a result of oxidative denaturation of hemoglobin by drugs or drug metabolites.[74-77] Although severe oxidant stress may cause hemolysis of normal RBC,[77] intraerythrocytic metabolic abnormalities or the presence of unstable hemoglobins may predispose the red cell to the effects of oxidant drugs.

In these patients, compatibility testing presents no problem and transfused red cells may survive normally in those cases in which an intraerythrocytic defect—e.g., G-6PD deficiency—is a predisposing factor to the hemolytic anemia.

REFERENCES

1. Mollison, P.L.: Blood Transfusion in Clinical Medicine. Fifth Edition. Blackwell Scientific Publications, Oxford. 1972, (a) p. 133, (b) p. 36, (c) p. 477, (d) p. 510, (e) p. 46-48, (f) pp. 550-552, (g) p. 581, (h) p. 446.
2. Hillman, R.S.: Blood loss anemia. Postgrad. Med. 64:88, 1978.
3. Williams, W.J., Beutler, E., Erslev, A.J., and Rundles, R.W., eds.: Hematology, 2nd Edition, McGraw-Hill, New York, 1977, p. 239.
4. Masourdis, S.P.: Clinical use of blood and blood products in hematology. In: Hematol-ogy, 2nd Ed. Williams, W.J., Beutler, E., Erslev, A.J., and Rundles, R.W., eds. McGraw-Hill, New York, 1977, pp. 1530-1546.
5. Metheny, D.: Clinical estimation of acute blood loss by the Tilt test. Am. Surg. 33:573, 1967.
6. Blackburn, E.K.: Indications for blood transfusion. Practitioner. 195:174, 1965.
7. Elwood, P.C. and Wood, M.M.: Effect of oral iron therapy on the symptoms of anaemia. Br. J. Prevent. Soc. Med. 20:172, 1966.
8. Elwood, P.C., Waters, W.E., Greene, W.J., Sweetnam, P., and Wood, M.M.: Symptoms and circulating haemoglobin level. J. Chron. Dis. 21:615, 1969.
9. Elwood, P.C. and Hughes, D.: A clinical trial of iron therapy on psychomotor function in anaemic women. Br. Med. J. iii:254, 1970.
10. Morrow, J.J., Dagg, J.H., and Goldberg, A.: A controlled trial of iron therapy in sideropenia. Scot. J. Med. 13:78, 1968.
11. Wood, M.M. and Elwood, P.C.: Symptoms of iron deficiency anaemia. A community survey. Br. J. Prevent. Soc. Med. 20:117, 1968.
12. Milinan, N.: Blood transfusion requirements before and after bilateral nephrectomy in patients undergoing chronic haemodialysis. Acta. Med. Scand. 195:479, 1974.
13. Todd, D.: Diagnosis of haemolytic states. Clin. Haematol. 4:63, 1975.
14. Pirofsky, B.: Immune haemolytic disease: The autoimmune haemolytic anaemias. Clin. Haematol. 4:167, 1975.
15. Rausen, A.R., LeVine, R., Hsu, T.C.S., and Rosenfield, R.E.: Compatible transfusion therapy for paroxysmal cold hemoglobinuria. Pediatr. 55:275, 1975.
15a. Pirofsky, B.: Clinical aspects of autoimmune hemolytic anemia. Sem. Hematol. 13:251, 1976.
16. Habibi, B.: Autoimmune hemolytic anemia in children. Am. J. Med. 56:61, 1974.
17. Bell, C.A., Zwicker, H., and Sacks, H.J.: Autoimmune hemolytic anemia: Routine serologic evaluation in a general hospital population. Am. J. Clin. Pathol. 60:903, 1973.
18. Leddy, J.P. and Swisher, S.N.: Acquired immune hemolytic disorders (including drug-induced immune hemolytic anemia). In: Immunological Diseases, Third Edition. Samter, M., ed. Little, Brown, Boston, Vol. 1, 1978, p. 1187.

18a. Petz, L.D. and Garratty, G.: Acquired Immune Hemolytic Anemias, Churchill Livingstone, N.Y., 1980.

18b. Allen, N.K.: Hyland Reference Manual of Immunohematology. Hyland, Los Angeles, CA, 1963, Fig. 18.

19. Dorner, I.M., Parker, C.W., and Chaplin, H.: Autoagglutination developing in a patient with acute renal failure. Br. J. Haematol. 14:383, 1968.

20. Petz, L.D. and Garratty, G.: Laboratory correlations in immune hemolytic anemias. In: Laboratory Diagnosis of Immunologic Disorders. Vyas, G.N., Stites, D.P., and Brecher, G., eds. Grune & Stratton, 1975, p. 139.

21. Morel, P.A., Bergren, M.O., and Frank, B.A.: A simple method for the detection of alloantibody in the presence of warm autoantibody. Transfusion (abstr.) 18:388, 1978.

22. Bove, J.R., Holburn, A.M., and Mollison, P.L.: Non-specific binding of IgG to antibody-coated red cells (the Matuhasi-Ogata phenomenon). Immunol. 25:793, 1973.

23. Matuhasi, T.: Plasma protein and antibody fractions observed from the serological point of view. Proc. 15th Gen. Assem. Jap. Med. Congr., Tokyo 4:80, 1959.

24. Ogata, T. and Matuhasi, T.: Problems of specific and cross reactivity of blood group antibodies. Proc. 8th Congr. Int. Blood Transf., Tokyo. Karger, Basel/New York, 1960, p. 208.

25. Ogata, T. and Matuhasi, T.: Further observations on the problem of specific and cross reactivity of blood group antibodies. Proc. 9th Congr. Int. Soc. Blood Transf., Mexico. Karger Basel/New York, 1962, p. 528.

26. Giblett, E.R.: Blood group alloantibodies: an assessment of some laboratory practices. Transfusion 17:299, 1977.

26a. Croucher, B.E.E.: Differential diagnosis of delayed transfusion reaction. In: A Seminar on Laboratory Management of Hemolysis. Bell, C.A., ed. Las Vegas, NV, 1979, pp. 151-158.

26b. Beattie, K.M.: Laboratory evaluation and management of antibody specificities in warm autoimmune hemolytic anemia. In: A Seminar on Laboratory Management of Hemolysis. Bell, C.A., ed. Las Vegas, NV, 1979, pp. 105-128.

27. Mollison, P.L.: Measurement of survival and destruction of red cells in hemolytic syndromes. Br. Med. Bull. 15:59, 1959.

28. Salmon, C.: Autoimmune hemolytic anemia. In: Immunology. Back, J.F., Sivenson, R.S., and Schwartz, R.S., eds. John Wiley & Sons, New York, 1978, p. 675.

29. von dem Borne, A.E.G., Engelfriet, C.P., and Beckers, D.O., et al.: Autoimmune anaemias. Biochemical studies of red cells from patients with autoimmune haemolytic anaemia with incomplete warm antibodies. Clin. Exper. Immunol. 8:377, 1971.

30. Holländer, L.: Study of the erythrocyte survival time in a case of acquired haemolytic anaemia. Vox Sang. 4:164, 1954.

31. Crowley, L.V. and Bouroncle, B.A.: Studies on the specificity of autoantibodies in acquired hemolytic anemia. Blood 11:700, 1956.

32. Wiener, A.S., Gordon, E.B., and Russow, E.: Observations on the nature of the auto-antibodies in a case of acquired hemolytic anemia. Ann. Intern. Med. 47:1, 1957.

33. Ley, A.M., Mayer, K., and Harris, J.P.: Observations on a "specific autoantibody." Proc. 6th Congr. Int. Soc. Blood Trans., Boston, 1958, p. 148.

34. Högman, C., Killander, J., and Sjölin, S.: A case of idiopathic auto-immune haemolytic anaemia due to anti-e. Acta. Paediatr. (Uppsala) 49:270, 1960.

35. Standards for Blood Banks and Transfusion Services. Ninth Ed. Oberman, H., ed. Am. Assoc. Blood Banks, Washington, D.C., 1978.

36. Rosenfield, R.E. and Jagathambal: Transfusion therapy for autoimmune hemolytic anemia. Sem. Hematol. 13:311, 1976.

37. Garratty, G., Petz, L.D., and Hoops, J.K.: The correlation of cold agglutinin titrations in saline and albumin with haemolytic anemia. Br. J. Haematol. 35:587, 1977.

38. Mollison, P.L., Johnson, C.A., and Prior, D.M.: Dose-dependent destruction of A_1 cells by anti-A_1. Vox Sang. 35:149, 1978.

39. Stroup, M. and MacIlroy, M.: Evaluation of the albumin antiglobulin technic in antibody detection. Transfusion 5:184, 1965.

40. Deutsch, H.F. and Morton, J.I.: Dissociation of human serum macroglobulins. Science 125:600, 1957.

41. Grubb, R. and Swahn, B.: Destruction of some agglutinins but not of others by two sulfhydryl compounds. Acta. Path. Microbiol. Scand. 43:305, 1958.

42. Pirofsky, B. and Rosner, E.R.: DTT test: A new method to differentiate IgM and IgG

erythrocyte antibodies. Vox Sang. 27:480, 1974.

42a. Olson, P.R., Weiblen, B.J., O'Leary, J.J., Moscowitz, A.J., and McCullough, J.: A simple technique for the inactivation of IgM antibodies using dithiothreitol. Vox Sang. 30:149, 1976.

43. Freedman, J., Masters, C.A., Newlands, M., and Mollison, P.L.: Optimal conditions for the use of sulphydryl compounds of dissociating red cell antibodies. Vox Sang. 30:231, 1976.

44. Van Loghem, J.J., Peetom, F., and Van der Hart, M., et al.: Serological and immunochemical studies in hemolytic anemia with high-titer cold agglutinins. Vox Sang. 8:33, 1963.

45. Woll, J.E., Smith, C.M., and Nusbacher, J.: Treatment of acute cold agglutinin hemolytic anemia with transfusion of adult i RBCs. J.A.M.A. 229:1779, 1974.

46. Walford, R.I. and Taylor, P.: An in vivo crossmatching procedure for selected problem cases in blood banking. Transfusion 4:372, 1964.

47. Mayer, K., Bettigole, R.E., and Harris, J.P., et al.: Test in vivo to determine donor compatibility. Transfusion 8:28, 1968.

48. Silvergleid, A.J., Wells, R.P., Hafleigh, E.B., and Korn, G., et al.: Compatibility test using ^{51}Chromium-labeled red blood cells in crossmatch positive patients. Transfusion 18:8, 1978.

49. International Committee for Standardization in Haematology: Recommended method for radioisotope red-cell survival studies. Br. J. Haematol. 45:659, 1980.

50. Mollison, P.L.: Blood Transfusion in Clinical Medicine. Sixth Edition. Blackwell Scientific Publications. Oxford, London, Edinburgh, Melbourne, 1979.

50a. Chaplin, H.: Special problems in transfusion management of patients with autoimmune hemolytic anemia. In: A Seminar on Laboratory Management of Hemolysis. Bell, C.A., ed., Las Vegas, NV, 1979, pp. 135-149.

51. Peters, B., Reid, M.E., Ellisor, S.S., and Avoy, D.R.: Red cell survival studies of Lu^b incompatible blood in a patient with anti-Lu^b. (Abstr.) Transfusion 18:623, 1978.

52. Mayer, K., Chin, B., Magnes, J., Harris, J.P., and Tegoli, J.: Further experiences with the in vivo crossmatch and transfusion of Coombs incompatible red cells. In: XVII Congress of International Society of Hematology and XV Congress of International Society of Blood Transfusion Book of Abstracts, July 23-29, 1978, p. 49.

53. Chaplin, H., Jr.: Personal Communication.

54. Dacie, J.V.: The Haemolytic Anemias. 2nd ed. London, Churchill, Ltd., London, 1962, pp. 673-676.

55. Wallace, J.: Blood Transfusion for Clinicians. Churchill Livingstone, New York, 1977, pp. 154-155.

56. Johnsen, H.E., Brostrom, K., and Madsen, M.: Paroxysmal cold haemoglobinuria in children: 3 cases encountered within a period of 7 months. Scand. J. Haematol. 20:413, 1978.

57. Evans, R.S., Bingham, M., and Turner, E.: Autoimmune hemolytic disease: observations of serological reactions and disease activity. Ann. N.Y. Acad. Sci. 124:422, 1965.

57a. Evans, R.S., Turner, E., Bingham, M., and Woods, R.: Chronic Hemolytic Anemia Due to Cold Agglutinins. II. The role of C' in red cell destruction. J. Clin. Invest. 47:4, 1968.

58. Goldfinger, D., Connelly, M., Kellum, S., and Rosenbaum, D.: Transfusion of frozen autologous red blood cells in patients with positive direct antiglobulin tests. Blood 54 (Suppl. 1):123a, 1979.

59. Parr, G.V.S. and Ballard, J.O.: Autologous blood transfusion with methyldopa induced positive direct antiglobulin test. (Correspondence) Transfusion 20:119, 1980.

60. Snyder, E.L. and Spivack, M.: Clinical and serologic management of patients with methyldopa-induced positive antiglobulin tests. Transfusion 19:313, 1979.

61. Petz, L.D. and Fudenberg, H.H.: Immunologic mechanisms in drug-induced cytopenias. In: Progress in Hematology. Vol. IX. Brown, E.B., ed. Grune & Stratton, New York, 1975, p. 185.

62. Petz, L.D.: Drug-induced immune haemolytic anaemia. Clin. Haematol. 9:455, 1980.

63. Garratty, G. and Petz, L.D.: Drug-induced immune hemolytic anemia. Am. J. Med. 58:398, 1975.

64. Levine, B.B. and Redmond, A.: Immunochemical mechanisms of penicillin induced Coombs positivity and hemolytic anemia in man. Int. Arch. Allergy Appl. Immunol. 31:594, 1976.

65. Ries, C.A., Rosenbaum, T.J., Garratty, G., Petz, L.D., and Fudenberg, H.H.: Penicillin-induced immune hemolytic anemia. J.A.M.A. 233:432, 1975.

66. Jackson, F.N. and Jaffe, J.P.: Fatal penicillin-induced hemolytic anemia. Ltr. to the Editor. J.A.M.A. 242:2286, 1979.

67. Petz, L.D.: Immunologic reactions of humans to cephalosporins. Postgrad. Med. J. 47:(Suppl.)64, 1971.

68. Petz, L.D.: Immunologic cross-reactivity between penicillins and cephalosporins: A review. J. Infect. Dis. 137:S74, 1978.

69. Abraham, G.N., Petz, L.D., and Fudenberg, H.H.: Immunohaematological cross-allergenicity between penicillin and cephalothin in humans. Clin. Exp. Immunol. 3:343, 1968.

70. Spath, P., Garratty, G., and Petz, L.D.: Studies on the immune response to penicillin and cephalothin in humans. II. Immunohematologic reactions to cephalothin administration. J. Immunol. 107:860, 1971.

71. Nesmith, L.W. and Davis, J.W.: Hemolytic anemia caused by penicillin: Report of a case in which antipenicillin antibodies cross-reacted with cephalothin sodium. J.A.M.A. 203:27, 1968.

72. Moake, J.L., Butler, C.F., Hewell, G.M., Cheek, J., and Spruell, M.A.: Hemolysis induced by cefazolin and cephalothin in a patient with penicillin sensitivity. Transfusion 18:369, 1978.

73. Jaffe, J.P.: Personal Communication.

74. Beutler, E.: Drug-induced hemolytic anemia. Pharmacol. Rev. 21:73, 1969.

75. Girdwood, R.H.: Blood Disorders Due to Drugs and Other Agents. Excerpta Medica, Amsterdam, 1973.

76. de Gruchy, G.C.: Drug-Induced Blood Disorders. Blackwell Scientific Publications, Oxford, London, Edinburgh, Melbourne, 1975.

77. Nagel, R.L. and Ranney, H.M.: Drug-induced oxidative denaturation of hemoglobin. Sem. Hematol. 10:269, 1973.

32

Congenital Hemolytic Anemias

Denis R. Miller, M.D., and Patricia V. Giardina, M.D.

The congenital hemolytic anemias (CHA) comprise a diverse group of hereditary abnormalities involving one of the three main components of the erythrocyte—the membrane, hemoglobin, or intracellular enzymes. In compensated states of hemolysis, increased destruction, peripherally or within the bone marrow itself, is matched by an increased rate of erythropoiesis, as evidenced by erythroid hyperplasia, reticulocytosis, and increased iron turnover. Factors associated with a further increased rate of red cell destruction (e.g., infection, hypersplenism) and those associated with decreased erythropoiesis (e.g., nutritional deficiencies and toxic, chemical, or infectious agents) will upset the precarious balance. The resultant uncompensated hemolytic state will require transfusion therapy.

Ineffective erythropoiesis may accompany many congenital hemolytic anemias, particularly those characterized by defective synthesis of heme or globin as in the sideroblastic anemias and the thalassemia syndromes, respectively. Associated nutritional deficiencies of iron, vitamin B_{12}, or folic acid will induce ineffective erythropoiesis or dyserythropoiesis in patients with an underlying intrinsic red cell defect and add to the severity of uncompensated hemolysis.[1] In addition to acquired states of dyserythropoiesis, a number of congenital dyserythropoietic anemias have been described and are associated with intra-medullary destruction of erythroid precursors and shortened survival of circulating mature erythrocytes—in essence, a double defect of inefficient erythroid production and increased peripheral destruction of the defective product. Table 32-1 shows an abbreviated classification and outline of congenital hemolytic anemias of relevance to the clinical practice and application of transfusion therapy. The clinical, hematologic, and biochemical features, genetics, and pathophysiology of these inherited defects are presented in several recent comprehensive reviews.[1-7]

Hereditary defects of one component of the red cell may affect the structure, function, and integrity of another, resulting in an increased rate of red cell destruction and shortened erythrocyte survival. Classical examples are: (1) membrane lesions of the irreversibly sickled erythrocyte containing polymerized Hb S; or (2) the rigid, echinocytic, potassium-depleted, dehydrated pyruvate kinase (PK)-deficient erythrocyte.

Pathophysiologic mechanisms of red cell destruction in the congenital hemolytic anemias follow a number of common pathways[8] (Fig. 32-1). Altered intracellular metabolism, particularly that associated with metabolic depletion of adenosine triphosphatase (ATP) and accumulation of calcium results in alterations in cation permeability and transport, transformation of erythrocytes from deform-

Table 32-1. Congenital Hemolytic Anemias of Relevance to the Clinical Practice of Blood Transfusion

I. Defects of membrane
    A. Membrane protein anomalies
        1. Hereditary spherocytosis
        2. Hereditary elliptocytosis
        3. Hereditary stomatocytosis
          a. with hydrocytosis
          b. with xerocytosis
        4. Hereditary pyropoikilocytosis
        5. Membrane lipid anomalies
          a. High phosphatidylcholine

II. Defects of hemoglobin
    A. Structural anomalies
        1. Hb S, Hb C, etc.
    B. Unstable hemoglobin hemolytic anemias
    C. Synthetic anomalies
        1. Thalassemia syndromes
        2. α-thalassemia - Hb H disease
        3. β-thalassemia

III. Defects of enzymes (metabolic defects)
    A. Embden-Meyerhoff pathway anomalies: hexokinase, glucose phosphate isomerase, triose phosphate isomerase, 2,3-diphosphoglycerate mutase, phosphoglycerate kinase, pyruvate kinase
    B. Pentose phosphate shunt defects: glucose-6-phosphate dehydrogenase, glutathione reductase(?), glutathione peroxidase (?), glutathione synthetase
    C. Deficiencies of nucleotide metabolism: adenylate kinase, pyrimidine 5'-nucleotidase, adenosine triphosphatase, adenosine deaminase

able biconcave discs to crenated or echinocytic discs, and, finally, to rigid spherocytes and stomatocytes with a decreased surface area-to-volume ratio and marked susceptibility to entrapment and destruction in spleen, liver, or bone marrow. Destruction of red cells in pyruvate kinase (PK) deficiency and hereditary spherocytosis and other membrane protein defects follows this pathway (E in Fig. 32-1).

Certain structurally abnormal hemoglobins, such as Hb S and Hb C, polymerize or crystallize intracellularly, resulting in increased viscosity or rigidity, loss of membrane deformability, and membrane fragmentation (Pathway A, Fig. 32-1). The end-stage cell, a rigid poikilocyte, is entrapped and destroyed in the reticuloendothelial system or in the microvasculature of the capillary bed.

A third pathway (Pathway B, Fig. 32-1) of destruction of intrinsically defective erythrocytes is associated with inbalanced synthesis of globin chains, unstable hemoglobinopathies, or defects of the pentose phosphate shunt. Heinz body formation is a feature

common to these three disorders. The end-stage cell is a rigid poikilocyte with altered cation transport and membrane permeability. In fact, abnormalities of sodium-potassium permeability and transport, and water content have been described[9] in every general type of congenital hemolytic anemia (Table 32-2). Thus, the severity of hemolysis in many of these disorders is related to an associated membrane disorder.

ALTERED OXYGEN AFFINITY IN CONGENITAL HEMOLYTIC ANEMIAS

In certain congenital hemolytic disorders, the severity of the anemia and, as a corollary, transfusion requirements, may be modulated or intensified by the effects of altered metabolism on hemoglobin function. Enzymatic deficiencies of erythroid glycolysis associated with high or low concentrations of 2,3-diphosphoglycerate (2,3-DPG) influence the affinity of hemoglobin for oxygen.[10] In PK-deficiency hereditary hemolytic anemia the

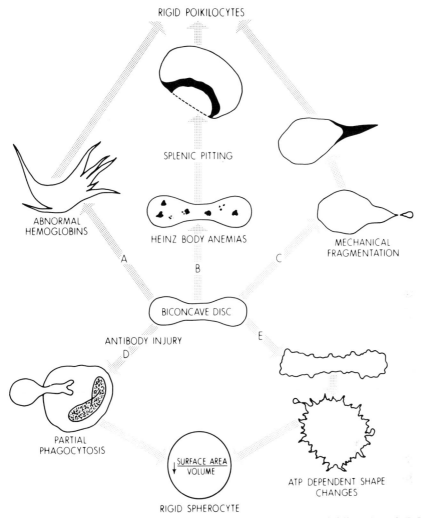

Fig. 32-1. Pathophysiologic pathways of erythrocyte fragmentation and rigidity. (Weed, R.I.: Plenary Session Papers XII Congress International Society of Hematology, 1968, p. 85.)

concentration of 2,3-DPG is markedly elevated, and in hexokinase (HK) deficiency it is markedly decreased, because of the location of the respective enzymatic deficiencies. As expected, the oxygen dissociation curve in PK deficiency is shifted to the right, and in HK deficiency it is displaced to the left (Fig. 32-2). The rightward shift in the oxygen dissociation curve in PK deficiency allows the delivery of as much oxygen from 9 g of Hb/dl as would be delivered by 15 g/dl at a similar rate of blood flow. In HK deficiency, in spite of the decreased 2,3-DPG content, a compensatory increase in red cell mass does not occur because of the rapid hemolytic rate. A block in glycolysis at the PK step results in increased concentrations of a number of glycolytic intermediates proximal to the PK reaction. Most important is the raised level of 2,3-DPG to 2 to 4 times normal. Increased levels of 2,-3-DPG decrease oxygen affinity and increase the P_{50} O_2, shifting the oxygen dissociation curve to the right. The net result is increased oxygen delivery to the tissues, providing physiological compensation to the moderately severe anemia.

Table 32-2. Examples of Abnormalities of Cation Transport, Permeability, and Hydration in Congenital Hemolytic Anemias

Disorder	Abnormality	Reference
Membrane defects		
Hereditary spherocytosis	Increased Na^+ flux and transport	Jacob and Jandl[133]
Hereditary elliptocytosis	Increased Na^+ FLUX	Peters et al.[134]
Hereditary stomatocytosis	Increased Na^+ and decreased K^+ with increased osmotic fragility	Zarowsky et al.[135]
	Increased Na^+, slightly decreased K^+, decreased osmotic fragility	Miller et al.[136]
Hemoglobin defects		
HbSS disease	K^+ loss in excess of Na^+ gain at low PO_2	Tosteson et al.[137]
β-thalassemia	Increased Na^+; increased K^+ permeability	Nathan[138]
Enzyme defects		
Pyruvate kinase deficiency	Increased K^+ and H_2O loss; xerocytosis	Nathan et al[139]
		Nathan and Shohet[140]

A change in the concentration of 2,3-DPG allows the red cell to adjust the supply of oxygen to the tissues in response to hypoxia.[11] Like hemoglobin concentration, oxygen affinity is inversely correlated with 2,3-DPG concentration. A change in the level of 2,3-DPG of 1mM/liter of RBC causes a shift of the P_{50} O_2 value of 3.8 mm Hg.[12] Alternate compensatory mechanisms for hypoxemia depend upon an increase in red cell mass secondary to erythropoietin-induced stimulation of the bone marrow.[13] This process takes several days and is ineffective when anemia is due to a primary or secondary decrease in red cell production or when accelerated destruction is too rapid for compensation to be achieved by maximal marrow hyperplasia.

A number of unstable hemoglobin hemolytic anemias (e.g., Hb Köln and Hb Zürich) are associated with increased oxygen affinity.[14,15] Decreased oxygen delivery results in increased erythropoietin production, increased erythropoiesis, an expansion of the red cell mass and, in some patients, erythrocytosis, obviating the requirement for transfusion except in the severest forms of unstable hemoglobinopathies such as Hb Hammersmith or Hb Olmstead.[16]

The α-thalassemias, Hb H disease with tetramers of β-chains (β_4) and Hb Barts with tetramers of γ-chains (γ_4) are associated with very high oxygen affinities (low P_{50} O_2). Certain structurally unstable hemoglobins (e.g., Hb Köln) shift the oxygen dissociation curve to the left throughout the physiologic range of PO_2. Lacking α-chains, β_4 and γ_4 do not interact with normal hemoglobin, preventing a significant alteration of the oxygen dissociation curve in the physiologic range of PO_2. In Hb H disease, oxygen delivery by Hb A, which makes up 85 to 90 percent of the red cell hemoglobin, is not affected, and there is little alteration in the P_{50} O_2. Hence, in these α-thalassemia syndromes, the additional erythropoietic stimulus induced by a leftward shift of the oxygen dissociation curve is absent, and the compensatory increase in red cell mass, already blunted by ineffective erythropoiesis, is not prominent. Compensation, as traditionally judged in terms of hemoglobin compensation, is incomplete; however, compensation in terms of oxygen delivery is probably similar in α-thalassemia and unstable hemoglobin syndromes as a result of the differences in oxygen affinity.

The oxygen affinity of Hb F is greater than that of adult hemoglobin Hb A. This is partially related to the greater affinity of deoxy Hb A than deoxy Hb F for 2,3-DPG and ATP. The differences in oxygen affinity of intraerythrocytic Hb A and Hb F are not related to erythrocyte 2,3-DPG, since the red

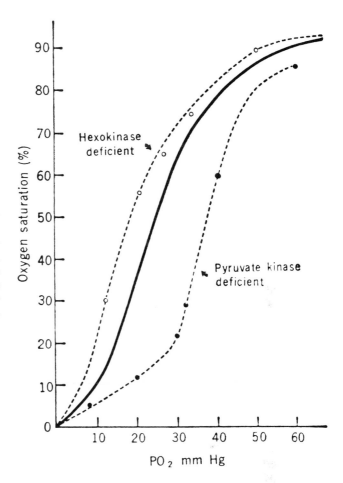

Fig. 32-2. Oxygen dissociation curves in normal individuals (*solid line*), hexokinase deficiency (*dashed line, open circles*) and pyrurate kinase deficiency (*dashed line, closed circles*). (Delivoria-Papadopoulos, M.: Oxygen-hemoglobulin dissociation curves: Effect of inherited enzyme defects of the red cell. Science 165:601–602, 1969. Copyright 1969 by the American Association for the Advancement of Science.)

cells of full-term newborns have the same 2,-3-DPG concentrations as those of normal adults.

In congenital hemolytic anemias, such as β-thalassemia major, in which a high concentration of Hb F is present, hemoglobin oxygen affinity is not reduced despite an increase in red cell 2,3-DPG. In the presence of large proportions of Hb F in the red cell, a beneficial compensatory right shift of the oxygen dissociation curve does not occur due to the failure of 2,3-DPG to interact with the γ-chain of Hb F as it does with the β-chain of Hb A.

These physiologic compensatory alterations must be considered in evaluating patients as candidates for acute or chronic transfusion therapy. It is now obvious that the

traditional and conventional method for quantifying the severity of anemia—the level of Hb—is obsolete, and that modulating effects on the oxygen dissociation curve—including 2,3-DPG, intracellular pH, MCHC, extracellular and intracellular Pi, temperature, extracellular pH, intracellular Hb, and overall metabolic activity—all play a role in determining oxygen delivery and adaptation to anemia.

Associated Medical Conditions

The transfusion requirements of patients with congenital hemolytic anemia will be dependent upon related extrinsic factors as well as the specific inborn error of cell metabolism, structure, and function. Physiological events in early infancy, other medical problems, associated organ dysfunction, endocrine disturbances, and nutritional deficiencies must be considered in designing therapeutic strategies for these patients.

Transfusion requirements in infants with congenital hemolytic syndromes are frequently maximal during the first 6 to 12 months of life. So-called physiologic anemia or erythroid hypoplasia of infancy is responsible for this transfusion dependency in infants with severe hemolytic anemia.[17] Compared to older children, the normal newborn has an increased red cell mass, hemoglobin level, and packed red blood cell volume. After the first week of life, the high level of hemoglobin declines progressively and reaches a nadir of 10 to 11 g/dl for full-term infants and 8 to 9 g/dl for prematures at 6 to 10 weeks of age.

Siep's[18] carefully controlled studies of reticulocyte counts in early infancy and the ferrokinetics studies of Garby[19] showed that erythrocyte production falls precipitously after the first week of life and remains low until about 8 to 10 weeks of age. Factors contributing to this state of decreased erythropoiesis include decreased erythropoietin production, short survival of the fetal red cell, and the rapid expansion of blood volume that accompanies the period of rapid somatic growth during early infancy. After the second day of life, erythropoietin is no longer detected in the plasma or urine until 6 to 8 weeks of age.[20] Improved oxygenation occurs when the lungs replace the placenta as the source of oxygen transport and arterial oxygenation increases from 45 percent to 95 percent. Clark[21] has suggested that, in addition to decreased erythropoietin production, an erythropoiesis-inhibiting factor in the plasma and urine contributes to the physiologic anemia. The degree and rapidity of decline of hemoglobin levels in premature infants is more profound and exaggerated than in full-term babies.[22] Although full-term infants respond to hypoxic stress with an erythropoietic burst,

premature infants lack this capability. Whereas there is a significant inverse correlation between erythropoietin levels and anemia after the third month of age, the levels of hemoglobin or packed cell volume at which erythropoietin production and erythropoiesis are turned on are much lower from birth to 3 months of age than in later infancy, childhood, or adult life.[23] The response to anemia in premature infants is aberrant in that no erythropoietin is detected in them, but it is readily measurable in older children with a similar degree of anemia.[24] Any disturbances, and particularly congenital hemolytic anemia syndromes that add further stress to an already overburdened and tenuous equilibrium, are invariably associated with severe transfusion-dependent anemia in the early weeks and months of life. Additional factors include iron deficiency, folate depletion, and vitamin E deficiency. Gastrointestinal disturbances and increased dietary polyunsaturated fatty acids will compound the severity of physiologic and hemolytic anemia and increase transfusion requirements. When transfusions are necessary during the phase of physiologic anemia, small amounts of blood should be given, the object being to increase the level of hemoglobin to approximately 8 g/dl. Transfusing to higher levels of hemoglobin may delay spontaneous recovery by suppressing normal erythropoiesis.

Complicating medical conditions such as chronic infections, chronic inflammatory disorders, malignant neoplastic disease, and chronic renal disease will have serious adverse effects upon a preexisting congenital hemolytic anemia and markedly increase transfusion requirements. Typically, the anemia of these chronic disorders share in common the following features: mild-to-moderate anemia; slightly decreased red blood cell survival; decreased serum iron and iron-binding capacity; increased tissue iron stores and serum ferritin; abnormal ferrokinetics; decreased marrow sideroblasts; relative bone marrow unresponsiveness to erythropoietin; and, in chronic renal disease, inappropriately decreased erythropoietin levels. The following conditions will exacerbate the severity of a preexisting congenital hemolytic state and increase transfusion requirements: cardiopulmonary insufficiency; hypothyroidism and hypopituitarism; acquired autoimmune hemolytic anemia associated with frequent and chronic transfusion therapy; hypersplenism; and severe, intercurrent life-threatening infections (septicemia, pneumonia, meningitis), particularly in post-splenectomy patients. Accordingly, a thorough medical evaluation of all organ systems is required before embarking upon transfusion therapy for these patients. Transfusions in these secondary anemias are considered in Chapters 29 and 30. Perinatal and neonatal transfusion therapy is discussed in Chapter 33.

COMMON FEATURES OF CONGENITAL HEMOLYTIC ANEMIAS

Hyperbilirubinemia and Anemia in the Neonatal Period

The normal newborn's erythrocytes are biochemically, structurally, and functionally unlike their adult type counterparts.[25] Significant variations have been detected in membrane phospholipid and fatty acid composition (increased sphingomyelin, increased lipid phosphorus and cholesterol, and decreased lecithin); cation transport and permeability (decreased active flux); biophysical properties (decreased deformability); hemoglobin content and function (increased Hb F with increased O_2 affinity, decreased methemoglobin reductase, and increased susceptibility to oxidative denaturation and Heinz body formation); and metabolic activity (decreased GSH stability and GSH peroxidase, increased lability of ATP and 2,3-DPG, decreased phosphofructokinase, and relatively decreased glycolysis). Given a congenitally defective erythrocyte, exaggerated hemolysis in the newborn period with extreme indirect

hyperbilirubinemia is not surprising. This is particularly true in congenital defects of the membrane and glycolytic enzymes. Profound hyperbilirubinemia (indirect bilirubin >15 mg/dl) necessitating exchange transfusion to prevent kernicterus has been reported in infants with deficiencies of G6PD, hexokinase (HK), glucose phosphate isomerase (GPI), phosphoglycerate kinase (PGK), pyruvate kinase (PK), and in the hereditary membrane anomalies of spherocytosis, elliptocytosis, and stomatocytosis.[26] The incidence of enzyme deficiency as a cause of neonatal hyperbilirubinemia is high, particularly in Greece and in Hong Kong.[27] Doxiadis et al.[28] reported that isoimmunization was excluded in one-third of full-term infants with severe neonatal jaundice. Many of these infants had Mediterranean type G6PD deficiency that may have been the causative factor in hyperbilirubinemia and kernicterus. A similar relationship has been reported from India, Thailand, Malaysia, South Africa, Nigeria, and Italy.[29] Nearly 75 percent of white infants with G6PD deficiency and with chronic congenital hemolytic anemia have a history of neonatal jaundice.[30]

G6PD deficiency was present in 65 percent of severely jaundiced newborn Thai infants.[31] In the United States, G6PD deficiency in black premature infants, but not in full-term infants, is associated with an increased incidence of hyperbilirubinemia and a greater frequency of exchange transfusions.[32] The incidence of neonatal jaundice in black Africans is much higher than it is in black Americans, despite the fact that both have the same A− variant of G6PD, suggesting additional genetic or environmental factors.[33]

It is noteworthy that, although an increase in neonatal jaundice has been observed in Greece, it could not be documented in Israel.[34] The G6PD variant prevalent in these regions is the same, G6PD Mediterranean, and the reason for the discrepancy is unclear.

Many infants with G6PD deficiency are most threatened in the neonatal period because of the danger of kernicterus and death.

Appropriate diagnostic studies in susceptible infants must be performed, and appropriate therapy, including exchange transfusion, should be initiated promptly. Clinically apparent jaundice occurs in the first 24 to 48 hours of life and rapidly may reach levels of 30 to 40 mg/dl. Severe hyperbilirubinemia, kernicterus, and death have occurred in infants discharged from the hospital during the first week of life only to return moribund a few days later. The indications for exchange transfusion are similar to those in infants with hemolytic disease of the newborn due to Rh or other blood group incompatibility with one major caveat—donors should be screened for G6PD deficiency and G6PD-deficient blood excluded.

Extreme hemolysis, hyperbilirubinemia, and kernicterus do not occur in most infants with hemoglobinopathies and thalassemia syndromes, particularly if the molecular defect involves the β-chain. Since 70 to 90 percent of the neonate's hemoglobin is Hb F, clinical manifestations of β-chain defects such as $\beta°$-thalassemia or sickle cell disease are not obvious until γ production is switched to β-chain synthesis. However, infants with inherited defects of α- or γ-chains will manifest symptoms of hemolysis in the newborn period. Unstable hemoglobinopathies involving the α- and/or γ-chain will also present in the newborn period with Heinz body hemolytic anemia. Hemoglobinopathies and thalassemia syndromes that are clincally apparent in the newborn period are listed in Table 32-3. Severe anemia, rather than hyperbilirubinemia, is the major clinical problem in the thalassemia syndromes, but homozygous α-thalassemia or Hb Bart's

hydrops fetalis syndrome is incompatible with life. Death is due to hypoxia and congestive heart failure. In one case in which the diagnosis was suspected antenatally, Caesarian section and exchange transfusion were not successful in prolonging life beyond the first few hours.[35] Generally, most infants with homozygous α-thalassemia are stillborn.

Hypoplastic Crisis

The hypoplastic or aplastic crisis is a feature common to all congenital hemolytic anemias. Patients most at risk of developing this potentially life-threatening complication are those with decreased red cell survival, barely compensated hemolysis with moderately severe anemia (Hb 7 to 9 g/dl), and maximally increased red cell production (5 to 8 times normal). Any compromise of the patient's maximal compensatory response rapidly results in profound anemia (Hb <5.0 g/dl), with weakness, listlessness, fever, tachypnea, tachycardia and diaphoresis. The aplastic crisis is caused by diminished red cell production superimposed on the usual increased destruction rather than increased rate of red cell destruction.

Infections, frequently of viral etiology, temporarily injure the erythron by an obscure mechanism. Red cell production ceases for one to three weeks and crises may occur in more than one affected family member, further supporting the infectious origin of the event.[36,37] Profound reticulocytopenia in the peripheral blood and virtual absence of erythroid precursors in the bone marrow are observed during the crisis.[38] Previously ele-

Table 32-3. Defects of Hemoglobin in the Newborn

Site of Defect	Diseases	Age of Onset
α-chain	Hb Da, I	Birth
	homozygous α-thalassemia	Birth
	Hb H	After 3 mos.
	various unstable Hb	Birth
β-chain	Hb S,C,E	After 3 mos.
γ-chain	Hb F Alexandra, Roma, Aegena, Texas	Birth
γ,δ,β	γ,δ,β thalassemia trait	Birth

vated levels of indirect bilirubin decrease, normoblasts disappear from the peripheral blood, and, rarely, the platelet and white blood cell counts diminish, reflecting a generalized effect on pluripotential stem cells rather than a sole effect on erythroid precursors. If aplastic crisis remains unrecognized and untreated, the level of hemoglobin may drop to 2 g/dl or less, with death resulting from congestive heart failure.

Most crises of erythroid aplasia terminate spontaneously after one to two weeks. The recovery phase is heralded by a brisk reticulocytosis, sometimes reaching 50 percent or greater, followed by a return of hemoglobin to pre-aplasia levels. Hematologic values during aplastic crises vary, depending upon the phase of the crisis. Diagnostic studies performed during the recovery phase can easily be misinterpreted as an exacerbation of acute hemolysis superimposed upon the underlying congenital defect.

Regardless of the specific type of congenital hemolytic anemia, transfusion of fresh packed red blood cells (PRBC) is the mandatory treatment. The rationale for using fresh PRBCs is to assure normal levels of 2,-3-DPG and normal oxygen delivery to the tissues. Cells should be transfused slowly in severely anemic patients (2 to 3 ml/kg of body weight over 4 hours every 6 to 8 hours) to avoid cardiac decompensation and until the hemoglobin is increased at least 5 g/dl.[39] Oxygen is indicated in dyspneic patients. Patients with evidence of high-output, hypoxic congestive failure should be closely monitored with a central venous catheter. A partial exchange transfusion can be carried out during the transfusion by withdrawing blood as donor PRBCs are administered. Prompt but cautious restoration of oxygen-carrying capacity is the key. Patients with prolonged aplasia may require maintenance transfusion therapy for the duration of the aplastic crisis. Patients diagnosed in the recovery phase with severe anemia but a high reticulocyte count may need a single transfusion to rescue them from congestive failure or prevent it.

Indications and Contraindications of Transfusions in CHA

The primary role of transfusion therapy in children and adults with congenital hemolytic anemia syndromes is palliative—the temporary restoration of red cell mass and oxygen-carrying capacity to levels that will obviate the signs and symptoms of chronic anemia and permit normal growth and development of the child. Acute events such as severe intercurrent infections and transient hypoplasia require special consideration. A rational transfusion program must be individualized with regard to:

1. the patient's underlying diagnosis, age, coexisting medical problems, nutritional status, and physiological adaptation to anemia;
2. the status of splenic function;
3. the long-range objectives and complications of chronic transfusion therapy;
4. the product to be used; and
5. the level of hemoglobin to be achieved posttransfusion.

In the following discussion of transfusion therapy in congenital hemolytic anemias, the focus will be on these universal considerations. Whereas these principles must be considered in all patients with transfusion-dependent congenital hemolytic anemias, unique problems of specific disorders will be reviewed comprehensively.

TRANSFUSION IN RED CELL MEMBRANE DEFECTS

Hereditary Spherocytosis, Elliptocytosis, and Stomatocytosis

Indications for transfusion therapy in congenital hemolytic anemias caused by perturbations of membrane structure and function are similar: neonatal hyperbilirubinemia; prolonged physiologic anemia superimposed upon the baseline hemolytic state; aplastic crisis induced by infection and/or nutritional deficiencies; pregnancy; and preoperative preparation for major surgical procedures. The spectrum of severity of hemolytic anemia varies from patient to patient regardless of diagnosis, although the degree of severity remains fairly constant among affected family members with these dominantly inherited disorders.

Chronic transfusion therapy is rarely, if ever, required in these otherwise uncomplicated, compensated hemolytic states, except during early infancy when the level of hemoglobin should be maintained above 8 g/dl. Because 2,3-DPG levels in reticulocytes are higher than in mature erythrocytes, the predicted P_{50} O_2 in patients with hereditary membrane defects should be increased. Paradoxically, the red cell content of 2,3-DPG in hereditary spherocytosis is low before splenectomy, perhaps the result of increased catabolism of 2,3-DPG in the acidic environment of the spleen.[39a] However, the P_{50} O_2 in patients with compensated hemolysis is normal,[40] suggesting that overt tissue hypoxia is not present.

Transfusions are rarely required beyond the first year or two of life, when the hemoglobin level in the compensated hemolytic state is usually between 8 and 13 g/dl. Only 10 to 15 percent of patients with hereditary elliptocytosis have a significant hemolytic anemia, but the hemoglobin invariably is above 9 to 10 g/dl, obviating transfusions except with aplastic or hyperhemolytic crisis, which are usually precipitated by severe intercurrent infection. The diagnosis of hereditary spherocytosis as well as other membrane defects may be delayed until adulthood in many patients who may be admitted to the hospital for evaluation of severe anemia complicating pregnancy,[41] cholelithiasis, or presumed aplastic anemia. Transfusion therapy may be required in these patients, particularly if preexisting iron, folate, or vitamin B_{12} deficiency, chronic renal disease, or hypothyroidism complicate the hemolytic anemia and cause decompensation of the precarious balance between red cell production and destruction. In each patient requiring supportive transfusion therapy, PRBC is the product of choice. To avoid suppression of erythropoiesis, the clinician should avoid transfusing to a level of hemoglobin above 8 to 9 g/dl. In the absence of hypersplenism and in the postsplenectomy state, compatible donor erythrocytes survive normally in the transfused host.

Rarer Membrane Disorders

A rare and recently described hereditary membrane defect, pyropoikilocytosis,[42] is moderately severe, and transfusions may be required early in life or with associated complicating disorders.

High phosphatidylcholine hemolytic anemia, transmitted as an autosomal dominant condition, is mild, and transfusions are not required.[43]

TRANSFUSION IN HEMOGLOBIN DEFECTS

Structural Disorders

Sickle Cell Anemia. The indications for transfusion therapy in sickle cell disease include severe vasoocclusive or painful crises refractory to conventional medical management, severe infection associated with the functional asplenia syndrome, acute splenic sequestration, stroke, hypoplastic crises, pregnancy, surgery,[44] acute lung syndrome, liver infarction, chronic leg ulcers, and priapism.[45] Frequently, patients with severe vasoocclusive crises fail to respond to general supportive measures, including: analgesia; treatment of any complicating infection; correction of fluid, electrolyte, acid-base imbalance, and hypoxia; and provision for adequate oxygenation. Thus, transfusions should be seriously considered in prolonged painful crises unresponsive or refractory to comprehensive but conservative medical management. Transfusions are not given to treat the anemia because hematologic deterioration does not occur in most vasoocclusive crises. The objective of transfusion therapy is to dilute the patient's sickle cells and decrease the resistance of blood by reducing the numbers of circulating sickle cells and the concentration of Hb S. If the proportion and number of sickle cells in the circulation can be reduced effectively, pain, tissue hypoxia, and further necrosis can be ameliorated. In vitro, the resistance of sickle cell blood is reduced when a cell mixture of Hb A and Hb S contains less than 40 percent sickle cells.[46] Clinically, when vasoocclusion occurs, the level of Hb S usually exceeds 50 percent.

When at least 60 percent of the patient's red cells are replaced by normal Hb A-containing cells, the progression of symptoms usually ceases. To achieve this objective, two therapeutic methods are available:

1. Transfusion of fresh PRBCs *from non-sickle cell donors,* 10 to 15 ml/kg can be given every 12 hours until the hemoglobin level has inceased to 12 to 13 g/dl. At this point, simple dilution will have decreased significantly the proportion of the patient's sickle cells. At this level of hemoglobin, erythropoiesis also will be inhibited. Sickle cells, because of their shortened survival, will disappear rapidly from the circulation. Thereafter, small, packed red cell transfusions given every 2 to 3 weeks will maintain the level of Hb S below 40 percent, suppress Hb S synthesis, and insure that the majority of circulating red cells will be normal. The adequacy of chronic or replacement transfusion therapy can be quantified by periodic determinations of Hb S. Isoimmunization, hepatitis, and iron overload are potential risks of prolonged transfusion therapy. Obviously, specific indications must be present before embarking upon any program of chronic transfusion therapy.

2. Simple transfusion, however, is time-consuming and increases the risk of fluid overload and congestive heart failure. For these reasons, limited or partial exchange transfusions have been advocated as an alternate, more rapid, and efficient means to decrease the concentration of Hb S.[47-49] Partial exchange transfusion in sickle cell anemia has been utilized in patients with painful crises, heart disease,[50] cerebrovascular accidents,[51,52] and during pregnancy.[53,54] Lanzkowsky et al.[55] performed 40 partial exchange transfusions in 17 children with serious complications of sickle cell anemia by transfusing 15 ml/kg of PRBCs and simultaneously withdrawing by gravity 20 ml/kg of whole blood from the opposite antecubital vein. The exchange was repeated 24 hours later in patients with acute lung syndrome, acute liver crisis, acute papillary necrosis, pneumococcal meningitis, persistent painful crisis, priapism, and preoperatively. The mean value for packed red cell volume rose from 23 percent before the exchange transfusion to 41 percent at the end of the second exchange, and the mean level of Hb S decreased from 94 percent before transfusion to 28 percent after the second exchange. Exchange transfusion lowers the serum bilirubin level and may reduce the late sequelae in acute liver crisis with attendant intralobular necrosis, infarction, and abscess formation leading to fibrosis and cirrhosis.[56,57] Similarly, PaO_2 increased after exchange transfusion in patients with the acute lung syndrome unresponsive to oxygen therapy.

Infection. Transfusions are indicated in sickle cell anemia patients with potentially overwhelming fatal pneumococcal infections (sepsis, pneumonia, and meningitis) related to functional hyposplenia. Pearson[58] defined functional asplenia as defective splenic reticuloendothelial activity of anatomically enlarged spleens of young children, generally under 3 years of age. The enhanced susceptibility to infections caused by pneumococci, *H. influenzae,* and *E. coli* is related to decreased phagocytosis and clearance of these organisms in functionally asplenic patients.[59] Defective phagocytic function of the spleen is manifested by the presence of Howell-Jolly bodies, Heinz bodies, and membrane pits in circulating red cells. Pearson et al.[60] showed that altered intrasplenic perfusion, demonstrated by ^{99m}Tc sulfur colloid scanning of the spleen, can be reversed temporarily by transfusion therapy. Intrasplenic sickling and decreased phagocytosis by macrophages in the splenic cords and lining of the splenic sinuses account for the decreased uptake of ^{99m}Tc label.

Thus, in patients with sepsis, pneumonia, meningitis, or other life-threatening infections during the first three or four years of life, transfusion therapy is indicated, in addition to appropriate antibiotics and general supportive measures. Exchange transfusion may also provide deficient opsonins, immunoglobulins, and other components of immunologic warfare, and remove bacteria and endotoxins.

Splenic Sequestration Crisis. Infants and children with homozygous sickle cell anemia whose spleens have not undergone total infarction and fibrosis ("autosplenectomy") and children with other sickle cell syndromes (e.g., sickle cell-β-thalassemia) associated with persistent splenomegaly are at grave risk of sudden acute splenic sequestration crisis. During this crisis, the spleen enlarges massively, the level of hemoglobin drops precipitously, and hypovolemic shock and death may ensue with startling rapidity. Within hours, the hemoglobin may drop from stable levels of 7 to 8 g/dl to 2 g/dl or less.[61,62]

Prompt whole blood transfusions will correct hypovolemia, reverse the shock, permit the recirculation of red cells sequestered in the spleen, and cause regression of the massive splenomegaly. Splenectomy should be considered to prevent further crises.

Stroke. Stroke is a devastating complication of sickle cell anemia and occurs in approximately 6 percent of sickle cell patients of all ages.[63] Infarction and attendant structural and functional defects are significantly more common during the first two decades of life.

Two-thirds of the patients suffering from one stroke will have a recurrence, usually within 36 months. Factors such as prior illness patterns, hemoglobin levels, fetal hemoglobin content, or previous neurological symptoms do not identify the patient at risk of developing a stroke. Unfortunately, 20 percent of these patients with stroke die. Survivors are often left with residual neurological and intellectual deficits and never regain totally their prestroke status.

Cerebral angiography is hazardous, but, with careful preparation consisting of repeated packed RBC transfusions over a one- to three-week period or exchange transfusion immediately before the procedure, the risk of intravascular sickling can be reduced and an accurate diagnosis can be established.[64] Computerized tomography should obviate many of the risks inherent in performing cerebral angiography.

Emergency transfusion therapy should be instituted to decrease the concentration of Hb S to 20 percent or less by simple packed RBC or exchange transfusions. Recent reports[65,66] of chronic transfusion therapy for one year or more suggest that this approach decreases the risk of recurrence and hastens the angiographic and clinical improvement of these patients who were maintained at a concentration of hemoglobin above 10 g/dl with Hb S levels below 30 percent. The optimal duration of chronic transfusion therapy has not been established. In a series of 35 patients with strokes observed in Los Angeles, the mean interval between strokes was 28 months, with 80 percent of the subsequent strokes recurring before 36 months, and all developing within 4 years of the initial insult. Thus, it seems unlikely that lifelong transfusion therapy, as required in thalassemia major, is indicated, particularly with the associated risks of isoimmunization, hepatitis, anaphylaxis, and transfusion hemosiderosis. Chelation therapy with subcutaneous deferoxamine should prevent this complication in patients enrolled in a transfusion program with a finite duration of 3 to 4 years.[65] Controlled studies with more patients are needed to resolve these questions.

Pregnancy. Pregnancy is another serious threat to the teenager or young woman with sickle cell anemia or Hb S/C disease. Mortality as high as 20 percent has been reported in poorly supervised pregnancies, but good medical care will decrease the frequency of serious complications and death.[66] Fetal prematurity and stillbirth rates are also unacceptably high.[67] A chronic transfusion program beginning during the last trimester or earlier may reduce placental insufficiency resulting from infarction and lower the rate of prematurity, stillbirth, and maternal morbidity and mortality.[68]

Leg Ulcers; Priapism. Chronic, indolent leg ulcers, unresponsive to the usual conservative therapy of frequent changes of dressing, immobilization, and treatment of superficial infection, may respond to multiple transfusions. The painful symptoms and devastating sequelae of priapism may be lessened by transfusion.[45]

Other Hemoglobinopathies

Specific indications for transfusion therapy in other clinically severe, structural hemoglobinopathies include hypoplastic crises, preparation for surgical procedures, and pregnancy. Whereas most of these disorders are less severe than sickle cell disease, uncompensated hemolysis accompanying certain severe unstable hemoglobinopathies with increased oxygen affinity may require periodic transfusion therapy.

TRANSFUSION THERAPY IN THALASSEMIA SYNDROMES

Considerable progress has been made recently in transfusion therapy of patients with homozygous β-thalassemia. Historically, treatment had been mainly supportive and consisted of intermittent whole blood or PRBC transfusions to control severe anemia. Such a transfusion program was effective in moderately correcting severe anemia to a "safe" hemoglobin level of 7 to 9 g/dl to avoid symptoms of anemia. The objective of more recent transfusion programs aimed at maintaining a minimal hemoglobin level of 10 g/dl, "hypertransfusion" therapy, is to decrease the effects of chronic anemia and prevent abnormal growth and development.[69] Another approach is to maintain a hemoglobin level greater than 12 g/dl. This "supertransfusion" program is designed to suppress completely intramedullary and extramedullary hematopoiesis. When the program is initiated from infancy, its goals include normal growth and development, normal daily functioning, and psychological well-being. This "supertransfusion" approach also reduces total blood volume and plasma iron turnover such that transfusion requirements and iron loading are actually reduced.[70] The classical thalassemic facies with orthodontic malocclusion, pathologic bone changes, and related fractures resulting from marrow expansion and unsuppressed intramedullary hematopoiesis can be avoided with a transfusion regimen designed to maintain a higher level of hemoglobin. The inhibition of erythropoiesis also reduces gastrointestinal iron absorption to normal, further reducing iron overload induced by chronic transfusions.[71] Although the mechanism of increased iron absorption in anemic, iron-replete patients is not clear, increased plasma iron turnover associated with ineffective erythropoiesis is thought to play a role.[72] Propper and Nathan[70] have shown that increasing the level of hemoglobin diminishes the amount of dietary iron absorbed from the gastrointestinal tract and reduces the rate of plasma iron turnover in the thalassemic patient.

The rationale for maintaining a higher level of hemoglobin is also supported by the experimental study of Necheles.[73] Mice given excess parenteral iron but not made anemic, did not develop cardiac hemosiderosis. However, mice concomitantly made anemic had iron deposited in the myocardium. Thus, a higher transfusion program may avert deposition of iron in parenchymal tissue by preventing the anemia that leads to tissue hypoxia and focal tissue necrosis.

A higher transfusion program has many advantages in contributing to the greater well-being and normal daily life-style of the thalassemic patient. The more normal red cell volume achieved decreases cardiac work and increases exercise tolerance. Thus, "normal" daily activity is achieved. Less cardiomegaly, adenopathy, and hepatosplenomegaly are observed with a higher transfusion program. Established splenomegaly may be reversible with hypertransfusion due to suppression of extramedullary hematopoiesis. The risk of cord compression (albeit rare) secondary to massive extramedullary hematopoiesis in paravertebral lymph nodes is also lessened. There appears to be little question that higher transfusion regimens improve the quality of life of the thalassemic patient.

BLOOD PRODUCTS

The functional integrity of hemoglobin in the transfused red cells is an important consideration in selecting the best product. Red cells banked in ACD preservative are depleted of 2,3-DPG and have high oxygen affinity.[74] An inverse correlation of red cell mass and DPG concentration occurs in the absence of metabolic alterations which may alter oxygen affinity directly through the Bohr effect, or indirectly by affecting glycolysis. In metabolically normal recipients, transfused red cells replenish 2,3-DPG in 36 to 48 hours, and oxygen affinity returns to normal.[75] De Furia and coworkers[76] found inappropriately low values for $P_{50} O_2$ and low levels of 2,3-DPG in patients with homozygous β-thalassemia treated with a transfusion program designed to maintain the level of hemoglobin above 8 g/dl with ACD-banked blood. Other factors[77] known to affect hemo-

globin function within the red cell—ATP, ΔpH, MCHC, and base excess—were within normal limits. Increased oxygen affinity in transfused thalassemic patients was not due to an increased level of Hb F, which has a higher oxygen affinity than Hb A. However, in transfusion-dependent patients with thalassemia intermedia, a significant correlation existed between the concentration of Hb F and $P_{50} O_2$. Thus, in the absence of hemoglobin dysfunction per se, the metabolic integrity of the red cells in chronically transfused patients was in question. Subtle changes related to blood banking and aging may impair the synthesis of increased amounts of DPG in response to anemia.

The metabolic and functional defects of blood in chronically transfused patients may have contributed to their morbidity and poor clinical status prior to the use of hypertransfusion and supertransfusion regimens and better-preserved CPD-stored or frozen-thawed red blood cells. Firstly, relatively high oxygen affinity may contribute to tissue hypoxia, cell membrane damage, and, ultimately, fibrosis. Secondly, the high oxygen affinity per se stimulates erythropoietin production and endogenous production of defective cells. The ideal transfusion program must supply erythrocytes with normal metabolism and hemoglobin function *and* totally suppress erythropoiesis.

An ideal, although expensive, program for the transfusion-dependent patient with homozygous thalassemia uses washed frozen-thawed red cells. This product is less contaminated by donor plasma proteins, leukocytes, and other agents such as viruses. These contaminating particles are a major concern in the treatment of chronically transfused patients. Febrile reactions in patients receiving frozen-thawed red cells are reduced, and a corresponding reduction in antileukocyte antibody also occurs. The fever/chill reactions and the fatal "pulmonary transfusion-anaphylaxis syndrome"[78] attributed to autoleukocyte and HLA antibodies may also be obviated with the use of frozen-thawed washed red blood cells. Most of the urticarial-anaphylactoid reactions from the infusion of donor plasma proteins such as the IgA molecule can also be avoided by using frozen-thawed washed cells.

When transfusing frozen-thawed cells, the use of a fine-mesh, 10-micron microaggregate filter further reduces the amount of leukocyte antigenic material infused. Patients who have had previous febrile and urticarial reactions should be pretreated with antipyretics (e.g., Tylenol), antihistamines (e.g., Benadryl), and occasionally glucocorticosteroids (e.g., hydrocortisone).

Hemolytic transfusion reactions due to isoimmunization also can be reduced by use of frozen-thawed red cells. Although nearly 50 percent of the chronically transfused thalassemia patients in our clinic have antibodies to red cell antigens, half of these do not have identifiable antigenetic specificity. It is occasionally difficult to find compatible donors for these patients with "nonspecific" red cell antibodies. The use of frozen-thawed processing provides compatible units by preselection of the donor or precrossmatching, thereby decreasing the chance of using incompatible blood and avoiding delays in finding compatible units. Donor cells may be separated in aliquots from donor units, frozen, and stored at a regional center. Thus, multiple units can be crossmatched and compatible units can be selected, frozen, and stored for use in individual patients at a later date. Isoimmunization to minor blood groups (e.g., Kell, Duffy, C, K, E) as well as the ubiquitous cold (12° C) anti-I are encountered in larger clinics.

Although still an investigational procedure, transfusion of the younger 50 percent of donor red cells, separated by counterflow cell centrifugation, appears promising in that red cell survival is prolonged, transfusion requirements are decreased, and iron overload is reduced.[79]

The incidence of infection from hepatitis B virus (HBV) has also decreased in our clinic population with the use of frozen-thawed cell transfusions.[80] In uncontrolled, nonrandomized studies encompassing the administration of 25,000 units of frozen-thawed red cells, the incidence of posttransfusioin hepatitis appears to be lower than that in historical controls treated with standard red cells.[81-84] The only prospective randomized, double-blind study of hepatitis and frozen-thawed red cells was reported by Tullis et al.[85] The incidence of hepatitis was lower in patients receiving red cells resuspended in albumin rather than plasma.

In Greece, where the prevalence of HBV infection (detected by HBsAg or anti-HBs) in a general population of healthy blood donors was 17.3 percent, 90.5 percent of 148 multiply transfused patients with thalassemia had evidence of serum hepatitis which increased with age and the number of blood transfusions administered. In contrast, the prevalence of antibody to hepatitis A virus (HAV) was significantly lower in patients than in controls (12.8 percent vs. 59.9 percent) and decreased with the number of blood transfusions from a donor population with anti-HAV antibodies.[86] Since better screening techniques for serum hepatitis in donors are now available, it is difficult to determine whether the reduced incidence of serum hepatitis is due to virus removal by the cell processing or whether such processing can render the hepatitis virus noninfectious. Unfortunately, no single method of preparation is foolproof or absolutely safe. In chimpanzees, hepatitis B has been transmitted via frozen-thawed red cells.[87]

CLINICAL TRANSFUSION PROGRAM

A regular hypertransfusion program is best administered on an outpatient basis in a comprehensive care center. This reduces the costs to the patient and can obviate a cumbersome, inconvenient, and expensive two- or three-day inpatient hospital stay. In addition to the daytime outpatient services available, evening clinics can be adapted for students and employed patients.

A supertransfusion program designed to maintain a pretransfusion level of hemoglobin greater than 12 g/dl is achieved by administering frozen-thawed red cells to patients every 3 to 4 weeks. The usual volume transfused is 10 to 20 ml/kg body weight. As body size increases, transfusion of 1 to 2 units (approximately 220 ml per unit of frozen-thawed red cells) are infused every 2 to 3 weeks. Transfusions are administered at a rate of 1 to 2 ml/min with one unit of cells given over a period of 90 to 120 minutes. Patients are premedicated with antipyretics, antihistamines, or steroids as determined by prior transfusion reactions. Microaggregate blood filters are also used for patients with previous severe febrile or urticarial reactions. If a febrile, urticarial, or more serious reaction occurs, the transfusion is immediately terminated and an infusion of isotonic saline solution is initiated with a new administration setup. The unit of blood and the patient's blood and urine specimens are sent to the laboratory for evaluation. If febrile reaction occurs, a blood culture is performed and appropriate antipyretics are administered. If an urticarial reaction develops, epinephrine and antihistamines are administered. More severe hemolytic reactions require hydration, diuresis, possible steroid therapy, and inpatient observation and monitoring. Additional details regarding the diagnosis and management of transfusion reactions are presented in Chapter 40.

IRON METABOLISM AND OVERLOAD IN TRANSFUSION THERAPY

Regular transfusion therapy is essential for survival in most patients with homozygous β-thalassemia. As a result of the multiple blood transfusions, transfusional hemosiderosis develops. There is a progressive increase in the burden of body iron, as nearly 160 mg of iron accumulate with each unit of transfused blood. Continual iron accumulation leads to hyperpigmentation due to deposition of both melanin and iron in the dermis. Iron accumulation in other tissues such as heart, liver, pancreas, other endocrine glands, and the gonads results in fibrosis and organ dysfunction. Diabetes mellitus, hepatic insufficiency, and endocrine disturbances may occur. The most serious complications are bizarre atrial and ventricular arrhythmias and cardiac failure.

Iron distribution in the iron overloaded thalassemic state is a function of the reticuloendothelial system (RES), iron consumption and release, the iron transport system, the rate of erythropoiesis, iron storage, and iron excretion. The RES appears to play a primary role in the distribution of iron. The RES removes senescent erythrocytes from circulation. It stores some portion of the iron from heme catabolism as ferritin and the remainder return to the plasma for delivery to the erythroid precursors cells, liver parenchymal cells, and other tissues.

Iron from the RES passes into the circulation by two pathways: (1) a fast pathway with halftime of 23 minutes, and (2) a slow pathway with a halftime of 7 days. As the quantity of erythrocytes taken up by the RES increases, a proportional increase in the amount of iron released occurs; the exact mechanism controlling the release of iron from the RE cells is not clearly understood.[88] Apparently the rate of erythropoiesis also has a role in controlling iron released from the RES, since suppression of erythropoiesis by hypertransfusion decreased the proportion of iron released from the RES.[89] This is probably mediated by the rate of plasma iron turnover. Thus, in terms of iron metabolism, hypertransfusion should actually reduce the proportion of iron delivered to parenchymal tissues that are most susceptible to iron damage and favor retention of iron in the RES where it is less toxic.

SERUM FERRITIN

There is indirect evidence that hypertransfusion favors RES iron storage. The concentration of ferritin in the serum is generally thought to be an index of body iron stores and is derived from the RE cells. It also correlates well with the number of transfusions the patient has received.[90-94] A comparison of serum ferritin concentration in two groups of thalassemic patients from our clinic population was made: one chronically maintained at a pretransfusion hemoglobin level of 8.5 g/dl and the other at 10.0 g/dl. At the same age, hypertransfused patients have higher concentrations of serum ferritin than those maintained at a lower level of hemoglobin. When expressed as a function of the number of transfusions administered, the relationship persisted—i.e., the hypertransfused patient who had received a given number of transfusions had a higher level of serum ferritin than the nonhypertransfused patient who received the same number of transfusions (Fig. 32-3). Since serum ferritin is primarily RE in origin, these data demonstrate that hypertransfusion favors RE storage rather than tissue redistribution of iron. Thus, the patient should benefit clinically from a hypertransfusion program.[95]

IRON CHELATION IN THALASSEMIA

Because of the marked iron overload that occurs in β-thalassemia, it is theoretically advantageous to remove excess iron stores by means of iron chelators. Ideally, an iron-chelating agent should bind strongly to iron but not to other cations, and it should not interfere with intracellular iron metabolism.[96]

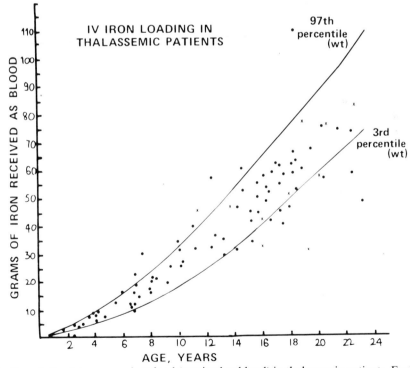

Fig. 32-3. Cumulative intravenous iron load (received as blood) in thalassemic patients. Each point represents the present status of a single patient. Dead patients are indicated by crosses. (Modell, B., Owen, M. & Kaye, S.B.: Clinical experience with the use of deferoxamine in the United Kingdom. Reproduced from Chelation Therapy in Chronic Iron Overload. Symposia Specialists, Miami, 1977.)

Deferoxamine (DFO) is currently the most efficacious iron chelator available.

Deferoxamine is a member of the hydroxamic acid class of iron chelators produced by *Streptomyces pilosis*. Iron excretion in response to DFO treatment is directly related to the load of the body iron. Indeed, iron stores must reach a level at least 10 times normal before significant iron chelation is achieved. The exact mechanism of DFO-induced iron chelation is not entirely understood. Under ideal conditions—i.e., in the absence of competing ions and at an optimal pH—the B value (the stability product) of the transferrin-Fe^{3+} complex is approximately 10^{36}, while that for DFO is 10^{31}.[97] However, under physiologic conditions, in the presence of competing cations, the effective binding constants of transferrin and DFO are 10^{24} and $10^{24.5}$, respectively. Theoretically, DFO should remove iron from transferrin; yet, in vivo this does not occur. If ^{59}Fe is attached to transferrin and intravenously injected and then DFO is injected, no ^{59}Fe is excreted. However, if DFO is injected first and followed by intravenous ^{59}Fe, DFO effectively competes with transferrin and ^{59}Fe excretion occurs.[98] It is not clear why DFO does not remove iron from transferrin. It may be related to the short circulating half-life of DFO, which is only 75 minutes.

DFO and all other hydroxamic acids are not absorbed by the gastrointestinal tract, since they do not readily penetrate cell membranes.[99] It appears that DFO competes with transferrin for a pool of iron at cell membranes (probably reticuloendothelial) that is small at any given time but is in equilibrium with low molecular weight complexes of iron.

The nature of these low-molecular-weight complexes is not well understood. The consensus is that their function involves the transport of iron through membranes and into and out of macromolecules or membrane-bound receptors. A small pool of low-molecular-weight complexes in the cytosol is in equilibrium with transferrin or chelating agents outside the cell and ferritin inside the cell.[100,101] In the RE cells, this iron pool is capable of inducing ferritin synthesis.[102] The fall in serum ferritin concentration associated with DFO use is most likely a reflection of the shift in the equilibrium toward the outside of the RE cell. Thus, the major source of iron excreted in response to DFO appears to be RE in origin.[103] It seems likely that DFO does not enter the cell but rather that its physiological iron-binding constant enables it to compete with transferrin for iron entering the plasma from any tissue. The net effect is an increase in the amount of iron which leaves the cell and an increase in iron excretion.

The use of DFO to minimize the problem of iron toxicity in thalassemia is still under investigation. DFO has been used in various treatment regimens since 1960. Despite years of experience with DFO, the best way to give the drug has only recently been established. Although DFO was first introduced in 1960, its use was virtually abandoned by 1969 because intramuscular administration was incapable of achieving zero or negative iron balance. A renewal of interest in DFO began in 1974 when Barry and ncoworkers[104] reported that persistent use of DFO over a given 1-year period decreased the rate of iron accumulation in thalassemic patients. The concentrations of both liver iron and serum ferritin were significantly reduced by a daily regimen of 500 mg of DFO given intramuscularly in conjunction with 2 gm intravenously at the time of transfusion. Histopathologic evaluation of serial liver biopsies demonstrated that progressive hepatic fibrosis did not occur. Subsequent evaluation of these patients showed that longevity is improved by DFO therapy.[105]

Since 1974, further research activity has led to other routes of administration and an improvement of the efficacy of DFO. It was observed[106] that maximal urinary iron excretion occurred when the drug was administered as a slow, constant intravenous infusion. More recent investigations have confirmed Smith's study.[107-109] As with intramuscular DFO, the response to intravenous DFO in thalassemia is a function of the body iron load. Our studies have shown that patients aged 10 years or less have almost no increment in iron excretion after receiving infusions of DFO in a dose above 20 mg/kg/24 h, suggesting that children in this age group should receive no more than this dose of DFO. In contrast, patients 11 to 15 or 16 or older increased their urinary excretion after receiving infusions of DFO in doses up to 60 to 80 mg/kg/24 h, respectively (Fig. 32-4). Given the greater potential benefit of chelation therapy to older children who are at risk of cardiac and endocrine dysfunction, higher doses of the drug seem justifiable.

The development of a small, portable battery-operated infusion pump has made effective subcutaneous chelation therapy possible on an outpatient basis. Dose for dose, the response to subcutaneous (SC) DFO infusions is significantly greater than intramuscular DFO and is 80 to 90 percent as effective as IV DFO. Furthermore, at a dose of 20 mg/kg, the response to an 8- or 16-hour infusion was 80 percent of that for a 24-hour IV infusion, and a daily 8-hour SC infusion (during sleep) of 20 to 40 mg/kg was sufficient therapy to achieve negative iron balance in thalassemic children as young as 5 years of age. To date, toxicity associated with DFO has been confined to symptoms at the injection site consisting of local and reversible pruritis, erythema, and swelling. These symptoms are minimized, but not abolished, by the addition of 1 mg of hydrocortisone to each ml of DFO solution.

Although this regimen will undoubtedly prevent many of the sequelae of hemosiderosis if begun early enough, whether or not it is capable of dramatically improving the clinical condition of patients with severe iron overload is unanswered. In our experience,[109] iron chelation therapy has been given to 63 patients with homozygous β-thalassemia from 5 to 30 years old as SC DFO at 20 mg/kg via a portable pump, 8 hours daily for 5 to 7 days/week for 2 to 3 years. Urinary iron excretion increased with increasing patient age and varied from 4 to 90 mg/day. Most younger patients achieved iron balance and

AVERAGE URINARY IRON EXCRETION: AGE OF PATIENT VS DOSE OF DFO

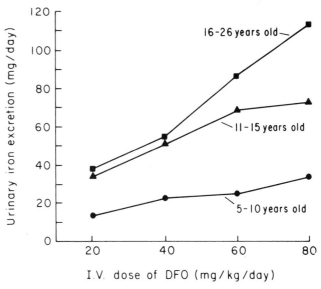

Fig. 32-4. Intravenous deferoxamine dose-response as a function of age. (Graziano, J. H. et al.: J. Pediatr. 92:649, 1978.)

the older patients negative balance. Serum ferritin levels decreased, particularly in patients with high initial values, and a progressive decrease in serum transaminase levels occurred with increasing time on chelation. Arthropathy and hyperpigmentation improved, but the duration of treatment is insufficient to demonstrate improved cardiac function or at least no progression of dysfunction. The optimal age at which chelation therapy should be initiated is not currently resolved. During the first 4 to 5 years of therapy, the efficiency of SC DFO does not exceed 30 percent. It is not known whether chelation therapy during the early years, despite its low efficiency, is beneficial.[109]

TRANSFUSION THERAPY IN THALASSEMIA INTERMEDIA

Approximately 10 percent of patients with homozygous β-thalassemia are doubly heterozygous for β-thalassemia traits (e.g., β-thalassemia and Hb Lepore trait) have a moderately severe anemia but are able to maintain a hemoglobin level of 6 to 9 g/dl without chronic transfusion therapy. Many patients survive into adulthood and have normal maturation and development.[110] Iron overload with hemosiderosis, diabetes mellitus, and congestive heart failure may develop in the fourth or fifth decade of life.[111] Patients with thalassemia intermedia have a functional degree of anemia more severe than would be predicted. Because of high levels of HbF, with its increased oxygen affinity, and inappropriately low levels of 2,3-DPG, the result is high oxygen affinity with P_{50} O_2 values of 20 to 26 mm Hg.[112]

In the asymptomatic patient, transfusions are not necessary; but, in patients with grotesque facies, severe osteoporosis, recurrent fractures, progressive cardiomegaly, or massive splenomegaly, a transfusion program with DFO chelation as outlined above should be instituted to suppress erythropoiesis and prevent further iron overload.

TRANSFUSION THERAPY IN RBC ENZYMOPATHIES

Clinical acumen, investigative imagination, serendipity, and advances in biochemical methods have led to the identification of 11 different hereditary erythrocyte enzyme deficiencies associated with congenital hemolytic anemia[2,3] (Table 32-4). In one disorder, a 40- to 70-fold increase in the target enzyme, adenosine deaminase, is present.[113] Other reported enzyme deficiencies are of uncertain or doubtful significance in that some are acquired defects related to an underlying nutritional deficiency (e.g., GSH reductase deficiency with riboflavin deficiency,[114] some are epiphenomena of another deficiency (e.g., secondary ribose phosphate pyrophosphokinase deficiency with a primary deficiency of pyrimidine 5′ nucleotidase),[115] and in some insufficient clinical and biochemical evidence was provided to establish an unequivocal re-

Table 32-4. Classification of Red Cell Enzyme Deficiencies

A. Deficiencies of Embden-Meyerhof Pathway
   1. Hexokinase (HK)
   2. Glucose phosphate isomerase (GPI)
   3. Phosphofructokinase (PFK)
   4. Triose phosphate isomerase (TPI)
   5. Phosphoglycerate kinase (PGK)
   6. 2, 3-diphosphoglycerate mutase (2, 3-DPGM)
   7. Pyruvate kinase (PK)

B. Deficiencies of hexose monophosphate shunt
   1. G-6-PD
      a. Drug-induced hemolytic anemia
      b. Chronic hemolytic anemia
   2. GSH synthetase
      a. γ-glutamyl cysteine synthetase
      b. GSH synthetase

C. Deficiencies (or excess) of enzymes of nucleotide metabolism
   1. Adenylate kinase (AK)
   2. Pyrimidine 5′-nucleotidase
   3. ATPase
   4. Increased adenosine deaminase

D. Deficiencies of uncertain or doubtful significance
   1. Phosphogluconate dehydrogenase
   2. Glutathione reductase
   3. Glutathione peroxidase
   4. Glyceraldehyde phosphate dehydrogenase
   5. 2, 3-DPG phosphatase
   6. Enolase

lationship between the purported enzyme deficiency and the hemolytic anemia. The latter cases are in limbo until additional details of metabolic investigations or other well-documented cases are described.

Hemolytic disease associated with a deficiency of erythrocytic enzymes may be caused by the decreased production of an enzyme, production of a functionally abnormal or unstable enzyme, or a combination of both defects. During the past few years, the marked heterogeneity of enzyme deficiency diseases has become apparent. This genetic polymorphism has accounted for over 100 variants of G6PD, eight variants of PK, and a few variants of HK, GPI, and PFK, each isoenzyme differing from other mutants in kinetics, electrophoretic migration, stability, and allosteric activation. Thus, the indications and requirements for transfusions vary not only with the different enzyme disorders, but even within a specific enzyme disorder in which tremendous clinical and biochemical heterogeneity exists. For example, anemia in PK deficiency varies from mild, well-compensated hemolysis to severe, uncompensated transfusion-dependent hemolytic disease. The specific congenital metabolic defects associated with hemolytic anemia, and their severity, neonatal manifestations, and transfusion requirements are presented in Table 32-5. As with all congenital hemolytic anemias, indications for transfusion therapy include neonatal hyperbilirubinemia, aplastic crises or hyperhemolysis precipitated by infection, pregnancy, refractory leg ulcers, and preparation for surgery. Only unique features or situations related to specific transfusion therapy in the enzyme disorders will be presented in this section, in order of their prevalence.

TRANSFUSION THERAPY IN ENZYME DEFICIENCIES

G6PD Deficiency. The severity and degree of hemolysis and anemia in G6PD deficiency, both in the absence and presence of stress, depend primarily and critically on the slope of the decline in enzyme activity as a function of red cell age, which is characteristic for each variant of G6PD.[30] In G6PD A⁻ deficiency, common in blacks, or in the Mediterranean variant, the activity falls below the critical level after 90 to 100 days, or 75 percent of the normal red cell life span, when only 0.2 percent of the original enzyme activity remains. Deficient cells are then removed by the RES. With oxidant stress induced by certain drugs, infections, or acidosis, the level of G6PD activity required to protect the red cell is 10 times higher than in the basal stae, or 2 percent of original activity. Accordingly, older cells are more susceptible to hemolysis. In G6PD A⁻ under stress about 40 percent of the circulating red cells will be destroyed intravascularly, but under more severe stress progressively younger cells will be affected. Transfusions are the exception rather than the rule in an acute drug-induced hemolytic crisis in a black patient with G6PD A⁻ when the hemoglobin rarely drops below 8 to 9 g/dl. However, with underlying medical problems, or with evidence of congestive failure or renal failure caused by the precipitous destruction of G6PD-deficient cells, transfusion therapy with PRBC will be required.

Controversy exists concerning the screening for and use of G6PD-deficient blood for transfusions. Based upon a hemolytic reaction occurring in a single patient who received presumed G6PD-deficient blood,[116] some authors have recommended that donors be screened for G6PD deficiency and that G6PD-deficient blood be avoided in emergencies and for surgery.[117,118] McCurdy and Morse[119] followed 23 patients who received 24 units of G6PD-deficient blood and were unable to show deleterious effects. Excluding G6PD-deficient blood for transfusions does not appear to be justifiable, except in exchange transfusions of newborns, in whom any excess bilirubin load would be intolerable.

Table 32-5. Hemolytic Anemias due to Congenital Metabolic Defects

Enzyme Deficiency	References	Severity of anemia (Hb range, g/dl)	Neonatal jaundice	Transfusion requirement	Associated findings
Embden-Myerhof Pathway					
Hexokinase	Keitt[141] Valentine et al.[142]	variable (4.5-nl)	+	+	↓2,3-DPG ↑O₂ affinity
Glucosephosphate isomerase	Paglia and Valentine[143]	mild to fatal (4.2 to 12.3)	(? kernicterus)	↓ρ splenectomy	glycogenosis ? x-linked
Phosphofructokinase	Tarui et al.[144] Waterbury[145]	mild		–	multisystem disorder (cardiac and neurologic) dysfunction
Triose phosphate isomerase	Schneider et al.[126]	moderate (5 to 10)	severe	+	x-linked; death in infancy; mental retardation
Phosphoglycerate kinase	Valentine et al.[146]	variable (3 to 13.7)	+	+ρ splenectomy	fatal at 3 mos ↑O₂ affinity
2,3-Diphosphoglycerate mutase	Schröter[129]	profound mild	+	+	↑2,3-DPG,
Pyruvate kinase	Rosa et al.[147] Tanaka et al.[148]	variable (3 to 14)	+	↓ρ splenectomy	↓O₂ affinity
Hexose monophosphate shunt					
Glucose 6-phosphate dehydrogenase drug induced chronic	Beutler[149]	self-limited 20% < 10	premature +	with favism rarely	Favism N. Europ. backgrd. Drug- and fava-induced hemolysis
GSH synthetase	Prins[150]	mild	–	–	neurologic sx
Nucleotide metabolism Adenylate kinase ATP ase <	Szeinberg et al.[151] Harvald et al.[152]	variable → mild (> 10.9)	+ → –	± → –	c̄ G6PD deficiency ↓K⁺, ↑Na⁺
Pyrimidine 5′ nucleotidase	Valentine et al.[115]	moderate (8 to 10)	+	–	Ribose phosphate pyrophosphokinase deficiency
↑Adenosine deaminase	Valentine et al.[113]	mild	–	–	↓ATP

Favism. Favism or acute hemolytic anemia after eating broad beans (*Vicia fava*) or inhaling the pollen of the bean blossom occurs almost exclusively in persons with G6PD Mediterranean deficiency.[120] The clinical spectrum ranges from mild disease to massive hemolysis, acute renal failure, and death within 48 to 72 hours after exposure to the dangerous bean or its pollen. Infants and young children are at particularly high risk. Symptoms usually begin within seconds after pollen inhalation and hours after a fava bean meal. In Kattamis' series,[120] 80 percent of hospitalized patients had levels of hemoglobin below 6 g/dl. The lowest recorded hemoglobin was 1 g/dl! Prior to the days of modern transfusion therapy, a mortality of 8 percent was recorded.[121] Prompt recognition of the problem and emergency transfusion therapy are mandatory in extreme hemolytic crises. Appropriate diagnostic studies, including a quantitative assay for G6PD, should be performed prior to rather than after transfusion.

Pyruvate Kinase Deficiency. Pyruvate kinase (PK) deficiency hereditary hemolytic anemia is a heterogenous disorder with a wide clinical spectrum ranging from severe neonatal anemia and hemolysis requiring exchange transfusions, occasionally progressing to kernicterus[122,26] to a fully compensated mild hemolytic process first diagnosed in grandmothers with gallstones. Severe anemia requiring transfusion therapy occurs either in early infancy as a complication of marrow hypoplasia or later during pregnancy. The requirement for transfusion is either eliminated or markedly decreased following splenectomy.

Because of the raised levels of 2,3-DPG, decreased oxygen affinity, and increased delivery of oxygen to the tissues, stable patients with PK deficiency generally tolerate anemia and vigorous exercise with relatively few symptoms.[10]

Glucose Phosphate Isomerase Deficiency. Severe and fatal anemia has been reported in three patients in a family in which transfusions and/or splenectomy were refused.[123] Aplastic crisis with profound anemia (hemoglobin 2.1 g/dl) and neonatal hyperbilirubinemia requiring exchange transfusion have been reported.[124,125]

Hexokinase Deficiency. The enzyme hexokinase phosphorylates glucose and is a key rate-limiting step of glycolysis. In hexokinase deficiency, glycolysis is diminished, the levels of 2,3-DPG are low, and the oxygen affinity of hemoglobin is increased. The resultant decreased delivery of oxygen to the tissues is partly responsible for the disproportionate severity of symptoms relative to the degree of anemia. Oski et al.[10] found that vigorous physical exertion in HK deficiency was associated with a prompt fall in central venous oxygen tension to a level close to that below which oxidative phosphoxylation can no longer proceed. Cardiac output also doubled. Thus, HK-deficient patients are not able to tolerate strenuous physical activity and must modify their life-styles. Transfusion therapy may be indicated in patients with clinical symptoms of anemia, exercise intolerance, or delayed growth and development. Long-term transfusion therapy has been required in some patients to maintain a level of hemoglobin above 7 to 8 g/dl.

Triose Phosphate Isomerase Deficiency. TPI deficiency is a multisystem disorder involving erythrocytes, skeletal and cardiac muscles, and the central nervous system. The hematologic disorder is most severe in early infancy, when transfusions are required to prevent death. Beyond this period, fatalities have been related to sudden cardiac arrest.[126,127] or a progressive, debilitating neuromuscular disease. Associated sickle cell trait and G6PD deficiency may add to the clinical severity of this disorder.

Phosphoglycerate Kinase Deficiency. This X-linked, moderately severe hemolytic disorder is associated with mental retardation, impaired speech, emotional lability, and progressive extrapyramidal tract disease.[128] In some, but not all, patients, transfusion

Table 32-6. Acquired Erythrocyte Enzyme Deficiencies in Dyshematopoietic Disorders

Disorder	Enzyme Deficiency	References
Congenital dyserythropoietic anemia		
Types I, II, III	GSH reductase, AK,acetylcholinesterase (ACE)	Verwilghen et al.[153] Valentine et al.[154]
Type IV	PFK, PK, AK	Valentine et al.[155] Miller et al.[156]
Fe deficiency	GSH peroxidase	MacDougall[157]
Primary refractory anemia	PFK, DPGM, PK, AK	Boivin[132]
Fanconi's anemia	HK	Lohr et al.[158]
Idiopathic aplastic anemia	PFK, DPGM, PK, AK	Boivin[159]
Preleukemia and acute leukemia	PFK, DPGM, PK, AK	Boivin[132]
P. Vera	PGI, PFK, G3PD, DPGM, PGM	Boivin[132]
Myelofibrosis	PGI, PGM	Boivin[132]
PNH	PFK, PGM, PK, ACE	Miller et al.[160] Boivin[132]

therapy has been required before splenectomy after which partial but not complete improvement is observed.

2,3-Diphosphoglycerate Mutase Deficiency. Direct evidence for 2,3-DPGM deficiency was provided by Schröter.[129] The patient was severely affected, transfusion-dependent, and died at 3 months of age, by which time 80 transfusions had been given. The rapid destruction of transfused red cells suggested an additional extrinsic mechanism of hemolysis. In multiply transfused patients, the risk of isoimmunization to minor blood group antigens increases with the number and frequency of transfused units. Cartier et al.[130] reported decreased levels of 2,3-DPG and increased oxygen affinity of hemoglobin, adding an additional physiologic handicap to the existing hypoxia in severely affected patients.

Pyrimidine 5'-Nucleotidase Deficiency. A relatively recent newcomer to the list of congenital hemolytic anemias, pyrimidine 5'-nucleotidase deficiency is associated with raised levels of ATP, decreased ribose phosphate pyrophosphokinase, raised levels of GSH, and prominent basophilic stippling in the red cells.[115] No unique transfusion requirements are associated with this disorder. Of interest is that the disorder may also be acquired as a result of lead intoxication.[131]

Other Deficiencies. Other acquired deficiencies of erythrocytic enzymes have been reported[132,3] in association with secondary dyserythropoiesis, congenital dyserythropoietic anemias, preleukemic states, and frank hematologic malignancies; these deficiencies are listed in Table 32-6. Generally, partial deficiencies are detected. Whereas the relationship between the acquired enzymopathy and the severity of anemia has not been established, it is conceivable that red cell survival could be compromised further and transfusion requirements increased as a result of these acquired metabolic defects.

REFERENCES

1. Lewis, S.M. and Verwilghen, R.L.: Diserythropoiesis: definition, diagnosis and assessment. In: Dyserythropoiesis. Lewis, S.M. and Verwilghen, R.L., eds. London, Academic Press, 1977, p. 3.
2. Beutler, E.: Hemolytic Anemia in Disorders of Red Cell Metabolism. Plenum, New York, 1978.
3. Miller, D.R.: Hemolytic anemia: metabolic defects. In: Smith's Blood Diseases of Infancy and Childhood. Miller, D.R., Pearson, H.A., Baehner, R.L., and McMillan, C.W., eds. C. V. Mosby, St. Louis, 1978, p. 313.
4. Bunn, H.F., Forget, B.G., and Ranney, H.M.: Human Hemoglobins. W.B. Saunders, Philadelphia, 1977.

5. Serjeant, G.R.: The Clinical Features of Sickle Cell Disease. American Elsevier, New York, 1974.

6. Weatherall, D.J. and Clegg, J.B.: The Thalassemia Syndromes. Blackwell Scientific Publications, Oxford, 1972.

7. Chang, H. and Miller, D.R.: Hemolytic anemia: Membrane defects. In: Smith's Blood Diseases of Infancy and Childhood. Edited by Miller, D.R., Pearson, H.A., Baehner, R.L., and McMillan, C.W., eds. C.V. Mosby, St. Louis, 1978, p. 287.

8. Weed, R.I.: The cell membrane in hemolytic disorders. In: Plenary Session Papers, XII Congress International Society of Hematology, International Society of Hematology, New York, 1968, p. 81.

9. Orringer, E.P. and Parker, J.C.: Ion and water movements in red blood cells. In: Progress in Hematology, vol. VIII. Brown, E.R., ed. Grune & Stratton, New York, 1973, p. 1.

10. Oski, F.A., Marshall, B.E., Delivoria-Papadopoulos, M., and Gottlieb, A.J.: Exercise with anemia: the role of the left-shifted or right-shifted oxygen hemoglobin equibilirubin curve. Ann. Intern. Med. 74:44, 1971.

11. Benesch, R.: How do small molecules do great things? N. Engl. J. Med. 280:1179, 1969.

12. Duhm, J. and Gerlach, E.: Metabolism and function of 2,3-diphosphoglycerate in red blood cells. In: The Human Red Cell in Vitro. Greenwalt, T.J. and Jamieson, G.A., eds. Grune & Stratton, New York, 1974, p. 111.

13. Beutler, E.: A "shift to the left" or "a shift to the right" in the regulation of erythropoiesis. Blood 33:496, 1969.

14. Bellingham, A.J. and Huehns, E.R.: Compensation in haemolytic anaemias caused by abnormal haemoglobins. Nature (London) 218:924, 1968.

15. de Furia, F.G. and Miller, D.R.: Oxygen affinity in hemoglobin Köln disease. Blood 39:398, 1972.

16. White, J.M.: The unstable haemoglobin disorders. Clin. Haematol. 3:333, 1974.

17. O'Brien, R.T. and Pearson, H.A.: Physiologic anemia of the newborn infant. J. Pediatr. 79:132, 1971.

18. Siep, M.: The reticulocyte level and the erythrocyte production judged from reticulocyte studies in newborn infants during the first week of life. Acta. Paediatr. 44:355, 1955.

19. Garby, L., Sjolin, S., and Viulle, J.C.: Studies on erythrokinetics in infancy. III. Disappearance from plasma and red cell uptake of radioactive iron injected intravenously. Acta. Paediatr. 52:537, 1963.

20. Halvorsen, S.: Plasma erythropoietin levels in cord blood and in blood during the first weeks of life. Acta Paediatr. 52:425, 1963.

21. Clark, A.C.L.: Erythropoiesis in the newborn. III. Urinary inhibition—is it an oestrogen? Aust. Paediatr. J. 10:270, 1974.

22. Sisson, T.R.C., Whalen, L.E., and Tilek, A.: Blood volume of infants. II. The premature infant during the first years of life. J. Pediatr. 55:430, 1959.

23. Stockman, J.A., Garcia, J.F., and Oski, F.A.: The anemia of prematurity: factors governing the erythropoietin response. N. Engl. J. Med. 296:647, 1977.

24. Buchanon, G.R. and Schwartz, A.D.: Impaired erythropoietin response in anemic premature infants. Blood 44:347, 1974.

25. Oski, F.A. and Komazawa, M.: Metabolism of the erythrocytes of the newborn infant. Sem. Hematol. 12:49, 1975.

26. Gilman, P.A.: Hemolysis in the newborn infant resulting from deficiencies of red blood cell enzymes: diagnosis and management. J. Pediatr. 84:625, 1974.

26a. Austin, R.F. and Desforges, J.F.: Hereditary elliptocytosis: an unusual presentation of hemolysis in the newborn associated with transient morphologic abnormalities. Pediatr. 44:1969, 1969.

26b. Stamey, C.C. and Diamond, L.K.: Congenital hemolytic anemia in the newborn. Am. J. Dis. Child. 94:616, 1957.

26c. Trucco, J.I. and Brown, A.K.: Neonatal manifestations of hereditary spherocytosis. Am. J. Dis. Child. 113:263, 1967.

27. Jim, R.T.S. and Chu, F.K.: Hyperbilirubinemia due to glucose-6-phosphate dehydrogenase in a newborn Chinese infant. Pediatr. 31:1046, 1963.

28. Doxiadis, S.A., Fessas, P.H., and Valoes, T.: Glucose-6-phosphate dehydrogenase deficiency: a new aetiological factor of severe neonatal jaundice. Lancet 1:297, 1961.

29. Doxiadis, S.A., Valoes, T., Karaklis, A., and Stavrakakis, D.: Risk of severe jaundice in

glucose-6-phosphate dehydrogenase deficiency of the newborn. Lancet 2:1210, 1964.

30. Luzzatto, L.: Inherited haemolytic states: glucose-6-phosphate dehydrogenase deficiency. Clin. Haematol. 4:83, 1975.

31. Phornphatkul, C., Whitaker, J.A., and Worathumrong, N.: Severe hyperbilirubinemia in Thai newborns in association with erythrocyte G6PD deficiency. Clin. Pediatr. 8:275, 1969.

32. Eshaghpour, E., Oski, F.A., and Williams, M.: The relationship of erythrocyte glucose-6-phosphate dehydrogenase deficiency to hyperbilirubinemia in Negro premature infants. J. Pediatr. 70:595, 1967.

33. Bienzle, U., Effiong, C., and Luzzatto, L.: Erythrocyte glucose-6-phosphate dehydrogenase deficiency (G6PD type A⁻) and neonatal jaundice. Acta Paediatr. Scand. 65:701, 1976.

34. Szeinberg, A., Oliver, M., Schmidt, R., Adam, A., and Sheba, C.: Glucose-6-phosphate dehydrogenase deficiency and haemolytic disease. Arch. Dis. Child. 38:23, 1963.

35. Weatherall, D.J., Clegg, J.B., and Wong, H.B.: The haemoglobin constitution of infants with haemoglobin Bart's hydrops foetalis syndrome. Br. J. Hematol. 18:357, 1970.

36. Leikin, S.L.: The aplastic crisis of sickle cell disease: occurrence in several of families within a short period of time. Am. J. Dis. Child. 93:128, 1957.

37. Markenson, A.L., Chandra, M., Lewy, J.E., and Miller, D.R.: Sickle cell anemia, the nephrotic syndrome and hypoplastic crisis in a sibship. Am. J. Med. 64:719, 1978.

38. Charney, E. and Miller, G.: Reticulocytopenia in sickle cell disease. Aplastic episodes in the course of sickle cell disease in children. Am. J. Dis. Child. 107:450, 1964.

39. Pearson, H.A.: Sickle cell syndromes and other hemoglobinopathies. In: Smith's Blood Diseases of Infancy and Children, 4th edition. Miller, D.R., Pearson, H.A., Baehner, R.L., and McMillan, C.W., eds. C.V. Mosby, St. Louis, 1978.

39a. Palek, J., Mircevova, L., and Brabec, V.: 2,-3-DPG metabolism in hereditary spherocytosis. Br. J. Haematol. 17:59, 1969.

40. Fernandez, L.A. and Erslev, A.J.: Oxygen affinity and compensated hemolysis in hereditary spherocytosis. J. Lab. Clin. Med. 80:780, 1972.

41. Kohler, H.G., Meynell, M.J., and Cooke, W.T.: Spherocytic anemia, complicated by megaloblastic anemia of pregnancy. Br. Med. J. 1:779, 1960.

42. Zarkowsky, H.S., Mohandas, N., Speaker, C.B., and Shohet, S.B.: A congenital hemolytic anemia with thermal sensitivity of the erythrocyte membrane. Br. J. Haematol. 29:537, 1975.

43. Jaffé, E.R. and Gottfried, E.L.: Hereditary nonspherocytic hemolytic disease associated with an altered phospholipid composition of erythrocytes. J. Clin. Invest. 47:1375, 1968.

44. Spigelman, A. and Warden, M.J.: Surgery in patients with sickle cell disease. Arch. Surg. 104:761, 1972.

45. Karayalcin, G., Imran, M., and Rosner, F.: Priapism in sickle cell disease: Report of five cases. Am. J. Med. Sci. 264:289, 1972.

46. Lessin, L.S., Kurantsin-Mills, J., Kulg, P.P., and Weems, H.B.: Determination of rheologically optimal mixtures of AA and SS erythrocytes. Blood 50 (suppl. 1):111, 1977.

47. Brody, J.I., Goldsmith, M.H., and Park, S.K.: Symptomatic crisis of sickle cell anemia treated by limited exchange transfusion. Ann. Intern. Med. 72:327, 1970.

48. Charache, S.: The treatment of sickle cell anemia. Arch. Intern. Med. 133:698, 1974.

49. Anderson, R., Cassell, M., Mullinax, G.L., and Chaplin, H., Jr.: Effect of normal cells on viscosity of sickle cell blood: *In vitro* studies and report of six years experience with a prophylactic program of "partial exchange transfusion." Arch. Intern. Med. 111:286, 1963.

50. Sommer, A., Kontras, S.B., and Craenen, J.M.: Partial exchange transfusion in sickle cell anemia complicated by heart disease. J.A.M.A. 215:484, 1971.

51. Russell, M.O., Goldberg, H.I., Reis, L., Friedman, S., Slater, R., Reivich, M., and Schwartz, E.: Transfusion therapy for cerebrovascular abnormalities in sickle cell disease. J. Pediatr. 88:382, 1976.

52. Lusher, J.M., Haghighat, H., and Khalifa, A.S.: A prophylactic transfusion program for children with sickle cell anemia complicated by CNS infarction. Am. J. Hematol. 1:265, 1976.

53. Morrison, J.C. and Wiser, W.L.: The effect of partial exchange transfusion on the infants of

patients with sickle cell anemia. J. Pediatr. 89:286, 1976.

54. Ricks, P.: Further experience with exchange transfusion in sickle cell anemia and pregnancy. Am. J. Obstet. Gynecol. 100:1087, 1968.

55. Lanzkowsky, P., Shende, A., Karayalcin, G., Kim, Y-J, and Aballi, A.: Partial exchange transfusion in sickle cell anemia. Am. J. Dis. Child. 132:1206, 1978.

56. Bogoch, A., Casselman, W.G.B., Margolies, M.P., and Bockus, H.L.: Liver disease in sickle cell anemia: A correlation of clinical, biochemical, histologic and histochemical observations. Am. J. Med. 19:583, 1955.

57. Green, T.W., Conley, C.L., and Berthrong, M.: The liver in sickle cell anemia. Bull. Johns Hopkins Hosp. 92:99, 1953.

58. Pearson, H.A., Spencer, R.P., and Cornelius, E.A.: Functional asplenia in sickle cell anemia. N. Engl. J. Med. 281:923, 1969.

59. Lukens, J.N.: Hemoglobin S., the pneumococcus, and the spleen. Am. J. Dis. Child. 123:6, 1972.

60. Pearson, H.A., Cornelius, E.A., Schwartz, A.D., Zelson, J.H., Wolfson, S.L., and Spencer, R.P.: Transfusion-reversible functional asplenia in young children with sickle cell anemia. N. Engl. J. Med. 283:334, 1970.

61. Jenkins, M.E., Scott, R.B., and Baird, R.L.: Studies in sickle cell anemia. XVI. Sudden death during sickle cell anemia crisis in young children. J. Pediatr. 56:30, 1960.

62. Seeler, R.A. and Shwiaki, M.Z.: Acute splenic sequestration crisis (ASSC) in young children with sickle cell anemia. Clin. Pediatr. 11:701, 1972.

63. Powars, D., Wilson, B., Imbus, C., Pegelow, C., and Allen, J.: The natural history of stroke in sickle cell disease. Am. J. Med. 65:461, 1978.

64. Stockman, J.A., Nigro, M.A., Mishkin, M.M., and Oski, F.A.: Occlusion of large cerebral vessels in sickle cell anemia. N. Engl. J. Med. 287:846, 1972.

64a. Davis, K.R., Traveras, J.M., and New, R.F.J.: Cerebral infarction diagnosis by computerized tomography. Am. J. Roentgenol. 124:643, 1975.

65. Cohen, A. and Schwartz, E.: Excretion of iron in response to deferoxamine in sickle cell anemia. J. Pediatr. 92:659, 1978.

66. Eisenstein, M.I., Posner, A.C., and Friedman, S.: Sickle cell anemia in pregnancy. Am. J. Obstet. Gynecol. 72:622, 1956.

67. Freeman, M.G. and Ruth, G.J.: SS disease-SC disease-CC disease: obstetric considerations and treatment. Clin. Obstet. Gynecol. 12:134, 1969.

68. Pritchard, J.A., Scott, D.E., Whalley, P., Cunningham, F.G., and Mason, R.A.: The effects of maternal sickle cell hemoglobinopathies and sickle cell trait on reproductive performance. Am. J. Obstet. Gynecol. 117:662, 1971.

68a. Modell, B.: Management of thalassemia major. Br. Med. Bull. 32:270, 1976.

69. Wolman, I.J.: Transfusion therapy in Cooley's anemia: Growth and health as related to long range hemoglobin levels. A progress report. Ann. N.Y. Acad. Sci. 119:736, 1964.

70. Propper, R. and Nathan, D.G.: Persistent maintenance of normal hematocrits in thalassemia major. Blood 50:116, 1977.

71. Heinrich, H.C., Gabbe, E.E., and Oppitz, K.H.: Absorption of inorganic and food iron in children with heterozygous and homozygous B-thalassemia. Z. Kinderheilkd. 115:1, 1973.

72. Cavill, I., Worwood, M., and Jacobs, A.: Internal regulation of iron absorption. Nature 256:328, 1975.

73. Necheles, T.F., Chung, S., Sabbah, R., and Whitten, D.: Intensive transfusion therapy in thalassemia major: An eight year follow up. Ann. N.Y. Acad. Sci. 232:179, 1974.

74. Bunn, H.F., May, M.H., Kocholaty, W.F., and Shields, C.: Hemoglobin function in stored blood. J. Clin. Invest. 48:311, 1969.

75. Beutler, E. and Wood, L.: The *in vitro* regeneration of red cell 2,3-diphosphoglyceric acid after transfusion of stored blood. J. Lab. Clin. Med. 74:300, 1969.

76. de Furia, F.G., Miller, D.R., and Carale, V.C.: Red blood cell metabolism and function in transfused β-thalassemia. Ann. N.Y. Acad. Sci. 232:323, 1974.

77. Bellingham, A.J., Detter, J.C., and Lenfant, C.: The role of hemoglobin oxygen affinity and red cell 2,3 DPG in the management of diabetic ketoacidosis. Trans. Am. Assoc. Phys. 83:113, 1971.

78. Wolf, C.F.W. and Canale, V.: Fatal pulmo-

nary hypersensitivity reaction to HL-A incompatible blood transfusion: report of a case and review of the literature. Transfusion 16:135, 1976.

79. Corash, L., Seaman, C., Reibman, T., Tytun, A., and Piomelli, S.: Qualitatively Improved Red Cell Transfusion: A New Approach to Therapy of Chronic Anemia. Proc. 16th Int. Congr. Hematol., Kyoto, Japan, 1976, p. 91.

80. Stevens, C.E., Gilbert, J.A., Miller, D.R., Dienstag, J.L., Purcell, R.H., and Szmuness, W.: Serologic evidence of hepatitis A and B virus infections in thalassemia patients: A retrospective study. Transfusion 18:356, 1978.

81. Haynes, L.L., Tullis, J.L., and Pyle, H.M.: Clinical use of glycerolized frozen blood. J.A.M.A. 173:1657, 1960.

82. Huggins, C.E.: Frozen blood. Eur. Surg. Res. 1:3, 1969.

83. Bryant, L.R. and Wallace, M.E.: Experiences with frozen erythrocytes in a private hospital. Transfusion 14:481, 1974.

84. Sumida, S. and Sumida, M.: Transfusion of frozen red cells and serum hepatitis. Cryobiology 11:538, 1974.

85. Tullis, J.L., Hinman, J., and Sproul, M.T.: Incidence of posttransfusion hepatitis in previously frozen blood. J.A.M.A. 214:719, 1970.

86. Papaevangelou, G., Frösner, G., Economidou, J., Parcha, S., and Roumeliotou, A.: Prevalence of hepatitis A and B infections in multiply transfused thalassaemic patients. Brit. Med. J. 1:689, 1978.

87. Alter, H.J., Tabor, E., Meryman, H.T., Hoofnagle, J.H., Kahn, R.A., Holland, P.V., Gerety, R.J., and Barker, L.F.: Transmission of hepatitis B virus infected by transfusion of frozen-deglycerolized red blood cells. N. Engl. J. Med. 298:637, 1978.

88. Lipschitz, D.A., Dugard, J., Simon, M.O., Bothwell, T.H., and Charlton, R.W.: The site of action of desferrioxamine. Br. J. Haematol. 20:395, 1971.

89. Noyes, W.D., Bothwell, T.H., and Finch, C.A.: The role of the reticuloendothelial cell in iron metabolism. Br. J. Haematol. 6:43, 1960.

90. Siimes, M.A., Addiego, J.E., and Dallman, P.R.: Ferritin in serum: diagnosis of iron deficiency and iron overload in infants and children. Blood 43:581, 1974.

91. Jacobs, A.: Serum ferritin in iron metabolism and thalassemia. Bergsma, D., Cerami, A., Peterson, C.M., and Graziano, J.H., eds. Alan R. Liss, New York, 1976, p. 97.

92. Addison, G.M., Beamish, M.R., Hales, C.N., Hodgkins, M., Jacobs, A., and Llewellin, P.: An immunoradiometric assay for ferritin in the serum of normal subjects and patients with iron deficiency and iron overload. J. Clin. Pathol. 25:236, 1972.

93. Jacobs, A., Miller, F., and Worwood, M.: Ferritin in the serum of normal subjects and patients with iron deficiency and iron overload. Br. Med. J. 4:206, 1972.

94. Letsky, E.A., Miller, F., Worwood, M., and Flynn, D.M.: Serum ferritin in children with thalassemia regularly transfusesd. J. Clin. Pathol. 27:652, 1974.

95. Graziano, J.H. and Cerami, A.: Chelation therapy for the treatment of thalassemia. Sem. Hematol. 14:127, 1977.

96. Waxman, H.S. and Brown, E.B.: Clinical usefulness of iron chelating agents. Prog. Hematol. 6:338, 1969.

97. Aasa, R., Malmastrom, G.B., Saltman, P., and Vanngard, T.: The specific binding of iron (III) and copper (II) to transferrin and conalbumin. Biochim. Biophys. Acta 75:203, 1963.

98. Hedenberg, L.: Studies on iron metabolism with desferrioxamine in man. Scand. J. Haematol. (Suppl.)6:3, 1969.

99. Grady, R.W., Graziano, J.H., Akers, H.A., and Cerami, A.: The development of new iron-chelating drugs. J. Pharmacol. Exp. Ther. 196:478, 1976.

100. White, G.P., Bailey-Wood, R., and Jacobs, A.: The effect of chelating agents on cellular iron metabolism. Clin. Sci. Mol. 50:145, 1976.

101. May, P.M., Williams, D.R., and Linder, P.W.: The biological significance of low molecular weight iron (III) complexes. In: Metal Irons in Biological Systems. Vol. 7. Sigel, H., ed. Plenum Press, New York, 1978.

102. Lipschitz, D.A., Simon, M.O., Lynch, S.R., Dugard, J., Bothwell, T.H., and Charlton, R.W.: Some factors affecting the release of iron from reticuloendothelial cells. Br. J. Haematol. 21:289, 1971.

103. Graziano, J.: Iron metabolism and chelation therapy in hemosiderosis. Curr. Top. Hematol. 1:127, 1978.

104. Barry, M., Flynn, D.M., Letsky, E.A., and Risdon, R.A.: Long-term chelation therapy in thalassemia major: Effect on liver iron concentration, liver histology, and clinical progress. Br. Med. J. 2:16, 1974.

105. Modell, C.B.: Total management of thalassemia. Arch. Dis. Child. 52:489, 1977.

106. Smith, R.S.: Chelating agents in the diagnosis and treatment of iron overload in thalassemia. Ann. N.Y. Acad. Sci. 119:776, 1964.

107. Propper, R.D., Shurin, S.B., and Nathan, D.G.: Reassessment of the use of desferrioxamine B in iron overload. N. Engl. J. Med. 294:1421, 1976.

107a. Propper, R., Cooper, B., Rufo, R.R., Nienhuis, A.W., Anderson, W.F., Bunn, H.F., Rosenthal, A., and Nathan, D.G.: Continuous subcutaneous administration of deferoxamine in patients with iron overload. N. Engl. J. Med. 297:418, 1977.

108. Nienhuis, A.W., Delea, C., Aamodt, R., Bartter, F., and Anderson, W.F.: Evaluation of desferrioxamine and ascorbic acid for the treatment of chronic iron overload. In: Iron Metabolism and Thalassemia. Bergsma, D., Cerami, A., Peterson, C.M., and Graziano, J.H., eds. Alan R. Liss, New York, 1976, p. 177.

108a. Graziano, J.H., Markenson, A., Miller, D.R., Chang, H., Bestak, M., Meyers, P., Pisciotto, P., and Rifkind, A.: Chelation therapy in B-thalassemia major. I. Intravenous and subcutaneous deferioxamine. J. Pediatr. 92:648, 1978.

109. Markenson, A.L., Graziano, J.H., Ehlers, K.H., Saenger, P., and Hilgartner, M.W.: Clinical improvement on chronic subcutaneous desferrioxamine therapy in B-thalassemia. Ped. Res. 13:436 (abstract 664), 1979.

109a. Weiner, M., Karpatkin, M., Hart, D., Seaman, C., Vora, S.K., Henry, W.L., and Piomelli, S.: Cooley anemia: High transfusion regimen and chelation therapy, results and perspective. J. Pediatr. 92:653, 1978.

110. Pearson, H.A.: Thalassemia intermedia: genetic and biochemical considerations. Ann. N.Y. Acad. Sci. 119:390, 1964.

111. Bannerman, R.M., Keusch, G., Kreimer-Birnbaum, M., Vance, V.K., and Vaughan, S.: Thalassemia intermedia with iron overload, cardiac failure, diabetes mellitus, hypopituitarism and porphyrinuria. Am. J. Med. 42:476, 1967.

112. de Furia, F.G., Miller, D.R., and Canale, V.C.: Red blood cell metabolism and function in transfused B-thalassemia. Ann. N.Y. Acad. Sci. 232:323, 1974.

113. Valentine, W.N., Paglia, D.E., Tartaglia, A.P., and Gilsanz, F.: Hereditary hemolytic anemia with increased red cell adenosine deaminase (45- to 70-fold) and decreased adenosine triphosphate. Science 195:783, 1977.

114. Flatz, J.: Population study of erythrocyte glutathione reductase activity. I. Stimulation of the enzyme by flavin adenine dinucleotide and by riboflavin supplementation. Humangenetik 11:278, 1971.

115. Valentine, W.N., Fink, K., Paglia, D.E., Harris, S.R., and Adams, W.S.: Hereditary hemolytic anemia with human erythrocyte pyrimidine 5'-nucleotidase deficiency. J. Clin. Invest. 54:866, 1974.

116. Van Der Sar, A., Schouten, H., and Struyker Boudier, A.M.: Glucose-6-phosphate dehydrogenase deficiency in red cells. Incidence in the Curacao population, its clinical and genetic aspects. Enzyme 27:289, 1964.

117. Stuckey, W.J.: Hemolytic anemia and erythrocyte glucose-6-phosphate dehydrogenase deficiency. Am. J. Med. Sci. 251:104, 1966.

118. Tizianello, A., Pannacciulli, I., Salvidio, E., and Gay, A.: Erythrocytic glucose-6-phosphate dehydrogenase deficiency as a problem in the selection of blood donors. Vox Sang. 8:47, 1963.

119. McCurdy, P.R. and Morse, E.E.: Glucose-6-phosphate dehydrogenase deficiency and blood transfusion. Vox Sang. 28:230, 1975.

120. Kattamis, C.A., Kyriazakow, M., and Chaidas, S.: Favism. Clinical and biochemical data. J. Med. Genet. 6:34, 1969.

121. Luisada, L.: Favism: singular disease affecting chiefly red blood cells. Medicine 20:229, 1941.

122. Bowman, H.S. and Procopio, F.: Hereditary non-spherocytic hemolytic anemia of the pyruvate kinase deficient type. Ann. Intern. Med. 58:567, 1963.

123. Hutton, J.J. and Chilcote, R.R.: Glucose phosphate isomerase deficiency with hereditary nonspherocytic hemolytic anemia. J. Pediatr. 85:494, 1974.

124. Baughan, M.A., Valentine, W.N., Paglia, D.E., Ways, R.O., Simon, E.R., and De Marsh, Q.B.: Hereditary hemolytic anemia associated with glucosephosphate isomerase (GPI) deficiency—a new enzyme defect of human erythrocytes. Blood 32:236, 1968.

125. Paglia, D.E., Holland, P., Baughan, M.A., and Valentine, W.N.: Occurrence of defective hexosephosphate isomerization in human erythrocytes and leukocytes. N. Engl. J. Med. 280:66, 1969.

126. Schneider, A.S., Valentine, W.N., Hattori, M., and Heins, H.L., Jr.: Hereditary hemolytic anemia with triose phosphate isomerase deficiency. N. Engl. J. Med. 272:229, 1965.

127. Angelmann, H., Brain, M.E., and MacIver, J.E.: A case of triosephosphate isomerase deficiency with sudden death. In: Abstracts of Thirteenth International Congress of Hematology, Munich, 1970.

128. Konrad, P.N., McCarthy, D.J., Mauer, A.M., Valentine, W.N., and Paglia, D.E.: Erythrocyte and leukocyte phosphoglycerate kinase deficiency with neurologic disease. J. Pediatr. 82:456, 1973.

129. Schröter, W.: 2,3-Diphosphoglyceratstoffwechsel und 2,3-Diphosphoglyceratmutase-Mangel in Erythrocytin. Blut 20:1, 1970.

130. Cartier, P., Labie, D., Leroux, J.P., Najman, A. and I. Demaugre, F.: Deficit familial en diphosphoglycerate-mutase: Etude hematologique et biochemique. Nouv. Rev. Fr. Hematol. 12:269, 1972.

131. Valentine, W.N., Paglia, D.E. Fink, K., and Madokoro, G.: Lead poisoning, association with hemolytic anemia, basophilic stippling, erythrocyte pyrimidine 5′-nucleotidase deficiency, and intraerythrocytic accumulation of pyrimidines. J. Clin. Invest. 58:926, 1976.

132. Boivin, P.: Red cell enzyme abnormalities in dyserythropoietic anaemias. In: Dyserythropoiesis. Lewis, S.M. and Verwilghen, R.L., eds. Academic Press, London, 1977, p. 222.

133. Jacob, H.S. and Jandl, J.H.: Increased cell membrane permeability in the pathogenesis of hereditary spherocytosis. J. Clin. Invest. 43:1704, 1964.

134. Peters, J.C., Rowland, M., Israels, L.G., and

135. Zarkowsky, H.S., Oski, F.A., Sha'afi, R., Shohet, S.B., and Nathan, D.G.: Congenital hemolytic anemia with high sodium, low potassium red cells. I. Studies of membrane permeability. N. Engl. J. Med. 278:573, 1968.

136. Miller, D.R., Rickles, F.R., Lichtman, M.A., Week, R.I., and Reed, C.F.: A new variant of hereditary hemolytic anemia with stomatocytosis and erythrocyte cation abnormality. Blood 38:184, 1971.

137. Tosteson, D.C., Shea, E., and Darling, R.C.: Potassium and sodium of red blood cells in sickle cell anemia. J. Clin. Invest. 31:406, 1952.

138. Nathan, D.G.: Thalassemia: a syndrome of deficient globin synthesis, cell membrane deformities, and erythroproliferation. Am. J. Med. 41:815, 1966.

139. Nathan, D.G., Oski, F.A., Sidel, V.W., Garner, F.H., and Diamond, L.K.: Studies of erythrocyte spicule formation in haemolytic anaemia. Br. J. Haematol. 12:385, 1966.

140. Nathan, D.G. and Shohet, S.B.: Erythrocyte nontransport defects and hemolytic anemia: "Hydrocytosis" and "dessicocytosis." Sem. Hematol. 7:381, 1970.

141. Keitt, A.S.: Hemolytic anemia with impaired hexokinase activity. J. Clin. Invest. 48:1997, 1969.

142. Valentine, W.N., Oski, F.A., Paglia, D.E., Baughan, M.A., Schneider, A.S., and Naiman, J.L.: Hereditary hemolytic anemia with hexokinase deficiency, role of hexokinase in erythrocyte aging. N. Engl. J. Med. 276:1, 1967.

143. Paglia, D.E. and Valentine, W.N.: Hereditary glucose phosphate isomerase deficiency, a review. Am. J. Clin. Pathol. 62:740, 1974.

144. Tarui, S., Okuno, G., and Ikura, Y.: Phosphofructokinase deficiency in skeletal muscle: a new type of glycogenosis. Biochim. Biophys. Res. Commun. 19:517, 1965.

145. Waterbury, L. and Frankel, E.P.: Phosphofructokinase deficiency in congenital nonspherocytic hemolytic anemia. Clin. Res. 17:347, 1969.

146. Valentine, W.N., Hseih, H., Paglia, D.E., Anderson, H.M., Baughan, M.A., Jaffé, E.R., and Garson, O.M.: Hereditary hemolytic

Zipursky, A.: Erythrocyte sodium transport in hereditary elliptocytosis. Canad. J. Physiol. 44:817, 1966.

anemia associated with phosphoglycerate kinase deficiency in erythrocytes and leukocytes. N. Engl. J. Med. 280:528, 1969.

147. Rosa, R., Najean, Y., Prehu, M., Beuzard, Y., and Rosa, J.: Total deficiency of red cell diphosphoglycerate mutase (DPGM). Blood 50 (Suppl. 1):84, 1977.

148. Tanaka, K.R., Valentine, W.N., and Miwa, S.: Pyruvate kinase (PK) deficiency hereditary non-spherocytic hemolytic anemia. Blood 19:267, 1962.

149. Beutler, E.: Abnormalities of the hexose monophosphate shunt. Semin. Hematol. 8:311, 1971.

150. Prins, H.K., Oort, M., Loos, J.A., Zürcher, C., and Beckers, T.: Congenital monospherocytic hemolytic anemia, associated with glutathione deficiency of the erythrocytes. Blood 27:145, 1966.

151. Szeinberg, A., Kahana, D., Gavendo, S., Zaidman, J., and Ben-Ezzer, J.: Hereditary deficiency of adenylate kinase in red blood cells. Acta. Haematol. 42:111, 1969.

152. Harvald, B., Hanel, K.H., Squires, R., and Trap-Jensen, J.: Adenosine-triohosphatase deficiency in patients with non-spherocytic haemolytic anaemia. Lancet 2:18, 1964.

153. Verwilghen, R.L., Lewis, S.M., Dacie, J.V., Crookston, J.H., and Crookston, M.: HEMPAS-congenital dyserythropoietic anaemia (type II). Q. J. Med. 42:257, 1973.

154. Valentine, W.N., Crookston, J.H., Paglia, D.E., and Konrad, P.N.: Erythrocyte enzymatic abnormalities in HEMPAS (Hereditary erythroblastic multinuclearity with a positive acidified serum test). Br. J. Haematol. 23:107, 1972.

155. Valentine, W.N., Konrad, P.N., and Paglia, D.E.: Dyserythropoiesis, refractory anemia and "preleukemia": metabolic features of erythrocytes. Blood 41:857, 1973.

156. Miller, D.R., Lieberman, P., and Meyers, P.A.: A variant of congenital dyserythropoietic anemia. Pediatr. Res. 13:436 (abstract 666), 1979.

157. MacDougall, L.G.: Red cell metabolism in iron deficiency. The relationship betwen glutathione peroxidase, catalase, serum vitamin E, and susceptibility of iron-deficient red cells to oxidative hemolysis. J. Pediatr. 80:775, 1972.

158. Lohr, G.W., Waller, H.D., Anschutz, F., and Knopp, A.: Hexokinasemangel in Blutzellen bei einer Sippe met familiarer Panmyelopathie. Klin. Wschr. 43:870, 1965.

159. Boivin, 1965.

160. Miller, D.R., Baehner, R.L., and Diamond, L.K.: Paroxysmal nocturnal hemoglobinuria in childhood and adolescence. Pediatr. 39:675, 1966.

ACKNOWLEDGMENTS

The authors are grateful for the indefatigable and expert secretarial assistance of Ms. Jessie Ross, Anna Triano, and Yolanda Marquez; and to our colleagues Drs. Alicejane Markenson, Joseph Graziano, Margaret Hilgartner, and Robert Grady for their many contributions to the treatment of our patients with thalassemia.

This paper was supported by Children's Blood Foundation, the National Foundation, Cooley's Anemia Volunteers. NIH Grants Nos. CA14557, HL19898 and RR-47 (General Clinical Research Centers Program of the Division of Research Resources).

33

Perinatal and Neonatal Transfusion

Martin Klemperer, M.D.

The major uses of transfusion therapy in the fetus and in the neonate have, in the past, been for the treatment of hematologic diseases. More recently, the use of blood products has been extended to include them in treatment programs for hyaline membrane disease, sepsis, and disseminated intravascular coagulation in the critically ill neonate. The objectives of this chapter are to review: (1) the hematophysiology of the newborn; (2) the causes and prevention of maternal alloimmunization by the fetus; (3) the treatment of hemolytic disease of the newborn; and (4) transfusion therapy of the newborn, employing whole blood or separated blood products such as red blood cells, white blood cells, platelets, and plasma.

HEMATOPHYSIOLOGY OF THE NEWBORN AND NEONATE

The blood volume of the newborn infant is significantly greater in proportion to body weight than that in the older child or adult, and it is greatly affected by the amount of blood received postpartum from placental transfusion. The average blood volume of the full-term infant at birth is 85 ml/kg, while that of the premature infant is 108 ml/kg.[1,2] Since the placenta contains approximately 75 to 150 ml of blood, a delay in clamping the umbilical cord may transfuse the newborn with up to an additional 100 ml of blood.[3] Usher and coworkers[4] have studied the effect of placental transfusions upon the blood volume of the newborn. At birth the blood volume is 78 ml/kg, and increases above this level are mainly the result of a delay in cord clamping. The amount of blood transfused varies with the delay in clamping past delivery. One half of the volume is transfused within the first minute after birth, and 90 percent is transfused within 10 minutes after birth. Since the placental vessels of the premature infant hold relatively more blood than those of the full-term infant, the incremental increase in blood volume with delayed clamping will be greater in the preterm newborn.

After birth, the blood volume decreases rapidly as a result of transudation of blood plasma. By the end of the first 4 hours of life, the blood volume decreases, on average, from 126 ml/kg to 89 ml/kg, and the venous hematocrit increases from 48 percent to 64 percent. These changes in circulating blood volume and in venous hematocrit do not occur when the cord is clamped immediately after birth.[4]

Walker and Turnbull[5] have studied the hemoglobin levels in blood obtained from therapeutically aborted fetuses and premature infants. Fetuses at approximately 10 weeks gestation had hemoglobin levels of 9.0 g/dl, and at 38 weeks gestation the hemoglobin was 15.2 g/dl. Oski and Naiman[1] note that by 34 weeks gestation cord blood hemoglobin is 15.0 g/dl. Hemoglobin levels of small-for-gestational-age infants born between 36 and 46 weeks gestation are reported to be higher than those of comparable normal infants, 17.1 ± 2.1 g/dl versus 16.2 ± 2.3 g/dl.[6] This polycythemia is believed to be secondary to placental insufficiency, which is common to this group of infants. Burnan and Morris have reported that cord hemoglobin values of premature males are higher than those of premature females.[7] However, this has not been corroborated by other studies.[8,9]

The maturation from embryo to newborn is accompanied by the synthesis of six distinct hemoglobins, three of which are present in cord blood. Gower 1 ($\zeta_2\epsilon_2$), Gower 1 ($\alpha_2\epsilon_2$), and Hemoglobin Portland ($\zeta_2\delta_2$) are embryonic hemoglobins and are not present

normally in cord blood. The fetal hemoglobins, Barts (γ_4) and F ($\alpha_2\gamma_2$), and the adult hemoglobins, A ($\alpha_2\beta_2$) and A_2 ($\alpha_2\delta_2$), are present in the cord blood of premature and term infants.[10] (Fig. 33-1).

Fetal hemoglobin is the principal hemoglobin of the preterm or term infant, constituting 60 to 85 percent of cord hemoglobin. The oxygen affinity of fetal hemoglobin is greater than that of the adult hemoglobins A or A_2. This increased affinity is in part due to the lesser interaction of fetal hemoglobin with 2,3-diphosphoglycerate (2,3-DPG), which binds reversibly with hemoglobin.[11,12] 2,3-DPG is an intermediate product of glycolytic metabolism of the red cell. The 2,3-DPG-hemoglobin complex has a lesser oxygen affinity than does uncomplexed hemoglobin.[13,14]

The oxygen-hemoglobin equilibration curve in the newborn is determined by the concentrations of fetal and adult hemoglobins and by the concentration of erythrocyte

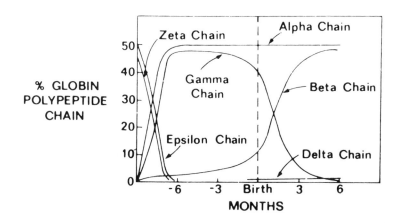

	HEMOGLOBIN	GLOBIN POLYPEPTIDES	% IN CORD BLOOD
EMBRYONIC	GOWER -1	Zeta-2, Epsilon-2 ($\zeta_2\epsilon_2$)	0
	GOWER -2	Alpha-2, Epsilon-2 ($\alpha_2\epsilon_2$)	0
FETAL	BARTS	Gamma-4 (γ_4)	<1%
	Hgb F	Alpha-2, Gamma-2 ($\alpha_2\gamma_2$)	60-85%
ADULT	Hgb A	Alpha-2, Beta-2 ($\alpha_2\beta_2$)	15-40%
	Hgb A_2	Alpha-2, Delta-2 ($\alpha_2\delta_2$)	<1%

Fig. 33-1. Fetal and infant globin production (*top*); cord blood hemoglobin composition (*bottom*). (Glader, B.E., and Platt, O.: Haemolytic disorders of infancy. Clinics in Haematol. 7:35, 1978.)

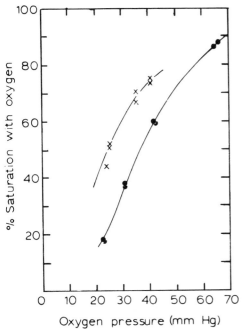

Fig. 33-2. The oxygen dissociation curves of fetal (--x--x) and maternal (•--•) blood. (Lehmann, H. and Huntsman, R.G.: Man's Haemoglobins. Elsevier/North-Holland, Inc., Amsterdam, 1966.)

2,3-DPG. Preterm infants are born with a higher concentration of fetal hemoglobin and a lower erythrocyte 2,3-DPG concentration than are term infants; therefore, preterm infants have a greater hemoglobin oxygen affinity. This shift of the oxygen-hemoglobin to the left (Fig. 33-2) is advantageous to the developing fetus, since the hemoglobin is saturated at a lower oxygen tension than it is in the adult. However, after birth increased oxygen binding may be relatively detrimental because oxygen release at this tissue level may be decreased; this question has not been resolved at the time of this writing.

DISORDERS REQUIRING EXCHANGE TRANSFUSION FOR NEONATAL HYPERBILIRUBINEMIA

The use of exchange transfusion was introduced by Hart,[15] modernized by Waller-

stein,[16] and popularized by Diamond and his coworkers[17,18] as therapy for hyperbilirubinemia secondary to hemolytic disease of the newborn, which at that time was due most frequently to maternal Rh-alloimmunization. More recently, exchange transfusion has been used also in treating neonates with alloimmune* thrombocytopenic purpura, severe respiratory distress syndrome, and disseminated intravascular coagulation (DIC).

Hemolytic Disease of the Newborn

Hemolytic disease of the newborn is a direct consequence of immune destruction of fetal erythrocytes which results from transplacental passage of maternal alloantibodies. The maternal antibodies are the product of a normal immune response to a foreign substance—in this case, antigenic fetal red cells or donor red cells—and must be of the IgG class if they are to cross the placenta and enter the fetal circulation.[19,20] Although hemolytic disease caused by ABO incompatibility occurs with twice the frequency of that caused by Rh incompatibility, ABO hemolytic disease usually is less severe and has not been associated with intrauterine and neonatal death or with the amount of major morbidity which is caused by Rh hemolytic disease.

The diverse presentations resulting from immune hemolysis in the fetus and in the newborn were proposed by Diamond and coworkers[21] to be caused by a single pathophysiologic process. This unifying concept was basic to the present understanding of the spectrum of disease secondary to alloimmune* hemolysis. In 1939 Levine and Stetson[22] described a red cell agglutinin in the

* Alloimmune is used in place of isoimmune since it is more accurate. In the present terminology of immunogenetics, isoimmune refers to an immune response provoked by a graft between genetically identical or near-identical individuals. Alloimmune refers to the response provoked by a graft between genetically dissimilar individuals of the same species.

serum of a mother who had given birth to an erythroblastic infant. This agglutinin had a spectrum of reactivity similar to that which Landsteiner and Weiner raised in rabbits against rhesus monkey erythrocytes.[23] This case report established the immunological nature of hemolytic disease of the newborn. A major advance in diagnosing hemolytic disease of the newborn was introduced in 1945 by Coombs and coworkers.[24,25] The Coombs' antiglobulin test enabled the detection and quantification of maternal immunization by fetal red cells during pregnancy and delivery. The use of antiglobulin serum to demonstrate the presence of specific antibody, immunoglobulin, on the surface of red cells or in an individual's serum vastly extended the precision and scope of blood grouping and provided a reproducible method for screening maternal sera for antibody directed against paternally derived fetal erythrocyte antigens.

Maternal Screening

The ability to detect immunoglobulin specifically directed against fetal blood group antigens is basic to every therapeutic maneuver aimed at reducing the morbidity and mortality which may result from alloimmunization. In the discussion which follows, the terms "Rh-positive" and "Rh-negative" will refer to the presence or absence of the red cell antigen, D, as determined by reactions with antiserums containing anti-D. This specificity is also referred to as Rho in the Weiner nomenclature. In the Fisher-Race nomenclature, D and d are allelic gene products, and three red cell genotypes—DD, Dd, and dd— are postulated.[26] The Rh-positive individual, therefore, can be DD or Dd. These genotypes cannot be distinguished directly, since anti-d has not been found. Rh-negative individuals are dd. Although other Rh system antigens can provoke antibody production during pregnancy, they are less potent immunizers than D and only infrequently cause hemolytic disease of the newborn.

All pregnant women should be typed for major blood group and the D antigen at their initial obstetrical visit. If an individual is D-positive, an initial screen for agglutinating and nonagglutinating antibodies of other specificities should be performed. If this is negative, further serological studies are not indicated unless there has been a history of prior alloimmunization. The serum of Rh-negative women should be screened for the presence of both saline agglutinins, which are usually IgM antibodies, and for nonagglutinating anti-D antibodies, employing the indirect antiglobulin test as evidence of Rh alloimmunization. Since IgG is the only immunoglobulin which is transferred across the placenta, only nonagglutinating IgG antibodies are involved in the pathobiology of hemolytic disease of the newborn. Such antibodies are not transferred transplacentally to any great extent until 12 to 16 weeks gestation.[19] Therefore, repeat screening for the presence of maternal sensitization need not be performed before 16 weeks gestation. Repeat examinations of D-negative women should be carried out again at 28 to 32 weeks; if anti-D antibodies are not found at that time, no further screening is indicated until postdelivery, when blood typing and a direct antiglobulin test should be performed on a sample of cord blood.

Women who have demonstrable anti-D at 12 to 16 weeks gestation should have anti-D titers performed monthly until 24 weeks. Should the titer of anti-D rise significantly, amniocentesis should be performed at 22 to 24 weeks to define the severity of intrauterine fetal disease more accurately. Although maternal antibody titer does correlate roughly with the severity of fetal hemolytic disease, the correlation is too imprecise to rely on this determination alone.[27,28] The mother's previous obstetrical history, together with the maternal antibody titer, are more reliable predictors of disease severity in the infant and can be used as a guide for the performance of amniocentesis to define more accurately the degree of the fetal hemolytic process.

Recently introduced techniques for quantifying maternal anti-D appear to be stronger in their correlation with the severity of hemolytic disease than are test-tube titers. Employing an automated assay, Fraser and Tovey[29] have reported that 472 of 490 women with IgG anti-D of less than 1 $\mu g/ml$ had mildly affected newborns. Those with IgG anti-D greater than 10 $\mu g/ml$ had severely affected newborns. IgG anti-D is almost universally of the subclasses IgG_1 and IgG_3.[30-32] Schanfield[33] reported that the infants of women with IgG_1 anti-D had more severe hemolytic disease than did infants in whom the maternal anti-D was of IgG_3 subclass.

Paternal Testing (Determination of Probable Rh Genotype)

If a woman is Rh-negative, it is valuable to know if the child's father is Rh-negative, and, if not, whether he is homozygous or heterozygous for the D antigen. If the father is D-positive, a statistical approximation of his genotype can be made by typing his red cells for the other principal antigens of the Rh system—C, c, E, and e. By serotypically determining his phenotype, the probability of his having a given genotype can be calculated from the frequencies of the genotypes in the U.S. population. For example, if the Rh phenotype is CCDee, the probable genotypes are CDe/CDe or CDe/Cde, with a respective incidence of 90 percent and 4 percent. Thus, the chances are 20:1 that the individual is CDe/CDe. If the infant is affected with hemolytic disease of the newborn, the odds are 99 to 1 that the father is homozygous at the D-locus.[34]

Although red cells homozygous for D will take up more anti-D than do red cells heterozygous for D, the genotype cannot be determined precisely by this method in random subjects.[34] Therefore, the serotypic determination of the probable Rh genotype remains the most practical means of evaluating paternal zygosity for D.

Antibodies Associated with Hemolytic Disease of the Newborn

Although Rh hemolytic disease of the newborn remains the model for alloimmune hemolytic disease and is clinically the most significant because of its severity, hemolytic disease due to matero-fetal ABO incompatibility occurs about twice as frequently.[17,35] The actual incidence has not been well defined; the criteria for diagnosing ABO hemolytic disease are not as clear-cut as those for Rh-related disease. The finding of IgG anti-A or anti-B in a pregnant woman is not firm evidence of significant alloimmunization. Many individuals, particularly those of blood type O, have IgG anti-A or anti-B with no history of previous blood transfusions or pregnancies. Since IgG is transmitted across the placenta, the finding of anti-A or anti-B in the cord blood is confirmatory but not diagnostic for allosensitization of the newborn. The direct antiglobulin test is frequently only weakly positive in these cases. The reason for this is poorly understood. The density of A and B antigens on the red cells of newborn infants is less than that of adults,[36] but this does not appear to explain the lack of strong antiglobulin reactions. Only rarely is the Coombs test negative with modern, commercially available antiglobulin reagents. If occurrence of jaundice within the first 24 hours of life is used as a denominator, the incidence of ABO hemolytic disease would be approximately 1 in 140 live births with this potential.[37] Obviously this is an underestimate, since it would not include minimally affected newborn infants whose liver function was capable of adequately conjugating and excreting the excess bilirubin derived from hemoglobin degradation.

Rh_o and ABO alloimmunization account for approximately 97 to 98 percent of the cases of hemolytic disease of the newborn. The next most frequent red cell antigens associated with rare cases of hemolytic disease of the newborn are: C, E, K (Kell), Fy^a (Duffy), and Jk^a (Kidd).[17,34]

MANAGEMENT OF HEMOLYTIC DISEASE OF THE NEWBORN

Any pregnant woman who has given birth previously to an infant with hemolytic disease of the newborn or who has serologic evidence of red cell alloimmunization must be examined at regular intervals, the length of which are dependent upon the rate of rise in antibody titer. In the case of Rh hemolytic disease, the severity of disease in previously affected infants and the results of maternal antibody titers are of value in predicting the probable outcome of the present pregnancy.[28] The first affected infant generally is affected less severely than subsequent infants, and the severity generally increases with each succeeding pregnancy. However, it has been noted that, within families, if one infant is mildly affected, subsequent infants are more likely to be mildly affected.[17,38,39]

Although a schedule for following maternal sensitization has been given in the section on screening for maternal antibody, it must be stressed that each case must be evaluated individually. Newly introduced methods of quantifying and characterizing serum anti-D antibody possibly correlate more closely with the severity of the hemolytic process than do estimations based on the standard tube titrations of maternal anti-D in use in most laboratories.[29,33,40,41] However, other investigators have reported that quantitation of maternal antibody has no advantage over antibody titrations in predicting the severity of disease.[42,43] The possible poor correlation of quantitation of maternal IgG anti-D with severity of hemolytic disease may be explained by the findings of Schanfield, who notes that, although there is a high level of correlation if the maternal antibody is of IgG_1 subclass, only poor correlation exists if the antibody is of IgG_3 subclass or a mixture of IgG_1 and IgG_3.[44]

Should the titer or quantity of maternal antibody reach the critical level (that amount associated with significant fetal morbidity or with intrauterine or neonatal death), amniocentesis should be performed to estimate

better the severity of fetal hemolytic disease. The critical level of antibody will vary among laboratories and therefore must be established for each laboratory and each time new reagents are employed for antibody titration or quantification. Frazer and Tovey[29,40] have proposed the following criteria as indications for amniocentesis:

1. In the first affected pregnancy, if the maternal antibody level is 1.5 $\mu g/ml$ or greater, amniocentesis should be performed before 35 weeks gestation.

2. In pregnancies subsequent to one in which an infant had been affected, if the maternal antibody level is 1.0 $\mu g/ml$ or greater, amniocentesis should be performed before 35 weeks gestation.

3. In a pregnancy subsequent to one in which an infant was moderately affected, amniocentesis should be performed at 28 weeks even if the antibody level remains below 1.0 $\mu g/ml$.

4. In any pregnancy which was preceded by a severely affected infant, amniocentesis is advised at 22 weeks gestation.

An additional factor in the correlation of maternal antibody with Rh hemolytic disease must be mentioned. Rising titers of anti-D IgG do not always indicate gestation of a D-positive fetus. In one study, maternal antibody levels were determined in 300 mothers with a history of previous hemolytic disease of the newborn. In 71 women who later give birth to D-negative infants, the concentration of antibody was greater than 1.0 $\mu g/ml$. In 58 of these women, the level remained constant or fell. However, in 13 women the antibody concentration increased significantly.[29] Hopkins[45] noted a significant increase in anti-D titer, greater than 4 doubling tube dilutions, in 4 of 239 D-sensitized women bearing a D-negative fetus.

Amniocentesis

Amniotic fluid normally is colorless or pale straw-colored. When a fetus is affected with hemolytic disease, the depth of color will increase, and in severe cases it becomes bright yellow. The pigments are derived from hemoglobin degradation and are most probably bilirubin.[46] A significant advance in the management of hemolytic disease of the newborn was made possible by documenting a correlation between the quantity of bilirubin in the amniotic fluid and the severity of intrauterine fetal disease.[47,48,48a] The use of amniotic fluid analysis for determining the severity of hemolytic disease and guiding its management was popularized by Liley in 1961.[49]

Amniotic fluid is analyzed spectrophotometrically over the spectral range of 350 to 700 nm, and the optical density rise at 450 to 460 nm is determined. The height of that peak correlates with the concentration of bilirubin in the amniotic fluid. In the course of a normal pregnancy, this value falls steadily between 26 weeks and term. In following a presumably affected fetus, serial samples of amniotic fluid are analyzed, and the optical densities at 450 nm are plotted on a graph which defines the degree of fetal risk (Fig. 33-3). At least two samples should be obtained and plotted in order to verify the results and to establish whether or not the optical densities are constant, increasing, or decreasing.[50]

The quality and treatment of the samples

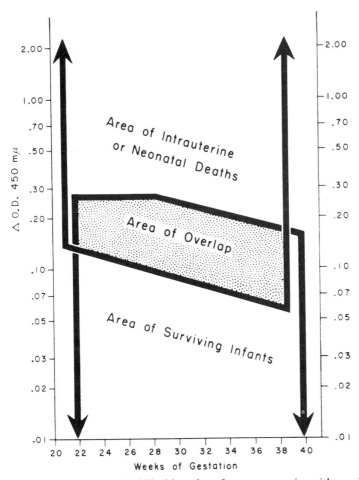

Fig. 33-3. Distribution of amniotic fluid bilirubin values from pregnancies with surviving infants and pregnancies resulting in death *in utero* or in the neonatal period. The area of overlap is critical to the following of amniotic fluid bilirubin levels during pregnancy. (Queenan, J.T. and Goetschel, E.: Amniotic fluid analysis for erythroblastosis fetalis. Obstet. Gynecol. 32:120, 1968.)

of amniotic fluid must be optimal because of their importance in determining the course of action during pregnancy. Samples should be protected from light, which oxidizes the bile pigments, resulting in a spuriously low optical density. The sample should be free from meconium and fetal or maternal blood, since these increase the optical density at 450 nm.[51]

Recently, Fraser and Tovey[29] reported the value of quantifying anti-D in the amniotic fluid. They have noted that such quantifications are of great help in distinguishing between moderately affected fetuses and mildly or unaffected fetuses (Table 33-1). They found a positive correlation between severity of disease and increasing antibody concentration. All of 28 fetuses were severely affected or stillborn when amniotic fluid antibody concentrations were greater than 5.0 μg/ml.

Intrauterine Transfusion

If analyses of amniotic fluid pigments are indicative of severe hemolytic disease, intrauterine fetal transfusion is considered. Because of the difficulties imposed by the small size of the fetus and the poor success rate, intrauterine transfusions usually are postponed until 26 weeks gestation.[52,53] In cases where intrauterine transfusion is performed at 26 weeks gestation or later, fetal survival in recent years has been 84.6 percent, with a mortality rate of 2.2 percent per procedure; however, if fetal hydrops is present, the success

rate falls to 25 percent.[52] Blood employed in intrauterine transfusions must be carefully crossmatched against maternal serum. There is no general agreement about the optimal red cell product, except that it should consist of packed red cells to ensure the greatest hemoglobin yield per ml transfused. Hamilton[54] employs fresh washed maternal red cells if the mother's hemoglobin is greater than 10 g/dl. Others recommend frozen or fresh washed donor red cells.[55] The blood volume of the fetus at different gestational ages varies, and therefore the volume of packed cells administered increases with gestational age (Table 33-2). After intrauterine transfusion, amniotic fluid analysis is of no further value, since the procedure leads to leakage of fetal blood, maternal blood, or transfused red cells into the amniotic fluid. Usually, intrauterine transfusions are repeated every 2 to 4 weeks until delivery.

Intrauterine transfusions are not without risk to both the mother and the fetus. Maternal complications include premature labor,[56] infection,[53] hepatitis,[57] placental separation,[57] sensitization to non-Rh antigens,[58] and central nervous system embolization.[59] Fetal complications are more common and include perforation of various structures such as bowel, stomach, bladder, thorax, spinal cord, cranium, and pericardium.[59a] Graft-versus-host disease in the newborn has been a rare complication of intrauterine transfusion.[60-62] It is not known whether such infants were immunologically normal or were affected by an immunological deficiency state which made

Table 33-1. Rh Antibody Levels in Amniotic Fluid Samples (602 Cases)

Degree of haemolytic disease	<0.1	0.1 - 0.2	0.2 - 0.6	0.6 - 1.0	1.0 - 5.0	5.0+	Totals
Rh negative	58	5	3	1	3	0	70
Mild	127	25	3	1	0	0	156
Mild to moderate	33	43	12	1	0	0	89
Moderate to severe	1	23	64	10	0	0	98
Severe to stillbirth	0	1	69	67	24	28	189
							602

Fraser, I.D. and Tovey, G.H.: Observations on Rh iso-immunization: past, present and future. Clin Haematol: 5:149, 1976.)

Table 33-2. Volume of Intrauterine Transfusion by Gestational Age

Week of Gestation	Approximate Blood Volume (in ml)	Packed Cells Given (in ml)
24	100	40
25	110	50
26	120	70
27	140	80
28	150	90
29	175	100
30	200	100
31	220	100
32	240	100–120

(Werch, A.: Prenatal evaluation of hemolytic disease of the fetus. In: A Seminar on Perinatal Blood Banking, 31st Annual Meeting of the American Association of Blood Banks, American Association of Blood Banks, 1978.)

them susceptible to graft-versus-host disease. One means of avoiding this rare complication—irradiating the red cells prior to administration at a dose of 1500 r—should be done if feasible.

The objective of intrauterine transfusion is to replace the fetal D-positive cells with D-negative cells which are not affected by maternal anti-D and should therefore have a normal survival. The performance of intrauterine transfusions decreases fetal anemia and possibly hydrops. It enables some previously doomed fetuses to be delivered in good enough condition to allow control hyperbilirubinemia by exchange transfusion if necessary. Hyperbilirubinemia in utero is not a major problem, since the placenta is an effective organ for fetal bilirubin exchange.

Exchange Transfusion

After birth, exchange transfusion remains the major effective method of managing significant hyperbilirubinemia in newborns with hemolytic disease. The objectives of exchange transfusion are:

1. to remove antibody-coated red cells, which, when destroyed, provide the source of neurotoxic bilirubin, and to replace them with red cells compatible with the mother.

2. to correct anemia.

3. to remove bilirubin.

4. to remove antibody that will combine with newly formed red cells of the infant.

Since both the IgG and bilirubin are distributed in significant amounts extravascularly, the effectiveness of exchange transfusion in their removal is determined to some extent by their rate of equilibration with the intravascular compartment.

The indications for exchange transfusions are based on criteria for the infant's hemoglobin concentration and degree of hyperbilirubinemia. A suitable guide for exchange transfusion is given in Table 33-3. In the majority of infants, exchange transfusions are performed to prevent neurotoxic hyperbilirubinemia, not to correct anemia. Development of kernicterus is a disaster in an affected infant, many of whom survive in a severely handicapped state. All newborns at risk must be monitored closely by bilirubin determinations obtained at 4- to 8-hour intervals, with the objective of keeping the serum unconjugated bilirubin levels below 20 mg/dl in term infants and below 15 mg/dl in premature infants.

PREVENTION OF MATERNAL Rh-ALLOIMMUNIZATION

The preceding section has described methods of salvaging infants affected with hemolytic disease of the newborn. A more effective, highly economical, and less hazardous solution to this problem has been provided by our recently acquired ability to prevent Rh sensitization in Rh-negative women. Prior to an effective means of preventing Rh sensitization, hemolytic disease of the newborn caused 10,000 deaths annually and was a major cause of severe mental retardation in the United States.[63] The routine administration of commercially available, high-titered IgG anti-D globulin has the potential for virtually eliminating Rh hemolytic disease.[29,43,64] However, the success already

Table 33-3. Guidelines for Exchange Transfusion for Rh Hemolytic Disease of the Newborn

Findings	Observe	Consider Exchange	Do Exchange
AT BIRTH:			
History or course of action in previous offspring	No exchange transfusion	Exchange transfusion was necessary or kernicterus was observed	Death or near death from erythroblastosis
Maternal Rh antibody titer	<1:64	>1:64	
Clinical situation	Apparently normal	Induced or spontaneous delivery of premature infant	Jaundice, fetal hydrops
Cord hemoglobin	>14 g/dl	12–14 g/dl	<12 mg/dl
Cord bilirubin	<4 mg/dl	4–5 mg/dl	>5 mg/dl
AFTER BIRTH:			
Capillary blood hemoglobin	>12 g/dl	<12 g/dl	<12 g/dl and falling in first 24 hours
Serum bilirubin	<18 mg/dl	18–20 mg/dl	20 mg/dl in first 48 hours or 22 mg/dl on two successive determinations at 6- to 8-hour intervals after 48 hours. Clinical signs suggesting kernicterus at any time or at any bilirubin level

(McKay, R.J., Jr.: Current status of exchange transfusion in newborn infants. Pediatr. 33:763, 1964. Copyright American Academy of Pediatrics 1964.)

attained is leading to complacency in diagnosing and carefully observing pregnant women who are sensitized to other possibly important red cell antigens. Women alloimmunized to Rh or other antigens by previous transfusions will continue to present problems of hemolytic disease of the newborn. Although the absolute number of affected infants is small at present, hemolytic disease of the newborn caused by non-D antigens is now becoming a major cause of severe disease.

Mechanism of Maternal Alloimmunization by Pregnancy

It has been well documented that during pregnancy fetal cells do enter the maternal circulation and provide a source of antigen which may be recognized by the mother as "nonself." The introduction by Kleihauer and coworkers of a sensitive method of identifying fetal hemoglobin F containing cells by their relative stability to acid hemolysis has enabled detection of as little as 0.05 ml of fetal blood in the maternal circulation.[65] Because of its simplicity, the Kleihauer-Betke technique remains the most commonly used method for detecting fetal red cells in the maternal circulation and has not been replaced by more sensitive assays employing fluorescence-labeled antihemoglobin F.[66,66a]

Cohen and coworkers reported that fetal cells were present in one of 15 women by the third month of pregnancy and in 50 percent of women at term with ABO-compatible fetuses.[67] Zipursky and coworkers reported the presence of fetal red cells in the maternal circulation at 9 weeks gestation.[68] When an immunofluorescent technique was employed to detect Hgb F containing cells in the circulation of 15 pregnant women, all had an increased number of HgF-positive cells from 16 to 30 weeks gestation.[69]

The demonstration of an increase in HgF

containing cells as direct evidence for fetal-maternal bleeds has been challenged by Pembrey and coworkers.[70] They noted that HgF may be of maternal origin since analysis of the γ^{15} peptide yielded glycine:alanine ratios in the range of adult HgF rather than in the fetal HgF range. When hemoglobin synthesis was measured by ^{14}C-labeled L-leucine incorporation in vitro, they noted that maternal reticulocytes synthesized HgA and HgF in the ratios found in the peripheral blood.

In the course of most pregnancies, the amount of fetal blood that enters the maternal circulation at any one time is probably less than 0.1 ml. It is during delivery that larger amounts, greater than 0.2 ml, enter the circulation.[71] It is these larger boluses of antigen that are causative in maternal sensitization. Immunogenic doses of fetal red cells have been reported as a consequence of spontaneous[72] or induced abortions,[73] amniocentesis,[73a] ectopic pregnancy,[74,75] Cesarean section,[73a] and manual removal of the placenta.[76]

The lower incidence of Rh sensitization in pregnancies in which the father was "ABO-incompatible" with the mother was first noted by Levine.[77] Later studies[17,78,79] have confirmed these findings (Table 33-4). However, Vos reported that such protection was not complete and that ABO incompatibility protected only against the formation of high-titered Rh antibodies.[79a] The protective effect of ABO incompatibility was postulated to be due to the rapid clearance from the maternal circulation of incompatible fetal red cells.

The natural protective effect of ABO in-compatibility was a major conceptual stimulus for the passive immunization of Rh-negative mothers at risk for developing anti-D antibody. Since the introduction of Rh-immune globulin in the early 1960s, a steady decline in the incidence of alloimmunization in Rh-negative mothers has been reported; as a consequence, there has been a corresponding decrease in the incidence of Rh hemolytic disease[80] (Figs. 33-4, 33-5). The success observed with the use of prophylactic anti-D immunoglobulin is solid evidence that, in most instances, the potentially immunizing doses of fetal red cells are transferred at the time of delivery. If the major antigenic challenge occurred earlier in gestation, immune globulin given after delivery would not abrogate the antibody response. The routine administration of immune anti-D after delivery has reduced the incidence of Rh sensitization to less than 1 percent in multiparous Rh-negative mothers.[80] Prior to the use of immune anti-D, the incidence of sensitization in Rh-negative mothers after the delivery of the second Rh-positive infant was 13 to 17 percent.[80,81]

The standard method for the prevention of sensitization to the D antigen is administration of 300 μg of Rh-immune globulin intramuscularly to all unsensitized Rh-negative women within 72 hours of delivery of an Rh-positive infant. Obviously, since abortions are another common immunizing event, Rh-immune globulin should be used administered to an Rh-negative woman after abortion of an Rh-positive fetus. If Rh-immune globulin has not been administered within 72 hours, it should be administered late rather than withheld whenever its use is indicated. This

Table 33-4. Effect of ABO Compatibility and Rh Dose on the Risk of Sensitization by Pregnancy in Rh-Negative Women

Husband's zygosity for Rh	ABO compatibility of husband		ABO type of husband known (%)
	Incompatible (%)	Compatible (%)	
Heterozygous	1	3	2
Homozygous	4-5	11	9
Zygosity unknown	2-3	7-8	5

(Allen, F.H., Jr. and Diamond, L.K. 1958. Erythroblastosis fetalis. Little Brown & Co., Boston, 1958.)

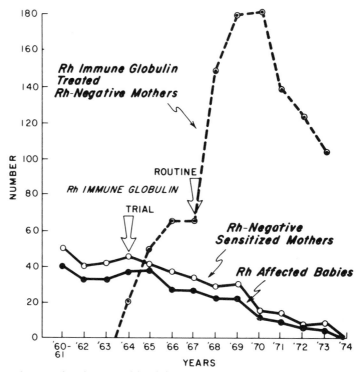

Fig. 33-4. Effect of preventive therapy with Rh immune globulin on the incidence of maternal sensitization and Rh hemolytic disease of the newborn. (Freda, V., Gorman, J.G., Pollack, W., and Bowe, E.: Prevention of Rh hemolytic disease: ten years' clinical experience with Rh immune globulin. Reprinted, by permission of N. Engl. J. Med. 292:1014, 1975.)

dose will prevent sensitization by a bleed of up to 10 ml of Rh-positive red cells.[82] If very large numbers of Rh-cells are found in the maternal circulation, immune anti-D should be given at a dose of 50 μg/2.5 ml D-positive red cells.[83] This topic is discussed in further detail in Chapter 40.

OTHER INDICATIONS FOR EXCHANGE TRANSFUSION

Hemolytic States Other Than Rh-related Disease

A major objective of exchange transfusion is the control of hyperbilirubinemia. Obviously, in hemolytic disease of the newborn caused by alloimmunization to red cell antigens other than D, the criteria for exchange transfusion are similar to those for Rh disease. Exchange transfusion has also been employed to treat the hyperbilirubinemia associated with intrinsic red cell defects, such as hereditary spherocytosis and severe glucose-6-phosphate dehydrogenase deficiency. Hyperbilirubinemia caused by sepsis, enclosed hemorrhage, and congenital viral and protazoal infections also has been controlled by exchange transfusion.

Severe Respiratory Distress Syndrome

Several authors have reported significantly increased survival of infants with severe respiratory distress syndrome when treated with exchange transfusion. The precise causes for the increased survival with ex-

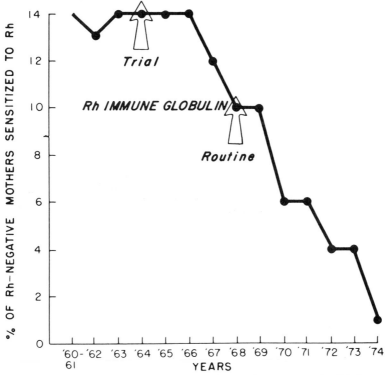

Fig. 33-5. Decreasing incidence of sensitized Rh-negative mothers seen at the Rh Antepartum Clinic, Columbia-Presbyterian Medical Center, from 1960 to 1974. (Freda, V.J., Gorman, J.G., Pollack, W., and Bowe, E.: Prevention of Rh hemolytic disease: ten years' clinical experience with Rh immune globulin. Reprinted, by permission of N. Engl. J. Med. 292:1014, 1975.)

change transfusion have not been identified. However, several mechanisms have been postulated:

1. Premature infants have higher HgF and lower 2,3-DPG levels than do adults. Their hemoglobin affinity for oxygen is greater than that of the adult, and, therefore, less oxygen is released at the tissue level at a given tissue oxygen tension. Exchange transfusions with fresh adult blood or 2,3-DPG enriched blood might improve oxygen delivery.[84,85]

2. Gottuso and coworkers reported a rise in arterial oxygen concentration shortly after exchange transfusion.[86] They noted a significant decrease in the ratio of oxygen requirements to the PaO_2 within 7 hours of the procedure. The authors postulated that the improved pulmonary ventilation and alveolar perfusion were due to the removal of substances which might produce pulmonary hypoperfusion. Friedman and coworkers reported that, during the acute phase of the respiratory distress syndrome, plasma concentrations of prostaglandins E and F is reduced significantly.[87]

3. DeLemos and coworkers attributed the improved survival in infants with the respiratory distress syndrome who underwent exchange transfusion to the correction of coagulation abnormalities which result in a significant incidence of fetal pulmonary and/or cerebral hemorrhage.[88] Gottuso and coworkers noted the correction of the partial thromboplastin time (PTT) with exchange transfusion but could not find a significant correlation with survival of affected infants.[86] Exchange transfusion in the therapy of severe respiratory distress syndrome appears in pre-

liminary reports to improve survival.[88a] However, it must be considered an investigational technique at this time.

Disseminated Intravascular Coagulation

Disseminated intravascular coagulation is an acquired coagulopathy with many causes, in which plasma fibrinogen is decreased and circulating fibrin split products are increased. Frequently, Factors II, V, VIII and blood platelets are decreased. When these substances fall to a level insufficient to maintain hemostasis, a hemorrhagic diathesis is present. Exchange transfusion has been reported to be effective in the management of disseminated intravascular coagulation. Presumably, exchange transfusion should remove fibrin degradation products and provide plasma clotting factors and platelets.[89] It must be stressed that the most concerted efforts of the physician should be to diagnose and treat the underlying cause of disseminated intravascular coagulation. The use of exchange transfusion must be regarded as a nonspecific therapy.

Other Conditions

Exchange transfusion may be indicated in the following other conditions:

1. Neonatal polycythemia: Partial exchange transfusion with fresh frozen plasma should lower the hematocrit to less than 60 percent. A suitable volume calculation in ml is:

$$\frac{[85 \text{ (blood vol/kg)} \times \text{weight in kg}] \times \text{observed HCT} - \text{desired HCT}}{\text{observed HCT}}$$

2. Fetal hydrops: Partial exchange transfusion with packed fresh red cells should preferably be anticoagulated with heparin. In most instances, the initial exchange should be

a one-volume exchange (calculated on wt in kg × 85) at the most. During the exchange, elevated venous pressure should be corrected gradually by removing more blood than is infused—e.g., remove aliquots of 20 ml and infuse 10 ml aliquots. Albumin should *not* be administered, since this will increase the circulating blood volume.

3. Removal of toxic substances which cross the placenta—e.g., diazepam, magnesium sulfate.

TECHNIQUE OF EXCHANGE TRANSFUSION

The method of exchange transfusion has remained unchanged during the more than 20 years since it was described completely by Allen and Diamond.[17,18] Improvements have been made in equipment, and a commercially obtainable exchange transfusion tray—Sterile Exchange Transfusion Tray by Pharmaseal Laboratories of Glendale, CA—is used most frequently. Because of the decreasing use of exchange transfusions, fewer individuals are experienced in the procedure. It must be emphasized that exchange transfusions should be performed or supervised by individuals who are experienced in the technique.

When an exchange transfusion is being performed to treat hemolytic disease of the newborn, blood should be crossmatched against maternal serum whenever possible. If the antibody specificity is known and blood that is ABO-compatible with the infant can be obtained, it should be used rather than type O blood which contains anti-A and anti-B. If the antibody is directed against a high-incidence red cell antigen (e.g., the e antigen of the Rh complex) and a compatible donor is not available, washed maternal cells resuspended in AB plasma can be used.

Heparinized blood is thought by some to be preferable because it avoids the acidosis and other metabolic changes associated with citrated blood. Citrated blood, however, is widely used. Heparinized blood must be used within 24 hours and thus must be drawn immediately prior to use. In a well-planned procedure, the donor can be crossmatched with the mother's serum, and the necessary tests of the donor for hepatitis and serology can be performed in advance. The donor can then be bled into heparin when a decision is made to perform an exchange transfusion.

Frequently, an exchange transfusion is performed without prepartum planning or on an infant who is too critically ill to wait until a donor can be located and bled. Under these circumstances, CPD blood less than 3 days old should be used. Such blood has a low plasma potassium concentration and has adequate concentrations of red cell 2,3-DPG.[89a]

Prior to exchange transfusion, a nasogastric tube should be passed and the gastric contents aspirated. The tube should be left in place and aspirated periodically throughout the procedure to prevent regurgitation and aspiration of the stomach contents. The heart rate and electrocardiogram should be followed continually on a cardiac monitor. The infant should be kept warm, and the blood that is given should be warmed and kept at 37° C by employing a thermally regulated warming bath.

For most purposes a single unit of donor blood is sufficient, and no more than a two blood volume exchange should be performed. This amount will remove approximately 85 percent of the infant's blood. The percentage may be approximated by the nomogram shown as Figure 33-6 or by the equation:

$$\% \ R = \left[\frac{V - S}{V} \right]^n$$

where R = percentage of infant's blood remaining, V = estimated blood volume, S = the volume of each aliquot removed and replaced, and n = the number of cycles performed in the exchange transfusion.[17]

Proper placement of the umbilical catheter is vital to the success of an exchange transfusion. The catheter is inserted into the umbilical vein and gently passed through the ductus venosus into the inferior vena cava. A ligature laced around the umbilical stump and gently

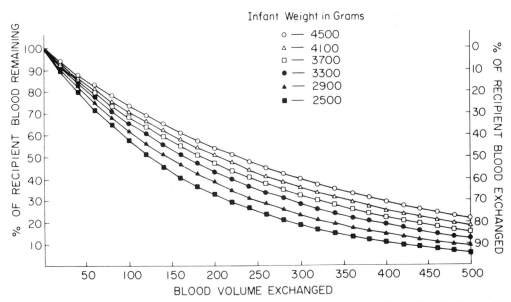

Fig. 33-6. The predicted percentage of blood exchange based on infant weight. A blood volume of 75 ml/kg has been assumed and the percentage is based on the equation $\% \ R = \left[\frac{V - S}{V} \right]^n$. (Bucholtz, D.H.: Blood transfusion: merits of component therapy. J. Pediatr. 84:1, 1974.)

pulled caudally helps in advancing the catheter. *Under no circumstances should the catheter be forced.* When the catheter is in the inferior vena cava, blood may be removed and infused easily. If this does not occur, replacement by slow advancement or withdrawal of the catheter should be carried out until a free flow of blood is established. The catheter then can be held in place by gently tightening the umbilical ligature. *Under no circumstances should blood be infused forcefully.* The aliquot volumes exchanged are usually 20 ml for term infants and 10 ml for premature infants. Exchange transfusion should be completed in 1 to 1.5 hours.

When citrated blood is used, agitation and tachycardia may occur periodically during the procedure. Calcium gluceptate or gluconate should be administered slowly via the umbilical catheter to correct these physical changes. When heparinized blood is employed, protamine should be administered at the completion of the procedure. Since heparinized blood contains 4.5 IU/ml, the amount of heparin remaining can be calculated by multiplying the infant's blood volume by the percent of blood exchanged times 4.5. For each of 100 IU of heparin remaining, 0.5 to 0.75 mg protamine should be given. Recently, frozen red cells suspended in albu-

min or in heparinized, recalcified fresh frozen plasma have been reported to be useful in exchange transfusion.[90,90a] Such a preparation has the benefits of delivering red cells with good levels of 2,3-DPG without the presence of citrate. Until more information is available, routine use of this procedure cannot be advised.

When exchange transfusions are performed on infants in good physical condition, the mortality rate is less than 1 percent.[1] Numerous complications have been reported and have been reviewed by Odall et al.[91] The complications of exchange transfusion are listed in Table 33-5.

TRANSFUSION THERAPY IN THE YOUNG INFANT

The selection of the most suitable blood product for transfusion therapy in the neonate and young infant is best determined by the nature of the disease process which has made transfusion necessary. Transfusion with whole blood is required for all infants who are anemic and in hypovolemic shock. In the majority of other circumstances, transfusion with packed red blood cells is preferable in order to correct anemia without increasing the risk of volume overload.

A major problem in supplying blood for neonatal transfusion therapy is the small volume of each individual transfusion. Several solutions to this problem have been developed. Previously, the required volume of fresh whole blood, usually less than 50 ml, was withdrawn from a unit of whole blood and used to transfuse the infant. Since the unit of blood, once entered, has an expiration time of 24 hours, the remaining portion must be discarded unless another suitable recipient can be found. In larger newborn services, several infants can be crossmatched and transfused from a single unit, thus decreasing the amount of blood wasted.

Another means of supplying blood for small-volume transfusions is the walking donor program.[92,93] These programs have

Table 33-5. Complications of Exchange Transfusion

Cardiac
   Arrhythmias
   Arrest
   Myocardial infarction

Vascular
   Volume depletion
   Volume overload
   Anemia
   Thrombosis, esp. portal vein
   Embolization with air or thrombi
   Perforation of vessels

Coagulation
   Overheparinization
   Thrombocytopenia

Infection
   Bacterial, e.g., sepsis, omphalitis
   Viral, e.g., hepatitis, cytomegalovirus

Miscellaneous
   Incompatible blood transfusion
   Injury to donor cells, mechanical, thermal
   Hypovolemia

depended heavily upon the use of hospital personnel as donors; in cases of emergency, they have required the use of banked whole blood prior to the administration of freshly drawn blood. However, transfusions from walking donors may not provide the optimal blood product for the following reasons: (1) hepatitis screening may at times be overlooked; (2) crossmatching may not be adequate; and (3) blood may be overheparinized. It is also difficult to obtain packed red blood cells from blood drawn into a syringe.[94] The walking donor program may also put hospital personnel at an increased risk of hepatitis exposure.

The development of the "multiple blood pack" has provided a more practical method for supplying small-volume transfusions. A unit of blood is collected into a CPD quadruple blood pack. With this closed system, the unit can then be separated into four 125-ml units. Each of these smaller units can be subdivided into still smaller aliquots, but these must then be used within 24 hours. More than one neonate can be crossmatched with the same donor so that each unit can be utilized more efficiently. Crossmatching of the recipient neonate does not need to be repeated as long as a single series of transfusions from the multiple bag system of a single donor comprises the only blood products used. A derivative method for obtaining blood for small-volume transfusions is the collection of 225 ml into a CPD "triple pack" with the volume of anticoagulant reduced for the smaller amount of blood drawn. This closed system provides two small units of packed red blood cells. The same donor can be bled an additional 225 ml within a few days if this is necessary.[95]

The most recent innovation in neonatal transfusion therapy has been the use of frozen red cells.[96] This blood product has a "shelf life" of years and, when prepared from fresh red cells, has normal concentrations of 2,3-DPG.[90,97] Red cells from a single donor can be glycerolized and frozen in a closed system which contains three polyolefin freezing bags.[98] Frozen red cells appear to be the op-

timal product for the treatment of perinatal or neonatal anemia. This blood product has normal levels of 2,3-DPG, contains few platelets and white cells, and does not contain anticoagulant. In addition, if a long-term transfusion requirement is predicted, the infant can receive blood from one or at most a limited number of donors, which eliminates exposure to a wide range of red cell, white cell, and platelet antigens.

AMOUNT OF TRANSFUSATE

In the severely anemic infant who is not volume depleted, partial exchange transfusion remains the most rapid method for correction of anemia. In severely anemic neonates who are not exchanged, the lower the hemoglobin, the smaller the volume of transfusate. Thus, a child with a hemoglobin of 3 g/dl should receive 3 ml/lb of packed red cells, and one with a 5 g/dl, 5 ml/lb. In the more common circumstances where anemia is not so profound, the amount to be transfused can be calculated as follows:

$$\frac{(\text{circulating blood vol}) \times (\text{incremental increase in hemoglobin})}{\text{Hemoglobin gm/dl of blood product}}$$

Example: A 3.0-kg infant has a hemoglobin of 8 g/dl, and it is desired to raise the hemoglobin to 12 g/dl. If frozen-thawed red cells are used,

$$\frac{(3.0 \times 85) \times (12 - 8)}{25} = \frac{1020}{25} =$$
40.8 ml of frozen-thawed cells.

Or, if packed red cells were used,

$$\frac{(3.0 \times 8.5) \times (12 - 8)}{20} =$$
$$\frac{1020}{20} = 51 \text{ ml packed cells.}$$

Calculations should be used to determine the volume of transfusion necessary, rather than using a "safe figure" such as 10 to 15 ml per pound, a dosage which should be used only as an estimate of the maximum volume per transfusion. If there is any question about the cardiovascular stability of the infant, several small transfusions rather than a single large transfusion should be employed.

The newborn infant suffering from anemia and hypovolemic shock from acute blood loss presents a medical emergency. Such infants should be well oxygenated and should have an umbilical catheter inserted. As soon as possible, a volume expander should be infused rapidly at 20 ml/kg; for this purpose, group O, Rh-negative whole blood (do not wait for a complete crossmatch), or 5 percent albumin is preferable to isotonic saline. If the infant continues to be hypotensive with a low venous pressure, another 10 to 20 ml/kg of whole blood should be administered. The site and cause of hemorrhage should be determined as quickly as possible.

Since newborn infants, particularly prematures, have a relatively small circulating blood volume, blood samples obtained for laboratory studies may constitute a source of significant blood loss. An individual record of the time and volume of each blood aliquot removed for the laboratory must be kept. When the total volume removed is 7 ml/kg, replacement therapy usually is indicated. Severely ill infants may require replacement when 5 ml/kg has been removed.

PLATELET TRANSFUSION THERAPY

The newborn infant, particularly the premature infant, may have minor defects in platelet function and in vascular hemostatic function. Platelet counts in both premature and full-term infants are within the usual normal range,[99] and in premature infants the incidence of platelet counts below 100,000/μl during the first month of life is less than 3.6 percent.[100] In the newborn, platelet aggregation in response to ADP, collagen, and thrombin is below that of adults.[99, 101] Vascu-

lar integrity as determined by capillary fragility tests appears to be normal in full-term infants but abnormal in premature infants.[101] Nevertheless, there is no evidence that these minor hemostatic defects have any clinical significance in healthy full-term or premature infants.

Platelet therapy in the neonate should be governed primarily by symptomatic bleeding and not by the isolated laboratory finding of thrombocytopenia. Careful, repeated observations are most important to the management of any thrombocytopenic infant. Efforts must be made to define the cause of thrombocytopenia prior to the administration of platelets. Table 33-6 lists the major causes of neonatal thrombocytopenic purpura.

In most instances, thrombocytopenia is caused by nonimmunologic mechanisms and can be treated if necessary by infusion of ABO- and Rh-compatible platelet concentrates. Each unit consists of 30 to 50 ml of plasma containing approximately 7×10^{10} platelets. Since the volume of the transfusate may be critical in transfusing neonates, concentrates may have to be split into two doses. Another approach is to concentrate the plate-

Table 33-6. Causes of Neonatal Thrombcytopenic Purpura

A. Normal physical examination
  1. Immunologic
    a. Maternal alloimmunization—alloimmune neonatal thrombocytopenic purpura
    b. Maternal autoimmunization—chronic ITP in mother, or after splenectomy
  2. Drug induced—thiazides, tolbutamide
  3. Infections—bacterial sepsis

B. Associated with hepatosplenomegaly
  1. Infectious
    a. Viral—congenital rubella, congenital cytomegalovirus
    b. Protozoal—congenital toxoplasmosis
    c. Spirochetal—congenital syphilis
    d. Bacterial
  2. Noninfectious
    a. associated with alloimmune hemolytic disease
    b. congenital leukemia

C. Associated with congenital anomalies
  1. giant hemangioma
  2. bilateral absence of the radii

D. Associated with multiple exchange transfusions

lets after recentrifugation. Since bleeding due to thrombocytopenia alone is uncommon at platelet counts above 50,000/μl transfusion therapy should not be aimed at keeping platelets much above this level.

NEONATAL PURPURA

Neonatal alloimmune purpura is a relatively rare disorder with a pathogenesis identical to hemolytic disease of the newborn, except that target is the platelet rather than the red cell. The platelet antigen, Pl^{A1}, is most frequently involved.[102] Since this platelet antigen is present in 98 percent of the population, Pl^{A1}-negative donors are rare. Although there is no general agreement as to therapy, the following plan appears to be rational:

If the newborn infant is mildly affected, prednisone at a dose of 60 mg/m^2 may be administered for 2 weeks and then stopped. If a Pl^{A1}-negative donor cannot be found, severely affected infants should be transfused with washed maternal platelets suspended in group AB, Rh-negative plasma. Usually, only one transfusion is necessary.[102]

In cases of neonatal purpura associated with maternal autoimmune thrombocytopenic purpura, the management is similar to that of alloimmune thrombocytopenic purpura with the following major exception: The causative platelet antibodies bind to almost all platelets; therefore, compatible donors should not be sought. If platelet therapy is necessary, an exchange transfusion should be performed to decrease the amount of antibody present in the infant, and then platelet concentates should be administered as necessary.

The proper treatment of disseminated intravascular coagulation in which thrombocytopenia occurs in the neonatal period is not well defined. Agreement has been reached that the underlying disease process must be defined and treated vigorously. A diversity of opinion persists in recommendations for supportive therapy. Exchange transfusion and

heparinization have been recommended.[1,89] Heparinization of the newborn has its risks since the clearance of heparin is markedly prolonged and bleeding secondary to the persistence of heparin may occur.[103] Possibly the most judicious means of treating this entity is to treat the cause and to supply platelets and fresh plasma as necessary to control hemorrhage.

GRANULOCYTE TRANSFUSIONS

The use of granulocyte concentrates obtained by leukophoresis does have a therapeutic rationale in the treatment of the neutropenic and septic neonate. Since the volume of current donor granulocyte preparations is too large to be given as a single infusion, the packs should be split so that aliquots of the white cells may be given every 6 or 12 hours. The volume to be transfused is governed by the fluid requirements of the infant. Since the intravascular life-span of mature neutrophils is 6 to 12 hours, the efficacy of transfusions cannot be determined by the rise in the absolute neutrophil count; rather, it must be indicated by the clinical state of the infant. Transfusions often need to be continued for a minimum of 4 days. The donor should be ABO- and Rh-compatible with the recipient. Since the need for prolonged or repeated white cell support is slight, non-HLA-matched donors are suitable. There have been no reported controlled trials of granulocyte transfusions in neonatal infants. Therefore, the use of this blood product cannot be regarded as accepted medical practice.

COAGULATION FACTOR REPLACEMENT

The majority of newborns with hereditary deficiencies of coagulation factors do not present with hemorrhage during the neonatal period. Therefore, if a newborn infant presents with bleeding, it must be assumed that the infant has a severe factor deficiency. Deficiencies of Factors XIII and IX account for approximately 99 percent of all heritable coagulation deficiencies presenting in the neonatal period.[104] Therefore, assays for these factors should be the first performed if a single-factor deficiency is suspected.

The precise nature of the coagulopathy should be defined as quickly as possible. A careful family history should be obtained and the prior administration of vitamin K in adequate dose, 1 mg, must be documented. If vitamin K has not been administered, 1 mg should be given intravenously while identification of the defect is being carried out. Vitamin K deficiency is reflected by decreased levels of Factors II, VII, IX, and X. Inherited factor deficiencies will involve a single factor.

Fresh frozen plasma contains all of the clotting factors at a concentration of approximately 1 unit activity/ml. Since only 10 to 15 ml/kg should be given as a single dose, the maximum expected rise in factor activity is approximately 15 percent. This dose can be repeated every 12 hours and may be sufficient to control bleeding. If bleeding is severe, factor concentrates should be used. Factor VIII may be administered at a dose of 30 to 50 units/kg at 12- 24-hour intervals. Factor IX should be administered at a dose of 50 to 100 units/kg once daily. More frequent administration usually is not necessary. Table 33-7 lists the available preparations and their activities per ml of Factor VIII and Factor IX. If therapy must be instituted before the precise factor deficiency is delineated, samples of ci-

trated plasma should be frozen so that a definitive diagnosis can be established later.

REFERENCES

1. Oski, F.A. and Naiman, J.L.: Hematologic problems in the newborn. 2nd Ed., W.B. Saunders Co., Philadelphia, 1971.
2. Schulman, I., Smith, C.H., and Stern, G.S.: Studies on the anemia of prematurity. Am. J. Dis. Child. 88:567, 1955.
3. Colozzi, A.E.: Clamping of the umbilical cord: its effect on the placental transfusion. New Engl. J. Med. 250:629, 1954.
4. Usher, R., Shephard, M., and Lind, J.: The blood volume of the newborn infant and placental transfusion. Acta. Paediatr. 52:497, 1963.
5. Walker, J. and Turnbull, E.P.N.: Haemoglobin and red cells in the human fetus and their relation to the oxygen content of the blood in the vessels of the umbilical cord. Lancet 2:312, 1953.
6. Humbert, J.R., Abelson, H., Hathaway, W.E., and Battoglia, F.C.: Polycythemia in small for gestational age infants. J. Pediatr. 75:812, 1969.
7. Burnam, D. and Morris, A.F.: Cord haemoglobin in low birthweight infants. Arch. Dis. Child. 49:382, 1974.
8. Cook, C.D., Brodie, H.R., and Allen, D.W.: Measurement of fetal hemoglobin in newborn infants. Correlation with gestational age and intrauterine anoxia. Pediatr. 20:272, 1957.
9. Marks, J., Gairdner, D., and Roscoe, J.D.: Blood formation in infancy. Part III. Cord blood. Arch. Dis. Child. 30:117, 1955.
10. Glader, B.E. and Platt, O.: Haemolytic disorders of infancy. Clin. Haematol. 7:35, 1978.
11. Allen, D.W., Wyman, J., Jr., and Smith, C.A.: The oxygen equilibrium of fetal and adult human hemoglobin. J. Biol. Chem. 203:81, 1953.
12. Bauer, C., Ludwig, I., and Ludwig, M.: Different effects of 2,3-diphosphoglycerate and adenosine triphosphate on the oxygen affinity of adult and foetal human hemoglobin. Life Sci. 7(I):1333, 1968.
13. Benesch, R. and Benesch, R.E.: The effect of organic phosphates from the human

Table 33-7. Preparations of Factor VIII and of Factor IX

Factor	Preparation	Units/ml
VIII	Fresh frozen plasma	1
	Cryoprecipitate	5-10
	Profilate (Abbott)	20-25
	Factorate (Armour)	20-25
	Koate (Cutter)	25
	Hemofil (Hyland)	25
	Humafac (Parke-Davis)	13-40
IX	Fresh frozen plasma	1
	Konyne (Cutter)	25
	Proplex (Hyland)	17-18

erythrocyte on the allosteric properties of hemoglobin. Biochem. Biophys. Res. Commun. 26:162, 1967.

14. Chanutin, A. and Curnish, R.R.: Effect of organic and inorganic phosphates on the oxygen equilibrium of human erythrocytes. Arch. Biochem. Biophys. 121:96, 1967.

15. Hart, A.P.: Familial icterus of the newborn and its treatment. Can. Med. Assoc. J. 15:1008, 1925.

16. Wallerstein, H.: Treatment of severe erythroblastosis by simultaneous removal and replacement of blood of the newborn infant. Science 103:583, 1946.

17. Allen, F.H., Jr. and Diamond, L.K.: Erythroblastosis Fetalis. Little, Brown & Co., Boston, 1958.

18. Diamond, L.K., Allen, F.H., Jr., and Thomas, W.O., Jr.: Erythroblastosis fetalis. VII. Treatment with exchange transfusion. N. Engl. J. Med. 244:39, 1951.

19. Gitlin, D.: Maternofetal immunoglobulin transfer mechanisms. Immunology in Obstetrics and Gynaecology: Proceedings of the First International Congress. Padua Centaro and Carretti, N., eds., Excerpta Medica, Amsterdam, 1974.

20. Gitlin, D., Kumate, J., Urrusti, J., and Morales, C.: The selectivity of the human placenta in the transfer of plasma proteins from mother to fetus. J. Clin. Invest. 43:1938, 1964.

21. Diamond, L.K., Blackfan, K.D., and Baty, J.M.: Erythroblastosis fetalis and its association with universal edema of the fetus, icterus gravis neonatorum, and anemia of the newborn. J. Pediatr. 1:269, 1932.

22. Levine, P. and Stetson, R.E.: An unusual case of intra-group agglutination. J.A.M.A. 113:126, 1939.

23. Landsteiner, K. and Weiner, A.S.: An agglutinable factor in human blood recognized by immune sera for rhesus blood. Proc. Soc. Exp. Biol. Med. 43:223, 1940.

24. Coombs, R.R.A., Mourant, A.E., and Race, R.R.: A new test for the detection of weak and "incomplete" Rh agglutinins. Br. J. Exp. Pathol. 26:255, 1945.

25. Coombs, R.R.A., Mourant, A.E., and Race, R.R.: Detection of weak and "incomplete" Rh agglutinins: a new test. Lancet 2:15, 1945.

26. Race, R.R.: The Rh genotypes and Fischer's theory. Blood 3(Suppl. 2):27, 1948.

27. Kelsall, G.A. and Vos, G.H.: The antibody titre in maternal and infant's serum as an indication for treatment in haemolytic disease of the newborn. Med. J. Austral. 1:349, 1952.

28. Walsh, R.J. and Ward, H.K.: Haemolytic disease of the newborn: an analysis of family histories and serological findings. Aust. Ann. Med. 8:262, 1959.

29. Fraser, I.D. and Tovey, G.H.: Observations of Rh iso-immunization: past, present and future. Clin. in Haematol. 5:149, 1976.

30. Devey, M.E. and Voak, D.: A critical study of the IgG subclasses of Rh anti-D antibodies formed in pregnancy and in immunized volunteers. Immunology 27:1073, 1974.

31. Morell, A.S., Kvaril, F., and Rufener, J.L.: Characterization of Rh antibodies formed after incompatible pregnancies and after repeated booster injections. Vox Sang. 24:323, 1973.

32. McKay, R.J., Jr.: Current status of exchange transfusion in newborn infants. Pediatr. 33:763, 1964.

33. Schanfield, M.S.: Correlation between severity of Rh hemolytic disease of the newborn and IgG subclass and allotype. Transfusion 16:528, 1976.

34. Mollison, P.L.: Blood transfusion in clinical medicine. 6th edition, Blackwell Scientific Publications, Oxford, 1979.

35. Valentine, G.H.: ABO incompatibility and haemolytic disease of the newborn. Arch. Dis. Child. 33:185, 1958.

36. Economidou, J., Hughes-Jones, N.C., and Gardner, B.: Quantitative measurements concerning A and B antigen sites. Vox Sang. 12:321, 1967.

37. Hsia, D.Y.-Y. and Gellis, S.S.: Studies on erythroblastosis due to ABO incompatibility. Pediatr. 13:503, 1954.

38. Davies, B.S., Gerrard, J., and Waterhouse, J.A.H.: The pattern of haemolytic disease of the newborn. Arch. Dis. Child. 28:466, 1953.

39. Walker, W. and Murray, S.: Haemolytic disease of the newborn as a family problem. Br. Med. J. 1:187, 1956.

40. Fraser, I.D. and Tovey, G.H.: Estimation of antibody protein in amniotic fluid to predict severity of rhesus haemolytic disease. J. of Obstet. and Gynaecol. of the Br. Commonwealth 79:981, 1972.

41. Morley, G., Gibson, M., and Ettingham, D.: The use of discriminant analysis in relating material anti-D levels to the severity of haemolytic disease of the newborn. Vox Sang. 32:90, 1977.

42. Hughes-Hones, N.C., Ivona, J., Ellis, M., and Walker,W.: Anti-D concentration in mother and child in haemolytic disease of the newborn. Vox Sang. 21:135, 1971.

43. Walker, W.: Haemolytic anemia in the newborn infant. Clinics in Haematol. 4:145, 1975.

44. Schanfield, M.S.: Personal communication, 1979.

45. Hopkins, D.F.: Maternal anti-Rh (D) and the D-negative fetus, Am. J. Obstet. and Gynecol. 108:268, 1970.

46. Brazie, J.V., Bowes, W.A., Jr., and Ibbot, F.A.: An improved, rapid procedure for the determination of amniotic fluid bilirubin and its uses in the prediction of the course of Rh-sensitized pregnancies. Am. J. Obstet. Gynecol. 104:80, 1969.

47. Bevis, D.C.A.: Blood pigments in haemolytic disease of the newborn. J. Obstet. Gynaecol. Br. Emp. 63:68, 1956.

48. Walker, A.H.C.: Liquor amnii studies in the prediction of haemolytic disease of the newborn. Br. Med. J. 2:376, 1957.

48a. Bowman, J.M. and Pollock, J.M.: Amniotic fluid spectroscopy and early delivery in the management of erythroblastosis fetalis. Pediatrics 35:815.

49. Liley, A.W.: Liquor amnii analysis in the management of the pregnancy complicated by rhesus sensitization. Am. J. Obstet. Gynecol. 82:1359, 1961.

50. Queenan, J.T.: Amniotic fluid analysis. Clin. Obstet. Gynecol. 14:505, 1971.

51. Liley, A.W.: Errors in the assessment of hemolytic disease from amniotic fluid. Am. J. Obstet. Gynecol. 86:485, 1963.

52. Hamilton, E.G.: Intrauterine transfusion: safeguard or peril? Obstet. and Gynecol. 50:255, 1977.

53. Queenan, J.T.: Intrauterine transfusions: a cooperative study. Am. J. Obstet. Gynecol. 104:397, 1969.

54. Hamilton, E.G.: Intrauterine transfusion for Rh disease: a status report. Hosp. Pract. 13#8:113, 1978.

55. Werch, A.: Prenatal evaluation of hemolytic disease of the fetus. A seminar on perinatal blood banking, 31st Annual Meeting of the American Associaation of Blood Banks, 1978.

56. Bowes, W.A., Jr.: Intrauterine transfusion: indications and results. Clin. Obstet. Gynecol. 14:561, 1971.

57. Mandelbaum, B.: Fetal transfusions. Int. J. Gynaecol. Obst. 7:71, 1969.

58. Simpson, M.B., Jr., Pryzbydik, J.A., Denham, M.A., and Radcliffe, J.H.: Appearance of maternal anti-Jk[a] antibody following intrauterine transfusions and amniocentesis. Obstet. and Gynecol. 52:616, 1978.

59. Friesen, R.F.: Complications of intrauterine transfusions. Clin. Obstet. Gynecol. 14:572, 1971.

59a. Barnes, P.H., McInnis, A.C., Friesen, R.F., and Bowman, J.M.: Maternal mishap following fetal transfusion. Can. Med. Assoc. J. 92:1277, 1965.

60. Böhm, N., Kleine, W., and Enzel, U.: Graft-versus-host disease in two newborns after repeated blood transfusions because of rhesus incompatibility. Beitr. Pathol. 160:381, 1977.

61. Naiman, J.L., Punnett, H.H., Lischner, H.W., Destiné, M.L., and Arey, J.B.: Possible graft-versus-host reaction after intra-uterine transfusion for Rh erythroblastosis fetalis. N. Engl. J. Med. 281:697, 1969.

62. Parkman, R., Mosier, D., Umansky, I., Cochran, W., et al.: Graft-versus-host disease after intrauterine and exchange transfusions for hemolytic disease of the newborn. N. Engl. J. Med. 290:359, 1974.

63. Freda, V.J.: Rh immunization: experience with full-term pregnancies. Clin. Obstet. Gynecol. 14:594, 1971.

64. Gorman, J.V., Freda, V.J., and Pollack, W.: Intramuscular injection of a new experimental gammaglobulin preparation containing high levels of Rh antibody as a means of preventing sensitization to Rh. Proc. Ninth Cong. Int. Soc. Haematol. 2:545, 1962.

65. Kleihauer, E., Braun, H., and Betke, K.: Demonstration von fetalem hämoglobin in den erythrocyten einen blutausstrichs. Klin. Wochenschr. 35:637, 1957.

66. Cohen, F. and Zuelzer, W.W.: Identification of blood group antigens by immunofluorescence and its application to the detection of

the transplacental passage of erythrocytes in mother and child. Vox Sang. 9:75, 1964.

66a. Hosoi, T.C. 1958. Serological identification of fetal blood in the maternal circulation. Yokohama Med. Bull. 9:61, 1958.

67. Cohen, F., Zuelzer, W.W., Gustafson, D.C., and Evans, M.M.: Mechanisms of isoimmunization. I. The transplacental passages of fetal erythrocytes in homospecific pregnancies. Blood 23:621, 1964.

68. Zipursky, A., Pollack, J., Neelands, P., Chown, B., et al.: The transplacental passage of foetal red blood cells and the pathogenesis of Rh immunization during pregnancy. Lancet 2:489, 1963.

69. Popat, N., Wood, W.G., Weatherall, D.J., and Turnbull, A.C.: Pattern of maternal F-cell production during pregnancy. Lancet 2:377, 1977.

70. Pembrey, M.E., Weatherall, D.J., and Clegg, J.B.: Maternal synthesis of haemoglobin F in pregnancy. Lancet 1:1350, 1973.

71. Woodrow, J.C. and Finn, R.: Transplacental haemorrhage. Br. J. Haematol. 12:297, 1966.

72. Queenan, J.T., Gadow, E.C., and Lopes, A.C.: Role of spontaneous abortions of Rh-immunization. Am. J. Obstet. Gynecol. 110:128, 1971.

73. Queenan, J.T., Shah, S., Kubarych, S.F., and Holland, B.: Role of induced abortion in Rh-immunization. Lancet 1:815, 1971.

73a. Zipursky, A., Pollack, J., Chown, B., and Israels, L.G. 1963. Transplacental foetal haemorrhage after placental injury during delivery or amniocentesis. Lancet 2:493, 1963.

74. Katz, J. and Marcus, R.G.: The risk of Rh isoimmunization in ruptured tubal pregnancy. Br. Med. J. 3:667, 1972.

75. Liedholm, P.C.: Feto maternal hemorrhage in ectopic pregnancy. Acta Obstet. Gynecol. Scand. 50:367, 1971.

76. Queenan, J.T. and Nakomoto, J.: Postpartum immunization: the hypothetical hazard of manual removal of the placenta. Obstet. Gynecol. 23:392, 1964.

77. Levine, P.: Serological factors as possible causes in spontaneous abortions. J. Hered. 34:71, 1943.

78. Murray, S., Knox, E.G., and Walker, W.: Rhesus haemolytic disease of the newborn and the ABO groups. Vox Sang. 10:6, 1965.

79. Nevanlinna, H.R. and Vainio, T.: The influence of mother-child, ABO incompatibility on Rh immunization. Vox Sang. 1:26, 1956.

79a. Vos, G.H. 1965. The frequency of ABO-incompatible combinations in relation to maternal rhesus antibody values in Rh immunized women. Am. J. Hum. Genet. 17:202.

80. Freda, V.J., Gorman, J.G., Pollack, W., and Bowe, E.: Prevention of Rh hemolytic disease: ten years' clinical experience with Rh immune globulin. N. Engl. J. Med. 292:1014, 1975.

81. Woodrow, J.C. and Donohue, W.T.A.: Rh-immunization by pregnancy: results of a survey and their relevance to prophylactic therapy. Br. Med. J. 4:139, 1968.

82. Pollack, W., Ascari, W.Q., Kochesky, R.J., O'Connor, R.R., et al.: Studies on Rh prophylaxis: I. Relationship between doses of anti-Rh and size of antigenic stimulus. Transfusion 11:333, 1971.

83. Crispen, J.: Immunosuppression of small quantities of Rh-positive blood with MIC RhoGAM in Rh-negative male volunteers. Proceedings of Symposium on Rh Antibody Mediated Immunosuppression, Ortho Research Institute, Raritan, New Jersey, 1976.

84. Delivoria-Papadopolous, M., Miller, L.D., Branca, B., Foster, R.E., et al.: Effect of exchange transfusion on altering mortality in: (1) infants weighing less than 1250 grams at birth and (2) infants with severe respiratory distress syndrome. Pediat. Res. 7:291, 1973.

85. Delivoria-Papadopolous, M., Miller, L.D., Foster II, R.E., and Oski, F.A.: The role of exchange transfusion in the management of low birth weight infants with and without severe RDS. J. Pediatr. 89:279, 1976.

86. Gottuso, M.A., Williams, M.I. and Oski, F.A.: The role of exchange transfusion in the management of low birth weight infants with or without severe respiratory distress syndrome. J. Pediatr. 89:279, 1976.

87. Friedman, Z. and Demers, L.M.: Essential fatty acids, prostaglandins and respiratory distress syndrome of the newborn. Pediatr. 61:341, 1978.

88. deLemos, R.A., McLaughlin, G.W., Koch, H.F., and Diserens, H.W.: Abnormal partial thromboplastin time and survival in respira-

tory distress syndrome: effect of exchange transfusion. Pediatr. Res. 7:396, 1973.

88a. Anday, E.A., Sacks, L.M., Kumar, S.P., and Delivorea-Papadopoulos, M.: The role of exchange transfusion with settled cells on altering mortality in very low birth weight infants less than 1100 grams with severe respiratory distress syndrome at birth. Pediatr. Res. (Abst.)12:518, 1978.

89. Gross, S.A. and Melhorn, D.K.: Exchange transfusions with citrated whole blood for disseminated intravascular coagulation. J. Pediatr. 78:415, 1971.

89a. Bailey, D.N. and Bove, J.R.: Chemical and hematological changes in stored CPD blood. Transfusion 15:244, 1975.

90. Umlas, J. and Gootblatt, S.: The use of frozen blood in neonatal exchange transfusion. Transfusion 16:636, 1976.

90a. Kevy, S.V., Jacobson, M., and Button, L.: Clinical uses of frozen-thawed erythrocytes in pediatrics. Clinical Uses of Frozen-Thawed Red Blood Cells. Alan R. Liss, Inc., New York, 1976.

91. Odell, G.B., Bryan, W.B., and Richard, M.D.: Exchange transfusion. Ped. Clin. North Am. 9:605, 1962.

92. Blankenship, W.J., Goetzman, B.W., Gross, S., and Hattersley, P.G.: A walking donor program for an intensive care nursery. J. Pediatr. 86:583, 1975.

93. Janis, K.M. and McBride, J.W.: Management of massive blood losses in small infants: incremental transfusions of fresh unanticoagulated adult blood. Anesthesiology 34:298, 1971.

94. Oberman, H.A.: Replacement transfusion in the newborn infant: a commentary. J. Pediatr. 86:586, 1975.

95. Konugres, A.A.: Transfusion therapy for the neonate. A Seminar on Perinatal Blood Banking. Bell, C.A., ed., American Association of Blood Banks, Washington, D.C., 1978.

96. Huggins, C.E.: A general system for the preservation of blood by freezing. In: Long-Term Preservation of Red Blood Cells. National Academy of Sciences, National Research Council Bull., 1965.

97. Valeri, C.R. and Runck, A.H.: Long term frozen storage of human red blood cells: studies in vivo and in vitro of autologous red blood cells preserved up to six years with high concentrations of glycerol. Transfusion 9:5, 1969.

98. Staples, J.W. and Fritz, G.E.: Development and use of pediatric frozen red cell packs. Transfusion 16:566, 1976.

99. Bleyer, W.A., Hakami, N., and Shepard, T.H.: The development of hemostatis in the human fetus and the newborn infant. J. Pediatr. 79:838, 1971.

100. Aballi, A.J., Puapondlh, Y., and Desposito, F.: Platelet counts in thriving premature infants. Pediatr. 42:685, 1968.

101. Mull, M.M. and Hathaway, W.E.: Altered platelet function in newborns. Pediatr. Res. 4:229, 1970.

102. McIntosh, S., O'Brian, R.T., Schwartz, A.D., and Pearson, H.A.: Neonatal iso-immune purpura. Response to platelet infusions. J. Pediatr. 82:1020, 1973.

103. Abildgaard, C.F.: Recognition and treatment of intravascular coagulation. J. Pediatr. 74:163, 1969.

104. Glader, B.E. and Buchanan, G.R.: The bleeding neonate. Pediatrics 58:548, 1976.

34

Therapeutic Cytapheresis and Plasma Exchange

Jacob Nusbacher, M.D.

Cell separators were introduced into blood banks in the late 1960s for the collection of granulocytes from normal donors.[1] All cell separators are centrifuges through which large quantities of donor blood can be "processed" rapidly. These centrifuge systems separate blood into cells and plasma on the basis of their differing specific gravities. In its simplest form, donor whole blood entering the cell separator is divided into three portions—red blood cells, plasma, and a buffy-coat (leukocyte) interface. For granulocyte collection—a procedure termed leukapheresis—the interface is automatically transferred to a bag while the red blood cells and plasma are returned to the donor. Procedural modifications permit "harvesting" of platelets rather than granulocytes—a technique termed plateletpheresis—while other modifications enable collection of both granulocytes and platelets together, other blood cells, or plasma.

Although originally designed for cell acquisition from normal donors, cell separator technology was soon applied therapeutically. The earliest uses were in the treatment of chronic myelocytic leukemia where a leukapheresis procedure could produce an immediate and significant fall in the patient-donor's white blood cell count while simultaneously providing a product for transfusion into a septic granulocytopenic recipient. Other therapeutic cytapheresis applications followed quickly. Virtually every pathological condition associated with an abnormally high leukocyte or platelet count has been treated by a cytapheresis technique. These are sometimes designated by the specific cell that is removed—e.g., therapeutic lymphapheresis, therapeutic eosinapheresis, etc. In recent years, therapeutic cytapheresis has been used to remove lymphocytes from certain patients with normal counts because it is suspected that the cell plays an important pathogenic role in the patient's illness.

Of perhaps greater significance, and certainly of more frequent use, has been the application of cell separator techniques for removing large amounts of plasma. Such patients are known or presumed to have abnormal plasma constituents that play important roles in disease pathogenesis or in producing secondary symptoms. In these procedures, many liters of plasma are removed rapidly and replaced immediately with an "inert" or normal material, usually Normal Serum Albumin or fresh frozen plasma, thereby effecting a rapid reduction in the patient's endogenous, pathological plasma factor. This technique, often called "therapeutic plasmapheresis," is more accurately described as therapeutic "plasma exchange" because not only is plasma being removed from the patient-donor, but another material is being returned simultaneously as replacement.

Therapeutic plasma exchange has been performed in an astonishing large number of diverse pathological conditions. At the time of this writing, a literature search revealed about 100 different conditions that have been treated by this form of therapy. New case reports accrue weekly. As might be expected, most conditions in which plasma exchange has been attempted have not been amenable to more conventional forms of therapy and often have a poor prognosis. Many of these conditions are uncommon. Therefore, it is not surprising to find that there are no randomized prospective studies demonstrating the efficacy of plasma exchange for any condition so treated. Because it is unlikely that investigators will publish cases in which a new form of therapy produces no beneficial effect, the current literature is comprised primarily of case reports demonstrating efficacy. This analysis is not meant as criticism, but merely points out the difficulty in assessing the future role of this new therapy in medical practice.

THERAPEUTIC CYTAPHERESIS

Leukapheresis

The treatment of malignant leukocytosis by leukapheresis will achieve a reduction in the peripheral blood white count regularly. The frequency and intensity of leukapheresis required to achieve this result, as well as the duration of cytoreduction, depend primarily upon the balance between: (1) the proliferative rate of the malignant cell; (2) the total body burden of leukocytes at the time of the procedure; and (3) the efficiency of the leukapheresis procedure. Leukemias associated with slow cell proliferation are likely to be more amenable to sustained cytoreduction than those with more rapid cell kinetics. However, it is often difficult to predict, even within a single disease class, the intensity and frequency of leukapheresis necessary to reduce the peripheral blood count to any predetermined level. Thus, treatment protocols are usually individualized to suit the specific patient.

The goal of treatment should be clear before embarking on leukapheresis therapy. Given our current understanding of the pathogenesis of leukemia, it is unlikely that this form of therapy is capable, by itself, of removing all cells of the malignant clone and achieving a cure. However, where chronic leukapheresis has been attempted in lieu of chemotherapy, such as in the treatment of chronic myelogenous leukemia (CML), patient survival has been comparable to chemotherapy. Some investigators have suggested that rapid cell removal could serve as a method of "priming" a patient for chemotherapy by inducing cell division and making these cells more susceptible to chemotherapy regimens. Such speculation remains to be proven. Most frequently, leukapheresis has been used as an adjunct to conventional therapy or where standard treatment is undesirable or demonstrably ineffective. These applications of leukapheresis seem rational and often achieve the desired result; therefore, they are likely to remain an important part of the management of leukemia patients.

Chronic Leukemia. A number of investigators have treated chronic myelogenous leukemia (CML) by therapeutic leukapheresis, both in lieu of standard chemotherapy and as initial therapy prior to chemotherapeutic induction.[2-6] The magnitude of peripheral blood cytoreduction achieved by leukapheresis is related to the patient's white blood cell count, the duration of the procedure, and whether red blood cell sedimenting agents were used to increase collection efficiency.[3] In the usual procedure, a 25 to 35 percent reduction in the white blood cell count is achieved per procedure, but this effect usually lasts for only a few days.[2,4,5] Thus, frequent leukapheresis procedures are required, perhaps 2 to 3 times per week, so that the rate of peripheral blood leukocyte replenishment is exceeded by the rate of cell removal. With frequent leukapheresis, a reduction of 80 percent of the initial leukocyte count can be achieved.[3] After achieving such reductions in the peripheral leukocyte count, leukapheresis is usually required less frequently to maintain the count at that level.

Intensive leukapheresis for the treatment of CML has been found to be a safe procedure that produces rapid relief of symptoms such as sweating, malaise, and pain due to splenomegaly.[4] Significant reduction in organomegaly also has been observed, and problems due to hyperuricemia that might occur with conventional chemotherapy are obviated.[3,4] Unfortunately, there are significant drawbacks to this form of therapy. The need for frequent, time-consuming procedures, especially during the early phases of treatment, interferes with the patient's normal activities when compared with standard busulfan therapy. Also, leukapheresis procedures are very expensive to perform.

Treatment of patients with CML by leukapheresis has not been associated with bone marrow remission. Transformation into blastic crisis has not been prevented or delayed, and longevity has not been improved.[3] Thus, routine management of these patients with leukapheresis is not established, especially since conventional therapy is reasonably effective and safe. However, there are circumstances wherein leukapheresis is a valuable therapeutic tool for treating CML. These include the concomitant presence of severe thrombocytopenia which may make chemotherapy more hazardous, pregnancy,[7] the presence of severe symptomatic hyperuricemia, and the presence of hyperleukocytic leukostasis which requires very rapid cytoreduction.[8]

Patients with chronic lymphocytic leukemia (CLL) have also been treated by leukapheresis.[9,10] As in the case in CML, the quantity of leukocytes removed is related to the patient's preleukapheresis lymphocyte count and the duration of the procedure. As a rule, sedimenting agents are not necessary in lymphocyte collections because the specific gravity of lymphocytes differs from that of red blood cells to a greater degree than is the case with myeloid cells.

Intensive leukapheresis for CLL has resulted in decrease in the patient's peripheral blood lymphocyte count and reduced splenomegaly, lymph node size, and degree of bone marow infiltration in the majority of patients.[9] However, it is not clear whether secondary hematological abnormalities—anemia or thrombocytopenia—also improve regularly after leukapheresis for CLL, although we have had occasion to observe this in some patients.[11] This uncertainty may be due, at least in part, to the unavoidable removal of large quantities of platelets and some red blood cells during leukapheresis. At present, it is not known whether chronic leukapheresis for CLL is more efficacious than standard chemotherapy, and it is unlikely that an answer to this question will be forthcoming soon, given the chronicity of this disorder.

The drawbacks to leukapheresis for CLL are similar to those cited for CML-expense and patient inconvenience. At present, when treatment is indicated, chemotherapy is still the modality of choice. Leukapheresis is usually reserved for patients who are refractory to standard therapy, and for those who have severe thrombocytopenia or other associated conditions that preclude conventional treatment.

Acute Leukemia. It is now well-recognized that patients with acute leukemia (and occasionally those with CML) who have very high peripheral blood blast counts require urgent cytoreduction to prevent the complications of hyperleukocytic leukostasis.[12,13] Such patients are prone to develop pulmonary or cerebral insufficiency resulting from vascular occlusion by leukocytes.[14,15] Intracerebral hemorrhage is also frequent in these patients.[14] In one study,[12] it was demonstrated that death during the first week after the diagnosis of acute myelogenous leukemia (AML) is 5 times higher when the peripheral blood blast count is greater than $100 \times 10^9/L$ than when it is less than this number.

Leukapheresis has been reported to achieve rapid cytoreduction and dramatic improvement in symptoms attributable to leukostasis. In one case report of a patient with AML and a white blood cell count of $172,000/\mu l$ (97 percent blasts), leukapheresis was performed after the patient's white blood cell count was unresponsive to intravenous hydroxyurea.[13] The leukocyte count was reduced to $40,000/\mu l$, and the patient's neurological symptoms all resolved during the procedure. A patient with CML, a high white blood count, and papilledema also responded to leukapheresis therapy;[8] we have treated two other CML patients with similar responses.[11] Thus, it is likely that leukapheresis has a place in the treatment of acute and chronic myelogenous leukemia when the white blood cell count is very high (greater than $100,000/\mu l$) and rapid-acting chemotherapy is undesirable or ineffective.

Other Leukemias. Intensive leukapheresis of a patient with Sezary syndrome has been reported to result in a marked reduction of the white blood cell count and in complete resolution of the skin infiltration typical of this condition.[16] When the leukapheresis procedures were discontinued, the patient's white blood cell count increased and skin lesions returned. Repeated leukapheresis again improved the dermatological findings. Two other patients with Sezary syndrome have also been reported to benefit from leukapheresis although, in these cases, chemotherapy was given concomitantly.[17] In a similar manner, a patient with leukemic reticuloendotheliosis (hairy cell leukemia) was reported to show marked improvement in blood counts, reduction of lymph node size, and clearing of skin lesions after intensive short-term leukapheresis.[18] The improvement was sustained for nearly two years—the reported period of observation—with no further therapy.

Stem Cell Collection. The presence of pluripotential stem cells in the peripheral blood of normal individuals is well recognized. In untreated patients with CML, the concentration of granulocyte/monocyte precursor cells (CFU-C) in the peripheral blood exceeds that present in the marrow. Goldman et al.,[19] in an imaginative experiment, performed leukapheresis on two patients with CML and stored the collected cells frozen in liquid nitrogen. When the inevitable acute blastic transformation occurred in these patients some time later, the patients were treated with vigorous chemotherapy which was followed by reinfusion of the previously collected (stem) cells. Marrow repopulation and restoration of the disease to its chronic form was achieved for at least six months. It remains to be seen how long such restitution lasts before the advent of another acute blastic phase, and whether restitution can be achieved effectively a number of times.

It is likely that harvesting peripheral blood stem cells by leukapheresis will be evaluated more fully for the management of patients with other forms of malignant neoplasms, even in cases where peripheral blood leukocyte counts are normal. It has been demonstrated recently[20,21] that precursor cells, as measured by CFU-C assay, can be collected from normal donors as a by-product of leukapheresis and plateletpheresis procedures in quantities that approach the theoretical number required for bone marrow repopulation if five to ten procedures are performed. Furthermore, it was found[21] that after a single plateletpheresis procedure (wherein 30 percent of peripheral blood progenitor cells are collected concomitantly) there occurs a doubling of both erythroid and myeloid precursors in the donor's peripheral blood 48 to 72 hours later. These studies point to the feasibility of applying cell separator technology as an instrument for facilitating autologous marrow reconstitution after chemotherapy.

Plateletpheresis

Markedly elevated platelet counts associated with a variety of myeloproliferative disorders or after splenectomy are known to predispose patients to life-threatening thrombotic and/or hemorrhagic complications. Conventional therapy with either cytotoxic drugs or ^{32}P may take days to weeks before the platelet count is reduced sufficiently. Plateletpheresis, however, has been demonstrated to be highly effective in achieving a rapid reduction in the platelet count.

In one study, Taft et al.[22] reported acute reduction of the platelet count by plateletpheresis in five patients with severe thrombocytosis (platelet count $>1 \times 10^6/\mu l$). All patients had symptoms attributable to the elevated platelet count, including symptoms of cerebral ischemia, pulmonary embolism, angina pectoris, and gastrointestinal bleeding. A single plateletpheresis procedure, with removal of about 2 to 9×10^{12} platelets, and a mean reduction in platelet count of 52 percent (range 33 to 81 percent), resulted in relief of symptoms. In most of these patients, between 2 and 6 plateletpheresis procedures performed over a 1- to 3-week period were required to keep the platelet counts low until cytotoxic therapy could take effect. Other investigators report similar results.[17]

Long-term plateletpheresis has been performed on a number of patients with markedly elevated platelet counts.[23,24] The results of such therapy were variable. Although the platelet count was reduced after each procedure, in some cases severe thrombocytosis returned quickly and as many as five procedures per week were required to maintain counts at less than 1 million.[24] In one instance,[23] the necessary frequency of plateletpheresis procedures diminished after an initial intensive course of therapy. It appears that conventional therapy is preferable to plateletpheresis for the chronic management of patients with thrombocythemia, unless such therapy is contraindicated.

As with leukapheresis, the number of platelets removed during each plateletpheresis procedure and the magnitude of platelet count reduction are related to patient's initial platelet count and the volume of blood "processed" through the cell separator.[25,26] There is also evidence that, during plateletpheresis, there is mobilization of platelets into the circulation, probably from the spleen.[26] Thus, patients with thrombocytosis and massive splenomegaly may require intensive plateletpheresis to achieve a significant and sustained reduction in platelet count.

Immediate plateletpheresis appears to be indicated in patients with a significant elevation in platelet count and signs or symptoms attributable to thrombocytosis. Cytotoxic therapy should be started concomitantly to achieve a long-lasting effect. It is not clear whether plateletpheresis is also indicated as a prophylactic measure in the asymptomatic patient, and, if so, at what level of platelet count it is indicated.

Red Blood Cell Exchange

Exchange transfusions have been used infrequently in the treatment of sickle cell disease. Indications for exchange have included priapism,[27] unrelenting painful crises,[28] pregnancy,[29] and preparation for surgery.[30] The rationale of this treatment is to break the cycle of hypoxia and sickling that occurs in homozygous S disease by removing erythrocytes containing hemoglobin S and replacing them with normal erythrocytes containing hemoglobin A. The effectiveness of exchange, while likely, is difficult to assess fully because the patient usually received other therapy concomitant with the exchange.

The difficulty in performing large volume exchanges for sickle cell disease with standard bag techniques has limited its use. With cell separators, however, it is a simpler procedure and it has been possible to achieve a hemoglobin A concentration of greater than 90 percent in a 3½-hour procedure.[30] It is likely that whole blood exchange transfusion or red blood cell exchange will now be performed more frequently in these patients.

Red blood cell exchange using cell separators has also been performed in preparing a patient with paroxysmal nocturnal hemoglobulinemia (PNH) for cardiac surgery[31] and in treating a patient with severe posttransfusion falciparum malaria.[32] In the latter case, the patient had developed progressive cerebral deterioration despite medical treatment. Exchange transfusion was done, the entire procedure taking slightly more than 3 hours, in which a 6-liter exchange was accomplished. The patient became alert and fully oriented during the exchange.

PLASMA EXCHANGE

Plasmapheresis using simple collection bag methods has been used successfully in treating the hyperviscosity syndrome associated with various paraproteinemias, particularly Waldenstrom's macroglobulinemia.[33-37] Other therapeutic applications of this method of plasmapheresis have been few, primarily because it is difficult to remove or exchange large quantities of plasma in a simple efficient manner with this technique. The development of cell separators has now made such therapeutic applications possible. As a result, automated plasma exchange has been attempted in treating almost every condition in which there is a known or presumed abnormal plasma factor that contributes to the etiology or pathogenesis of that disease. Unfortunately, although beneficial results have been reported in many conditions, the absence of well-controlled, randomized studies makes it difficult to determine efficacy clearly. This section will review the physiology and kinetics of plasma exchange and point out the potentially beneficial applications of this form of therapy.

The Physiology of Plasma Exchange

In an idealized model of a plasma (or whole blood) exchange for removing an abnormal plasma factor, the volume of plasma removed is simultaneously and completely replaced with another solution which is devoid of the plasma substance in question. If a number of assumptions are made—i.e., mixing in the patient is complete and instantaneous, the patient's blood volume does not change, and there is no mobilization of the putative plasma substance from extravascular sources—then the concentration of the plasma substance being removed in a continuous exchange can be calculated from the following formula:

$$X_t = X_o e^{\frac{-b}{v}t}$$

Where X_o = the concentration of the substance in question in the patient's blood before exchange; X_t = the concentration of the substance in question remaining in the patient's blood after time t; t = the time (duration) of the exchange; b = the volume of blood exchanged; and v = the patient's blood volume.[38]

This formula describes the curve illustrated in Fig. 34-1. Table 34-1 tabulates the degree of theoretical exchange achieved after continuous flow exchanges of 1 to 3 plasma volumes. In practice, it is useful to compare the measured efficiency of removal of abnormal plasma constituents during exchange with the theoretical model. In this way, the movement of the abnormal plasma constituent across body compartments and its synthetic rate after removal can be evaluated. Such measurements also aid in determining the necessary volume and frequency of exchanges.

As might be expected, actual comparisons of changes in plasma factors before and after exchange often vary from the theoretical model. For example, Flaum et al.,[39] in evaluating coagulation factors in eleven 4-liter

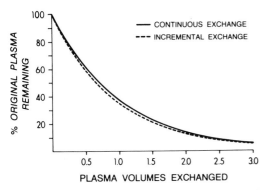

Fig. 34-1. Comparison of the percent of original plasma remaining after plasma exchange by the continuous exchange and incremental exchange approach. (Modified from Collins, J.A.: Problems associated with the massive transfusion of stored blood. Surgery 75:274, 1974.)

plasma exchanges using Normal Serum Albumin or Plasma Protein Fraction (PPF) as replacement fluid, found reductions in all factors studied. However, there was considerable disparity in the level of decrements noted among the different factors. They also found that, at 4 hours after exchange, some hemostatic factors—Factor IX, ristocetin cofactor, and Factor VIII procoagulant activities—had returned to normal, while all were normal by 24 hours. Similarly, Russell et al.[40] evaluated patients with hyperviscosity syndrome treated by plasma exchange and found a disparity between the predicted reduction in paraprotein, based on a mathematical model, and the observed changes. Undoubtedly, such discrepancies result from a variety of factors mentioned above, and therefore assist in gaining a better understanding of the physiology of both the disease under treatment and the exchange procedure.

The usual volume of plasma exchanged varies among different institutions and perhaps with different patients. There appear to be two distinct approaches. Because the efficiency of exchange is greatest early in the procedure (Fig. 34-1), some investigators perform limited exchanges of about one plasma volume per procedure. Reequilibration or new synthesis of the pathological substance into the vascular space is permitted to occur before another procedure is performed. Other investigators perform more extensive plasma exchanges of as much as three plasma volumes, attempting to remove as much pathological material as possible during any procedure. The former approach has the advantage of greatest efficiency per time expended and is less likely to result in secondary hazards such as severe depletion of coagulation factors; however, it may result in the necessity of performing a greater number of exchange procedures on any patient. The latter approach will, of course, achieve a greater total reduction in the abnormal plasma constituent per procedure—a consideration which may be important in the critically ill patient—and might promote more effective mobilization of pathological material from tissues into the vascular space. At present, it is difficult to generalize as to which approach is more desirable, and each patient requiring exchange should be evaluated individually. In general, however, the former approach of limited 1-plasma-volume exchanges will suffice for most circumstances.

The replacement solution for plasma exchanges has been either Normal Serum Albumin, PPF, or plasma. These provide, by their oncotic properties, support in maintaining intravascular volume. In practice, it usually has not been necessary to replace the patient's plasma completely with these protein solutions, and crystalloid solutions are often used concomitantly. Albumin and PPF have the advantage of not transmitting hepatitis and

Table 34-1. Percent of Original Plasma Remaining after Continuous Flow Exchange.*

Plasma Volume Exchanged	Percent Original Plasma Remaining
1	36.8 (34.9)
2	13.5 (12.2)
3	5 (4.2)

* Numbers in parentheses indicate results with intermittent exchange. (After Collins, J.A.: Problems associated with the massive transfusion of stored blood. Surgery 75:274, 1974.)

do not require matching for ABO compatibility when compared with plasma. However, they are far more expensive than plasma. There does not seem to be any advantage in using PPF instead of albumin, and the former may induce hypotension when given rapidly. The use of plasma as replacement solution is beneficial when replacement of depleted coagulation factors is required. In these cases, fresh frozen plasma (FFP) is the product of choice.

While it is generally assumed that the effectiveness of plasma exchange is due to *removal* of abnormal plasma constituents, there is evidence in a few conditions that replacement with plasma is required specifically to achieve clinical benefit. Furthermore, in many conditions of unknown etiology treated by plasma exchange, it is difficult to ascertain whether the replacement fluid was simply that—replacement—or a positive factor in achieving the clinical result. The relative effectiveness of using plasma versus other colloid solutions as the replacement material requires careful evaluation.

When performing a plasma exchange, the patient's blood must be anticoagulated while ex vivo in the cell separator. Three anticoagulant protocols are used: citrate alone, heparin alone, or a combination of the two. Citrate anticoagulation is given as a continuous drip infusion immediately after blood leaves the patient's arm in a ratio of 1 ml citrate solution to 8 ml blood. Acid-Citrate-Dextrose (ACD), Citrate-Phosphate-Dextrose (CPD), and Sodium Citrate solutions all have been used. Citrate anticoagulation will often result in symptoms of hypocalcemia in the patient, especially when rapid flow rates are used. These are easily relieved by slowing the rate of reinfusion. With citrate anticoagulation, the patient is never anticoagulated. Alternatively, heparin is an effective anticoagulant for plasma exchange procedures but has the potential risk of hemorrhage because anticoagulation occurs in vivo. Some investigators use a combination of a low dose of heparin and simultaneously a reduced concentration of citrate, which may minimize the problems occurring with either anticoagulant alone.[41]

Conditions Treated by Plasma Exchange

It would be difficult and undesirable to give a complete account of all conditions reported to benefit from plasma exchange. As discussed earlier in this chapter, there are virtually no randomized, controlled studies demonstrating efficacy of plasma exchange for any condition. In many, only a few case reports showing benefit are available. Therefore, the ensuing discussion will attempt to highlight those circumstances in which therapeutic plasma exchange appears to be best established or most promising.

Hyperviscosity Syndrome Associated with the Paraproteinemias. Increased blood viscosity resulting from paraproteins present in the plasma of patients with Waldenstrom's macroglobulinemia and, infrequently, in patients with multiple myeloma, is a well-recognized clinical problem. The manifestations of hyperviscosity syndrome include bleeding from mucous membranes, retinal vein engorgement, retinal bleeding, visual disturbances, neurological abnormalities, and cardiac failure. While chemotherapy directed at the paraprotein-producing cell is the standard therapy in these patients, several weeks may pass before paraprotein levels fall and symptoms of hyperviscosity abate.

Nearly two decades ago, it was demonstrated that simple (bag) plasmapheresis is an effective, but tedious, method for treating the hyperviscosity syndrome.[33-37] In recent years, plasma exchange using cell separators has been performed effectively for this purpose.[40,42,43] With automated equipment, removal (exchange) of large quantities of paraproteinemic plasma can be achieved rapidly and with relative ease. Russel et al.[40] described their experience of 313 continuous-flow plasma exchanges (range 1 to 45 performed on 60 patients) with various paraproteinemic states. They found that the quantity of paraprotein removed was greater than what was predicted on the basis of the mathematical model for exchange. This was attributed to two factors: mobilization of paraprotein from the extravascular space and demonstrable contraction of the patient's blood volume during the procedure. They also found little difference in efficiency between plasma exchanges performed for IgG or IgA multiple myeloma and those performed for (IgM) macroglobulinemia. Clinical evaluation demonstrated that plasma exchange is an effective therapeutic modality for alleviating most signs and symptoms attributable to the presence of paraproteins. However, they could discern no long-term benefit in uremic myeloma patients.

Thrombotic Thrombocytopenic Purpura (TTP). Effective treatment for TTP has eluded medical practice. This syndrome, characterized by thrombocytopenic purpura, microangiopathic hemolytic anemia, neurological abnormalities, and fever has been reported to have a mortality of 80 percent.[44] While occasional remissions have been reported after treatment with corticosteroids, splenectomy, dextran, and combinations of these, no modality has emerged as the effective treatment of choice.

In recent years, there have been a number of reports describing the efficacious use of plasma exchange in the treatment of TTP.[45-48] More than 70 percent of nearly 40 reported cases have recovered after plasma exchange. However, it is very difficult to judge adequately the value of plasma exchange in TTP for the following reasons:

1. There are no randomized trials. This is to be expected, and unlikely to be altered, because of the seriousness and rarity of this condition and the apparent reported benefit of the procedure.

2. Virtually all patients were given ancillary treatment with some of the more conventional therapies cited above. For example, in one report there was some evidence that administration of antiplatelet agents—aspirin and dipyridamole—played an important role in the successful outcome of plasma exchange.[48]

3. The volume and frequency of exchange varies widely among the reported cases.[47]

Recovery has been reported with as little as one exchange of 2 liters, but other patients have required as many as 12 exchanges with a total exchange volume of 28 liters to achieve a successful result.

Perhaps the most significant factor determining the outcome of plasma exchange in TTP is the use of plasma as the exchange fluid. There are reports suggesting that plasma infusion per se, without exchange, is effective.[49] There is also evidence that the plasma of patients with TTP contains a platelet-aggregating factor which is inhibited by normal plasma.[50] Thus, plasma exchange may not be required in treating this disorder, although the volumes of plasma that seem to be required in some patients make exchange necessary in order to avoid volume overload. Furthermore, it may be speculated that plasma exchange, if indeed efficacious for TTP, serves to both *remove* a pathological plasma constituent—the platelet-aggregating factor—while simultaneously *providing* a therapeutic material—normal plasma—in adequate dose. It is likely that these issues will be resolved with further investigation of the plasma abnormality present in these patients.

Removal of Alloantibody. Although alloantibody generally protects patients against exogenous immunogens, there are circumstances where removal of alloantibody or reduction in alloantibody titer may be desirable. Rhesus immunization is perhaps the ideal example of this, because removal of antibody from the pregnant mother would have a beneficial effect on the severity of fetal hemolytic disease. There are a number of reports describing the use of conventional (bag) plasmapheresis in the antenatal management of Rhesus immunization. In the largest series, Fraser et al.[51] performed plasmapheresis combined with intrauterine transfusions on 44 immunized pregnant women, and plasmapheresis alone on another 52 women. In the former group, the success rate (fetal salvage) was 61 percent, as compared with a previous series of women treated with intrauterine exchange alone, where the success rate was only 33 percent. The fetal salvage rate in the group treated with plasmapheresis alone was 72 percent, but these women had, as a group, less severely affected children with previous pregnancies. Although the volume of plasma removed per procedure was modest in this group (1 to 4 liters per week), there was significant reduction in maternal antibody concentration after plasmapheresis in most cases, and this appeared to correlate with a successful outcome of the pregnancy.

Plasma exchange using a cell separator also has been performed for the treatment of Rhesus immunization. Graham-Pole et al.[52] described eight pregnant women with a past history of Rhesus immunization and severely affected fetuses, including 17 previous fetal deaths, who were treated with continuous-flow plasma exchange beginning at 16 to 27 weeks gestation. Between 4 and 19 liters were exchanged weekly, the mean total exchange volume being 124 liters. Comparison of values before and after the course of plasma exchange revealed a mean reduction in circulating Rh antibody of greater than 50 percent (16.7 mg/L to 7.6 mg/L) and a reduction in amniotic fluid optical density when compared with previously affected pregnancies.

While it is not clear what is the precise role of plasma exchange or plasmapheresis in treating maternal immunization, it is likely that this technique will be best used in the severely immunized mother, especially early in pregnancy when intrauterine exchange is difficult to perform and hazardous to the fetus. However, a note of caution seems warranted because of the report of Isbister et al.,[53] who observed the formation of Rh-specific autoantibodies in two women following large-volume plasma exchange for Rhesus immunization.

Plasma exchange also has been used to remove circulating alloantibody which pre-vented efficacious infusion of therapeutic agents. Among these applications are: the removal of leukocyte antibodies to permit granulocyte transfusion;[54] the removal of Factor VIII inhibitors;[17,55,56] and the depletion of ABO alloagglutinins preparatory to ABO-incompatible bone marrow transplantation.[57,57a-c]

A rare, but apparently useful, application of plasma exchange has been in the treatment of posttransfusion purpura.[58,59] In this condition, the presence of PlA1 antibodies in a recipient of platelet transfusion causes destruction of donor PlA1-positive platelets (98 percent of the population is positive for PlA1). In addition, the recipient's own platelets, which are PlA1-negative, seem to be caught up in the antigen-antibody reactions and are removed from the circulation. Plasma or whole blood exchange has resulted in rapid improvement of the platelet count in a number of reported instances.

Removal of Autoantibody. Pathological conditions resulting from the presence of autoantibodies or immune complexes comprise the most diverse group now being treated by plasma exchange. A considerable number of hematological, renal, and neurological diseases have been reported to benefit from plasma exchange, usually in circumstances where conventional treatment has been ineffective. As a number of these conditions are of unknown etiology, quite common, but difficult to treat, it is likely that, at least in the near future, plasma exchange will continue to be used as adjunctive therapy in this group of patients.

Autoimmune hemolytic anemias of both the warm-reactive[54] and cold agglutinin[60] types have been treated with plasma exchange. Data supporting the effectiveness of plasma exchange in warm autoantibody AHA are very limited. The patient reported by Branda[54] may well have been developing a spontaneous remission of the disease. Patten reported experience in a patient with the Evans Syndrome type of AHA who had only transient benefit from repeated plasma exchanges. This patient subsequently died, unresponsive to repeated plasma exchanges.[54a] Rosenfield and Jagathambal have commented that plasma exchange has not been useful in their experience in patients with the warm autoantibody type of AIHD,[54b] a view consistent with the experience of Petz[54c] and Swisher.[54d]

We have had the opportunity to treat a patient with cold agglutinin disease and severe Raynaud's phenomenon whose peripheral vascular manifestations improved markedly after plasma exchange.[11] There is considerably more reported experience in this situation than in the case of warm autoantibody AIHA.[54c] The procedure is more difficult in the presence of high-titered cold agglutinins, and is thus more time-consuming and expensive. Cold agglutinin titers can be temporarily reduced by plasma exchange, but the clinical aspects of the illness may not be changed very much.[54b-c]

In summary, the response of patients with AIHA to plasma exchange is usually brief and incomplete. This effect may occasionally be useful in anticipation of response to more definitive therapy.

While plasma exchange has been used in these autoimmune hematological conditions as therapy directed at a secondary manifestation of the disease, its application in the treatment of idiopathic (autoimmune) thrombocytopenic purpura (ITP) may be associated with more long-lasting results. Branda et al.[61] described three patients with ITP treated with plasma exchange. One patient with the chronic form failed to respond, but satisfactory responses—apparent complete remissions—were observed in two patients who had the disease for only several months. We have had the opportunity to treat by plasma exchange 14 consecutive patients with ITP—five with the chronic form and nine with acute disease.[62] In the former group, all of whom had had splenectomy for their disease, there were no responses to plasma exchange. In the group of patients with acute ITP, we observed prompt and

complete responses in four patients, obviating the need for splenectomy. We also noted that the good responses were all temporally associated with the use of plasma as the exchange fluid; the use of albumin was not associated with any increase in platelet counts. Such observations must be considered preliminary, however, and require randomized prospective studies for confirmation.

Among the neurological disorders that have been treated with plasma exchange, myasthenia gravis has been the subject of a number of reports.[63-67] This serious condition, characterized by weakness and fatigability of skeletal muscle, has been associated with the finding of antibodies to acetylcholine receptors (AChR) in the serum of most patients, the presence of IgG and complement on postsynaptic membrane, and the ability to passively transfer the disease to experimental animals by infusion of plasma from an affected patient or to a fetus in utero via placental transfer. Clinical improvement has been noted with immunosuppressive therapy and thoracic duct drainage, and correlates with a reduction in circulating antibodies to AChR. Thus, the immunological nature of this condition is well established.

Plasma exchanges of approximately one plasma volume, using nonplasma materials as exchange fluid, have been reported to cause clinical improvement in myasthenic patients, improvement in objective measures of muscular function, reduction in the doses of drugs required after plasmapheresis, and reduction in circulating AChR antibody levels.[63] Unfortunately, most of these patients were also treated with immunosuppressive drugs, and it is difficult to gain a clear differentiation of the contributory roles of these different therapeutic ingredients. Measurement of serum AChR antibody levels show more rapid decline in patients treated with exchange and immunosuppression when compared with immunosuppression alone over a relatively short period of observation,[63] but more prolonged assessment revealed no differences between the two groups.[64] Because fall in AChR antibody titer is associated with clinical improvement, this issue is of some importance.

The role of plasma exchange in treating myasthenia gravis remains to be defined precisely. It is probable that exchange therapy is a useful adjunct in the rapid control of severe symptoms and, perhaps, in patients who do not respond to drug therapy. Its role as a long-term therapeutic modality requires further study.

Renal Disease. A variety of renal conditions, known or presumed to result from autoimmune phenomena or the presence of immune complexes, have been reported to benefit by plasma exchange. In one study,[68] Goodpasture's syndrome—a condition characterized by renal glomerular damage, pulmonary hemorrhage, and the presence of antiglomerular-basement-membrane antibody in the plasma—was treated by immunosuppression combined with plasma exchange in seven patients. The exchange volume was 4 liters with nonplasma fluids being used as the exchange material. They found that the three patients who still had residual renal function benefited from this regimen, while those who were anuric at presentation did not show improved renal function. Pulmonary hemorrhage, however, was rapidly reversed by plasma exchange in the five patients in whom this was the major presenting feature. Antiglomerular-basement-membrane antibody levels fell in all patients but completely disappeared in the three patients who presented with some renal function. Other case reports suggest similar beneficial effects from plasma exchange plus immunosuppression.[69]

Plasma exchange combined with drug therapy has also proved successful in treating nephritides thought to be related to the presence of immune complexes such as fulminant crescentic nephritis[70,71] and lupus erythematosus.[72] In both conditions, reduction of circulating immune complexes and clinical improvement occurred in the majority of patients and was temporally related to the exchange procedure. We have also observed a patient with lupus cerebritis who recovered rapidly after plasma exchange, but this patient received medical treatment as well.[11]

Miscellaneous Conditions Treated with Plasma Exchange. *Raynaud's Disease.* Five patients with Raynaud's disease were treated with plasma exchange. Treatment consisted of one 2- to 2.5-liter exchange weekly for 5 weeks. The exchange fluid consisted of either plasma or plasma plus PPF. All patients showed marked reduction in the frequency and intensity of acute symptoms, and all digital ulcers but one healed during treatment. Ultrasonic velocimetry measurements also improved in all patients. Although symptomatic regression occurred after treatment, all patients were still improved 6 months after plasma exchange therapy. These interesting observations require confirmation in a randomized prospective study.[73]

Metabolic Errors. Perhaps the most conceptually satisfying application of plasma exchange is in the treatment of patients with hereditary errors of metabolism. In these conditions, the accumulation of a metabolite leads to "toxic" effects which are often fatal. Plasma exchange would theoretically deplete the metabolite in question from the blood and, if mobilization from tissue occurs, could arrest or reverse clinical manifestations. Two reported cases of patients with heredopathic atactica polyneruritiformis (Refsum's disease) are examples of the use of plasma exchange in these conditions.[74,75] In the one patient that we observed,[74] there was marked improvement in neurological function and depletion of the offending lipid, phytanic acid, from tissue (including nerves) as well as from blood after a course of intensive plasma exchanges of 2 to 3 one plasma volume exchanges per week. The frequency of exchanges were subsequently reduced, but more than one hundred procedures were performed within one year. The patient has subsequently remained clinically stable on a regimen of dietary restriction without further exchanges.

In a similar manner, plasma exchange has been used in treating homozygous familial hypercholesterolemia. In one report,[76] exchanges with PPF were performed every three weeks on two women with this condition. It was demonstrated that plasma cholesterol and low-density lipoproteins were reduced after 4 to 8 months on this regimen, and that mobilization of cholesterol from tissue into plasma occurred. This treatment also was associated with cessation of angina pectoris. However, it is not known whether plasma exchange would arrest the development of coronary atheromata or whether patient survival would be significantly prolonged.

REFERENCES

1. Freireich, E.J., Judson, G., and Levin, R.H.: Separation and collection of leukocytes. Cancer Res. 24:1516, 1965.
2. Morse, E.E., Carbone, P.P., and Freireich, E.J., et al.: Repeated leukapheresis of patients with chronic myelocytic leukemia. Transfusion 6:175, 1966.
3. Vallejos, G.S., McCredie, K.B., and Britten, G.M., et al.: Biological effects of repeated leukapheresis of patients with chronic myelogenous leukemia. Blood 42:925, 1973.
4. Lowenthal, R.M., Buskard, N.A., and Goldman, J.M., et al.: Intensive leukapheresis as initial therapy for chronic granulocytic leukemia. Blood 46:835, 1975.
5. Huestis, D.W., Price, M.J., and White, R.F., et al.: Leukapheresis of patients with chronic granulocytic leukemia (CGL), using the Haemonetics Blood Processor. Transfusion 16:255, 1976.
6. Huestis, D.W., Corrigan, J.J., and Johnson, H.V.: Leukapheresis of a five-year-old girl with chronic granulocytic leukemia. Transfusion 15:489, 1975.
7. Caplan, S.N., Coco, F.V., and Berkman, E.M.: Management of chronic myelocytic leukemia in pregnancy by cell pheresis. Transfusion 18:120, 1978.
8. Stirling, M.L., Parker, A.C., and Keller, A.J., et al.: Leukapheresis for papilloedema in

9. Curtis, J.E., Hersh, E.M., and Freireich, E.J.: Leukapheresis therapy of chronic lymphocytic leukemia. Blood 39:163, 1972.
10. Hocker, P., Pitterman, E., and Gobets, M., et al.: Treatment of patients with chronic myeloid leukemia (CML) and chronic lymphocytic leukemia (ClL) by leukapheresis with a continuous flow blood cell separator. In: Leukocytes: Separation, Collection and Transfusion. Goldman, J.M. and Lowenthal, R.M., eds. Academic Press, London, 1975, p. 510.
11. Nusbacher, J.: Unpublished observations.
12. Harris, A.L.: Leukostasis associated with blood transfusion in acute myeloid leukaemia. Br. Med. J. 1:1169, 1978.
13. Eisenstadt, R.S. and Berkman, E.M.: Rapid cytoreduction in acute leukemia. Management of cerebral leukostasis by cell pheresis. Transfusion 18:113, 1978.
14. Fritz, R.D., Forkner, G.E., and Freireich, E.J., et al.: The association of fatal intracranial hemorrhage and "blastic crisis" in patients with acute leukemia. N. Engl. J. Med. 261:59, 1959.
15. McKee, L.C. and Collins, R.D.: Intravascular leukocyte thrombi and aggregates as a cause of morbidity and mortality in leukemia. Medicine 53:463, 1974.
16. Edelson, R., Facktor, M., and Andrews, A., et al.: Successful management of the Sezary syndrome. N. Engl. J. Med. 291:293, 1974.
17. Pineda, A.A., Brzica, S.M., and Taswell, H.F.: Continuous- and semicontinuous-flow blood centrifugation systems: therapeutic applications, with plasma-, platelet-, lympha-, and eosinapheresis. Transfusion 17:407, 1977.
18. Fay, J.W., Moore, J.O., and Logue, G.L., et al.: Leukopheresis therapy of leukemic reticuloendotheliosis (hairy cell leukemia). Blood 54:747, 1979.
19. Goldman, J.M., Catovsky, D., and Galton, D.A.G.: Reversal of blast-cell crisis in C.G.L. by transfusion of stored autologous buffy-coat cells. Lancet 1:437, 1978.
20. Nguyen, B.T. and Perkins, H.A.: Quantitation of granulocyte-macrophage progenitor cells (CFU-C) in plateletpheresis and leukapheresis concentrates. Blood Transf. Immunohaematol. 22:489, 1979.
21. Abboud, G.N., Brennan, J.K., and Lichtman,

chronic granulocytic leukaemia. Br. Med. J. 2:676, 1977.

M.A., et al.: Quantification of erythroid and granulocytic precursor cells in plateletpheresis residues. Transfusion 20:9, 1980.

22. Taft, E.G., Babcock, R.B., and Scharfman, W.B., et al.: Plateletpheresis in the management of thrombocytosis. Blood 50:927, 1977.

23. Panlilio, A.L. and Reiss, R.F.: Therapeutic plateletpheresis in thrombocythemia. Transfusion 19:147, 1979.

24. Goldfinger, D., Thompson, R., and Lowe, C., et al.: Long-term plateletpheresis in the management of primary thrombocytosis. Transfusion 19:336, 1979.

25. Szymanski, L.O., Patti, K., and Kliman, A.: Efficacy of Latham blood processor to perform plateletpheresis. Transfusion 13:405, 1973.

26. Nusbacher, J., Scher, M.L., and MacPherson, J.L.: Plateletpheresis using the Haemonetics Model 30 cell separator. Vox Sang. 33:9, 1977.

27. Lanzowsky, P., Shende, A., and Karayalcin, G., et al.: Partial exchange transfusion in sickle cell anemia. Am. J. Dis. Child. 132:1200, 1978.

28. Brody, J.I., Goldsmith, M.H., and Park, S.K., et al.: Symptomatic crisis of sickle cell anemia treated by limited exchange transfusion. Ann. Intern. Med. 72:327, 1970.

29. Ricks, P.: Further experience with exchange transfusion in sickle cell anemia and pregnancy. Am. J. Obstet. Gynecol. 100:1087, 1968.

30. Kernoff, L.M., Botha, M.C., and Jacobs, P.: Exchange transfusions in sickle cell disease using a continuous-flow blood cell separator. Transfusion 17:269, 1977.

31. Cundall, J.R., Moore, W.H., and Jenkins, D.E.: Erythrocyte exchange in paroxysmal nocturnal hemoglobinuria prior to cardiac surgery. Transfusion 18:626, 1978 (abstr.).

32. Yarrish, R.L., Janas, J.S., and Nosanchuk, J.S., et al.: Transfusion-acquired falciparum malaria: treatment with exchange transfusion following delayed diagnosis. Submitted for publication.

33. Skoog, W.A., Adams, W.S., and Coburn, J.W.: Metabolic balance study of plasmapheresis in a case of Waldenstrom's macroglobulinemia. Blood 19:425, 1962.

34. Solomon, A. and Fahey, J.L.: Plasmapheresis therapy in macroglobulinemia. Ann. Intern. Med. 58:789, 1963.

35. Lawson, N.S., Nosanchuk, J.S., and Oberman, H.A., et al.: Therapeutic plasmapheresis in treatment of patients with Waldenstrom's macroglobulinemia. Transfusion 8:174, 1968.

36. Luxemberg, M.N. and Mausolf, F.A.: Retinal circulation in the hyperviscosity syndrome. Am. J. Ophthal. 70:588, 1970.

37. Lindsely, H., Teller, D., and Noonan, B., et al.: Hyperviscosity syndrome in multiple myeloma. A reversible, concentration-dependent aggregation of the myeloma protein. Am. J. Med. 54:682, 1973.

38. Collins, J.A.: Problems associated with the massive transfusion of stored blood. Surgery 75:274, 1974.

39. Flaum, M.A., Cuneo, R.A., and Applebaum, F.R., et al.: The hemostatic imbalance of plasma-exchange transfusion. Blood 54:694, 1979.

40. Russell, J.A., Toy, J.L., and Powles, R.L.: Plasma exchange in malignant paraproteinemias. Exp. Hematol (Suppl.)5:105, 1977.

41. MacPherson, J.L., Nusbacher, J., and Bennett, J.M.: The acquisition of granulocytes by leukapheresis: a comparison of continuous flow centrifugation and filtration leukapheresis in normal and corticosteroid-stimulated donors. Transfusion 16:221, 1976.

42. Powles, R., Smith, C.R., and Hamilton Fairley, G.: Method of removing abnormal protein rapidly from patients with malignant paraproteinemias. Br. Med. J. 2:664, 1971.

43. Buskard, N.A., Galton, D.A.G., and Goldman, J.M., et al.: Plasma exchange in the long-term management of Waldenstrom's macroglobulinemia. Canad. Med. Assoc. J. 117:135, 1977.

44. Amorosi, E.L. and Ultmann, J.E.: Thrombotic thrombocytopenic purpura: report of 16 cases and review of the literature. Medicine 45:139, 1966.

45. Bukowski, R.M., King, J.W., and Hewlett, J.S.: Plasmapheresis in the treatment of thrombotic thrombocytopenic purpura. Blood 50:413, 1977.

46. Pisciotta, A.V., Garthwaite, T., and Darin, J., et al.: Treatment of thrombotic thrombocytopenic purpura by exchange transfusion. Am. J. Hematol. 3:73, 1977.

47. Taft, E.G.: Thrombotic thrombocytopenic purpura and dose of plasma exchange. Blood 54:842, 1979.

48. Myers, T.J., Wakem, C.J., and Ball, E.D., et al.: Thrombotic thrombocytopenic purpura: combined treatment with plasmapheresis and antiplatelet agents. Ann. Intern. Med. 92:149, 1980.

49. Byrnes, J.J. and Khurana, M.: Treatment of thrombotic thrombocytopenic purpura with plasma. N. Engl. J. Med. 297:1386, 1977.

50. Lian, E.C.Y., Harkness, D.R., and Byrnes, J.J., et al.: Presence of a platelet aggregating factor in the plasma of patients with thrombotic thrombocytopenic purpura (TTP) and its inhibition by normal plasma. Blood 53:333, 1979.

51. Fraser, I.D., Bothamley, J.E., and Bennett, M.O., et al.: Intensive antenatal plasmapheresis in severe rhesus immunization. Lancet 1:6, 1976.

52. Graham-Pole, J., Barr, W., and Willoughby, M.L.N.: Continuous-flow plasmapheresis in management of severe rhesus disease. Br. Med. J. 1:1185, 1977.

53. Isbister, J.P., Ting, A., and Seeto, K.M.: Development of Rh-specific maternal autoantibodies following intensive plasmapheresis for Rh immunization during pregnancy. Vox Sang. 33:353, 1977.

54. Branda, R.F., Moldow, G.F., and McCullough, J.J., et al.: Plasma exchange in the treatment of immune disease. Transfusion 15:570, 1975.

54a. Patten, E., Reuter, F.P., Castle, R., and Mercer, C.: Evans' syndrome: benefit from plasma exchange. Transfusion 18:383, 1978.

54b. Rosenfield, R.E., Jagathambal: Transfusion therapy for autoimmune hemolytic anemia. Sem. Hematol. 13:311, 1976.

54c. Petz, L.D. and Garratty, G.: Acquired immune hemolytic anemias. Churchill Livingstone, New York, 1980, pp. 418-420 and 424-425.

54d. Swisher, S.N.: Unpublished observations.

55. McCullough, J.J., Fortuny, I.E., and Kennedy, B.J., et al.: Rapid plasma exchange with the continuous flow centrifuge. Transfusion 13:94, 1973.

56. Pitterman, E., Hocker, P., and Lechner, K., et al.: Plasmapheresis with the continuous flow blood cell separator in the treatment of macroglobulinaemia, multiple myeloma, haemophilia and hyperlipidemia. In: Leukocytes: Separation, Collection and Transfusion.

Goldman, J.M., and Lowenthal, R.M., eds. Academic Press, London, 1975, p. 561.

57. Berkman, E.M., Caplan, S., and Kim, G.S.: ABO-incompatible bone marrow transplantation: preparation by plasma exchange and in vivo antibody absorption. Transfusion 18:504, 1978.

57a. Buckner, C.D., Clift, R.A., Sanders, J.E., Williams, B., Gray, M., Storb, R., and Thomas, E.D.: ABO-incompatible marrow transplants. Transplantation 26:233, 1978.

57b. Hershko, C., Gale, R.P., Ho, W., and Fitchen, J.: ABH antigens and bone marrow transplantation. Br. J. Haematol. 44:65, 1980.

57c. Biggs, J.C., Concannon, A.J., Dodds, A.J., Isbister, J.P., Kesteven, P., and Ma, D.F.: Allogeneic bone marrow transplantation across the ABO barrier. Med. J. Aust. 2:173, 1979.

58. Cimo, P.L. and Aster, R.H.: Post-transfusion purpura. Successful treatment by exchange transfusion. N. Engl. J. Med. 287:290, 1972.

59. Abramson, N., Eisenberg, P.D., and Aster, R.H.: Post-transfusion purpura: immunologic aspects and therapy. N. Engl. J. Med. 291:1163, 1974.

60. Taft, E.G., Propp, R.P., and Sullivan, S.A.: Plasma exchange for cold agglutinin hemolytic anemia. Transfusion 17:173, 1977.

61. Branda, R.F., Tate, D.Y., McCullough, J.J., et al.: Plasma exchange in the treatment of fulminant idiopathic (autoimmune) thrombocytopenic purpura. Lancet 1:688, 1978.

62. Marder, V.J., Nusbacher, J., Anderson, F.W.: One year followup of plasma exchange therapy in 14 patients with idiopathic thrombocytopenic purpura. Transfusion (in press).

63. Dau, P.C., Lindstrom, J.M., and Cassel, C.K., et al.: Plasmapheresis and immunosuppressive drug therapy in myasthenia gravis. N. Engl. J. Med. 297:1134, 1977.

64. Newsome-Davis, J., Wilson, S.G., and Vincent, A., et al.: Long-term effects of repeated plasma exchange in myasthenia gravis. Lancet 1:464, 1979.

65. Newsome-Davis, J., Ward, G.D., and Wilson, S.G., et al.: Plasmapheresis: short- and long-term benefits? In: Plasmapheresis and the Immunobiology of Myasthenia Gravis. Dau, P.C., ed. Houghton Mifflin, Boston, 1979, p. 199.

66. Lisak, R.P., Abramsky, O., and Schotland, D.L.: Plasmapheresis in the treatment of

myasthenia gravis: preliminary studies in 21 patients.In: Plasmapheresis and the Immunobiology of Myasthenia Gravis. Dau, P.C., ed. Houghton Mifflin, Boston, 1979, p. 209.

67. Dau, P.C., Lindstrom, J.M., and Cassel, C.K., et al.: Plasmapheresis in myasthenia gravis and polymyositis. In: Plasmapheresis and the Immunobiology of Myasthenia Gravis. Dau, P.C., ed. Houghton Mifflin, Boston, 1979, p. 229.

68. Lockwood, C.M., Rees, A.J., and Pearson, T.A., et al.: Immunosuppression and plasmaexchange in the treatment of Goodpasture's syndrome. Lancet 1:711, 1976.

69. Misiani, R., Bertani, T., and Licini, R., et al.: Asphyxia in Goodpasture's syndrome: early treatment by immunosuppression and plasma exchange. Lancet 1:552, 1978.

70. Lockwood, C.M., Rees, A.J., and Pinching, A.J., et al.: Plasma-exchange and immunosuppression in the treatment of fulminant immune-complex crescentic nephritis. Lancet 1:63, 1977.

71. Harmer, D., Finn, R., and Goldsmith, H.J., et al.: Plasmapheresis in fulminating crescentic nephritis. Lancet 1:679, 1979.

72. Verrier Jones, J., Fraser, I.D., and Bothamley, J., et al.: A therapeutic role for plasmapheresis in the management of acute systemic lupus erythematosus. Plasma Therapy 1:33, 1979.

73. Talpos, G., Horricks, M., and White, J.M., et al.: Plasmapheresis in Raynaud's disease. Lancet. 1:416, 1978.

74. Penovich, P.E., Hollander, J., and Nusbacher, J., et al.: Note on plasma exchange therapy in Refsum's disease. In: Advances in Neurology. Karp, R.A.P., Rosenberg, R.N., and Schut, L.J., eds. Raven Press, New York, 1978, p. 151.

75. Gibberg, F.B., Billimoria, J.D., and Page, N.G.R., et al.: Heredopathia atactica polyneuritiformis (Refsum's disease) treated by diet and plasma exchange. Lancet 1:575, 1979.

76. Thompson, G.R., Lowenthal, R., and Myant, N.B.: Plasma exchange in the management of homozygous familial hypercholesterolaemia. Lancet 1:1208, 1975.

35

Clinical Use of Blood Substitutes

Scott N. Swisher, M.D., and Lawrence D. Petz, M.D.

ARTIFICIAL BLOOD SUBSTITUTES

Blood substitutes have long been a subject of scientific interest. To date, they have had little practical impact on clinical practice in the United States. The widespread availability of blood and plasma products has not been a stimulus to basic research and clinical investigation into these problems, except for the work of a small group of investigators dedicated to this area. The interests of the military medical services and those concerned with treatment of mass casualties and accident victims have been the main centers of interest in these problems in the past. More recently, the problems of surgical treatment of members of the Jehovah's Witnesses, whose religious beliefs proscribe use of human blood or its products, have added some impetus to investigations in this field. Public awareness of this research area has increased greatly since late 1979, following extensive news coverage of a few early human trials of oxygen-carrying blood substitutes.

Blood substitutes are of two general types: (1) those designed to provide colloid osmotic activity for maintenance or expansion of the plasma volume, and (2) those which are able to transport oxygen. Substitute materials for platelet and leukocyte activities have not been considered in any major way as yet. Because substitutes for human serum albumin have been under active investigation much longer, they are better known and evaluated than are materials which might substitute for the oxygen-carrying capacity of hemoglobin.

PLASMA SUBSTITUTES

During, and for a period following World War II, much attention was given to the role of artificial colloid materials administered intravenously in the management of acute blood loss and shock. More recent investigation has grown out of research carried on during the war in Vietnam. This newer knowledge deemphasized the administration of colloid materials for maintenance of blood volume and emphasized the use of crystalloid solutions. (This topic is more fully discussed in Chapters 22 and 23.) The major research and development activities as well as clinical investigation of plasma protein substitutes thus dates to the era of 1945 to about 1970. Since then, the use of some of these materials has been considered or adopted for other purposes, such as the possible effects of low-molecular-weight dextrans on perfusion of the microcirculation or the use of hydroxyethyl starch in leukapheresis procedures.

A number of nonmetabolizable artificial plasma substitutes have been investigated in the past. The artificial polymer polyvinyl-pyrollidone (PVP) employed in Germany and in other parts of Europe is an example of such a compound. Acaccia has also been studied less extensively. The efficacy of PVP as it was used then is unclear. However, its utility was rendered moot by the discovery that much of the PVP was stored for very long periods in the reticuloendothelial system. Although no hazard has been identified in connection with long storage, further use of PVP has been abandoned as unacceptable. Interest in PVP as a cryoprotective agent for freezing of red cells developed in researach carried on by the Union Carbide Corporation in the 1960s.[4,5] This approach had to be abandoned because of the unacceptability of this material for intravenous administration. Frozen blood storage systems in which PVP was removed after storage appeared to have little advantage over the well-developed systems employing glycerol.

A wide variety of other materials have been tried or in some instances used on a substantial scale as plasma volume expanders. These include a large number of modified animal sera, human ascitic fluid, products based upon human donor red cells or placental blood, casein, pectin, and Isinglass. Two relatively new materials, the levans and polymannuronic acid (Alginon), may become more widely used if they are further developed. All of the other materials mentioned have largely been abandoned or are not in use in the U.S. because of significant unfavorable reactions. None are discussed further here. Two general monographs and a symposium on the subject of blood substitutes and artificial plasma volume expanders will be found useful to interested readers.[1-3]

Table 35-1 summarizes the characteristics of the principal candidate materials employed currently as artificial plasma expanders. Since there is relatively little use of any of these materials for this purpose in the United States at present, they will not be dis-

cussed in great detail here. Clearly, none have advantages over human albumin products from the practical point of view. Interest might be regenerated in their use in connection with mass casualty management, but this seems unlikely.

It should be noted that, in other countries, significant interest exists in at least one artificial plasma expander. Kissmeyer-Neilsen in Switzerland has proposed an approach to integrate the use of serum albumin products with modified fluid gelatin (MFG) in such a way that the country might become self-sufficient in the supply of plasma derivatives.[6,7] There is little interest in this approach in the United States and Canada today. There appears to be a decline in the use of serum albumin at present in these countries, and indeed in Western Europe. The amount of albumin products now available appears to be at least equal to the real need. The use and characteristics of available albumin products are discussed in detail in Chapters 22 and 23.

Gelatins

Gelatin was the first of the artificial colloids still in use for the treatment of shock during World War I.[8] It was not until the modern era of investigation of shock in man after World War II that interest in these materials redeveloped. Three derivative products of gelatin listed in Table 35-1 have been developed between 1951 and 1962.[9-12] Problems associated with gelatin at lower temperatures of early preparations resulted in decreased interest in gelatin products in U.S. They were rejected by the U.S. military forces for this reason. At present, the low temperature fluidity of modern gelatin preparations is quite satisfactory, but their use and further development has taken place largely in Europe.[7,13]

Like all other artificial colloids used as plasma expanders, gelatins are polydisperse—i.e., variable in molecular size and configuration. This is in contrast to albumin, which is essentially homogenous (monodis-

Table 35-1. Characteristics of Principal Plasma Expander Colloids

Material	Solution Concentration	Source Material	Chemical Structure	M_n*	Excretion Route	Intravascular Persistence	Comments
Gelatins			*Protein*				
1) Oxypolygelatin (OPG)	1) 5-6%	Hydrolysis of animal collagen	1) Condensed with glyoxal and oxidized with H_2O_2	23,300	All largely renal excretion; some proteolytic metabolism	About as for MFG	Gelatins are now largely prepared by European firms and marketed in Europe.
2) Modified fluid gelatin (MFG)	2) 3-4%		2) Degraded and coupled with polycarboxylic acid anhydrides	22,600		50% of volume persists 4 to 5 hours postinfusion	OPG may be most antigenic in man.
3) Urea-linked gelatin (ULG)	3) 3-4% (All with electrolytes)		3) Cross-linked with diisocyanate (urea bridges)	24,500	75% excreted 1 wk.	About as for MFG	MFG most widely used at present
Dextrans			*Complex Carbohydrate*				
1) D-70 "high molecular weight"	1) 6%	Bacterial synthesis by *Leukonostoc mesenteroides* from sucrose substrate	Polymers of D-glucopyranose linked -(1-6); partial acid hydrolysis with fractionation by molecular size	1) 35,000 to 40,000	Largely renal excretion; some metabolism to CO_2	Longer than gelatins; 50% of volume persist 8 hours postinfusion	1) Used primarily for plasma volume expansion. *M_w nominal 70,000.
2) D-40 "low molecular weight"	2) 10% (Both with electrolytes)			2) 25,000	55% excreted in urine in 4 hours	Shorter than D70	2) Also used for "flow promotion" in capillary bed and anti-thrombotic prophylaxis. *M_w nominal 40,000
Starch			*Commplex Carbohydrate*				
Hydroxyethyl Starch (HES) (hetastarch)	6% with electrolyte	Waxy maize starch (amylopectin)	Highly branched glucose polymer; hydroxyethylation with ethylene oxide to slow rate of enzymatic hydrolysis in vivo	See text	Renal excretion and metabolism ? other routes of excretion	HES 25/75 about same as albumin	Several preparations with variable intrinsic viscosity and degree of hydroxyethylation. HES 25/75 resembles D70 HES 16/43 resembles D40 (See text)

* M_n = number average molecular weight; M_w = weight average molecular weight. M_w is larger than M_n for polydisperse colloids.

Note: The data for this table have been assembled from multiple sources in the literature; much of it has been obtained from References 1 and 2. There is a great deal of variation in figures reported for molecular weight, excretion rate, and intravascular persistence. Some of this is explained by methodological differences and experimental variability. Reported differences in concentration suggest that a number of different formulations have been studied from time to time, and that the formulation of even a trade-name product may also have changed periodically. Thus, the characteristics of these materials given in Table 35-1 should not be regarded as specific for any product. Rather, they are general descriptions of preparations that have been in clinical use.

perse), except for the presence of variable, usually small amounts of dimer and oligomers which are found in the usual clinical preparations of this protein. Variability in molecular weight as well as molecular configuration of a polydisperse colloid affect its intravascular persistence and pattern of elimination as well as its viscosity and oncotic effect. A simple description of all of these physiochemical characteristics is not possible. Number average molecular weight (M_N) is somewhat more informative for purposes of comparison of colloids than is weight average molecular weight (M_w). Other notations such as those used to describe preparations of hydroxyethyl starch, discussed in more detail later in this chapter, employ intrinsic viscosity measurements as one of the descriptors.

Although their use has been largely abandoned in the U.S., gelatin preparations, particularly modified fluid gelatin (MFG), have been widely used in Europe. They are of intermediate effectiveness in plasma volume expansion, superior to electrolyte solutions but less effective in this respect than long-persisting artificial colloids such as Dextran 70. That gelatins have found a clinical role in Europe is attested to by the report of Nahas et al. in 1978 which shows that over 2.2 million units of 500 ml were given to about 1 million patients in France during the period from 1973 to 1976. In 1976, fluid gelatins constituted 58.7 percent of all artificial plasma expanders employed in France, where the use of electrolyte solutions alone for volume expansion is not widely practiced.[13]

Undesirable Effects

There is little question that modern preparations of gelatin are effective plasma volume expanders. They are alleged to share two problems common to all artificial colloids: (1) alteration of the hemostatic mechanism[14,15] and (2) transient effects on renal tubular function.[13] The effect of colloids on hemostasis is discussed in more detail in connection

with the use of dextrans. Neither of these effects seems to be clinically significant in the French experience.[13] Lundsgaard-Hansen and Tschirren cite evidence that gelatins have neither of these undesirable characteristics, other opinions notwithstanding.[7]

Most artificial colloids also have at least some antigenic potential in man. Hydroxyethyl starch appears to be nonantigenic. The incidence of significant reactions of anaphylactic type to gelatin products appears to be comparable to that of other artificial colloids. Wide ranges of reaction frequencies are reported for all such colloids, ranging 2.5/10,-000 units to 1/300,000 units for dextran. Nahas et al. estimate the frequency of such reactions to gelatin to be in the range of 1/40,000 to 1/100,000 units. In many instances, the immunological basis of such reactions is doubtful or unproven. The risk of anaphylaxis is thus not great, and very large volumes of MFG—15 to 20 liters—have been given without event to numbers of patients.[13] Nevertheless, concerns about safety appear to be the principal factor mitigating against the wider use of gelatin as well as other artificial colloid materials in the U.S. at present. In spite of this, the use of fluid gelatins for volume expansion should be reconsidered in the U.S., particularly if albumin should become limited in supply or too costly. Its use in the management of mass casualties should also be reevaluated, since human serum albumin is no longer being stockpiled in this country.

Dextran

Experimental evaluations of dextrans as a plasma volume expander in man began in 1944.[16] A clinical product, D70, was introduced for this purpose in 1947, and in 1961 so-called "low-molecular-weight" dextran, D40, was available for use in situations characterized by low perfusion of the capillary bed.[17] These materials largely displaced interest in gelatin products in the U.S., where they became the principal artificial colloids in clinical use over the next decade. It has been estimated that over 60 million units of dextran have been used, primarily for volume expansion, since its introduction.[18]

Volume Expansion Effects

Dextrans appeared to be preferable to gelatin because they would not gel at lowered temperatures and were thus better adapted for military and emergency use. D70 has a powerful volume expansion effect, at least as great or greater than albumin, and a relatively long intravascular persistence.[19] Only 30 to 40 percent of D70 is excreted in the urine during the first 12 hours after infusion.[20] There is a substantial body of physiological research documenting its efficacy in this respect. Investigations which compare its efficacy with other colloids such as albumin on outcomes in patients so treated are lacking in the early literature. Indeed, this controversy regarding the relative efficacy of colloids of all types and crystalloids in the management of patients still persists (see Ch. 20 through 24). Nevertheless, there was a substantial use of dextran for blood volume expansion in the U.S. until relatively recently, when its use was largely replaced by albumin.

Low-molecular-weight dextran, D40, has a higher oncotic effect per gram of infused material than D70. Because about 63 percent of the molecules of D40 are below 50,000 M_w, the approximate renal excretion threshold size, this colloid has a much shorter intravascular persistence. Arturson et al. showed that 60 to 70 percent of an infused dose was excreted in the urine over 12 hours, with about 50 percent lost in 5 hours.[20] In spite of relatively short intravascular persistence, D40 appears to produce satisfactory temporary plasma volume support.

Capillary Flow Promotion

Greater investigative interest in D40 dextran was based upon the proposal that this colloid improved perfusion of the capillary bed in the clinical setting of trauma, shock, or sepsis. Much interest in the problem of intravascular red cell aggregation and capillary perfusion was generated by the work of Knisley in 1945 and 1951.[21,22] As a result of observations indicating red cell disaggregation by administration of the smaller size range of dextran molecules in experimental shock, Gelin and Ingelman suggested the use of a specially prepared low-molecular-weight dextran for this purpose in 1961.[17] Because D70 preparations contain a significant proportion of molecules in this small size range, similar effects on capillary circulation were also found for this preparation. Interest in the use of D70 for volume expansion gradually waned as concern about its adverse effect on hemostasis grew; some use of D40 as a red cell disaggregating agent still persisted. It is still used in some disorders for this purpose in the U.S.—for example, as an empirical measure in treatment of thrombotic thrombocytopenic purpura, although its efficacy in this disorder is unproven.

Antithrombotic Effects

The possible role of dextran in prevention of thrombosis may be related to the red cell disaggregating effect of dextran and/or to its still poorly understood interference with blood coagulation and hemostasis. Thorén et al. have been among the principal advocates of this use of dextran and continue to use it as a measure to reduce the incidence of postoperative deep vein thrombosis and pulmonary embolism. Thorén has recently assembled the evidence supporting this use of D70.[18] He reports the combined results of 11 studies, largely from Europe, in which 1722 patients were given D70 prophylactically with 6 fatal cases of pulmonary embolism, and 1801 untreated controls with 36 such fatalities, all verified at autopsy ($P < 0.001$). Similar data for D40 were also found. Thorén has also summarized the information regarding the possible mechanism of this effect, which still remains obscure. Other European authors have reviewed this topic with similar conclusions.[23-25] In spite of this opinion, dextran is not used to any great extent for this purpose in the United States at present. In a sense, the use of dextrans for capillary flow promotion or antithrombotic effects is not related to their incorporation into a strategy of transfusion of blood or blood products. Nevertheless, these pharmacological uses are of some interest and may warrant reevaluation in the United States, where the use of low-dose heparin therapy has been widely practiced for prevention of postoperative venous thrombosis and pulmonary embolism. It is notable that controversy still surrounds the efficacy of this practice also. We have only recently appreciated the difficulties involved in conducting adequately controlled experiments on the therapy or prevention of venous thrombosis and pulmonary embolism. Many of the studies cited in support of the antithrombotic effect of dextran can be criticized on the basis of the experimental design employed.

Undesirable Effects

Immunological. Disadvantages of dextran as an artificial plasma colloid include anaphylactoid reactions of variable severity in common with all other colloid solutions. As discussed in relation to gelatin solutions, various reports give widely different incidence figures for these reactions. Mild reactions include rashes, fever, tachycardia, hypotension, or respiratory symptoms and may occur in about 5 percent or more of patients, according to Thompson.[26] Other authors report incidence figures 2 to 3 orders of magnitude lower.[17,26] One can only conclude that the true incidence of these reactions is uncertain, but probably less than 1 percent since the bulk of the reports cluster around low-incidence figures. One source of confusion in the literature is the fact that some reports are based upon reactions encountered per 100 infusions; others report the percentage of patients given infusions who react unfavorably.

By contrast, it is generally agreed that the incidence of severe reactions, including the few which are lethal, is very low; on the basis of a number of estimates, it appears to be in the range of 8 per 100,000 infusions.[6,17,25,26] In contrast with the infrequency of severe anaphylactoid reactions, preformed dextran-reactive hemagglutinating antibodies are found quite frequently; such antibodies have been demonstrated in more than two-thirds of patients in one study. Some of these dextran-reactive hemagglutinating antibodies may be the result of exposure to other natural complex carbohydrate immunogens by other routes.[18] They do not appear to be involved in anaphylactic reactions.[28] High-molecular-weight dextrans are immunogenic as demonstrated by Kabat et al., but clinical materials are not immunogenic as a rule.[29-32] Thus, it is not clear what component of a dextran solution may be responsible for the clinically observed reactions. A bacterial by-product of the biosynthesis process might be responsible. It is also of note that reaction rates of the same order of magnitude are reported for human plasma and plasma derivatives.

Viscosity Related. Dextrans have high intrinsic viscosity. Their concentration in the urine may become very high after administration of D40 with elevation of urine viscosity. This produces diuresis and a type of transient tubular obstruction and change in renal function, particularly when renal perfusion is reduced.[26] This may be associated with transient oliguria and decreased renal function. As Thorén and others have pointed out, this phenomenon, easily demonstrable in dogs, is more difficult to evaluate in clinical practice, since dextran D40 is frequently given in the presence of other factors which may cause or contribute to renal failure.[18,20] It is generally agreed that dextrans by themselves do not include significant renal damage.

Hemostatic Defects Caused by Dextran and Other Artificial Colloids

Concern about the effect of dextrans on the hemostatic mechanism was initiated by the report of Carbone et al. in 1951.[33] They observed an increase in bleeding time in about 5 percent of otherwise normal subjects given dextran. Many studies since that time have confirmed and amplified this observation.[15] Several of these reports involved clinically significant hemostatic defects secondary to dextran administration.[34,35] By 1958 it had been shown that nearly half of patients given one liter or more of clinical dextran showed increased bleeding time, and daily administration or administration of larger volumes resulted in abnormalities of bleeding in virtually all patients. Coexistent thrombocytopenia aggravates the bleeding tendency, as does simultaneous administration of dicumarol or aspirin.[36-38] Other artificial colloids have similar but less marked effects. The problem may be most severe and thus significant in severely traumatized patients.

The mechanism of bleeding due to dextran administration has been investigated extensively. The subject was recently reviewed by Alexander, who has made important contributions to this work.[15,14] Although the mechanism of increased bleeding after dextran administration is still incompletely understood, Alexander makes a convincing case that it is comparable to an induced form of von Willebrand's disease. This is based upon the demonstration of defects in platelet function, Factor VIII, and von Willebrand factor activities, as well as capillary changes, all resembling those seen in von Willebrand's disease. This may be caused by slow macromolecular precipitation of fibrinogen (Factor I), fibrin monomer, Factor VIII, including von Willebrand factor as well as direct effects upon platelet and endothelial surfaces. Hemodilution of coagulant proteins does not account for the effects.[15] These mechanisms may account for the antithrombogenic effects

of dextrans as well, although this remains unproven.

Concern over induction of abnormal bleeding undoubtedly was the principal factor which caused the decline in clinical use of dextran in the United States. Increased availability of human albumin products certainly was contributory to the declining usage. The bleeding tendency was rarely found to be severe with limited administration of dextran, and its use in significant quantities as a plasma volume expander continued in other countries, even though increased availability of albumin has also recently decreased the use of dextran there as well. The use of D70 is declining rapidly, although D40 usage persists for its other possible indications.

Hydroxyethyl Starch (HES)

This family of substances are the most recently introduced artificial intravascular colloids. One of the principal advantages of HES is that its molecular size and rate of elimination can be relatively precisely controlled. A further advantage lies in its enzymatic degradability by α amylases which are widespread in tissues; this results in only small amounts of long-term storage of the compound. Enzymatic hydrolysis of the starch, normally quite rapid, is decreased by hydroxyethylation with ethylene oxide in alkaline solutions. The degree of hydroxyethylation can be controlled over a wide range of molecular substitution ratios. For a given molecular weight, hydroxyethyl starches are much less filterable through the glomerulus or capillaries than are dextrans because of their "dense" molecular configuration.[26]

These polydisperse colloids are described in terms of their intrinsic viscosity, the limiting viscosity of a polymer in a solution as the concentration is extrapolated to zero. The molecular substitution ratio of hydroxyethyl groups is the second pertinent description. Thus, hetastarch which has been used clinically in the U.S. is described as HES-25/75; the intrinsic viscosity is 25 ml/g and the ratio of hydroxyethyl groups to anhydroglucose units is .75. Other colloids are under investigation, including HES-16/43 and HES-90/50. The effects of HES-25/75 resemble those of dextran 70, and HES-16/43 behaves much as D40.[26]

Volume Expansion Effects

Hydroxyethyl starch, HES-25/75, is an effective plasma volume expander with somewhat longer intravascular persistence than the comparable dextran. Administration of a single unit of HES-25/75 resulted in excretion of 39 percent of the dose in the urine in 24 hours, compared to 45 percent of D70 dextran.[39,40] The incidence of anaphylactoid reactions and abnormalities of hemostasis may be somewhat lower than is the case with other artificial colloids. Significant tissue injury secondary to transient storage in the reticuloendothelial system or uptake by renal tubular cells has not been observed or demonstrated physiologically. HES appears to be nonantigenic in man,[41-43] and it does not appear to have an antithrombogenic effect.[26]

Use of HES in Leukopheresis

One of the more important uses of HES has been in the collection of donor granulocytes by continuous flow or cyclic machine centrifugation (see Ch. 9). In this application, it acts to increase red cell sedimentation and speed centrifugal separation. Many leukapheresis donors have been so treated without untoward reactions. The large amounts given to some of these repeated donors constitutes substantial evidence of its safety. Although an ideal system of donor granulocyte procurement or therapeutic leukapheresis would involve no modification of the donor, the use of HES for this purpose appears to be acceptably safe at present.

The clinical utility of HES has not been fully explored as yet. Although these polymers are under active clinical investigation, it will require extensive clinical use under a wide variety of conditions to determine their ultimate utility and place in transfusion practice. When these materials have been fully developed, HES may well prove to be the colloid of choice for most purposes, if any of the artificial colloids again attain widespread use as plasma volume expanders.

OXYGEN-CARRYING BLOOD SUBSTITUTES

Hemoglobin Solutions

Early efforts to develop a substitute for the oxygen-carrying capacity of intact red cells focused upon stroma-free solutions of human hemoglobin, in some instances altered in ways designed to retain the materials intravascularly. It is of interest that hemoglobin solutions were first proposed as plasma volume expanders.[44-49] Improved intravascular retention has been approached by linking the hemoglobin molecule to another macromolecule or cross-linking the hemoglobin to reduce the amount of rapidly eliminated hemoglobin monomer. Hemoglobins of animal origin have been considered in the past, but the antigenicity of these proteins certainly limits their usefulness.

Hemoglobin solutions have their oxygen dissociation curve shifted to the left. As a result, they off-load oxygen less effectively in tissue sites of low oxygen tension. This results from the loss of the intracellular organophosphates, principally 2,3-diphosphoglyceric acid, which complexes with oxyhemoglobin in the red cell and increases the rate of oxygen dissociation. In an effort to correct this functional alteration, pyridoxal phosphate hemoglobin was synthesized. The synthetic was found to improve oxygen delivery but to be of little practical use because of its short intravascular persistence time.[56,51]

Hemoglobin solutions which may have long intravascular persistence may not maintain the hemoglobin iron in the reduced ferrous state. Within the red cell, the conversion of hemoglobin to methemoglobin with iron in the ferric state occurs spontaneously at a slow rate, about 1 percent per day. It is reduced to the ferrous state primarily by the diaphorase enzyme system linked to NADH. When this enzyme system and a source of NADH are no longer available to the hemoglobin free in plasma, a slow conversion to methemoglobin with loss of oxygen-carrying capacity would be expected to occur. A solution to this problem does not exist at present, although it may not be a significant consideration if hemoglobin solutions were to be administered for only a brief time.[52]

Hemoglobin solutions have one distinct advantage over chemicals which transport oxygen in solution: they also provide oncotic activity which obviates the need for administration of an additional artificial substance for this purpose. Since human hemoglobin solutions must start with donations of blood, as a practical matter it is usually as easy to use the red cells themselves. Salvaged red cells from outdated units of blood might be employed as a source of human hemoglobin. Loss of blood by outdating is still substantial in the United States, and this source of blood might be employed effectively at the logistic costs of shipping the units with appropriate documentation to manufacturing facilities. An unknown risk of hepatitis transmission by hemoglobin solutions is present, but it is probable that they would be icterogenic, particularly if they were processed in large pools. Still undefined are the long-term stability of hemoglobin solutions under a variety of field and storage conditions, as well as their acute and chronic effects in man. At the time of this writing, there exists no satisfactory procedure of chemical modification of hemoglobin to retain it in the vascular system in a fully functional state. Also, emergence of an entirely different approach to the problem of oxygen-carrying blood substitutes—the use

of inert chemical compounds with high oxygen solubility—has preempted most of the current research interest in this topic. For these reasons, major developmental efforts to produce useful hemoglobin solutions have been largely abandoned.

Perfluorochemical Compounds

At the outset, it should be pointed out that the use of these compounds in man remains highly investigative at the present time. Based upon the expected time required for governmental approval of other new drugs in the U.S., it will be at least several years from this writing before these compounds are approved for any general use in this country, even if major adverse effects are not encountered. Nevertheless, this topic deserves some discussion here because of the high level of public interest it has generated.

A large number of chemical compounds, generically known as perfluorochemicals, have been investigated in animals as oxygen transport compounds. Suitable compounds should have a number of characteristics:

1. A high solvent capacity for dissolved oxygen.
2. Chemical inertness, including inability to be metabolized.
3. Low or absent acute or chronic toxicity (related to 2).
4. Persistence in the circulation for a useful period but with virtually complete excretion ultimately.
5. Compatibility with other materials needed to maintain osmotic and oncotic pressure, electrolyte activity and pH, metabolism, and CO_2 transport.

Perfluorochemicals are a large class of chemical compounds which are composed primarily of carbon and fluorine. Some also contain oxygen and/or nitrogen. Many other related compounds are known which are not strictly perfluorochemicals in that they con-

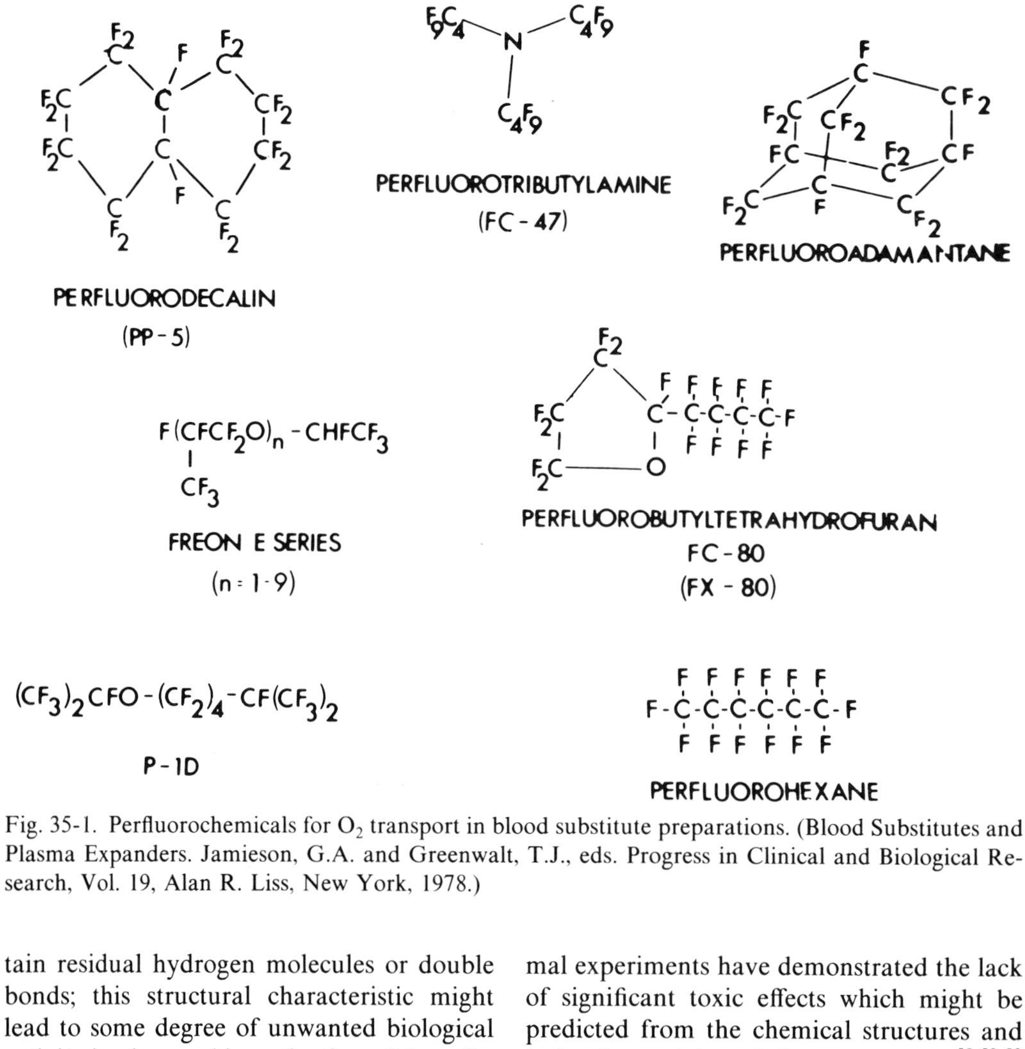

Fig. 35-1. Perfluorochemicals for O_2 transport in blood substitute preparations. (Blood Substitutes and Plasma Expanders. Jamieson, G.A. and Greenwalt, T.J., eds. Progress in Clinical and Biological Research, Vol. 19, Alan R. Liss, New York, 1978.)

tain residual hydrogen molecules or double bonds; this structural characteristic might lead to some degree of unwanted biological activity in vivo, and investigation of them for their usefulness is incomplete.

Figure 35-1 shows the structure of two of the most widely investigated compounds. They vary widely in their patterns of tissue retention. Perfluorodecalin is retained in tissues for a relatively short time, whereas perfluorotributylamine is retained as small droplets in tissues for a long time.[50] Tissue storage does not apparently evoke a histologically visible tissue reaction, but functional appraisals of possible tissue damage over long periods have not been adequately documented as yet. Short-term toxicological studies utilizing cell cultures, tissue perfusions, and acute ani-

mal experiments have demonstrated the lack of significant toxic effects which might be predicted from the chemical structures and lack of reactivity of the compounds.[50,52,53]

These compounds must be administered as a highly stable emulsion to prevent confluence of droplets and embolic blockade of vessels. This requires an emulsifying agent and emulsion stabilizers. Emulsion droplets of about 0.2μ diameter are employed in current investigations, with larger droplets removed by filtration. The emulsifiers, such as Pluronic F68, also contribute some oncotic pressure activity, but in general an artificial plasma volume expander such as hydroxyethyl starch must also be added to elevate the oncotic pressure adequately. Osmotic activity is provided by the usual plasma electrolytes, and pH is buffered by bicarbonate. The stability of the emulsion determines the usable life of the preparation. In some instances, it is necessary to freeze the freshly prepared emulsion to prevent breakdown and to assemble the final preparation just prior to use. It is apparent that there will be technical requirements for administration of these materials beyond that needed for intravenous solutions if and when they become available for use.[50]

None of the compounds investigated to date combines an ideal long intravascular persistence with low long-term storage. This has led to efforts to prepare mixtures of compounds with long and short intravascular persistence in an effort to reduce the amount of compound retained in tissues.

Table 35-2 gives the composition of Fluosol D-A, a commercial product manufactured by the Green Cross Corporation in Osaka, Japan. This material has been administered to a significant number of patients in Japan, and more recently to a few patients in the U.S.[54] Its function in vivo seems to meet the expected properties predicted from the in vitro characteristics. It is administered as a finely divided stabilized water emulsion and appears to remain largely in this physical state in vivo. It must be kept frozen until used. Other formulations are under active evaluation, and ultimately several with somewhat variable characteristics may be available.

Intracellular hemoglobin carries out other functions in addition to the transport of oxygen by virtue of its unique reversible oxygen binding. It provides a substantial part of the buffering capacity of whole blood. It is involved in the transport of CO_2 from tissue sites to the lung. For these reasons, the solubility of CO_2 in fluorocarbon compounds is also of importance. They are adequate in this respect, although they do not enter into the overall buffering systems of whole blood because of their chemical inertness. This requires the administration of buffer and careful monitoring of pH of the "blood" water phase.

The therapeutic usefulness of Fluosol D-A remains to be evaluated in studies of therapeutic outcome for patients when it is employed in a comparative way with standard red cell transfusions in a variety of clinical problems. These data, along with longer-term evaluations of untoward effects, will form the basis of approval of these substances for therapeutic use in the U.S.

Perfluorochemicals have been investigated primarily in a physiological context in which animals are rendered virtually bloodless and are sustained with artificial blood substitutes. Figure 35-2 illustrates such an experiment. These are strenuous tests, much different in character from investigation of therapeutic utility in clinical medicine. Erythropoiesis progressively replaces the oxygen transport of the bloodless animals as the perfluorochemical is eliminated.[50,53,55] Geyer has emphasized that the critical minimum oxygen transport capacity of the blood must be maintained during the recovery phase of these experiments, or the animals will die. This may require continuing infusions until sufficient red cells have reappeared to take over oxygen transport.[50] The compounds provide an interesting approach to the problem of blood replacement under what will certainly be rather sharply limited circumstances. This point is emphasized most

Table 35-2. Composition of Fluosol D-A*

Perfluorodecalin	14.0/W/V%
Perfluorotripropylamine	6.0/W/V%
Pluronic F68	2.7W/V%
Yolk phospholipids	0.4W/V%
Glycerol	0.8W/V%
NaCl	0.48W/V%
KCl	0.027W/V%
$MgCl_2$	0.015W/V%
$CaCl_2$	0.022W/V%
$NaHCO_3$	0.168W/V%
Glucose	0.144W/V%
Hydroxyethyl starch	3.0W/V%
pH: 7.4–7.6	

* Green Cross Corp, Osaka, Japan
(After Geyer, R.: Substitutes for blood and its components. In: Blood Substitutes and Plasma Expanders: Progress in Clinical and Biological Research, Vol. 19. Jamieson and Greenwalt, eds. Alan R. Liss, New York, 1978.)

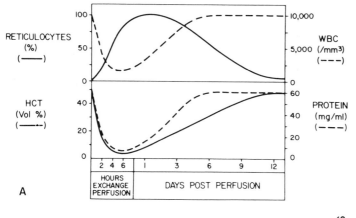

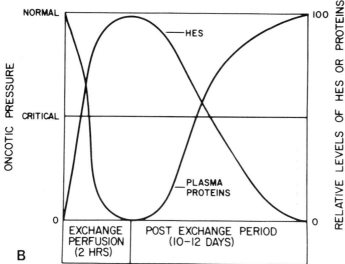

Fig. 35-2. Course of the removal and return of blood components of rat perfuse-exchanged with perfluorochemical blood substitute. (Geyer, R.: Substitutes for blood and its components. In: Blood Substitutes and Plasma Expanders. Jamieson, G.A. and Greenwalt, T.J., eds. Progress in Clinical and Biological Research, Vol. 19, Alan R. Liss, New York, 1978.)

strongly by researchers actively working in the field. The predicted early demise of the blood bank seems quite premature.

Uses of artificial blood substitutes for purposes other than emergency support of oxygen transport may, in fact, be of greater ultimate importance. Blood "wash out" in certain toxic states may prove feasible and useful. Antibodies and drugs may have markedly different in vivo kinetics and distribution when administered in the presence of these compounds. In vitro organ perfusion for transplantation may be an early use. Finally, it is already clear that these materials will provide an important experimental tool, useful in a wide variety of investigations.[52, 56-59]

HUMAN SERUM ALBUMIN PRODUCTS

INTRODUCTION

Human serum albumin products are by far the most commonly employed plasma volume expanders in use in the U.S. and Canada. In a sense, these products are also "artificial" in that they are produced from human plasma by a manufacturing process referred to as fractionation. The alternative to fractionated human serum albumin—unfractionated whole human plasma—is much less useful because (1) it contains isoagglutinins; (2) it contains proteins such as fibrinogen which may be unwanted; and (3) most importantly, it cannot be heat-sterilized to render it free of the hepatitis virus. Pooled, lyophilized human plasma used during World War II resulted in a seriously high incidence of hepatitis before albumin became available. Albumin products have great logistic advantages as well. They are stable under reasonable storage conditions and can be concentrated to 25 percent solutions for shipment to areas where diluent can be prepared locally. Thus, these products had great appeal to the military medical services and to civil defense and disaster management authorities for treatment of war casualties and civilian disaster victims. As albumin products became available, interest in the artificial colloids of nonhuman origin promptly waned. Clinical use diminished rapidly as did further research and development in the field in the U.S.

Growth in the use of albumin was essentially controlled only by the available supply. Although albumin was first introduced as a plasma volume expander, a wide variety of other uses were soon proposed. Many of these uses were justified on strictly empirical grounds—i.e., if the patient's serum albumin level was low, it could frequently be raised by albumin infusions. Data indicating that this therapy had a beneficial effect on the clinical outcome of the treated patients was frequently lacking. Many early studies of the efficacy of albumin were poorly designed and inadequately executed or analyzed by modern standards. Indeed, it is only recently that the community of clinical investigators fully realized the difficulties and sources of error inherent in studying a problem of efficacy of this sort. The primary problem is the inherent great variability in the treated patient population, which makes it almost impossible to obtain comparable groups of treated and control patients, or groups treated in two different ways. Thus, it is not surprising that much of the available information about the efficacy of albumin therapy in a wide variety of circumstances remains inconclusive, even today.

Military medical research has been of great value in studies of the problems of trauma and shock. These patient populations are more homogeneous and their management can be standardized more readily, in spite of the great vicissitudes of doing such studies in the theater of a war. The subjects of military medical research are primarily young males in excellent physical condition. Although this provides a limitation of some degree on the translation of war-time experience to civilian practice involving children, females, the elderly, and the otherwise ill, the general principles clarified by these studies are nonetheless transferrable, and have been found to be of real value in civilian practice of traumatology and major surgery. One can only admire investigators who have contributed this knowledge under such demanding conditions.[60-62] (See also Ch. 21.)

As supplies of albumin increased, its marketing promoted uses for which there was little or no supporting evidence. These uncritical uses have led to a number of efforts to define appropriate and inappropriate uses of these products.[63-65] Several of these studies were motivated by issues of supply, sources of commercially obtained plasma, and costs.[63] The major effort in this regard was made by the Division of Blood Diseases and Resources, National Heart and Lung Institute of The National Institutes of Health, when in February of 1975 they sponsored a conference on the scientific basis of the clinical uses of albumin. The proceedings of this conference have been published and provide a valuable document in this area.[66] In early 1977, Tullis, who summarized the conference, published two papers on the physiology and use of albumin, based largely on the results of the 1975 conference. These papers provided the first scientifically based comprehensive guidelines to the appropriate use of albumin materials.[67,68] In the time since they were published, it has become clear that these guidelines, felt to be overly restrictive by some when first published, are actually quite liberal.

The increased use of crystalloid solutions alone for the initial resuscitation of the severely hypovolemic patient, followed by whole blood, has also resulted in some decrease in the use of albumin products[69] (see Ch. 21). Thus, at this writing, the use of albumin products in the U.S. is in flux. It is difficult to predict what role these materials will have in therapy as other changes in medical practice occur. As the misuses of albumin decline and its use in shock management is replaced, other potential uses appear. For example, the practice of plasma exchange by mechanical plasmapheresis procedures is growing rapidly and consuming significant amounts of albumin products, a use barely envisioned at the time of the 1975 conference or the preparation of Tullis' paper (see Ch. 34). It is probable that human albumin products will be useful in clinical practice for some time to come; it is to be hoped that new uses will be documented before they become established practices of doubtful validity, as has been too often the case in the past with these materials. The guidelines for albumin use provided in this chapter are based primarily on those of Tullis, with some modifications reflecting the authors' interpretations of the available data and more recent developments in the field.

Characteristics of Albumin and Its Physiology

Human albumin is a highly soluble, symmetrical, slightly heterogeneous protein which weighs about 67,000 daltons (584 amino acid residues) with 17 internal disulfied bridges. It carries a high net negative charge of -19. The high negative charge results in albumin binding a large number of compounds including drugs. Albumin contains a large amount of aspartic and glutamic acids and is relatively deficient in leucine and tryptophan, particularly the latter.[66,67] It is synthesized in the liver, normally at from one-third to one-half maximal rate, which is thought to be controlled largely by the oncotic pressure of the interstitial fluid. The synthesis of albumin is rapid, but hepatic reserves of albumin are small.[70]

Albumin is responsible for 80 percent of the colloid oncotic pressure (COP) of the plasma, normally about 27 mmHg; reduction of COP to about 20 mmHg, corresponding to a *total* serum protein of about 5.2 g percent, has been regarded as a "critical value" leading to an excessively expanded interstitial volume (about $+50$ percent).

Albumin is a dynamic protein. Total body stores approximate 300 g in a 70-kg adult, of which 60 to 65 percent is extravascular in skin, muscle, and gut primarily.[66,67] These pools have been regarded as "reserves," but it is more probable that albumin here is part of a complex regulatory process of fluid exchange involving hydrostatic and osmotic forces. The various extravascular pools equilibrate with intravascular albumin at various rates, but generally rapidly. About 15 g of albumin (4 to 5 percent) are metabolized and synthesized daily in the normal steady state. Small amounts are normally lost in the gut. A wide variety of factors influence both the synthesis and degradation of albumin. Albumin production is decreased by malnutrition, hormonal influences, and a wide range of diseases, particularly chronic liver disease. Refeeding results in the onset of albumin synthesis in minutes in the presence of adequate hepatic function.[71]

Albumin Products Available

Three manufactured albumin products are available in the U.S.: human serum albumin, 5% solution; human serum albumin, 25% solution; and plasma protein fraction (PPF). PPF contains at least 83% albumin as a 5% solution in electrolyte with the remainder of the protein made up of alpha and beta globulins and traces of many other plasma proteins. Twenty-five percent human serum albumin is usually diluted to 5 percent in electrolyte solution before infusing. The current cost of these materials is in the neighborhood of $28 to $35 per unit (early 1980).

Plasma protein fraction yields somewhat more useful protein per liter of starting plasma in the fractionating process. The nonalbumin proteins are probably quickly removed from the circulation because of heat denaturation. All these products are freed of hepatitis virus by heating after chemical stabilization of the protein with the additives caprylate and/or acetyltryptophanate. Variable amounts of albumin dimers and oligomers result from the fractionation process and storage. The functional significance of these and their in vivo persistence is unknown. Shelf life depends on storage temperature; 3 years are permitted at below $37°C$ and 5 years at 2 to $10°C$. After expiration of storage life, albumin can be "reworked," although this practice was largely confined to military and civil defense stock piles of albumin. Albumin is no longer stockpiled in large amounts in the U.S. for these purposes.

Newer Methods of Fractionation of Plasma Proteins

All of the albumin products manufactured in the U.S. and Canada are produced by variations of the basic Cohn process, developed by the late E. J. Cohn and colleagues during World War II.[72] This process also yielded fibrinogen and gamma globulin. Fibrinogen has recently been removed from the market because of its high risk of transmitting hepatitis. More recently added process modifications permit harvesting of Factor VIII by cryoprecipitation prior to the fractionation process itself. The Cohn process, now almost 40 years old, is based upon differential precipitation of proteins by varying concentrations of alcohol, and pH in the cold. Its great advantage lies in its proven safety. Albumin products withstand virus inactivation by heat. The gamma globulins, for poorly understood

reasons, are rarely if ever capable of transmitting hepatitis.

A number of new methods of plasma protein fractionation employing a variety of physiocochemical principles have been developed.[73-76] Several of these, particularly column chromatographic separation techniques, have the potential for isolating a number of presently unavailable plasma proteins of possible therapeutic value. Examples of such proteins are C_1 esterase inhibitor, α 1 antitrypsin, antithrombin III, α 2 macroglobulin, metal- and enzyme-binding proteins, transport proteins, and many others. Presumably, these new methods would yield albumin products at least as good or better than present products.

Unfortunately, commercial development of these products is financially unfeasible at the present time.[76] Pilot scale quantities of the proteins are needed to investigate their usefulness. The course of such clinical investigations is prolonged, made very difficult because of present restrictions on investigation of any sort of human subjects, and extremely costly. By the time regulatory approval could be obtained, the investment even in a potentially very useful and marketable product is so high as to be practically unrecoverable in a reasonable period. Thus, we are left with a limited method, far behind the state of the art, useful only because it is proven to be relatively safe. The resolution of this profound paradox—that is, large amounts of public and privately donated monies have gone into support of the basic research that developed these new methods that cannot now be used—is a major challenge for society as a whole and for government, the biomedical research establishment, and industry in particular.

The Rational Use of Albumin Products

Blood Volume Expansion. This is the primary indication for administration of albumin, although authorities on the management of trauma and shock differ as to its value. About 50 percent of the injected volume of albumin solution remains after 4 hours as the albumin redistributes itself into the extravascular space. This phenomenon is the reverse aspect of the physiological process by which albumin "reserves" enter the vascular space to restore blood volume and COP of plasma; redistribution of albumin permits early treatment of hypovolemia with crystalloid solutions[77] (see Ch. 21).

Albumin Loss.   After adequate fluid replacement, the burn patient who loses large amounts of albumin probably profits from liberal albumin administration begun 24 hours after injury (Ch. 21). Other acute albumin losses—acute nephrosis, ascites, protein-losing enteropathy—can be appropriately replaced with albumin infusions at least in the short term, until recovery or improvement can be effected. The value of this therapy on patient outcomes is not as well established as in shock and burns.

Other Uses of Albumin Products

1. **In Bypass Pump Priming.**   Particularly when marked hemodilution is used, albumin may be needed to maintain the plasma COP above the critical level.

2. **In Adult Respiratory Distress Syndrome.**   This poorly understood disorder may be improved by albumin infusion, providing a great increase in pulmonary capillary permeability has not occurred. Control of overhydration of the shocked patient may be more important[78] (Ch. 21).

3. **As a "Chemical Buffer."**   Due to its high net negative charge, many drugs and chemicals are bound to albumin. In the case of hyperbilirubinemia of newborns, therapeutic albumin may bind additional bilirubin and reduce the incidence of kernicterus.[79] Information about this potential use of albumin is still very incomplete for most other drugs and chemicals.[80]

4. **In Postsurgical or Posttrauma Patients.**   These patients tend to become hypoproteinemic due to malnutrition, reduced albumin synthesis, and increased catabolism. Short-term administration of albumin may be appropriate, but its efficacy in improving patient outcomes has not been unequivocally established.[81]

Comment: There is no appropriate indication for administration of only 1 or 2 units of albumin to an adult. The albumin-depleted patient requires replacement of both the intravascular albumin and the larger amount which is stored in the extravascular space. When albumin is really needed, it is frequently given in inadequate amounts.

5. **As a Medium in Which to Resuspend Sedimented Red Cells for Transfusion.**   This is wasteful, expensive, and less effective than the use of whole blood; its use should be limited to emergencies and a few highly specialized circumstances, such as a bleeding patient with IgA hypersensitivity.

6. **As a Replacement Colloid for Plasma Replacement by Mechanical Plasmapheresis.**   This is a relatively new use, the efficacy of which is still in doubt (see Ch. 21). Opinion remains divided over the question of plasma replacement with albumin products or with fresh frozen plasma. It will be some time before this matter is settled, and it is possible that albumi products will be best for some indications, and plasma for others.

Misuses of Albumin Products

1. **Malnutrition.**   Use of albumin in this case is inefficient, expensive and may defer proper measures to restore caloric and amino acid intake. Albumin is of absolutely no value in "toning up the system," a use once proposed to one of the authors. Only about 45 percent of infused albumin as a total protein source enters the body protein pool of protein-depleted isocaloric patients.[82]

2. **Situations of Chronic Albumin Loss.**   Such situations—i.e., chronic nephrosis and

cirrhosis of the liver—are not improved by long-term albumin administration.

Adverse Effects of Albumin Administration

Albumin products are inherently surprisingly safe. Only a few significant adverse effects are reported in the literature. Some of these are due to technical accidents during manufacture. Probably more frequent are adverse effects due to inappropriate or incorrect administration.[66,67] From 1970 to 1974, total reported reactions involved 1.53 percent of all lots released, but only 0.47 percent involved three or more patients.[83]

Bacterial Contamination. Rarely, a lot of an albumin product has been found to be contaminated with bacteria, particularly with *pseudomonas* spp. These lots have produced febrile reactions, transient bacteremia, shock, and possible sepsis in the recipient.[84] Human Serum Albumin, 25%, is a good culture medium for a number of organisms. Not only does it support growth, but it appears to stabilize certain organisms and preserve viability.[85]

It is important to note that the heating step in manufacture of albumin products, 60° C for 10 hours, is done to inactivate the hepatitis viruses, not to insure bacterial sterility, which would require autoclaving.[83] Albumin cannot withstand these temperatures. Extreme care in preventing contamination during manufacture and filtration prior to bottling are required to prevent contamination. All lots released by the Bureau of Biologics are tested for contamination and pyrogenicity.[83] In spite of these precautions, bacterial contamination can occur and should be considered in any patient who has an episode of fever, particularly with shaking chills during or shortly after albumin administration. It is important that samples of the administered material and other vials of the same lot be preserved for investigation. Both the manufacturer and the Bureau of Biologics should be notified of such reactions.

Pyrogenic Reactions. Reactions characterized by chills and fever constitute about 75 percent of all reported reactions. It is difficult to be sure that the cause of these reactions was in fact due to albumin administration, or that they were truly pyrogenic in nature. The fact that only a single patient may be reported as reacting to a single lot of albumin suggests that most such reactions are of other origin. These reactions are rarely severe but, if suspiciously related to albumin product administration, they should be reported to the manufacturer for appropriate investigation.

Hepatitis. When properly heated and protected from subsequent contamination, Human Serum Albumin and PPF are unable to transmit hepatitis.[86] Nevertheless, an outbreak of hepatitis traceable to PPF prepared by one manufacturer occurred in 1973.[87] It is probable that a defect in the heating process accounted for this episode, but this was never proven. It is of interest that serum albumin products prepared simultaneously by this manufacturer from similar source plasma were not infective. The requirement to screen for hepatitis B surface antigen (HBsAg) and eliminate those plasmas that are positive has resulted in a sharp decline in the amount of this antigen detectable in albumin products. This may contribute to safety of the product, but it also reduces the amount of passively transferred HBsAg given to recipients, which may cause diagnostic confusion. In spite of the unlikelihood of such an event, it is well to remember that all safeguards can fail and that these products are not unqualifiedly free of hepatitis viruses.

Hypotension. It has been known for some time that rapid administration of PPF is frequently associated with transient hypotension. Attention was focused on this problem by the report of Bland in 1973.[88] Rarely, lots of Human Serum Albumin were thought to evoke a similar reaction. The topic was investigated in great detail following an episode in which somewhat more severe hypotension was found to follow administration of PPF prepared by one manufacturer in 1977. Although this reaction was thought to be due to the presence of bradykinin in trace amounts, these investigations demonstrated that pre-kallikrein activator (PKA) present in PPF and in a few lots of Human Serum Albumin was responsible. The PKA activates the production of bradykinin from the recipient's own kinin system. This problem has now been resolved by changes in the manufacturing process which result in inactivation of PKA.[89] This topic is discussed in more detail in Chapter 23.

Other Reactions.   A number of other reactions have been reported in relation to administration of albumin products. Of these, urticaria is the most believable. Many such reports may involve coincidences which do not involve a cause-and-effect relationship.

Risks Due to Improper Administration.   Excessive administration of albumin should be avoided. If the concentration of albumin is raised artificially above about 5.5 g percent in the plasma, a hyperoncotic state is induced which, in the absence of available extracellular fluid, results in increased albumin catabolism and decreased hepatic synthesis. If there is excessive extracellular fluid, excessive albumin administration will result in a rise in intravascular volume and possible pulmonary edema. The same effect can occur if excessive amounts of albumin and crystalloid are given simultaneously. These adverse reactions are more frequent and severe in patients with intrinsic heart disease who have lowered cardiac functional reserves. Both rate of administration and amount given are important. Pulmonary edema can occur in both the clinical context of treatment of hypovolemia with rapid fluid and albumin administration, and in the treatment of other hypoalbuminemic states at a more leisurely pace. Careful, frequent evaluation of the patient, with preliminary calculation of the replacement need in both amount and rate, will minimize these adverse reactions.

Cost of Albumin

The cost of albumin may account for 10 percent or more of a modern hospital pharmacy budget. Much of this is wasted due to misuse. Alexander et al.[90] recently reported that, in a VA hospital, 41 percent of all the albumin used was inappropriate, and only 29 percent of that given to surgical patients was appropriate, on the basis of the relatively liberal criteria prepared by Tullis. There probably is declining use of albumin in the U.S. today. Historical national consumption has been about 350 kg/million population; by comparison, Canadian use is about 150 kg/M. Countries of Western Europe appear to use even more albumin than does the U.S.

Whether declining usage of albumin will continue will depend upon many factors, including valid new uses. It is probable, however, that forces which are exerting pressures for health care cost controls will continue to reduce the misuse of this valuable product, possibly by providing cost reimbursement for only selected indications. This would be unfortunate and probably excessively rigid and restrictive. Much to be preferred would be the thoughtful prescription of these products based upon careful analysis of the clinical problem and knowledge of albumin physiology and proven therapeutic indications.

REFERENCES

1. Gruber, U.F.: Blood Replacement. Springer Verlag, Berlin, Heidelberg, New York, 1969.
2. Jamieson, G.A. and Greenwalt, T.J., eds.: Blood Substitutes and Plasma Expanders: Progress in Clinical and Biological Research, Vol. 19, Alan R. Liss, New York, 1978.
3. Artificial Blood, A Symposium. Fed. Proc. 34:1428, 1975.
4. Rinfret, A.P.: Some Aspects of Preservation of Blood by Rapid Freeze-Thaw Procedures. Fed. Proc. 22:94, 1963.
5. Richards, V., Braverman, M., Floridia, R., Persidsky, M., and Lowenstein, J.: Initial clinical experiences with liquid nitrogen pre-

served blood, employing PVP as a protective additive. J. Surg. 108:311, 1964.

6. Lundsgaard-Hansen, P., Bucher, U., Tschirren, B., Haase, S., Kueke, B., Lüdi, H., Stankiewicz, L.A., and Hässig, A.: Red cells and gelatin as the core of a unified program for the national procurement of blood components and derivatives. Prediction, performance and impact on supply of albumin and Factor VIII. Vox Sang. 34:261, 1978.

7. Lundsgaard-Hansen, P. and Tschirren, B.: Modified Fluid Gelatin as a Plasma Substitute. In: Blood Substitutes and Plasma Expanders: Progress in Clinical and Biological Research, Vol. 19. Jamieson, G.A. and Greenwalt, T.J., eds., Alan R. Liss, New York, 1978, p. 227.

8. Hogan, J.J.: Intravenous use of colloidal (gelatin) solutions in shock. J.A.M.A. 64:721, 1915.

9. Campbell, D.H., Koepfli, J.B., Pauling, L., Abrahamson, N., Dandliker, W., Feigen, G.A., Lanni, G., and LeRosen, A.: The preparation and properties of a modified gelatin (Oxypolygelatin) as an oncotic substitute for serum albumin. Tex. Rep. Biol. Med. 9:235, 1951.

10. Tourtelotte, D. and Williams, H.E.: Acylated Gelatins and Their Preparations. U.S. Patent No. 2:817, 1958 (cited in Ref. 4).

11. Ibid., Chemical Modifications of Gelatin for Use as Plasma Volume Expander. In: Stainsby, G.: Recent Advances in Gelatin and Glue Research. Pergamon Press, London, 1957, p. 246.

12. Schmidt-Thome, J., Mager, A., and Schöne, H.H.: Zur chemie einer neuen, plasmaexpanders. Arzneim. Forsch. 12:378, 1962.

13. Nahas, G.G., Vourch, G., and Tannieres, M.L.: The Current Use in France of Modified Fluid Gelatins as Plasma Expanders. In: Blood Substitutes and Plasma Expanders: Progress in Clinical and Biological Research, Vol. 19. Jamieson, G.A. and Greenwalt, T.J., eds. Alan R. Liss, New York, 1978, p. 259.

14. Alexander, B., Odake, K., Lawler, D., and Swanger, M.: Coagulation, Hemostasis, and Plasma Expanders: A Quarter Century Enigma. Fed. Proc. 34:1429, 1975.

15. Alexander, B.: Effects of Plasma Expanders on Coagulation and Hemostasis: Dextran, Hydroxyethyl Starch, and Other Macromolecules Revisited. In: Blood Substitutes and

Plasma Expanders: Progress in Clinical and Biological Research, Vol. 19. Jamieson, G.A. and Greenwalt, T.J., eds. Alan R. Liss, New York, 1978, p. 293.

16. Grönwall, A. and Ingelman, B.: Untersuchunger über Dextran und sein Verhalten by Parenteraler Zufuhr. Acta. Physiol. Scand. 7:97, 1944.

17. Gelin, L.-E. and Ingelman, B.: Rheomacrodex—A New Dextran Solution for Rheological Treatment of Impaired Capillary Flow, Acta. Chir. Scand. 122:294, 1961.

18. Thorén, L.: Dextran as a plasma volume substitute. In: Blood Substitutes and Plasma Expanders: Progress in Clinical and Biological Research, Vol. 19. Jamieson, G.A. and Greenwalt, T.J., eds. Alan R. Liss, New York, 1978, p. 265.

19. Arturson, G. and Wallenius, G.: The intravascular persistence of dextran of different molecular sizes in normal humans. Scand. J. Clin. Lab. Invest. 16:76, 1964.

20. Arturson, G. and Wallenius, G.: The renal clearance of dextran of different molecular sizes in normal humans. Scand. J. Clin. Lab. Invest. 16:81, 1964.

21. Kniseley, M.H., Eliot, T.S., and Bloch, E.H.: Sludged blood in traumatic shock. I. Microscopic observations on the precipitation and agglutination of blood flowing through the vessels in crushed tissues. Arch. Surg. 51:221, 1945.

22. Kniseley, N.H.: An annotated bibliography on sludged blood. Postgrad. Med. 10:15, 1951.

23. Gruber, U.F.: Blood Replacement. Springer Verlag, Berlin, Heidelberg, New York, 1969, p. 87.

24. Steinmann, E., Duckert, F., and Gruber, U.F.: Wert von dextran 70 zur thromboembolie prophylaxe in der Allgemeinen. Chirurgie, Orthopädie, Urologie, und Gynakologie. Schweiz Med. Wochenschr. 105:1637, 1975 (English Absts.)

25. Verstraete, M.: The prevention of postoperative deep vein thrombosis and pulmonary embolism with low dose subcutaneous heparin and dextran. Surg. Gynecol. Obstet. 143:981, 1976.

26. Thompson, W.L., Jr.: Hydroxyethyl starch. In: Blood Substitutes and Plasma Expanders: Progress in Clinical and Biological Research,

Vol. 19. Jamieson, G.A. and Greenwalt, T.J., eds. Alan R. Liss, New York, 1978, p. 283.

27. Ring, J. and Messmer, K.: Incidence and severity of anaphylactoid reactions to colloid volume substitutes. Lancet i:466, 1977.

28. Hedin, H., Richter, W., and Ring, J.: Dextran-induced anaphylactoid reactions in man: Role of dextran reactive antibodies. Int. Arch. Allergy Appl. Immunol. 52:145, 1976.

29. Kabat, E.A. and Berg, D.: Dextran—an antigen in man. J. Immunol. 70:514, 1953.

30. Allen, P.Z. and Kabat, E.A.: Persistence of circulating antibodies in human subjects immunized with dextran, levan, and blood group substances. J. Immunol. 80:495, 1958.

31. Kabat, E.A., Turino, G.M., Tarrow, A.B. and Maurer, P.H.: Studies on the immunochemical basis of allergic reactions to dextran in man. J. Clin. Invest. 36:1160, 1957.

32. Kabat, E.A. and Bezer, A.E.: The effect of variations in molecular weight on the antigenicity of dextran in man. Arch. Biochem. 78:306, 1958.

33. Carbone, J.V., Furth, F.W., Scott, R., and Crosby, W.H.: A hemostatic defect associated with dextran infusion. Proc. Soc. Exp. Biol. Med. 85:101, 1954.

34. Bronwell, A.W., Artz, C.P., and Sako, Y.: Evaluation of blood loss from a standardized wound after dextran. Surg. Forum 5:809, 1954.

35. Horvath, S.M., Hamilton, L.H., Spurr, G.B., Allbaugh, E.B., and Hutt, B.K.: Plasma expanders and bleeding time. J. Appl. Physiol. 7:614, 1955.

36. Adelson, E., Crosby, W.H., and Roeder, W.: Further studies of a hemostatic defect caused by intravenous dextran. J. Lab. Clin. Med. 45:441, 1955.

37. Adelson, E.: Bleeding time prolongation after dextran infusion. Bibl. Haematol. 7:275, 1958.

38. Brodman, R.F., Sarg, M., Veith, F.J., and Spaet, T.: Dextran 40-induced coagulopathy confused with von Willebrand Disease. Arch. Surg. 112:321, 1977.

39. Metcalf, W., Dargan, E.L., Hehre, E.J., Levitsky, S., and DiBuono, T.J.: Clinical physiological characterization of a new dextran. Surg. Gynecol. Obstet. 115:199, 1962.

40. Metcalf, W., Papadopoulas, A., Tufaro, R., and Barth, A.: A clinical physiologic study of hydroxyethyl starch. Surg. Gynecol. Obstet. 131:255, 1970.

41. Salvaggio, J., Kayman, H., and Leskowitz, S.: Immunologic responses of atopic and normal individuals to aerosolized dextran. J. Allergy 38:31, 1966.

42. Brickman, R.D., Murray, G.F., Thompson, W.L., and Ballinger, W.F.: The Antigenicity of Hydroxyethyl Starch in Humans. J.A.M.A. 198:1277, 1966.

43. Maurer, P.H. and Berardinelli, B.: Immunologic studies with hydroxyethyl starch (HES), a proposed plasma expander. Transfusion 8:265, 1968.

44. Rabiner, S.F., Helbert, J.R., Lopas, H., and Friedman, L.H.: Evaluation of a stroma-free hemoglobin solution for use as a plasma expander. J. Exp. Med. 126:1127, 1967.

45. Rabiner, S.F.: Hemoglobin solution as a plasma expander. Fed. Proc. 34:1454, 1975.

46. Mok, W., Chen, D., and Mazur, A.: Cross-linked hemoglobin as potential plasma protein extenders. Fed. Proc. 34:1458, 1975.

47. Tam, S.-C., Blumenstein, J., and Wong, J. T.-F.: Soluble dextran-hemoglobin complex as a potential blood substitute. Proc. Natl. Acad. Sci. (USA) 73:2128, 1976.

48. Horowitz, B. and Mazur, A.: Oxygen equilibrium and structural studies of amidinated human hemoglobin. In: Blood Substitutes and Plasma Expanders: Progress in Clinical and Biological Research, Vol. 19. Jamieson, G.A. and Greenwalt, T.J., eds. Alan R. Liss, New York, 1978, p. 149.

49. Blumenstein, T., Tam, S.-C., Chang, J.E., and Wong, J. T.-F.: Experimental transfusion of dextran hemoglobin. In: Blood Substitutes and Plasma Expanders: Progress in Clinical and Biological Research, Vol. 19. Jamieson, G.A. and Greenwalt, T.J., eds. Alan R. Liss, New York, 1978, p. 250.

50. Geyer, R.: Substitutes for blood and its components. In: Blood Substitutes and Plasma Expanders: Progress in Clinical and Biological Research, Vol. 19. Jamieson, G.A. and Greenwalt, T.J., eds. Alan R. Liss, New York, 1978, p. 1.

51. Messmer, K.: cited by Geyer, R.: Substitutes for blood and its components. In: Blood Substitutes and Plasma Expanders: Progress in Clinical and Biological Research, Vol. 19.

Jamieson, G.A. and Greenwalt, T.J., eds. Alan R. Liss, New York, 1978.

52. Sloviter, H.A.: Perfusion of the brain and other isolated organs with dispersed perfluoro compounds. In: Blood Substitutes and Plasma Expanders: Progress in Clinical and Biological Research, Vol. 19. Jamieson, G.A. and Greenwalt, T.J., eds. Alan R. Liss, New York, 1978, p. 27.

53. Clark, L.C.: Perfluorodecalin as a red cell substitute. In: Blood Substitutes and Plasma Expanders: Progress in Clinical and Biological Research, Vol. 19. Jamieson, G.A. and Greenwalt, T.J., eds. Alan R. Liss, New York, 1978, p. 69.

54. Maugh, T.H.: Blood substitute passes its first test. Science 206:205 (October 12), 1979.

55. Zucali, J.R., Mirand, E.A., and Gordon, A.S.: Erythropoiesis and artificial blood substitution with a perfluorocarbon-polyol, J. Lab. Clin. Med. 94:742, 1979.

56. Hall, C.A., and Rappazzo, M.: Organ perfusion with perfluorocarbon. In: Blood Substitutes and Plasma Expanders: Progress in Clinical and Biological Research, Vol. 19. Jamieson, G.A. and Greenwalt, T.J., eds. Alan R. Liss, New York, 1978, p. 41.

57. Wada, J., Paloheimo, S., Thalmann, I., Bohne, B.A., and Thalmann, R.: Maintenance of Cochlear Function with Artificial Oxygen Carriers. Laryngoscope 89:1457, 1979.

58. Franke, H., Málynsz, M., and Runge, D.: Improved Sodium and PAH Transport in the Isolated Fluorocarbon-perfused Rat Kidney. Nephron. 22:423, 1978.

59. Steinberg, H., Fisher, A.B., and Sloviter, H.A.: Accelerated Removal of Platelets During Perfusion of Isolated Lungs with Perfluoro Erythrocyte Substitute. Proc. Soc. Exp. Biol. Med. 162:179, 1979.

60. Beecher, H.K., Burnett, C.H., Shapiro, S.L., Simeone, F.L., Smith, L.D., Sullivan, E.R., and Mallory, T.B.: The Physiologic Effects of Wounds. Med. Dept. U.S. Army; Surgery in WW II. Office of the Surgeon General, Dept of Army, Washington, D.C., 1952.

61. Simmons, R.L., Heisterkamp, C.A., and Doty, D.B.: Post-resuscitative Blood Volumes in Combat Casualties. Surg. Gynecol. Obstet. 128:1193, 1969.

62. Collins, J.A., Simmons, R.L., James, P.M., Bredenberg, C.E., Anderson, R.W., and Heis-

terkamp, C.A.: Acid-base Status of Seriously Wounded Combat Casualties. I. Before Treatment. Ann. Surg. 171:595, 1970.

63. Sgouris, J.T. and Dorsey, H.W.: Survey of the Use of Plasma Expanders in the United States. In: Proceedings of the Workshop on Albumin, 1975. Sgouris, J.T. and René, A., eds. National Heart and Lung Institute, National Institutes of Health, Department of Health, Education and Welfare, Bethesda, MD, 1976, pub. #76-925, p. 137.

64. Lundh, B.: The Consumption of Albumin at the University Hospital, Lund, Sweden. In: Proceedings of the Workshop on Albumin, 1975. Sgouris, J.T. and René, A., eds. National Heart and Lung Institute, National Institutes of Health, Department of Health, Education and Welfare, Bethesda, MD, 1976, pub. #76-925, p. 239.

65. Report of Panel 6 on Safety and Efficacy of Blood and Blood Derivatives. Swisher, S.N., Chrmn. and Ed., Bureau of Biologics, Food and Drug Administration, The Federal Register. (In press.)

66. Sgouris, J.T. and René, A., eds.: Proceedings of the Workshop on Albumin, 1975. Pub. #76-925, National Heart and Lung Institute, National Institutes of Health, Department of Health, Education and Welfare, Bethesda, MD, 1976.

67. Tullis, J.L.: Albumin. 1. Background and Use. J.A.M.A. 237:335, 1977.

68. Tullis, J.L.: Albumin. 2. Guidelines for Clinical Use. J.A.M.A. 237:460, 1977.

69. Carey, L.C., Cloutier, C.T., and Lowery, B.D.: The Use of Balanced Electrolyte Solution for Resuscitation. In: Body Fluid Replacement in the Surgical Patient. Fox, C.L. and Nahas, G.G., eds., Grune and Stratton, New York, 1970, p. 200.

70. Urban, J., Inglis, A.S., and Edwards, K.: Chemical Evidence for the Difference Between Albumins from Microsomes and Serum and a Possible Precursor Product Relationship. Biochem. Biophys. Res. Comm. 61:444, 1974.

71. Rothschild, M.A., Oratz, M., and Mongelli, J.: Effects of a Short-Term Fast on Albumin Synthesis: Studies *in vivo*, in the Perfused Liver, and on Amino Acid Incorporation by Hepatic Microsomes. J. Clin. Invest. 47:2591, 1968.

72. Cohn, A.J., Oncley, J.L., Strong, L.E.,

Hughes, W.L., Mulford, D.J., Ashworth, J.N., Melin, M., and Taylor, H.L.: A System for the Separation into Fractions of the Protein and Lipoprotein Components of Biological Tissues and Fluids. J. Am. Chem. Soc. 68:459, 1946.

73. Polson, A., Potgieter, G.M., Largier, J.F., Mears, G.E.F., and Joubert, F.J.: The Fractionation of Protein Mixtures by Linear Polymers of High Molecular Weight. Biochim. Biophys. Acta. 82:463, 1964.

74. Watt, J.G.: Automatically Controlled Continuous Recovery of Plasma Protein Fractions for Clinical Use. A Preliminary Report. Vox Sang. 18:42, 1970.

75. Condie, R.M., Hull, B.L., Howard, R.J., Fryd, D., Simmons, R.L., and Najarian, J.S.: Treatment of Life-Threatening Infections in Renal Transplant Recipients with High Dose IV Human IgG. Transplant. Proc. 11:66, 1979.

76. Proceedings of the International Workshop on Technology for Protein Separation and Improvement of Blood Plasma Fractionation. Sandberg, H.E., ed., National Institutes of Health, U.S. Dept. of Health, Education and Welfare, Washington, D.C., pub. #NIH 78-1422, 1978.

77. Collins, J.A. and Howland, W.: Generic statement on albumin and PPF. In: Report of Panel 6 on Safety and Efficacy of Blood and Blood Derivatives. Swisher, S.N., Chrmn. and Ed., Bureau of Biologics, Food and Drug Administration, The Federal Register. (In press.)

78. Collins, J.A.: The Acute Respiratory Distress Syndrome. Adv. in Surg. 11:171, 1977.

79. Cornely, A. and Wood, B.: Albumin Administration in Exchange Transfusion for Hyperbilirubinaemia. Arch. Dis. Childhood. 43:151, 1968.

80. Koch-Wesser, J. and Sellers, E.M.: Binding of Drugs to Serum Albumin. N. Engl. J. Med. 294:311, 1976.

81. Davison, A.M.: The Use of Albumin Concentrates in Hypoproteinaemic States. Clin. in Hematol. 5:135, 1976.

82. Waterhouse, C., Bassett, S.H., and Holler, J.: Metabolic Studies on Protein Depleted Patients Receiving a Large Part of Their Nitrogen Intake from Human Serum Albumin Administered Intravenously. J. Clin. Invest. 28:245, 1949.

83. Barker, L.F.: Albumin Products and the Bureau of Biologics. In: Proceedings of the

Workshop on Albumin, 1975. Sgouris, J.T. and René, A., eds. National Heart and Lung Institute, National Institutes of Health, Department of Health, Education and Welfare, Bethesda, MD, 1976, pub. #76-925, p. 22.

84. Steere, A.C.: Adverse Reactions to Albumin Caused by Bacterial Contamination. In: Proceedings of the Workshop on Albumin, 1975. Sgouris, J.T. and René, A., eds. National Heart and Lung Institute, National Institutes of Health, Department of Health, Education and Welfare, Bethesda, MD, 1976, pub. #76-925, p. 278.

85. Hochstein, H.D. and Seligmann, E.B.: Microbial Contamination in Albumin. In: Proceedings of the Workshop on Albumin, 1975. Sgouris, J.T. and René, A., eds. National Heart and Lung Institute, National Institutes of Health, Department of Health, Education and Welfare, Bethesda, MD, 1976, pub. #76-925, p. 284.

86. Hoofnagle, J.H. and Barker, L.F.: Hepatitis B Virus and Albumin Products. In: Proceedings of the Workshop on Albumin, 1975. Sgouris, J.T. and René, A., eds. National Heart and Lung Institute, National Institutes of Health, Department of Health, Education and Welfare, Bethesda, MD, 1976, pub. #76-925, p. 305.

87. Pattison, C.P., Klein, C.A., Leger, R.T., Maynard, J.E., Berquist, K.R., Hoofnagle, J.H., Barker, L.F., Bryan, J.A., and Smith, D.E.: Field Studies of Type B Hepatitis Associated with Transfusion of Plasma Protein Fraction. In: Proceedings of the Workshop on Albumin, 1975. Sgouris, J.T. and René, A., eds. National Heart and Lung Institute, National Institutes of Health, Department of Health, Education and Welfare, Bethesda, MD, 1976, pub. #76-925, p. 315.

88. Bland, J.H.L., Laver, M.B., and Lowenstein, E.: Vasodilator Effect of Commercial 5 Percent Plasma Protein Fraction Solutions. J.A.M.A. 224:1721, 1973.

89. Alving, B.M., Hojima, Y., Pisano, J.J., Mason, B.L., Buckingham, R.E., Mozen, M.M., and Finlayson, J.S.: Hypotension Associated with Prekallikrein Activator (Hageman-Factor Fragments) in Plasma Protein Fraction. N. Engl. J. Med. 299:66, 1978.

90. Alexander, M.R., Ambre, J.J., Liskow, B.I., and Trost, D.C.: Therapeutic Use of Albumin, J.A.M.A. 241:2527, 1979.

36

Viral Hepatitis and Other Infections Transmitted by Transfusion; Use of Active and Passive Immunization

Lewellys F. Barker, M.D.

INTRODUCTION

In the early days of transfusion therapy, when blood was directly transfused from donors to recipients without storage, transmission of syphilis was recognized as a serious hazard. In many years of experience with refrigerated banked blood, however, this complication has virtually disappeared; so has the once serious risk of massive bacterial contamination of banked blood, which has been relegated to the annals of medical history since the adoption of fully assembled and sterilized plastic blood collection and component separation sets. Transmission of hepatitis viruses, on the other hand, has remained a serious complication of transfusion therapy since its recognition in the early 1940s, so that the risk of viral hepatitis must always be considered in weighing the risks against the benefits of treating patients with blood and blood products. This situation prevails despite much progress towards our understanding and control of viral hepatitis. Other infectious diseases may be transmitted by blood transfusion, but for the most part they do not represent frequent or serious hazards of modern transfusion therapy.

POSTTRANSFUSION HEPATITIS

Background

The first clear description of hepatitis transmission by human serum is in a report by Lürman in Germany in 1885.[1] In 1883, a large number of shipyard workers in Bremen received smallpox vaccine made from human lymph; of 1289 vaccinees, 191 became jaundiced during succeeding months. In retrospect, one of the donors of the lymph used to make the vaccine must have been a hepatitis B virus carrier. In the first few decades of this century, the disease, which became known as serum hepatitis, was seen in recipients of antisyphilitic treatment and other types of injection therapy due to contamination of needles and syringes with patients' blood. Large outbreaks occurred in the late 1930s and early 1940s in recipients of yellow fever vaccine, which contained pooled human plasma to stabilize the yellow fever vaccine virus.[2] In 1943, Beeson described jaundice occurring several months after transfusions with blood or plasma.[3]

During the next 20 years, studies in volunteers and observations of recipients of blood transfusions provided the major advances in our understanding of posttransfusion hepatitis.[2,4-7] The volunteer studies provided information on virus size, stability, and titer; they also supported epidemiologic evidence that there were two viruses, which are currently termed hepatitis A virus for the agent of infectious or epidemic hepatitis and hepatitis B virus for the agent of serum or posttransfusion hepatitis.[4] The agents were shown to be immunologically distinct, since individuals who recovered from one were fully susceptible to the other; and, in the case of hepatitis A virus, immune serum globulin was shown to be useful for prophylaxis.

There was clearly an asymptomatic carrier state for hepatitis B virus, but not for hepatitis A virus, which tended to produce explosive outbreaks as a result of virus spread by contaminated food or water in the characteristic fecal-oral mode of transmission of enteric pathogens. Epidemiologic studies during this period demonstrated a much higher posttransfusion hepatitis risk associated with blood collected by commercial blood banks from paid donors than with blood collected from volunteer donors.[7]

Agents, Antigens, and Antibodies

Hepatitis B. In 1963, Blumberg and coworkers described a new antigen first found in the serum of an Australian aborigine, which they called Australia antigen.[8] They employed the agar gel immunodiffusion technique of Ouchterlony, using serum from multiply transfused hemophiliacs as a source of antibody, to find the antigen in patients with leukemia, Down's syndrome, and viral hepatitis.

Between 1968 and 1969, a series of reports by Prince, Okochi and Murakami, and others[9-12] established that the Australia antigen, now known as hepatitis B surface antigen (HBsAg), was closely associated with posttransfusion hepatitis. Within a few years it became clear that HBsAg was a component of hepatitis B virus (HBV), which was visualized by Dane and coworkers using electron microscopy in serum containing HBsAg.[13]

Hepatitis B virus is a DNA virus, 42 nm in diameter, with a nucleocapsid core and a lipoprotein coat (Figs. 36-1 and 36-2A). The nucleocapsid cores, 27 nm in diameter, replicate in the nuclei of infected hepatocytes (Fig. 36-3) and possess their own distinct antigenic specificity, termed hepatitis B core antigen (HBcAg).[14] The virion contains DNA polymerase activity and a circular, predominantly double-stranded DNA molecule.[15] The DNA molecule has a single-stranded region which accounts for about one quarter of its length and probably provides the template for the DNA polymerase.

The lipoprotein coat of HBV is produced in the cytoplasm of hepatocytes; it forms a 7-nm thick outer shell or surface component of the virus particles and carries the HBsAg specificity (Fig. 36-1). In acute and chronic hepatitis B infections, there is a massive excess of HBsAg produced over that which coats intact virus particles. Release of this excess HBsAg into the bloodstream may result in serum HBsAg levels of 10 μg/ml or higher, thereby making direct detection of HBsAg possible, even by the relatively insensitive immunodiffusion technique. HBsAg in serum is particulate, consisting predominantly of 20-nm diameter spherical particles (Fig. 36-2B) but also of filaments 20-nm in diameter and variable in length. Purified HBsAg contains carbohydrate, as well as protein and lipid, and has been split into seven polypeptides with HBsAg specificity.[16] Chronic hepatitis B carriers may have HBsAg particle counts in serum of 10^{13} or more per ml, and titrations of HBV in chimpanzees have revealed 10 to 100 million infectious HBV particles per ml of serum.[17] As a rule, the concentration of HBsAg particles in serum exceeds the number of infectious HBV particles by many thousand-fold.

HBsAg possesses a group or common antigenic determinant (*a*) and at least two allelic pairs of subtype determinants (*d/y*) and

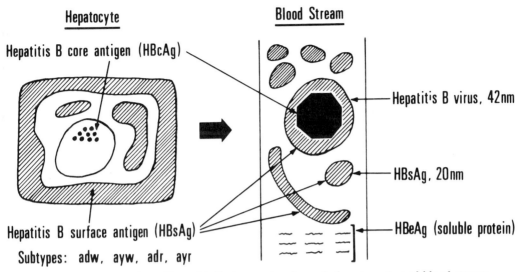

Fig. 36-1. Schematic drawing of hepatitis B virus and antigens in hepataocyte and blood stream.

(w/r).[18,19] Further antigenic analysis revealed four variants of the *w* determinants, two of which are associated with *ad* and all four of which are associated with *ay*. The subtyping of HBsAg has provided a valuable tool for epidemiologic studies, which have revealed pronounced geographic patterns of distribution and clustering in outbreaks.[20] The *adw* and *ayw* subtypes account for approximately 80 and 20 percent of HBsAg positive reactions, respectively, among U.S. volunteer blood donors.[21] The *adw* subtype predominates throughout North and South America, northern Europe, and Australia; *ayw* is the

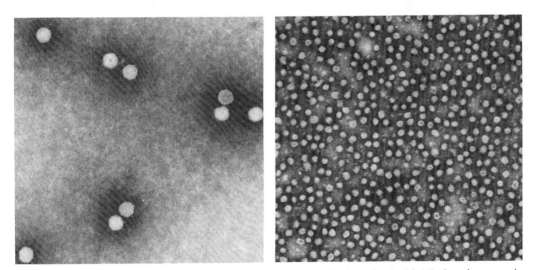

Fig. 36-2. (a) Electron micrograph of purified HBV virions negatively stained with 1% phospho-tungstic acid, 100,000× magnification. (b) Electron micrograph of purified hepatitis B surface antigen, 20 nm forms, negatively stained with 1 percent phospho-tungstic acid, 100,000× magnification; preparation is a sample of experimental hepatitis B vaccine. (Both figures kindly provided by Dr. John Gerin.)

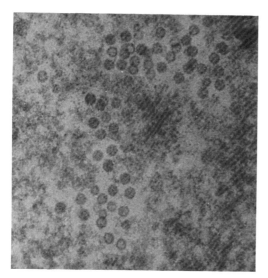

Fig. 36-3. Hepatitis B virus nucleocapsid core particles in the nucleus of hepatocyte in biopsy of an HBsAg carrier, stained with alcoholic uranyl acetate and counterstained with lead citrate, 84,-000× magification. (Figure kindly provided by Mr. Philip P. McGrath.)

commonest subtype in northern and western Africa, southeastern Europe, the Middle East, the Soviet Union, and the Indian subcontinent; and the *adr* subtype is predominant in Japan and much of southeastern Asia.[20] Clinical manifestations of hepatitis B do not appear to correlate with the subtype of the infecting virus, and there is evidence of cross-protection between subtypes, indicating that an immune response to the group antigen is adequate to provide substantial protective immunity.

A third antigen found in approximately 25 percent of sera containing HBsAg is termed the hepatitis B e antigen (HBeAg).[22] HBeAg usually appears transiently during acute hepatitis, but it often remains detectable in carriers with chronic active hepatitis.[23] Presence of HBeAg correlates with high HBsAg levels and high HBV infectivity.[24-26] Unlike HBsAg and HBcAg, which are integral parts of HBV virions, HBeAg is a soluble protein found separate from HBsAg and HBV particles. The exact nature of HBeAg is not clear, al-

though it may be present in a masked location in HBV particles and may be an enzyme or other product of HBV-infected cells which plays a role in viral replication or assembly. In some sera, it is also possible to detect the DNA polymerase specifically associated with HBV particles which, like HBeAg, is a useful marker for the presence of large numbers of infectious HBV particles in HBsAg positive serum.[24,25]

Antibodies against HBsAg (anti-HBs) and HBcAg (anti-HBc) develop in most people (80 to 90 percent) who recover from hepatitis B infections.[23,27-28] Anti-HBc is also present in almost all people with chronic hepatitis B infections, whereas anti-HBs is not usually detectable in these individuals.[28] In those HBsAg carriers who do have detectable anti-HBs, the subtype specificities of the coexisting HBsAg and anti-HBs have been found to differ. Multiply transfused patients such as hemophiliacs and thalassemics have a high prevalence of anti-HBs as a result of their repeated exposure to HBV-contaminated blood and blood products. Hyperimmunization by HBsAg is presumed to account for their high serum anti-HBs titers, which made their sera invaluable for the original detection of HBsAg by immunodiffusion. Anti-HBe is present in most HBsAg-positive sera which do not contain detectable HBeAg.

Over the years following the discovery that HBsAg was a specific immunologic marker for HBV infection, numerous serologic methods have been developed for detection of antigens and antibodies associated with hepatitis B. Table 36-1 provides a summary of these test methods and their relative sensitivity.[29,30]

Absence of a susceptible cell culture system has impeded the study of HBV infection and replication in vitro, although it has been possible to establish cell lines from hepatomas which support HBsAg production and provide a model for the study of HBsAg synthesis in vitro.[31] Chimpanzees are highly susceptible to HBV, however, and these animals develop the same biochemical, histologic, and

Table 36-1. Serological Methods for Detecting Hepatitis B Antigens and Antibodies

Method	Relative sensitivity[a] for detecting:				
	HBsAg	Anti-HBs	HBcAg	Anti-HBc	HBeAg and Anti-HBe
Solid phase radioimmunoassay	++++	++++	++++	++++	+++
Radioimmunoprecipitation	++++	++++		++++	
Enzyme-linked immunoassay	++++		++++	++++	+++
Reversed passive hemagglutination	+++				
Immune adherence hemagglutination	+++	+++	+++	+++	
Passive hemagglutination	++[b]	+++			
Reserved passive latex agglutination	++				
Immune electron microscopy	+++	+++	+++	++	
Immunofluorescence microscopy	++	++	+++	++	
Complement fixation	++	++	+	+	
Rheophoresis	++	++	+	+	+
Counterelectrophoresis	++	++	+	+	
Agar gel immunodiffusion	+	+			+

[a] Estimated relative sensitivity from least (+) to most (++++) sensitive.
[b] HBsAg detected by inhibition of passive hemagglutination.
(Gerety, R.J., Tabor, E., Hoofnagle, J.H., Mitchell, F.D., and Barker, L.F.: Tests for HBV-associated antigens and antibodies. In: Viral Hepatitis. Vyas, G.N., Cohen, S.N., and Schmid, R., eds. Franklin Institute Press, Philadelphia, 1978.
(Feinstone, S.M., Barker, L.F., and Purcell, R.H.: Hepatitis A and B. In: Diagnostic Procedures for Viral, Rickettsial and Chlamydial Infections, 5th Ed. Lennette, E.H. and Schmidt, N.J. eds. Am. Public Health Assoc., Washington, D.C., 1979.)

serologic changes indicative of acute and chronic HBV infection as seen in humans. Studies of hepatitis B in chimpanzees have provided data on many aspects of HBV behavior, such as virus infectivity, virus titers, virus physical properties, virus inactivation, safety testing of vaccines, efficacy of passive and active immunization, immunopathology, routes of virus transmission, and methods for attempting to treat or interrupt the virus carrier state.[32]

Hepatitis A. Hepatitis A virus (HAV) is a 27-nm RNA virus with many characteristics of enteroviruses. Its discovery by Feinstone, Kapikian, and Purcell using immune electron microscopy led to the rapid development of sensitive methods for antibody (anti-HAV) detection and extensive seroepidemiologic studies of type A hepatitis.[30,33] Several such studies revealed that HAV does not play an important role in the etiology of posttransfusion hepatitis, as serial bleedings from non-B hepatitis cases following transfusion consistently showed no evidence of HAV infection.[34-36] Viremia in type A hepatitis is generally of short duration, but it may precede the onset of clinical hepatitis.[37] Thus, it is possible to collect blood from a donor in the incubation period of type A hepatitis and transmit the virus to the recipient of the blood, if the blood is transfused before the donor develops clinical hepatitis and the blood bank learns about the donor's illness. This is a rare combination of events, and, since there does not appear to be a chronic carrier state for HAV, the risk of HAV transmission by blood transfusion is extremely low.

Hepatitis A virus infection can be transmitted experimentally to marmoset monkeys and chimpanzees. It is the only human hepatitis virus which has been propagated successfully in vitro in tissue culture.

Non-A, Non-B Hepatitis. The existence of an agent or agents other than HBV which cause many cases of posttransfusion hepatitis became increasingly clear with the application of sensitive methods for detecting HBV antigens and antibodies.[34-36,38,40] The diagnosis of non-A, non-B hepatitis will remain one of exclusion, however, until specific tests are available for the etiologic agent(s). Again, the chimpanzee model has proved invaluable in demonstrating that the sera of blood donors implicated in non-A, non-B transmission and patients with acute and chronic non-A, non-B hepatitis contain a transmissible agent.[41,42] Virus-like particles, 25 to 27 nm in diameter, have been found in material known to contain a non-A, non-B hepatitis virus, but it is not yet clear whether the visualized particles are the non-A, non-B agent.[43]

A precipitating antigen-antibody reaction has been described in acute and convalescent phase sera from patients and chimpanzees with non-A, non-B hepatitis, but it is not clear whether the antigen detected is specific for non-A, non-B hepatitis and, if so, whether it is a viral antigen like HBsAg or more like the HBeAg, which appears to be separable from HBV particles or their components.[44] A variety of nonspecific serum markers of non-A, non-B hepatitis, such as elevated liver enzyme levels, elevated carcinoembryonic antigen levels and antigen-antibody (immune) complexes, have also been described.[45] Specific immunologic markers for non-A, non-B hepatitis remain elusive at this time, however, so that most of our knowledge of the agent(s) comes from experimental studies in chimpanzees and from prospective studies of transfused patients (vide infra).

Observation of more than one acute episode of non-A, non-B hepatitis in patients has raised the possibility that there may be more than one etiologic agent or immunologically distinct non-A, non-B serotypes.[46] Two different kinds of cytopathology have been found by electron microscopic examination of the livers of chimpanzees infected with different inocula containing non-A, non-B agents,[47] but specific serologic tests will probably be required to determine whether there are multiple antigenic types or agents responsible for non-A, non-B hepatitis.

Clinical Features

Hepatitis B. Acute HBV infection may produce a wide spectrum of clinical manifestations, ranging from a totally asymptomatic course to severe, fulminant disease with a fatal outcome (Fig. 36-4).[48] Although recovery without sequelae is the rule in hepatitis B infections, chronic infection develops in 5 to 10 percent of adults and in a much higher percent of infants and young children.[23] Chronic HBV infection with circulating HBsAg may be asymptomatic with little or no liver function abnormalities and liver biopsy findings of mild chronic persistent hepatitis, or it may be more severe, with biopsy findings of chronic active hepatitis and possible progression to postnecrotic cirrhosis or hepatocellular carcinoma. Studies in countries with both a high and low incidence of hepatocellular carcinoma have revealed a strong

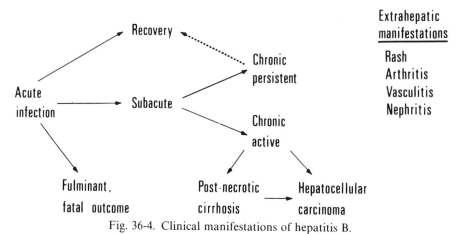

Fig. 36-4. Clinical manifestations of hepatitis B.

correlation between this malignancy and chronic hepatitis B infection.[49] A fulminant, fatal course of posttransfusion hepatitis B appears to be more common in elderly patients, whereas asymptomatic acute and chronic infections are particularly common in infants and children.

The first detectable abnormality in acute hepatitis B is usually the appearance of HBsAg in the patient's serum; the amount of infectious virus in the inoculum influences the interval between exposure and appearance of HBsAg, which may be as short as 2 weeks with a high-titer inoculum and as long as 3 or 4 months with a low-titer inoculum. Liver enzyme elevations, jaundice in some cases, and other signs and symptoms tend to appear close to the time of peak serum HBsAg levels, as shown in a schematic illustration (Fig. 36-5) of the typical course of events in an acute, self-limited case.[23] In self-limited acute hepatitis B infections, HBsAg remains detectable for a period ranging from a few days to several months. In most cases, anti-HBc becomes detectable during the acute illness, often while HBsAg is still present.[23]

Several types of extrahepatic tissue injury may occur in patients with hepatitis B. A transient, serum sickness-like prodromal phase manifested by a variable combination of rash, urticaria, polyarthralgia, and acute arthritis is the most common syndrome of extrahepatic manifestations of hepatitis B. The prodromal syndrome occurs a few days to a few weeks before jaundice and may also occur in anicteric cases. Typical polyarteritis nodosa with fever, rash, polyarthralgia, myalgia, and urticaria progressing to peripheral neuropathy, hypertension, and renal damage is a relatively uncommon extrahepatic manifestation of hepatitis B. There have also been cases of glomerulonephritis described in patients with chronic hepatitis B. In all of these syndromes, circulating immune complexes and deposits of HBsAg associated with immunoglobulin and complement at the sites of tissue injury provide persuasive evidence that the host immune response to HBV is responsible for the extrahepatic tissue damage and consequences.[50]

Anti-HBs generally becomes detectable after HBsAg disappears, but in some cases the appearance of anti-HBs, signalling recovery from the acute illness, may be delayed for many weeks or months after HBsAg becomes undetectable.[51,52] During this period, anti-HBc may be the only detectable marker indicating a recent HBV infection.[53] In some cases, neither HBsAg nor anti-HBs is detectable in the serum, using present methods, at any time during acute illness or convales-

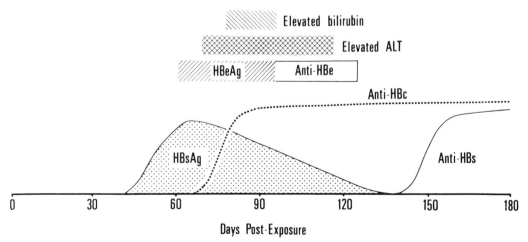

Fig. 36-5. Serological and biochemical events in acute hepatitis B.

cence. In such cases, appearance of anti-HBc may be the only indicator and is therefore the most reliable indicator that the patient experienced an HBV infection. In individuals who have had a prior HBV infection, reexposure may produce an anamnestic rise in anti-HBs titer without any evidence of reinfection, such as new appearance of HBsAg or a rise in anti-HBc titer.[52] These individuals are almost always protected against reinfection by their acquired immunity.

In chronic HBV infection, depicted schematically in Figure 36-6, HBsAg remains detectable for many years, perhaps for the entire life of the individual. Some individuals do recover from the chronic carrier state, however, so that life-long persistence of HBsAg is not inevitable in carriers. Anti-HBc is present in almost all chronic HBsAg carriers; those with high HBsAg titers may have HBeAg and DNA polymerase present, as well. Serum enzyme elevations and liver biopsy abnormalities characteristic of chronic persistent or chronic active hepatitis are common in carriers.[54] The carrier state develops most often in individuals who acquire their HBV infections early in life, particularly in the perinatal period, or at a time when they have depressed immune responses due to underlying diseases or immunosuppressive therapy. There are also many immunologically intact individu-als who become carriers, however, suggesting a selective tolerance for HBsAg.

Non-A, Non-B Hepatitis. Prospective studies of posttransfusion hepatitis in recipients of blood tested and found nonreactive for HBsAg by radioimmunoassay indicate that about 90 percent of the hepatitis cases under these circumstances are neither type A nor type B, so they are designated non-A, non-B (Table 36-2).[34-36,38-40] In early studies, prior to the introduction of routine HBsAg testing of all blood units, there were indications that HBV infection would not account for many hepatitis cases in transfused patients, as only 20 to 30 percent of the posttransfusion hepatitis cases in those studies could be shown to be type B.[10,45,55]

The clinical features of non-A, non-B hepatitis in transfused patients are similar in their protean nature to those of hepatitis B.[45] Table 36-3 provides a comparison of several features of these two forms of posttransfusion hepatitis from the prospective studies summarized in Table 36-2. The mean incubation period tended to be slightly longer for type B cases than for the non-A, non-B cases, and the proportion of icteric cases was slightly higher for the B cases. However, because the type B cases occurred in patients who received blood that was nonreactive for HBsAg by radioimmunoassay, it is likely that they

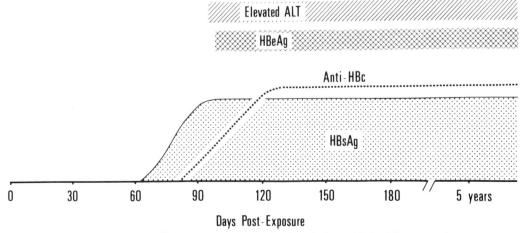

Fig. 36-6. Serological and biochemical events in chronic hepatitis B/HBsAg carrier state.

Table 36-2. Occurrence of Types B and Non-A, Non-B Posttransfusion Hepatitis in Prospectively Followed Recipients of Blood Tested for HBsAg by Radioimmunoassay

Study[a]	No. Transfused Patients	No. Hepatitis Cases (%) B	non-A, non-B	Total Cases (%)
A[39]	969	4 (0.4)	119 (12.3)	123 (12.7)
B[36]	595	10 (1.7)	65 (10.9)	75 (12.6)
C[40]	364	3 (0.8)	28 (7.3)	31 (8.5)
D[35]	388	3 (0.8)	27 (6.9)	30 (7.7)
Total	2316	20 (0.9)	239 (10.3)	259 (11.2)

[a] Blood used in studies A and B collected from both volunteer and paid donors; in studies C and D, from volunteer donors only.

were exposed to relatively low doses of HBV, and higher HBV doses might have produced shorter incubation periods and more icteric cases in the hepatitis B group. The acute form of non-A, non-B disease, then, may be somewhat milder than acute type B hepatitis, but both forms commonly lead to subacute or chronic sequelae. There are reports of more than one episode of non-A, non-B hepatitis in the same individual, but it is not yet possible to be sure whether these represent exacerbations and remissions of a chronic infection with periods of latency or serial infections with multiple non-A, non-B agents.[45,46]

In non-A, non-B hepatitis, chronic active hepatitis is inclined to follow anicteric acute episodes with high alanine aminotransferase (ALT, SGPT) levels and to resolve towards normal liver function tests over a period of a few years in most patients.[56] Whether or not chronic non-A, non-B hepatitis will lead to postnecrotic cirrhosis or hepatocellular carcinoma in some cases is not yet known, but present evidence suggests that the chronic

sequelae of non-A, non-B infections, although commonplace, are less severe than those of hepatitis B.

Blood Donor Testing and Epidemiology

Hepatitis B Surface Antigen Testing. Recognition that a positive serum test for HBsAg is diagnostic of acute or chronic hepatitis B virus infection and that HBsAg-positive blood has an overwhelming probability of carrying infectious HBV led to the rapid introduction of specific testing of donated blood.[29] The likelihood that identification and removal of HBsAg-positive units would reduce the risk of hepatitis B transmission by transfusion was first reported by Prince and by Okochi and Murakami; it was confirmed by additional studies that showed a much greater relative risk of type B hepatitis in recipients of HBsAg-positive blood than in recipients of HBsAg-negative blood.[9,10,12]

Table 36-3. Characteristics of Posttransfusion Hepatitis Observed in Prospectively Followed Recipients of Blood Tested for HBsAg by Radioimmunoassay

	Hepatitis B	Hepatitis non-A, non-B
Mean incubation period (weeks)[a]	11.8, 10.3, 16.6	8.4, 6.3, 8.2
Icteric cases[b] (%)	6/20 (30) (range 0–100)	45/239 (18.8) (range 0–31)
Chronic cases[b] (%)	7/20 (35) (range 0–33)	67/239 (28.1) (range 10–55)

[a] Incubation periods from studies A, B, and D in Table 36-2.
[b] Icteric and chronic cases from studies A, B, C, and D in Table 36-2.

In early 1971, as soon as standardized reagents were available in sufficient quantity for large-scale HBsAg testing, testing of every donated unit of blood or plasma became a legal requirement in the U.S. Initially, virtually all blood testing laboratories used the counterelectrophoresis method, which is somewhat more sensitive and rapid than the agar gel method used for the original discovery and studies of HBsAg (Table 36-1). Since mid-1975, the U.S. Food and Drug Administration has required that HBsAg testing of blood be done with one of the most sensitive and reliable available methods, termed "third generation." These methods presently include radioimmunoassay, enzyme-linked immunosorbent assay, and reversed passive hemagglutination (Table 36-1). The average, overall prevalence of HBsAg in blood collected from volunteer donors in the U.S. is approximately one per thousand, so that currently as many as 10,000 HBsAg-positive units may be detected among the 10 million-plus units collected annually from volunteer donors. In the American Red Cross from 1975 through 1978, 15,954 HBsAg-reactive units were detected among 19,140,169 units tested, giving a prevalence of 0.83 per 1,000 donations.[57] A number of studies found a 5 to 10 times higher prevalence of HBsAg-positive reactions in blood collected from paid donors by commercial blood banks than in volunteer donor blood.[36,39,40,58-60]

In studying the epidemiology of hepatitis B in blood donors, it is important to note that the prevalence of HBsAg-positive reactions is 3 to 9 times higher in first-time donors than in repeat donors.[57,60,61] Repeat donors have a lower prevalence of HBsAg because they are a selected population of individuals who have been previously tested for HBsAg, in contrast with first-time donors, who have not been previously tested. As the overwhelming majority of donors with HBsAg are chronic carriers, the lower HBsAg prevalence in the repeat donors largely reflects acute or newly acquired HBV infections in the donor population. Epidemiologic studies of factors that correlate with the chronic HBsAg carrier state in donors are therefore best conducted on first-time donors. Further valuable epidemiologic information can be obtained by testing donor blood for anti-HBs and anti-HBc. Presence of these antibody markers does not disqualify donors from repeat donations, so that these markers provide a more complete picture of a population's experience with HBV than would HBsAg testing alone.

Hepatitis B Epidemiology. The number of HBsAg carriers throughout the world has been estimated to be on the order of 120 million.[49] In the United States alone, there may be about 900,000 chronic carriers of HBsAg. The most extensively tested population of normal people in this country and elsewhere are those individuals who present themselves to be blood donors. The blood donor population cannot be considered as representative of the general population, but it has nevertheless proven of great value in providing numerous clues to the epidemiology of hepatitis B.

Studies of blood donors and other groups in the United States have provided many clues to risk factors for exposure to HBV and for persistence of HBV infection manifested by the HBsAg carrier state (Table 36-4).[49,61] In first-time donors, there is a one-and-a-half to three-fold higher HBsAg prevalence in males than in females, a higher prevalence in both sexes between the ages of 20 and 50 than below 20 or above 50, and higher prevalences among blacks and orientals than among whites. The age at which hepatitis B infection occurs is important, in that newborn infants and young children are far more likely to become chronic carriers than adults.[62] Transmission of hepatitis B is favored by close contact, so that families and institutions where there are infected individuals are high-risk settings for HBV infection.[63,64] Sexual partners of acutely infected individuals and newborn infants of infected mothers appear to be at particularly high risk. The risk for newborn infants is greatly increased when the serum of the HBsAg-positive mother also contains the HBeAg.[26] Siblings, parents, and other members of the household are also at

Table 36-4. Hepatitis B Risk Factors

A. *Increased Risk of Exposure*

Multiple transfusions of blood and plasma products

Other percutaneous exposure to blood or serum—e.g., tattooing, narcotics abuse

Sexual contact with an infected person

Household contact with an infected person

Lower socioeconomic class

Health care workers (medical, dental, laboratory)

B. *Increased Risk of Persistence*

Inherited or acquired decrease in immunologic responsiveness

Early age at time of exposure

Male sex

Race: Non-Caucasian

Genetic (?)

C. *Increased Risk of Exposure and Persistence*

Infants of infected mothers

Institutional care for retardation

high risk of infection, however, in families where one member of the household is a chronic carrier of HBsAg.[63]

Health care workers, either medical or dental, are in a setting where risk of exposure is greater than for the general population, and accidental needle sticks or other forms of inoculation as well as service in certain specialized areas, such as renal hemodialysis and oncology units, carry a particularly high risk. Multiple transfusions of blood or plasma are among the highest exposure risk factors, as are other forms of percutaneous exposure to infectious blood, including tattooing and illicit narcotics use.

Although the prevalences of anti-HBs and anti-HBc generally follow the same epidemiologic patterns as HBsAg, these antibodies are detected 30 to 100 times more frequently than HBsAg in various populations that have been tested for these hepatitis B markers.[49] In the case of sex, there are similar prevalences of anti-HBs in first-time male and female blood donors, contrasted with a higher prevalence of HBsAg in the males than in the females.[61] This finding suggests that males are more likely to develop chronic infections when exposed to HBV, and females are more likely to have self-limited infections. These sex differences support the hypothesis that ge-

netic factors may predispose infected people to develop chronic HBV infections. Attempts to link other genetic markers, such as red blood cell or HLA phenotypes, to the HBsAg carrier state have given mixed results which are inconclusive.[49]

Testing Donors for Non-A, Non-B Hepatitis. The absence of an established specific test for non-A, non-B hepatitis has impeded our understanding of the epidemiology of this form of hepatitis, which accounts for most posttransfusion cases in recipients of HBsAg nonreactive blood.[45] Prospective studies have shown that donor bloods with abnormal elevations of alanine aminotransferase (ALT) are associated with non-A, non-B hepatitis in recipients.[36] However, since ALT is not specific for non-A, non-B hepatitis, it is not surprising that many bloods with elevated ALT levels do not cause posttransfusioin hepatitis in recipients. Elevated levels of carcinoembryonic antigen (CEA) have been found in patients with non-A, non-B hepatitis,[65] but, in view of the nonspecificity of the CEA test and the number of conditions that cause CEA elevations, this test does not appear to provide a promising approach to donor screening for non-A, non-B hepatitis.

Of great interest are several immunologic tests which have given positive reactions in implicated donors and in transfused patients with non-A, non-B hepatitis. These include agar gel diffusion, counterelectrophoresis, radioimmunoassay, and immunofluorescence microscopy.[44,45] The practical applicability of these methods will remain unclear, however, until there is sufficient standardization and confirmation of their specificity to assure that they are useful for routine blood donor testing in order to detect and remove units of blood capable of transmitting non-A, non-B hepatitis.

Control of Posttransfusion Hepatitis: Status and Prospects

Risk Factors—Amount of Exposure. The prospects for better control of posttransfusion

Table 36-5. Posttransfusion Hepatitis Risk Factors

Source of blood: volunteer vs. paid donors

Markers in blood: HBsAg, (ALT)

Number of units transfused

High risk pooled plasma derivatives
    (Factor VIII, Factor IX concentrates)

(Hospitalization)

hepatitis can be analyzed by reviewing the major risk factors (Table 36-5) and considering what additional steps can be taken to reduce the risk. An important risk factor which has been identified in studies before and after the arrival of HBsAg testing is the number of units transfused. The increase in the attack rate of posttransfusion hepatitis as the number of units transfused increases is much less readily apparent when the blood comes from volunteer donors than when the blood is from paid donors.[39] Therefore, the judicious use of whole blood and components is of utmost importance in the prevention of posttransfusion hepatitis.

Certain plasma derivatives which contain coagulation factors and are made from large pools of plasma collected from thousands of donors carry a particularly high risk of transmitting hepatitis (Table 36-6). One such blood product, fibrinogen made from pooled plasma, has been removed from transfusion practice in the United States because the risk of posttransfusion hepatitis was judged to exceed the benefits associated with it.[66] In uncommon situations, such as congenital afibrinogenemia, where fibrinogen is considered

to be of therapeutic value, small pools of cryoprecipitate from single donations, which are rich in fibrinogen, are now recommended instead of the pooled plasma product. The use of small pools of plasma or plasma components to reduce the risk of posttransfusion hepatitis also applies to situations such as the need to reverse the effect of dicumarol for emergency surgery, where replacement of the prothrombin complex is a one-time or infrequent requirement. Severe cases of congenital Factor VIII or Factor IX deficiency are less amenable to posttransfusion hepatitis risk reduction by use of single-donor as opposed to pooled plasma products. These patients have a lifelong requirement for replacement therapy which inevitably results in eventual exposure to large numbers of donors. Thus, it is not surprising that comparison of groups of hemophilia cases after prolonged treatment with either cryoprecipitated antihemophilic factor from single donations or antihemophilic factor concentrates from pooled plasma have shown high prevalences of hepatitis B markers and liver enzyme elevations in the different groups.

Hospitalization without Transfusion. In one of the prospective studies of posttransfusion hepatitis, a control group of patients who were hospitalized but received no blood or blood products was followed to determine whether hospitalization alone was a risk factor that contributed to the total cases of hepatitis following blood transfusion.[36] During the study period, 2.2 percent of these hospital-

Table 36-6. Classification of Blood Components and Derivatives vis-à-vis Risk of Posttransfusion Hepatitis

1. High risk: Certain pooled plasma derivatives
       —Factor VIII (antihemophilic factor) concentrate
       —Factor IX (prothrombin complex) concentrate
       —Fibrinogen (no longer available)
2. "Average" or lower risk: whole blood and components of single units of blood or single-donor pheresis products
       —red blood cell concentrates
       —platelet concentrates
       —leukocyte concentrates
       —fresh frozen plasma
       —cryoprecipitated antihemophilic factor/fibrinogen
3. "Safe" plasma derivatives
       —normal serum albumin and plasma protein fraction (heated 10 hours at 60°C)
       —immune serum globulin and specific immune globulins

ized, nontransfused patients developed hepatitis. Of the 16 hepatitis episodes, one was asymptomatic, anicteric hepatitis B and the remaining 15 were anicteric cases of non-A, non-B hepatitis. As the hepatitis attack rate was 12.6 percent in the transfused patients (Table 36-2), it is clear that most episodes of hepatitis after transfusion are caused by viruses in the blood and blood products and are not due to other kinds of exposure during hospitalization.

Donor Testing and Selection. Presence of HBsAg in donor blood carries an overwhelming risk of posttransfusion hepatitis for the recipient; therefore, all donor units are now tested by one of the most sensitive available methods, and reactive units are not transfused. HBsAg-positive donors are interdicted from future donations because most are chronically infected and there is insufficient information on recovery from the chronic carrier state to know when such recovered donors' blood might be safe. Despite the universal application of sensitive HBsAg testing, there is still a residual risk of posttransfusion hepatitis B. Several studies have suggested that the presence of anti-HBc alone, in the absence of detectable HBsAg or anti-HBs, might identify some donors whose blood can transmit HBV.[67,68] In the case of non-A, non-B hepatitis, there is evidence of risk associated with bloods containing high ALT levels, as mentioned earlier. There are unanswered questions regarding the effectiveness, practicality, and reliability of the use of anti-HBc or ALT testing of donor blood, however, so that these approaches have not been adopted for routine use.

Permanent exclusion of prospective blood donors with a history of hepatitis was introduced as a measure to reduce the risk of posttransfusion hepatitis long before the availability of serologic tests for hepatitis B antigen and antibody markers. A study of prospective volunteer donors who were disqualified because of a positive history of hepatitis revealed a three-fold higher prevalence of hepatitis B markers when compared to a control group of donors with no history of viral hepatitis; the total prevalence of HBV markers was 19 percent in the former group and 6.3 percent in the controls.[69] In the prospective donors with a history of hepatitis, anti-HBs and anti-HBc are the most common hepatitis B markers, and their presence together is considered indicative of recovery from hepatitis B. Although 81 percent of prospective donors with a history of hepatitis do not have any hepatitis B markers, there remains a chance that donor exclusion based on a history of hepatitis is a useful measure for excluding some donors who have experienced non-A, non-B hepatitis and may be carriers of a non-A, non-B agent.

Exclusion of donors whose blood has been implicated in posttransfusion hepatitis cases following one- or two-unit transfusions is another long-standing practice which has been widely applied to attempt to reduce the risk of posttransfusion hepatitis. As in the case of donors with a history of hepatitis, a minority of such implicated donors (23 percent) were found to have any serologic markers of hepatitis B in one study, leaving 77 percent as possible transmitters of non-A, non-B hepatitis.[69] However, the fact that a great many cases of both type B and non-A, non-B hepatitis are asymptomatic and go unrecognized raises the likelihood that determination of either a history of hepatitis or of donor implication in posttransfusion hepatitis cases are of limited effectiveness. Specific markers for non-A, non-B hepatitis will be necessary for a more critical evaluation of these measures.

There are several other approaches to reducing the risk of posttransfusion hepatitis that are applicable to both hepatitis B and non-A, non-B. The need to select donors from low-risk population groups is fundamental to the effort to achieve an all-volunteer donor system, as commercial blood banks have traditionally recruited paid donors largely from the ranks of the unemployed and destitute members of the population. These paid donors have proven not only to have markedly higher prevalences of HBsAg, anti-HBs, and anti-HBc than volunteer donors, but also to be much higher-risk donors for transmission of non-A, non-B hepatitis.[36,39,40] In fact, in the absence of a reliable, specific test for non-A, non-B hepatitis, avoidance of paid donors from lower socioeconomic levels has been shown in multiple studies to be the best available means of lowering the non-A, non-B hepatitis risk of transfused blood. Avoidance of blood from high-risk paid donors already proved the most effective measure for lowering the risk of type B post-transfusion hepatitis, even with the availability of sensitive testing, which detects the majority of hepatitis B carriers in the donor population.[35,36,39,40]

Treatment of Blood and Blood Products. Washing of red blood cells to remove plasma or, in the case of frozen red cells, to remove plasma and glycerol, provides a method for reducing the level of hepatitis virus contamination in such red cell preparations. A study in chimpanzees of blood contaminated with a known amount of HBV showed that a standard red cell freezing and washing procedure did not remove all of the virus, although prolongation of the hepatitis B incubation period in the animals suggested that a substantial reduction in virus titer was achieved.[70] Although cell washing still holds some promise of improving the safety of red blood cells, the benefits would be lost in the event that the patient required other components such as platelet concentrates or plasma.

In addition, there have been efforts to apply various forms of physical and chemical treatment, particularly to the very high-risk plasma derivatives containing coagulation factors, to inactivate or remove the hepatitis viruses in these products. No satisfactory method has been established for this purpose, with the exception of heating albumin products for 10 hours at 60° C; such heating appears to be reliable when properly used for inactivation of HBV in albumin products, but it cannot be applied to the heat labile coagulation factor products. Although immuno-

globulin products prepared from pooled plasma are not subjected to any physical or chemical treatment other than cold ethanol fractionation, they appear to be generally free of infectious hepatitis B virus, with rare reported exceptions.[71]

Treatment of Viral Hepatitis. Experimental treatment of hepatitis with antiviral drugs and with biologicals such as interferon and transfer factor has been attempted in chronic carriers of hepatitis B.[20] Although there have been encouraging results reported with interferon and interferon inducers, this work is too preliminary to make any predictions about the future prospects for successful therapeutic intervention in cases of acute and chronic hepatitis.

PASSIVE AND ACTIVE IMMUNIZATION

Immunoglobulin in Hepatitis Prophylaxis

Hepatitis A. Immune Serum Globulin (ISG) is the official name for the nonspecific immunoglobulin product which is prepared by cold ethanol fractionation of large pools of plasma from normal donors. Testing of many batches of ISG has revealed that modest antibody titers against hepatitis A virus are always present, reflecting the high prevalence of anti-HAV in the adult population. Numerous studies over many years have demonstrated that administration of ISG before or shortly after exposure to HAV confers passive protection against clinical manifestations of type A hepatitis in 80 to 90 percent of exposed, susceptible persons.[72] Asymptomatic HAV infection resulting in long-lasting active immunization may occur under the passive protection provided by ISG. The recommended dose of ISG varies depending on whether it is being used for preexposure or postexposure prophylaxis. Prevention of illness in persons at risk of type A hepatitis is the most common indication for ISG administration; the other major indication is as replacement therapy for protection against infections in patients with both inherited and acquired immunoglobulin deficiency states.

Hepatitis B. The role of passive immunization in providing protection against type B hepatitis is much less clear than in the case of type A hepatitis. A number of studies of prophylaxis of posttransfusion hepatitis with ISG were done before the availability of tests for HBsAg and anti-HBs.[73] The results of these studies were generally not encouraging with regard to effectiveness, and ISG is not recommended for this purpose. In these studies, it was not possible to distinguish between hepatitis B cases and non-A, non-B cases or to determine the anti-HBs content of the ISG preparations that were tested.

Application of tests for anti-HBs makes it possible to select plasma from donors with high anti-HBs titers to manufacture the specific immunoglobulin product, Hepatitis B Immune Globulin (HBIG). This product is available from several licensed producers whose batches meet a uniform requirement for anti-HBs potency. Since the introduction of HBsAg testing led to elimination of all HBsAg-positive plasmas from plasma pools for fractionation, all current batches of ISG contain low titers of anti-HBs, on the order of 1:100 to 1:1000, in comparison with anti-HBs titers of 1:100,000 or greater in HBIG batches tested by sensitive methods such as radioimmunoassay or passive hemagglutination.

There are numerous possible clinical indications for administration of immunoglobulin to provide passive immunity against hepatitis B, but they fall into three major groups:

1. Postexposure prophylaxis.
2. Preexposure prophylaxis.
3. Treatment of acute or chronic hepatitis B.

Based on data from clinical trials, the best established indication for HBIG administration is postexposure prophylaxis after a single acute exposure to HBV, as may occur in an accidental inoculation (needle-stick), oral ingestion, or a splash with HBsAg-positive blood in hospital or medical laboratory settings. Three separate studies showed HBIG to be more effective than ISG in such postexposure prophylaxis situations.[74-76] In one of these studies,[76] appearance of cases 8 to 12 months after exposure in HBIG recipients but not in ISG recipients suggested that the HBIG effect was more to delay the onset rather than to prevent hepatitis B; another of the studies[74] showed partial protection from the ISG preparation when compared with no treatment at all. In the third study,[75] late cases did not occur in HBIG recipients, and the greater protective effect of HBIG than of ISG was particularly clear in individuals who were exposed to HBeAg-positive blood.[75] A fourth study of postexposure prophylaxis with HBIG[77] showed substantially better protection when the immunoglobulin was given in two separate doses—the first dose as close as possible to exposure and the second dose approximately one month later—than when the entire dose was given at the time of exposure. The Public Health Service Center for Disease Control has recommended postexposure prophylaxis following single acute exposure as the main indication for HBIG, to be given in two doses one month apart, and further recommended use of ISG in these situations if HBIG is not available.[72]

Postexposure prophylaxis has also been evaluated in spouses of acutely infected persons, in newborn infants of infected mothers, and in patients accidentally transfused with HBsAg-positive blood. Preexposure prophylaxis has been evaluated in several endemic settings, including renal dialysis units and custodial institutions for retarded children. Although there have been indications of HBIG efficacy in some of these studies, ISG containing lower levels of anti-HBs may be preferred in situations where prolonged exposure provides an opportunity to acquire active immunity under the protective cover of partial passive immunity.[72]

HBIG treatment has not proven to be an effective therapy in acute fulminant cases of hepatitis B or in the chronic hepatitis B carrier state. There is relatively little reported experience with the use of HBIG in patients who have received transfusions of HBsAg-positive blood by accident, but it is unlikely that HBIG would provide much protection in these uncommon misfortunes.

Non-A, Non-B Hepatitis. Although passive immunization may be of some value in protecting against non-A, non-B hepatitis, this possibility will be difficult to evaluate without specific tests for antibodies against non-A, non-B in immunoglobulin preparations to determine their potency and in exposed persons to determine their susceptibility. Nevertheless, in two randomized studies in which ISG or placebo was administered to transfused patients, there was a tendency towards reduced severity of non-A, non-B hepatitis in the ISG recipients as measured by incidence of icteric cases.[39,78] The studies did not produce evidence of an overall reduction in non-A, non-B hepatitis cases, most of which were anicteric. The use of passive immunization against non-A, non-B posttransfusion hepatitis is not currently recommended.

Active Immunization

In 1971, Krugman reported that active immunization against hepatitis B could be accomplished by injection of HBsAg-positive serum after boiling to destroy infectious HBV.[79] The recipients of this first experimental vaccine developed anti-HBs and protective immunity against type B hepatitis. Subsequently, experimental vaccines have been prepared by purifying HBsAg from carriers' plasma and treating this material with formalin to inactivate any live virus that might find its way into the product (Fig. 36-2A).[80,81] Tests of multiple batches of these experimental vaccines in chimpanzees have shown that the vaccines are free of infectious HBV, evoke substantial anti-HBs responses, and protect the animals against challenge with known amounts of infectious HBV.

Initial small-scale trials of these experimental inactivated hepatitis B vaccines in people have further established absence of infectious HBV in the preparations and provided data on the necessary dose and timing of injections to obtain anti-HBs responses in the majority of vaccine recipients. Large-scale trials in progress in several populations at high risk of acquiring hepatitis B will provide the ultimate test of the safety and effectiveness of experimental hepatitis B vaccines.[82] These trials are designed to compare experimental vaccines with placebo preparations in randomized subjects. The results of these studies will become known early in the 1980s.

In the event that inactivated hepatitis B vaccine proves to be safe and effective for preventing type B hepatitis, there are a number of high-risk groups that may benefit from active immunization (Table 36-4). Just how useful vaccination will be in preventing type B hepatitis in transfused patients remains to be determined. Patients who are at risk of severe posttransfusion hepatitis B because of factors such as their age or their need to be transfused with large numbers of units, including those patients who require prolonged replacement therapy with coagulation factors, will undoubtedly be among the candidates considered for active immunization against hepatitis B.

OTHER INFECTIONS TRANSMITTED BY TRANSFUSION

Malaria

Although naturally transmitted malaria has been eradicated in the United States, this serious protozoal infection is still endemic in many countries in Central and South America, Africa, and Asia.[83] Malaria in the United States, therefore, occurs almost exclusively in immigrants and visitors from endemic areas or in travelers returning to this country after exposure in endemic areas. Malaria poses two related problems in blood transfusion. The first problem is transmission of the disease by donor blood to transfused patients; this is a very uncommon complication of transfusion in malaria-free countries. The second problem is determination of the appropriate measures needed to avoid accepting blood donors who are likely to transmit malaria without rejecting an unduly large number of voluntary blood donors.

Parasites and Disease. The four species of malaria parasites that infect man—*Plasmodium falciparum, P. vivax, P. ovale,* and *P. malariae*—can all survive in refrigerated donor blood and have all caused cases of transfusion-induced malaria. A survey of approximately 1200 cases of transfusion malaria reported in the world literature between 1950 and 1970 revealed the following distribution in those cases where the diagnosis was known: *P. malariae,* 697 cases; *P. vivax,* 278 cases; *P. falciparum,* 60 cases; and *P. ovale,* 2 cases.[84] During the period from 1967 to 1971, there was a sharp increase in the incidence of transfusion malaria cases in the U.S., which accompanied a dramatic rise in the number of malaria cases with onset in this country to a peak of 4,247 in 1970 (Table 36-7).[83] Almost all of the latter cases occurred in military personnel returning from exposure in a maleria-endemic zone in Southeast Asia. At the same time that the incidence of transfusion malaria increased, there were a number of cases of the most malignant form of malaria, caused by *P. falciparum,* in contrast with earlier U.S. experience, in which most cases were relatively benign, caused by *P. malariae.*

The diagnosis of transfusion-related malaria should be considered in any patient who develops a spiking fever after receiving a transfusion containing red cells (including frozen and deglycerolized red cells), platelet concentrates, or even fresh frozen plasma, which may contain a few red cells. The fever may be synchronous, occurring at 48- to 72-hour intervals, or it may be asynchronous, as often happens in primary attacks. The incubation periods for 33 cases of transfusion malaria in the U.S. varied widely according to species and ranged from 6 to 106 days (Table 36-8).[85]

The paroxysmal fever of malaria, often accompanied by chills and other systemic symptoms, reflects the lysis of parasite-infected red blood cells and the release of free parasites into the bloodstream. Identification of the parasites in the blood provides the diagnosis. Falciparum malaria may have a rapid, lethal course, and drug-resistant strains have become common since their discovery in 1961. In the case of falciparum malaria, therefore, treatment must be provided immediately with the combination of drugs considered optimal at the time.[86] A three-day course of chloroquine is generally adequate treatment for the other forms of malaria.

Donor Selection and Prevention. All prospective blood donors are questioned regarding past history of malaria or recent travel or residence in areas where malaria is endemic. Travelers returning from malaria areas are deferred for six months—unless they took antimalarial drug prophylaxis, in which case they are deferred as blood donors for three years after discontinuing the drug. Immigrants or visitors from endemic areas are deferred for three years after leaving the en-

Table 36-7. Relationship of Transfusion Malaria Cases to Total Malaria Cases in U.S., 1961–1977

Years	All Malaria Cases		Transfusion Malaria Cases	
	Total	Average Number per Year	Total	Average Number per Year
1961–1965	673	134	4	0.8
1967–1971	17,040	3,408	32	6.4
1973–1977	1,879	376	9	1.8

Malaria Surveillance Annual Summary, 1977. Center for Disease Control. Issued July 1978.

Table 36-8. Incubation Periods for Transfusion Malaria

Species	Cases	Incubation in Days Average	(Range)
P. falciparum	12	16.0	(8–29)
P. malariae	9	57.2	(6–106)
P. vivax	10	19.6	(8–30)
P. ovale	1	23.0	—

demic area; subsequently they may be accepted, provided they have not had any malaria symptoms or received antimalarial treatment during the three-year period. Prospective donors with a history of malaria are deferred for three years after their last symptoms and cessation of therapy. Known malaria carriers or persons known to have had quartan malaria, caused by *P. malariae,* are permanently excluded.

The above procedures, if followed, should prevent transmission of any cases of the most dangerous and malignant form of malaria, as all reported cases of naturally acquired falciparum malaria have their onset within one month of exposure in individuals who are not on antimalarial prophylaxis.[85] Although asymptomatic cases of falciparum malaria may occur in residents of endemic areas and in persons on antimalarial prophylaxis, spontaneous recovery within one year is the rule; in such circumstances, persistence of asymptomatic *P. falciparum* beyond three years is considered most unlikely.[86] Although the onset of *P. vivax* infections may rarely occur more than six months after exposure in the absence of any antimalarial prophylaxis, and persistence of *P. vivax* and *P. ovale* may rarely extend beyond three years after recovery, transmission of either of these forms of malaria is highly unlikely if the donor selection rules are followed. The rules do leave a small risk, however, of *P. malariae* transmission, as this form may persist in the bloodstream. for many years without producing symptoms.

In the event that a case of transfusion malaria does occur, it is usually possible to identify the infected donor by indirect fluo-

rescent antibody testing after the fact. Many such donors give no history of malaria, but, with the exception of rare *P. malariae* cases, they have usually been accepted within a shorter time after exposure than the existing rules would allow.[85] The possibility that such errors will occur in donor selection underscores the importance of suspecting the diagnosis of malaria in patients who become febrile after blood transfusions.

Syphilis

The spirochete, *Treponema pallidum,* is incapable of surviving refrigerated storage in banked blood at 4 to 6°C or in plasma at −20°C for more than 48 to 72 hours.[87,88] This lability of *T. pallidum* is probably the major reason for the almost complete disappearance of syphilis transmission by blood transfusion since the introduction of modern blood banking storage procedures in the late 1930s. When blood was transfused shortly after collection from the donor and without refrigerated storage, transmission of syphilis was a serious and not uncommon complication.[89] Although a case of syphilis transmission by fresh platelet concentrates demonstrated the continuing risk of this complication associated with use of fresh blood components,[90] the move to an all-volunteer donor system in the U.S. has probably made a further contribution to lowering the risk of transfusion syphilis to the vanishing point.

During the period when refrigerated storage of blood was becoming standard practice, serological testing of donor blood for syphilis became mandatory practice in the U.S. The role of the serological test for syphilis (STS) in preventing transfusion syphilis has been questioned and is controversial for several reasons. In primary syphilis, the STS or reagin test is only positive in 25 percent of cases at the onset and 50 percent of cases by the second week; almost all cases are positive by the fourth week, but in some cases the reagin test remains negative in primary and later stages of definite treponemal infection.[91] As spirochetemia is most prominent in early primary syphilis, when the STS is frequently nonreactive, the fallibility of the test for preventing transfusion syphilis is readily apparent.

The STS or reagin test has another shortcoming when applied to large-scale testing of healthy people, and that is the preponderance of biologic false positive (BFP) reactions. In volunteer donors, these BFP reactions may account for 80 to 90 percent of positive reactions, in contrast with venereal disease clinics where the preponderance of positive STS tests are specific for *T. pallidum* infection. Furthermore, most BFP reactions in healthy volunteer blood donors are likely to be acute and transient. These acute BFP reactions are associated with a variety of benign conditions, such as a recent viral infection or immunization, or no apparent explanation in many instances, whereas chronic BFP reactions are sometimes associated with serious underlying chronic disease such as systemic lupus erythematosus and dysproteinemias.[92] The only known consequence of transfusing STS-positive blood or plasma after refrigerated storage for seven or more days is the transient appearance of reagin in the recipient.[89,93]

In view of the possibility of transmitting syphilis with STS-negative blood and the small likelihood of transmission by STS-positive blood after refrigerated storage, further consideration of the mandatory requirement to do STS testing on all blood units would seem appropriate. Although the risk of syphilis transmission by fresh components does exist, use of healthy volunteer donors is probably the best means of preventing this complication, just as is the case for posttransfusion hepatitis.

Other Viruses

Cytomegalovirus and Epstein-Barr Virus. Asymptomatic chronic infection with cytomegaloviruses (CMV) and Epstein-Barr virus (EBV), both members of the herpes virus family, is so common in healthy adults that these agents can almost be viewed as normal flora. Both CMV and EBV are viruses which survive best within cells and are thought to exist in latent form in the leukocytes of many, if not all, people with antibodies indicative of earlier infection.[94] EBV is the agent which causes infectious mononucleosis with a positive heterophil antibody response, and CMV is capable of producing a heterophil antibody-negative syndrome which closely resembles infectious mononucleosis in many other respects.

An infectious mononucleosis-like syndrome noted to occur one to two months after open-heart surgery has become known as the postperfusion syndrome or posttransfusion mononucleosis. Suspicion of a viral etiology of this syndrome led to investigations which implicated CMV in the more common, heterophil-negative cases of the postperfusion syndrome and EBV in less common, heterophil-positive cases.[95,96] Both agents have produced posttransfusion mononucleosis in the absence of extracorporeal perfusion, although transfusion of large volumes of relatively fresh blood appears to be a risk factor for the CMV-associated syndrome.

Attempts to isolate CMV from donor blood and thereby demonstate the carrier state in healthy donors have been generally unsuccessful, in contrast with a number of reports of CMV isolation from transfused patients with the mononucleosis-like syndrome.[94] EBV, on the other hand, is almost always found in lymphoblastoid cell lines established from the blood of healthy donors with antibodies to EBV.

The evidence for transmission of CMV and EBV by blood transfusion is most convincing when the recipient goes from a sero-negative state prior to transfusion to sero-positive accompanied by the mononucleosis-like illness several weeks posttransfusion. A common variation on this pattern, however, is the appearance of a rise in the antibody titer to CMV after transfusion without any symptoms or signs of illness. In these patients, the possibility exists that their own latent CMV infection has been activated by the blood transfusions or by other events such as treatment for their underlying illness or major surgery. Virus isolation and serology notwithstanding, it has been difficult to establish whether the antibody responses indicative of CMV infection in transfused patients with preexisting CMV antibodies are due to the introduction of exogenous virus or activation of endogenous virus.

Renewed interest in the transmissibility of CMV and EBV by blood transfusion occurred with the recognition of non-A, non-B hepatitis as the commonest form of posttransfusion hepatitis. Analysis of serial sera from prospectively followed, transfused patients who developed non-A, non-B hepatitis has revealed very few with serologic evidence of infection with CMV or EBV.[34-36] Therefore, although these agents are capable of producing liver damage which bears a close clinical resemblance to viral hepatitis, they do not appear to be responsible for more than a very small proportion of cases of non-A, non-B posttransfusion hepatitis.

Other Latent and Slow Viruses. Two chronic, lethal degenerative diseases of the central nervous system, kuru and Creutzfeld-Jakob disease (CJD) are clearly caused by transmissible agents which are presumed to be viruses, albeit atypical.[97] Kuru has only been recognized in the highlands of New Guinea, but CJD, which has numerous syn-

onyms, is found worldwide, as shown in a 1979 survey which described 1453 cases.[98]

Person-to-person transmission of CJD has occurred as a result of corneal transplantation in one case and from the use of intracerebral stereotactic electrodes in two other cases.[99,100] Although there is a possibility that these and similar agents may circulate in the bloodstream of healthy persons or persons who are incubating the diseases but are as yet asymptomatic, there is no evidence of transmission of these agents by blood transfusion to date. They, therefore, pose only a hypothetical hazard at present, but one which bears watching and will, like hepatitis B, be more amenable to scientific evaluation when specific tests are available to identify the agents and possible carriers.

Other Parasites and Bacteria

Trypanosomiasis. Chagas' disease is endemic in many countries in Central and South America. Chronic infection with *Trypanosoma cruzi* may be asymptomatic, in which case it can be diagnosed by a specific complement fixation (CF) reaction or other serologic tests. The CF test is positive in 4.7 to 9 percent of prospective donors in areas where it is used as a screening test.[84] Other measures used to reduce the risk of *T. cruzi* transmission by transfusion include refrigerated storage for 10 days or more and addition of gentian violet to the blood. The parasites can survive for several weeks in stored blood, however, and transmission by blood transfusion is considered a serious risk in endemic areas.[101]

African trypanosomiasis or sleeping sickness is less likely to be transmitted by blood transfusion because most patients have acute or chronic symptoms which would disqualify them as blood donors. There are some cases of chronic asymptomatic infection, and rare episodes of transmission of these parasites by blood transfusion have been reported.[101]

Leishmaniasis. Visceral leishmaniasis (kala-azar) occurs in parts of Central and South America, southern Europe, Africa, and Asia. The leishmania parasites may circulate in monocytes and polymorphonuclear leukocytes, but reports of transmission by blood transfusion are extremely rare.[101]

Toxoplasmosis. Serologic surveys have shown that infection with *Toxoplasma gondii* is commonplace throughout the world. Although the parasitemia is generally confined to the acute illness, *T. gondii* can persist in the bloodstream of asymptomatic, chronically infected individuals and can survive for many weeks in blood stored at 4 to 6 ° C.[101] Despite the potential risk of *T. gondii* transmission by blood transfusion, the only reported cases involved transfusions of leukocyte concentrates to patients with malignancies who were receiving chemotherapy, suggesting that heavy exposure of patients with depressed immune responses is necessary for this mode of transmission to occur.

Filariasis. Microfilariae circulate in large numbers in the blood of chronically infected people in the tropics and survive in refrigerated stored blood. Transmission of microfilariae by transfusion may produce allergic reactions in the recipients, but a passage of the microfilariae from man through an insect vector and back to man is necessary for development of the adult worms. Therefore, transmission of microfilariae is not a serious complication of blood transfusion.[101]

Bacteria. Although low-level bacterial contamination may be rather common in freshly collected blood, reports of transmission of bacteria by blood transfusion have been rare since the introduction of plastic blood containers with sterile plastic tubing and satellite containers. Bacterial contamination is probably most likely to result from the introduction of small cores of skin into the blood from the venipuncture site; airborne contamination of the needle, preexisting contamination of the collection set, or bacteremia in blood donors are other possible sources of contamination.

In the era of glass bottles for blood storage, there were a number of cases of severe, and sometimes fatal, reactions in patients transfused with blood which contained massive bacterial contamination. Gram-negative bacteria, particularly coliform and pseudomonas species, were the most common agents in fatal cases.[102] Although bacterial contamination remains a serious potential hazard, the bactericidal capacity of fresh blood stored in the refrigerator and even of platelet concentrates stored at 22 ° C appears to be adequate in almost all instances to eliminate bacteria from blood which is collected, processed, and stored in closed, sterile plastic containers.[103]

REFERENCES

1. Lürman, A.: Eine icterusepidemie. Berlin Klin Wschr 22:20, 1885.
2. Zuckerman, A.J.: The chronicle of viral hepatitis. Abstr. Hygiene. 54:1113, 1979.
3. Beeson, P.B.: Jaundice occurring one to four months after transfusion of blood or plasma. Report of seven cases. J.A.M.A. 121:1332, 1943.
4. Neefe, J.R., Stokes, J., Jr., and Gellis, S.S.: Homologous serum hepatitis and infectious (epidemic) hepatitis; Studies in volunteers bearing on immunological and other characteristics of the etiological agents. Am. J. Med. 1:3, 1946.
5. Neefe, J.R., Norris, R.F., Reinhold, J.G., Mitchell, C.B., and Howell, D.S.: Carriers of hepatitis virus in the blood and viral hepatitis in whole blood recipients. Studies on donors suspected as carriers of hepatitis virus and as sources of posttransfusion viral hepatitis. J.A.M.A. 154:1066, 1954.
6. Murray, R., Diefenbach, W.C.L., Ratner, F., Leone, N.C., and Oliphant, J.W.: Carriers of hepatitis virus in the blood and viral hepatitis in whole blood recipients. 2. Confirmation of carrier state by transmission experiments to volunteers. J.A.M.A. 154:1072, 1954.
7. Allen, J.G. and Sayman, W.A.: Serum hepatitis from transfusions of blood. J.A.M.A. 180:1079, 1962.
8. Blumberg, B.S., Alter, H.J., and Visnich, S.:

A "new" antigen in leukemia sera. J.A.M.A. 191:541, 1965.

9. Prince, A.M.: An antigen detected in the blood during the incubation period of serum hepatitis. Proc. Nat. Acad. Sci. 60:814, 1968.

10. Okochi, K. and Murakami, S.: Observations on Australia antigen in Japan. Vox Sang. 15:374, 1968.

11. London, W.T., Sutnick, A.I., and Blumberg, B.S.: Australia antigen and acute viral hepatitis. Ann. Intern. Med. 70:55, 1969.

12. Gocke, D.J., Greenberg, H.B., and Kavey, N.B.: Correlation of Australia antigen with posttransfusion hepatitis. J.A.M.A. 212:877, 1970.

13. Dane, D.S., Cameron, C.H., and Briggs, M.: Virus-like particles in serum of patients with Australia-antigen associated hepatitis. Lancet 1:659, 1970.

14. Almeida, J.D., Rubinstein, D., and Stott, E.J.: New antigen-antibody system in Australia-antigen-positive hepatitis. Lancet 2:1225, 1971.

15. Robinson, W.S.: Genome of hepatitis B virus. Ann. Microbiol. 31:357, 1977.

16. Shih, J.W-K. and Gerin, J.L.: Proteins of hepatitis B surface antigen. J. Virol. 21:347, 1977.

17. Barker, L.F., Maynard, J.E., Purcell, R.H., Hoofnagle, J.H., Berquist, K.R., London, W.T., Gerety, R.J., and Krushak, D.H.: Hepatitis B virus infection in chimpanzees: titration of subtypes. J. Infect. Dis. 132:451, 1975.

18. Le Bouvier, G.L.: The heterogeneity of Australia antigen. J. Infect. Dis. 123:671, 1971.

19. Bancroft, W.H., Mundon, F.K., and Russell, P.K.: Detection of additional antigenic determinants of hepatitis B antigen. J. Immunol. 109:842, 1972.

20. Advances in Viral Hepatitis. WHO Tech. Rep. Ser. 602, WHO, Geneva, 1977.

21. Dodd, R.Y., Holland, P.V., Ni, L.Y., Smith, H.M., and Greenwalt, T.J.: Regional variation in incidence and subtype ratio in the American Red Cross donor population. Am. J. Epidemiol. 97:111, 1973.

22. Magnius, L. and Espmark, J.A.: New specificities in Australia antigen positive sera distinct from the Le Bouvier determinants. J. Immunol. 109:1017, 1972.

23. Krugman, S., Overby, L.R., Mushahwar, I.K., Ling, C-M., Frösner, G.G., and Dein-hardt, F.: Viral hepatitis, type B. Studies on natural history and prevention re-examined. N. Engl. J. Med. 300:101, 1979.

24. Hindman, S.H., Gravelle, C.R., Murphy, B.L., Bradley, D.W., Budge, W.R., and Maynard, J.E.: "e" antigen, Dane particles, and serum DNA polymerase activity in HBsAg carriers. Ann. Intern. Med. 85:458, 1976.

25. Alter, H.J., Seeff, L.B., Kaplan, P.M., McAuliffe, V.J., Wright, E.C., Gerin, J.L., Purcell, R.H., Holland, P.V., and Zimmerman, H.J.: Type B hepatitis: the infectivity of blood positive for e antigen and DNA polymerase after accidental needlestick exposure. N. Engl. J. Med. 295:909, 1976.

26. Okada, K., Kamiyama, I., Inomata, M., Imai, M., Miyakawa, Y., and Mayumi, M.: e antigen and anti-e in the serum of asymptomatic carrier mothers as indicators of positive and negative transmission of hepatitis B virus to their infants. N. Engl. J. Med. 294:746, 1976.

27. Lander, J.J., Alter, H.J., and Purcell, R.H.: Frequency of antibody to hepatitis-associated antigen as measured by a new radioimmunoassay technique. J. Immunol. 106:1166, 1971.

28. Hoofnagle, J.H., Gerety, R.J., and Barker, L.F.: Antibody to hepatitis B virus core in man. Lancet 2:869, 1973.

29. Gerety, R.J., Tabor, E., Hoofnagle, J.H., Mitchell, F.D., and Barker, L.F.: Tests for HBV-associated antigens and antibodies. In: Viral Hepatitis. Vyas, G.N., Cohen, S.N., and Schmid, R., eds. Franklin Institute Press, Philadelphia, 1978, p. 121.

30. Feinstone, S.M., Barker, L.F., and Purcell, R.H.: Hepatitis A and B. In: Diagnostic Procedures for Viral, Rickettsial and Chlamydial Infections, 5th Ed. Lennette, E.H. and Schmidt, N.J., eds. Am. Public Health Assoc., Washington, D.C., 1979, p. 879.

31. Aden, D.P., Fogel, A., Plotkin, S., Damjanov, I., and Knowles, B.B.: Controlled synthesis of HBsAg in a differentiated human liver carcinoma-derived cell line. Nature 282:615, 1979.

32. Barker, L.F., Maynard, J.E., Purcell, R.H., Hoofnagle, J.H., Berquist, K.R., and London, W.T.: Viral hepatitis, type B, in experi-

mental animals. Am. J. Med. Sci. 270:189, 1975.

33. Feinstone, S.M., Kapikian, A.Z., and Purcell, R.H.: Hepatitis A detection by immune electron microscopy of a virus-like antigen associated with acute illness. Science 182:1026, 1973.

34. Feinstone, S.M., Kapikian, A.Z., Purcell, R.H., Alter, J., and Holland, P.V.: Transfusion-associated hepatitis not due to viral hepatitis Type A or B. N. Engl. J. Med. 292:767, 1975.

35. Alter, H.J., Purcell, R.H., Feinstone, S.M., Holland, P.V., and Morrow, A.G.: Non-A, non-B hepatitis: a review and interim report of an ongoing prospective study. In: Viral Hepatitis. Vyas, G.N., Cohen, S.N., and Schmid, R., eds. Franklin Institute Press, Philadelphia, 1978, p. 359.

36. Aach, R.D., Lander, J.J., Sherman, L.A., Miller, W.V., Kahn, R.A., Gitnick, G.L., Hollinger, F.B., Werch, J., Szmuness, W., Stevens, C.E., Kellner, A., Weiner, J.M., and Mosley, J.W.: Transfusion-transmitted viruses: interim analysis of hepatitis among transfused and nontransfused patients. In: Viral Hepatitis. Vyas, G.N., Cohen, S.N., and Schmid, R., eds. Franklin Institute Press, Philadelphia, 1978, p. 383.

37. Krugman, S., Ward, R., and Giles, J.P.: The natural history of infectious hepatitis. Am. J. Med. 32:717, 1962.

38. Prince, A.M., Brotman, B., Grady, G.F., Kuhns, W.J., Hazzi, C., Levine, R.W., and Millian, S.J.: Post-transfusion viral hepatitis caused by an agent or agents other than hepatitis B virus or hepatitis A virus. Impact on efficiency of present screening methods. In: Transmissible Disease and Blood Transfusion. Greenwalt, T.J. and Jamieson, G.A., eds. Grune and Stratton, New York, 1975, p. 129.

39. Seeff, L.B., Wright, E.C., Zimmerman, H.Z., Hoofnagle, J.H., Dietz, A.A., Felsher, B.F., Garcia-Pont, P.H., Gerety, R.J., Greenlee, H.B., Kiernan, T., Leevy, C.M., Nath, N., Schiff, E.R., Schwartz, C., Tabor, E., Tamburro, C., Vlahcevic, Z., Zemel, R., and Zimmon, D.S.: Posttransfusion hepatitis, 1973-1975: a Veterans Administration Cooperative Study. In: Viral Hepatitis. Vyas, G.N., Cohen, S.N., and Schmid, R., eds.

Franklin Institute Press, Philadelphia, 1978, p. 371.

40. Goldfield, M., Bill, J., and Colosimo, F.: The control of transfusion-associated hepatitis. In: Viral Hepatitis. Vyas, G.N., Cohen, S.N., and Schmid, R., eds. Franklin Institute Press, Philadelphia, 1978, p. 405.

41. Alter, H.J., Purcell, R.H., Holland, P.V., and Popper, H.: Transmissible agent in non-A, non-B hepatitis. Lancet 1:459, 1978.

42. Tabor, E., Gerety, R.J., Drucker, J.A., Seeff, L.B., Hoofnagle, J.H., Jackson, D.R., April, M., Barker, L.F., and Tamondong, G.P.: Transmission of non-A, non-B hepatitis from man to chimpanzee. Lancet 1:463, 1978.

43. Bradley, D.W., Cook, E.H., Maynard, J.E., McCausland, K.A., Ebert, J.W., Dolana, G.H., Petzel, R.A., Kantor, R.J., Heilbrunn, A., Fields, H.A., and Murphy, B.L.: Experimental infection of chimpanzees with antihemophilic (Factor VIII) materials: recovery of virus-like particles associated with non-A, non-B hepatitis. J. Med. Virol. 2:253, 1979.

44. Shirachi, R., Shiraishi, H., Tateda, A., Kikuchi, K., and Ishida, N.: Hepatitis "C" antigen in non-A, non-B, posttransfusion hepatitis. Lancet 2:853, 1978.

45. Aach, R.D. and Kahn, R.A.: Posttransfusion hepatitis. Current perspectives. Ann. Intern. Med. 92:539, 1980.

46. Mosley, J.W., Redeker, A.G., Feinstone, S.M., and Purcell, R.H.: Multiple hepatitis viruses in multiple attacks of acute viral hepatitis. N. Engl. J. Med. 296:75, 1977.

47. Shimizu, Y.K., Feinstone, S.M., Purcell, R.H., Alter, H.J., and London, W.T.: Non-A, non-B hepatitis: Ultrastructural evidence for two agents in experimentally infected chimpanzees. Science 205:197, 1979.

48. Redeker, A.G.: Viral hepatitis: clinical aspects. Am. J. Med. Sci. 270:9, 1975.

49. Szmuness, W.: Recent advances in the study of the epidemiology of hepatitis B. Am. J. Pathol. 81:629, 1975.

50. Gocke, D.J.: Immune complex phenomena associated with hepatitis. In: Viral Hepatitis. Vyas, G.N., Cohen, S.N., and Schmid, R., eds. Franklin Institute Press, Philadelphia, 1978, p. 277.

51. Lander, J.J., Holland, P.V., Alter, H.J., Chanock, R.M., and Purcell, R.H.: Antibody to hepatitis-associated antigen. Frequency

and pattern of response as detected by radioimmunoprecipitation. J.A.M.A. 220:1079, 1972.

52. Barker, L.F., Peterson, M.R., Shulman, N.R., and Murray, R.: Antibody responses in viral hepatitis, type B. J.A.M.A. 223:1005, 1973.

53. Hoofnagle, J.H., Gerety, R.J., Ni, L.Y., and Barker, L.F.: Antibody to hepatitis B core antigen: a sensitive indicator of hepatitis B virus replication. N. Engl. J. Med. 290:1336, 1974.

54. Klatskin, G.: Persistent HB antigenemia: associated clinical manifestations and hepatic lesions. Am. J. Med. Sci. 270:33, 1975.

55. Gocke, D.J.: A prospective study of post-transfusion hepatitis. The role of Australia antigen. J.A.M.A. 219:1165, 1972.

56. Berman, M., Alter, H.J., Ishak, K.G., Purcell, R.H., and Jones, E.A.: The chronic sequelae of non-A, non-B hepatitis. Ann. Intern. Med. 91:1, 1979.

57. Baastians, M.J.S., Dodd, R.Y., Nath, N., Pineda-Tamondong, G., Sandler, S.G., and Barker, L.F.: Hepatitis-associated markers in the American Red Cross volunteer blood donor population. I. Trends in HBsAg detection, 1975 to 1978. Vox Sang. (in press, 1980).

58. Kliman, A.: Australia antigen in volunteer and paid blood donors. N. Engl. J. Med. 284:109, 1971.

59. Cherubin, C.E. and Prince, A.M.: Serum hepatitis specific antigen (SH) in commercial and volunteer sources of blood. Transfusion 11:25, 1971.

60. Szmuness, W., Prince, A.M., Brotman, B., and Hirsch, R.L.: Hepatitis B antigen and antibody in blood donors: an epidemiologic study. J. Infect. Dis. 127:17, 1973.

61. Szmuness, W., Hirsch, R.L., Prince, A.M., Levine, R.W., Harley, E.J., and Ikram, H.: Hepatitis B surface antigen in blood donors: further observations. J. Infect. Dis. 131:111, 1975.

62. Schweitzer, I.L.: Vertical transmission of hepatitis B surface antigen. Am. J. Med. Sci. 270:287, 1975.

63. Szmuness, W., Prince, A.M., Hirsch, R.L., and Brotman, B.: Familial clustering of hepatitis B infection. N. Engl. J. Med. 289:1162, 1973.

64. Szmuness, W. and Prince, A.M.: The epidemiology of serum hepatitis (SH) infections: a controlled study in two closed institutions. Am. J. Epidemiol. 94:585, 1971.

65. Gitnick, G.L., Brezina, M.L., and Mullen, R.L.: Application of alanine aminotransferase, carcinoembryonic antigen and cholyl glycine levels to the prevention and evaluation of acute and chronic hepatitis. In: Viral Hepatitis. Vyas, G.N., Cohen, S.N., and Schmid, R., eds. Franklin Institute Press, Philadelphia, 1978, p. 431.

66. Bove, J.: Fibrinogen—is the benefit worth the risk? Transfusion 18:129, 1978.

67. Lander, J.J., Gitnick, G.L., Gelb, L.H., and Aach, R.D.: Anticore antibody screening of transfused blood. Vox Sang. 34:77, 1978.

68. Hoofnagle, J.H., Seeff, L.B., Bales, Z.B., and Zimmerman, H.J.: Type B hepatitis after transfusion with blood containing antibody to hepatitis B core antigen. N. Engl. J. Med. 298:1379, 1978.

69. Tabor, E., Hoofnagle, J.H., Smallwood, L.A., Drucker, J.A., Pineda-Tamondong, G.C., Ni, L.Y., Greenwalt, T.J., Barker, L.F., and Gerety, R.J.: Studies of donors who transmit posttransfusion hepatitis. Transfusion 19:725, 1979.

70. Alter, H.J., Tabor, E., Meryman, H.T., Hoofnagle, J.H., Kahn, R.A., Holland, P.V., Gerety, R.J., and Barker, L.F.: Transmission of hepatitis B virus infection by transfusion of frozen-deglycerolized red blood cells. N. Engl. J. Med. 298:637, 1978.

71. Tabor, E. and Gerety, R.J.: Transmission of hepatitis B by immune serum globulin. Lancet 2:1293, 1979.

72. Immune globulins for protection against viral hepatitis. Morbidity and Mortality Weekly Report 26:425. Center for Disease Control, 1977.

73. Ginsberg, A.L.: Immune serum globulin for the prevention of posttransfusion hepatitis: a reassessment after 30 years of controversy. In: Viral Hepatitis. Vyas, G.N., Cohen, S.N., and Schmid, R., eds. Franklin Institute Press, Philadelphia, 1978, p. 477.

74. Krugman, S., Giles, J.P., and Hammond, J.: Viral hepatitis, type B (MS-2 strain): prevention with specific hepatitis B immune serum globulin. J.A.M.A. 218:1665, 1971.

75. Seeff, L.B., Wright, E.C., Zimmerman, H.J., Alter, H.J., Dietz, A.A., Felsher, B.F., Fin-

kelstein, J.D., Garcia-Pont, P., Gerin, J.L., Greenlee, H.B., Hamilton, J., Holland, P.V., Kaplan, P.M., Kiernan, T., Koff, R.S., Leevy, C.M., McAuliffe, V.J., Nath, N., Purcell, R.H., Schiff, E.R., Schwartz, C.C., Tamburro, C.H., Vlahcevic, Z., Zemel, R., and Zimmon, D.S.: Type B hepatitis after needle-stick exposure: prevention with hepatitis B immune globulin. Ann. Intern. Med. 88:285, 1978.

76. Grady, G.F., Lee, V.A., Prince, A.M., Gitnick, G.L., Fawaz, K.A., Vyas, G.N., Levitt, M.D., Senior, J.R., Galambos, J.T., Bynum, T.E., Singleton, J.W., Clowdus, B.F., Akdamar, K., Aach, R.D., Winkelman, E.I., Schiff, G.M., and Hersh, T.: Hepatitis B immune globulin for accidental exposures among medical personnel: final report of a multicenter controlled trial. J. Infect. Dis. 138:625, 1978.

77. Klein, H.G., Alter, H.J., and Holland, P.V.: Postexposure immunoglobulin prophylaxis of hepatitis B: a comparison of two dosage schedules. In: Viral Hepatitis. Vyas, G.N., Cohen, S.N., and Schmid, R., eds. Franklin Institute Press, Philadelphia, 1978, p. 483.

78. Knodell, R.G., Conrad, A.L., Ginsberg, M.E., Bell, C.J., and Flannery, E.P.: Efficacy of prophylactic gamma-globulin in preventing non-A, non-B posttransfusion hepatitis. Lancet 1:1557, 1976.

79. Krugman, J., Giles, J.P., and Hammond, J.: Viral hepatitis, type B (MS-2 strain): studies on active immunization. J.A.M.A. 217:41, 1971.

80. Buynak, E.B., Roehm, R.R., Tytell, A.A., Bertland, A.U., Lampson, G.P., and Hilleman, M.R.: Vaccine against human hepatitis B. J.A.M.A. 235:2832, 1976.

81. Purcell, R.H. and Gerin, J.L.: Hepatitis B vaccines: On the threshold. Am. J. Clin. Pathol. 70:159, 1978.

82. Szmuness, W.: Large-scale efficacy trials of hepatitis B vaccines in the USA: baseline data and protocols. J. Med. Virol. 4:327, 1979.

83. Malaria Surveillance Annual Summary, 1977. Center for Disease Control. Issued July 1978.

84. Bruce-Chwatt, L.J.: Blood transfusion and tropical disease. Trop. Dis. Bull. 69:825, 1972.

85. Dover, A.S. and Schultz, M.G.: Transfusion-induced malaria. Transfusion 11:353, 1971.

86. Miller, L.H.: Transfusion malaria. In: Transmissible Disease and Blood Transfusion. Greenwalt, T.J. and Jamieson, G.A., eds. Grune and Stratton, New York, 1975, p. 241.

87. Turner, T.B. and Diseker, T.H.: Duration of infectivity of Treponema pallidum in citrated blood stored under conditions obtaining in blood banks. Bull. Johns Hopkins Hosp. 68:269, 1941.

88. Ravitch, M.M. and Chambers, J.W.: Spirochaetal survival in frozen plasma. Bull. Johns Hopkins Hosp. 71:299, 1942.

89. Ravitch, M.M., Farmer, T.W., and Davis, B.: Use of blood donors with positive serologic tests for syphilis—with a note on the disappearance of passively transferred reagin. J. Clin. Invest. 28:18, 1949.

90. Chambers, R.W., Foley, H.T., and Schmidt, P.J.: Transmission of syphilis by fresh blood components. Transfusion 9:32, 1969.

91. Spangler, A.S., Jackson, J.H., Fiumara, N.J., and Warthin, T.A.: Syphilis with a negative blood test reaction. J.A.M.A. 189:87, 1964.

92. Catterall, R.D.: Systemic disease and the biological false positive reaction. Br. J. Vener. Dis. 48:1, 1972.

93. Walker, R.H.: The disposition of STS reactive blood in a transfusion service. Transfusion 5:452, 1965.

94. Lang, D.L.: Transfusion and perfusion-associated cytomegalovirus and Epstein-Barr virus infections: Current understanding and investigations. In: Transmissible Disease and Blood Transfusion. Greenwalt, T.J. and Jamieson, G.A., eds. Grune and Stratton, New York, 1975, p. 153.

95. Kaariainen, L., Klemola, E., and Paloheimo, J.: Rise of cytomegalovirus antibodies in an infectious-mononucleosis-like syndrome after transfusion. Br. Med. J. 1:1270, 1966.

96. Gerber, P., Walsh, J.H., and Rosenblum, E.N.: Association of EB-virus infection with the post-perfusion syndrome. Lancet 1:593, 1969.

97. Herzberg, L., Gibbs, C.J., Asher, D.M., Gajdusek, D.C., and French, E.L.: Slow, latent, and chronic viral infections of the central nervous system. In: Transmissible Disease

and Blood Transfusion. Greenwalt, T.J. and Jamieson, G.A., eds. Grune and Stratton, New York, 1975, p. 197.

98. Masters, C.L., Harris, J.O., Gajdusek, C., Gibbs, C.J., Bernoulli, C., and Asher, D.M.: Creutzfeld-Jakob disease: patterns of worldwide occurrence and the significance of familial and sporadic clustering. Ann. Neurol. 5:177, 1979.

99. Duffy, P., Wolf, J., Collins, G., Devoe, A.G., and Streeter, B.: Possible person-to-person transmission of Creutzfeld-Jakob disease. N. Engl. J. Med. 290:692, 1974.

100. Bernoulli, C., Siegfried, J., Baumgartner, G., Regli, F., Rabinowicz, T., Gajdusek, D.C., and Gibbs, C.J.: Danger of accidental person-to-person transmission of Creutzfeld-Jakob disease by surgery. Lancet 1:478, 1977.

101. Wolfe, M.S.: Parasites other than malaria, transmissible by blood transfusion. In: Transmissible Disease and Blood Transfusion. Greenwalt, T.S. and Jamieson, G.A., eds. Grune and Stratton, New York, 1975, p. 267.

102. Pittman, M.: A study of bacteria implicated in transfusion reactions and bacteria isolated from blood products. J. Lab. Clin. Med. 42:273, 1953.

103. Myhre, B.A., Walker, L.J., and White, M.L.: Bacteriocidal properties of platelet concentrates. Transfusion 14:116, 1974.

37

Other Adverse Effects of Transfusion

Paul V. Holland, M.D.

INTRODUCTION

While transfusion of blood and its components is usually a safe and effective, albeit temporary, form of therapy, untoward effects can occur. These adverse effects are usually called transfusion reactions, but this term does not cover all of the potentially deleterious effects which may accompany the admininistration of blood or blood products. Some of the adverse effects are preventable but some cannot be avoided. Thus, every physician should be aware of the possible and probable risks of blood transfusions and weigh these against the potential therapeutic benefits.

This chapter deals with adverse effects of transfusion other than disease transmission. The types of adverse reactions are subdivided here according to whether they are immediate or delayed, and whether they are immunologically mediated or not. Each adverse effect is discussed in terms of its etiology, its treatment, and possible preventive measures. In addition, this chapter will attempt to answer such questions as: What clinical findings merit a detailed workup for the manifold causes of adverse effects of transfusion? When should the blood transfusion be stopped, and can it be restarted? What are the relative merits of different modes of treatment for certain types of reactions—e.g., the

usefulness of fluids, various diuretic agents, and heparin in patients undergoing a hemolytic transfusion reaction?

EVALUATION OF SUSPECTED ADVERSE EFFECTS OF A TRANSFUSION

When any unexpected or untoward sign or symptom occurs during or shortly after a transfusion of blood or one of its components, consider that it might have been caused by the blood product, until proven otherwise. Only a high index of suspicion will allow adverse reactions to be diagnosed. In general, stopping the transfusion to minimize the amount of blood infused will also minimize the adverse effect, and may obviate some of the potentially disastrous consequences. *So, the first rule is stop the transfusion.* But the corollary is: *Keep the intravenous line open with a slow infusion of normal saline (0.9% NaCl).* If the patient's signs or symptoms are not due to the transfusion, it can be restarted. Or, if urticaria (hives) is the *only* adverse manifestation of the transfusion, infusion of the blood product can be resumed after administration of an antihistaminic drug.

One of the most devastating adverse effects

Table 37-1. Initial Signs and Symptoms of a Hemolytic Transfusion Reaction

Mild	Major
Fever	Dyspnea
Chills	Chest pain
Back pain	Hemoglobinemia
Flushing	Hemoglobinuria
Hypotension	Oliguria or Anuria
	Shock
	Generalized oozing

of a transfusion is acute intravascular hemolysis. This dreaded reaction is usually heralded by a fever, with or without chills, but can initially be manifested by a variety of symptoms (Table 37-1). The physician's first efforts should be directed at ruling this diagnosis in or out. If a hemolytic transfusion reaction is not occurring, then a less urgent approach to the patient's transfusion problem can be undertaken. If the patient is undergoing a hemolytic reaction, prompt diagnosis and therapy may be life-saving. To immediately rule a hemolytic transfusion reaction in or out, a carefully drawn, anticoagulated sample of blood from the patient should be evaluated for (1) evidence of free hemoglobin in the plasma, and (2) antibody coated on the red cells (Table 37-2). After centrifugation of the blood sample, look for the presence of pink or red staining of the supernatant plasma. As little as 50 mg/dl of free hemoglobin can be detected by the naked eye (Fig. 37-1). If the plasma is yellow or straw-colored but a hemolytic reaction is still suspected, have the Blood Bank perform a direct antiglobulin (Coombs) test on the same blood

sample. This test takes only minutes to perform and can detect the presence of antibody-coated red cells. If these two observations are negative, it is extremely unlikely that a patient is undergoing a hemolytic reaction. If both are positive, hemolysis has occurred and should be treated (see section on Management of Hemolytic Transfusion Reactions). If hemolysis is present, the most likely cause is an error somewhere from the initial drawing of the patient's blood sample for crossmatching, to the actual hanging of the unit. Check first to see that the right blood has been given to the correct patient.

A hemolytic transfusion reaction may still be strongly suspected, even when the patient's plasma does not have free hemoglobin and the direct antiglobulin test on his red cells is negative. The former may be due to rapid clearance of the free hemoglobin from the plasma and the latter due to removal of all of the antibody-coated cells from the circulation by the reticuloendothelial system. A sample of urine should be tested for the presence of hemoglobinuria. Further, one may measure the patient's plasma haptoglobin level on the pretransfusion specimen and on a sample obtained as soon as practical after the implicated transfusion. If the pretransfusion level is within the normal range (usually 100 to 150 mg/dl), and the posttransfusion level is negligible, hemolysis is likely to have occurred. After transfusion of several units of blood, even of banked blood close to its day of expiration, the patient's plasma haptoglobin is usually ±50 percent of its initial, pretransfu-

Table 37-2. Initial Steps to Perform for a Suspected Hemolytic Transfusion Reaction

Stop the transfusion, *but:*
1. Keep the intravenous line open with normal saline solution (0.9% NaCl).
2. Draw an anticoagulated blood sample, then
   a. spin and observe supernatant for free hemoglobin in plasma (pink or red instead of straw color).
   b. perform direct antiglobulin (Coombs) test on the patient's red cells.
3. If both tests are negative and hemolysis is still suspected, measure pretransfusion and posttransfusion haptoglobin levels.
4. If there is free hemoglobin in the plasma and/or the direct Coombs test is positive, proceed as follows:
   a. send transfused blood unit to Blood Bank along with clotted sample of patient's blood; then
   b. institute therapy to prevent shock, renal failure, and disseminated intravascular clotting as indicated (see text and Table 37-4).

Fig. 37-1. Increasing levels of free hemoglobin in plasma of patients with hemolytic transfusion reactions. The patient's postreaction plasma should be compared to the pretransfusion plasma specimen.

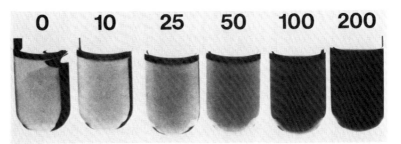

sion level.[1] Remember, however, that non-immunologically caused hemolysis—e.g., infusion of distilled water and large retroperitoneal hematomas—can lower the serum haptoglobin level significantly.[1]

IMMEDIATE TRANSFUSION REACTIONS

Adverse reactions to the transfusion of blood or its components which occur during the infusion, or within an hour or two of its completion, are termed "immediate." A listing of the possible adverse reactions of blood which can occur "immediately" is given in Table 37-3. These are divided into whether or not they are immunologically mediated. The most likely etiology for each category is also listed. As the most dreaded transfusion reaction is that in which there is immune hemolysis of the donor's or patient's blood, this will be discussed first.

HEMOLYTIC TRANSFUSION REACTIONS

Hemolysis of donor blood by preformed antibodies in a patient's plasma can have disastrous consequences for that patient. On the other hand, the effect of transfusing antibodies in a donor's plasma directed against the patient's red cells is not usually so deleterious. The patient may initially have no signs or symptoms when incompatible blood is being destroyed in his circulation but, more likely, has at least some mild complaints, and

may even begin with major problems. There is no pathognomonic sign, symptom, or set of signs and symptoms which accompanies a hemolytic transfusion reaction. A patient often experiences a vague uneasiness, back pain, or chills during the early stages of a hemolytic transfusion reaction. Fever is one of the most common initial manifestations of immune hemolysis, being present in 35 of 47 cases reported by Pineda, Brzica, and Taswell;[2] about half the time, the fever is accompanied by chills. Generalized flushing, nausea, and lightheadedness occur less commonly. Red or wine-colored urine may be the first sign the patient notices; while dramatic, it is usually painless.

More severe hemolytic transfusion reactions may begin with dyspnea, flank pain, or hypotension. These can progress to shock with all of its consequences, including oliguria or even complete renal shutdown. Rarely, generalized oozing or frank bleeding may be the first sign of disseminated intravascular coagulation (DIC) triggered by an incompatible transfusion. In patients who are anesthetized or unconscious for other reasons, shock, anuria or a bleeding diathesis may be the presenting findings of a hemolytic reaction.

DIAGNOSIS

When a hemolytic transfusion reaction is suspected, either on the basis of a patient's signs and symptoms or when frank hemoglobinuria is noted, immediate steps should be taken to diagnose this condition, determine

Table 37-3. Immediate Adverse Effects of Transfusion

A. Immunologic Reactions	Usual Etiology
1. Hemolysis *with symptoms*	Red cell incompatibility
2. Anaphylaxis	Antibody to IgA
3. Febrile, nonhemolytic	Antibody to donor leukocyte antigens
4. Urticaria	Antibody to plasma proteins
5. Noncardiogenic pulmonary edema	Antibody to leukocytes of patient
B. Nonimmunologic Effects	
1. Congestive heart failure	Volume overload
2. Marked fever with shock	Bacterially contaminated blood
3. Hypothermia	Rapid infusion of cold blood
4. Hemolysis *without symptoms*	Physical or chemical destruction of blood, (e.g., freezing, over-heating, addition of hemolytic drug or water)
5. Emboli	
a.) Particulate	Microemboli in stored blood
b.) Air	Air infusion in line
6. Hyperkalemia	Rapid infusion of multiple units of bank blood
7. Hypocalcemia	Massive transfusion of citrated blood

its etiology, and minimize its consequences. As noted already, the infusion of blood should be stopped, for the morbidity and mortality of a hemolytic reaction are roughly proportional to the amount of incompatible blood infused. The risk of a severe reaction is much higher if more than 200 ml of incompatible blood has been transfused (proportionately less in children). However, marked symptoms and signs are often produced after transfusion of 5 to 20 ml of ABO-incompatible blood and may even occur after transfusion of 0.7 ml.[3] Because hypotension often accompanies a hemolytic reaction and may progress to frank shock, the intravenous line should be kept open with a saline infusion (0.9% normal saline).

Next, check to see that the patient has been receiving blood intended for him or her. One of the most common reasons for the transfusion of incompatible blood is a clerical error, primarily the infusion of the wrong patient's blood. Check the name and blood group on the donor unit against the recipient's name and blood group. An error may result in a major ABO incompatibility between patient and donor; this type of reaction is most likely to result in acute renal shutdown, DIC, and death.[4] Once this "clerical" check has been performed, draw an anticoagulated (e.g., EDTA) and an unanticoagulated sample of blood from the patient and send these, along with the offending unit of blood, to the Blood Bank for workup of a suspected hemolytic transfusion reaction. The anticoagulated specimen can be tested for free plasma hemoglobin, either visually or by a spectrophotometer for quantitation, as well as for evidence of circulating but antibody-coated red cells, by the direct antiglobulin test. The clotted sample can be recrossmatched with the red cells from the bag of donor blood, and can be used for chemical tests—e.g., haptoglobin level, bilirubin, and creatinine. The Blood Bank can determine if the unit of blood being transfused to the patient is incompatible with the postreaction patient's serum and should recrossmatch with the prereaction serum specimen, too.

The most useful tests to document the occurrence of an immune-mediated hemolytic transfusion reaction are the plasma hemoglobin level, the direct antiglobulin test, and the serum haptoglobin level. Additional confirmatory tests may also be used to verify a hemolytic transfusion reaction, but they are less specific, and less often positive, in the presence of immune hemolysis. Figure 37-2 illustrates laboratory tests which have been used when a hemolytic reaction, either acute or delayed, is suspected, and their frequency of yielding a useful result. Depending on the degree of hemolysis and the method of testing, the serum bilirubin level may be artifac-

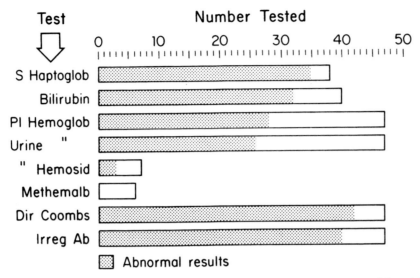

Fig. 37-2. Usefulness of tests for red blood cell destruction during an acute or a delayed hemolytic transfusion reaction. *S Haptoglob* = serum haptoglobin; *Pl Hemoglob* = plasma hemoglobin; *Hemosid* = hemosiderin; *Methemalb* = methemalbumin; *Irreg Ab* = irregular antibodies. (Reprinted, by permission, from Pineda, A.A., Brzica, S.M., Jr., and Taswell, H.F.: Hemolytic transfusion reaction: a recent experience in a large blood bank. Mayo Clin. Proc. 53:382, 1978.)

tually low; this may be one of the reasons why the bilirubin does not always rise after a hemolytic reaction.[5] One should also determine if the patient's hemoglobin or hematocrit has risen as expected after a transfusion; e.g., in a 70-kg adult, an increase of about 1 g/dl of hemoglobin, or 3 percent for hematocrit, should be expected for each unit of blood or packed cells.

MANAGEMENT

Once it has been determined that a transfusion of incompatible blood has occurred, prophylactic therapy should be begun (Table 37-4). The morbidity of a hemolytic transfusion reaction is due to renal failure (acute tubular necrosis) and/or bleeding. Renal failure in this case is usually due to hypotension, probably mediated by complement activation[3] caused by the red cell antigen-antibody reaction. The bleeding is caused by consumption of clotting factors (disseminated intravascular coagulation [DIC]) also initiated by the red cell antigen-antibody reac-

tion.[6] With hypotension or shock, blood is shunted away from the kidneys with resultant renal cortical ischemia. This is the main mechanism responsible for the acute renal failure which can accompany an acute hemolytic transfusion reaction. Free hemoglobin, released by destroyed red cells, can be found in the tubules of the kidneys; but this is not responsible for oliguria or anuria. Hemoglobin is not directly toxic to the kidneys and has been used experimentally as a universal blood substitute, provided it is free of red cell membranes (stroma) with their contained antigens.[7] Hemoglobin-free but incompatible red cell stroma infusions have provoked acute renal failure, both transiently and with acute tubular necrosis.[8]

To prevent the renal failure which may accompany a hemolytic transfusion reaction, therapy should be directed toward maintaining adequate perfusion of the kidneys. Following an acute hemolytic transfusion reaction, the urine output must be monitored. If hypotension or shock can be adequately treated, renal perfusion can usually be maintained and renal failure obviated. Thus,

Table 37-4. Treatment of Immediate, Adverse Effects of Blood Transfusion

Sign or Symptom	Treatment
Congestive Heart Failure	1. Slow the transfusion 2. IV diuretic (e.g., 40 mg furosemide)
Urticaria alone	1. Diphenhydramine or tripelennamine 50 mg im or po 2. May restart blood slowly after 15-30 minutes. 3. Consider prophylactic antihistamine before next transfusion
Fever *without* hemolysis	1. ASA 600 mg po or acetaminophen 650 mg po 2. Do not restart transfusion 3. Consider prophylactic antipyretic therapy next time and/or white cell poor blood product
Anaphylaxis, asthma	1. Epinephrine 0.4 ml of 1:1,000 sq (or give 0.1 ml diluted in 10 ml saline over 5 min IV if severe shock)

Hemoglobinuria, shock, oliguria
 	
If ABO incompatibility and > 200 ml blood infused and/or evidence of diffuse bleeding
	1. To prevent renal failure
	  a) 1000 ml 0.9% NaCl over 1-2 hr
	  b) Diuretic therapy—furosemide 20 to 80 mg IV or ethacrynic acid
	  c) Continue fluids and diuretics to maintain urine flow over 100 ml/hr
	  d) Prevent overhydration—see text
	2. To prevent disseminated intravascular coagulation
	  a) Obtain baseline clotting studies then give
	  b) heparin 5000 u IV stat, then 1,500 u/hr by constant iv infusion maintain heparinization for 6-24 hr
	  c) Use albumin 5%, to maintain blood pressure as necessary; give platelets and/or fresh frozen plasma as needed for clotting deficiencies

fluids, primarily in the form of normal saline (0.9% NaCl), should be the first therapeutic modality employed. Adequate hydration (but not overhydration) should be continued in order to keep urine flow at or over 100 ml/hr in adults.

To improve blood flow to the kidneys and increase urine output, specific diuretic agents should also be given. Both ethacrynic acid and furosemide can improve renal blood flow at the same time that they promote a diuresis. These should be used in place of mannitol, which has been traditionally recommended during a hemolytic transfusion reaction. The clinical evidence to support the use of mannitol as an osmotic diuretic in this situation is not convincing.[9] Further, if mannitol is ineffective, it can result in hypervolemia, congestive heart failure, and even pulmonary edema. Improving renal blood flow by using ethacrynic acid or furosemide is a more rational means of preventing renal failure, even though no controlled trials have been conducted to prove this therapy, either. Pressor agents are contraindicated because they de-

crease blood flow to the kidneys and may aggravate renal failure accompanying the transfusion reaction.

If, in spite of these measures, progressive oliguria occurs, care should be taken to prevent overhydration of the patient. Pulmonary edema can occur if uncontrolled fluid administration is permitted. The management problem now becomes that of acute tubular necrosis, a problem which should be entrusted to a physician well versed in its management. Dialysis may be required acutely to correct fluid and electrolyte imbalance if these have developed, and more chronically if the renal failure is of long duration.

DISSEMINATED INTRAVASCULAR COAGULATION

Disseminated intravascular coagulation (DIC), with its potential for causing a bleeding diathesis, can also result from a hemolytic transfusion reaction. The only possibly effective prophylactic therapy for DIC is heparinization. However, heparin itself can result in bleeding and may be contraindicated in a patient undergoing surgery or already bleeding because of the preexisting condition for which the transfusion was being given. Thus, the decision to give heparin prophylactically for a hemolytic transfusion reaction, which may or may not result in DIC, is difficult. The factors to consider regarding heparinization are the severity of the reaction and the patient's clinical status. The most severe hemolytic transfusion reactions are those due to (1) ABO incompatibilities, and (2) infusion of more than 200 ml of mismatched blood. These are also the situations which are likely to result in DIC and death due to an incompatible transfusion.[4] Unless strong contraindications exist, heparin therapy should be begun, as outlined in Table 37-4. In an adult, a loading dose of 5,000 u of heparin should be given intravenously (IV), followed by a continuous IV infusion of 1,500 u/hr.[6] This should be continued for 6 to 24 hours. In patients with relative contraindications to heparin therapy (e.g., postsurgical cases), half this dose may be given. A continuous infusion of heparin can be slowed or stopped and adds a margin of safety. If bleeding develops, heparin reversal with protamine should be considered. This program of management is also appropriate for the patient in whom DIC has already developed.

Consideration should be given to transfusion of the patient with compatible blood if, indeed, the patient was seriously in need of the offending transfusion in the first place. Many physicians are reluctant to do this. They are concerned about a second hemolytic episode. However, if the Blood Bank has resolved the cause of the donor-recipient incompatibility, a transfusion at this point is as safe as any transfusion.

PREVENTION

The prevention of hemolytic transfusion reactions is difficult. These reactions occur so rarely—approximately once for every 6,000 units of blood transfused in a well-run blood bank[2]—that it is difficult to establish effective means to prevent them completely. Those reactions due to errors, such as initially drawing a blood sample from the wrong patient for crossmatching, or transfusing Mary Smith's blood to John Jones, can only be obviated by careful attention to details—e.g., having two individuals check patient identification. Transfusion therapy should be used judiciously, only when absolutely needed, and then to stabilize the patient and *not* necessarily to normalize his hemoglobin level or hematocrit. Each blood transfusion carries a risk of about 1 percent of immunizing a patient to one of the "minor" blood group factors.[10] While crossmatching with a recently obtained blood sample from a patient will usually identify unexpected red cell antibodies, blood bank techniques are not perfect and will not identify all cases of incompatibility. Rarely, hemolytic reactions can occur after a blood transfusion even though it appeared compatible by all available methods and no unusual antibodies were demonstrable.[11] All clinicians who employ transfusions should be aware of the manifold presentations of hemolytic transfusion reactions. Clinicians should be prepared to diagnose this type of reaction quickly and should know how and when to institute prophylactic therapy to minimize the severe complication which can result.

ANAPHYLACTIC TRANSFUSION REACTIONS

Anaphylactic, or anaphylactoid, reactions to the transfusion of blood or blood components are exceedingly rare. They are dramatic, however, and can result in death unless recognized and treated promptly. The onset of shock, loss of consciousness and/or severe gastrointestinal symptoms can occur after the infusion of only a few ml of blood or plasma. Symptoms usually begin with nausea, abdominal cramps, emesis, and diarrhea. Transient hypertension is followed by profound hypotension. Generalized flushing and, occasionally, chills may be present, but *fever is virtually never found.* In fact, the rapid onset of gastrointestinal symptoms and/or shock in the absence of fever distinguishes the anaphylactic reaction from that due to leukocyte incompatibility, hemolysis, or sepsis.

The most common cause of anaphylactic or anaphylactoid reactions is the presence of antibodies to IgA.[12] Such antibodies are found in patients with IgA deficiency who have become sensitized to this immunoglobulin (e.g., due to prior transfusion or pregnancy). IgA-deficient patients may make IgG and/or IgM antibodies to IgA, which can fix complement. Upon reexposure to even minute quantities of IgA, patients lacking IgA who have antibody to it may experience an anaphylactic reaction.

The immediate treatment of an anaphylactic reaction to blood or plasma is to stop the transfusion and administer epinephrine. Once again, keep the intravenous line open with normal saline, for severe hypotension is the most significant manifestation of an IgA-anti-IgA transfusion reaction. Epinephrine, 0.4 ml of a 1:1,000 solution, should be given subcutaneously as quickly as possible. If tissue perfusion is already compromised due to presence of shock, give instead 0.1 ml of the 1:1,000 epinephrine diluted to 10 ml with normal saline intravenously over 5 minutes. *Under no circumstances should the transfusion be restarted.*

To make the diagnosis of an IgA-anti-IgA reaction as the cause of an anaphylactic transfusion reaction, measure the serum IgA level in the patient. Only about one in 700 individuals is IgA-deficient, so the absence of IgA in a patient who has had an anaphylactic transfusion reaction is virtually diagnostic. The demonstration of specific anti-IgA antibodies is much more difficult, requires sophisticated research laboratory techniques, and is not usually necessary in this situation.

To prevent anaphylactic transfusion reactions in sensitized, IgA-deficient patients, the patients must be transfused with blood products that lack IgA. Since most blood products contain IgA in hazardous quantities, provision of IgA-deficient blood or components is not easy. Whole blood may be obtained from IgA-deficient blood donors, but few blood donors are so identified. Registries of such donors are available—e.g., the American National Red Cross in Washington, D.C., the Irwin Memorial Blood Bank in San Francisco, and the Canadian National Red Cross in Toronto. It is more practical, however, to use red blood cells which have been completely freed of the IgA in the plasma. This can be accomplished by washing of the red cells. Usually, extensive washing in a mechanical cell washer is adequate, but, rarely, frozen-thawed red cells are necessary. The frozen-thawed red cells are essentially free of IgA by virtue of their method of preparation, and can be safely transfused to even highly immunized, IgA-deficient patients.

Alternatively, such patients can be their own donors (see Ch. 15). For anticipated, elective transfusions, IgA-deficient patients can donate blood, which can be stored for several weeks in the Blood Bank in a liquid state, or frozen and held for years in the freezer. With autologous blood, both red cells and IgA-deficient plasma are available for the patient. A variation of this is to perform plasmapheresis of the IgA-deficient patient. The autologous plasma can be stored in the frozen state and given later, along with well-washed donor red cells, for the patient who needs both volume replacement and red cells during an anticipated surgical procedure.

Minute quantities of IgA are present in most albumin preparations, and even more IgA is present in plasma protein fraction; these blood products should not be given to sensitized, IgA-deficient patients. In an emergency, crystalloid solutions may be necessary, along with frozen-thawed red cells, for the IgA-deficient patient who has not had the opportunity to set aside autologous blood or plasma. Patients with IgA deficiency who have antibodies to IgA should wear or carry some type of medical alert device to notify emergency room physicians of their condition.

There are other causes, less well defined, of anaphylactic transfusion reactions. These may be due to traces of an allergen in the donor's plasma to which the recipient is exquisitely sensitive. The immediate management of these reactions is as described previously. If IgA deficiency can be ruled out (by demonstration of normal IgA and absence of anti-IgA), the subsequent investigation of the problem is difficult or impossible. If the patient requires subsequent transfusion, it may be necessary to try another donor with careful observation and full preparation for the management of anaphylaxis.

NONCARDIOGENIC PULMONARY EDEMA

If congestive heart failure occurs during a blood transfusion, it is almost always due to hypervolemia, especially in the very young, the very old, or patients with long-standing anemia. However, very rarely, transfusion can provoke a form of noncardiogenic pulmonary edema.[13] This type of pulmonary edema may have an immunologic basis.[14] Noncardiogenic pulmonary edema should be suspected in the following cases: (1) patients who would not be expected to develop congestive heart failure due to hypervolemia and (2) transfused patients under anesthesia who unexpectedly manifest poor oxygenation of their tissues. The reaction may occur after the infusion of relatively small quantities of blood or plasma. Signs of pulmonary edema without the findings of cardiac failure, confirmed by a characteristic chest radiograph (Fig. 37-3), usually establish this diagnosis. Chills, fever, cyanosis, and hypotension occur in the more severe cases.

When an etiology can be defined, noncardiogenic pulmonary edema induced by a transfusion is usually due to passively transfused antibodies to leukocytes. These are

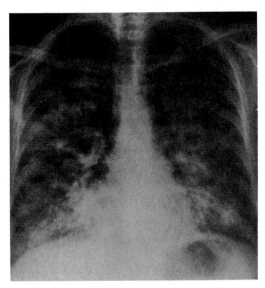

Fig. 37-3. Chest radiograph from a patient with a pulmonary "hypersensitivity" reaction induced by non-HLA leukoagglutinins. (Thompson, J.S., Severson, C.D., Parmely, M.J., Marmorstein, B.L., and Simmons, A.: Pulmonary "hypersensitivity" reactions induced by transfusion of non-HLA leukoagglutinins. N. Engl. J. Med. 284:1120, 1971. Reprinted by permission.)

usually leukoagglutinins in the donor's blood which have been induced by prior transfusions or pregnancy. If the leukocyte antibodies react specifically with antigenic determinants on a transfused patient's leukocytes, leukoagglutination may occur with trapping of white cell aggregates in the pulmonary microcirculation. It is this "filtering" action of the vasculature of the lungs which invokes the reaction which is, in essence, an allergic reaction occurring in the lungs.[15]

The treatment of noncardiogenic pulmonary edema begins with stopping the transfusion. Because of the rarity of this condition, further therapy has been empirical and has included diuretics, such as ethacrynic acid or furosemide; oxygen by mask; corticosteroids; and epinephrine. Most patients have resolution of their symptoms within 12 to 24 hours and clearance of the bilateral pulmonary infiltrates found on chest radiograph within a few days.

Donors with leukocyte antibodies are a hazard only for patients who have the specific leukocyte antigens that can react with them—a situation that occurs extremely rarely. Screening of all blood donors for leukocyte antibodies is not practical. A policy of rejecting multiparous blood donors, or those with prior transfusions who might have leukocyte antibodies, would result in an unacceptable loss of donors. Recognition of the entity of noncardiogenic pulmonary edema and differentiation of it from hypervolemic cardiac failure are the most important aspects of this very uncommon entity.

FEVER WITHOUT HEMOLYSIS

Fever without hemolysis is one of the most common adverse effects of transfusion. Ahrons and Kissmeyer-Nielsen[16] estimated that febrile, nonhemolytic (FNH) transfusion reactions occur after about 1 percent of transfusions. More recently, Goldfinger and Lowe, after careful evaluation of 6,359 reported reactions, concluded that the incidence of non-RBC-mediated reactions was 0.49 percent.[17] Although the authors did not distinguish between FNH and other types of nonhemolytic reactions, most such reactions can be assumed to have been FNH. As the name implies, FNH reactions are manifested by fever, with or without chills, but without red cell hemolysis. The fever may be mild to severe but does not usually occur until most of the unit of blood or component has been transfused, and sometimes not for an hour or two after completion of the transfusion.

Recipients who have been transfused repeatedly with blood products are those who tend to experience FNH reactions. These individuals have become sensitized to leukocyte antigens, especially HLA determinants on lymphocytes, granulocytes and/or platelets.[18] The reaction of the patient's antibodies, primarily with the granulocytes in a donor's blood, gives rise to the characteristic febrile reaction. The specificity of white cell antibodies in the recipient, combined with the number or concentration of granulocytes in the blood product, determines the frequency and severity of FNH reactions in immunized patients.

Fever is the hallmark and most important sign of a FNH transfusion reaction. It can be treated by antipyretics such as acetylsalicylic acid or acetaminophen. However, there are two important considerations whenever a patient develops a febrile reaction to a blood product. First, the fever may be the initial manifestation of something more serious than a FNH reaction; fever may be the presenting sign of an immune-mediated hemolytic reaction[2] or a response to a blood product contaminated with bacteria.[19] Thus, the transfusion should be stopped so that these conditions can be ruled in or out. Second, prevention of subsequent FNH reactions is a more important consideration than their immediate management. If a patient experiences one FNH reaction, the odds are 1 in 8 that he will have a similar reaction to the next blood transfusion.[20] Thus, the use of granulocyte-poor blood products should not be automatic or mandatory after a single FNH reaction. If, however, a patient has had two or more FNH reactions, it is reasonable to try to prevent further occurrences by asking the Blood Bank to provide products which are relatively free of contaminating granulocytes.

Diluting red cells with saline and then sedimenting them, or washing them in a cell washer, can remove sufficient granulocytes to obviate FNH reactions in virtually all patients. There is some loss of red cells with all procedures for these purposes.[20a] If recipients have high levels of antileukocyte antibodies, the most effective method of preparing granulocyte-poor red cells is to use frozen-thawed RBC which have very low concentrations of granulocytes; this product will obviate FNH reactions even in highly sensitized recipients.

If the febrile reactions occur after platelet transfusions, this is likely to be a result of alloimmunization and to be associated with poor posttransfusion platelet count increments. The best management of this problem is to use HLA-matched platelets (see Chs. 26 and 27).

URTICARIA

While urticaria is one of the most frequent adverse effects of a transfusion, hives are generally only a mild and bothersome complication. This allergic reaction to blood or blood components may accompany 1 to 2 percent of transfusions. This may be an underestimate, however, because hives are considered such a common and insignificant adverse effect of transfusion that they are often not reported to the Blood Bank.

Urticarial reactions, if they are unaccompanied by any other adverse effects, are the only type of transfusion reactions where the blood product can continue to be infused. Usually an antihistamine is administered while the flow of blood is slowed or temporarily stopped. After 15 to 30 minutes, when the hives have faded, the blood may be slowly transfused once again. In patients who frequently experience urticarial reactions, pretreatment with an antihistamine is warranted before each transfusion.

In most clinical situations, the etiology of urticarial reactions is never ascertained. This type of reaction is mild and doesn't warrant a detailed investigation. Recurrent hives occasionally are due to antibodies in patients directed against antigenic determinants on donor serum proteins, such as IgA allotypes.[12] Prevention of this type of reaction is more important than its exact etiology. Removal of plasma proteins from blood products may avert urticarial reactions—e.g., with washed or frozen red cells. Usually, however, pretreatment with an antihistamine is adequate to prevent the appearance of hives in patients who have frequently experienced urticaria.

NONIMMUNOLOGIC TRANSFUSION REACTIONS

CONGESTIVE HEART FAILURE

Heart failure induced by the transfusion of blood or its components is a common, yet preventable, adverse effect of a transfusion. Its true frequency is unknown, since it is often not recognized and certainly rarely reported to the Blood Bank. Hypervolemia with secondary congestive failure can potentially occur in any patient who is transfused too rapidly.[21] In practice, transfusion-induced heart failure occurs primarily in certain patients. The very young, the elderly, patients with established cardiac disease, and those patients with expanded plasma volumes (especially when associated with chronic, long-standing anemia) are the most likely to develop heart failure with transfusions. In these patients, the usual transfusion rate of about 200 ml of blood per hour may be excessive. They cannot accommodate this rapid expansion of their blood volume and may experience congestive heart failure.

The therapy of transfusion-induced congestive heart failure is essentially that of congestive heart failure of any etiology. The transfusion should be stopped or infused extremely slowly. Rapid-acting diuretics such as furosemide or ethacrynic acid should be given intravenously. At the same time, patients should be placed in a sitting position, given oxygen by mask, and given IV morphine if necessary. If frank pulmonary edema has developed, phlebotomy of 200 to 400 ml of blood may be necessary; but these patients are usually anemic to begin with, so this should not be done without serious consideration. The shed blood can be anticoagulated, the plasma removed, and the red cells reinfused after cardiac compensation has been reestablished.

Once again, prevention is the key to handling this transfusion-induced reaction. In susceptible patients, transfusions should be administered slowly (1 ml/kg body weight/hr)[21] and in the most concentrated form available. Packed red cells or red cells suspended in a minimal amount of saline should be used to raise the hematocrit of infants, the elderly, or those with chronic anemias. Plasmapheresis or partial exchange with packed RBC may also be considered at the time of transfusion to reduce the patient's expanded plasma volume and permit more rapid infusion of red cells.

TRANSFUSION OF BACTERIALLY CONTAMINATED BLOOD

During phlebotomy or in the preparation of components from whole blood, it is possible for bacteria to enter the product. If bacteria grow, then a subsequent septic transfusion can occur. Fortunately, this potentially adverse effect of a transfusion is extremely infrequent. However, when blood products heavily contaminated with bacteria are transfused, a devastating transfusion reaction can occur. Endotoxin, produced by certain gram-negative bacteria which are able to grow at refrigerator temperatures, initiates the reaction. Patients may experience high fever, shock, hemoglobinuria, renal failure and DIC.[19] Thus, contaminated blood products can provoke any of the signs and symptoms usually attributed to hemolytic transfusion reactions. Of note is the fact that the shock is usually of the "warm" type with flushing and dryness of the skin and may be accompanied by either abdominal pain with cramps and diarrhea, and/or pain in the extremities with generalized muscle aches.

Prompt recognition of a reaction due to contaminated blood is essential. As soon as this possibility is considered, the blood product should be stopped and examined for evidence of bacterial contamination. This can be done either by gross observation, which may reveal an unusual color to the blood product or clots in the bag, or by a gram stain of the bag's contents. If the diagnosis of a septic transfusion is likely, both the patient's blood and the blood product should be cultured, for both aerobic and anerobic organisms and at multiple incubation temperatures. The IV solution should also be cultured because this, too, is a potential source of organisms.[22] Broad spectrum antibiotic coverage should then be instituted. Usually, two or three antibiotics, to cover a variety of gram-negative organisms, are administered intravenously pending determination of the responsible organism and its sensitivities. Fluids and vasopressors should be used to maintain blood pressure if necessary. If DIC is evident, heparin therapy should generally be instituted at once.

HEMOLYSIS DUE TO PHYSICAL OR CHEMICAL CAUSES

Red blood cells intended for transfusion may be inadvertently hemolyzed by physical or chemical means. Freezing of whole blood or packed cells without a cryoprotective agent such as glycerol, or heating of red cells to greater than 50° C will result in hemolysis. Drugs, as well as hyper- or hypotonic solutions, when mixed with or simultaneously infused with red cells, may also cause lysis; *normal saline (0.9% NaCl) is the only solution that should be added to or infused with blood.*[23] Certain exceptions to this rule are acceptable only in emergencies (see Ch. 18). Asymptomatic hemoglobinuria is the most usual result of transfusing hemolyzed but compatible red cells. Patients do not experience fever, chills, hypotension, or any of the other signs or symptoms associated with an immune hemolytic reaction or transfusion of bacterially hemolyzed blood.

Most patients clear the free hemoglobin without difficulty, but disseminated intravascular clotting is at least a theoretical possibility after transfusion of lysed, compatible red cells. Shulman et al.[24] showed that infusions of compatible red cell stroma caused no problems in humans, but Quick[25] demonstrated that lysed erythrocytes can release procoagulant materials; even hemolyzed autologous red cells could induce DIC. DIC after infusion of lysed, compatible red cells has rarely been observed clinically; thus, heparin therapy should be withheld pending some evidence of intravascular clotting. Fluids should be given and careful observation maintained if hemolyzed blood has been administered.

Clinicians should attempt to prevent inadvertent hemolysis of red cells; when this occurs, there is always the worry that the patient may have had an immune hemolytic reaction. Documentation of the hemolysis and ruling out of an immune basis for it should always be undertaken in these situations. Care to see that refrigerated blood is not accidentally placed in a freezer or heated excessively by a blood warmer[26] will prevent most cases of physical hemolysis of blood. A strict rule of never adding a drug or any intravenous solution to blood except 0.9% NaCl will eliminate chemical or osmotic hemolysis. Also, patients undergoing prostate surgery have inadvertently received distilled water intravenously from the bladder irrigation fluid, which has resulted in intravascular hemolysis.[1]

EMBOLISM—AIR OR MICROEMBOLI

With the widespread use of plastic bags instead of glass bottles, the hazard of air embolism has virtually disappeared from transfusion of blood. Mechanical means of infusing blood rapidly work primarily by placing pressure on the outside of the blood bag, so air embolism is not very likely. When air is pumped into the blood container to speed infusion, air embolus is a distinct possibility; therefore, this should never be done.

Patients who receive air intravenously may experience acute cardiopulmonary insufficiency. The air tends to lodge in the right ventricle and prevent blood from entering the pulmonary artery. Acute cyanosis, pain, cough, dyspnea, shock, and cardiac arrhythmia may result; death may supervene unless immediate action is taken. Having the patient lie head down on his left side will usually displace the air bubble away from the pulmonary valve. This also places the patient in an optimal position for removal of the air by aspiration using a transthoracic needle inserted below the second or third rib just to the right of the sternum.

Microemboli form in blood while it is stored in the Blood Bank refrigerator. White cells and platelets, plus some fibrin and entangled red cells, make up most of this microscopic debris, which accumulates during the storage of blood despite the anticoagulant-preservative in which it is kept. These microemboli can be demonstrated by using special filters with openings smaller than the usual blood filter of 170-micron pore size. Since most of the microemboli pass through the standard blood bank filter, this material may be trapped in the lungs after transfusion. The main questions, however, are how clinically important this is, and what, if anything, should be done to prevent it. While microemboli do form in bank blood, there is little clinical information documenting their deleterious effect, except in the massively transfused patient.[27] Special "micropore" blood filters are on the market and can be shown to remove microaggregates missed by standard blood filters. Whether such filters are needed or are of significant benefit for all transfusions remains to be shown; thus, the routine use of micropore filters for all transfusions cannot be recommended. They should probably be utilized in only those patients who are receiving massive transfusions of blood. Differences of opinion on this matter still exist (see Chs. 10, 22, 23, and 24). It must be realized, however, that micropore filters remove functional platelets from fresh blood and increase the osmotic fragility of red cells in the process of removing microaggregates.[28]

MASSIVE TRANSFUSION EFFECTS

Patients who receive large volumes of blood may experience some untoward effects of these multiple transfusions. "Massive" transfusion here refers to the infusion of a minimum of 10 units of blood in an adult, or replacement of one blood volume, within a 24-hour period. Despite its anticoagulant-preservative, blood does age while sitting in the Blood Bank refrigerator. As part of the aging process, the pH of the blood, already slightly acid due to the citrate, falls somewhat; potassium leaks from the red cells; and some labile clotting components deteriorate. In addition, the 2,3-diphosphoglycerate (2,3-DPG) level falls gradually. The effect of the loss of this last compound within the red cells is that hemoglobin binds oxygen more tightly and gives it up less well to the body's tissues.

Massive transfusion can have physical, chemical, and/or physiologic effects on a patient. Rapid transfusion of banked blood right out of the refrigerator (at 1 to 6°C) can cause hypothermia in patients, or at least hypothermic effects on the heart.[29] To affect the heart adversely by lowering its temperature, very rapid infusion of multiple units of blood is usually necessary (e.g., 50 to 100 ml of blood per minute). If transfusion at this rapid pace is contemplated, then the blood should be warmed to body temperature (but not above 37°C) during the transfusion. Chemical effects of massive transfusion of stored blood can be due to its lack of free calcium ion (complexed by the citrate anticoagulant), gradually increasing acidity, and progressive hyperkalemia. Because citrate is rapidly metabolized in the body, it is extremely difficult for a patient to develop significant hypocalcemia, even during massive transfusion. Prolongation of clotting time due to complexing of plasma calcium has been infrequently reported with massive transfusion.[30] Cardiac effects of transfusion-induced hypocalcemia are more theoretical than real; the arrhythmias that are observed are more often due to the cold blood than to the decreased calcium.[29] To minimize the possibility of transfusion-induced hypocalcemia, some clinicians recommend infusion of 10 ml of 10 percent calcium chloride after every few units of banked blood. However, this is generally regarded as unnecessary, and extreme hypercalcemia has been induced by this means[31] (see Ch. 23).

The plasma level of potassium may increase 0.5 to 1 meq/l per day of shelf storage.[32] Thus, another possible adverse effect during massive transfusion is hyperkalemia due to rapid infusion of plasma with an elevated potassium level which has been leaked from the red cells; however, this is rarely of clinical consequence, except perhaps in patients with renal insufficiency or preexisting hyperkalemia. Massive transfusion may actually result in hypokalemia in patients.[33] This may be due to the fact that, in the circulation, the transfused red blood cells will take up potassium to replace that which has been lost during storage.

Additional effects of massive transfusion may result from (1) shifting of the oxygen dissociation curve of hemoglobin so that it binds O_2 more tightly, or from (2) depletion of labile clotting factors. Massive transfusion of banked blood, with low 2,3-DPG levels of its red cells, may temporarily impair tissue oxygenation. The 2,3-DPG is regenerated in vivo by the red cells and is usually nearly normal within 24 hours of the transfusion. How real a problem this is at a clinical level remains unclear, since there is little useful information on this point. Similarly, as blood ages during storage, platelets, Factor VIII (anti-hemophilic factor) and Factor V (labile factor) deteriorate. Infusion of large quantities of bank blood might result in a deficiency of one or more of these factors in massively transfused patients. (The management of potential coagulation factor deficiencies occurring during massive transfusion is discussed in Chapters 21 through 24.)

A point to be kept in mind during massive transfusion is the possible adverse effect of rapid infusion of plasma protein fraction

(PPF) or, rarely, albumin solution in this situation. Some lots of these protein fractions have had vasoactive substances which provoke hypotension.[34] This may not be immediately recognized in the urgency of the clinical situation, for often the patient is already hypotensive due to blood loss. Slowing the infusion rate of the protein solution which has a hypotensive effect is usually sufficient to handle this problem. Recently produced lots of PPF have been free of this undesirable property.

DELAYED TRANSFUSION EFFECTS

Adverse effects due to blood transfusion can occur some time after completion of the infusion. The delay can be days, months, or years later. Immunologic or nonimmunologic mechanisms may be responsible (see Table 37.5). These potential late hazards should always be kept in mind when a blood transfusion is given, even if no untoward effects have occurred during the actual infusion.

ALLOIMMUNIZATION

As no two humans, except identical twins, have the same genetic makeup, a blood transfusion exposes a patient to numerous "foreign" antigens. Those antigens which the patient does not possess are potentially immunogenic. Antibodies in the recipient may develop to any of the components of blood and may be formed days, weeks, or months after the transfusion.

Even though blood is crossmatched and given as ABO- and Rh_o (D)-compatible to a patient, a recipient may still develop an antibody to any of hundreds of red cell antigens. Immunization to red cell antigens can also occur during pregnancy. If a red cell antibody is formed, or recalled in an anamnestic fashion while there are circulating donor red cells, a delayed hemolytic transfusion reaction can result. Most often, this is completely asymptomatic and only noted by a more rapid fall in the patient's hemoglobin level than expected. This can be documented in some cases by the presence of a mixed field positive direct antiglobulin (Coombs) test which agglutinates the antibody-coated donor cells but not the recipient's cells. After all donor cells are removed by the reticuloendothelial system, free antibody may be demonstrated in the patient's serum by the indirect antiglobulin test. On occasion, the delayed hemolytic reaction can be so brisk as to evoke symptoms, usually fever and hemoglobinemia, and may even result in renal shutdown[35] and death.[36] The clinical course of a patient who experienced a delayed hemolytic transfusion reaction with consequent renal failure is illustrated in Figure 37-4.

An unusual presentation of a delayed hemolytic reaction is a serum sickness-like picture.[37] When this occurs in a patient with sickle-cell anemia who has been recently transfused, a sickle-cell crisis might be sus-

Table 37-5. Delayed Transfusion Reactions

Types of Reactions	Usual Etiology
A. *Immunologic*	
1. Hemolysis	Anamnestic antibody to red cell antigen
2. Serum sickness-like	Developing red cell antigen incompatibility[37]
3. Graft-vs.-host disease	Functional lymphocytes in transfused blood
4. Posttransfusion purpura	Development of antiplatelet antibody (usually anti-Pl[A1])
B. *Nonimmunologic*	
1. Iron overload	Multiple transfusions (100+) in chronically anemic patients without blood loss
2. Disease transmission	
a. Hepatitis	Non-A, non-B agent but occasionally type B (probably never type A)
b. Protozoa	Malaria Parasites

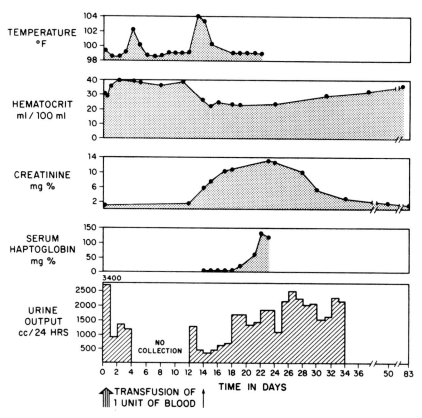

Fig. 37-4. Hospital course of a patient who experienced a delayed hemolytic transfusion reaction with acute renal failure due to an anamnestic antibody response to the red cell antigen Jk[b]. (Holland, P.V. and Wallerstein, R.D.: Delayed hemolytic transfusion reaction with acute renal failure. J.A.M.A. 204:1007, 1968. Reprinted by permission.)

pected incorrectly instead of a delayed hemolytic transfusion reaction.

Isoimmunization of patients to "minor" red cell antigens has another potential effect. In patients who have developed antibodies to multiple red cell antigens, it may be difficult to find compatible blood which lacks these factors. Thus, the presence of irregular or unexpected antibodies induced by prior transfusion may severely limit subsequent safe transfusion. Even blood products only minimally contaminated with red blood cells, such as platelet concentrates, can evoke antibodies to red cell antigens; however, this risk is lower in immunosuppressed patients.[38]

Three things concerning delayed hemolytic transfusion reactions must be kept in mind: First, the risk of sensitizing a recipient to a "minor" red cell antigen is about 1 percent for each unit of blood transfused. Second, the onset of a delayed hemolytic reaction may be quite insidious, if not virtually unnoticed, save for the gradual recurrence of anemia. Third, fever is the most common sign and symptom of a delayed hemolytic transfusion reaction, especially one which occurs one to two weeks after a transfusion.[2] Fever occurring even 10 to 14 days after a blood transfusion may, rarely, be due to transfusion-induced malaria.[39]

Alloimmunization to platelets, white cells, and plasma proteins after blood transfusions may also occur. Antibodies to platelets may cause not only febrile transfusion reactions[40] but also immune destruction of transfused platelets. Very rarely, posttransfusion purpura with severe thrombocytopenia has been induced by transfusion of blood.[40a] In this situation, which usually occurs in women who have been immunized during pregnancy, an antibody to transfused platelets, anti-Pl^{A1}, causes thrombocytopenia even though the patient's platelets lack the Pl^{A1} antigen.[41] This may result from cross-reactivity of the antibody with the patient's own platelets or somehow a "nonspecific" destruction of the patient's Pl^{A1}-negative platelets.

Antibodies to white cells, especially to HLA determinants, are the primary cause of febrile, nonhemolytic transfusion reactions. It was thought for some time that blood transfusions, with their propensity to evoke alloimmunization to white cells, had another deleterious effect: decreased survival of a cadaver kidney transplant. It now appears that, as long as the donor kidney is ABO-compatible with the recipient and a crossmatch between recipient serum and donor histocompatibility antigens is negative, blood transfusion may actually enhance the survival of a cadaver kidney transplant.[42] (See Ch. 29.) As previously mentioned, alloimmunization to IgA determinants is responsible for many urticarial reactions and most anaphylactic transfusion reactions.[12]

DELAYED EFFECTS OF TRANSFUSED WHITE BLOOD CELLS

Several very unusual complications of blood transfusion can occur due to the presence of viable, mononuclear cells in whole donor blood. Donors who have had exposure to tuberculosis and are PPD-positive can transfer delayed hypersensitivity to recipients by the lymphocytes in their donation. If a patient has developed a positive skin test to tuberculin, consider whether this might have been caused by a blood transfusion in the previous few months.[43]

A blood donor's lymphocytes can react against those of a recipient and be the cause of a transient, atypical lymphocytosis after transfusion[44] or even provoke a full-blown graft-versus-host (GVH) disease. The indications for irradiation of blood products to prevent lymphoid engraftment and subsequent graft-versus-host (GVH) disease are not clearly defined. A dose of 600 to 1000 rads of radiation to lymphoid cells will inhibit the production of DNA, as shown by the mixed lymphocyte reaction and by mitogen stimulation tests. To insure a margin of safety, a dose of 1500 rads has arbitrarily been chosen for irradiation of cellular blood products when necessary, although up to 5000 rads will not compromise their functional qualities.[44a]

Potential disadvantages of irradiation of blood products exist, but their significance is as yet unclear. Although in vivo evidence is still inadequate, in vitro studies indicate that platelet and granulocyte function are not impaired; survival of transfused red cells remains normal.[44a] Clinical studies have not determined whether irradiated granulocytes are as effective as nonirradiated cells; such a study would be difficult, considering the problems inherent in the evaluation of the effectiveness of granulocytes in any case. The widespread use of irradiated blood products for recipients of bone marrow transplants during periods of prolonged granulocytopenia has led to the belief that irradiated granulocytes function adequately, although such data are not definitive.

An additional theoretical disadvantage is the potential for subsequent malignant transformation of irradiated lymphocytes which may survive in the recipient. There have been no reported examples suggesting such an occurrence.

Indications for the use of irradiated cellular blood products to prevent GVH are beclouded by the fact that the definitive diagnosis of GVH is very difficult. Many of the reported cases of GVH following transfusion are not accepted as conclusive by other investigators. On the other hand, GVH is so difficult to distinguish from other clinical syndromes that it is possible that there are a large number of unreported cases. Thus, the incidence of GVH following transfusion in settings other than bone marrow transplantation and severe congenital immune deficiency disorders is not well documented. Anecdotal reports of GVH following transfusion of nonirradiated cellular blood products have been described[45-47] in patients who are being treated for malignancies (leukemias, lymphomas, and carcinomas) with immunosuppressive drugs; in intrauterine transfusion; and after exchange transfusion of full-term infants. More than one-half of the reported cases of GVH have been in patients who received granulocyte concentrates and one-fourth of the granulocye concentrates were from donors with chronic granulocytic leukemia.

On the basis of the available data, there is agreement that cellular blood products should be irradiated prior to their administration to recipients of bone marrow transplants until immune functions have been reconstituted; also, patients with some congenital immune deficiencies require irradiated blood products. Less clear are the indications for irradiation prior to intrauterine transfusion and the transfusion of neonates. Some pediatric departments irradiate all blood used for exchange transfusion in newborns, for intrauterine transfusions, and for transfusion of premature infants, but this practice is not widespread. The present consensus is that, in spite of the rare reports of GVH following transfusion in patients with malignancy who are being treated with immunosuppressive drugs, routine irradiation of blood products in this setting is not indicated. However, if the granulocyte concentrates are prepared from patients who have chronic granulocytic leukemia, these should probably be irradiated.

NONIMMUNOLOGIC, DELAYED COMPLICATIONS OF BLOOD TRANSFUSION

DISEASE TRANSMISSION

Blood donors may carry a variety of pathogens in their blood, despite their apparent healthy status. Viral hepatitis of at least two types can be transmitted unwittingly by asymptomatic blood donor carriers. Hepatitis is still a potential hazard of transfusion of blood and most of its components, despite the best efforts of the blood bank. Hepatitis viruses and other transmissible agents in blood are discussed at length in Chapter 36.

IRON OVERLOAD—TRANSFUSION HEMOSIDEROSIS

Every pint of blood contains approximately 250 mg iron complexed with its hemoglobin. While this is not a problem for most transfused patients and may actually be a boon to those in need of iron, it poses a threat to chronically transfused patients who do not have continuing blood losses. In individuals with congenital hemolytic anemias or long-standing aplastic anemia, the iron load of chronic transfusion therapy can become deleterious over a period of time. Transfusion hemosiderosis may be manifest after the transfusion of 100 units of blood in these chronically transfused patients. Unless some means is taken to remove the excess iron from the body, it accumulates in critical organs such as the liver, heart, and endocrine glands, and eventually causes failure of these organs. Iron chelation therapy is being attempted to reduce accumulated body iron, but it is a slow, tedious process of uncertain therapeutic efficacy.[48]

Transfusions should be kept to a minimum in this patient population, specifically to reduce the likelihood of transfusion hemosiderosis. Also, supertransfusion with neocytes has been reported to be effective in decreasing the rate of iron accumulation in thalassemia.[49]

REFERENCES

1. Fink, D.J., Petz, L.D., and Black, M.D.: Serum Haptoglobin: A valuable diagnostic aid in suspected hemolytic transfusion reactions. J.A.M.A. 199:615, 1967.
2. Pineda, A.A., Brzica, S.M., Jr., and Taswell, H.F.: Hemolytic transfusion reaction: recent experience in a large blood bank. Mayo Clin. Proc. 53:378, 1978.
3. Mollison, P.L.: Blood Transfusion in Clinical Medicine, 5th Ed. Blackwell Scientific Publications, London, 1979, pp. 567-568.
4. Schmidt, P.J.: Clinical-Pathological concepts of hemolytic transfusion reactions. In: Immunobiology of the Erythrocyte. Sandler, S.G. and Jamieson, G.A., eds. Alan R. Liss, Inc., New York, 1980.
5. Watson, D.: A note on the haemoglobin error in some nonprecipitation diazo-methods for bilirubin determinations. Clin. Chim. Acta. 5:613, 1960.
6. Goldfinger, D.: Acute hemolytic transfusion reactions—a fresh look at pathogenesis and considerations regarding therapy. Transfusion. 17:85, 1977.
7. Rabiner, S.F., Helbert, J.R., Lopas, H. and Friedman, L.H.: Evaluation of a stroma-free hemoglobin solution for use as a plasma expander. J. Exp. Med. 126:1127, 1967.
8. Schmidt, P.J. and Holland, P.V.: Pathogenesis of the acute renal failure associated with incompatible transfusion. Lancet ii:1169, 1967.
9. Barry, K.G. and Crosby, W.H.: The prevention and treatment of renal failure following transfusion reactions. Transfusion 3:34, 1963.
10. Lostumbo, M.M., Holland, P.V., and Schmidt, P.J.: Isoimmunization after multiple transfusions. N. Engl. J. Med. 175:141, 1966.
11. Stewart, J.W. and Mollison, P.L.: Rapid destruction of apparently compatible cells. Br. Med. J. 1:1247, 1959.
12. Vyas, G.N., Holmdahl, L., Perkins, H.A., and Fudenberg, H.H.: Serologic specificity of human anti-IgA and its significance in transfusion. Blood 34:573, 1969.
13. Carilli, A.D., Ramanamurty, M.V., Chang, Y., Shin, D., and Sethi, V.: Noncardiogenic pulmonary edema following blood transfusion. Chest 74:310, 1978.
14. Thompson, J.S., Severson, C.D., Parmely, M.J., Marmorstein, B.L., and Simmons, A.: Pulmonary "hypersensitivity" reactions induced by transfusion of non-HLA leukoagglutinins. N. Engl. J. Med. 284:1120, 1971.
15. Kernoff, P.B.A., Durrant, I.J., Rizza, C.R., and Wright, F.W.: Severe allergic pulmonary edema after plasma transfusion. Br. J. Haematol. 23:777, 1972.
16. Ahrons, S. and Kissmeyer-Nielsen, F.: Serological investigations of 1,358 transfusion reactions in 74,000 transfusions. Dan. Med. Bull. 15:259, 1968.
17. Goldfinger, D. and Lowe, C.: Prevention of transfusion reactions, using saline washed red blood cells. Blood (Suppl.)54:125a, 1979.
18. Thulstrup, H.: The influence of leukocyte and thrombocyte incompatibility on non-haemolytic transfusion reactions: a retrospective study. Vox Sang. 21:233, 1971.
19. Braude, A.I.: Transfusion reactions from contaminated blood: their recognition and treatment. N. Engl. J. Med. 258:1289, 1958.
20. Kevy, S.V., Schmidt, P.J., McGinniss, M.H., and Workman, W.G.: Febrile, non-hemolytic transfusion reactions and the limited role of leukoagglutinins in their etiology. Transfusion 2:7, 1962.
20a. Meryman, H.T., Bross, J., and Lebovitz, R.: The preparation of leukocyte-poor red blood cells: A comparative study. Transfusion 20:285, 1980.
21. Marriott, H.L. and Kekwick, A.: Volume and rate in blood transfusion for the relief of anemia. Br. Med. J. 1:1043, 1940.
22. Elin, R.J., Lundberg, W.B., and Schmidt, P.J.: Evaluation of bacterial contamination in blood processing. Transfusion 15:260, 1975.
23. Ryder, S.E. and Oberman, H.A.: Compatibility of common intravenous solutions with CPD blood. Transfusion 15:250, 1975.
24. Shulman, N.R., Weinrach, R.S., Libre, E.P., and Andrews, H.L.: The role of the reticuloendothelial system in the pathogenesis of idiopathic thrombocytopenic purpura. Trans. Assoc. Am. Phys. 78:374, 1965.
25. Quick, A.J.: Influence of erythrocytes on the coagulation of blood. Am. J. Med. Sci. 239:101, 1960.

26. Staples, P.J. and Griner, P.F.: Extracorporeal hemolysis of blood in a microwave blood warmer. N. Engl. J. Med. 285:217, 1971.

27. Reul, G.J., Greenberg, S.D., Lefrak, E.A., McCollum, W.B., Beall, A.C., Jr., and Jordan, G.L.: Prevention of posttraumatic pulmonary insufficiency; fine screen filtration of blood. Arch. Surg. 106:386, 1973.

28. Marshall, B.E., Wurzel, H.A., Ellison, N., Neufeld, G.R., and Soma, L.R.: Microaggregate formation in stored blood: III. Comparison of Bentley, Fenwal, Pall and Swank micropore filtration. Circul. Shock. 2:249, 1975.

29. Boyan, C.P. and Howland, W.S.: Cardiac arrest and temperature of bank blood. J.A.M.A. 183:58, 1963.

30. Aggeler, P.M., Perkins, H.A., and Watkins, H.B.: Hypocalcemia and defective hemostasis after massive blood transfusion. Report of a case. Transfusion 7:35, 1967.

31. Wolf, P.L., McCarthy, L.J., and Hafleigh, B.: Extreme hypercalcemia following blood transfusion combined with intravenous calcium. Vox Sang. 19:544, 1970.

32. Bailey, D.N. and Bove, J.R.: Chemical and hematological changes in stored CPD blood. Transfusion 15:244, 1975.

33. Greenwalt, T.J., Polesky, H.J.F., Rath, C.E., Chaplin, H., Rosenfield, R.E., and Schmidt, P.J., eds.: General Principles of Blood Transfusion. 2nd ed. Am. Med. Assoc., Chicago, 1977, p. 14.

34. Alving, B.M., Hojima, Y., Pisano, J.J., Mason, B.L., Buckingham, R.E., Mozen, M.M., and Finlayson, J.S.: Hypotension associated with prekallikrein activator (Hageman-factor fragments) in plasma protein fraction. N. Engl. J. Med. 299:66, 1978.

35. Holland, P.V. and Wallerstein, R.D.: Delayed hemolytic transfusion reaction with acute renal failure. J.A.M.A. 204:1007, 1968.

36. Hillman, N.M.: Fatal delayed hemolytic transfusion reaction due to anti-c +E. Transfusion 19:548, 1979.

37. Diamond, W.J., Brown, F., Bitterman, P., Klein, H., Davey, R.J., and Winslow, R.M.: Delayed hemolytic transfusion reaction presenting as sickle cell crisis. Ann. Intern. Med. 93:231, 1980.

38. Goldfinger, D. and McGinniss, M.H.: Rh-incompatible platelet transfusions—risks and consequences of sensitizing immunosup-

pressed patients. N. Engl. J. Med. 284:942, 1971.

39. Miller, L.H.: Transfusion malaria and immigrant blood donors. J. Infect. Dis. 133:727, 1976.

40. Brittingham, T.E. and Chaplin, H., Jr.: Febrile transfusion reactions caused by sensitivity to donor leukocytes and platelets. J.A.M.A. 165:819, 1957.

40a. Morrison, F.S. and Mollison, P.L.: Post-transfusion purpura. N. Engl. J. Med. 275:243, 1966.

41. Shulman, N.R., Aster, R.H., Leitner, A., and Hiller, M.C.: Immunoreactions involving platelets. V. Post-transfusion purpura due to a complement-fixing antibody against a genetically controlled platelet antigen. A proposed mechanism for thrombocytopenia and its relevance in "autoimmunity." J. Clin. Invest. 40:1597, 1961.

42. Opelz, G. and Terasaki, P.I.: Improvement of kidney-graft survival with increased numbers of blood transfusions. N. Engl. J. Med. 299:799, 1978.

43. Mohr, J.A., Killebrew, L., Muchmore, H.G., Felton, F.G., and Rhoades, E.R.: Transfer of delayed hypersensitivity: the role of blood transfusion in humans. J.A.M.A. 207:517, 1969.

44. Schechter, J.P., Soehnlen, F., and McFarland, W.: Lymphocyte response to blood transfusion in man. N. Engl. J. Med. 287:1169, 1972.

44a. Button, L.N., DeWolf, W.C., Newburger, P.E., Jacobson, M.S., and Kevy, S.V.: The effects of irradiation upon blood components. Transfusion (in press for 1981).

45. Ford, J.M., Lucey, J.J., Cullen, M.H., Tobins, J.S., and Lister, T.A.: Fatal graft-versus-host disease following transfusion of granulocytes from normal donors. Lancet ii:1167, 1976.

46. Rosen, R.D., Huestis, D.W., and Corrigan, J.J.: Acute leukemia and granulocyte transfusion: fatal graft-versus-host reaction following transfusion of cells obtained from normal donors. J. Pediatr. 93:268, 1978.

47. Cohen, D., Weinstein, H., and Mihm, M., and Yankee, R.: Non-fatal graft-versus-host-disease occurring after transfusion with leukocytes and platelets obtained from normal donors. Blood 53:1053, 1979.

48. Hoffbrand, A.V., Gorman, A., Laulicht, M., Garidi, M., Economidou, J., Georgipoulou,

G., Hussain, M., A.M., and Flynn, D.M.: Improvement in iron status and liver function in patients with transfusional iron overload with long-term subcutaneous desferrioxamine. Lancet i:947, 1979.

49. Propper, R.D., Button, L.N., and Nathan, D.G.: New approach to the transfusion management of thalassemia. Blood 55:1, 1980.

38

Gamma Globulin Therapy in Altered Host Defense States

Donald B. Kaufman, M.D.

Gamma globulin therapy is essentially the replacement of immunoglobulin (Ig)—or, more accurately, antibody (ab)—with a source of pooled human immunoglobulins. There are several preparations available for use in man. The potential uses of gamma globulin include passive immune prophylaxis against infecting organisms in susceptible, but otherwise healthy, individuals (e.g., rabies, hepatitis, rubella), and treatment and prophylaxis in patients who have altered host defense mechanisms. Prevention of hemolytic disease of the newborn due to Rh_o (D) incompatibility is also accomplished by administration of gamma globulin containing anti Rh_o (D) to the mother of the Rh_o (D) infant.

Unfortunately, gamma globulin is one of the most frequently misused therapeutic agents currently available. This inappropriate use is not without its serious side effects. It is, therefore, essential that any discussion of immunoglobulin therapy be preceded by a discussion of the immunoglobulins themselves, and of the immune system; this basic understanding can make therapy more rational and less likely to produce undesirable side effects.

After discussions of the immunoglobulins and the basic immune system that pertain to Ig therapy, this chapter will discuss gamma globulin itself, its constituents, its several preparations, and its rational, appropriate therapeutic uses.

IMMUNOGLOBULINS

Immunoglobulins are a collection of protein molecules which exist in the blood and are the effector molecules of the humoral limb of the immune system. As the effector limb or mediators of the humoral system, they are known as antibodies. These antibodies are highly specific proteins which are the products of the B lymphocytes and plasma cells and can either be cell-bound or circulating. The major function of antibodies, the humoral limb of the immune system, is in their contribution to immunity against bacterial infections, although they also may have effects on viruses, parasites, and some fungi.

In man, five specific classes of immunoglobulins have been discovered, each with a specific structure and function. These classes are designated G, M, A, D, and E, preceded by the abbreviation Ig—e.g., IgG, thus designating its immunoglobulin function. They are occasionally referred to by the prefix γ (gamma), indicating their electrophoretic mobility as gamma globulins.[1,2,3]

These immunoglobulins may exist free in

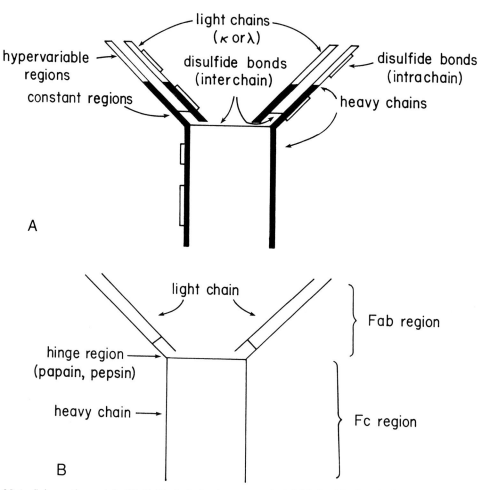

Fig. 38-1. Schematic model of IgG (4-chain basic structure). (*A*) Major biochemical components of the immunoglobulin chains. (*B*) Principal fragments of the immunoglobulin molecule.

the serum (IgG, IgM) or in the secretions (IgA), or they may be cell bound (IgE), where they exert their major function. However, receptors for most of the immunoglobulins exist on the surface of B lymphocytes, the major surface receptor being for IgM. Table 38-1 lists some of the major properties of each of the classes of immunoglobulins.

Structure

The biologic properties and antigenic differences of the immunoglobulin molecules are determined by their specific heavy chains.

These heavy chains are designated γ, μ, α, δ, ϵ for G, M, A, D, and E. Each Ig molecule has two identical heavy chains and two identical light chains. The light chains are designated κ (kappa), λ (lambda) (Fig. 38-1A). The light chains occur in all five classes of Ig, creating ten possible combinations of heavy and light chains, all of which are normally found in any individual. Only one type of light chain, either κ or λ, is found on any given antibody molecule. There are structural differences in immunoglobulins which are genetically determined or inherited. These genetically determined structural differences are referred to as allotypic markers; for example, Gm for

Table 38-1. Physical Properties of Immunoglobulins

Class	Adult mean Conc. mg/100ml	∿MW	Sed. Coef.	Half-Life	Heavy Chain	# Classes Subclass	Localization
IgG (γG)	1240	150,000	7	25	γ	4	Extra cell-44% intravasc.
IgA (γA)	280	170,000	7, 10, 14	6	α	2	Exocrine
IgM (γM)	120	900,000	19	5	μ	1	80% vasc.
IgD (γD)	3	150,000	7	2.8	δ	2	Vasc. 73%
IgE (γE)	.03	200,000	8	1.5	ε	1	Exocrine

heavy chain IgG, or Km (also known as Inv) for κ or λ chains. These allotypic markers are isoantigens and, as such, antibodies to them can be formed. They may also be related to antibody specificity. A related example of such isoantigens would be the anti-A and anti-B substances normally present in the serum of individuals. Minor changes in the amino acid sequence of the variable region of the immunoglobulin chains (Fig. 38-1A) are responsible for the different Gm and/or Km allotypic markers of different individuals. Two other chains, J and the secretory component of IgA, are responsible for polymerizing molecules such as IgM (four heavy and four light chains) and IgA (dimer), and in the case of IgA responsible for transmucosal passage.[3-7]

The antibody molecules have also been structurally designated as having several different fragments. These fragments are defined by the way in which proteolytic enzymes such as pepsin or papain break up the molecule. The two principal fragments are the Fc portion, which is the complement-fixing portion and is necessary for placental transfer, and the Fab portion, which is the antibody combining site. Important biological properties of the immunoglobulin in molecules are determined by these two polypeptide fragments (Fig. 38-1B). Four different subclasses of IgG designated 1, 2, 3, and 4 have been described, and two each of IgA and IgD. Again, these differences are related to changes in amino acid sequences. In some cases, important biologic differences have been attributed to these relatively minor antigenic differences, which subdivide immunoglobulins into these classes.

Ig Concentrations and Role

All of the immunoglobulins are found in the serum, but not all exert their major function in the circulation. The mean serum concentrations vary for each of the classes of immunoglobulins according to age, with some minor variation due to sex and race. The normal concentrations found in the literature will vary slightly from author to author, due to variability in purity of the antibodies and the accuracy and sensitivity of the assay used to measure them.[8,9] The concentration of these immunoglobulins is usually measured as Mg% or mg/dl. Recently, the use of Iu (international units) has been proposed to provide more uniformity, but unfortunately this has not been widely adopted. Some properties of the immunoglobulins are given in Table 38-2, and the average concentrations found in man are listed in Table 38-3. Immunoglobulins are usually measured by radial immunodiffusion on commercially available plates—a technique which, while more than adequate for clinical use, is neither highly accurate nor precisely reproducible. The Mancini or end-point determination is the most accurate of the available immunodiffusion techniques. It should also be noted that these immunodiffusion techniques measure only total Ig and do not measure the subclasses of Ig. More recently the use of nephelometry, which uses light dispersion as a probe for antigen-antibody reactions, has been introduced. Nephelometry is rapid and accurate and has many applications, but it has not yet been perfected.

All immunoglobulins are present and functional at birth.[10] The majority of IgG

Table 38-2. Biologic Properties of the Immunoglobulins

	IgG	IgA	IgM	IgD	IgE
Gram + bacteria	++++	+	+	+	?
Gram—bacterial	++	+	++++	?	?
Viruses	+	++	+	?	?
Parasites	+	+	—	?	+?
Reagins	?+	—	—	—	++++
C'activation	+	alternate pathway	++	?	alternate pathway
Opsonic activity	+	?	++	?	?

present at birth is usually transferred maternal antibody and provides the majority of humoral protection for the first several months of neonatal life. IgG is the most abundant of all the immunoglobulins. It achieves significant concentrations in both the intra- and extravascular space and is found in the mucous membrane secretions. It has the longest half-life of all the Ig's (~ 23 days); it crosses the placenta; and all but one of its subclasses, IgG_4, binds and activates complement. Receptors for IgG exist on monocytes, lymphocytes, and platelets. Its major contribution to the immune system lies in its protective function against infecting agents that have blood-borne dissemination, principally of the gram-positive bacterial type, but also against other types of bacteria, some viruses, and fungi. Because of its ability to diffuse between intra- and extravascular spaces and its high precipitating capacity, IgG is effective in neutralizing toxins in both blood and tissues.

IgA is the second most abundant serum Ig; its major contribution appears to be in immu-

nity at mucous membrane surfaces. It has very high concentrations in the lymphoid tissues of the gastrointestinal, respiratory, and genitourinary systems.[3,11,12] Its particular construction and combination with secretory piece endow the molecule with protection against proteolytic enzymes. In the secretions IgAs (secretory IgA) is found as a dimer 1 or 2 molecules linked together. It apparently activates complement via the alternate pathway and provides protection to the newborn via maternal colostrum. IgA antibodies appear to be the important "first line of defense" because of their secretory location. Its decrease or absence of IgA in the GI secretions of some newborns has been linked to the development of allergy. Of all the immunoglobulins, IgA has the most potent antiviral effects.

IgM is the largest molecule of the five classes; because of its size, it is restricted to the intravascular space. IgM has, on a molar basis, greater opsonizing, bactericidal, and agglutinating capacities than IgG and is highly efficient in binding and activating complement. IgM antibodies assume their

Table 38-3. Approximate Concentration of Ig's [range (mean)]* mg/ml

	Immunoglobulin Class				
Age	G	A	M	D	E ng/ml
Newborn	640–1700 (1135 ± 200)	10	3–30 (10 ± 3)	1	
1–3 mos	200– 920 (423 ± 150)	5–57 (25 ± 16)	18–70 (35 ± 17)	1	
4–6	206–1200 (412 ± 70)	8–120 (30 ± 15)	19–96 (45 ± 15)	1	
7–12	220–1530 (567 ± 200)	10–130 (37 ± 20)	18–130 (34 ± 20)	1–2(1)	
1–2 yr.	260–1390 (702 ± 200)	17–120 (51 ± 24)	20–116 (58 ± 22)	1–2(1)	
2–4	360–1500 (800 ± 233)	25–210 (80 ± 35)	20–120 (60 ± 20)	1–3(1–3)	62–308 (152 ± 66)
4–6	500–1500 (865 ± 250)	40–230 (100 ± 45)	31–170 (65 ± 25)	1–2.5(1.4)	63–490 (210 ± 100)
6–9	700–1750 (1240 ± 280)	30–210 (100 ± 50)	35–150 (62 ± 25)	1–6.5(2.1)	65–530 (254 ± 162)
9–16	700–1750 (1240 ± 280)	60–250 (140 ± 60)	35–196 (65 ± 30)	1–9.1(2.5)	50–800 (257 ± 180)
Adult	700–1750 (1240 ± 280)	60–340 (175 ± 60)	40–220 (98 ± 40)	1–55(3.6)	60–850 (300 ± 200)

* Values derived are from a compilation of the literature and our own laboratory—Normal values will depend on the laboratory and technique used.

greatest importance in the first few days of an immune response. IgM levels rise, peak, and decline more rapidly than IgG; the initial antibody response is in IgM, followed by an IgG response. Anamnestic or secondary responses are primarily IgG. IgM is thought to have a greater role in protection against gram-negative bacteria than against gram-positive.

IgE only normally exists in trace in amounts in the serum. It is primarily a cytophilic, or homocytotrophic, antibody and is found attached to cells and at the mucous membrane surfaces. IgE also can apparently activate the alternate complement pathway. While IgE is known to be involved in allergic reactions, the protective role of IgE antibodies is less clearly understood.[13, 14]

The biological role of IgD is not understood at this time. It is found as a surface receptor on lymphoid cells, and it may play a role in the initiation of the immune response. It is found only in trace amounts in the serum and, like IgE, it cannot be measured accurately by radial immunodiffusion because this method is too insensitive.[9, 13]

In addition to the immunologic properties of antibodies outlined above and in Table 38-2, they are important in the following immune functions: chemotaxis, phagocytosis, vasoactive amine release, lysosomal-mediated injury, and, therefore, in acute hypersensitivity reactions, serum sickness, transplantation immunity, and autoimmune reactions. Thus an absence or decrease in immunoglobulins, and therefore antibodies, is involved in a variety of immunodeficiency and inflammatory states which lead to clinically significant illness.

IMMUNODEFICIENCY STATES

The concept of immunodeficiency (ID) was first introduced in 1952 by Bruton,[14a] who reported the first case of agammaglobulinemia in a four-year-old boy with repeated bacterial infections. Since that time, a great deal of progress has been made in de-

fining and understanding immunodeficiency states, and many different disease entities have been described. Current emphasis lies in attempting to define these diseases as defects of particular cell types or populations. This approach is useful from both a diagnostic and a therapeutic point of view.

It is beyond the scope of this chapter to define the great variety of immune deficiency diseases, their diagnosis, and their therapy. Rather, an overview of the problem and a guide to considering therapy will be presented. A more complete review of the various immunodeficiency diseases can be found in the general references cited[3, 15] and in the National Foundation Birth Defect Series.[16] In considering its defects, the immune system can be divided into three major systems: the humoral, mentioned in connection with immunoglobulins; the cell-mediated; and the nonspecific system, which includes phagocytic and complement defects. Each system may act separately or in concert with another.

Immunodeficiency states or states of altered host susceptibility to infection may be classified as either primary or secondary. Those deficiency states which are classified as primary are the classical immune deficiency states; they are principally deficiencies in B cells or humoral immunity leading to antibody deficiency states, or are cellular immunity defects (T cell) leading to host deficiencies responsible for delayed hypersensitivity and immunity to viral and fungal infections. They may also include defects in nonspecific immune functions such as chemotaxis, opsonization, complement, and phagocytosis (Table 38-4). All of these defects may be either congenital or acquired and are most often, but not exclusively, found in children. Secondary deficiencies may be manifest by the same above-described mechanisms and present the same clinical symptoms, but they are secondary to other processes such as malignancy, infections (viral), drugs, or nutritional abnormalities.

In this chapter, we shall limit our discussion of ID states to those disorders amenable

Table 38-4. Infections Associated with ADS

	Primary Defense Mechanism
Pneumonococcus	Antibody
Streptococcus	
Hemophilus	
Meningococcus	
Pseudomonas	
Pneumocystis	
Hepatitis Virus	
	Bactericidal Function
Staphlococcus	(leucocytes, C', chemotaxis)
Klebsiella	
Serratia	
Aerobacter	
Candida	
Aspergillus	

to gamma globulin replacement therapy—i.e., those altered host defense mechanisms principally involved with antibody deficiency states or immunoglobulin defects (humoral immunity).

B Cell Deficiency

Antibodies provide the primary defense against virulent encapsulated bacteria and certain viruses, prevent recurrence of viral and certain bacterial infections, detoxify proteins and toxins and produce surface Ig as specific receptors of lymphocytes. B cells are primarily responsible for the production of antibody. Secretion of immunoglobulins and antibodies is the major function of the B cells after they have differentiated into plasma cells. Antibodies are produced after the cells have been stimulated by an antigenic challenge. This may be provided by bacteria, virus, cellular components, or a variety of other foreign substances. In the production of antibodies, macrophages and T cells are important and often essential. Certain antigens require T cell help before antibody production can begin. The T cells interact with the B cells to provide help, augmentation, or suppression of certain antibody responses. This is mediated in part by specific subpopulations of T cells.

By and large, cellular immune deficiency

states are not amenable to replacement therapy with gamma globulin. This may even be true when there is a secondary deficit in antibody production, particularly if that deficit is related to a lack of T cell help in antibody production. Since evidence of true benefit of Ig therapy is difficult to establish in these situations, there still exists controversy in this area.

Hypogammaglobulinemia (Antibody Deficiency)

In general, the accepted criterion for the diagnosis of an immunoglobulin deficiency state is an IgG level of less than 200 mg/dl after one year of age and less than 100 mg/dl under one year of age. Values *less than one fifth* of the age-related norms for the other immunoglobulins, principally IgA and IgM, are considered to be clinically significant. With the exception of IgA, isolated deficiencies of the other Ig classes are extremely rare.[17] The primary cause of such apparent deficiencies is most frequently laboratory error.

In certain situations, abnormal levels of IgG are secondary to more general protein loss such as in protein-losing enteropathy or altered metabolic states. Although low, such values may not indicate clinical deficiency, since the host is perfectly capable of mounting and maintaining an adequate antibody response. Synthetic rates of Ig in these situations are usually normal. In other circumstances where IgG levels may be intermediate, although below the normal age-related range (i.e., around 400 mg/dl where normal values are = 600 to 1000 mg/dl), there is usually no clinically significant deficiency present.

In the above situations and other questionable states, the diagnosis of antibody deficiency can be documented reliably only by measuring specific antibody production. IgM antibody can be measured easily by assaying isohemagglutinin titers. Such titers are, in part, age related. In addition, other naturally occurring antibodies such as ASO or streptozyme (an antigenic mixture of most of the streptococcal enzymes) can be measured in most hospital laboratories. Where available, IgG activity can be measured by the simple expedient of a Schick test in a diphtheria-immunized individual. Rubella antibody titers in known immunized patients are also available in many laboratories. IgG and IgM responses can also be determined by measuring salmonella O and H flagellar antigens after immunization with typhoid vaccine. All of the above assays are readily available in most clinical laboratories and can usually give an adequate picture of an individual's antibody-forming capabilities.

By far the most accurate, reproducible, and informative measure of antibody production can be obtained with the use of bacteriophage ϕX 174. This standard antigenic preparation has been used for approximately 10 years to assess immunologic responses in healthy individuals and those with a variety of primary immunodeficiency diseases. Ochs and co-workers[18] developed a classification of seven different antibody responses. Their method has proven extremely useful and in some cases predictive of responsiveness to gamma globulin therapy. Where any serious question exists as to the necessity and efficacy of gamma globulin therapy, use of this assay is highly recommended; its use can avoid the potential hazards of gamma globulin therapy and the prolonged and even life-time commitment to such therapy. This test could be invaluable in the rare situation where an antibody deficiency exists because of an abnormality of one of the IgG subclasses, but where total IgG levels may be normal.[19,20] A high degree of suspicion is necessary in subclass deficiency cases because subclass-specific antiimmunoglobulin determination is not readily available clinically. In any case, it is necessary to document true specific antibody deficiency in most situations before diagnosing an antibody deficiency state (ADS). Gamma globulin therapy is rarely useful in IgG subclass deficiency states.

Finally, defective humoral immunity may be found in association with severe trauma, shock, or major surgery, nutritional deprivation, and malignancy. In addition, certain disease states which may be treated with potent immunosuppressive drugs, parimarily antimetabolites such as azathioprine, or alkylators such as cyclophosphamide provide still other examples of immunodeficiency of a complex nature. In general, corticosteroids have little effect on antibody synthesis but can profoundly affect cellular immunity and the inflammatory response.

Other Deficiency States

Other immunodeficiency states which may include defects of phagocytosis, opsonization, or abnormal functions of other parts of the reticuloendothelial system (RES) may not be amenable to replacement therapy because the action of antibacterial antibody is based primarily on opsonization; therefore, an intact RES is a requirement for response even in antibody deficiency syndromes (ADS). Other primary immune defects not associated with ADS but in which significant bacterial infections occur are defects in chemotaxis and complement. In certain situations, some of these disorders may be responsive to replacement therapy, particularly those chemotactic defects associated with serum inhibitors or other blocking factors.[21-23] Only a trial of therapy can usually determine this (Table 38-5).

Diagnosis

The most important aid in diagnosing an ADS or other IDS is the clinical history. The diagnosis should be suspected where one finds (1) a family history of such diseases; (2) repeated or recurrent documented bacterial infections (at least three); (3) unusual infect-

Table 38-5. Some ID Conditions Potentially Amenable to Replacement Therapy

Hypogammaglobulinemia
  Decreased Ig Synthesis
    Congenital and acquired hypogammaglobuline-mia
    Selective Ig deficiency—dysgammaglobuline-mia
    Chronic lymphocytic leukemia
    Ataxia Telangiectasia (when associated with hypogammaglobulinemia)
    Wiskott—Aldrich (IgM) (plasma)
  Excessive Loss
    Nephrotic Syndrome (plasma—Ig loss not usually a problem)
    Gastrointestinal loss (lymphatic abn, ulcerating condition, unknown causes)

Hypercatabolism
  Familial hypercatabolic hypoproteinuria

Phagocytic Dysfunction
  Hyper IgE syndrome
  Lazy leucocyte syndrome
  Miscellaneous chemotactic deficiencies

Complement abnormalities
  (usually C_3 and C_5 deficiencies)

ing organisms; or (4) states known to be associated with such disorders, such as unexplained hematological disorders of leukocytes. The appropriate diagnostic laboratory tests can then be performed to confirm and define the deficiency state (Table 38-6).

While concentrations of immunoglobulins are the primary means for diagnosing ADS, they cannot be used as the sole criteria for a diagnosis. Reports of people with selective deficiencies of a single Ig class without any evidence of associated disease are abundant. IgA may be undetectable in up to 0.5 percent of the normal population. Since the concentration of Ig is the net result of synthesis, catabolism, and loss, the interpretation of an Ig level must take into account these metabolic factors. Normal Ig levels also do not exclude ADS; patients with high or normal levels as well as patients with isolated subclass deficiencies can sometimes fail to respond to one or more specific antigens, or classes of antigens. Antibody response to antigenic stimulation should be tested if an ID is strongly suspected. Only when a diagnosis is made should therapy with immunoglobulin replacement be considered.

GAMMA GLOBULIN

All too often, gamma globulin is administered not because of any proven beneficial effect to the patient but because the physician feels the need to do something. In principle, therapy should be considered when individuals lack adequate humoral protection (Ig's or Ab) to prevent or overcome an imminent or manifest infection. Such a situation can occur on occasion in a nonimmunodeficient individual. When gamma globulin is used, it is necessary to bear in mind that not all corresponding antibodies have protective properties, and not all preparations may contain the needed protective antibodies. On the other hand, very small amounts of protective viral neutralizing and antitoxin antibodies can provide protection of a nonimmunized host. The latter is true only if the antibodies are provided before the onset of viremia.

Table 38-6. Diagnostic Tests for Antibody Deficiency States

Tests to Evaluate Antibody Function (Initial Screening)

1. Quantification of immunoglobulin levels by radial immunodiffusion
2. Measurement of antibodies to naturally occurring or widely distributed antigens in nature—e.g., issogglutinins (IgM), ASO, Schick Test (DPT), IgG, antiviral antibody—polio, measles (IgG)
3. Measurement of specific antibody responses: de novo sensitization salmonella O (IgM), H (IgG), pneumococcal vaccine, bacteriophage.

Tests for Phagocytic and Complement Defects (Screening Only)

1. WBC count and differential—neutrophil count
2. Stimulated and unstimulated NBT
3. Complement—C_3, C_4, C_5 by radial immunodiffusion
4. Total hemolytic complement

Composition of ISG

Gamma globulin, also referred to as immune serum globulin (ISG), is a pooled product derived primarily from Cohn fractionation (alcohol) of human donor blood plasma. As such, it contains most of the antibodies found in whole blood. On occasion, it may be derived from convalescent or immune plasma, and even from placental blood plasma. The standard preparation contains only 16% gamma globulin and must be given intramuscularly (IM) or subcutaneously (SC). It is generally derived from a pool of not less than 1,000 donors, and more than 90 percent of the Ig present is IgG. Some special preparations may contain as much as 20 mg/ml respectively of IgA and IgM with a total gamma globulin in the range of 165 mg/ml.[24,25]

Due to both the method of preparation and the half-life of the immunoglobulins (Table 38-1), it is apparent why commercial gamma globulin is 90% IgG. Procedures to enrich the preparation with IgA and IgM can produce unwanted side effects and are of questionable benefit. It is doubtful if injected IgA without J chain and transport piece can be transported to the mucous membranes where its effect is exerted. The half-life of IgM is so short as to raise the question of any potential prophylactic benefit from injection of this immunoglobulin, particularly since most practical injection schedules are at 3 to 4-week intervals. Finally, transfer of IgA antibodies to IgA-deficient individuals could lead to significant hazards due to isoimmunization of the recipient and hazardous reactions on subsequent exposure.

The uptake of injected IgG is extremely variable. The Fc fragment of the immunoglobulin is important in the catabolism and function of the various preparations. With the traditional preparations there is significant breakdown and catabolism at the site of injection, thus reducing the potential efficacy of the ISG. In several studies, the amount of IgG in the serum 3 to 4 days after IM or SC injection was 30 percent of a similar dose injected intravenously (IV).[25-28]

Usage and Problems

For effective prophylaxis or therapy, the following factors are critical:

1. variety and concentration of protective antibodies in the available preparation.
2. ability to inject a biologically active form, in adequate amounts, without risk to the patient.
3. biologic half-life of the preparation.
4. loading dose.

Intramuscular or subcutaneous injection is, therefore, a problem where high doses, rapid onset of effect, and high blood levels are required.

All of the preparations tend to aggregate into dimers and polymers leading to significant reactions (Table 38-7). In addition, the risk of sensitization of the patient increases with increased use, particularly for gamma

Table 38-7. Reactions to ISG Therapy

Clinical Reactions	Mechanisms
Cardiovascular and/or respiratory shock	Aggregates, complement activation, Kallikrein-Kinin activation
(Cyanosis, hypotension, cough, dyspnea, wheezing)	Accidental IV injection
Urticaria, rash, adenopathy	Aggregates ⎱ complement activation
Fever (usual IV use)	Aggregates ⎰ contact activated factors
Loss of antibody activity	Fragmentation
Sensitization, encephalopathy	Anti-Gm, Anti-IgA, Ab to aggregates
Development of anti-A and anti-B antibodies	A & B contamination of placental sources
Pain	Volume of injection
	Bradykinin

globulin of placental origin which is contaminated with blood group substances. Isoimmunization due to *Gm* factors, as previously discussed, also occurs. In addition to isoimmunization with allo- and idiotypic antigens, the presence of antiimmunoglobulin antibodies, principally IgA, can lead to sensitization and anaphylactic-like reactions.[27,29,30]

Most of the older literature refers to high-molecular-weight components and aggregated gamma globulin as the major causes of reactions, primarily due to the anticomplementary activity of the commercial preparation (complement activation). This may be true only in part. Recent work has indicated that ISG contains numerous contact-activated factors such as occur in the kallikrein-kinin system and the coagulation system. Significant amounts of prekallikrein activator, kallikrein, and Factor XI have been found in ISG.[31] The vasoactive amines and coagulant factors released by contact activation (Hageman factor being a common component to the activation of complement, fibrinolysis, coagulation, and kallikrein) appear to have a significant role in ISG reactions. One example may be the pain associated with injection of gamma globulin, which could be due to bradykinin release. Therefore, while the historically related activation of C′ by aggregated gamma globulin may be significant, other factors may be of equal or greater importance in the adverse reactions associated with ISG administration.[32,33]

The incidence of reactions is difficult to assess but has been variously estimated by different authors to be between 0 and 25 percent. Reliable estimates are difficult to establish for a variety of reasons, such as what constitutes a reaction in the opinion of the physician reporting. In one Medical Research Council of Britain (MRC) study, Soothill reported reactions in 18 percent of patients with hypogammaglobulinemia although this comprised only 0.2 percent of the doses given.[29,34,35]

One of the more common long-term effects has to do with isoimmunization. Patients without immunodeficiency or with only partial deficiency may develop anti-Ig antibodies following gamma globulin administration. Such antibodies do occur but are rare in patients with severe immunodeficiency. In most instances, the anti-Ig antibodies are not associated with clinical reactions, with the exception of anti-IgA class-specific antibody. Antibody formation is due to the polymorphism of immunoglobulins and corresponds to the various genetically determined idiotypic, allotypic, and isotypic antigenic determinants of the Ig molecules.

Ropers et al. reported incidences of isoimmunization of 50 percent in non-ID patients, 30 percent in partial ID, and 4 percent in severe ID, exclusive of patients with IgA deficiency.[35] These data agree with those of several other authors. Of interest is the fact that the most severe reactions occurred in patients with severe ID (excluding IgA), a finding consistent with those of Barandum.[25] The cause of this is unknown, but it has been postulated that patients with severe ID may have persistent circulating bacterial antigens, making them more susceptible to reactions. Alternatively, they may have abnormalities of the alternate complement activation pathway.

The development of isoimmunization and severe reactions is quite common in cases of IgA deficiency.[36,37] It is possible to measure IgA antibodies in these patients; their frequency and titers can vary considerably. Because of this potential for reactions, it is our practice to avoid, wherever possible, the administration of immunoglobulin and to have patients who have IgA deficiency wear a "medic-alert" Tm tag warning of the potential hazards of blood or blood product administration.

Finally, IM injection is extremely painful and is, in part, related to the volume injected, a particular problem in the older patient. Neovascularization occurs at the injection site after many years of injections, and accidental IV injection with catastrophic results have occurred.

Some advantages of the gamma globulin

Table 38-8. Indications for Passive Immunization with ISG

Indication	Application	Procedure
Prophylaxis	Prevention or treatment of certain infectious diseases	ISG or HIG*
	Critically ill patients	ISG, plasma
Replacement Therapy	Immunedeficiency syndromes (hypogammaglobulinemia primarily)	ISG
Suppression of Primary Immune Response	Prevention of Rh_o (D) isoimmunity	Rh_o (D) Ig
	Transplantation	ALS or ATG

* HIG = hyperimmune globulin

preparations in current use are the fact that they are concentrates, readily available, stable in long-term storage, and hepatitis-free.

Despite all of the associated problems, there is general agreement that ISG therapy is effective in the immunodeficiency states where thymic independent B cell dysfunction occurs: agammaglobulinemia, hypogammaglobulinemia, dysgammaglobulinemia, deficient specific Ab response. There are several other situations in which ISG also appears to be efficacious (Table 38-8).

The efficacy of ISG therapy has been verified by the studies by Gitlin and Janeway, the MRC, Barandun et al., as well as our own experience and that of numerous clinical immunologists over the years. It is accepted therapy in transient hypogammaglobulinemia of infancy, dysgammaglobulinemia or agammaglobulinemia, and common variable immunodeficiency (acquired hypogammaglobulinemia). ISG therapy is advocated for some patients with selective deficiency of IgG subclasses, but here its efficacy is not established. While not considered definitive treatment in cellular and combined immune disorders, its use may be rational, though controversial. In these situations, its benefit, if any, is probably confined to its more immediate prophylactic properties.

Dosage

Even in clinical situations where ISG is efficacious, it is not 100 percent effective. It reduces the frequency of actue infections but does not abolish them. It does not affect chronic infections, and it rarely influences chronic pulmonary and gastrointestinal infectious diseases. In some severe cases of ADS, a rapidly progressive demyelinating disease of the central nervous system leading to death occurs; it is not improved by ISG and, in fact, could possibly be related to anti-Ig antibody development.

The aim of therapy for ADS is to raise the IgG level to between 200 to 400 mg% from the patient's baseline IgG level. This level appears to be necessary to maintain a beneficial effect. One need not attempt to maintain normal serum levels. These recommended levels can usually be obtained with the usual recommended dosage schedule of 0.6 ml/kg IM every 3 or 4 weeks, but will vary somewhat, depending on the initial baseline Ig level. A loading dose of 1.2 to 1.6 ml/kg is necessary to obtain adequate levels before maintenance therapy can be instituted. If larger doses are necessary to achieve these effective levels, it is recommended that a more frequent injection schedule be utilized—e.g., every 2 weeks. We routinely measure Ig levels at 3 weeks postinjection and determine our dosage and schedule based on these values (see Table 38-9).

Uses

Immune serum globulin does not appear to have any benefit in IgM or IgA deficiency, in Ataxia Telangiectasia, or in Wiskott-Aldrich syndrome. To reiterate, it is only of unequivocal benefit in B cell deficiency syndromes.

Common misuses of ISG therapy are in cases of recurrent infections without immunodeficiency, such as upper respiratory in-

Table 38-9. Passive Immunization with ISG in Antibody Deficiency States

Primary ADS	Indication	Dose
Either congenital, transient or acquired Dysgammaglobulinemia	Replacement or therapy ISG	1.4 mg/kg loading dose 0.7 ml/kg monthly
Associated with cellular immune Dysfunction		(.2 to .7 ml/kg) (100–200 mg/kg)
Secondary ADS Drugs, neoplasia, burns	ISG	1.4 ml/kg (150 to 250 mg/kg)

fections, asthma, and bronchitis, tonsillitis and pyelonephritis, in putative hypogammaglobulinemia based upon serum protein electrophoresis only, and in patients with border-line low gamma globulins (e.g., 1 or 2 SD below the mean) but without true antibody deficiency. In all of these situations, not only is ISG therapy of no benefit and not indicated, but it is contraindicated because of the reactions that can occur.

Non-ADS Uses

Uses of ISG, other than the treatment of ADS, are those involving suppression of the primary immune response for Rh_o (D) hemolytic disease of the newborn, immune prophylaxis for certain viral diseases, and tetanus treatment or prophylaxis in patients sensitive to horse serum.[38-40] These usages usually involve only a single injection of gamma globulin. The preparation used may be either pooled ISG, as in the case of hepatitis; or specialized hyperimmune serum, as in the case of Zoster immune globulin (ZIG) for varicella; or anti-Rh_o, (Rh_o Gam^{Tm}) for prevention of Rh_o (D) isoimmunizations. Table 38-10 lists these accepted applications of ISG therapy. For a complete listing of all the products available for passive immunization and their dosages, the reader is referred to Fudenberg et al.[3] Of the various preparations available for passive immunization against viruses or bacteria, or for inhibition of the primary immune response, only the following have proven effective; the benefit of any others has either not been established or is minimal:

Vaccinia (VIG or ZIG), rubella, tetanus, hepatitis A, and Rh_o (D) immunoglobulin. In order for the ISG or hyperimmune serum to be effective in viral disease, it must be administered before the organism can infect cells—that is, before the onset of viremia. This requires it to be present within 48 hours after intimate exposure to the infecting organism such as measles or chickenpox. The use of rabies hyperimmune human ISG offers high promise but is in limited supply. The same is true for antibody against hepatitis B. Mumps and pertussis immune serum globulin appear to be of little benefit.

Hemolytic Disease

Rh_o (D) immune serum prophylaxis has provided a significant therapeutic tool for prevention of hemolytic disease of the newborn. Almost all neonatal deaths due to hemolytic disease are a result of Rh incompatibility. The morbidity and mortality have dropped respectively from 40 and 2.7/10,000 patients in 1970 to less than 18 and 0.7/10,000 patients in 1977. While some failures of prophylaxis do occur, it is felt that, with even better utilization, these figures can be reduced. Rh_o immune globulin is a highly effective product with few serious side effects. This topic is dealt with in greater detail in Chapter 33.

There are other poorly defined clinical situations in which secondary suppression of the immune system occurs and the use of gamma globulin may be beneficial. These situations may or may not have an associated transitory

Table 38-10. ISG Passive Immunization in Non-ADS

Disease	Preparation	Dose
Hepatitis A	ISG	.02 to 1 ml/kg
Hepatitis B	HIG	.06 ml/kg
Tetanus	HIG	250 to 500 iu prophylaxis
		5,000 to 1,000 treatment
Vaccinia	HIG	.3 ml/kg prophylaxis
		.6 ml/kg therapy
Varicella	HIG (ZIG)	5 ml
Rubella	HIG (ISG)	.05 to .2 ml/kg—(.5 to 1 ml/kg)
Rabies	HIG	20 iu
Rh_o (D)	Rh_o Ig	300 μg
Life Threatening Illness		
Septicemia	ISG	1 ml/kg (plasma better)
Toxemia		
Bacterial complication of viral illness		

ADS. While ISG may be of benefit, plasma therapy may be more efficacious, and its use will be discussed later. These situations include the therapy of infections in patients with secondary ADS due to drugs, lymphoreticular malignancies, severe burns, or extensive surgery. Some prophylactic benefit may also be obtained in these conditions. Other, less clear-cut indications are in cases of overwhelming septicemia and toxemia. These conditions tend to require a much higher dosage of immunoglobulin than is ordinarily required in most prophylactic situations; doses in the range of 150 to 250 mg/kg have been used. It should be emphasized that use of ISG in these cases is largely empirical and remains unvalidated by adequate studies.

I.V. Gamma Globulin (Other Forms of Immunoglobulin)

Because of the problems associated with the IM and SC administration of gamma globulin, attempts have been made to give gamma globulin by the IV route. A satisfactory IV preparation would eliminate the problems of volume of administration, pain, injection site catabolism, variable uptake, and injection site neovascularization. However, the danger of severe reactions from the anticomplementary effects of aggregated gamma globulin and from contact-activated factors is aggravated by IV injection. There-

fore, the standard preparations of ISG cannot be given intravenously.

The anticomplementary activity of ISG requires the structural integrity of the Fc fragment and the formation of immunoglobulin aggregates. Unfortunately, attempts to alter the Fc portion of the molecule have had deleterious effects on the functional integrity of the Ig molecules. The Fc fragment is critical in the normal catabolism of Ig as well as in its complement fixing, opsonization, and specific cytolytic properties; therefore, enzymatic treatment with pepsin, plasmin, and papain have not yielded suitable preparations for IV use due to cleavage and loss of the Fc fragment. Methods to prevent aggregation during plasma fractionation or to remove aggregates from the standard gamma globulin preparations have also been tried. Beta prioprolactone, rivanol, acid treatment, and gel filtration to remove aggregates have all been tried without comletely satisfactory results.[24-26] Most recently, Condie et al.[41] reported on an IV preparation in which the aggregates have been removed by a combination of pH control and silica dioxide stabilization plus gel filtration. Fifty-two patients were treated with this preparation. The results so far appear to be promising, but further work needs to be done in this area. One reason for the failure of the various IV preparations to reduce side effects may be related to the presence of contact-activated factors and the associated activation of the kallikrein, coagulation, and complement systems and not due to gamma globulin aggregation.

Plasma

An alternative possibility for therapy is the use of fresh-frozen plasma.[42,43] Plasma has the advantage of providing some complement components, nutrients, and other nonspecific factors in addition to immunoglobulin. It also does not produce the side effects of IgG concentrates. It does, however, carry the risk of volume overload and hepatitis transmission. It also carries with it a greater risk of isoimmunization.

Other potential problems associated with plasma infusion are the risk of graft-versus-host (GVH) disease in patients with cell-mediated immune deficiencies and immunization of the recipient to red cell, leukocyte, and platelet antigens. To minimize these problems, we employ a single related ABO-matched donor, usually the father, in a "buddy system" to prepare fresh-frozen plasma. These precautions, particularly freezing of the plasma, will usually serve to reduce or eliminate the dangers of GVH disease, administration of foreign blood cell antigens, and, with a single donor, reduce the risk of hepatitis. However, the risk of hepatitis from plasma cannot be completely eliminated, even with testing for the hepatitis B antigen or antibody. Elimination of leukocytes is achieved partially by freezing of the plasma and more effectively by irradiation. Irradiation will eliminate GVH reactions. We advise the use of irradiated plasma or blood in ID patients whenever available. In the IgA-deficient patient who receives fresh-frozen plasma, the same danger exists as with administration of blood or any other IgA-containing blood product.

The major benefits from the use of fresh-frozen plasma therapy have been demonstrated by several authors.[42,43] It has the advantage of containing IgM and IgA antibodies which, despite their mean half-lives of only 9.6 and 5.9 days, respectively, may provide some passive protection in the short term. Plasma does not cause the reactions that conventional gamma globulin does. Plasma has nutritional properties which may be of benefit in the severely ill and/or malnourished patient. It is easily given IV. It is, of course, of great benefit in those ADS patients who have reactions from ISG injection. Plasma contains other antibacterial factors which may be of benefit to patients with severe infections. One can also maintain higher Ig concentrations with one plasma injection given every 3 weeks than with one ISG injection given every 2 weeks.

There is evidence to suggest that plasma administration is of particular benefit in those with protein-losing enteropathy.[44,45] Buckley has described an ID patient who had cessation of intractable diarrhea after plasma infusions.[46] We have also observed similar benefits. Finally, it has been suggested that patients with opsonizing defects, complement defects (C_3 and C_5), and those with certain types of chemotactic defects where a plasma inhibitor exists, can benefit from plasma therapy as opposed to use of ISG. We have recently described the correction of chemotactic defects in patients with the idiopathic nephrotic syndrome of childhood by plasma therapy, presumably due to the replacement of factors in the alternate complement pathway.[47] Although unproven, plasma may be of benefit in those AD patients who show progressive or chronic pulmonary disease in the absence of any acute infections (Table 38-11).

It is our current practice to use fresh-frozen plasma for a single related donor in more severely affected hypogammaglobulinemic patients. Usually 10 to 20 ml/kg is administered IV at a rate between 10 to 100 ml/hr, depending on the size and physical condition of the patient. Ten ml/kg of plasma is roughly equivalent to 30 ml of ISG.

The future of immunoglobulin therapy will see the development of intravenous gamma globulin preparations. More and better prep-

Table 38-11. Use of Fresh-Frozen Plasma

Treatment of Choice

Wiskott-Aldrich Syndrome
(ID with eczema and thrombocytopenia)
ADS requiring large doses of ISG
ADS with reactions to ISG
Complement deficiencies (C_5, C_3)
  (opsonic defects)
Chemotactic defects

Possible Benefits

Severe unresponsive ADS
ID with diarrhea
ID with severe life threatening illness
Newborn with sepsis

arations for specific infectious disease such as diphtheria, malaria, rubella, and varicella and other viruses will be developed. It may also be anticipated that, as a better understanding of immunodeficiency develops, specific components such as complement factors will become available and their use defined. For the immediate future, the wider use of plasma and intravenous gamma globulin preparations can be expected.

REFERENCES

1. Smith, R.: Human immunoglobulins—a guide to nomenclature and clinical application. Pediatr. 37:822, 1966.
2. Merler, E., ed.: Immunoglobulins. Natl. Acad. Sci., Washington, D.C., 1970.
3. Fudenberg, H.H., Stites, D.P., Caldwell, J.L., and Wells, J.V., eds.: Basic and Clinical Immunology, 2nd ed. Lange Publ., Los Altos, CA, 1978.
4. Merler, E. and Rosen, F.: The structure and synthesis of immunoglobulin. N. Engl. J. Med. 275:480, 1976.
5. Kabat, E.: Structural Concepts in Immunology and Immunochemistry. Holt, Rinehart and Winston, Inc., N.Y., 1968.
6. Edelmann, G.: Antibody structure and molecular immunology. Science 180:830, 1973.
7. Nisonoff, A.: Molecules of Immunity in Immunobiology. Good, R.A. and Fisher, D.W., eds. Sinauer Assoc. Inc., Stanford, Connecticut, 1971.
8. Allansmith, M., McClellan, B.H., Butterworth, M., and Maloney, J.R.: The development of immunoglobulin levels in man. J. Pediatr. 72:276, 1968.
9. Buckley, R. and Fiscus, S.: Serum IgD and IgE concentrations in immunodeficiency. J. Clin. Invest. 55:157, 1975.
10. Rothberg, R.: Immunoglobulin and specific antibody synthesis during the first weeks of life of premature infants. J. Pediatr. 75:391, 1969.
11. Tomasi, T.: The Gamma A Globulins: First Line of Defense in Immunobiology. Good, R.A. and Fisher, D.W., eds. Sinauer Assoc. Inc., Stanford, Connecticut, 1971.
12. The Secretory Immunologic System. Dayton, et al., eds.: Dept. HEW. NICH-HD, 1969.
13. Ishizaka, K.: Structure and biologic activity of IgE. Hosp. Pract. Jan.:57, 1977.
14. Norman, P.: The Clinical Significance of IgE. Hosp. Pract. Aug.:41, 1975.
14a. Bruton, O.C., Apt, L., Gitlin, D., and Janeway, C.A.: Absence of serum gamma globulins. Am. J. Dis. Child. 84:632, 1952.
15. Immunodeficiency—Report of a WHO scientific group. *Clin. Immunol. Immunopathol.* *13*:296, 1978.
16. Immunodeficiency in man and animals. Bergsma, Good, Paul, eds. Birth Defect Series Natl. Fdn., Sinauer Assoc. Inc., Sunderland, Mass., 1975.
17. Stoelinga, G.B.A., VanMiester, P.J., and Sloff, J.: Antibody deficiency syndrome and autoimmune hemolytic anemia in a boy with isolated IgM deficiency-dysgamma type V. Acta. Pediatr. Scand. 58:352, 1969.
18. Ochs, H., Davis, S., and Wedgewood, R.: Immunologic response to bacteriophage ϕX 174 in immunodeficiency diseases. J. Clin. Invest. 50:2559, 1971.
19. Oxelius, V.A.: Chronic infections in a family with hereditary deficiency of IgG_2 and IgG_4. Clin. Exp. Immunol. 17:19, 1974.
20. Yount, W., Hong, R., Seligman, M., Good, R.A., and Kunkel, H.G.: Imbalance in gamma globulin subgroups and gene defects in patients with primary hypogammaglobulinemia. J. Clin. Invest. 49:1957, 1970.
21. Miller, M.E. and Nilsson, V.K.: A familial defect of the phagocytic-enhancing activity of serum related to dysfunction of the 5th complement component (C_5). N. Engl. J. Med. 282:354, 1970.

22. Jacobs, J. and Miller, M.: Fatal familial leiners disease, a deficiency of opsonic activity of serum complement. Pediatr. 49:225, 1972.

23. Soriano, R., South, M.A., Goldman, A.S., and Smith, C.W.: Defective neutrophil motility in a child with recurrent bacterial infections and disseminated CMV. J. Pediatr. 83:951, 1973.

24. Hitzig, W. and Muntener, U.: Conventional immunoglobulin therapy. In: Immunodeficiency in Man and Animals, Natl. Fdn., Sinauer Assoc., Inc., Sunderland, Mass., 1975, p. 339.

25. Barandun, S., Skvaril, F., and Morell, A.: Prophylaxis and treatment of diseases by means of immunoglobulins. Mong. Allerg. 9:39, 1975.

26. Janeway, C., Merler, E., Rosen, F., Salmon, S., and Crain, J.: Gamma globulin: Metabolism of gamma globulin fragments in normal and agammaglobulinemic persons. N. Engl. J. Med. 278:919, 1968.

27. Kleinman, P. and Webster, M.: Repeated reactions following IM injection of gamma globulin. J. Pediatr. 83:827, 1973.

28. Smith, G., Mollinson, D., Griffiths, B., and Mollison, P.: Uptake of IgG after intramuscular injection. Lancet 1:1208, 1972.

29. Steihm, E.R. and Fudenberg, H.H.: Antibodies to gamma globulin in infants and children exposed to isologous gamma globulin. Pediatr. 25:229, 1965.

30. Henny, C. and Ellis, E.: Antibody production to aggregated human gamma globulin in acquired hypogammaglobulinemia. N. Engl. J. Med. 278:827, 1973.

31. Alving, B.M., Tankersley, D.L., Mason, B.L., Rossi, F., Arronson, D.L., and Finlayson, J.S.: Contact activated factors: Contaminants of immunoglobulin preparations with vasoactive and coagulant properties. Thromb. Hemostasis 42:253, 1979.

32. Christian, C.L.: Studies of aggregated γ-globulin. II. Effect *in vivo*. J. Immunol. 84:117, 1960.

33. Ishizaka, T., Ishizaka, K., Salmon, S., and Fudenberg, H.: Biologic activity of aggregated gamma globulin. J. Immunol. 79:82, 1967.

34. Soothill, J.F.: Reactions to immunoglobulins. In: Hypogammaglobulinemia in United Kingdom. MRC Special Series Report #310, 1971.

35. Ropers, C., Griscilli, C., Homberg, J.C., and Salmon, C.: Anti-immunoglobulin antibodies in immunodeficiencies: Their influence on intolerance reactions to γ-globulin administration. Vox Sang. 27:294, 1974.

36. Amman, A.J. and Hong, R.: Selective IgA deficiency: Presentation of 30 cases and review of literature. Medicine 50:223, 1971.

37. Vyas, G.N. and Fudenberg, H.H.: Immunobiology of human anti IgA: A serologic and immunogenetic study of immunization to IgA in transfusion and pregnancy. Clin. Genet. 1:45, 1970.

38. Schiff, G.M.: Titered lots of immune globulin: Efficacy in the prevention of rubella. Am. J. Dis. Child. 118:322, 1969.

39. Conrad, M., Young, A., Conrad, P., et al.: Prophylactic use of gamma globulin to prevent endemic viral hepatitis. J. Clin. Invest. 50:210, 1971.

40. Burnell, P., Ross, A., Miller, L., and Kuo, B.: Prevention of varicella by Zoster immune globulin. N. Engl. J. Med. 280:1191, 1969.

41. Condie, R.M., Hall, B.L., Howard, R.J., Fryd, D., Simmons, R.L., and Najarian, J.S.: Treatment of life threatening infections in renal transplant recipients with high dose IV human IgG. Transplant. Proc. 11:66, Issue #1, March, 1979.

42. Buckley, R.: Plasma therapy in immunodeficiency diseases. Am. J. Dis. Child. 124:376, 1972.

43. Steihm, E.R., Vaerman, J., and Fudenberg, H.H.: Plasma infusions in immunologic deficiency states: Metabolic and therapeutic studies. Blood 28:918, 1966.

44. Bender, H.J. and Reynolds, R.: Control of diarrhea in 2° hypogammaglobulinemia by fresh frozen plasma infusion. N. Engl. J. Med. 277:802, 1967.

45. Norman, M.E., Hansell, J.R., Holtzapple, P., Parks, J., and Waldmann, T.A.: Malabsorption and protein losing enteropathy in a child with x linked agammaglobulinemia. Clin. Immunol. Immunopathol. 4:157, 1975.

46. Buckley, R.: Plasma therapy in immunodeficiency diseases. In: Immunodeficiency in Man and Animals, Natl. Fdn., Sinauer Assoc., Sunderland, Mass., 1975.

47. Anderson, D.C., Kaufman, D.B., Hassett, C., and Smith, W.C.: Assessment of chemotaxis and C_3 PA in idiopathic nephrotic syndrome of childhood. Abstr. Soc. Ped. Res., 1978.

39

Immunoprophylaxis of Rh_o Alloimmunization with Rh_o Immune Globulin

Jacob Nusbacher, M.D., and Scott N. Swisher, M.D.

INTRODUCTION

Hemolytic disease of the newborn due to anti-Rh_o (D) was a significant problem prior to the advent of immunoprophylaxis in 1968. It is remarkable that less than 30 years elapsed from the time that the immunological nature of the disorder was recognized until the introduction of effective preventive measures. Milestones in the understanding and management of this problem include: the discovery of the Rh_o (D) antigen; elucidation of the pathogenesis of the disease; the development of exchange transfusion in the neonate; the development of intrauterine diagnosis by amniocentesis; and intrauterine transfusions. Despite these formidable achievements, it was estimated that, in 1968, 2.7 deaths per 10,000 live births occurred in the United States as a result of this condition.[1] In addition, life-long residual brain damage secondary to kernicterus resulted in significant morbidity in many children who did not die.

The pathogenesis of Rh hemolytic disease of the newborn is well known. In a primigravid Rh-negative woman who has not been exposed previously to Rh-positive blood, primary immunization occurs most frequently during labor and delivery—particularly during the third stage of labor, when Rh-positive fetal red blood cells (RBC) cross the placenta and enter the maternal circulation in substantial numbers. The risk of immunization is related to the magnitude of fetomaternal hemorrhage. In the presence of ABO compatibility between mother and fetus, the risk is 3 percent when less than 0.1 ml of fetal RBC are present in the mother, 25 percent when 0.25 to 1 ml are present, and 65 percent when more than 5 ml are present. Perhaps 75 percent of delivering women have less than a 0.1 ml fetomaternal hemorrhage, while only 0.3 percent have fetomaternal hemorrhage of greater than 15 ml. Thus, the overall risk of Rh immunization in ABO compatible pregnancies is 13 to 15 percent per Rh incompatible pregnancy. In ABO incompatible pregnancies, the risk is 2 to 3 percent.[2]

POSTPARTUM IMMUNOPROPHYLAXIS

A major development in the prevention of this problem occurred in the late 1960s when it was demonstrated by a number of investigators that active immunization of Rh-negative mothers carrying Rh-positive fetuses could be prevented by the administration to the mother of an intramuscular injection of

Rh$_o$ immune globulin within 72 hours after delivery.[3-6] With use of the standard dose of 300 micrograms of Rh$_o$ antibody, there has been a 90 percent reduction of the immunization rate, from about 15 percent to about 1.5 percent.[2,7]

The recommended 72-hour postpartum limit for Rh$_o$ immune globulin resulted from a feature of the experimental design employed in the original studies on this material.[7] This time limit appears valid for optimal protection. If the Rh$_o$ antibody has not been administered within this period, it should still be administered later, because protection, albeit to a lesser degree, may still be achieved at little risk.[8]

Failures of Immunoprophylaxis

The reasons for failure to achieve complete prophylaxis are not entirely clear and may reflect, in part, a lack of understanding of the mechanism by which the prophylactic effect is achieved. Failures may result from a number of factors:

1. Immunization may have already occurred during pregnancy. Fetomaternal hemorrhages have been noted as early as during the early portion of the second trimester and increase in size and frequency as gestation proceeds.[2] Thus, some women may be immunized early in pregnancy. In recognition of this, some investigators have administered Rh$_o$ immune globulin during pregnancy in either a single dose (300 μg) at 28 or 34 weeks gestation, or twice at both 28 and 34 weeks gestation.[9] The evidence to date suggests that as many as 65 to 90 percent of all prophylaxis failures may be eliminated by antepartum administration of Rh$_o$ immune globulin.[10,11] Infants born after antenatal Rh$_o$ antibody treatment of the mother show no evidence of increased red cell destruction which might result from the passive antibody administration; however, many do manifest a positive direct antiglobulin test of their red cells.

2. A large fetomaternal bleed may have occurred, and the standard 300 μg dose is therefore inadequate. Studies indicate that 300 μg of Rh antibody is sufficient to prevent immunization when up to 15 ml of Rh-positive red cells have been infused into Rh-negative subjects.[12,13] As only 0.3 percent of all pregnancies will have fetomaternal bleeds of greater than 15 ml, this mechanism cannot account for more than a small number of all the Rh$_o$ immune globulin prophylactic failures.[2] In most pregnancies, the standard dose of anti-Rh$_o$ is probably more than is necessary. However, it is desirable for each clinical service to evaluate every Rh-incompatible delivery for the possibility of a large fetomaternal hemorrhage by using either an indirect antiglobulin test or a quantitative Kleihauer-Betke stain on postpartum maternal blood. If a large fetomaternal hemorrhage is demonstrated, the dose of anti-Rh$_o$ should be increased proportionately.

3. It is possible that the intramuscular route of administration may not assure adequate uptake of antibody into the circulation. While there is no direct evidence on this point, European investigators have been using intravenous administration of a preparation of anti-Rh$_o$ especially prepared for intravenous use.[14] The World Health Organization has recommended that only half the usual dose is necessary if the intravenous route of administration is used.

4. Rh-negative women born of Rh-positive mothers may have been actively immunized by a *maternofetal* bleed when they were born ("grandmother theory"). When these women deliver an Rh-positive fetus, Rh$_o$ immune globulin would not be effective because of their prior immunization as infants. Studies suggest this possibility, and a maternofetal bleed rate of 5 to 11 percent has been observed.[15-18] Other studies have not confirmed these findings.[19-21] Further studies are necessary to confirm the validity of the "grandmother theory." If proven, Rh-negative female children born of Rh-positive mothers might receive Rh$_o$ immune globulin to prevent such immunization and later occurrence of hemolytic disease in their children. Present information does not justify the

use of anti-Rh₀ immunoprophylaxis in this situation.

While not a factor strictly relevant to the Rh₀ immune globulin prophylaxis failure rate, it is noteworthy that failure to administer Rh₀ immune globulin still occurs. Estimates by the Center for Disease Control indicate that only 80 percent of women who should receive immunoprophylaxis actually do so.[1] Clearly, further educational efforts are needed in the total program aimed at eliminating Rh₀ hemolytic disease of the newborn.[22]

OTHER ASPECTS OF Rh₀ IMMUNE GLOBULIN USE

Other situations in which Rh₀ immune globulin administration has been considered include:

Abortion

In cases of abortion, a risk of maternal immunization exists. The overall rate of maternal alloimmunization has been estimated to be between 3 and 5.5 percent where the Rh type of the fetus is unknown.[23,24] The method of inducing abortion may influence this rate; hypertonic saline abortion results in a three times greater frequency of transplacental hemorrhage than does curettage abortion.[23] The risk of immunization also increases directly with gestational age. On the basis of these considerations, Rh immunoprophylaxis has gained general acceptance in cases of abortion. While controlled studies demonstrating the effectiveness of immunoprophylaxis in abortion cases have not been performed, the argument for use of Rh₀ immune globulin in these cases is very compelling.

Transfusion

Another major clinical circumstance where Rh₀ immune globulin may be used is when Rh₀ (D)-negative patients have accidentally received a transfusion of Rh₀ (D)-positive blood. Studies in volunteers have shown up to an 80 percent immunization rate in these circumstances. Administration of 20 μg of Rh₀ immune globulin for each 1 ml of red blood cells transfused affords total protection against immunization.[12,13] Other reports substantiate these initial observations.[25-28]

Rh₀ immune globulin need not be administered to every Rh₀-negative patient who receives a transfusion of Rh₀-positive blood. Immunization to the Rh₀ antigen is usually of little consequence, as it only precludes future transfusion of Rh₀-positive blood, a circumstance that is undesirable in the first instance. Immunoprophylaxis with Rh₀ immune globulin should be reserved, in these cases, for women in the childbearing age and in other rare circumstances where future transfusion with Rh₀-positive blood is likely to occur.

After Transfusion of Blood Components Containing Rh-Positive Erythrocytes to Rh-Negative Recipients

Transfusion of platelet or granulocyte concentrates is usually associated with infusion of substantial numbers of red cells. Primary immunization to the Rh antigen may be prevented with Rh₀ immune globulin in those patients in whom it is desirable to do so—e.g., women in childbearing age if donors and recipients are not compatible for the Rh₀ antigen. There is no evidence that cryoprecipitate from Rh-positive individuals can immunize Rh-negative recipients.

After Amniocentesis or Abdominal Trauma to an Rh-Negative Woman during Pregnancy

There is evidence that abdominal trauma, particularly amniocentesis, can be associated with fetomaternal bleeding.[29-34] It appears rational in these circumstances to administer intrapartum Rh₀ immune globulin, although controlled studies are not available to support this use.

Intrapartum Administration to All Rh-Negative Women

Current evidence from a number of studies indicates that primary Rh_o alloimmunization may be largely prevented by routine administration of anti-Rh_o to Rh-negative women during pregnancy. Protection is not complete, however, as determined by postpartum Rh antibody detection.[2, 10, 11] Furthermore, few data exist on the outcome of future Rh-positive pregnancies in women given intrapartum prophylaxis. While it is now generally assumed that intrapartum prophylaxis will reduce the incidence of Rh immunization, such a program would be directed at the 1.5 percent of at-risk women who currently fail to be protected by present postpartum prophylaxis. If such a program were instituted, the number of doses of Rh_o immune globulin required would increase two- to three-fold, and the impact on health care costs and on immunized plasmapheresis donors, the source of antibody-containing plasma, would therefore be great. The advisability of routine antepartum prophylaxis has been seriously questioned recently.[37, 38]

Administration of Anti-Rh_o to D^u Women

There are case reports of women with the D^u antigen ("Rh_o variant") who developed "anti-D" with resulting hemolytic disease of the newborn. This must be a rare event. At present, there is no evidence that administration of Rh_o immune globulin to these women is protective; much of the administered anti-Rh_o antibody would be absorbed by maternal red cells.[34] Of greater concern is the clinical situation where the mother's Rh status is unknown prior to delivery. In this case, a postpartum maternal blood typing as D^u might indicate the presence of a large fetomaternal hemorrhage of Rh-positive cells in an Rh-negative woman. In such cases, Rh_o immune globulin should, of course, be given.

PREPARATION OF Rh_o IMMUNE GLOBULIN

Rh_o immune globulin is manufactured from human plasma containing anti-Rh_o (D) antibody. The plasma is obtained from paid donors who have been immunized accidentally or deliberately. The plasma undergoes fractionation, and the globulin fraction is obtained. The material is tested for specificity and potency in vitro, in the latter case, by comparison with an FDA, Bureau of Biologics reference material. The final product may be diluted with serum globulin which does not contain anti-Rh_o (D) to bring the product to a standard concentration of anti-Rh_o. Stabilizing and antibacterial materials also are added.

Regulations require that at least 200 ml each of plasmas (or sera) from 20 different donors be represented in the original plasma pool. While this is an apparently arbitrary number, it does permit some confidence that all specificities of the Rh_o (D) mosaic and antibodies of different affinity constants are represented in the final material. There are also limits for the presence of red cell antibodies other than anti-Rh_o (D).

REACTIONS TO Rh_o IMMUNE GLOBULIN

Rh_o immune globulin has not been associated with severe or systemic reaction. Localized reaction at the site of intramuscular injection is probably the most frequent adverse side effect. A variety of complications have been reported in association with the administration of Rh_o immune globulin, but causal relationships are not always clear. Urticaria, temperature elevation, fever, myalgia, hyperbilirubinemia, splenomegaly, and rare sensitivities after repeated injections have been observed. Transmission of hepatitis has not been associated with this product.

Rh₀ immune globulin administered during pregnancy to an Rh-negative woman carrying an Rh-positive fetus has not been associated with iatrogenic Rh hemolytic disease in the fetus, although some infants show a positive direct antiglobulin test.[2,10,11,35] Even when anti-Rh₀ is administered to Rh-positive adults, there appears to be little hazard.[36]

CONTRAINDICATIONS TO THE USE OF Rh₀ IMMUNE GLOBULIN

Rh₀ immune globulin should not be given to:

1. Rh₀-positive individuals.
2. Rh-negative individuals known to be already immunized to the Rh antigen.
3. Rh-negative pregnant women where the fetus is known to be Rh-negative.

CONCLUSION

The use of immunoprophylaxis with anti-Rh₀ to prevent Rh₀ alloimmunization to this highly immunogenic red cell antigen in a variety of clinical circumstances represents one of the major triumphs of the fields of hematology, immunology, pediatrics, obstetrics, and gynecology and the U.S. biologics industry of this century. The principles developed in the course of this research may be applicable to prevention of other undesirable alloimmunizations in the future. The major task for clinicians in the immediate future is to increase the appropriate use of this powerful preventive tool in situations where it is useful, particularly the primigravid postpartum Rh₀-negative woman who has delivered an Rh₀-positive child.

REFERENCES

1. Rh Hemolytic Disease Surveillance, 1974. Center for Disease Control, August, 1976.

2. Bowman, J.M.: Rh erythroblastosis fetalis 1975. Sem. Hematol. 12:189, 1975.

3. Freda, V.J., Gorman, J.G., and Pollack, W., et al.: Prevention of Rh isoimmunization. Progress report of the clinical trial in mothers. J.A.M.A. 199:390, 1967.

4. Pollack, W., Gorman, J.G., Freda, V.J., Ascari, W.Q., Allen, A.E., and Baker, W.J.: Results of clinical trials of Rh₀GAM in women. Transfusion 8:151, 1968.

5. Chown, B., et al.: Prevention of primary Rh-immunization. First report of western Canadian trial, 1966-1968. Can. Med. Assoc. J. 100:1021, 1969.

6. Clarke, C.A., Donohue, W.T.A., McConnell, R.B., et al.: Further experimental studies in the prevention of Rh-haemolytic disease. Br. Med. J. 1:979, 1963.

7. Freda, V.J., Gorman, J.G., Pollack, W., and Bowe, E.: Prevention of Rh hemolytic disease. Ten years' clinical experience with Rh₀GAM immune globulin (human). In: Rh Antibody Mediated Immunosuppression. Ortho Research Institute of Medical Sciences, Raritan, N.J., 1975, pp. 71-75.

8. Samson, D. and Mollison, P.L.: Effect of primary Rh immunization of delayed administration of anti-Rh. Immunology 28:349-357, 1975.

9. Bowman, J.M. and Pollack, J.M.: Antenatal prophylaxis of Rh isoimmunization: 28-weeks' gestation service program. Can. Med. J. 118:627, 1978.

10. Davey, M.G.: Antenatal administration of anti-Rh: Australia 1969-1975. In: Rh Antibody Mediated Immunosuppression. Ortho Research Institute of Medical Sciences, Raritan, N.J., 1975, pp. 59-62.

11. Bowman, J.: Winnipeg antenatal prophylaxis trial. In: Rh Antibody Mediated Immunosuppression. Ortho Research Institute of Medical Sciences, Raritan, N.J., 1975, pp. 55-58.

12. Pollack, W., Ascari, W.Q., Kochesky, R.J., O'Connor, R.R., Ho, T.Y., and Tripodi, D.: Studies on Rh prophylaxis. I. Relationship between doses of anti-Rh and size of antigenic stimulus. Transfusion 11:333, 1971.

13. Pollack, W., Ascari, W.Q., Crispen, J.F., O'Connor, R.R., and Ho, T.Y.: Studies on Rh prophylaxis. II. Rh immune prophylaxis after transfusion with Rh-positive blood. Transfusion 11:340, 1971.

14. Hoppe, H.H., Mester, T., Hennig, W., and

Krebs, H.J.: Prevention of Rh-immunization. Modified production of IgG anti-Rh for intravenous application by ion exchange chromatography (IEC). Vox Sang. 25:308, 1973.

15. Taylor, J.F.: Sensitization of Rh-negative daughters by their Rh-positive mothers. N. Engl. J. Med. 276:547, 1967.

16. Bowen, F.W. and Renfield, M.: The detection of anti-D in Rh_o (D)-negative infants born of Rh_o (D)-positive mothers. Pediatr. Res. 10:213, 1976.

17. Scott, J.R.: Immunologic risks to fetuses from maternal to fetal transfer of erythrocytes. In: Rh Antibody Mediated Immunosuppression. Ortho Research Institute of Medical Sciences, Raritan, N.J., 1975, pp. 19-22.

18. Hindemann, P.: Maternofetal transfusion during delivery and Rh-sensitization of the newborn. Lancet i:46, 1973.

19. deAlmeida, J.M.R. and Roasdo, L.: Rh blood group of grandmother and incidence of erythroblastosis. Arch. Dis. Child. 47:609, 1972.

20. Jennings, E.R.: Maternal-fetal hemorrhage: Its incidence and sensitizing effects. In: Rh Antibody Mediated Immunosuppression. Ortho Research Institute of Medical Sciences, Raritan, N.J., 1975, pp. 23-32.

21. Scott, J.R., Beer, A.E., Guy, R., Liesch, M., and Elbert, G.: Pathogenesis of Rh immunization in primigravidas. Fetomaternal versus maternofetal bleeding. Obstet. & Gynecol. 49:9-14, 1977.

22. Tovey, L.A.D., Murray, J., and Stevenson, B.J., et al.: Prevention of Rh haemolytic disease. Br. Med. J. 2:106, 1978.

23. Queenan, J.T., Kubarych, S., Shah, S., and Holland, B.: Role of Induced Abortion in Rhesus Immunization. Lancet i:815, 1971.

24. Freda, V.J., Gorman, J.G., Galen, R.S., and Treacy, N.: The threat of Rh immunization from abortion. Lancet ii:147, 1970.

25. Bowman, J.M. and Chown, B.: Prevention of Rh immunization after massive Rh-positive transfusion. Can. Med. Assoc. J. 99:385, 1968.

26. Keith, L., Cuva, A., Houser, K., and Webster, A.: Suppression of primary Rh immunization by anti-Rh. Transfusion 10:42, 1970.

27. Keith, L.G. and Houser, G.H.: Anti-Rh im-

mune globulin after a massive transfusion accident. Transfusion 11:176, 1971.

28. Bowman, H.S., Mohn, J.F., and Lambert, R.M.: Prevention of maternal Rh immunization after accidental transfusion of D (Rh_o)-positive blood. Vox Sang. 22:385, 1972.

29. Queenan, J.T. and Adams, D.W.: Amniocentesis: A Possible Immunizing Hazard. Obstet. & Gynecol. 24:250, 1964.

30. Zipursky, A., et al.: Transplacental foetal hemorrhage after placental injury during delivery or amniocentesis. Lancet ii:493, 1963.

31. Aickin, D.R.: The significance of rises in Rhesus antibody titre following amniocentesis. Am. J. Obstet. & Gynecol. 78:149, 1971.

32. Henry, G., et al.: Rh-immune globulin after amniocentesis for genetic diagnosis. Obstet. & Gynecol. 48:557, 1976.

33. Wang, M.Y.F.W., et al.: Fetomaternal hemorrhage from diagnostic transabdominal amniocentesis. Am. J. Obstet. & Gynecol. 97:1123, 1967.

34. Schneider, J.: German Trials. In: Rh Antibody Mediated Immunosuppression. Ortho Research Institute of Medical Sciences, Raritan, N.J., 1975, pp. 63-66.

35. Pollack, J., et al.: Rh prophylactic treatment during pregnancy. Vox Sang. 26:26, 1974.

36. Chown, B., et al.: The effect of anti-D IgG on D-positive recipients. Can. Med. Assoc. J. 102:1161, 1970.

37. Tovey, G.H.: Should antiD immunoglobulin be given antenatally? Lancet 2:466, 1980.

38. Nusbacher, J. and Bove, J.R.: Rh Immunoprophylaxis: Is antepartum therapy desirable? N. Engl. J. Med. 303:935, 1980.

ACKNOWLEDGMENT

This paper is based upon material prepared by Dr. Jacob Nusbacher for the report of Panel 6, Safety and Efficacy Review of Blood and Blood Products, Bureau of Biologics, Food and Drug Administration, S. N. Swisher, Chairman, published in the Federal Register (In Press).

Index

Page numbers followed by f indicate figures; numbers followed by t indicate tables